The APRN's Complete Guide to Prescribing Pediatric Drug Therapy

2019

Mari J. Wirfs, PhD, MN, RN, APRN, ANP-BC, FNP-BC, CNE, began her career with an ASN (1968, Dekalb College), and subsequently completed a BSN (1970, Georgia State University), MS (1975, Emory University), Post-Masters Certificates in Primary Care of the Family Adult (1997) and (1998, LSU Health Sciences Center), and PhD in Higher Education Administration and Leadership (1991, University of New Orleans). She is a nationally certified Adult Nurse Practitioner (1997, American Nurses Credentialing Center), Family Nurse Practitioner (1998, American Academy of Nurse Practitioners), and Certified Nurse Educator (2008, National League for Nursing). Her career spans 50 years inclusive of collegiate undergraduate and graduate nursing education and clinical practice in critical care, pediatrics, psychiatric–mental health nursing, and advanced practice primary care nursing. During her academic career, she has achieved the rank of professor with tenure in two university systems. She is a frequent guest lecturer on a variety of advanced practice topics to professional groups and general health care topics to community groups.

Dr. Wirfs was a founding member of the medical staff in the establishment of Baptist Community Health Services, a community-based nonprofit primary care clinic founded post-hurricane Katrina in the New Orleans Lower Ninth Ward. Since 2002, Dr. Wirfs has served as clinical director and primary care provider at the Family Health Care Clinic, serving faculty, staff, students, and their families at New Orleans Baptist Theological Seminary (NOBTS). She is also adjunct graduate faculty, teaching neuropsychology and psychopharmacology, in the NOBTS Guidance and Counseling program. She is a long-time member of the National Organization of Nurse Practitioner Faculties (NONPF), Sigma Theta Tau International Honor Society of Nursing, and several academic honor societies.

Dr. Wirfs has completed, published, and presented six quantitative research studies focusing on academic leadership, nursing education, and clinical practice issues, including one for the Army Medical Department conducted during her 8 years reserve service in the Army Nurse Corps. Her publications include co-authored family primary care certification review books and study materials. Her first prescribing guide, ***Clinical Guide to Pharmacotherapeutics for the Primary Care Provider***, was published by Advanced Practice Education Associates (APEA) from 1999 to 2014. ***The APRN's Complete Guide to Prescribing Drug Therapy*** (launched in 2016), ***The APRN's Complete Guide to Prescribing Pediatric Drug Therapy*** (launched in 2017), and ***The PA's Complete Guide to Prescribing Drug Therapy*** (launched in 2017) are published by Springer Publishing Company. Each book is accompanied by the ebook version with quarterly electronic updates. These prescribing guides are currently under development by Springer Publishing as downloadable APPs with projected availability in 2019.

The APRN's Complete Guide to Prescribing Pediatric Drug Therapy was awarded second place, **Book of the Year 2017,** in the Child Health Category, by the ***American Journal of Nursing***, official publication of the American Nurses Association. The panel of judges included the founder of the nurse practitioner role and first nurse practitioner program, Dr. Loretta C. Ford, Professor Emerita. Dr. Wirfs was the recipient of the **2018 AANP Nurse Practitioner State Award for Excellence from Louisiana** by the **American Association of Nurse Practitioners**. This prestigious award is given annually to a dedicated nurse practitioner in each state who demonstrates excellence in their area of practice.

The APRN's Complete Guide to Prescribing Pediatric Drug Therapy

2019

Mari J. Wirfs, PhD, MN, RN, APRN, ANP-BC, FNP-BC, CNE

SPRINGER PUBLISHING COMPANY
NEW YORK

Springer Publishing Company, LLC
11 West 42nd Street
New York, NY 10036
www.springerpub.com

Acquisitions Editor: Margaret Zuccarini
Composition: Exeter Premedia Services Private Ltd.

ISBN: 978-0-8261-5107-0
e-book ISBN: 978-0-8261-5108-7

18 19 / 5 4 3 2 1

This book is a quick reference for health care providers practicing in primary care settings. The information has been extrapolated from a variety of professional sources and is presented in condensed and summary form. It is not intended to replace or substitute for complete and current manufacturer prescribing information, current research, or knowledge and experience of the user. For complete prescribing information, including toxicities, drug interactions, contraindications, and precautions, the reader is directed to the manufacturer's package insert and the published literature. The inclusion of a particular brand name neither implies nor suggests that the author or publisher advises or recommends the use of that particular product or considers it superior to similar products available by other brand names. Neither the author nor the publisher makes any warranty, expressed or implied, with respect to the information, including any errors or omissions, herein.

Library of Congress Cataloging-in-Publication Data

Names: Wirfs, Mari J., author.
Title: The APRN's complete guide to prescribing pediatric drug therapy, 2019 / Mari J. Wirfs.
Other titles: Complete guide to prescribing pediatric drug therapy, 2019
Description: New York, NY: Springer Publishing Company, LLC, [2017] | Includes bibliographical references and index.
Identifiers: LCCN 2017002668| ISBN 9780826151070 | ISBN 9780826151087 (e-book)
Subjects: | MESH: Drug Therapy—nursing | Pediatric Nursing | Advanced Practice Nursing—methods | Handbooks
Classification: LCC RM170 | NLM WY 49 | DDC 615.5/8—dc23
LC record available at https://lccn.loc.gov/2017002668

Printed in the United States of America.

CONTENTS

SECTION II: APPENDICES

REVIEWERS

Kelley M. Anderson, PhD, FNP
Assistant Professor of Nursing, Georgetown University School of Nursing and Health Studies, Washington, DC

Kathleen Bradbury-Golas, DNP, RN, FNP-C, ACNS-BC
Associate Clinical Professor, Drexel University, Philadelphia, Pennsylvania, Family Nurse Practitioner, Virtua Medical Group, Hammonton and Linwood, New Jersey

Lori Brien, MS, ACNP-BC
Instructor, AG-ACNP Program, Georgetown University School of Nursing and Health Studies, Washington, DC

Jill C. Cash, MSN, APN
Nurse Practitioner, Logan Primary Care, West Frankfort, Illinois

Catherine M. Concert, DNP, RN, FNP-BC, AOCNP, NE-BC, CNL, CGRN
Nurse Practitioner—Radiation Oncology, Laura and Isaac Perlmutter Cancer Center, New York University Langone Medical Center; Clinical Assistant Professor, Pace University Lienhard School of Nursing, New York, New York

Aileen Fitzpatrick, DNP, RN, FNP-BC
Clinical Assistant Professor, Pace University Lienhard School of Nursing, New York, New York

Tracy P. George, DNP, APRN-BC, CNE
Assistant Professor of Nursing, Amy V. Cockroft Fellow 2016–2017, Francis Marion University, Florence, South Carolina

Norma Stephens Hannigan, DNP, MPH, FNP-BC, DCC, FAANP
Clinical Professor of Nursing, Coordinator, Accelerated Second Degree (A2D) Program/ Sophomore Honors Program, Hunter College, CUNY Hunter-Bellevue School of Nursing, New York, New York

Ella T. Heitzler, PhD, WHNP-BC, FNP-BC, RNC-OB
Assistant Professor, Georgetown University School of Nursing and Health Studies, Washington, DC

Melissa H. King, DNP, FNP-BC, ENP-BC
Director of Advanced Practice Providers, Director of TelEmergency, Department of Emergency Medicine, University of Mississippi Medical Center, Jackson, Mississippi

Jan Stockton, MSN, RN, ACNS-BC
Infectious Disease Clinical Nurse Specialist, The Christ Hospital Health Network, Cincinnati, Ohio

Michael Watson, DNP, APRN, FNP-BC
Lead Family Nurse Practitioner, Wadley Regional Medical Center, Emergency Department, Texarkana, Texas

FOREWORD

The 2019 edition of *The APRN's Complete Guide to Prescribing Pediatric Drug Therapy* provides current and clinically relevant information for advanced practice nurses working with the pediatric population. Written by a nurse educator with more than 20 years of experience as an APRN, the information is presented in a practical, accessible, and easily understandable format. The information has been critically reviewed by a geographically diverse group of expert clinicians and nurse educators to ensure that it contains the latest information about medications used to treat pediatric conditions.

A stand-out feature of *The APRN's Complete Guide to Prescribing Pediatric Drug Therapy* is that it is arranged alphabetically by diagnosis rather than by medication. It is portable, well-organized, and contains hundreds of entries that can be accessed quickly—making it easy to use in clinical settings. It presents material that APRNs need to know when working in a variety of clinical settings—including inpatient, outpatient, and specialty clinical areas.

In addition to providing comprehensive information on an abundance of prescription medications for the pediatric patient, the *Guide* has dosing and age-appropriate instructions for common over-the-counter medications used in pediatrics such as acetaminophen, diphenhydramine, ibuprofen, and naproxen. Pharmacologic treatment choices for common episodic conditions seen in the pediatric setting, such as fever and thrush, are provided, as well as treatment choices for chronic conditions such as type 1 and type 2 diabetes mellitus and options for medication therapy for mental and behavioral health conditions seen in pediatrics such as depression, anxiety, and attention deficit hyperactivity disorder.

Several features set this book apart from other drug therapy reference books, including **access to a free ebook with periodic content updates** to keep users current throughout the year; **quick prescribing reminders** that alert practitioners to important points to consider when prescribing certain medications to children, such as ibuprofen being contraindicated for children less than 6 months of age; and **medication listings that are cross-referenced** for different pediatric health conditions.

A particularly unique feature is the **Comments** section, which appears within many entries of the book. The Comments provide a wealth of information to assist APRNs in the proper prescribing of medications to children and adolescents and draw the prescriber's attention to essential factors regarding pediatric medication therapy, such as contraindications for certain ages, alternative indications for the use of certain medications, and potential medication interactions. The Comments section for some medications, such as treatments for gonorrhea and syphilis, reference national guidelines for treatment (e.g., the CDC Guidelines for treating sexually transmitted infections--authored by the Centers for Disease Control and Prevention).

The APRN's Complete Guide to Prescribing Pediatric Drug Therapy has ample **appendices** that cover topics ranging from contraceptive contraindications and recommendations and topical steroids by potency to a hemaglobin A1c-to-average daily serum blood glucose. The 2019 edition also includes several pages of resources that are of value to APRNs, such as the website addresses for the CDC *Morbidity and Mortality Weekly Report* the FDA website for approved drug products and recalls, as well as the FDA website for market withdrawals and safety alerts.

Another key feature is the **index,** which cross-references brand/trade and generic medications with FDA pregnancy category and controlled substance category. For example, this helpful section informs, at a glance, that Adderall (ampthetamine sulfate) is a pregnancy category C and also a DEA schedule II medication.

Overall, the unique format and comprehensive information provided in the 2019 edition of *The APRN's Complete Guide to Prescribing Pediatric Drug Therapy* makes it an excellent resource for APRNs working with pediatric patients across settings and specialties.

Mikki Meadows-Oliver, PhD, MSN, MPH, PNP-BC, RN, FAAN
Associate Professor
Coordinator of Global Nursing Education Programs
School of Nursing, University of Connecticut

PREFACE

The APRN's Complete Guide to Prescribing Pediatric Drug Therapy 2019 is a prescribing reference, organized in a concise and easy-to-read format, intended for use by health care providers in all clinical practice settings who are involved in the primary care management of pediatric patients with acute, episodic, and chronic health problems, and needs for health promotion and disease prevention. Comments are interspersed throughout, including such clinically useful information as laboratory values to be monitored, patient teaching points, safety information, and research notes. If pediatric indications for a drug have not been established *or* a drug is not recommended for a pediatric subgroup, this information is noted accordingly. Where manufacturers use the generic terms "pediatric" or "children," these terms generally refer to patients ≤12 years-of-age. "Adolescence" generally refers to 13-17 or 18 years-of-age. Patients ≥18 years-of-age may usually receive adult medication doses.

This reference is divided into two major sections. **Section I** presents drug treatment regimens for over 550 clinical diagnoses. Each drug is listed alphabetically by generic name, followed by the FDA pregnancy category (A, B, C, D, X), over-the-counter availability (OTC), DEA schedule (I, II, III, IV, V), generic availability (G), dosing regimens, brand/trade name(s), dose forms, whether tablets, caplets, or chew tabs are single-scored (*), cross-scored (**), or tri-scored (***), flavors of chewable, sublingual, buccal, and liquid forms, and information regarding additives (i.e., dye-free, sugar-free, preservative-free or preservative type, alcohol-free or alcohol content). Drugs that received FDA-approval *prior to June 30, 2015* retain their assigned A, B, C, D, or X pregnancy category classification, a one-letter classification system reflecting summary relative risk of fetal harm with maternal use during pregnancy. This simplified system was retired and replaced, *for drugs receiving FDA approval on or after June 30, 2015*, with descriptive narratives of fetal risk associated with maternal use during pregnancy, risks to the breastfed newborn, risks to human milk production, risks to male/female fertility, and risks in special populations (e.g., children, the elderly, end-organ dysfunction, genetic deficiencies). If there are not sufficient data from well-controlled studies or clinical observations to inform the prescriber of drug-associated risks, this is stated in the narrative. Full prescribing information for a specific drug, in the uniformly organized FDA format, is available in the manufacturer's package insert and at https://www.accessdata.fda.gov/scripts/cder/daf/index.cfm

Section II presents clinically useful information organized in table format, including: the JNC-8 and ASH recommendations for hypertension management, childhood immunization recommendations, brand/trade-name drugs (with contents) for the management of common respiratory symptoms, anti-infectives by classification, pediatric dosing by weight for liquid forms, glucocorticosteroids by potency and route of administration, and contraceptives by route of administration and estrogen and/or progesterone content. An alphabetical cross reference index of drugs by generic and brand/trade name, with FDA pregnancy category and controlled drug schedule, facilitates quick identification of drugs by alternate names and page location(s).

Selected diseases and diagnoses (e.g., angina, ADD/ADHD, growth failure, glaucoma, multiple sclerosis, cystic fibrosis) and selected drugs (e.g., antineoplastics, antipsychotics, antiarrhythmics, anti-HIV drugs, anticoagulants) are included as pediatric patients are frequently referred to primary care providers by specialists for follow-up monitoring and on-going management. Further, the shifting healthcare paradigm is such that with expanding roles and patient empowerment through education, initial diagnosis and initiation of treatment is increasing in primary care with measurable increases in access to quality healthcare and improved patient self-care. Several diseases are included that may not be prevalent in North America, but have been identified in other parts of the world. Certain endemic diseases for which there is no FDA-approved treatment are also included with known transmission and treatment interventions. Accordingly, this guide serves primary care providers internationally. We are in an era of rapidly expanding knowledge in the field of genomics and, as such, each new edition of this prescribing guide (and quarterly update) contains new drug classes and new FDA-approved drugs as well as brief synopses of recent published research findings with source reference(s).

For quick reference to weight-based dosing of liquid anti-infectives, the user is directed to the dose by weight table for that drug in the appendices. Potential safe, efficacious, prescribing and monitoring of drug therapy regimens for children and adolescents requires adequate knowledge about (a) the pharmacodynamics and pharmacokinetics of drugs, (b) concomitant therapies, and (c) individual characteristics of the patient (e.g., age, weight, current and past medical history, physical examination findings, hepatic and renal function, co-morbidities, and risk factors). Users of this clinical guide are encouraged to utilize the manufacturer's package insert, recommendations and guidance of specialists, standard of practice protocols, and the current research literature for more comprehensive information about specific drugs (e.g., special precautions, drug-drug and drug-food interactions, risk versus benefit, age-related considerations, potential adverse reactions, and appropriate patient-focused care).

ACKNOWLEDGMENTS

This publication, which we consider to be a "must have" for students, academicians, and practicing clinicians with prescriptive authority, represents the culmination of Springer Publishing Company's collaborative team effort. Margaret Zuccarini, Publisher, Emerita, Nursing; Joanne Jay, Vice President, Production and Manufacturing; and the Editorial Committee shared my vision for a handy pocket prescribing reference for new and experienced prescribers in primary care. Joanne Jay designed the contents for ease and efficiency of user navigation. The production team at Exeter Premedia Services, on behalf of Springer Publishing Company, understood the critical nature of exactness in this prescribing resource and faithfully managed the complex files as content was updated and cross-paginated for the final product. The work of the reviewers from academia and clinical practice was essential to the process and their contributions are greatly appreciated. I am proud of my association with these dedicated professionals and I thank them on behalf of the medical and advanced practice nursing community worldwide, for supporting the end goal of quality health care for all.

QUICK CHECK PRESCRIBING REMINDERS

ACE-Is and **ARBs** are contraindicated in the 2nd and 3rd trimesters of pregnancy. Addition of a daily ACE-I or ARB is strongly recommended for renal protection in patients with hypertension and/or diabetes. The "ACE inhibitor cough," a dry cough, is an adverse side effect produced by an accumulation of bradykinins that occurs in 5-10% of the population and resolves within days of discontinuing the drug.

Alcohol is contraindicated with concomitant ***narcotic analgesics***, ***benzodiazepines***, ***SSRIs***, ***antihistamines***, ***TCAs***, and other sedating agents due to risk of over-sedation.

Alpha-1 blockers have a potential adverse side effect of sudden hypotension, especially with first dose. Alert the patient regarding this "first-dose effect" and recommend the patient sit or lie down to take the first dose. Usually start at lowest dose and titrate upward.

Antidepressant monotherapy should be avoided until any presence of hypomania <u>or</u> positive family history for bipolar spectrum disorder has been ruled out because antidepressant monotherapy can induce mania in the bipolar patient.

Aspirin is contraindicated in children and adolescents with *Varicella* or other viral illness, and 3rd trimester of pregnancy.

Beta-blockers, by all routes of administration, are generally contraindicated in severe COPD, history of <u>or</u> current bronchial asthma, sinus bradycardia, and 2nd <u>or</u> 3rd degree AV block. Use a cardio-specific beta-blocker where appropriate in these cases.

Biosimilar means the biological product is FDA-approved based on data demonstrating that it is highly similar to an FDA-approved biological product, known as a reference product, and that there are no clinically meaningful differences between the biosimilar product and the reference product; e.g., **Cyltezo** (***adalimumab-adbm***) is biosimilar to **Humira** (***adalimumab***).

Calcium channel blockers may cause the adverse side effect of pedal edema (feet, ankles, lower legs) that resolves with discontinuation of the drug. The FDA is advising caution before prescribing the antibiotic ***clarithromycin*** to patients with heart disease because of a potential increased risk of heart problems or death that can occur years later. This recommendation is based on a review of the results of a 10-year follow-up study of patients with coronary heart disease from a large clinical trial that first observed this safety issue. Consider risk benefit and the use of other antibiotics in such patients.

Codeine is known to be excreted in breast milk. <12 years: not recommended; 12-<18: use extreme caution; not recommended for children and adolescents with asthma or other chronic breathing problem. The FDA and the European Medicines Agency (EMA) are investigating the safety of using ***codeine***-containing medications to treat pain, cough, and colds in children 12-<18 years because of the potential for serious side effects, including slowed <u>or</u> difficult breathing.

Corticosteroids increase blood sugar in patients with diabetes and decrease immunity; therefore, consider risk vs. benefit in susceptible patients, use lowest effective dose, and taper gradually to discontinue.

Check ***drug interactions*** (e.g., www.drugs.com/drug_interactions.php).

Check FDA drug recalls, market withdrawals, and safety alerts (http://www.fda.gov/Safety/Recalls/default.htm).

Contraceptives that are **estrogen-progesterone** combinations and **progesterone-only** are contraindicated in pregnancy (pregnancy category X)

Erythromycin may increase INR with concomitant ***warfarin***, as well as increase serum level of ***digoxin***, ***benzodiazepines***, and ***statins***.

Finasteride, a 5-alpha reductase inhibitor, is associated with low but increased risk of high-grade prostate cancer. Pregnant females should not touch broken tablets.

Fluoroquinolones and **quinolones** are contraindicated <18 years-of-age, pregnancy, and breastfeeding. *Exception:* In the case of anthrax, ***ciprofloxacin*** is indicated for patients <18 years-of-age and dosed based on mg/kg body weight. Risk of tendonitis or tendon rupture (ex: ***ciprofloxacin***, ***gemifloxacin***, ***levofloxacin***, ***moxifloxacin***, ***norfloxacin***, ***ofloxacin***).

Ibuprofen is contraindicated in children <6 months of age and in the 3rd trimester of pregnancy.

Live vaccines are contraindicated in patients who are immunosuppressed or receiving immunosuppressive therapy, including immunosuppressive levels of corticosteroid therapy.

The MEDWATCH drug event reporting form is available from U.S. Department of Health and Human Services, FDA Safety Information and Adverse Event Reporting Program, and the completed form may be faxed to 1-800-FDA-0178. www.fda.gov/downloads/AboutFDA/ReportsManualsForms/Forms/UCM163919.pdf

Metronidazole and **tinidazole** are contraindicated in the 1st trimester of pregnancy. Alcohol is contraindicated during treatment with oral forms and for 72 hours after therapy due to a possible ***disulfiram***-like reaction (nausea, vomiting, flushing, headache).

When prescribing **opioid analgesics**, presumptive urine **drug testing** (UDT) should be performed when opioid therapy for chronic pain is initiated, along with subsequent use as adherence monitoring, using in-office point of service testing, to identify patients who are non-compliant or abusing prescription drugs or illicit drugs (American Society of Interventional Pain Physicians [ASIPP]).

Oral **PDE5 inhibitors** are contraindicated in patients taking nitrates due to risk of hypotension or syncope (ex: ***avanafil***, ***sildenafil***, ***tadalafil***, ***vardenafil***).

Proton pump inhibitors (PPIs) should be discontinued, and should not be initiated, in patients with acute kidney injury (AKI) and chronic kidney disease (CKD). Chronic long-term use of PPIs carries a risk to renal function (consider risk-benefit and alternative treatment).

Statins are strongly recommended as adjunctive therapy for patients with diabetes, with or without abnormal lipids.

Sulfonamides (ex: ***sulfamethoxazole, trimethoprim***) are not recommended in pregnancy or lactation. *CrCl 15-30 mL/min:* reduce dose by 1/2; *CrCl <15 mL/min:* not recommended. Contraindicated with G6PD deficiency. A high fluid intake is indicated during sulfonamide therapy to avoid crystallization in the kidneys.

Tetracyclines are contraindicated in children <8 years-of-age, pregnancy, and breastfeeding (discolors developing tooth enamel). A side effect may be photo-sensitivity (photophobia). Do not take with antacids, calcium supplements, milk or other dairy, or within 2 hours of taking another drug (ex: ***doxycycline***, ***minocycline***, ***tetracycline***).

Tramadol is known to be excreted in breast milk. The FDA and the European Medicines Agency (EMA) are investigating the safety of using ***tramadol***-containing medications to treat pain in children 12-18 years because of the potential for serious side effects, including slowed or difficult breathing.

The **Transmucosal Immediate Release Fentanyl (TIRF) Risk Evaluation and Mitigation Strategy (REMS)** program is an FDA-required program designed to ensure informed risk-benefit decisions before initiating treatment, and while patients are treated to ensure appropriate use of TIRF medicines. The purpose of the TIRF REMS Access program is to mitigate the risk of misuse, abuse, addiction, overdose, and serious complications due to medication errors with the use of TIRF medicines. You must enroll in the TIRF REMS Access program to prescribe, dispense, or distribute TIRF medicines. To register, call the TIRF REMS Access program at 1-866-822-1483 or register online at www.tirfremsaccess.com/TirfUI/rems/home.action

SECTION I

PEDIATRIC DRUG THERAPY BY CLINICAL DIAGNOSIS

ACETAMINOPHEN OVERDOSE

ANTIDOTE/CHELATING AGENT

▷ ***acetylcysteine*** **(B)(G)** *Loading dose:* 150 mg/kg administered over 15 minutes; *Maintenance:* 50 mg/kg administered over 4 hours; then 100 mg/kg administered over 16 hours

Acetadote *Vial: soln for IV infusion after dilution:* 200 mg/ml (30 ml; dilute in D5W) (preservative-free)

Comment: ***acetaminophen*** overdose is a medical emergency due to the risk of irreversible hepatic injury. An IV infusion of ***acetylcysteine*** should be started as soon as possible and within 24 hours if the exact time of ingestion is unknown. Use a serum ***acetaminophen*** nomogram to determine need for treatment. Extreme caution is needed if used with concomitant hepatotoxic drugs.

ACNE ROSACEA

Comment: All acne rosacea products should be applied sparingly to clean, dry skin as directed. Avoid use of topical corticosteroids.

▷ ***ivermectin*** **(C)** apply bid

Soolantra *Crm:* 1% (30 gm)

Comment: **Soolantra** is a macrocyclic lactone. Exactly how it works to treat acne rosacea is unknown.

TOPICAL ALPHA-1A ADRENOCEPTOR AGONIST

▷ ***oxymetazoline hcl*** **(B)** <18 years: not recommended; ≥18 years: apply a pea-sized amount once daily in a thin layer covering the entire face (forehead, nose, cheeks, and chin) avoiding the eyes and lips; wash hands immediately

Rhofade *Crm* 1% (30 gm tube)

Comment: **Rhofade** acts as a vasoconstrictor. Use with caution in patients with cerebral or coronary insufficiency, Raynaud's phenomenon, thromboangiitis obliterans, scleroderma, or Sjögren's syndrome. **Rhofade** may increase the risk of angle closure glaucoma in patients with narrow-angle glaucoma. Advise patients to seek immediate medical care if signs and symptoms of potentiation of vascular insufficiency or acute angle closure glaucoma develop.

TOPICAL ALPHA-2 AGONIST

▷ ***brimonidine*** **(B)** <18 years: not recommended; ≥18 years: apply to affected area once daily

Mirvaso *Gel:* 0.33% (30, 45 gm tube; 30 gm pump)

Comment: For persistent erythema; constricts dilated facial blood vessels to reduce redness.

TOPICAL ANTIMICROBIALS

▷ ***azelaic acid*** **(B)** apply affected area bid

Azelex *Crm:* 20% (30, 50 gm)

Finacea *Gel:* 15% (30 gm); *Foam:* 15% (50 gm)

▷ ***metronidazole*** **(B)** apply affected area bid

MetroCream apply bid

Emol crm: 0.75% (45 gm)

MetroGel apply once daily

Gel: 1% (60 gm tube; 55 gm pump)

MetroLotion apply bid
Lotn: 0.75% (2 oz)

▶ ***sodium sulfacetamide*** (C)(G) apply 1-3 x daily
Klaron *Lotn:* 10% (2 oz)

▶ ***sodium sulfacetamide+sulfur*** (C)
Clenia Emollient Cream apply 1-3 x daily
Wash: sod sulfa 10%+sulfur 5% (10 oz)
Clenia Foaming Wash wash affected area once or twice daily
Wash: sod sulfa 10%+sulfur 5% (6, 12 oz)
Rosula Gel apply 1-3 x daily
Gel: sod sulfa 10%+sulfur 5% (45 ml)
Rosula Lotion apply tid
Lotn: sod sulfa 10%+sulfur 5% (45 ml) (alcohol-free)
Rosula Wash wash bid
Clnsr: sod sulfa 10%+sulfur 5% (335 ml)

ORAL ANTIMICROBIALS

▶ ***doxycycline*** (D)(G) <8 years: not recommended; ≥8 years, ≤100 lb: 2 mg/lb on first day in 2 divided doses, followed by 1 mg/lb/day in 1-2 divided doses; ≥8 years, >100 lb: 40-100 mg bid; *see page 605 for dose by weight table*
Acticlate *Tab:* 75, 150**mg
Adoxa *Tab:* 50, 75, 100, 150 mg ent-coat
Doryx *Tab:* 50, 75, 100, 150, 200 mg del-rel
Doxteric *Tab:* 50 mg del-rel
Monodox *Cap:* 50, 75, 100 mg
Oracea *Cap:* 40 mg del-rel
Vibramycin *Tab:* 100 mg; *Cap:* 50, 100 mg; *Syr:* 50 mg/5 ml (raspberry-apple) (sulfites); *Oral susp:* 25 mg/5 ml (raspberry)
Vibra-Tab *Tab:* 100 mg film-coat

▶ ***minocycline*** (D)(G) <8 years: not recommended; ≥8 years, ≤100 lb: 2 mg/lb on first day in 2 divided doses, followed by 1 mg/lb q 12 hours x 9 more days; ≥8 years, >100 lb: 200 mg on first day; then 100 mg q 12 hours x 9 more days
Dynacin *Cap:* 50, 100 mg
Minocin *Cap:* 50, 75, 100 mg; *Oral susp:* 50 mg/5 ml (60 ml) (custard) (sulfites, alcohol 5%)

ACNE VULGARIS

Comment: In their 2016 published report, researchers concluded different hormonal contraceptives have significantly varied effects on acne. Females (n=2,147) who were using a hormonal contraceptive at the time of their first consultation for acne comprised the study sample. Participants completed an assessment at baseline to report how the contraceptive affected their acne. Then the researchers used the Kruskal-Wallis test and logistic regression analysis to compare the outcomes by contraceptive type. On average, the vaginal ring and combined oral contraceptives (COCs) improved acne, whereas depot injections, subdermal implants, and hormonal intrauterine devices worsened acne. In the COC categories, ***drospirenone*** was the most helpful in improving acne, followed by ***norgestimate*** and ***desogestrel***, and then ***levonorgestrel*** and ***norethindrone***. Although triphasic progestin dosage had a positive effect on acne, ***estrogen*** dosage did not.

REFERENCE

Lortscher, D, Admani, S, Satur, N, & Eichenfield, LF. (2016). Hormonal contraceptives and acne: a retrospective analysis of 2147 patients. *Journal of Drugs in Dermatology, 15*(6), 670–674. http://jddonline.com/articles/dermatology/S1545961616P0670X

TOPICAL ANTIMICROBIALS

Comment: All topical antimicrobials should be applied sparingly to clean, dry skin.

▶ ***azelaic acid*** **(B)** apply to affected area bid
  Azelex *Crm:* 20% (30, 50 gm)
  Finacea *Gel:* 15% (30 gm); *Foam:* 15% (50 gm)

▶ ***benzoyl peroxide*** **(C)(G)** may discolor clothing and linens.
  Benzac-W initially apply to affected area once daily; increase to bid-tid as tolerated
    Gel: 2.5, 5, 10% (60 gm)
  Benzac-W Wash wash affected area bid
    Wash: 5% (4, 8 oz); 10% (8 oz)
  Benzagel apply to affected area one <u>or</u> more x/day
    Gel: 5, 10% (1.5, 3 oz) (alcohol 14%)
  Benzagel Wash wash affected area bid
    Gel: 10% (6 oz)
  Desquam X^{5} wash affected area bid
    Wash: 5% (5 oz)
  Desquam X^{10} wash affected area bid
    Wash: 10% (5 oz)
  Triaz apply to affected area daily bid
    Lotn: 3, 6, 9% (bottle), 3% (tube); *Pads:* 3, 6, 9% (jar)
  ZoDerm apply once <u>or</u> twice daily
    Gel: 4.5, 6.5, 8.5% (125 ml); *Crm:* 4.5, 6.5, 8.5% (125 ml); *Clnsr:* 4.5, 6.5, 8.5% (400 ml)

▶ ***clindamycin*** topical **(B)** <12 years: not recommended; ≥12 years: apply once daily
  Cleocin T (G) *Pad:* 1% (60/pck) (alcohol 50%); *Lotn:* 1% (60 ml); *Gel:* 1% (30, 60 gm); *Soln w. applicator:* 1% (30, 60 ml) (alcohol 50%)
  Clindagel *Gel:* 1% (42, 77 gm)
  Evoclin Foam: 1% (50, 100 gm) (alcohol)

▶ ***clindamycin+benzoyl peroxide*** topical **(C)** <12 years: not recommended; ≥12 years: apply once daily; ***benzoyl peroxide*** may discolor clothing and linens
  Acanya (G) apply qd-bid
    Gel: clin 1.2%+*benz* 2.5% (50 gm)
  BenzaClin (G) apply bid
    Gel: clin 1%+*benz* 5% (25, 50 gm)
  Duac apply daily in the evening
    Gel: clin 1%+*benz* 5% (45 gm)
  Onexton Gel apply once daily
    Gel: clin 1.2%+*benz* 3.75% (50 gm pump) (alcohol-free, preservative-free)

▶ ***dapsone*** topical **(C)(G)** <12 years: not recommended; ≥12 years: apply to affected area bid
  Aczone *Gel:* 5, 7.5% (30, 60, 90 gm pump)

▶ ***erythromycin+benzoyl peroxide*** **(C)** initially apply once daily; increase to bid as tolerated; ***benzoyl peroxide*** may discolor clothing and linens
  Benzamycin Topical Gel *Gel: eryth* 3%+*benz* 5% (46.6 gm/jar)

▶ ***sodium sulfacetamide*** **(C)(G)** apply tid
  Klaron *Lotn:* 10% (2 oz)

ORAL ANTIMICROBIALS

- ▶ ***doxycycline*** **(D)(G)** <8 years: not recommended; ≥8 years, ≤100 lb: 2 mg/lb on first day in 2 divided doses, followed by 1 mg/lb/day in 1-2 divided doses; ≥8 years, >100 lb: 100 mg bid; *see page 605 for dose by weight table*
  - **Acticlate** *Tab:* 75, 150**mg
  - **Adoxa** *Tab:* 50, 75, 100, 150 mg ent-coat
  - **Doryx** *Tab:* 50, 75, 100, 150, 200 mg del-rel
  - **Monodox** *Cap:* 50, 75, 100 mg
  - **Oracea** *Cap:* 40 mg del-rel
  - **Vibramycin** *Tab:* 100 mg; *Cap:* 50, 100 mg; *Syr:* 50 mg/5 ml (raspberry-apple) (sulfites); *Oral susp:* 25 mg/5 ml (raspberry)
  - **Vibra-Tab** *Tab:* 100 mg film-coat
- ▶ ***erythromycin base*** **(B)(G)** <45 kg: 30-50 mg in 2-4 divided doses x 7-10 days; ≥45 kg: 250 mg qid, 333 mg tid or 500 mg bid x 7-10 days; then taper to lowest effective dose
  - **Ery-Tab** *Tab:* 250, 333, 500 mg ent-coat
  - **PCE** *Tab:* 333, 500 mg
- ▶ ***erythromycin ethylsuccinate*** **(B)(G)** 30-50 mg/kg/day in 4 divided doses x 7-10 days; may double dose with severe infection; max 100 mg/kg/day or 400 mg qid; *see page 607 for dose by weight table*
  - **EryPed** *Oral susp:* 200 mg/5 ml (100, 200 ml) (fruit); 400 mg/5 ml (60, 100, 200 ml) (banana); *Oral drops:* 200, 400 mg/5 ml (50 ml) (fruit); *Chew tab:* 200 mg wafer (fruit)
  - **E.E.S.** *Oral susp:* 200, 400 mg/5 ml (100 ml) (fruit)
  - **E.E.S. Granules** *Oral susp:* 200 mg/5 ml (100, 200 ml) (cherry)
  - **E.E.S. 400 Tablets** *Tab:* 400 mg
- ▶ ***minocycline*** **(D)(G)** <8 years: not recommended; ≥8 years: initially 50-100 mg once daily; reduce dose after improvement
  - **Dynacin** *Cap:* 50, 100 mg
  - **Minocin** *Cap:* 50, 75, 100 mg; *Oral susp:* 50 mg/5 ml (60 ml) (custard) (sulfites, alcohol 5%)
  - **Minolira** *Tab:* 105, 135 mg ext-rel
  - **Solodyn** *Tab:* 55, 65, 80, 105, 115 mg ext-rel

  Comment: Once-daily dosing of **Minolira** or **Solodyn,** extended-release ***minocyclines,*** is approved for inflammatory lesions of non-nodular moderate-to-severe acne vulgaris for patients ≥12 years-of-age. The recommended dose of **Solodyn** is 1 mg/kg once daily x 12 weeks.
- ▶ ***tetracycline*** **(D)(G)** <8 years: not recommended; ≥8 years, ≤100 lb: 25-50 mg/kg/day in 2-4 divided doses; *see page 618 for dose by weight table;* ≥8 years, >100 lb: initially 1 gm/day in 2-4 divided doses; after improvement, 125-500 mg once daily
  - **Achromycin V** *Cap:* 250, 500 mg
  - **Sumycin** *Tab:* 250, 500 mg; *Cap:* 250, 500 mg; *Oral susp:* 125 mg/5 ml (100, 200 ml) (fruit) (sulfites)

  Comment: ***tetracycline*** is contraindicated <8 years-of-age, in pregnancy, and lactation (discolors developing tooth enamel). A side effect may be photosensitivity (photophobia). Do not give with antacids, calcium supplements, milk or other dairy, or within two hours of taking another drug.

TOPICAL RETINOIDS

Comment: Wash affected area with a soap-free cleanser; pat dry and wait 20 to 30 minutes; then apply sparingly to affected area; use only once daily in the evening. Avoid applying to eyes, ears, nostrils, and mouth.

▶ ***adapalene*** **(C)** <12 years: not recommended; ≥12 years: apply once daily at HS
  Differin *Crm:* 0.1% (45 gm); *Gel:* 0.1, 0.3% (45 gm) (alcohol-free); *Pad:* 0.1% 30/pck) (alcohol 30%); *Lotn:* 0.1% (2, 4 oz)

▶ ***tazarotene*** **(X)(G)** <12 years: not recommended; ≥12 years: apply once daily at HS
  Avage Cream *Crm:* 0.1% (30 gm)
  Tazorac Cream *Crm:* 0.05, 0.1% (15, 30, 60 gm)
  Tazorac Gel *Gel:* 0.05, 0.1% (30, 100 gm)

▶ ***tretinoin*** **(C)(G)** <12 years: not recommended; ≥12 years: apply to affected area once daily at HS
  Atralin Gel *Gel:* 0.05% (45 gm)
  Atralin Gel *Gel:* 0.05% (45 gm)
  Avita *Crm:* 0.025% (20, 45 gm); *Gel:* 0.025% (20, 45 gm)
  Renova *Crm:* 0.02% (40 gm); 0.05% (40, 60 gm)
  Retin-A Cream *Crm:* 0.025, 0.05, 0.1% (20, 45 gm)
  Retin-A Gel *Gel:* 0.01, 0.025% (15, 45 gm) (alcohol 90%)
  Retin-A Liquid *Soln:* 0.05% (alcohol 55%)
  Retin-A Micro Gel *Gel:* 0.04, 0.08, 0.1% (20, 45 gm)
  Tretin-X Cream *Crm:* 0.075% (35 gm) (parabens-free, alcohol-free, propylene glycol-free)

TOPICAL RETINOID+ANTIMICROBIAL COMBINATIONS

Comment: Wash affected area with a soap-free cleanser; pat dry and wait 20-30 minutes; then apply sparingly to affected area; use only once daily in the evening. Avoid eyes, ears, nostrils, and mouth.

▶ ***adapalene+benzoyl peroxide*** **(C)(G)** <18 years: not recommended; ≥18 years: apply a thin film to the affected area once daily; ***benzoyl peroxide*** may discolor clothing and linens
  Epiduo Gel *Gel: adap* 0.1%+*benz* 2.5% (45 gm)
  Epiduo Forte Gel *Pump gel:* adap 0.3%+benz 2.5% (15, 30, 45, 60 gm)

▶ ***tretinoin+clindamycin*** **(C)(G)** <18 years: not recommended; ≥18 years: apply a thin film to the affected area once daily
  Ziana *Gel:* tret 0.025%+clin 1.2% (30, 60 gm)

ORAL RETINOID

Comment: Oral retinoids are indicated only for severe recalcitrant nodular acne unresponsive to conventional therapy including systemic antibiotics.

▶ ***isotretinoin*** **(X)** <12 years: not recommended; ≥12 years: initially 0.5-1 mg/kg/day in 2 divided doses; maintenance 0.5-2 mg/kg/day in 2 divided doses x 4-5 months; repeat only if necessary 2 months following cessation of first treatment course
  Accutane *Cap:* 10, 20, 40 mg (parabens)
  Amnesteem *Cap:* 10, 20, 40 mg (soy)

Comment: ***isotretinoin*** is highly teratogenic and, therefore, female patients should be counseled prior to initiation of treatment as follows: Two negative pregnancy tests are required prior to initiation of treatment and monthly thereafter. Not for use in females who are or who may become pregnant or who are breastfeeding. Two effective methods of contraception should be used for 1 month prior to, during, and continuing for 1 month following completion of treatment. Low-dose *progestin* (mini-pill) may be an *inadequate* form of contraception. No refills; a new prescription is required every 30 days and prescriptions must be filled within 7 days. Serum lipids should be monitored until response is established (usually initially and again after 4 weeks). Bone growth, serum glucose, ESR, RBCs, WBCs, and liver enzymes should be monitored. Blood should not be donated during, or for 1 month after, completion of treatment. Avoid the sun and artificial UV light. ***isotretinoin*** should be discontinued if any of the following occurs: visual disturbances, tinnitus, hearing impairment, rectal bleeding, pancreatitis, hepatitis, significant decrease in CBC, hyperlipidemia (particularly hypertriglyceridemia).

ACROMEGALY

GROWTH HORMONE RECEPTOR ANTAGONIST

▶ ***pegvisomant*** **(B)** <12 years: not recommended; ≥12 years: *Loading dose:* 40 mg SC; *Maintenance:* 10 mg SC daily; titrate by 5 mg (increments or decrements, based on IGF-1 levels) every 4 to 6 weeks; max 30 mg/day

Somavert *Inj:* 10, 15, 20 mg

Comment: Prior to initiation of ***pegvisomant***, patients should have baseline fasting serum glucose, HgbA1c, serum K^+ and Mg^{++}, liver function tests (LFTs), EKG, and gall bladder ultrasound.

Cyclohexapeptide Somatostatin

▶ ***pasireotide*** **(C)** <12 years: not recommended; ≥12 years: administer SC in the thigh or abdomen; initial dose is 0.6 mg or 0.9 mg bid. Titrate dose based on response and tolerability; for patients with moderate hepatic impairment (Child-Pugh Class B), the recommended initial dosage is 0.3 mg twice daily and max dose 0.6 mg twice daily; avoid use in patients with severe hepatic impairment (Child-Pugh Class C)

Signifor LAR *Amp:* 0.3, 0.6, 0.9 mg/ml, single-dose, long-act rel (LAR) susp for inj

ACTINIC KERATOSIS

Comment: ***pasireotide*** is also indicated for destroying superficial basal cell carcinoma (sBCC) lesions.

▶ ***diclofenac sodium*** 3% **(C; D ≥30 wks)(G)** <12 years: not recommended; ≥12 years: apply to lesions bid x 60-90 days

Solaraze Gel *Gel:* 3% (50 gm) (benzyl alcohol)

Comment: Contraindicated with ***aspirin*** allergy. As with other NSAIDs, **Solaraze Gel** should be avoided in late pregnancy (≥30 weeks) because it may cause premature closure of the ductus arteriosus

Voltaren Gel <12 years: not recommended; ≥12 years: apply qid; avoid non-intact skin

Gel: 1% (100 gm)

▶ ***fluorouracil*** **(X)(G)** <12 years: not recommended; ≥12 years: apply to lesion(s) once daily-bid until erosion occurs, usually 2-4 weeks

Carac *Crm:* 0.5% (30 gm)

Efudex (G) *Crm:* 5% (25 gm); *Soln:* 2, 5% (10 ml w. dropper)

Fluoroplex *Crm:* 1% (30 gm); *Soln:* 1% (30 ml w. dropper)

▶ ***imiquimod*** **(B)**

Aldara (G) <18 years: not recommended; ≥18 years: rub into lesions before bedtime and remove with soap and water 8 hours later; treat 2 times per week; max 16 weeks

Crm: 5% (single-use pkts/carton)

Zyclara <12 years: not recommended; ≥12 years: rub into lesions before bedtime and remove with soap and water 8 hours later; treat for 2-week cycles separated by a 2-week no-treatment cycle; max 2 packs per application; max one treatment course per area

Crm: 3.75% (single-use pkts; 28/carton) (parabens)

▷ ***ingenol mebutate*** (C) <18 years: not recommended; ≥18 years: limit application to one contiguous skin area of about 25 cm^2 using one unit dose tube; allow treated area to dry for 15 minutes; wash hands immediately after application; may remove with soapy water after 6 hours; *Face and Scalp*: apply 0.015% gel to lesions daily x 3 days; *Trunk and Extremities*: apply 0.05% gel to lesions daily x 2 days

Picato *Gel:* 0.015% (3 single-use tubes), 0.05% (2 single-use tubes)

ALCOHOL DEPENDENCE & ALCOHOL WITHDRAWAL SYNDROME

ALCOHOL WITHDRAWAL SYNDROME

Comment: Total length of time of a given detoxification regimen and/or length of time of treatment at any dose reduction level may be extended based on patient-specific factors, including potential or actual seizure, hallucinosis, increased sympathetic nervous system activity (severe anxiety, unwanted elevation in vital signs). If any of these symptoms are anticipated or occur, revert to an earlier step in the dosing regimen to stabilize the patient, extend the detoxification timeline and consider appropriate adjunctive drug treatments (e.g., anticonvulsants, antipsychotic agents, antihypertensive agents, sedative hypnotic agents).

▷ ***clorazepate*** (D)(IV)(G) <18 years: not recommended; ≥18 years: *De-escalating dosage schedule: Day 1:* 30 mg initially, followed by 30-60 mg in divided doses; *Day 2:* 45-90 mg in divided doses; *Day 3:* 22.5-45 mg in divided doses; *Day 4:* 15-30 mg in divided doses; Thereafter, gradually reduce the daily dose to 7.5-15 mg; then discontinue when patient's condition is stable; max dose 90 mg/day

Tranxene *Tab:* 3.75, 7.5, 15 mg

Tranxene T-Tab *Tab:* 3.75*, 7.5*, 15*mg

▷ ***chlordiazepoxide*** (D)(IV)(G)

Librium <18 years: not recommended; ≥18 years: 50-100 mg q 6 hours x 24-72 hours; then q 8 hours x 24-72 hours; then q 12 hours x 24-72 hours; then daily x 24-72 hours

Cap: 5, 10, 25 mg

Librium Injectable <12 years: not recommended; ≥12 years: 50-100 mg IM or IV; then 25-50 mg IM tid-qid prn; max 300 mg/day

Inj: 100 mg

▷ ***diazepam*** (D)(IV)(G) <18 years: not recommended; ≥18 years: 2-10 mg q 6 hours x 24-72 hours; then q 8 hours x 24-72 hours; then q 12 hours x 24-72 hours; then daily x 24-72 hours

Diastat *Rectal gel delivery system:* 2.5 mg

Diastat AcuDial *Rectal gel delivery system:* 10, 20 mg

Valium *Tab:* 2*, 5*, 10*mg

Valium Injectable *Vial:* 5 mg/ml (10 ml); *Amp:* 5 mg/ml (2 ml); *Prefilled syringe:* 5 mg/ml (5 ml)

Valium Intensol Oral Solution *Conc oral soln:* 5 mg/ml (30 ml w. dropper) (alcohol 19%)

Valium Oral Solution *Oral soln:* 5 mg/5 ml (500 ml) (wintergreen spice)

▷ ***oxazepam*** (C) <18 years: not recommended; ≥18 years: 500 mg once daily x 1-2 weeks; then 250 mg once daily 10-15 mg tid-qid x 24-72 hours; decrease dose and/or frequency every 24-72 hours; total length of therapy 5-14 days; max 120 mg/day

Cap: 10, 15, 30 mg

ABSTINENCE THERAPY: GABA TAURINE ANALOG

▶ ***acamprosate*** (C)(G) <18 years: not recommended; ≥18 years: 666 mg tid; begin therapy during abstinence; continue during relapse; *CrCl 30-50 mL/min:* max 333 mg tid; *CrCl <30 mL/min:* contraindicated

Campral *Tab:* 333 mg ext-rel

Comment: **Campral** does not eliminate or diminish alcohol withdrawal symptoms.

AVERSION THERAPY

▶ ***disulfiram*** (X)(G) <18 years: not recommended; ≥18 years: 500 mg once daily x 1-2 weeks; then 250 mg once daily

Antabuse *Tab:* 250, 500 mg; *Chew tab:* 200, 500 mg

Comment: ***disulfiram*** use requires informed consent. Contraindications: severe cardiac disease, psychosis, concomitant use of ***isoniazid***, ***phenytoin***, ***paraldehyde***, and topical and systemic alcohol-containing products. Approximately 20% remains in the system for 1 week after discontinuation.

ALLERGIC REACTION: GENERAL

Oral 2nd Generation Antihistamines *see* **Drugs for the Management of Allergy, Cough, and Cold Symptoms** *page* 570
Topical Corticosteroids *see page* 542
Parenteral Corticosteroids *see page* 547

FIRST GENERATION PARENTERAL ANTIHISTAMINE

▶ ***diphenhydramine*** injectable (B)(G)

Benadryl Injectable <12 years: *See mfr pkg insert:* 1.25 mg/kg up to 25 mg IM x 1 dose; then q 6 hours prn; ≥12 years: 25-50 mg IM immediately; then q 6 hours prn *Vial:* 50 mg/ml (1 ml single-use); 50 mg/ml (10 ml multi-dose); *Amp:* 10 mg/ml (1 ml); *Prefilled syringe:* 50 mg/ml (1 ml)

FIRST GENERATION ORAL ANTIHISTAMINES

▶ ***diphenhydramine*** (B)(G) <2 years: not recommended; 2-6 years: 6.25 mg q 4-6 hours; max 37.5 mg/day; >6-12 years: 12.5-25 mg q 4-6 hours; max 150 mg/day; ≥12 years: 25-50 mg q 6-8 hours; max 100 mg/day

Benadryl (OTC) *Chew tab:* 12.5 mg (grape) (phenylalanine); *Liq:* 12.5 mg/5 ml (4, 8 oz); *Cap:* 25 mg; *Tab:* 25 mg; *Dye-free soft gel:* 25 mg; *Dye-free liq:* 12.5 mg/5 ml (4, 8 oz)

▶ ***hydroxyzine*** (C)(G) <6 years: 50 mg/day divided qid; ≥6 years: 50-100 mg/day divided qid 50-100 mg qid; max 600 mg/day

Atarax *Tab:* 10, 25, 50, 100 mg; *Syr:* 10 mg/5 ml (alcohol 0.5%)
Vistaril *Cap:* 25, 50, 100 mg; *Oral susp:* 25 mg/5 ml (4 oz) (lemon)

ALLERGIES: MULTI-FOOD

Comment: Eight food-types cause about 90% of food allergy reactions: ***Milk*** (mostly in children), ***Eggs, Peanuts, Tree nuts,*** (e.g., walnuts, almonds, pine nuts, brazil nuts, and pecans), ***Soy, Wheat*** (and other grains with gluten, including barley, rye, and oats), ***Fish*** (mostly in adults), ***Shellfish*** (mostly in adults). Combining ***omalizumab*** with oral immunotherapy (OIT, controlled regular exposure to small amounts of the allergenic food) significantly improves the effectiveness of OIT in children with multiple food allergies, according to the results of a recent study. Researchers conducted a blinded, phase 2 clinical trial including children aged 4 to 15 years who had multi-food allergies validated by double-blind, placebo-controlled food challenges. Participants were randomly assigned (3:1) to either receive ***omalizumab*** with multi-food OIT or placebo. ***omalizumab*** and placebo were administered for 16 weeks, with OIT beginning at 8 weeks. At week 36, a significantly greater proportion of the ***omalizumab***-treated participants passed double-blind, placebo-controlled food challenges, compared with placebo (83% vs 33%). No serious or severe adverse events were reported. Study conclusion: In multi-food allergic patients, ***omalizumab*** improves the efficacy of multi-food OIT and enables safe and rapid desensitization.

REFERENCE

Andorf, S, Purington, N, Block, WM, *et al.* (2018). Anti-IgE treatment with oral immunotherapy in multifood allergic participants: a double-blind, randomised, controlled trial. *The Lancet Gastroenterology & Hepatology, 3*(2), 85–94. doi:10.1016/s2468-1253(17)30392-8

IGE BLOCKER (IGG1K MONOCLONAL ANTIBODY)

➢ ***omalizumab*** **(B)** <12 years: not recommended; 30-90 kg + IgE >30-100 IU/ml 150 mg q 4 weeks; 90-150 kg + IgE >30-100 IU/ml or 30-90 kg + IgE >100-200 IU/ml or 30-60 kg + IgE >200-300 IU/ml 300 mg q 4 hours; >90-150 kg + IgE >100-200 IU/ml or >60-90 kg + IgE >200-300 IU/ml or 30-70 kg + IgE >300-400 IU/ml 225 mg q 2 weeks; >90-150 kg + IgE >200-300 IU/ml or >70-90 kg + IgE >300-400 IU/ml or 30-70 kg + IgE >400-500 IU/ml or 30-60 kg + IgE >500-600 IU/ml or 30-60 kg + IgE >600-700 IU/ml 375 mg q 2 weeks 150-375 mg SC every 2-4 weeks based on body weight and pre-treatment serum total IgE level; max 150 mg/injection site; ≥12 years: 150-375 mg SC every 2-4 weeks based on body weight and pre-treatment serum total IgE level; max 150 mg/injection site

Xolair *Vial:* 150 mg pwdr for SC injection after reconstitution (preservative-free)

AMEBIASIS

AMEBIASIS (INTESTINAL)

➢ ***diiodohydroxyquin (iodoquinol)*** **(C)(G)** <6 years: 40 mg/kg/day in 3 divided doses pc x 20 days; max 1.95 gm; 6-<12 years: 420 mg tid pc x 20 days; ≥12 years: 650 mg tid pc x 20 days

Tab: 210, 650 mg

➢ ***metronidazole*** **(not for use in 1st; B in 2nd, 3rd)(G)** <12 years: 35-50 mg/kg/day in 3 divided doses x 10 days; ≥12 years: 750 mg tid x 5-10 days

Flagyl *Tab:* 250*, 500*mg
Flagyl 375 *Cap:* 375 mg
Flagyl ER *Tab:* 750 mg ext-rel

Comment: Alcohol is contraindicated during treatment with oral ***metronidazole*** and for 72 hours after therapy due to a possible ***disulfiram***-like reaction (nausea, vomiting, flushing, headache).

➢ ***tinidazole*** **(not for use in 1st; B in 2nd, 3rd)** <3 years: not recommended; 3-12 years: 50 mg/kg daily x 3 days; take with food; max 2 gm/day; ≥12 years: 2 gm daily x 3 days; take with food

Tindamax *Tab:* 250*, 500*mg

▶ *paromomycin* 25-35 mg/kg/day in 3 divided doses x 5-10 days
Humatin *Cap:* 250 mg

AMEBIASIS (EXTRA-INTESTINAL)

▶ *chloroquine phosphate* (C)(G) <12 years: *see mfr pkg insert;* ≥12 years: 1 gm PO daily x 2 days; then 500 mg daily x 2 to 3 weeks or 200-250 mg IM daily x 10-12 days (when oral therapy is impossible); use with intestinal amebicide
Aralen *Tab:* 500 mg; *Amp:* 50 mg/ml (5 ml)

AMEBIC LIVER ABSCESS

ANTI-INFECTIVES

▶ ***metronidazole*** **(not for use in 1st; B in 2nd, 3rd)(G)** <12 years: not recommended; ≥12 years: 250 mg tid or 500 mg bid or 750 mg daily x 7 days
Flagyl *Tab:* 250*, 500*mg
Flagyl 375 *Cap:* 375 mg
Flagyl ER *Tab:* 750 mg ext-rel

Comment: Alcohol is contraindicated during treatment with oral ***metronidazole*** and for 72 hours after therapy due to a possible ***disulfiram***-like reaction (nausea, vomiting, flushing, headache).

▶ ***tinidazole*** **(not for use in 1st; B in 2nd, 3rd)** <3 years: not recommended; 3-12 years: 50 mg/kg once daily x 3-5 days; take with food; max 2 gm/day; ≥12 years: 2 gm once daily x 3-5 days; take with food
Tindamax *Tab:* 250*, 500*mg

AMENORRHEA: SECONDARY

▶ *estrogen+progesterone* (X)
Premarin (***estrogen***) 0.625 mg daily x 25 days; then 5 days off; repeat monthly
Provera (***progesterone***) 5-10 mg last 10 days of cycle; repeat monthly

▶ *human chorionic gonadotropin* 5,000-10,000 units IM x 1 dose following last dose of menotropins
Pregnyl *Vial:* 10,000 units (10 ml) w. diluent (10 ml)

▶ *medroxyprogesterone* (X) *Monthly:* 5-10 mg last 5-10 days of cycle; begin on the 16th or 21st day of cycle; repeat monthly; *One-time only:* 10 mg once daily x 10 days
Amen *Tab:* 10 mg
Provera *Tab:* 2.5, 5, 10 mg

▶ *norethindrone* (X) 2.5-10 mg daily x 5-10 days
Aygestin *Tab:* 5 mg

▶ *progesterone, micronized* (X)(G) 400 mg q HS x 10 days
Prometrium *Cap:* 100, 200 mg

Comment: Administration of ***progesterone*** induces optimum secretory transformation of the ***estrogen***-primed endometrium. Administration of ***progesterone*** is contraindicated with breast cancer, undiagnosed vaginal bleeding, genital cancer, severe liver dysfunction or disease, missed abortion, thrombophlebitis, thromboembolic disorders, cerebral apoplexy, and pregnancy.

ANAPHYLAXIS

Parenteral Corticosteroids *see page* 547
Oral Corticosteroids *see page* 546

▶ ***epinephrine*** **(C)(G)** <2 years: 0.05-0.1 ml; 2-6 years: 0.1 ml; ≥6-12 years: 0.2 ml; All: q 20-30 minutes as needed up to 3 doses; ≥12 years: 0.3-0.5 mg (0.3-0.5 ml of a 1:1000 soln) SC q 20-30 minutes as needed up to 3 doses

ANAPHYLAXIS EMERGENCY TREATMENT KITS

▶ ***epinephrine*** **(C)** <15 kg: 0.01 mg/kg SC or IM in thigh; may repeat if needed; 15-30 kg: 0.15 mg; ≥12 years, ≥30 kg: 0.3 ml IM or SC in thigh; may repeat if needed

Adrenaclick *Autoinjector:* 0.15, 0.3 mg (1 mg/ml; 1, 2/carton) (sulfites)

Auvi-Q *Autoinjector:* 0.15, 0.3 mg (1 mg/ml; 1/pck w. 1 non-active training device) (sulfites)

EpiPen *Autoinjector* 0.3 mg (epi 1:1000, 0.3 ml (1, 2/carton) (sulfites)

EpiPen Jr *Autoinjector* 0.15 mg (epi 1:2000, 0.3 ml) (1, 2/carton) (sulfites)

Symjepi *Prefilled syringe:* 0.3 mg (0.3 ml) single-dose for manual injection

Comment: **Symjepi** is intended for patients weighing ≥30 kg only. Each syringe is overfilled for stability purposes. More than half the solution remains in the syringe after use (and the syringe cannot be re-used).

Twinject *Autoinjector:* 0.15, 0.3 mg (epi 1:1000) (1, 2/carton) (sulfites)

▶ ***epinephrine+chlorpheniramine*** **(C)** infants-2 years: 0.05-0.1 ml SC or IM; 2-<6 years: 0.15 ml SC or IM plus 1 PO tab ***chlorpheniramine;*** 6-<12 years: 0.2 ml SC or IM plus 2 chewable ***chlorpheniramine*** tabs; ≥12 years: ***epinephrine*** 0.3 ml SC or IM plus 4 chewable ***chlorpheniramine*** tabs

Ana-Kit: *Prefilled injector:* 0.3 ml epi 1:1000 (2/carton) for self-injection plus 4 x chlor 2 mg chew tabs

ANEMIA OF CHRONIC KIDNEY DISEASE (CKD) & CHRONIC RENAL FAILURE (CRF)

ERYTHROPOIESIS STIMULATING AGENTS (ESAS)

▶ ***darbepoetin alfa*** (erythropoiesis stimulating protein) **(C)** <12 years: not recommended; ≥12 years: administer IV or SC q 1-2 weeks; do not increase more frequently than once per month; *Not currently receiving epoetin alpha:* initially 0.75 mcg/kg once weekly; adjust based on Hgb levels (target not to exceed 12 gm/dL); reduce dose if Hgb increases more than 1 gm/dL in any 2-week period; suspend therapy if polycythemia occurs; *Converting from epoetin alpha and for dose titration:* see mfr pkg insert

Aranesp *Vial:* 25, 40, 60, 100, 150, 200, 300, 500 mcg/ml (single-dose) for IV or SC administration (preservative-free, albumin [human] or polysorbate 80)

Aranesp Singleject, **Aranesp SureClick Singleject** *Prefilled syringe:* 25, 40, 60, 100, 150, 200, 300, 500 mcg (single-dose) for IV or SC administration (preservative-free, albumin [human] or polysorbate 80)

▶ ***peginesatide*** **(C)** <12 years: not established; ≥12 years: use lowest effective dose; initiate when Hgb <10 gm/dL; do not increase dose more often than every 4 weeks; if Hgb rises rapidly (i.e., >1 gm/dL in 2 weeks or >2 gm/dL in 4 weeks), reduce dose by 25% or more; if Hgb approaches or exceeds 11 gm/dL, reduce or interrupt dose and then when Hgb decreases, resume dose at approximately 25% below previous dose; if Hgb does not increase by >1 g/dL after 4 weeks, increase dose by 25%; if response inadequate after a 12-week escalation period, use lowest dose that will maintain Hgb sufficient to reduce need for RBC transfusion; discontinue if response does not improve; *Not currently on ESA:* initially 0.04 mg/kg as a single IV or SC dose once monthly; *Converting from epoetin alfa:* administer first dose 1 week after last ***epoetin alfa; Converting from darbepoetin alfa:*** administer first dose at next scheduled dose of ***darbepoetin alfa***

Omontys *Vial,* single use: 2, 3, 4, 5, 6 mg (0.5 ml) (preservative-free); *Vial,* multi-use: 10, 20 mg (2 ml) (preservatives); *Prefilled syringe:* 2, 3, 4, 5, 6 mg (0.5 ml) (preservative-free)

ERYTHROPOIETIN HUMAN, RECOMBINANT

- ***epoetin alpha*** **(C)** <1 month: not recommended; ≥1 month-12 years: individualize; *Dialysis:* initially 50 units/kg 3 x/week IV or SC; target Hct 30-36%; ≥12 years: individualize; initially 50-100 units/kg 3 x/week; IV (dialysis or non-dialysis) or SC (non-dialysis); usual max 200 units/kg 3 x/week (dialysis) or 150 units/kg 3 x/week (non-dialysis); target Hct 30-36%
  - **Epogen** *Vial:* 2,000, 3,000, 4,000, 10,000, 40,000 units/ml (1 ml) single-use for IV or SC administration (albumin [human]; preservative-free)
  - **Epogen Multidose** *Vial:* 10,000 units/ml (2 ml); 20,000 units/ml (1 ml) for IV or SC administration (albumin [human]; benzoyl alcohol)
  - **Procrit** *Vial:* 2,000, 3,000, 4,000, 10,000, 40,000 units/ml (1 ml) single-use for IV or SC administration (albumin [human]) (preservative-free)
  - **Procrit Multidose** *Vial:* 10,000 units/ml (2 ml); 20,000 units/ml, (1 ml) for IV or SC administration (albumin [human]; benzoyl alcohol)
- ***epoetin alpha-epbx*** **(C)** Evaluate iron status before and during treatment and maintain iron repletion; correct or exclude other causes of anemia before initiating treatment; *Patients with CKD: Initial dose (infants >1 month and children):* 50 units/kg 3 x/week; *Initial dose (≥18 years-of-age):* 50-100 units/kg 3 x/week; individualize maintenance dose; intravenous route recommended for patients on hemodialysis
  - *Patients on* **Zidovudine** *due to HIV-infection:* 100 units/kg 3 x weekly
  - *Patients with Cancer on Chemotherapy:* 40,000 units once weekly or 150 units/kg 3 x weekly (adults); 600 Units/kg IV once weekly (children >5 years)
  - *Surgery Patients:* 300 units/kg once daily for 15 days or 600 units/kg once weekly
    - **Retacrit** Retacrit *Vial:* 2,000, 3,000, 4,000, 10,000, 40,000 units/ml (1 ml), single-dose, for SC or IV infusion

Comment: **Retacrit** ***(epoetin alfa-epbx)*** is the first FDA-approved biosimilar to **Epogen/Procrit** ***(epoetin alfa)*** for the SC or IV infusion treatment of anemia caused by chronic kidney disease, chemotherapy, or ***zidovudine*** treatment for human immunodeficiency virus infection. **Retacrit** is also approved for use before and after surgery to reduce the potential need for blood transfusions due to blood loss during surgery. Common reported adverse side effects with **Retacrit** include high blood pressure, joint pain, muscle spasm, fever, and dizzyness. Contraindications to **Retacrit** include uncontrolled hypertension, pure red cell aplasia (PRCA) that begins after treatment with **Retacrit** or other erythropoietin protein drugs, and serious allergic reactions to **Retacrit** or other epoetin alfa products. BBW: Potential ESAs include increase the risk of myocardial infarction, stroke, venous thromboembolism, thrombosis of vascular access, and tumor progression or recurrence, and death (see mfr pkg insert for the full BBW). Therefore, use the lowest **Retacrit** dose sufficient to reduce the need for red blood cell (RBC) transfusions and DVT prophylaxis is recommended. The limited available data on ***epoetin alfa*** use in pregnancy are insufficient to determine a drug-associated risk of adverse developmental outcomes. There is no information regarding the presence of ***epoetin alfa*** products in human milk or effects on the breastfed infant. Safety and effectiveness in pediatric patients <1 month-of age have not been established.

☐ ANEMIA: FOLIC ACID DEFICIENCY

- ***folic acid*** **(A)(OTC)** 0.4-1 mg once daily

Comment: ***folic acid (vitamin*** B_9***)*** 400 mcg daily is recommended during pregnancy to prevent neural tube defects. Females who have had a baby with a neural tube defect should take 400 mcg every day, even when not planning to become pregnant, and if planning to become pregnant should take 4 mg daily during the month before becoming pregnant until at least the 12th week of pregnancy.

ANEMIA: IRON DEFICIENCY

Comment: Hemochromatosis and hemosiderosis are contraindications to iron therapy. ***Iron*** supplements are best absorbed when taken between meals and with ***vitamin C***-rich foods. Excessive ***iron*** may be extremely hazardous to infants and young children. All vitamin and mineral supplements should be kept out of the reach of children.

IRON PREPARATIONS

➢ *ferrous gluconate* (A)(G) <12 years: not recommended: ≥12 years: 1 tab once daily
Fergon (OTC) *Tab:* iron 27 mg (240 mg as gluconate)

➢ *ferrous sulfate* (A)(G)
Feosol Tablets (OTC) <6 years: use elixir; ≥6-12 years: 1 tab tid pc; ≥12 years: 1 tab tid-qid pc and HS
Tab: iron 65 mg (200 mg as sulfate)
Feosol Capsules (OTC) <12 years: not recommended; ≥12 years: 1-2 caps daily
Cap: iron 50 mg (169 mg as sulfate) sust-rel
Feosol Elixir (OTC) <1 year: not recommended; >1-11 years: 2.5-5 ml tid between meals; ≥12 years: 5-10 ml tid between meals
Fer-In-Sol (OTC) <4 years, use drops; ≥4 years: 5 ml once daily
Syr: iron 18 mg (90 mg as sulfate) per 5 ml (480 ml)
Fer-In-Sol Drops (OTC) <4 years: 0.6 ml daily; ≥4 years: use syrup
Oral drops: iron 15 mg (75 mg as sulfate) per 5 ml (50 ml)

ANEMIA: MEGALOBLASTIC/PERNICIOUS

Comment: Signs of ***vitamin B12*** deficiency include megaloblastic anemia, glossitis, paresthesias, ataxia, spastic motor weakness, and reduced mentation.

➢ ***vitamin B12 (cyanocobalamin)*** **(A)(G)** 500 mcg intranasally once a week; may increase dose if serum B12 levels decline; adjust dose in 500 mcg increments
Nascobal Nasal Spray *Intranasal gel:* 500 mcg/0.1 ml (1.3 ml, 4 doses) (citric acid, benzalkonium chloride)

Comment: **Nascobal Nasal Spray** is indicated for maintenance of hematologic remission following IM B12 therapy without nervous system involvement. Must be primed before each use.

ANGINA PECTORIS: STABLE

CALCIUM ANTAGONISTS

Comment: Calcium antagonists are contraindicated with history of ventricular arrhythmias, sick sinus syndrome, 2nd or 3rd degree heart block, cardiogenic shock, acute myocardial infarction, and pulmonary congestion.

➢ ***amlodipine*** (C)(G) <12 years: not recommended; ≥12 years: 5-10 mg daily
Norvasc *Tab:* 2.5, 5, 10 mg

➢ ***diltiazem*** (C)(G)
Cardizem <12 years: not recommended; ≥12 years: initially 30 mg qid; may increase gradually every 1-2 days; max 360 mg/day in divided doses
Tab: 30, 60, 90, 120 mg

Cardizem CD <12 years: not recommended; ≥12 years: initially 120-180 mg daily; adjust at 1- to 2-week intervals; max 480 mg/day
Cap: 120, 180, 240, 300, 360 mg ext-rel
Cardizem LA <12 years: not recommended; ≥12 years: initially 180-240 mg daily; titrate at 2 week intervals; max 540 mg/day
Tab: 120, 180, 240, 300, 360, 420 mg ext-rel
Cartia XT <12 years: not recommended; ≥12 years: initially 180 mg or 240 mg once daily; max 540 mg once daily
Cap: 120, 180, 240, 300 mg ext-rel
Dilacor XR <12 years: not recommended; ≥12 years: initially 180 mg or 240 mg once daily; max 540 mg once daily
Cap: 180, 240 mg ext-rel
Tiazac <12 years: not recommended; ≥12 years: initially 120-180 mg daily; max 540 mg/day
Cap: 120, 180, 240, 300, 360, 420 mg ext-rel

▶ ***nicardipine*** (C)(G) <12 years: not recommended; ≥12 years: initially 20 mg tid; adjust q 3 days; max 120 mg/day
Cardene *Cap:* 20, 30 mg

▶ ***nifedipine*** (C)(G)
Adalat CC <12 years: not recommended; ≥12 years: initially 30 mg once daily; usual range 30-60 mg tid; max 90 mg/day
Tab: 30, 60, 90 mg ext-rel
Procardia <12 years: not recommended; ≥12 years: initially 10 mg tid; titrate over 7-14 days: max 30 mg/dose and 180 mg/day in divided doses
Cap: 10, 20 mg
Procardia XL <12 years: not recommended; ≥12 years: initially 30-60 mg daily; titrate over 7-14 days; max dose 90 mg/day
Tab: 30, 60, 90 mg ext-rel

▶ ***verapamil*** (C)(G)
Calan <12 years: not recommended; ≥12 years: 80-120 mg tid; increase daily or weekly if needed
Tab: 40, 80*, 120*mg
Calan SR <12 years: not recommended; ≥12 years: initially 120 mg once daily; increase weekly if needed
Tab: 120, 180, 240 mg
Covera HS <12 years: not recommended; ≥12 years: initially 180 mg q HS; titrate in steps to 240 mg; then to 360 mg; then to 480 mg if needed
Tab: 180, 240 mg ext-rel
Isoptin SR <12 years: not recommended; ≥12 years: initially 120-180 mg in the AM; may increase to 240 mg in the AM; then 180 mg q 12 hours or 240 mg in the AM and 120 mg in the PM; then 240 mg q 12 hours
Tab: 120, 180*, 240*mg sust-rel

BETA-BLOCKERS

Comment: Beta-blockers are contraindicated with history of sick sinus syndrome (SSS), 2nd or 3rd degree heart block, cardiogenic shock, pulmonary congestion, asthma, moderate to severe COPD with FEV1 <50% predicted, patients with chronic bronchodilator treatment.

▶ ***atenolol*** (D)(G) <12 years: not recommended; ≥12 years: initially 25-50 mg daily; increase weekly if needed; max 200 mg daily
Tenormin *Tab:* 25, 50, 100 mg

- *metoprolol succinate* (C)(G) <12 years: not recommended; ≥12 years: initially 12.5-25 mg in a single-dose daily; increase weekly if needed; reduce if symptomatic bradycardia occurs; max 400 mg/day
  Toprol-XL *Tab:* 25*, 50*, 100*, 200*mg ext-rel
- *metoprolol tartrate* (C)(G) <12 years: not recommended; ≥12 years: initially 25-50 mg bid; increase weekly if needed; max 400 mg/day
  Lopressor *Tab:* 25, 37.5, 50, 75, 100 mg
- *nadolol* (C)(G) <12 years: not recommended; ≥12 years: initially 40 mg daily; increase q 3-7 days; max 240 mg/day
  Corgard *Tab:* 20*, 40*, 80*, 120*, 160*mg
- *propranolol* (C)(G)
  Inderal <12 years: not recommended; ≥12 years: initially 10 mg bid; usual range 160-320 mg/day in divided doses
  Tab: 10*, 20*, 40*, 60*, 80*mg
  Inderal LA <12 years: not recommended; ≥12 years: initially 80 mg daily in a single-dose; increase q 3-7 days; usual range 120-160 mg/day; max 320 mg/day in a single-dose
  Cap: 60, 80, 120, 160 mg sust-rel
  InnoPran XL <12 years: not recommended; ≥12 years: initially 80 mg q HS; max 120 mg/day
  Cap: 80, 120 mg ext-rel

NITRATES

Comment: Use a daily nitrate dosing schedule that provides a dose-free period of 14 hours or more to prevent tolerance. ***Aspirin*** and ***acetaminophen*** may relieve nitrate-induced headache. ***Isosorbide*** is not recommended for use in MI and/or CHF. Nitrate use is a contraindication for using phosphodiesterase type 5 inhibitors: ***sildenafil*** (**Viagra**), ***tadalafil*** (**Cialis**), ***vardenafil*** (**Levitra**).

- *isosorbide dinitrate* (C)
  Dilatrate-SR <12 years: not recommended; ≥12 years: 40 mg once daily; max 160 mg/day
  Cap: 40 mg sust-rel
  Isordil Titradose initially <12 years: not recommended; ≥12 years: 5-20 mg q 6 hours; maintenance 10-40 mg q 6 hours
  Tab: 5, 10, 20, 30, 40 mg
- *isosorbide mononitrate* (C)
  Imdur <12 years: not recommended; ≥12 years: initially 30-60 mg q AM; may increase to 120 mg daily; max 240 mg/day
  Tab: 30*, 60*, 120 mg ext-rel
  Ismo <12 years: not recommended; ≥12 years: 20 mg upon awakening; then 20 mg 7 hours later
  Tab: 20*mg
- *nitroglycerin* (C)(G)
  Nitro-Bid Ointment <12 years: not recommended; ≥12 years: initially 1/2 inch q 8 hours; titrate in 1/2 inch increments
  Oint: 2% (20, 60 gm)
  Nitrodisc <12 years: not recommended; ≥12 years: initially one 0.2-0.4 mg/hour patch for 12-14 hours/day
  Transdermal disc: 0.2, 0.3, 0.4 mg/Hr (30, 100/carton)
  Nitrolingual Pump Spray <12 years: not recommended; ≥12 years: 1-2 sprays on or under tongue; max 3 sprays/15 minutes
  Spray: 0.4 mg/dose (14.5 gm, 200 doses)

Nitromist <12 years: not recommended; ≥12 years: 1-2 sprays at onset of attack, on or under the tongue while sitting; may repeat q 5 minutes as needed; max 3 sprays/15 minutes; may use prophylactically 5-10 minutes prior to exertion; do not inhale spray; do not rinse mouth for 5-10 minutes after use

Lingual aerosol spray: 0.4 mg/actuation (230 metered sprays)

Nitrostat <12 years: not recommended; ≥12 years: 1 tab SL; may repeat q 5 minutes x 3

SL tab: 0.3 (1/100 gr), 0.4 (1/150 gr), 0.6 (1/4 gr) mg

Transderm-Nitro <12 years: not recommended; ≥12 years: initially one 0.2 mg/hour or 0.4 mg/hour patch for 12-14 hours/day

Transdermal patch: 0.1, 0.2, 0.4, 0.6, 0.8 mg/hour

NON-NITRATE PERIPHERAL VASODILATOR

▷ ***hydralazine*** (C)(G) <12 years: not recommended; ≥12 years: initially 10 mg qid x 2-4 days; then increase to 25 mg qid for remainder of first week; then increase to 50 mg qid; max 300 mg/day

Tab: 10, 25, 50, 100 mg

NITRATE & PERIPHERAL VASODILATOR COMBINATION

▷ ***isosorbide+hydralazine HCl*** (C) <12 years: not established; ≥12 years: initially 1 tab tid; max 2 tabs tid

Bidil *Tab:* isosorb 20 mg+hydral 37.5 mg

NON-NITRATE ANTIANGINAL

▷ ***ranolazine*** (C) <12 years: not recommended; ≥12 years: initially 500 mg bid; may increase to max 1 gm bid

Ranexa *Tab:* 500, 1000 mg ext-rel

Comment: **Ranexa** is indicated for the treatment of chronic angina that is inadequately controlled with other antianginals. Use with amlodipine, beta-blocker, or nitrate.

☐ ANGIOEDEMA, HEREDITARY (HAE, C1 ESTERASE INHIBITOR DEFICIENCY)

▷ ***C1 esterase inhibitor (human)*** <12 years: not established; ≥12 years: administer 60 International Units per kg body weight SC in the abdomen twice weekly (every 3 or 4 days); administer at room temperature within 8 hours after reconstitution; use a silicone-free syringe for reconstitution and administration; use either the Mix2Vial transfer set provided with HAEGARDA or a commercially available 566 double-ended needle and vented filter spike

Haegarda *Vial:* 2000, 3000 IU C1 INH pwdr for reconstitution, single-use

Comment: **Haegarda is** a plasma-derived concentrate of C1 esterase inhibitor [human], a serine proteinase inhibitor. Iindicated for routine prophylaxis to prevent HAE attacks in adults and adolescents. It is not indicated for treating acute attacks of HAE. **Haegarda** is the first C1 esterase inhibitor (human) SC injection approved for self-administration by the patient or caregiver after healthcare provider instruction. An international consensus panel states that human plasma-derived C1 esterase inhibitor is considered to be the therapy of choice for both treatment and prophylaxis of maternal hereditary angioedema during lactation. There are no prospective clinical data from **Haegarda** use in pregnant women. C1-INH is a normal component of human plasma. There is no information regarding the excretion of **Haegarda** in human milk or effect the breastfed infant. The developmental and health benefits of breastfeeding should be considered along with the mother's clinical need for **Haegarda** and any potential adverse effects on the breastfed infant from **Haegarda** or from the underlying maternal condition.

ANOREXIA/CACHEXIA

APPETITE STIMULANTS

▶ ***cyproheptadine*** **(B)(G)** <2 years: not recommended; ≥2-6 years: 2 mg bid-tid prn; max 12 mg/day; 7-14 years: 4 mg bid-tid prn; max 16 mg/day; >14 years: initially 4 mg tid prn; then adjust as needed; usual range 12-16 mg/day; max 32 mg/day

Periactin *Tab:* cypro 4*mg; Syr: cypro 2 mg/5 ml

▶ ***dronabinol*** (cannabinoid) **(B)(III)** <12 years: not recommended; ≥12 years: initially 2.5 mg bid before lunch and dinner; may reduce to 2.5 mg q HS or increase to 2.5 mg before lunch and 5 mg before dinner; max 20 mg/day in divided doses

Marinol *Cap:* 2.5, 5, 10 mg (sesame oil)

▶ ***megestrol*** (progestin) **(X)(G)** <12 years: not recommended; ≥12 years: 40 mg qid

Megace *Tab:* 20*, 40*mg

Megace ES *Oral susp (concentrate):* 125 mg/ml; 625 mg/5 ml (5 oz) (lemon-lime)

Megace Oral Suspension *Oral susp:* 40 mg/ml (8 oz); 820 mg/20 ml) (lemon-lime)

Megestrol Acetate Oral Suspension (G) 125 mg/ml

Comment: ***megestrol*** is indicated for the treatment of anorexia, cachexia, or an unexplained, significant weight loss in patients with a diagnosis of AIDS.

ANTHRAX (*BACILLUS ANTHRACIS*)

POSTEXPOSURE PROPHYLAXIS OF INHALATIONAL ANTHRAX AND TREATMENT OF INHALED AND CUTANEOUS ANTHRAX INFECTION

Comment: *B anthracis* spores are resistant to destruction, are easily spread by release into the air, and cause irreversible tissue damage and death. The most lethal form is inhalational anthrax. Even with the most aggressive treatment, the mortality rate is about 45%. People at risk are those who work in slaughterhouses, tanneries, and wood mills who are exposed to infected animals.

Immune Globulin

▶ ***bacillus anthracis immune globulin intravenous (human)*** <16 years: not established; 5-<10 kg: 1 vial; 10-<18 kg: 2 vials; 18-<25 kg: 3 vials; 25-<35 kg: 4 vials; 35-<50 kg: 5 vials; 50-<60 kg: 6 vials; ≥60 kg: 7 vials; ≥16 years: administer via IV infusion at a maximum rate of 2 ml/min; dose is weight-based as follows, but may be doubled in severe cases if weight >5 kg

Anthrasil *Vial:* (60 units) sterile solution of purified human immune globulin G (IgG) containing polyclonal antibodies that target the anthrax toxins of Bacillus anthracis for IV infusion

Comment: **Anthrasil** is indicated for the emergent treatment of inhaled anthrax in combination with appropriate antibacterial agents.

MONOCLONAL ANTIBODIES

Comment: ***obiltoxaximab*** and ***raxibacumab*** have no antibacterial activity; rather, they are monoclonal antibodies that neutralize toxins produced by *B. anthracis* by binding to the bacterium's protective antigen, preventing intracellular entry of key enzymatic toxin components. ***obiltoxaximab*** (**Anthim**) and ***raxibacumab*** are indicated for treatment of inhalational anthrax in combination with appropriate antibacterial drugs and for prophylaxis of inhalational anthrax when alternative therapies are unavailable or inappropriate. Vials must be refrigerated and protected from light. Do not shake the vials. Pre-medicate the patient with ***diphenhydramine***.

▶ ***obiltoxaximab*** <12 years: see mfr pkg insert for dosing based on kilograms body weight: ≥12 years: 16 mg/kg diluted in 0.9% NS via IV infusion over 90 minutes
  Anthim *Vial:* 600 mg in 6 ml (100 mg/ml) single-use, for dilution in 0.9% NS and IV infusion

▶ ***raxibacumab*** (**B**) ≤15 kg: 80 mg/kg; >15-50 kg: 60 mg/kg; >50 kg: 40 mg/kg diluted in 0.45% NS or 0.9% NS via IV infusion over 2 hours and 15 minutes; see mfr pkg insert for recommended volume of dilution according to weight-based dose
  Vial: 1700 mg/34 ml (50 mg/ml), single-use, for dilution and IV infusion

ANTIBACTERIAL AGENTS

▶ ***ciprofloxacin*** (**C**) <18 years: 20-40 mg/kg/day divided q 12 hours; ≥18 years: 500 mg or 10-15 mg/kg/day) q 12 hours for 60 days; max 1.5 gm/day; start as soon as possible after exposure
  Cipro (**G**) *Tab:* 250, 500, 750 mg; *Oral susp:* 250, 500 mg/5 ml (100 ml) (strawberry)
  Cipro XR *Tab:* 500, 1000 mg ext-rel
  ProQuin XR *Tab:* 500 mg ext-rel

▶ ***doxycycline*** (**D**)(**G**) <8 years: not recommended; ≥8 years, ≤100 lb: 2 mg/lb on first day in 2 divided doses, followed by 1 mg/lb/day in 1-2 divided doses; ≥8 years, >100 lb: 100 mg bid; *see page 605 for dose by weight table*
  Acticlate *Tab:* 75, 150** mg
  Adoxa *Tab:* 50, 75, 100, 150 mg ent-coat
  Doryx *Tab:* 50, 75, 100, 150, 200 mg del-rel
  Doxteric *Tab:* 50 mg del-rel
  Monodox *Cap:* 50, 75, 100 mg
  Oracea *Cap:* 40 mg del-rel
  Vibramycin *Tab:* 100 mg; *Cap:* 50, 100 mg; *Syr:* 50 mg/5 ml (raspberry-apple) (sulfites); *Oral susp:* 25 mg/5 ml (raspberry)
  Vibra-Tab *Tab:* 100 mg film-coat

Comment: ***doxycycline*** is contraindicated <8 years-of-age, in pregnancy, and lactation (discolors developing tooth enamel). A side effect may be photosensitivity (photophobia). Do not take with antacids, calcium supplements, milk or other dairy, or within 2 hours of taking another drug.

▶ ***minocycline*** (**D**)(**G**) <8 years: not recommended; ≥8 years, ≤100 lb: 2 mg/lb on first day in 2 divided doses, followed by 1 mg/lb q 12 hours x 9 more days; ≥8 years, >100 mg: 100 mg q 12 hours
  Dynacin *Cap:* 50, 100 mg
  Minocin *Cap:* 50, 75, 100 mg; *Oral susp:* 50 mg/5 ml (60 ml) (custard) (sulfites, alcohol 5%)

Comment: ***minocycline*** is contraindicated <8 years-of-age, in pregnancy, and lactation (discolors developing tooth enamel). A side effect may be photosensitivity (photophobia). Do not give with antacids, calcium supplements, milk or other dairy, or within two hours of taking another drug.

TREATMENT OF INHALATIONAL, GI, AND OROPHARYNGEAL ANTHRAX

▶ *ciprofloxacin* (C) <18 years: usually not recommended; 10-15 mg/kg IV q 12 hours (start as soon as possible); then switch to 10-15 mg/kg PO q 12 hours for 60 days; ≥18 years: 400 mg IV q 12 hours (start as soon as possible); then, switch to 500 mg PO q 12 hours for total 60 days max 1.5 gm/day

Cipro (G) *Tab:* 250, 500, 750 mg; *Oral susp:* 250, 500 mg/5 ml (100 ml) (strawberry); *IV conc:* 10 mg/ml after dilution (20, 40 ml); *IV pre-mixed:* 2 mg/ml (100, 200 ml)
Cipro XR *Tab:* 500, 1,000 mg ext-rel
ProQuin XR *Tab:* 500 mg ext-rel

Comment: ***ciprofloxacin*** is usually contraindicated <18 years-of-age, and during pregnancy and lactation. Risk of tendonitis or tendon rupture. Risk/benefit must be assessed in the case of anthrax. Infuse IV ***ciprofloxacin*** over 60 minutes.

▶ ***doxycycline*** (D)(G) <8 years: usually not recommended; ≥8 years, ≤100 lb: 2 mg/lb on first day in 2 divided doses, followed by 1 mg/lb/day in 1-2 divided doses for 10 days; ≥8 years, >100 lb: 100 mg bid day 1; then 100 mg daily x 10 days; *see page* 605 *for dose by weight table*

Acticlate *Tab:* 75, 150**mg
Adoxa *Tab:* 50, 75, 100, 150 mg ent-coat
Doryx *Tab:* 50, 75, 100, 150, 200 mg del-rel
Doxteric *Tab:* 50 mg del-rel
Monodox *Cap:* 50, 75, 100 mg
Oracea *Cap:* 40 mg del-rel
Vibramycin *Tab:* 100 mg; *Cap:* 50, 100 mg; *Syr:* 50 mg/5 ml (raspberry-apple) (sulfites); *Oral susp:* 25 mg/5 ml (raspberry)
Vibra-Tab *Tab:* 100 mg film-coat

Comment: ***doxycycline*** is usually contraindicated <8 years-of-age, in pregnancy, and lactation (discolors developing tooth enamel). Risk/benefit must be assessed in the case of anthrax. A side effect may be photosensitivity (photophobia). Do not take with antacids, calcium supplements, milk or other dairy, or within 2 hours of taking another drug.

▶ ***minocycline*** (D)(G) <8 years: not recommended; ≥8 years, ≤100 lb: 2 mg/lb on first day in 2 divided doses, followed by 1 mg/lb q 12 hours x 9 more days; ≥8 years, >100 lb: 100 mg q 12 hours

Dynacin *Cap:* 50, 100 mg
Minocin *Cap:* 50, 75, 100 mg; *Oral susp:* 50 mg/5 ml (60 ml) (custard) (sulfites, alcohol 5%)

Comment: ***minocycline*** is usually contraindicated <8 years-of-age, in pregnancy, and lactation (discolors developing tooth enamel). Risk/benefit must be assessed in the case of anthrax. A side effect may be photosensitivity (photophobia). Do not take with antacids, calcium supplements, milk or other dairy, or within 2 hours of taking another drug. Do not give with antacids, calcium supplements, milk or other dairy, or within two hours of taking another drug.

☐ ANXIETY DISORDER: GENERALIZED (GAD)/ANXIETY DISORDER: SOCIAL (SAD)

FIRST GENERATION ORAL ANTIHISTAMINE

▶ *diphenhydramine* (B)(G)

Benadryl (OTC) <2 years: not recommended; 2-6 years: 6.25 mg q 4-6 hours; max 37.5 mg/day; >6-12 years: 12.5-25 mg q 4-6 hours; max 150 mg/day; >12 years: 25-50 mg q 6-8 hours; max 100 mg/day

Chew tab: 12.5 mg (grape) (phenylalanine); *Liq:* 12.5 mg/5 ml (4, 8 oz); *Cap:* 25 mg; *Tab:* 25 mg; *Dye-free soft gel:* 25 mg
Dye-free liq: 12.5 mg/5 ml (4, 8 oz)

▶ *diphenhydramine* injectable **(B)(G)**
Benadryl Injectable <12 years: *See mfr pkg insert:* 1.25 mg/kg up to 25 mg IM x 1 dose; then q 6 hours prn; ≥12 years: 25-50 mg IM immediately; then q 6 hours prn
Vial: 50 mg/ml (1 ml single-use); 50 mg/ml (10 ml multi-dose); *Amp:* 10 mg/ml (1 ml); *Prefilled syringe:* 50 mg/ml (1 ml)

▶ ***hydroxyzine*** **(C)(G)** <6 years: 50 mg/day divided qid; ≥6-12 years: 50-100 mg/day divided qid; ≥12 years: 50-100 mg qid; max 600 mg/day
Atarax *Tab:* 10, 25, 50, 100 mg; *Syr:* 10 mg/5 ml (alcohol 0.5%)
Vistaril *Cap:* 25, 50, 100 mg; *Oral susp:* 25 mg/5 ml (4 oz) (lemon)

Comment: ***hydroxyzine*** is contraindicated in early pregnancy and in patients with a prolonged QT interval. It is not known whether this drug is excreted in human milk; therefore, ***hydroxyzine*** should not be given to nursing mothers.

AZAPIRONE

▶ ***buspirone*** **(B)** <6 years: not recommended; ≥6 years: initially 7.5 mg bid; may increase by 5 mg/day q 2-3 days; max 60 mg/day
BuSpar *Tab:* 5, 10, 15*, 30*mg

BENZODIAZEPINES

Comment: If possible when considering a benzodiazepine to treat anxiety, a short-acting benzodiazepine should be used only prn to avert intense anxiety and panic and for the least time necessary while a different non-addictive antianxiety regimen (e.g., SSRI, SNRI, TCA, ***buspirone***, beta-blocker) is established and effective treatment goals achieved. Benzodiazepines have a high addiction potential when they are chronically used and are common drugs of abuse. *Benzodiazepine withdrawal syndrome* may include restlessness, agitation, anxiety, insomnia, tachycardia, tachypnea, diaphoresis, and may be potentially life-threatening depending on the benzodiazepine and the length of use. Symptoms of withdrawal from short-acting benzodiazepines, such as ***alprazolam*** **(Xanax)**, ***oxazepam***, ***lorazepam*** **(Ativan)**, ***triazolam*** **(Halcion)**, usually appear within 6-8 hours after the last dose and may continue 10-14 days. Symptoms of withdrawal from long-acting benzodiazepines, such as ***diazepam*** **(Valium)**, ***clonazepam*** **(Klonopin)**, ***chlordiazepoxide*** **(Librium)**, usually appear within 24-96 hours after the last dose and may continue from 3-4 weeks to 3 months. People who are heavily dependent on benzodiazepines may experience *protracted withdrawal syndrome* (PAWS), random periods of sharp withdrawal symptoms months after quitting. A closely monitored medical detoxification regimen may be required for a safe withdrawal and to prevent PAWS. Detoxification includes gradual tapering of the benzodiazepine along with other medications to manage the withdrawal symptoms.

Short-Acting Benzodiazepines

▶ *alprazolam* **(D)(IV)(G)**
Niravam <18 years: not recommended; ≥18 years: initially 0.25-0.5 mg tid; may titrate every 3-4 days; max 4 mg/day
Tab: 0.25*, 0.5*, 1*, 2*mg orally-disint
Xanax <18 years: not recommended; ≥18 years: initially 0.25-0.5 mg tid; may titrate every 3-4 days; max 4 mg/day
Tab: 0.25*, 0.5*, 1*, 2*mg

Xanax XR <18 years: not recommended; ≥18 years: initially 0.5-1 mg once daily, preferably in the AM; increase at intervals of at least 3-4 days by up to 1 mg/day. Taper no faster than 0.5 mg every 3 days; max 10 mg/day. When switching from immediate-release ***alprazolam***, give total daily dose of immediate-release once daily.
Tab: 0.5, 1, 2, 3 mg ext-rel

▶ ***oxazepam*** (C)(IV)(G) <12 years: not recommended; ≥12 years: 10-15 mg tid-qid for moderate symptoms; 15-30 mg tid-qid for severe symptoms
Cap: 10, 15, 30 mg

Intermediate-Acting Benzodiazepines

▶ ***lorazepam*** (D)(IV)(G) <12 years: not recommended; ≥12 years: 1-10 mg/day in 2-3 divided doses
Ativan *Tab:* 0.5, 1*, 2*mg
Lorazepam Intensol *Oral conc:* 2 mg/ml (30 ml w. graduated dropper)

Long-Acting Benzodiazepines

▶ ***chlordiazepoxide*** (D)(IV)(G)
Librium <6 years: not recommended; 6-12 years: 5 mg bid-qid; increase to 10 mg bid-tid; ≥12 years: 5-10 mg tid-qid for moderate symptoms; 20-25 mg tid-qid for severe symptoms
Cap: 5, 10, 25 mg
Librium Injectable <12 years: not recommended; ≥12 years: 50-100 mg IM or IV; then 25-50 mg IM tid-qid prn; max 300 mg/day
Inj: 100 mg

▶ ***chlordiazepoxide+clidinium*** (D)(IV) <12 years: not recommended; ≥12 years: 1-2 caps tid-qid: max 8 caps/day
Librax *Cap: chlor* 5 mg+*clid* 2.5 mg

▶ ***clonazepam*** (D)(IV)(G) <18 years: not recommended; ≥18 years: initially 0.25 mg bid; increase to 1 mg/day after 3 days
Klonopin *Tab:* 0.5*, 1, 2 mg
Klonopin Wafers dissolve in mouth with or without water
Wafer: 0.125, 0.25, 0.5, 1, 2 mg orally-disint

▶ ***clorazepate*** (D)(IV)(G) <9 years: not recommended; ≥9 years: 30 mg/day in divided doses; max 60 mg/day
Tranxene *Tab:* 3.75, 7.5, 15 mg
Tranxene SD do not use for initial therapy
Tab: 22.5 mg ext-rel
Tranxene SD Half Strength do not use for initial therapy
Tab: 11.25 mg ext-rel
Tranxene T-Tab *Tab:* 3.75*, 7.5*, 15*mg

▶ ***diazepam*** (D)(IV)(G) <12 years: not recommended; ≥12 years: 2-10 mg bid to qid
Diastat *Rectal gel delivery system:* 2.5 mg
Diastat AcuDial *Rectal gel delivery system:* 10, 20 mg
Valium *Tab:* 2*, 5*, 10*mg
Valium Injectable *Vial:* 5 mg/ml (10 ml); *Amp:* 5 mg/ml (2 ml); *Prefilled syringe:* 5 mg/ml (5 ml)
Valium Intensol Oral Solution *Conc oral soln:* 5 mg/ml (30 ml w. dropper) (alcohol 19%)
Valium Oral Solution *Oral soln:* 5 mg/5 ml (500 ml) (wintergreen spice)

TRICYCLIC ANTIDEPRESSANTS (TCAs)

Comment: Co-administration of SSRIs and TCAs requires extreme caution.

- ▶ ***amitriptyline*** (C)(G) <12 years: not recommended; ≥12 years: 10-20 mg q HS
  Tab: 10, 25, 50, 75, 100, 150 mg
- ▶ ***amoxapine*** (C) <12 years: not recommended; ≥12 years: initially 50 mg bid-tid; after 1 week may increase to 100 mg bid-tid; usual effective dose 200-300 mg/day; if total dose exceeds 300 mg/day, give in divided doses (max 400 mg/day); may give as a single bedtime dose (max 300 mg q HS)
  Tab: 25, 50, 100, 150 mg
- ▶ ***clomipramine*** (C)(G) <10 years: not recommended; 10-<16 years: initially 25 mg daily in divided doses; gradually increase; max 3 mg/kg or 100 mg, whichever is smaller; >16 years: initially 25 mg daily in divided doses; gradually increase to 100 mg during first 2 weeks; max 250 mg/day; total maintenance dose may be given at HS
  Anafranil *Cap:* 25, 50, 75 mg
- ▶ ***desipramine*** (C)(G) <12 years: not recommended; ≥12 years: 100-200 mg/day in single or divided doses; max 300 mg/day
  Norpramin *Tab:* 10, 25, 50, 75, 100, 150 mg
- ▶ ***doxepin*** (C)(G) <12 years: not recommended; ≥12 years: 75 mg/day; max 150 mg/day
  Cap: 10, 25, 50, 75, 100, 150 mg; Oral conc: 10 mg/ml (4 oz w. dropper)
- ▶ ***imipramine*** (C)(G) <12 years: not recommended; ≥12 years:
  Tofranil initially 75 mg daily (max 200 mg); adolescents initially 30-40 mg daily (max 100 mg/day); if maintenance dose exceeds 75 mg daily, may switch to **Tofranil PM** for divided or bedtime dose
  Tab: 10, 25, 50 mg
  Tofranil PM initially 75 mg daily 1 hour before HS; max 200 mg
  Cap: 75, 100, 125, 150 mg
- ▶ ***nortriptyline*** (D)(G) <12 years: not recommended; ≥12 years: initially 25 mg tid-qid; max 150 mg/day
  Pamelor *Cap:* 10, 25, 50, 75 mg; *Oral soln:* 10 mg/5 ml (16 oz)
- ▶ ***protriptyline*** (C) <12 years: not recommended; ≥12 years: initially 5 mg tid; usual dose 15-40 mg/day in 3-4 divided doses; max 60 mg/day
  Vivactil *Tab:* 5, 10 mg
- ▶ ***trimipramine*** (C) <12 years: not recommended; ≥12 years: initially 75 mg/day in divided doses; max 200 mg/day
  Surmontil *Cap:* 25, 50, 100 mg

PHENOTHIAZINES

- ▶ ***prochlorperazine*** (C)(G)
  Compazine <12 years: not recommended; ≥12 years: 5 mg tid-qid
  Tab: 5 mg; *Syr:* 5 mg/5 ml (4 oz) (fruit); *Rectal supp:* 2.5, 5, 25 mg
  Compazine Spansule <12 years: not recommended; ≥12 years: 15 mg q AM or 10 mg q 12 hours
  Spansule: 10, 15 mg sust-rel
- ▶ ***trifluoperazine*** (C)(G) <12 years: not recommended; ≥12 years: 1-2 mg bid; max 6 mg/day; max 12 weeks
  Stelazine *Tab:* 1, 2, 5, 10 mg

SELECTIVE SEROTONIN REUPTAKE INHIBITORS (SSRIs)

Comment: Co-administration of SSRIs with TCAs requires extreme caution. Concomitant use of MAOIs and SSRIs is absolutely contraindicated. Avoid St. John's wort and other serotonergic agents. A potentially fatal adverse event is **serotonin syndrome**, caused by serotonin excess. Milder symptoms require HCP intervention to avert severe symptoms that can be rapidly fatal without urgent/emergent medical care.

Symptoms include restlessness, agitation, confusion, tachycardia, hypertension, dilated pupils, muscle twitching, muscle rigidity, loss of muscle coordination, diaphoresis, diarrhea, headache, shivering, piloerection, hyperpyrexia, cardiac arrhythmias, seizures, loss of consciousness, coma, death. Common symptoms of the *serotonin discontinuation syndrome* include flu-like symptoms (nausea, vomiting, diarrhea, headaches, diaphoresis); sleep disturbances (insomnia, nightmares, constant sleepiness); mood disturbances (dysphoria, anxiety, agitation); cognitive disturbances (mental confusion, hyperarousal); and sensory and movement disturbances (imbalance, tremors, vertigo, dizziness, electric-shock-like sensations in the brain often described by sufferers as "brain zaps").

▶ ***citalopram*** **(C)(G)** <12 years: not recommended; ≥12 years: initially 20 mg once daily; may increase after one week to 40 mg once daily; max 40 mg

  Celexa *Tab:* 10, 20, 40 mg; *Oral soln:* 10 mg/5 ml (120 ml) (peppermint) (sugar-free, alcohol-free, parabens)

▶ ***escitalopram*** **(C)(G)** <12 years: not recommended; 12-17 years: initially 10 mg daily; may increase to 20 mg daily after 3 weeks; ≥17 years: initially 10 mg daily; may increase to 20 mg daily after 1 week; *Hepatic impairment:* 10 mg once daily

  Lexapro *Tab:* 5, 10*, 20*mg

  Lexapro Oral Solution *Oral soln:* 1 mg/ml (240 ml) (peppermint) (parabens)

▶ ***fluoxetine*** (C)(G)

  Prozac <8 years: not recommended; 8-17 years: initially 10 mg/day; may increase after 1 week to 20 mg/day; range 20-60 mg/day; range for lower weight children, 20-30 mg/day; >17 years: initially 20 mg daily; may increase after 1 week; doses >20 mg/day should be divided into AM and noon doses; max 80 mg/day

    Cap: 10, 20, 40 mg; *Tab:* 30*, 60*mg; *Oral soln:* 20 mg/5 ml (4 oz) (mint)

  Prozac Weekly <12 years: not recommended; ≥12 years: following daily ***fluoxetine*** therapy at 20 mg/day for 13 weeks, may initiate **Prozac Weekly** 7 days after the last 20 mg ***fluoxetine*** dose

    Cap: 90 mg ent-coat del-rel pellets

▶ ***levomilnacipran*** **(C)** <12 years: not recommended; ≥12 years: swallow whole; initially 20 mg once daily for 2 days; then increase to 40 mg once daily; may increase dose in 40 mg increments at intervals of ≥2 days; max 120 mg once daily; *CrCl 30-59 mL/min:* max 80 mg once daily; *CrCl 15-29 mL/min:* max 40 mg once daily

  Fetzima *Cap:* 20, 40, 80, 120 mg ext-rel

▶ ***paroxetine maleate*** **(D)(G)**

  Paxil <12 years: not recommended; ≥12 years: initially 20 mg daily in AM; may increase by 10 mg/day at weekly intervals as needed; max 60 mg/day

    Tab: 10*, 20*, 30, 40 mg

  Paxil CR <12 years: not recommended; ≥12 years: initially 25 mg daily in AM; may increase by 12.5 mg at weekly intervals as needed; max 62.5 mg/day

    Tab: 12.5, 25, 37.5 mg cont-rel ent-coat

  Paxil Suspension <12 years: not recommended; ≥12 years: initially 20 mg daily in AM; may increase by 10 mg/day at weekly intervals as needed; max 60 mg/day

    Oral susp: 10 mg/5 ml (250 ml) (orange)

▶ ***paroxetine mesylate*** **(D)(G)** <12 years: not recommended; ≥12 years: initially 7.5 mg daily in AM; may increase by 10 mg/day at weekly intervals as needed; max 60 mg/day

  Brisdelle *Cap:* 7.5 mg

▶ ***sertraline*** **(C)(G)** <6 years: not recommended; 6-<12 years: initially 25 mg daily; max 200 mg/day; 12-17 years: initially 50 mg daily; max 200 mg/day; ≥17 years: initially 50 mg daily; increase at 1 week intervals if needed; max 200 mg daily; dilute oral concentrate immediately prior to administration in 4 oz water, ginger ale, lemon-lime soda, lemonade, or orange juice

  Zoloft *Tab:* 25*, 50*, 100*mg; *Oral conc:* 20 mg per ml (60 ml) (alcohol 12%)

SEROTONIN-NOREPINEPHRINE REUPTAKE INHIBITORS (SNRIs)

▶ ***desvenlafaxine*** (C)(G) <18 years: not recommended; ≥18 years: swallow whole; initially 50 mg once daily; max 120 mg/day

Pristiq *Tab:* 50, 100 mg ext-rel

▶ ***duloxetine*** (C)(G) <12 years: not recommended; ≥12 years: swallow whole; initially 30 mg once daily x 1 week; then, increase to 60 mg once daily; max 120 mg/day

Cymbalta *Cap:* 20, 30, 40, 60 mg del-rel

▶ ***venlafaxine*** (C)(G)

Effexor initially <18 years: not recommended; ≥18 years: 75 mg/day in 2-3 divided doses; may increase at 4 day intervals in 75 mg increments to 150 mg/day; max 225 mg/day

Tab: 37.5, 75, 150, 225 mg

Effexor XR <18 years: not recommended; ≥18 years: initially 75 mg q AM; may start at 37.5 mg daily x 4-7 days, then increase by increments of up to 75 mg/day at intervals of at least 4 days; usual max 375 mg/day

Tab/Cap: 37.5, 75, 150 mg ext-rel

▶ ***vortioxetine*** (C) <18 years: not established; ≥18 years: initially 10 mg once daily; max 30 mg/day

Brintellix *Tab:* 5, 10, 15, 20 mg

COMBINATION AGENTS

▶ ***chlordiazepoxide+amitriptyline*** (D)(G)

Limbitrol <12 years: not recommended; ≥12 years: 3-4 tabs/day in divided doses

Tab: chlor 5 mg+amit 12.5 mg

Limbitrol DS <12 years: not recommended; ≥12 years: 3-4 tabs/day in divided doses; max 6 tabs/day

Tab: chlor 10 mg+*amit* 25 mg

▶ ***perphenazine+amitriptyline*** (C)(G) <12 years: not recommended; ≥12 years: 1 tab bid-qid

Tab: **Etrafon 2-10** perph 2 mg+amit 10 mg

Etrafon 2-25 perph 2 mg+amit 25 mg

Etrafon 4-25 perph 4 mg+amit 25 mg

☐ APHASIA, EXPRESSIVE: STROKE-INDUCED

Comment: In a case report published in NEJM, a 52-year-old right-handed woman who sustained an ischemic stroke 3 years prior, the areas of infarction included the left insula, putamen, and superior temporal gyrus. Her stroke resulted in expressive aphasia, leaving her with no intelligible words, but with intact full language comprehension. ***zolpidem*** 10 mg was prescribed for insomnia. In repeated measures, it was found that the patient consistently demonstrated dramatic speech improvement, durable until HS, and return of the expressive aphasia in the AM. Subsequent single-photon-emission computed tomography (SPECT) scanning of this patient indicated that ***zolpidem*** increases flow in the Broca area of the brain, an area intimately involved with speech. From these observations, the authors concluded that a select subgroup of patients with aphasia, perhaps with subcortical lesions and spared but hypometabolic cortical structures, might benefit from this treatment. It may be worth trying ***zolpidem*** in patients who have been labeled with otherwise refractory chronic expressive aphasia. This finding raises the questions, could this intervention help patients earlier in the course, patients with milder disease, or patients with other ischemic central nervous system syndromes?

REFERENCE

Cohen, L, Chaaban, B, & Habert, M-O. (2004). Transient improvement of aphasia with zolpidem. *The New England Journal of Medicine, 350*(9), 949–950.

- ***zolpidem*** oral solution spray **(C)(IV)(G)** (imidazopyridine hypnotic) <18 years: not recommended; ≥18 years: 2 actuations (10 mg) immediately before bedtime; *Elderly, debilitated,* or *hepatic impairment:* 2 actuations (5 mg); max 2 actuations (10 mg)
  - **ZolpiMist** *Oral soln spray:* 5 mg/actuation (60 metered actuations) (cherry)
  - Comment: The lowest dose of ***zolpidem*** in all forms is recommended for persons >50 years-of-age and women as drug elimination is slower than in men.
- ***zolpidem*** tabs **(B)(IV)(G)** (pyrazolopyrimidine hypnotic) <18 years: not recommended; ≥18 years: 5-10 mg or 6.25-12.5 extrel q HS prn; max 12.5 mg/day x 1 month; do not take if unable to sleep for at least 8 hours before required to be active again; delayed effect if taken with a meal
  - **Ambien** *Tab:* 5, 10 mg

APHTHOUS STOMATITIS (MOUTH ULCER, CANKER SORE)

Comment: Aphthous ulcers are very painful sores with an inflamed base and non-viable tissue in the center that appears bacterial or viral. Although the sores are usually neither bacterial nor viral, herpetiform ulcers are most prevalent among the elderly). The sores may be single round/ovoid or several may be coalesced to form larger lesions, and located under the lip, on the buccal membrane, and/or on the tongue. Poor oral hygiene or an underlying immunity impairment can predispose the patient to ulcer formation (e.g., chronic illness, chemotherapy, poor nutrition, vitamin and mineral deficiencies, allergies, local trauma, stress, tobacco use, inflammatory bowel disease). They are frequently the result of local trauma (e.g., orthodontic-ware, chipped tooth) or allergy/irritation to a toothpaste or mouthwash ingredient (e.g. sodium lauryl sulfate). Changing toothpaste and applying dental wax to sharp edges are recommended until dental care is accessed. Debridement of the nonviable tissue by the direct application of salt (osmotic pulling pressure) for a few minutes, thus leaving a healthy tissue crater, speeds healing. Relief of the offending source of tissue trauma and application of a 5 mg prednisone tablet directly to the debrided ulcer are other remedies with reported success. These sores usually first appear in childhood or adolescence. Family history may have a role in the formation of recurrent aphthous stomatitis (RAS). When cases tend to occur in the same family (est 25-40% of the time), the ulcers earlier and with greater severity.

ANTI-INFLAMMATORY AGENTS

- ***dexamethasone*** elixir **(B)** <12 years: not recommended; ≥12 years: 5 ml swish and spit q 12 hours
  - *Elix:* 0.5 mg/ml
- ***triamcinolone acetonide*** <12 years: not recommended; ≥12 years: 0.1% dental paste **(G)** press (do not rub) thin film onto lesion at bedtime and, if needed, 2-3 x daily after meals; re-evaluate if no improvement in 7 days
  - **Oralone** *Dental paste:* 0.1% (5 gm)
- ***triamcinolone*** 1% in **Orabase (B)** <12 years: not recommended; ≥12 years: apply 1/4 inch to each ulcer bid-qid until ulcer heals
  - **Kenalog in Orabase** *Crm:* 1% (15, 60, 80 gm)

TOPICAL ANESTHETICS

- *benzocaine* topical gel (C)(G) apply tid-qid
- *benzocaine* topical spray (C)(G) 1 spray area every 2 hours as needed; retain for 15 seconds, then spit
  Cepacol Spray (OTC), Chloraseptic Spray (OTC)
- *lidocaine* viscous soln (B)(G) <3 years: not recommended; <3-11 years: 1.25 ml; apply with cotton-tipped applicator; may repeat after 3 hours; max 8 doses/day; ≥12 years: 15 ml gargle or swish, then spit; repeat after 3 hours; max 8 doses/day
  Xylocaine Viscous Solution *Viscous soln:* 2% (20, 100, 450 ml)
- *triamcinolone* (Kenalog) in **Orabase (C)** apply tid-qid

DEBRIDING AGENT/CLEANSER

- *carbamide peroxide 10%* **(OTC)** apply 10 drops to affected area; swish x 2-3 minutes, then spit; do not rinse; repeat treatment qid
  Gly-Oxide *Liq:* 10% (50, 60 ml squeeze bottle w. applicator)

ANTI-INFECTIVES

- *minocycline* (D)(G) <8 years: not recommended; ≥8 years: swish and spit 10 ml susp (50 mg/5 ml) or 1 x 100 mg cap or 2 x 50 mg caps dissolved in 180 ml water, bid x 4-5 days
  Dynacin *Cap:* 50, 100 mg
  Minocin *Cap:* 50, 75, 100 mg; *Oral susp:* 50 mg/5 ml (60 ml) (custard) (sulfites, alcohol 5%)

  Comment: ***minocycline*** is contraindicated <8 years-of-age, in pregnancy, and lactation (discolors developing tooth enamel). A side effect may be photosensitivity (photophobia). Do not give with antacids, calcium supplements, milk or other dairy, or within two hours of taking another drug.
- *tetracycline* (D)(G) <8 years: not recommended; ≥8 years: swish and spit 10 ml susp (125 mg/5 ml) or one 250 mg tab/cap dissolved in 180 ml water qid x 4-5 days
  Achromycin V *Cap:* 250, 500 mg
  Sumycin *Tab:* 250, 500 mg; *Cap:* 250, 500 mg; *Oral susp:* 125 mg/5 ml (100, 200 ml) (fruit) (sulfites)

  Comment: ***tetracycline*** is contraindicated <8 years-of-age, in pregnancy, and lactation (discolors developing tooth enamel). A side effect may be photosensitivity (photophobia). Do not give with antacids, calcium supplements, milk or other dairy, or within two hours of taking another drug.

ASPERGILLOSIS (*SCEDOSPORIUM APIOSPERMUM, FUSARIUM* SPP.)

INVASIVE INFECTION

- *isavuconazonium* (C) <18 years: not established; ≥18 years: swallow cap whole; *Loading dose:* 372 mg q 8 hours x 6 doses (48 hours); *Maintenance:* 372 mg once daily starting 12-24 hours after last loading dose
  Cresemba *Cap:* 186 mg; *Vial:* 372 mg pwdr for reconstitution (7/blister pck) (preservative-free)

  Comment: **Cresemba** is indicated for the treatment of invasive aspergillus and mucormycosis in patients ≥18 years old who are at high risk due to being severely compromised.
- *posaconazole* (D) <13 years: not recommended; ≥13 years: take with food; swallow tab whole; *Day 1:* 300 mg bid; then 300 mg once daily for duration of treatment (e.g., resolution of neutropenia or immunosuppression)

Noxafil *Tab:* 100 mg del-rel; *Oral susp:* 40 mg/ml (105 oz w. dosing spoon) (cherry)
Comment: **Noxafil** is indicated as prophylaxis for invasive aspergillus and candida infections in patients ≥13 years old who are at high risk due to being severely compromised.

- ***voriconazole*** **(D)(G)** <12 years: not recommended; ≥12 years: *PO:* <40 kg: 100 mg q 12 hours; may increase to 150 mg q 12 hours if inadequate response; ≥40 kg: 200 mg q 12 hours; may increase to 300 mg q 12 hours if inadequate; *IV:* 6 mg/kg q 12 hours x 2 doses; then 4 mg/kg q 12 hour; max rate 3 mg/kg/hour over 1-2 hours; response
  Vfend *Tab:* 50, 200 mg
  Vfend I.V. for Injection *Vial:* 200 mg pwdr for reconstitution (preservative-free)
  Vfend *Oral susp:* 40 mg/ml pwdr for reconstitution (75 ml)(orange)

ASTHMA

Parenteral Corticosteroids *see page* 547
Oral Corticosteroids *see page* 546

INHALED RACEPINEPHRINE (BRONCHODILATOR)

Comment: Inhalation racemic epinephrine is indicated for urgent/emergent acute bronchospasm rescue (e.g., acute asthma attack, laryngospasm, croup, epiglottitis, acute inflammation causing airway obstruction) Inhalational racemic epinephrine is only recommended for use during pregnancy when there are no alternatives and benefit outweighs risk.

- ***racepinephrine*** **(C)(OTC)(G)** <4 years: not recommended; ≥4 years: add 0.5 ml (contents of one vial) of solution to a hand-held rubber bulb nebulizer; administer 1 to 3 inhalations not more than every 3 hours. The use of this product by children should be supervised by an adult
  Pediatric: <4 years: not recommended; ≥4 years: same as adult
  Asthmanefrin *Starter kit:* 10 x 0.5 ml vials 2.25% solution for atomized inhalation w. EZ Breathe Atomizer; *Refills:* 30 x 0.5 ml vials 2.25% solution for atomized inhalation

INHALED BETA-2 AGONISTS (BRONCHODILATORS)

- ***albuterol sulfate*** **(C)(G)**
  AccuNeb Inhalation Solution <2 years: not recommended; 2-12 years: initially 0.63 mg or 1.25 mg tid-qid; 6-12 years: *Severe asthma* or *>40 kg* or *11-12 years:* initially 1.25 mg tid-qid by nebulizer; >12 years: not recommended
  Inhal soln: 0.63, 1.25 mg/3 ml (3 ml, 25/carton) (preservative-free)
  Albuterol Inhalation Solution (G) <2 years: not recommended; ≥2 years: 1 vial via nebulizer q 4-6 hours prn
  Inhal soln: 0.63 mg/3 ml (0.021%); 1.25 mg/3 ml (0.042%) (25/carton)
  Albuterol Inhalation Solution 0.5% (G) <4 years: not recommended; ≥4 years: 1 vial via nebulizer q 4-6 hours prn
  Inhal soln: 0.083% (25/carton)
  Albuterol Nebules (G) <12 years: use other forms; ≥12 years: 2.5 mg (0.5 ml of 5% diluted to 3 ml with sterile NS or 3 ml of 0.083%) tid-qid via nebulizer
  Inhal soln: 0.083% (25/carton)
  Proair HFA Inhaler <4 years: not established; ≥4 years: 1-2 inhalations q 4-6 hours prn; 2 inhalations 15 minutes before exercise as prophylaxis for exercise-induced asthma (EIA)
  Inhaler: 90 mcg/actuation (0.65 gm, 200 inh) (CFC-free)

Proair RespiClick <12 years: not established; ≥12 years: 1-2 inhalations q 4-6 hours prn; 2 inhalations 15-30 minutes before exercise as prophylaxis for exercise-induced asthma (EIA)

Inhaler: 90 mcg/actuation (8.5 gm, 200 inh)

Proventil HFA Inhaler <4 years: use syrup; ≥4 years: 1-2 inhalations q 4-6 hours prn; 2 inhalations 15 minutes before exercise as prophylaxis for exercise-induced asthma (EIA)

Inhaler: 90 mcg/actuation with a dose counter (6.7 gm, 200 inh)

Proventil Inhalation Solution <12 years: use syrup; ≥12 years: 2.5 mg diluted to 3 ml with normal saline tid-qid prn by nebulizer

Inhal soln: 0.5% (20 ml w. dropper); 0.083% (3 ml; 25/carton)

Ventolin Inhaler <2 years: not recommended; 2-4 years: use syrup; >4 years: 2 inhalations q 4-6 hours prn; 2 inhalations 15 minutes before exercise as prophylaxis for exercise-induced asthma

Inhaler: 90 mcg/actuation (17 gm, 220 inh)

Ventolin Rotacaps <4 years: not recommended; ≥4 years 1-2 caps q 4-6 hours prn; 2 inhalations 15 minutes before exercise as prophylaxis for exercise-induced asthma (EIA)

Rotacap: 200 mcg/dose (100 doses)

Ventolin 0.5% Inhalation Solution <2 years: not recommended; ≥2 years: initially 0.1-0.15 mg/kg/dose tid-qid prn; 10-15 kg: 0.25 ml diluted to 3 ml with normal saline by nebulizer tid-qid prn; >15 kg: 0.5 ml diluted to 3 ml with normal saline by nebulizer tid-qid prn

Inhal soln: 20 ml w. dropper

Ventolin Nebules <2 years: not recommended; ≥2 years: initially 0.1-0.15 mg/kg/dose tid-qid prn; 10-15 kg: 1.25 mg or 1/2 nebule tid-qid prn; >15 kg: 2.5 mg or 1 nebule tid-qid prn

Inhal soln: 0.083% (3 ml; 25/carton)

▶ ***isoproterenol*** **(B)** <12 years: not recommended; ≥12 years: *Rescue:* 1 inhalation prn; repeat if no relief in 2-5 minutes; *Maintenance:* 1-2 inhalations q 4-6 hours

Medihaler-1SO *Inhaler:* 80 mcg/actuation (15 ml, 30 inh)

▶ ***levalbuterol*** **(C)(G)** <12 years: not recommended; ≥12 years: initially 0.63 mg tid q 6-8 hours prn by nebulizer; may increase to 1.25 mg tid at 6-8 hour intervals as needed

Xopenex *Inhal soln:* 0.31, 0.63, 1.25 mg/3 ml (24/carton) (preservative-free)
Xopenex HFA *Inh:* 45 mg (15 gm, 200 inh) (preservative-free)
Xopenex Concentrate *Vial:* 1.25 mg/0.5 ml (30/carton) (preservative-free)

▶ ***metaproterenol*** **(C)(G)**

Alupent <6 years: use syrup; 6-12 years: via nebulizer 0.1-0.2 ml diluted with normal saline to 3 ml, up to q 4 hours prn; >12 years: 2-3 inhalations tid-qid prn; max 12 inhalations/day

Inhaler: 0.65 mg/actuation (14 gm, 200 doses)

Alupent Inhalation Solution <6 years: use syrup 6-12 years: via nebulizer 0.1-0.2 ml diluted with normal saline to 3 ml, up to q 4 hours prn; >12 years: 5-15 inhalations tid-qid prn or q 4 hours prn for acute attack

Inhal soln: 5% (10, 30 ml w. dropper)

▶ ***pirbuterol*** **(C)** <12 years: not recommended; ≥12 years: 1-2 inhalations q 4-6 hours prn; max 12 inhalations/day

Maxair *Autohaler:* 200 mcg/actuation (14 gm, 400 inh); *Inhaler:* 200 mcg/actuation (25.6 gm, 300 inh)

▶ ***terbutaline*** **(B)** <12 years: not recommended; ≥12 years: 2 inhalations q 4-6 hours prn

Inhaler: 0.2 mg/actuation (10.5 gm, 300 inh)

INHALED ANTICHOLINERGICS

➢ ***ipratropium bromide*** **(C)(G)** <12 years: not established; ≥12 years:
Atrovent 2 inhalations qid; additional inhalations as required; max 12 inhalations/day
Inhaler: 18 mcg/actuation (14 gm, 200 inh)
Atrovent Inhalation Solution 500 mcg tid-qid prn by nebulizer
Inhal soln: 0.02% (500 mcg in 2.5 ml; 25/carton)

Comment: ***ipratropium bromide*** is contraindicated with severe hypersensitivity to milk proteins.

INHALED CORTICOSTEROIDS

Comment: Inhaled corticosteroids are not for primary (rescue) treatment of acute asthma attack. After every inhalation of a steroid or steroid-containing medication treatment, rinse mouth to reduce risk of oral candidiasis. For twice daily dosing, allow 12 hours between doses.

➢ ***beclomethasone dipropionate*** **(C)(G)** <12 years: not established; ≥12 years: *Previously using only bronchodilators:* initiate 40-80 mcg bid; max 320 mcg bid; *Previously using inhaled corticosteroid:* initiate 40-160 mcg bid; max 320 mcg/day; *Previously taking a systemic corticosteroid:* attempt to wean off the systemic drug after approximately 1 week after initiating; rinse mouth after use
Qvar *Inhal aerosol:* 40, 80 mcg/metered dose actuation (8.7 gm, 120 inh) metered dose inhaler (chlorofluorocarbon [CFC]-free)

➢ ***budesonide*** **(B)**
Pulmicort Flexhaler <6 years: not recommended; 6-12 years: 1-2 inhalations bid; >12 years: initially 180-360 mcg bid; max 360 mcg bid; rinse mouth after use
Flexhaler: 90 mcg/actuation (60 inh); 180 mcg/actuation (120 inh)
Pulmicort Respules (G) <12 months: not recommended; 12 months-8 years: *Previously using only bronchodilators:* initiate 0.5 mg/day once daily or in 2 divided doses; may start at 0.25 mg daily; *Previously using inhaled corticosteroids:* initiate 0.5 mg once daily or in 2 divided doses; max 1 mg/day; *Previously taking oral corticosteroids*: initiate 1 mg/day daily or in 2 divided doses; >8-12 years: use flexhaler; rinse mouth after use; >12 years: use **Pulmicort Flexhaler**
Inhal susp: 0.25, 0.5, 1 mg/2 ml (30/carton)

➢ ***ciclesonide*** **(C)** <12 years: not recommended; ≥12 years: initially 80 mcg bid; max 320 mcg/day; rinse mouth after use; *Previously on inhaled corticosteroid:* initially 80 mcg bid; *Previously on oral steroid:* 320 mg bid
Alvesco *Inhal aerosol:* 80, 160 mcg/actuation (6.1 gm, 60 inh)

➢ ***flunisolide*** **(C)**
AeroBid, AeroBid-M <6 years: not recommended; 6-15 years: 2 inhalations bid; >15 years: initially 2 inhalations bid; max 8 inhalations/day; rinse mouth after use
Inhaler: 250 mcg/actuation (7 gm, 100 inh)
Aerospan HFA <6 years: not recommended; 6-11 years: 80 mcg bid; max 160 mcg bid; >11 years: initially 160 mcg bid; max 320 mcg bid
Inhaler: 80 mcg (5.1 gm, 60 doses; 80 mcg, 120 doses)

➢ ***fluticasone furoate*** **(C)** <12 years: not recommended; ≥12 years: *Currently not on inhaled corticosteroid:* usually initiate at 100 mcg once daily at the same time each day; may increase to 200 mcg once daily if inadequate response after 2 weeks; max 200 mcg/day; rinse mouth after use
Arnuity Ellipta *Inhal:* 100, 200 mcg/dry pwdr per inhalation (30 doses)

Comment: **Arnuity Ellipta** is not for primary treatment of status asthmaticus or acute asthma episodes. **Arnuity Ellipta** is contraindicated with severe hypersensitivity to milk proteins.

▶ ***fluticasone propionate*** (C)

ArmorAir <12 years: not established; ≥12 years: 1 inhalation bid (12 hours apart); initially 55 mcg bid; *Previously using an inhaled corticosteroid:* see mfr pkg insert; if insufficient response after 2 weeks, may increase the bid dose; max 232 mcg bid; after stability achieved, titrate to lowest effective dose; do not use with spacer or volume-holding chamber

Inhaler: 55, 113, 232 mcg/actuation (60 inh)

Flovent, Flovent HFA <11 years: use **Flovent Diskus**; ≥12 years: initially 88 mcg bid; *Previously using an inhaled corticosteroid:* initially 88-220 mcg bid; *Previously taking an oral corticosteroid:* 880 mcg bid; rinse mouth after use

Inhaler: 44 mcg/actuation (7.9 gm, 60 inh; 13 gm, 120 inh); 110 mcg/actuation (13 gm, 120 inh); 220 mcg/actuation (13 gm, 120 inh) (CFC-free)

Flovent Diskus <4 years: not recommended; 4-11 years: initially 50 mcg bid; max 100 mcg bid; rinse mouth after use; ≥11 years: may use **Flovent HFA**; initially 100 mcg bid; max 500 mcg bid; *Previously using an inhaled corticosteroid:* initially 100-250 mcg bid; max 500 mcg bid; *Previously taking an oral corticosteroid:* 1000 mcg bid

Diskus: 50, 100, 250 mcg/inh dry pwdr (60 blisters w. diskus)

▶ ***mometasone furoate*** (C)

Asmanex HFA <12 years: not recommended; ≥12 years: 220-440 mcg once daily or bid; max 880 mcg/day; rinse mouth after use

Inhaler: 100, 200 mcg/actuation (13 gm, 120 inh)

Asmanex Twisthaler <4 years: not recommended; 4-11 years: 110 mcg once daily in the PM; ≥12 years: may use **Asmanex HFA**; rinse mouth after use

Inhaler: 110 mcg/actuation (30 inh), 220 mcg/actuation (30, 60, 120 inh)

▶ ***triamcinolone*** (C)

Azmacort <6 years: not recommended; 6-12 years: 1-2 inhalations tid or 2-4 inhalations bid; >12 years: 2 inhalations tid-qid or 4 inhalations bid; rinse mouth after use

Inhaler: 100 mcg/actuation (20 gm, 240 inh)

LEUKOTRIENE RECEPTOR ANTAGONISTS (LRAs)

Comment: The LRAs are indicated for prophylaxis and chronic treatment, only. Not for primary (rescue) treatment of acute asthma attack.

▶ ***montelukast*** (B)(G) <12 months: not recommended; 12-23 months: one 4 mg granule pkt daily; 2-5 years: one 4 mg chew tab or granule pkt daily; >5-14 years: one 5 mg chew tab daily; >14 years: 10 mg once daily in the PM; for EIB, take at least 2 hours before exercise; max 1 dose/day

Singulair *Tab:* 10 mg

Singulair Chewable *Chew tab:* 4, 5 mg (cherry) (phenylalanine)

Singulair Oral Granules *Granules:* 4 mg/pkt; take within 15 minutes of opening pkt; may mix with applesauce, carrots, rice, or ice cream

▶ ***zafirlukast*** (B) <7 years: not recommended; 7-11 years: 10 mg bid 1 hour ac or 2 hours pc; >11 years: 20 mg bid, 1 hour ac or 2 hours pc

Accolate *Tab:* 10, 20 mg

▶ ***zileuton*** (C)(G) <12 years: not recommended; ≥12 years:

Zyflo <12 years: not recommended; ≥12 years: 1 tab qid (total 2400 mg/day)

Tab: 600 mg

Zyflo CR <12 years: not recommended; ≥12 years: 2 tabs bid (total 2400 mg/day)

Tab: 600 mg ext-rel

IGE BLOCKER (IGG1K MONOCLONAL ANTIBODY)

▶ ***omalizumab***(B) <12 years: not recommended; ≥12 years: 150-375 mg SC every 2-4 weeks based on body weight and pretreatment serum total IgE level; max 150 mg/injection site; 30-90 kg + IgE >30-100 IU/ml 150 mg q 4 weeks; 90-150 kg + IgE >30-100 IU/ml or 30-90 kg + IgE >100-200 IU/ml or 30-60 kg + IgE >200-300 IU/ml 300 mg q 4 hours; >90-150 kg + IgE >100-200 IU/ml or >60-90 kg + IgE >200-300 IU/ml or 30-70 kg + IgE >300-400 IU/ml 225 mg q 2 weeks; >90-150 kg + IgE >200-300 IU/ml or >70-90 kg + IgE >300-400 IU/ml or 30-70 kg + IgE >400-500 IU/ml or 30-60 kg + IgE >500-600 IU/ml or 30-60 kg + IgE >600-700 IU/ml 375 mg q 2 weeks

Xolair *Vial:* 150 mg pwdr for SC injection after reconstitution (preservative-free)

INHALED MAST CELL STABILIZERS (PROPHYLAXIS)

Comment: IMCSs are for prophylaxis and chronic treatment, only. Not for primary (rescue) treatment of acute asthma attack.

▶ ***cromolyn sodium*** (B)(G)

Intal <2 years: not recommended; 2-5 years: use inhal soln via nebulizer; >5 years: 2 inhalations qid via inhaler

Inhaler: 0.8 mg/actuation (8.1, 14.2 gm; 112, 200 inh) 2 inhalations qid; 2 inhalations up to 10-60 minutes before precipitant as prophylaxis; rinse mouth after use

Intal Inhalation Solution <2 years: not recommended; ≥2 years: 20 mg by nebulizer qid; 20 mg up to 10-60 minutes before precipitant as prophylaxis

Inhal soln: 20 mg/2 ml (60, 120/carton)

▶ ***nedocromil sodium*** (B)

Tilade <6 years: not recommended; ≥6 years: 2 sprays qid; rinse mouth after use

Inhaler: 1.75 mg/spray (16.2 gm; 104 sprays)

Tilade Nebulizer Solution 0.5% <2 years: not recommended; ≥2 years: initially 1 amp qid by nebulizer; 2-5 years: initially 1 amp tid by nebulizer; ≥5 years: 1 amp qid by nebulizer

Inhal soln: 11 mg/2.2 ml (2 ml; 60, 120/carton)

INHALED LONG-ACTING ANTICHOLINERGIC

▶ ***tiotropium (as bromide monohydrate)*** (C) <12 years: not recommended; ≥12 years: 2 inhalations once daily using inhalation device; do not swallow caps

Spiriva HandiHaler *Inhal device:* 18 mcg/cap pwdr for inhalation (5, 30, 90 caps w. inhalation device)

Spiriva Respimat *Inhal device:* 1.25, 2.5 mcg/actuation cartridge w. inhalation device (4 gm, 60 metered actuations) (benzalkonium chloride)

Comment: ***tiotropium*** is for prophylaxis and chronic treatment, only. Not for primary (rescue) treatment of acute attack. Avoid getting powder in eyes. Caution with narrow-angle glaucoma, BPH, bladder neck obstruction, and pregnancy. Contraindicated with allergy to ***atropine*** or its derivatives (e.g., ***ipratropium***).

INHALED ANTICHOLINERGIC+BETA-2 AGONIST

▶ ***ipratropium bromide+albuterol sulfate*** (C)

Combivent <12 years: not recommended; ≥12 years: 2 inhalations qid; additional inhalations as required; max 12 inhalations/day

Inhaler: ipra 18 mcg+albu 90 mcg/actuation (14.7 gm, 200 inh)

Duoneb <18 years: not recommended; ≥18 years: 1 vial via nebulizer 4-6 times daily prn

Inhal soln: ipra 0.5 mg (0.017%)+albu 2.5 mg (0.083%) per 3 ml (23/carton)

➢ *olodaterol* (C)

Striverdi Respimat <12 years: not established; ≥12 years: 12 mcg q 12 hours *Inhal soln:* 2.5 mcg/cartridge (metered actuation) 40 gm, 60 (actuations) (benzalkonium chloride)

Comment: **Striverdi Respimat** is contraindicated in persons with asthma without use of long-term control medication.

➢ *salmeterol* (C)(G) <4 years: not recommended; 4-12 years: 1 inhalation q 12 hours prn; 1 inhalation at least 30-60 minutes before exercise as prophylaxis for exercise-induced asthma; do not use extra doses for exercise-induced bronchospasm if already using regular dose; >12 years: 2 inhalations q 12 hours prn; 2 inhalations at least 30-60 minutes before exercise as prophylaxis for exercise-induced asthma; do not use extra doses for exercise-induced bronchospasm if already using regular dose

Serevent Diskus *Diskus (pwdr):* 50 mcg/actuation (60 doses/disk)

INHALED LONG-ACTING BETA-2 AGONIST (LABA)

Comment: LABA agents are not for primary (rescue) treatment of acute asthma attack. For twice daily dosing, allow 12 hours between doses.

➢ *arformoterol* (C) <12 years: not recommended; ≥12 years: 15 mcg bid via nebulizer

Brovana *Inhal soln:* 15 mcg/2 ml (2 ml; 30/carton)

Comment: ***arformoterol*** is indicated for the treatment of COPD but is used off-label for the treatment of asthma. It is used for prophylaxis and chronic treatment, only. Not for primary (rescue) treatment of acute attack.

➢ *formoterol fumarate* (C)

Foradil Aerolizer <5 years: not recommended; ≥5 years: 12 mcg q 12 hours *Inhaler:* 12 mcg/cap (12, 60 caps w. device)

Perforomist <12 years: not recommended; ≥12 years: 20 mcg q 12 hours *Inhal soln:* 20 mcg/2 ml (60/carton)

Comment: ***formoterol*** is for prophylaxis and chronic treatment, only. Not for primary (rescue) treatment of acute attack. Do not mix ***formoterol*** with other drugs. Use of ***formoterol*** is off-label for asthma.

➢ *olodaterol* (C) <12 years: not recommended; ≥12 years: 12 mcg q 12 hours

Striverdi Respimat *Inhal soln:* 2.5 mcg/cartridge (metered actuation) (40 gm, 60 metered actuations) (benzalkonium chloride)

Comment: **Striverdi Respimat** is contraindicated in persons with asthma without concomitant use of long-term control medication.

➢ *salmeterol* (C)(G) <4 years: not recommended; ≥4 years: 1 inhalation q 12 hours prn; 1 inhalation at least 30-60 minutes before exercise as prophylaxis for exercise-induced asthma; do not use extra doses for exercise-induced bronchospasm if already using regular dose 2 inhalations q 12 hours prn; 2 inhalations at least 30-60 minutes before exercise as prophylaxis for exercise-induced asthma; do not use extra doses for exercise-induced bronchospasm if already using regular dose

Serevent Diskus *Diskus (pwdr):* 50 mcg/actuation (60 doses/disk)

INHALED CORTICOSTEROID+LONG-ACTING BETA-2 AGONIST (LABA)

Comment: Inhaled corticosteroids and LABA agents are not for primary (rescue) treatment of acute asthma attack. For twice daily dosing, allow 12 hours between doses. After every inhalation of a steroid or steroid-containing medication treatment, rinse mouth to reduce risk of oral candidiasis.

▶ ***budesonide+formoterol*** (C) <12 years: not recommended; ≥12 years: 1 inhalation bid; rinse mouth after use

Symbicort 80/4.5 *Inhaler:* bud 80 mcg+for 4.5 mcg
Symbicort 160/4.5 *Inhaler:* bud 160 mcg+for 4.5 mcg

▶ ***fluticasone propionate+salmeterol*** (C)

Advair HFA *Not previously using inhaled steroid:* start with 2 inh 45/21 or 115/21 bid; if insufficient response after 2 weeks, use next higher strength; max 2 inh 230/50 bid; allow 12 hours between doses; *Already using inhaled steroid;* see mfr pkg insert

Advair HFA 45/21 <12 years: not recommended; >12 years: 1 inhalation bid; rinse mouth after use

Inhaler: flu pro 45 mcg+sal 21 mcg/actuation (CFC-free)

Advair HFA 115/21 <12 years: not recommended; >12 years: 1 inhalation bid; rinse mouth after use

Inhaler: flu pro 115 mcg+sal 21 mcg/actuation (CFC-free)

Advair HFA 230/21 <12 years: not recommended; >12 years: 1 inhalation bid; rinse mouth after use

Inhaler: flu pro 230 mcg+sal 21 mcg/actuation (CFC-free)

Advair Diskus *Not previously using inhaled steroid:* start with 1 inh 100/50 bid; *Already using inhaled steroid:* see mfr pkg insert; rinse mouth after use

Advair Diskus 100/50 <4 years: not recommended; ≥4 years: 1 inhalation bid; not a rescue inhaler; allow 12 hours between doses

Diskus: flu pro 100 mcg+sal 50 mcg/actuation (60 blisters)

Advair Diskus 250/50 <4 years: not recommended; 4-12 years: use 100/50 strength; >12 years: 1 inhalation bid; rinse mouth after use; not a rescue inhaler; allow 12 hours between doses

Diskus: flu pro 250 mcg+sal 50 mcg/actuation (60 blisters)

Advair Diskus 500/50 <4 years: not recommended; 4-12 years: use 100/50 strength; ≥12 years: 1 inhalation bid; rinse mouth after use; not a rescue inhaler; allow 12 hours between doses

Diskus: flupro 500 mcg+*sal* 50 mcg/actuation (60 blisters)

AirDuo RespiClick pwdr for oral inhalation; <12 years: not established; ≥12 years: *Not previously using an inhaled steroid:* 1 inh 55/14 bid; *Already using an inhaled steroid:* see mfr pkg insert; if insufficient response after 2 weeks, titrate with a higher strength; max inh 232/14 bid

AirDuo RespiClick 55/14 flu pro 55 mcg+sal (as xinafoate) 14 mcg dry pwdr/actuation (60 actuations)
AirDuo RespiClick 113/14 flu pro 113 mcg+sal (as xinafoate) 14 mcg dry pwdr/actuation (60 actuations)
AirDuo RespiClick *232/14* flu pro 232 mcg+sal (as xinafoate) 14 mcg dry pwdr/actuation (60 actuations)

▶ ***fluticasone furoate+vilanterol*** (C) <17 years: not established; ≥17 years: 1 inhalation 100/25 once daily at the same time each day

Breo Ellipta 100/25 *Inhal pwdr: flu* 100 mcg+*vil* 25 mcg dry pwdr per inhalation (30 doses)

Breo Ellipta 200/25 *Inhal pwdr: flu* 200 mcg+*vil* 25 mcg dry pwdr per inhalation (30 doses)

Comment: **Breo Ellipta** is contraindicated with severe hypersensitivity to milk proteins.

▶ ***mometasone furoate+formoterol fumarate*** (C) <12 years: not established; ≥12 years: 2 inhalations bid; not a rescue inhaler; rinse mouth after use;

Dulera 100/5 *Inhaler: mom* 100 mcg+*for* 5 mcg (HFA)
Dulera 200/5 *Inhaler: mom* 200 mcg+*for* 5 mcg (HFA)

INHALED ANTICHOLINERGIC+LONG-ACTING BETA AGONIST (LABA)

▶ *glycopyrrolate+formoterol fumarate* (C) ≥18 years: not established: >18 years: 2 inhalations bid (AM & PM)

Bevespi Aerosphere *Metered dose inhaler:* **9/4.8** *Inhal pwdr: gly 9 mcg+for 4.8 mcg* per inhal (10.7 gm, 120 inh)

ORAL BETA-2 AGONISTS (BRONCHODILATORS)

▶ *albuterol* (C)

Albuterol Syrup (G) <2 years: not recommended; 2-6 years: 0.1 mg/kg tid; initially max 2 mg tid; may increase gradually to 0.2 mg/kg tid; max 4 mg tid; >6-12 years: 2 mg tid-qid; may increase gradually; max 6 mg qid; ≥12 years: 2-4 mg tid-qid; may increase gradually; max 8 mg qid

Syr: 2 mg/5 ml

Proventil <6 years: use syrup; ≥6 years: 2-4 mg tid-qid prn

Tab: 2, 4 mg

Proventil Repetabs 4-8 mg q 12 hours prn

Repetab: 4 mg sust-rel

Proventil Syrup <2 years: not recommended; 2-6 years: 0.1 mg/kg tid prn; max initially 5 ml tid prn; may increase gradually to 0.2 mg/kg tid prn; max 10 ml tid; >6-14 years: 5 ml tid-qid prn; may increase gradually; max 60 ml/day in divided doses; >14 years: 5-10 ml tid-qid prn; may increase gradually; max 20 ml qid prn

Syr: 2 mg/5 ml

Ventolin <2 years: not recommended; 2-6 years: 0.1 mg/kg tid prn; max initially 2 mg tid prn; may increase gradually to 0.2 mg/kg tid; max 4 mg tid; >6-14 years: 2 mg tid-qid prn; may increase gradually; max 6 mg tid; >14 years: 2-4 mg tid-qid prn; may increase gradually; max 8 mg qid

Tab: 2, 4 mg; *Syr:* 2 mg/5 ml (strawberry)

VoSpire ER <6 years: not recommended; 6-12 years: 4 mg q 12 hours; max 24 mg/day q 12 hours; >12 years: 4-8 mg q 12 hours prn; max 32 mg/day divided q 12 hours; swallow whole

Tab: 4, 8 mg ext-rel

▶ *metaproterenol* (C)

Alupent <6 years: not recommended (doses of 1.3-2.6 mg/kg/day have been used); ≥6-9 years (<60 lb): 10 mg tid-qid prn; >9-12 years (>60 lb): 20 mg tid-qid prn; >12 years: 20 mg tid-qid prn

Tab: 10, 20 mg; *Syr:* 10 mg/5 ml

METHYLXANTHINES

Comment: Check serum theophylline level just before 5th dose is administered. Therapeutic theophylline level: 10-20 mcg/ml.

▶ *theophylline* (C)(G)

Theo-24 <45 kg: initially 12-14 mg/kg/day; max 300 mg/day; increase after 3 days to 16 mg/kg/day to max 400 mg; after 3 more days increase to 30 mg/kg/day to max 600 mg/day; ≥45 kg: initially 300-400 mg once daily at HS; after 3 days, increase to 400-600 mg once daily at HS; max 600 mg/day

Cap: 100, 200, 300, 400 mg ext-rel

Theo-Dur <6 years: not recommended; 6-15 years: initially 12-14 mg/kg/day in 2 divided doses; max 300 mg/day; then increase to 16 mg/kg in 2 divided doses; max 400 mg/day; then to 20 mg/kg/day in 2 divided doses; max 600 mg/day; ≥15 years: initially 150 mg bid; increase to 200 mg bid after 3 days; then to 300 mg bid after 3 more days

Tab: 100, 200, 300 mg ext-rel

Theolair-SR <12 years: not recommended; ≥12 years: 200-500 once daily
Tab: 200, 250, 300, 500 mg sust-rel
Uniphyl <12 years: not recommended; ≥12 years: 400-600 mg once daily
Tab: 400*, 600*mg cont-rel

METHYLXANTHINE+EXPECTORANT COMBINATION

▶ ***dyphylline+guaifenesin*** (C) <12 years: not recommended; ≥12 years: 1 tab qid
Lufyllin GG *Tab: dyphy* 200 mg+*guaif* 200 mg; *Elix: dyphy* 100 mg+*guaif* 100 mg per 15 ml

HUMANIZED INTERLEUKIN-5 ANTAGONIST MONOCLONAL ANTIBODY

▶ ***mepolizumab*** <12 years: not recommended; ≥12 years: 100 mg SC once every 4 weeks in upper arm, abdomen, or thigh
Nucala *Vial:* 100 mg pwdr for reconstitution, single use (preservative-free)
Comment: **Nucala** is an add-on maintenance treatment for severe asthma. There is a pregnancy exposure registry that monitors pregnancy outcomes in females exposed to **Nucala** during pregnancy. Healthcare providers can enroll patients or encourage patients to enroll themselves by calling 1-877-311-8972 or visiting www.mothertobaby.org/asthma

ASTHMA: SEVERE EOSINOPHILIA

Comment: ***tezepelumab*** is a human IgG2 monoclonal antibody that binds to thymic stromal lymphopoietin (TSLP), which is a cytokine produced in response to environmental and pro-inflammatory stimuli. It is an important potential mechanism because it works high up in the inflammatory cascade and appears to have a beneficial effect in patients across different asthma phenotypes. Currently available therapies for patients with severe asthma include anti-IgE therapy (***omalizumab***), anti-interleukin-5 monoclonal antibody ***mepolizumab***, interleukin-5 antagonist monoclonal antibody (IgG4 kappa) ***reslizumab***, and interleukin-5 receptor alpha-directed cytolytic monoclonal antibody (IgG1, kappa) ***benralizumab***.

HUMANIZED INTERLEUKIN-5 ANTAGONIST MONOCLONAL ANTIBODY

Interleukin-5 Antagonist Monoclonal Antibody (IgG1 Kappa)

▶ ***mepolizumab*** <12 years: not recommended; ≥12 years: 100 mg SC once every 4 weeks in upper arm, abdomen, or thigh
Nucala *Vial:* 100 mg pwdr for reconstitution, single-use (preservative-free)
Comment: **Nucala** is an interleukin-5 antagonist monoclonal antibody (IgG1 kappa). It is an add-on maintenance treatment for patients ≥12 years-of-age with severe asthma and with an eosinophilic phenotype. **Nucala** is also indicated for the treatment of patients >18 years-of-age with eosinophilic granulomatosis with polyangiitis (EGPA). **Nucala** is not for relief of acute bronchospasm or status asthmaticus. Hypersensitivity reactions (e.g., anaphylaxis, angioedema, bronchospasm, hypotension, urticaria, rash) have occurred after administration of **Nucala**; discontinue **Nucala** in the event of a hypersensitivity reaction. Herpes zoster infections have occurred in patients receiving **Nucala**. Consider vaccination if medically appropriate. Do not discontinue systemic or inhaled corticosteroids abruptly upon initiation of therapy with **Nucala**. Decrease corticosteroids gradually, if appropriate. Treat patients with pre-existing parasitic helminth infections before therapy with **Nucala**. If patients become infected while receiving treatment with **Nucala** and do not respond to anti-helminth treatment, discontinue **Nucala** until parasitic infection resolves. The most common adverse

reactions (incidence ≥5%) include headache, injection site reaction, back pain, and fatigue. Formal drug interaction trials have not been performed with **Nucala.** The data on pregnancy exposure are insufficient to inform on drug-associated risk. Monoclonal antibodies, such as ***mepolizumab***, are transported across the placenta in a linear fashion as pregnancy progresses; therefore, potential effects on a fetus are likely to be greater during the second and third trimester of pregnancy. There is a pregnancy exposure registry that monitors pregnancy outcomes in patients exposed to **Nucala** during pregnancy. Healthcare providers can enroll patients or enccourage patients to enroll themselves by calling 1-877-311-8972 or visiting www.mothertobaby.org/asthma. There is no information regarding the presence of ***mepolizumab*** in human milk or effects on the breastfed infant. To report suspected adverse reactions, contact GlaxoSmithKline at 1-888-825-5249 or FDA at 1-800-FDA-1088 or www.fda.gov/medwatch

Interleukin-5 Antagonist Monoclonal Antibody (IgG4 Kappa)

▶ ***resilumab*** <18 years: not established; ≥18 years: should be administered by a qualified healthcare professional and, in line with clinical practice, monitoring of patients after administration of biologic agents is recommended; recommended dose is 3 mg/kg once every 4 weeks via IV infusion over 20-50 minutes; do not administer as an IV push (IVP) or bolus

Cinqair *Vial:* 100 mg/10 ml (10 mg/ml) soln single-use (preservative-free)

Comment: **Cinqair** is an interleukin-5 antagonist monoclonal antibody (IgG4 kappa) indicated for add-on maintenance treatment of patients with severe asthma aged ≥18 years-of-age, and with an eosinophilic phenotype. Do not discontinue systemic or inhaled corticosteroids abruptly upon initiation of therapy with **Cinqair**. Decrease corticosteroids gradually, if appropriate. Treat patients with pre-existing parasitic helminth infection before therapy with **Cinqair**. If patients become infected while receiving **Cinqair** and do not respond to anti-helminth treatment, discontinue **Cinqair** until the parasitic infection resolves. The most common adverse reaction (incidence ≥2%) includes oropharyngeal pain. The data on pregnancy exposure from the clinical trials are insufficient to inform on drug-associated risk. Monoclonal antibodies, such as ***reslizumab***, are transported across the placenta in a linear fashion as pregnancy progresses; therefore, potential effects on a fetus are likely to be greater during the second and third trimester of pregnancy. ***reslizumab*** has a long half-life; this should be taken into consideration. In females with poorly or moderately controlled asthma, evidence demonstrates that there is an increased risk of preeclampsia in the mother and newborn prematurity, low birth weight, and small for gestational age. It is not known whether ***reslizumab*** is present in human milk or effects of ***reslizumab*** on the breastfed infant. To report suspected adverse reactions, contact Teva Pharmaceuticals at 1-888-483-8279 or FDA at 1-800-FDA-1088 or visit www.fda.gov/medwatch

IgE BLOCKER (IGG1K MONOCLONAL ANTIBODY)

▶ ***omalizumab*** **(B)** 150-375 mg SC every 2-4 weeks based on body weight and pre-treatment serum total IgE level; max 150 mg/injection site

<12 years: not recommended; 30-90 kg + IgE >30-100 IU/ml 150 mg q 4 weeks; 90-150 kg + IgE >30-100 IU/ml or 30-90 kg + IgE >100-200 IU/ml or 30-60 kg + IgE >200-300 IU/ml 300 mg q 4 hours; >90-150 kg + IgE >100-200 IU/ml or >60-90 kg + IgE >200-300 IU/ml or 30-70 kg + IgE >300-400 IU/ml 225 mg q 2 weeks; >90-150 kg + IgE >200-300 IU/ml or >70-90 kg + IgE >300-400 IU/ml or 30-70 kg + IgE >400-500 IU/ml or 30-60 kg + IgE >500-600 IU/ml or 30-60 kg + IgE >600-700 IU/ml 375 mg q 2 weeks

Xolair *Vial:* 150 mg pwdr for SC injection after reconstitution (preservative-free)

INTERLEUKIN-5 RECEPTOR ALPHA-DIRECTED CYTOLYTIC MONOCLONAL ANTIBODY (IGG1,KAPPA)

➢ ***benralizumab*** <12 years: not established; ≥12 years: should be administered by a qualified healthcare professional and, in line with clinical practice, monitoring of patients after administration of biologic agents is recommended; recommended dose is 30 mg SC every 4 weeks for the first 3 doses; then, once every 8 weeks thereafter; inject SC into the upper arm, abdomen, or thigh. Store in refrigerator; do not freeze; prior to administration, warm **Fasenra** by leaving carton at room temperature for about 30 minutes. Administer within 24 hours or discard into sharps container.

Fasenra *Prefilled syringe:* 30 mg/ml soln, single-dose (preservative-free)

Comment: ***benralizumab*** is an interleukin-5 receptor alpha-directed cytolytic monoclonal antibody (IgG1, kappa) produced in Chinese hamster ovary cells by recombinant DNA technology. **Fasenra** is indicated for the add-on maintenance treatment of patients with severe asthma ≥12 years-of-age, and with an eosinophilic phenotype. It is not for treatment of other eosinophilic conditions and not for relief of acute bronchospasm or status asthmaticus. Do not discontinue systemic or inhaled corticosteroids abruptly upon initiation of therapy with **Fasenra**; decrease corticosteroids gradually, if appropriate. Treat patients with pre-existing parasitic helminth infection before therapy with **Fasenra**. If patients become infected while receiving **Fasenra** and do not respond to anti-helminth treatment, discontinue **Fasenra** until the parasitic infection resolves. The most common adverse reactions (incidence ≥5%) include headache and pharyngitis. No formal drug interaction sytudies have been conducted. The data on pregnancy exposure from the clinical trials are insufficient to inform on drug-associated risk. Monoclonal antibodies such as ***benralizumab*** are transported across the placenta during the third trimester of pregnancy; therefore, potential effects on a fetus are likely to be greater during the third trimester of pregnancy. In women with poorly or moderately controlled asthma, evidence demonstrates that there is an increased risk of preeclampsia in the mother and neonate prematurity, low birth weight, and small for gestational age. The level of asthma control should be closely monitored in pregnant females and treatment adjusted as necessary to maintain optimal control. There is no information regarding the presence of ***benralizumab*** in human or animal milk, and the effects of ***benralizumab*** on the breastfed infant and on milk production are not known. To report suspected adverse reactions, contact Astra-Zeneca at 1-800-236-9933 or FDA at 1-800-FDA-1088 or visit www.fda.gov/medwatch

ATTENTION DEFICIT HYPERACTIVITY DISORDER (ADHD)

SELECTIVE NOREPINEPHRINE REUPTAKE INHIBITOR (SNRI)

➢ ***atomoxetine*** (C)(G) <6 years: not recommended; ≥6 years, <70 kg: initially 0.5 mg/kg/day: increase after at least 3 days to 1.2 mg/kg/day; max 1.4 mg/kg/day or 100 mg/day (whichever is less); ≥6 years, >70 kg: take one dose daily in the morning or in two divided doses in the morning and late afternoon or early evening; initially 40 mg/kg; increase after at least 3 days to 80 mg/kg; then after 2-4 weeks may increase to max 100 mg/day

Strattera *Cap:* 10, 18, 25, 40, 60, 80, 100 mg

Comment: **Strattera** is not associated with stimulant or euphoric effects. May discontinue without tapering. Common adverse effects associated with ***atomoxetine*** in children and adolescents included upset stomach, decreased appetite, nausea or vomiting, dizziness, tiredness, and mood swings. For adult patients, the most common adverse side effects included constipation, dry mouth, nausea, decreased appetite, sexual side effects, problems passing urine, and dizziness. Other adverse effects associated with atomoxetine included severe liver damage and potential for serious cardiovascular events. In addition, ***atomoxetine*** increases the risk of suicidal ideation in children and adolescents. Healthcare providers should monitor patients taking this medication for clinical worsening, suicidality, and unusual changes in behavior, particularly within the first few months of initiation or during dose changes.

STIMULANTS

▶ ***amphetamine, mixed salts of single entity amphetamine*** (C)(II)

Adzenys ER <6 years: not recommended; 6-17 years: take with or without food; individualize the dosage according to the therapeutic needs and response; 6-12 years: initially 6.3 mg (5 ml) once daily in the morning; max dose 18.8 mg (15 ml); ≥13 years: 12.5 mg (10 ml) once daily in the morning

Comment: Patients taking **Adderall XR** may be switched to **Adzenys ER** at the equivalent dose taken once daily; switching from any other amphetamine products (e.g., **Adderall** immediate-release), discontinue that treatment, and titrate with **Adzenys ER** using the titration schedule (see mfr pkg insert). To avoid substitution errors and overdosage, do not substitute for other amphetamine products on a mg-per-mg basis because of different amphetamine salt compositions and differing pharmacokinetic profiles. No dosage adjustments for renal or hepatic insufficiency are provided in the manufacturer's labeling.

Oral susp: 125 mg/ml ext-rel (450 ml) (orange)

Adzenys XT-ODT <6 years: not recommended; ≥6 years: take with or without food; individualize the dosage according to the therapeutic needs and response; initially 6.3 mg once daily in the morning; increase in increments of 3.1 mg or 6.3 mg at weekly intervals; max recommended dose 18.8 mg once daily (6-12 years-of-age) and 12.5 mg once daily (≥13 years-of-age)

Comment: Patients taking **Adderall XR** may be switched to **Adzenys XR-ODT** at the equivalent dose taken once daily; switching from any other amphetamine products (e.g., **Adderall** immediate-release), discontinue that treatment, and titrate with **Adzenys XR-ODT** using the titration schedule (see mfr pkg insert). To avoid substitution errors and overdosage, do not substitute for other amphetamine products on a mg-per-mg basis because of different amphetamine salt compositions and differing pharmacokinetic profiles. No dosage adjustments for renal or hepatic insufficiency are provided in the manufacturer's labeling.

ODT: 3.1, 6.3, 9.4, 12.5, 15.7, 18.8 mg orally-disint (orange) (fructose)

Dyanavel XR Oral Suspension <6 years: not recommended; ≥6 years: initially 2.5 mg or 5 mg once daily in the morning; may increase in increments of 2.5 mg to 5 mg per day every 4-7 days; max 20 mg per day; shake bottle prior to administration

Oral susp: 2.5 mg/ml (464 ml) ext-rel

Evekeo <3 years: not recommended; ≥3-5 years: initially 2.5 mg once or twice daily at the same time(s) each day; may increase by 2.5 mg/day at weekly intervals; max 40 mg/day; >5 years: initially 5 mg once or twice daily at the same time(s) each day; may increase by 5 mg/day at weekly intervals; max 40 mg/day

Tab: 5, 10 mg

Mydayis <13 years: not recommended; 13-17 years: initially 12.5 mg once daily in the morning; may titrate at weekly intervals; max 25 mg/day; >17 years: initially 12.5 mg once daily in the morning; may titrate at weekly intervals; max 50 mg/day

Cap: 12.5, 25, 37.5, 50 mg ext-rel

▶ ***dexmethylphenidate*** (C)(II)(G)

Focalin <6 years: not established; ≥6 years: initially 2.5 mg bid; allow at least 4 hours between doses; may increase at 1 week intervals; max 20 mg/day

Tab: 2.5, 5, 10*mg (dye-free)

Focalin ER <6 years: not established; ≥6 years: initially 5 mg weekly; usual dose 10-30 mg/day

Cap: 15, 30 mg ext-rel

Focalin XR <6 years: not established; ≥6 years: initially 5 mg weekly; usual dose 10-30 mg/day

Cap: 5, 10, 15, 20, 25, 30, 35, 40 mg ext-rel

▶ ***dextroamphetamine sulfate*** **(C)(II)(G)** <3 years: not recommended; ≥3-5 years: 2.5 mg daily; may increase by 2.5 mg daily at weekly intervals if needed; >5-12 years: initially 5 mg daily or bid; may increase by 5 mg/day at weekly intervals; usual max 40 mg/day; >12 years: initially 10 mg daily; may increase by 10 mg/day at weekly intervals; max 40 mg/day; may switch to daily dose with sust-rel spansules when titrated

Dexedrine *Tab:* 5*mg (tartrazine)

Dexedrine Spansule *Cap:* 5, 10, 15 mg ext-rel

Dextrostat *Tab:* 5, 10 mg (tartrazine)

▶ ***dextroamphetamine saccharate+dextroamphetamine sulfate+amphetamine aspartate+amphetamine sulfate*** **(C)(II)(G)**

Adderall <6 years: not indicated; ≥6-12 years: initially 5 mg daily; may increase by 5 mg/day at weekly intervals; >12 years: initially 10 mg daily; may increase weekly by 10 mg/day; usual max 60 mg/day in 2-3 divided doses; first dose on awakening; then q 4-6 hours prn

Tab: 5**, 7.5**, 10**, 12.5**, 15**mg, 20**, 30**mg

Adderall XR <6 years: not recommended; 6-12 years: initially 10 mg daily in the AM; may increase by 10 mg/day at weekly intervals; max 30 mg/day; 13-17 years: 10-20 mg by mouth daily in the AM; may increase by 10 mg/day at weekly intervals; max 40 mg/day; >12 years: initially 20 mg by mouth once daily in AM; may increase by 10 mg/day at weekly intervals; max: 60 mg/day; do not chew; may sprinkle on applesauce

Cap: 5, 10, 15, 20, 25, 30 mg ext-rel

▶ ***lisdexamfetamine dimesylate*** **(C)(II)** <6 years: not recommended; ≥6 years: 30 mg once daily in the AM; may increase by 10-20 mg/day at weekly intervals; max 70 mg/day

Vyvanse *Cap:* 20, 30, 40, 50, 60, 70 mg

Comment: May dissolve **Vyvanse** capsule contents in water; take immediately.

▶ ***methylphenidate (regular-acting)*** **(C)(II)(G)**

Methylin, Methylin Chewable, Methylin Oral Solution <6 years: not recommended; 6-12 years: initially 5 mg bid ac (breakfast and lunch); may increase 5-10 mg/day at weekly intervals; max 60 mg/day; >12 years: usual dose 20-30 mg/day in 2-3 divided doses 30-45 minutes before a meal; max 60 mg/day

Tab: 5, 10*, 20*mg; *Chew tab:* 2.5, 5, 10 mg; (grape) (phenylalanine); *Oral soln:* 5, 10 mg/5 ml (grape)

Ritalin <6 years: not recommended; ≥6 years: initially 5 mg bid ac (breakfast and lunch); may increase by 5-10 mg at weekly intervals as needed; max 60 mg/day; 10-60 mg/day in 2-3 divided doses 30-45 minutes ac; max 60 mg/day

Tab: 5, 10*, 20*mg

▶ ***methylphenidate (long-acting)*** **(C)(II)**

Concerta <6 years: not recommended; ≥6-12 years: initially 18 mg daily; max 54 mg/day; >12-17 years: initially 18 mg daily; max 72 mg/day or 2 mg/kg, whichever is less; >17 years: initially 18 mg q AM; may increase in 18 mg increments as needed; max 54 mg/day; do not crush or chew

Tab: 18, 27, 36, 54 mg sust-rel

Metadate CD (G) <6 years: not recommended; ≥6 years: initially 20 mg daily; may gradually increase by 20 mg/day at weekly intervals as needed; max 60 mg/day; do not crush or chew

Cap: 10, 20, 30, 40, 50, 60 mg immed- and ext-rel beads

Metadate ER <6 years: not recommended; ≥6-<12 years: use in place of regular-acting ***methylphenidate*** when the 8-hour dose of **Metadate-ER** corresponds to the titrated 8-hour dose of regular-acting ***methylphenidate;*** ≥12 years: 1 tab daily in the AM; do not crush or chew

Tab: 10, 20 mg ext-rel (dye-free)

QuilliChew ER <6 years: not recommended; ≥6 years: initially 1 x 10 mg chew tab once daily in the AM; may gradually increase by 20 mg/day at weekly intervals as needed; max 60 mg/day

Chew tab: 20*, 30*, 40 mg ext-rel

Quillivant XR <6 years: not recommended; ≥6 years: initially 20 mg once daily in the AM, with or without food; may be titrated in increments of 10-20 mg/day at weekly intervals; daily doses above 60 mg have not been studied and are not recommended; shake the bottle vigorously for at least 10 seconds to ensure that the correct dose is administered

Bottle: 5 mg/ml, 25 mg/5 ml pwdr for reconstitution; 300 mg (60 ml), 600 mg (120 ml), 750 mg (150 ml), 900 mg (180 ml)

Comment: **Quillivant XR** must be reconstituted by a pharmacist, not by the patient or caregiver.

Ritalin LA (G) 1 cap daily in the AM; <6 years: not recommended; ≥6 years: use in place of regular-acting ***methylphenidate*** when the 8-hour dose of **Ritalin LA** corresponds to the titrated 8-hour dose of regular-acting *methylphenidate*; max 60 mg/day

Cap: 10, 20, 30, 40 mg ext-rel (immed- and ext-rel beads)

Ritalin SR 1 cap daily in the AM; <6 years: not recommended; ≥6 years: use in place of regular-acting ***methylphenidate*** when the 8-hour dose of **Ritalin SR** corresponds to the titrated 8-hour dose of regular-acting **methylphenidate**; max 60 mg/day

Tab: 20 mg sust-rel (dye-free)

➢ ***methylphenidate*** (transdermal patch) **(C)(II)(G)** <6 years: not recommended; ≥6-17 years: initially 10 mg patch applied to hip 2 hours before desired effect daily in the AM; may increase by 5-10 mg at weekly intervals; max 60 mg/day; not applicable >17 years

Daytrana *Transdermal patch:* 10, 15, 20, 30 mg

➢ ***pemoline*** **(B)(IV)** <6 years: not recommended; ≥6 years: 18.75-112.5 mg/day; usually start with 37.5 mg in AM; may increase 18.75 mg/day at weekly intervals; max 112.5 gm/day

Cylert *Tab:* 18.75*, 37.5*, 75*mg

Cylert Chewable *Chew tab:* 37.5*mg

Comment: Check baseline serum ALT and monitor every 2 weeks thereafter.

CENTRAL ALPHA-2A AGONIST

➢ ***guanfacine*** **(B)(G)** <6 years: not recommended; ≥6-17 years: initially 1 mg once daily; may increase by 1 mg/day at weekly intervals; usual max 4 mg/day; not applicable >17 years

Intuniv *Tab:* 1, 2, 3, 4 mg ext-rel

Comment: Take **Intuniv** with water, milk, or other liquid. Do not take with a high-fat meal. Withdraw gradually by 1 mg every 3-7 days.

TRICYCLIC ANTIDEPRESSANTS (TCAs)

*see **Depression** page 108*

OTHER AGENTS

▶ *clonidine* (C)

Catapres <12 years: not recommended; ≥12 years: initially 0.1 mg bid; usual range 0.2-0.6 mg/day in divided doses; max 2.4 mg/day

Tab: 0.1*, 0.2*, 0.3*mg

Catapres-TTS <12 years: not recommended; ≥12 years: initially 0.1 mg patch weekly; increase after 1-2 weeks if needed; max 0.6 mg/day

Patch: 0.1, 0.2 mg/day (12/carton); 0.3 mg/day (4/carton)

Kapvay (G) <6 years: not recommended; ≥6-12 years: initially 0.1 mg at bedtime x 1 week; then 0.1 mg bid x 1 week; then 0.1 mg AM and 0.2 mg PM x 1 week; then 0.2 mg bid; withdraw gradually by 0.1 mg/day at 3-7 day intervals

Tab: 0.1, 0.2 mg

Nexiclon XR <12 years: not recommended; ≥12 years: initially 0.18 mg (2 ml) suspension or 0.17 mg tab once daily; usual max 0.52 mg (6 ml suspension) once daily

Tab: 0.17, 0.26 mg ext-rel; *Oral susp:* 0.09 mg/ml ext-rel (4 oz)

AMINOKETONES (FOR THE TREATMENT OF ADHD)

▶ ***bupropion HBr*** (C)(G) <18 years: not recommended; ≥18 years: initially 100 mg bid for at least 3 days; may increase to 375 or 400 mg/day after several weeks; then after at least 3 more days, 450 mg in 4 divided doses; max 450 mg/day, 174 mg/single dose

Aplenzin *Tab:* 174, 348, 522 mg

Comment: Safety and effectiveness in the pediatric population have not been established. When considering the use of **Aplenzin** in a child or adolescent, balance the potential risks with the clinical need.

▶ ***bupropion HCl*** (B)(G)

Forfivo XL <18 years: not recommended; ≥18 years: do not use for initial treatment; use immediate-release ***bupropion*** forms for initial titration; switch to **Forfivo XL** 450 mg once daily when total dose/day reaches 450 mg; may switch to **Forfivo XL** when total dose/day reaches 300 mg for 2 weeks and patient needs 450 mg/day to reach therapeutic target; swallow whole, do not crush or chew

Tab: 450 mg ext-rel

Wellbutrin <12 years: not recommended; ≥12 years: initially 100 mg bid for at least 3 days; may increase to 375 or 400 mg/day after several weeks; then after at least 3 more days, 450 mg in 4 divided doses; max 450 mg/day, 150 mg/single-dose

Tab: 75, 100 mg

Wellbutrin SR <12 years: not recommended; ≥12 years: initially 150 mg in AM for at least 3 days; may increase to 150 mg bid if well tolerated; usual dose 300 mg/day; max 400 mg/day

Tab: 100, 150 mg sust-rel

Wellbutrin XL <12 years: not recommended; ≥12 years: initially 150 mg in AM for at least 3 days; increase to 150 mg bid if well tolerated; usual dose 300 mg/day; max 400 mg/day

Tab: 150, 300 mg sust-rel

BACTERIAL ENDOCARDITIS: PROPHYLAXIS

Comment: Bacterial endocarditis prophylaxis is appropriate for persons with a history of previous infective endocarditis, persons with a prosthetic cardiac valve or prosthetic material used for valve repair, cardiac transplant patients who develop cardiac valvulopathy, congenital heart disease (CHD), unrepaired cyanotic CHD including palliative shunts and conduits, completely repaired congenital heart defect(s) with prosthetic material or device, whether placed by surgery or by catheter intervention, during the first 6 months after the procedure, repaired CHD with residual defects at the site or adjacent to the site of a prosthetic patch or prosthetic device (which may inhibit endothelialization), or any other condition deemed to place a patient at high risk.

DENTAL, ORAL, RESPIRATORY TRACT, ESOPHAGEAL PROCEDURES

- ***amoxicillin*** **(B)(G)** 50 mg/kg as a single-dose or 50 mg/kg (max 3 gm) 1 hour before procedure and (max 1.5 gm) 25 mg/kg 6 hours later; *see page* 588 *for dose by weight table* ≥40 kg: 2 gm PO 30-60 minutes before procedure as a single-dose or 3 gm 1 hour before procedure and 1.5 gm 6 hours later
  - **Amoxil** *Cap:* 250, 500 mg; *Tab:* 875*mg; *Chew tab:* 125, 200, 250, 400 mg (cherry-banana-peppermint) (phenylalanine); *Oral susp:* 125, 250 mg/5 ml (80, 100, 150 ml) (strawberry); 200, 400 mg/5 ml (50, 75, 100 ml) (bubble gum); *Oral drops:* 50 mg/ml (30 ml) (bubble gum)
  - **Trimox** *Tab:* 125, 250 mg; *Cap:* 250, 500 mg; *Oral susp:* 125, 250 mg/5 ml (80, 100, 150 ml) (raspberry-strawberry)
- ***ampicillin*** **(B)(G)** <12 years: 50 mg/kg PO/IM/IV 30-60 minutes before procedure; *see page* 592 *for oral dose by weight table;* ≥12 years: 2 gm PO/IM/IV 30-60 minutes before procedure
  - **Omnipen, Principen** *Cap:* 250, 500 mg; *Oral susp:* 125, 250 mg/5 ml (100, 150, 200 ml) (fruit)
- ***ampicillin+sulbactam*** **(B)(G)** <12 years: 50 mg/kg IV 30-60 minutes before procedure; ≥12 years: 2 gm IV 30-60 minutes before procedure
  - **Unasyn** Vial: 1.5, 3 gm
- ***azithromycin*** **(B)** <12 years: 15 mg/kg 30-60 minutes before procedure; max 500 mg; *see page* 593 *for dose by weight table;* ≥12 years: 500 mg 30-60 minutes before procedure
  - **Zithromax** *Tab:* 250, 500, 600 mg; *Oral susp:* 100 mg/5 ml (15 ml); 200 mg/5 ml (15, 22.5, 30 ml) (cherry)
- ***cefazolin*** **(B)** <12 years: 25 mg/kg IM/IV 30-60 minutes before procedure; ≥12 years: 1 gm IM/IV 30-60 minutes before procedure
  - **Ancef** *Vial:* 250, 500 mg; 1, 5 gm
  - **Kefzol** *Vial:* 500 mg; 1 gm
- ***ceftriaxone*** **(B)(G)** <12 years: 50 mg/kg IM/IV as a single-dose 30-60 minutes before procedure; ≥12 years: 1 gm IM/IV as a single-dose 30-60 minutes before procedure
  - **Rocephin** Vial: 250, 500 mg; 1, 2 gm
- ***cephalexin*** **(B)(G)** <12 years: 50 mg/kg as a single-dose 30-60 minutes before procedure; *see page* 601 *for dose by weight table*; ≥12 years: 2 gm as a single-dose 30-60 minutes before procedure
  - **Keflex** *Cap:* 250, 333, 500, 750 mg; *Oral susp:* 125, 250 mg/5 ml (100, 200 ml) (strawberry)
- ***clarithromycin*** **(C)(G)** <12 years: 15 mg/kg as a single-dose 30-60 minutes before procedure; *see page* 602 *for dose by weight table;* ≥12 years: 500 mg or 500 mg ext-rel as a single-dose 30-60 minutes before procedure
  - **Biaxin** *Tab:* 250, 500 mg
  - **Biaxin Oral Suspension** *Oral susp:* 125, 250 mg/5 ml (50, 100 ml) (fruit punch)
  - **Biaxin XL** *Tab:* 500 mg ext-rel

Comment: The FDA is advising caution before prescribing ***clarithromycin*** to patients with heart disease because of a potential increased risk of heart problems or death that can occur years later. This recommendation is based on a review of the results of a 10-year follow-up study of patients with coronary heart disease from a large clinical trial that first observed this safety issue. Consider risk benefit and the use of other antibiotics in such patients.

▷ ***clindamycin*** **(B)(G)** <12 years: 20 mg/kg (max 300 mg) 1 hour before procedure and 10 mg/kg (max 150 mg) 6 hours later; take with a full glass of water; *see page* 603 *for dose by weight table;* ≥12 years: 600 mg PO as a one-time single-dose or 300 mg 30-60 minutes before procedure and 150 mg 6 hours later; take with a full glass of water

Cleocin *Cap:* 75 (tartrazine), 150 (tartrazine), 300 mg
Cleocin Pediatric Granules *Oral susp:* 75 mg/ml (100 ml) (cherry)

▷ ***erythromycin estolate*** **(B)(G)** <12 years: 20 mg/kg 1 hour before procedure; then 10 mg/kg 6 hours later; *see page* 606 *for dose by weight table;* ≥12 years: 1 gm 1 hour before procedure; then 500 mg 6 hours later

Ilosone *Pulvule:* 250 mg; *Tab:* 500 mg; *Liq:* 125, 250 mg/5 ml (100 ml)

▷ ***penicillin v potassium*** **(B)(G)** <12 years: <60 lb: 1 gm 1 hour before procedure; then 500 mg 6 hours later or 1 gm 1 hour before procedure; then 500 mg q 6 hours x 8 doses; *see page* 616 *for dose by weight table;* ≥12 years: 2 gm 1 hour before procedure; then 1 gm 6 hours later or 2 gm 1 hour before procedure; then 1 gm q 6 hours x 8 doses

Pen-VK *Tab:* 250, 500 mg; *Oral soln:* 125 mg/5 ml (100, 200 ml); 250 mg/5 ml (100, 150, 200 ml)

BACTERIAL VAGINOSIS (BV)/*GARDNERELLA VAGINALIS*

PROPHYLAXIS AND RESTORATION OF VAGINAL ACIDITY

▷ ***acetic acid+oxyquinolone*** **(C)** <12 years: not recommended; ≥12 years: one full applicator intravaginally bid for up to 30 days

Relagard *Gel: acet acid* 0.9%+*oxyq* 0.025% (50 gm tube w. applicator)

Comment: The following treatment regimens for *bacterial vaginosis* are published in the **2015 CDC Sexually Transmitted Diseases Treatment Guidelines**. Treatment regimens are presented by generic drug name first, followed by information about brands and dose forms. BV is associated with adverse pregnancy outcomes, including premature rupture of the membranes, preterm labor, preterm birth, intra-amniotic infection, and postpartum endometritis. Therefore, treatment is recommended for all pregnant females with symptoms or positive screen.

RECOMMENDED REGIMENS

Regimen 1

▷ ***metronidazole*** 500 mg bid x 7 days or ***metronidazole er*** 750 mg once daily x 7 days

Regimen 2

▷ ***metronidazole*** gel 0.75% one full applicatorful (5 gm) once daily x 5 days

Regimen 3

▷ ***clindamycin*** cream 2% one full applicatorful (5 gm) intravaginally once daily at bedtime x 5 days

CDC ALTERNATE REGIMENS

Regimen 1

- *tinidazole* 2 gm once daily x 2 days

Regimen 2

- *tinidazole* 1 gm once daily x 5 days

Regimen 3

- *clindamycin* 300 mg bid x 7 days

Regimen 4

- *clindamycin* ovules 100 mg intravaginally once daily at bedtime x 3 days

Drug Brands and Dose Forms

- *clindamycin* (B)
  Cleocin (G) *Cap:* 75 (tartrazine), 150 (tartrazine), 300 mg
  Cleocin Pediatric Granules (G) *Oral susp:* 75 mg/5 ml (100 ml) (cherry)
  Cleocin Vaginal Cream *Vag crm:* 2% (21, 40 gm tubes w. applicator)
  Cleocin Vaginal Ovules *Vag supp:* 100 mg
- ***metronidazole*** **(not for use in 1st; B in 2nd, 3rd)**
  Flagyl *Tab:* 250*, 500*mg
  Flagyl 375 *Cap:* 375 mg
  Flagyl ER *Tab:* 750 mg ext-rel
  MetroGel-Vaginal, Vandazole *Vag gel:* 0.75% (70 gm w. applicator) (parabens)

  Comment: Alcohol is contraindicated during treatment with oral ***metronidazole*** and for 72 hours after therapy due to a possible ***disulfiram***-like reaction (nausea, vomiting, flushing, headache).
- ***tinidazole*** **(not for use in 1st; B in 2nd, 3rd)**
  Tindamax *Tab:* 250*, 500*mg

BELL'S PALSY

- ***prednisone*** (C)(G) <18 years: *see page* 547 for oral corticosteroid options; ≥18 years: 80 mg once daily x 3 days; then 60 mg daily x 3 days; then 40 mg daily x 3 days; then 20 mg x 1 dose; then discontinue
  Deltasone *Tab:* 2.5*, 5*, 10*, 20*, 50*mg

BILE ACID DEFICIENCY

BILE ACID

- ***ursodiol*** (B) <12 years: not recommended; ≥12 years: *Dissolution* of radiolucent non-calcified gallstones <20 mm diameter: 8-10 mg/kg/day in 2-3 divided doses; *Prevention:* 13-15 mg/kg/day in 4 divided doses
  Actigall *Cap:* 300 mg

  Comment: ***ursodiol*** decreases the amount of cholesterol produced by the liver and absorbed by the intestines. It helps break down cholesterol that has formed into stones in the gallbladder. ***ursodiol*** increases bile flow in patients with primary biliary cirrhosis. It is used to treat small gallstones in people who cannot have cholecystectomy surgery and to prevent gallstones in overweight patients undergoing rapid weight loss. ***ursodiol*** is not used for treating gallstones that are calcified.

BINGE EATING DISORDER

CENTRAL NERVOUS SYSTEM (CNS) STIMULANT

▶ ***lisdexamfetamine dimesylate*** (C)(II) <18 years: not established; ≥18 years: swallow whole or may open and mix/dissolve contents of cap in yogurt, water, orange juice and take immediately; 30 mg once daily in the AM; may adjust in increments of 20 mg at weekly intervals; target dose 50-70 mg/day; max 70 mg/day; *GFR 15-<30 mL/min:* max 50 mg/day; *GFR <15 mL/min, ESRD:* max 30 mg/day

Vyvanse *Cap:* 10, 20, 30, 40, 50, 60 70 mg

Comment: **Vyvanse** is not approved or recommended for weight loss treatment of obesity.

BIPOLAR DISORDERS

Comment: Bipolar I Disorder is characterized by one or more manic episodes that last at least a week or require hospitalization. Severe mania may manifest symptoms of psychosis. Bipolar II Disorder is characterized by one or more depressive episodes accompanied by at least one hypomanic episode. When one parent has Bipolar Disorder, the risk to each child of developing the disorder is estimated to be 15-30%. When both parents have the disorder, the risk to each child increases to 50-75%. Symptoms of mood disorders may be difficult to diagnose in children and adolescents because they can be mistaken for age-appropriate emotions and behaviors or overlap with symptoms of other conditions such as ADHD. However, since anxiety and depression in children may be precursors to Bipolar Disorder, these behaviors should be carefully monitored and evaluated. The cornerstone of treatment for Bipolar Disorder is mood stabilizers (***lithium*** and ***valproate***). Common adjunctive agents include antiepileptics, antipsychotics, and combination agents. Mounting evidence suggests that antidepressants aren't effective in the treatment of bipolar depression. A major study funded by the National Institute of Mental Health (NIMH) showed that adding an antidepressant to a mood stabilizer was no more effective in treating bipolar depression than using a mood stabilizer alone. Another NIMH study found that antidepressants work no better than placebo. If antidepressants are used at all, they should be combined with a mood stabilizer such as ***lithium*** or ***valproic acid***. Antidepressants, without a concomitant mood stabilizer, can increase the frequency of mood cycling and trigger a manic episode. Many experts believe that over time, antidepressant use as monotherapy (i.e., without a mood stabilizer) in people with Bipolar Disorder has a mood destabilizing effect, increasing the frequency of manic and depressive episodes. Drugs and conditions that can mimic Bipolar Disorder include thyroid disorders, corticosteroids, antidepressants, adrenal disorders (e.g. Addison's disease, Cushing's syndrome), antianxiety drugs, drugs for Parkinson's disease, vitamin B12 deficiency, neurological disorders (e.g., epilepsy, multiple sclerosis).

MOOD STABILIZERS

Lithium Salts Mood Stabilizer

▶ ***lithium carbonate*** (D)(G) <12 years: not recommended; ≥12 years: swallow whole; *Usual maintenance:* 900-1200 mg/day in 2-3 divided doses

Lithobid *Tab:* 300 mg slow-rel

Comment: Toxic and therapeutic levels of lithium are close. Draw blood for serum levels 8-12 hours after previous dose. Signs and symptoms of ***lithium*** toxicity can occur below 2 mEq/L and include blurred vision, tinnitus, weakness, dizziness, nausea, abdominal pains, vomiting, diarrhea to (severe) hand tremors, ataxia, muscle twitches, nystagmus, seizures, slurred speech, decreased level of consciousness, coma, death. Other potential adverse reactions may include dry mouth, metallic taste, polydipsia, polyuria, arrhythmias, renal toxicity, hypotension, lethargy, pseudotumor cerebri, extrapyramidal symptoms.

Valproate Mood Stabilizer

▶ *divalproex sodium* (D)(G) <12 years: not recommended; ≥12 years: take once daily; swallow ext-rel form whole; initially 25 mg/kg/day in divided doses; max 60 mg/kg/day

Depakene *Cap:* 250 mg; *Syr:* 250 mg/5 ml (16 oz)
Depakote *Tab:* 125, 250 mg
Depakote ER *Tab:* 250, 500 mg ext-rel
Depakote Sprinkle *Cap:* 125 mg

ANTIEPILEPTICS

▶ *carbamazepine* (D) <12 years: not recommended; ≥12 years: ext-rel oral forms should be swallowed whole; may open caps and sprinkle on applesauce (do not crush or chew beads); initially 400 mg/day in 2 divided doses; adjust in increments of 200 mg/day; max 1.6 gm/day. *Elderly:* reduce initial dose and titrate slowly; oral doses are preferred; IV administration is recommended when the patient is unable to swallow an oral form (see **Carnexiv**)

Carbatrol (G) *Cap:* 200, 300 mg ext-rel
Carnexiv *Vial:* 10 mg/ml (20 ml)

Comment: The total daily dose of **Carnexiv** is 70% of the total daily oral ***carbamazepine*** dose (see mfr pkg insert for dosage conversion table). The total daily dose should be equally divided into four 30-minute infusions, separated by 6 hours. Must be diluted prior to administration. Patients should be switched back to oral ***carbamazepine*** at their previous total daily oral dose and frequency of administration as soon as clinically appropriate. The use of **Carnexiv** for more than 7 consecutive days has not been studied.

Equetro (G) *Cap:* 100, 200, 300 mg ext-rel
Tegretol *Tab:* 200*mg; *Chew tab:* 100*mg; *Oral susp:* 100 mg/5 ml (450 ml; citrus-vanilla)
Tegretol XR (G) *Tab:* 100, 200, 400 mg ext-rel

Comment: ***carbamazepine*** is indicated in mixed episodes in bipolar I disorder.

▶ *lamotrigine* (C)(G) <12 years: not recommended; ≥12 years: *Not taking an enzyme-inducing antiepileptic drug (EIAED) (e.g.,* ***phenytoin, carbamazepine, phenobarbital, primidone, valproic acid****):* 25 mg once daily x 2 weeks; then 50 mg once daily x 2 weeks; then 100 mg once daily x 2 weeks; then target dose 200 mg once daily; *Concomitant* ***valproic acid:*** 25 mg every other day x 2 weeks; then 25 mg once daily x 2 weeks; then 50 mg once daily x 1 week; then target dose 100 mg once daily; *Concomitant EIAED, not* ***valproic acid****:* 50 mg once daily x 2 weeks; then 100 mg daily in divided doses; then increase weekly by 100 mg in divided doses to target dose 400 mg/day in divided doses daily

Lamictal *Tab:* 25*, 100*, 150*, 200*mg
Lamictal Chewable Dispersible Tab *Chew tab:* 2, 5, 25, 50 mg (black current)
Lamictal ODT *ODT:* 25, 50, 100, 200 mg
Lamictal XR *Tab:* 25, 50, 100, 200 mg ext-rel

Comment: ***lamotrigine*** is indicated for maintenance treatment of bipolar I disorder. See mfr pkg insert for drug interactions, interactions with contraceptives and hormone replacement therapy, and discontinuation protocol

ANTIPSYCHOTICS

Comment: Common side effects of antipsychotic drugs include drowsiness, weight gain, sexual dysfunction, dry mouth, constipation, blurred vision. *Neuroleptic Malignant Syndrome* (NMS) and *Tardive Dyskinesia* (TD) are adverse side effects (ASEs) most often associated with the older antipsychotic drugs. Risk is decreased with the newer "atypical" antipsychotic drugs. However, these syndromes can develop, although much less commonly, after relatively brief treatment periods at low doses. Given these considerations, antipsychotic drugs should be prescribed in a manner that is most likely to minimize the occurrence. NMS, a potentially fatal symptom complex, is characterized by hyperpyrexia, muscle rigidity, altered mental status and evidence of autonomic instability (irregular pulse or blood pressure, tachycardia, diaphoresis, and cardiac dysrhythmia). Additional signs may include elevated creatine phosphokinase (CPK), myoglobinuria (rhabdomyolysis), and acute renal failure (ARF). TD is a syndrome consisting of potentially irreversible, involuntary, dyskinetic movements that can develop in patients with antipsychotic drugs. Characteristics include repetitive involuntary movements, usually of the jaw, lips and tongue, such as grimacing, sticking out the tongue and smacking the lips. Some affected people also experience involuntary movement of the extremities or difficulty breathing. The syndrome may remit, partially or completely, if antipsychotic treatment is withdrawn. If signs and symptoms of NMS and/or TD appear in a patient, management should include immediate discontinuation of antipsychotic drugs and other drugs not essential to concurrent therapy, intensive symptomatic treatment, medical monitoring, and treatment of any concomitant serious medical problems. The risk of developing NMS and/or TD, and the likelihood that either syndrome will become irreversible, is believed to increase as the duration of treatment and the total cumulative dose of antipsychotic drugs administered to the patient increase. The first and only FDA-approved treatment for TD is ***valbenazine*** (**Ingrezza**) (*see page* 440)

- ***aripiprazole*** (C)(G) <10 years: not recommended; ≥10-17 years: initially 2 mg/day in a single-dose for 2 days; then increase to 5 mg/day in a single-dose for 2 days; then increase to target dose of 10 mg/day in a single-dose; may increase by 5 mg/day at weekly intervals as needed to max 30 mg/day; >17 years: initially 15 mg once daily; may increase to max 30 mg/day

    Abilify *Tab:* 2, 5, 10, 15, 20, 30 mg

    Abilify Discmelt *Tab:* 15 mg orally-disint (vanilla) (phenylalanine)

    Abilify Maintena *Vial:* 300, 400 mg ext-rel pwdr for IM injection after reconstitution; 300, 400 mg single-dose prefilled dual-chamber syringes w. supplies

    Comment: **Abilify** is indicated for acute and maintenance treatment of mixed episodes in bipolar I disorder, as monotherapy or as adjunct to ***lithium*** or ***valproic acid.***

- ***asenapine*** (C) <10 years: not established; 10-17 years: *Monotherapy:* initially 2.5 mg bid; may increase to 5 mg bid after 3 days; then to 10 mg bid after 3 more days; max 10 mg bid: >17 years: *Monotherapy:* 10 mg bid; *Adjunctive therapy:* 5 mg bid; may increase to max 10 mg bid; allow SL tab to dissolve on tongue; do not split, crush, chew, or swallow; do not eat or drink for 10 minutes after administration

    Saphris *SL tab:* 2, 5, 5, 10 mg (black cherry)

    Comment: **Saphris** is indicated for acute treatment of manic or mixed episodes in bipolar I disorder, as monotherapy or as adjunct to ***lithium*** or ***valproic acid***.

- ***cariprazine*** <12 years: not established: ≥12 years: administer dose once daily; initially 1.5 mg once daily; Day 2: increase to 3 mg; may further increase by 1.5-3 mg increments on subsequent days based on patient response and tolerability; usual range 3-6 mg once daily; max 6 mg/day; *Initiating a strong CYP3A4 inhibitor while taking* ***Vraylar***: decrease **Vraylar** dose by half; *Initiating* ***Vraylar*** *while taking a strong CYP3A4 inhibitor: Day 1:* 1.5 mg; *Day 2:* skip dose; *Day 3 and subsequent days:* 1.5 mg once daily; increase by 1.5-3 mg once daily; max 6 mg/day

Vraylar *Cap:* 1.5, 3, 4.5, 6 mg; 7-count (1 x 1.5 mg, 6 x 3 mg) mixed blister pck

Comment: **Vraylar** is an atypical antipsychotic with partial agonist activity at D2 and 5-HT1A receptors and antagonist activity at 5-HT2A receptors. It is indicated for acute treatment of mixed episodes in bipolar I disorder. There is a **Vraylar** pregnancy exposure registry that monitors pregnancy outcomes in females exposed to **Vraylar** during pregnancy. For more information, contact the National Pregnancy Registry for Atypical Antipsychotics at 1-866-961-2388 or visit https://womensmentalhealth.org/clinical-and-research-programs/pregnancyregistry.

➢ ***lurasidone*** **(B)** <18 years: not established: ≥18 years: initially 20 mg once daily; usual range 20 to max 120 mg/day; take with food; *CrCl <50 mL/min, moderate hepatic impairment (Child-Pugh 7-9):* max 80 mg/day; *Child-Pugh 10-15):* max 40 mg/day

Latuda *Tab:* 20, 40, 60, 80, 120 mg

Comment: **Latuda** is indicated for major depressive episodes associated with bipolar I disorder as monotherapy and as adjunctive therapy with ***lithium*** or ***valproic*** acid. Contraindicated with concomitant strong CYP3A4 inhibitors (e.g., ***ketoconazole, voriconazole, clarithromycin, ritonavir***) and inducers (e.g., ***phenytoin, carbamazepine, rifampin, St. John's wort***); see mfr pkg insert if patient taking moderate CYP3A4 inhibitors (e.g., ***diltiazem, atazanavir, erythromycin, fluconazole, verapamil***). The efficacy of **Latuda** in the treatment of mania associated with bipolar disorder has not been established.

➢ ***quetiapine fumarate*** **(C)(G)**

SeroQUEL <10 years: not recommended; ≥10-17 years: initially 25 mg bid, titrate q 2nd or 3rd day in increments of 25-50 mg bid-tid; max 600 mg/day in 2-3 divided doses: >17 years: initially 25 mg bid, titrate q 2nd or 3rd day in increments of 25-50 mg bid-tid; usual maintenance 400-600 mg/day in 2-3 divided doses

Tab: 25, 50, 100, 200, 300, 400 mg

SeroQUEL XR <18 years: not recommended; ≥18 years: swallow whole; administer once daily in the PM; *Day 1:* 50 mg; *Day 2:* 100 mg; *Day 3:* 200 mg; *Day 4:* 300 mg; usual range 400-600 mg/day

Tab: 50, 150, 200, 300, 400 mg ext-rel

➢ ***risperidone*** **(C)** *Tab:* initially 2-3 mg once daily; may adjust at 24 hour intervals by 1 mg/day; usual range 1-6 mg/day; max 6 mg/day; *Oral soln:* do not take with cola or tea; *M-tab:* dissolve on tongue with or without fluid; *Consta:* administer deep IM in the deltoid or gluteal; give with oral ***risperidone*** or other antipsychotic x 3 weeks; then stop oral form; 25 mg IM every 2 weeks; max 50 mg every 2 weeks

Risperdal <5 years: not established; 5-10 years: initially 0.5 mg once daily at the same time each day adjust at 24 hour intervals by 0.5-1 mg to target dose 2.5 mg/day; usual range 1-6 mg/day; max 6 mg/day; >10 years: *See generic* ***risperidone*** *above for dosing ≥10 years*

Tab: 0.25, 0.5, 1, 2, 3, 4 mg; *Oral soln:* 1 mg/ml (100 ml)

Risperdal Consta <18 years: not established; *See generic* ***risperidone*** *above for dosing* ≥18 years

Vial: 12.5, 25, 37.5, 50 mg pwdr for long-acting IM inj after reconstitution, single use w. diluent and supplies

Risperdal M-Tab <10 years: not established; ≥10 years: *See generic* ***risperidone*** *above for dosing ≥10 years*

Tab: 0.5, 1, 2, 3, 4 mg orally-disint (phenylalanine)

Comment: **Risperdal** tabs, oral solution, and M-tabs are indicated for the short-term monotherapy of acute mania or mixed episodes associated with bipolar I disorder, or in combination with ***lithium*** or ***valproic acid*** in patients >12 years-of-age. **Risperdal Consta** is indicated as monotherapy or adjunctive therapy to ***lithium*** or ***valproic acid*** for the maintenance treatment mania and mixed episodes in bipolar I disorder.

▶ ***ziprasidone*** (C)(G) <12 years: not recommended; ≥12 years: initially 40 mg bid; on day 2, may increase to 60-80 mg bid

Geodon *Cap:* 20, 40, 60, 80 mg

Comment: **Geodon** is indicated for acute and maintenance treatment of mixed episodes in bipolar I disorder, as monotherapy or as adjunct to ***lithium*** or ***valproic acid***.

COMBINATION AGENT

Thienobenzodiazepine+Selective Serotonin Reuptake Inhibitor (SSRI) Combination

▶ ***olanzapine+fluoxetine*** (C) <10 years: not recommended; 10-17 years: initially 1 x 3/25 cap once daily in the PM; max 1 x 12/50 cap once daily in the PM; >17 years: initially 1 x 6/25 cap once daily in the PM; titrate; max 1 x 12/50 cap once daily in the PM

Symbyax

Cap: **Symbyax 3/25** olan 3 mg+fluo 25 mg
Symbyax 6/25 olan 6 mg+fluo 25 mg
Symbyax 6/50 olan 6 mg+fluo 50 mg
Symbyax 12/25 olan 12 mg+fluo 25 mg
Symbyax 12/50 olan 12 mg+fluo 50 mg

Comment: **Symbyax** is indicated for the treatment of depressive episodes associated with bipolar I disorder and treatment-resistant depression (TRD).

BITE: CAT

TETANUS PROPHYLAXIS

▶ ***tetanus toxoid*** vaccine (C) 0.5 ml IM x 1 dose if previously immunized
Vial: 5 Lf units/0.5 ml (0.5, 5 ml); *Prefilled syringe:* 5 Lf units/0.5 ml (0.5 ml)
*see **Tetanus** page* 445 for patients not previously immunized

ANTI-INFECTIVES

▶ ***amoxicillin+clavulanate*** (B)(G)

Augmentin <40 kg: 40-45 mg/kg/day divided tid x 10 days or 90 mg/kg/day divided bid x 10 days; *see page* 590 *for dose by weight table;* ≥40 kg: 500 mg tid or 875 mg bid x 10 days

Tab: 250, 500, 875 mg; *Chew tab:* 125, 250 mg (lemon-lime); 200, 400 mg (cherry-banana) (phenylalanine); *Oral susp:* 125 mg/5 ml (banana), 250 mg/5 ml (75, 100, 150 ml) (orange); 200, 400 mg/5 ml (50, 75, 100 ml) (orange) (phenylalanine)

Augmentin ES-600 <3 months: not recommended; ≥3 months, <40 kg: 90 mg/kg/day divided q 12 hours x 10 days; *see page* 591 *for dose by weight table;* ≥40 kg: not recommended

Oral susp: 600 mg/5 ml (50, 75, 100, 125, 150, 200 ml) (strawberry cream) (phenylalanine)

Augmentin XR <16 years: use other forms; ≥16 years: 2 tabs q 12 hours x 7-10 days
Tab: 1000*mg ext-rel

▻ ***doxycycline*** **(D)(G)** <8 years: not recommended; ≥8 years, ≤100 lb: 2 mg/lb on first day in 2 divided doses, followed by 1 mg/lb/day in 1-2 divided doses x 10 days; ≥8 years, >100 lb: 100 mg bid x 10 days; *see page* 605 *for dose by weight table*

Acticlate *Tab:* 75, 150**mg
Adoxa *Tab:* 50, 75, 100, 150 mg ent-coat
Doryx *Tab:* 50, 75, 100, 150, 200 mg del-rel
Doxteric *Tab:* 50 mg del-rel
Monodox *Cap:* 50, 75, 100 mg
Oracea *Cap:* 40 mg del-rel
Vibramycin *Tab:* 100 mg; *Cap:* 50, 100 mg; *Syr:* 50 mg/5 ml (raspberry-apple) (sulfites); *Oral susp:* 25 mg/5 ml (raspberry)
Vibra-Tab *Tab:* 100 mg film-coat

Comment: ***doxycycline*** is contraindicated <8 years-of-age, in pregnancy, and lactation (discolors developing tooth enamel). A side effect may be photosensitivity (photophobia). Do not take with antacids, calcium supplements, milk or other dairy, or within 2 hours of taking another drug.

▻ ***penicillin v potassium*** **(B)(G)** <12 years: 25-75 mg/kg day divided q 6-8 hours x 3 days; *see page* 616 *for dose by weight table;* ≥12 years: 500 mg PO qid x 3 days

Pen-VK *Tab:* 250, 500 mg; *Oral soln:* 125 mg/5 ml (100, 200 ml); 250 mg/5 ml (100, 150, 200 ml)

BITE: DOG

TETANUS PROPHYLAXIS

see ***Tetanus*** *page* 445 for patients not previously immunized

▻ ***tetanus toxoid*** vaccine **(C)** 0.5 ml IM x 1 dose if previously immunized
Vial: 5 Lf units/0.5 ml (0.5, 5 ml); *Prefilled syringe:* 5 Lf units/0.5 ml (0.5 ml)

ANTI-INFECTIVES

▻ ***amoxicillin+clavulanate*** **(B)(G)**

Augmentin <40 kg: 40-45 mg/kg/day divided tid x 10 days or 90 mg/kg/day divided bid x 10 days; *see page* 590 *for dose by weight table;* ≥40 kg: 500 mg tid or 875 mg bid x 10 days
Tab: 250, 500, 875 mg; *Chew tab:* 125, 250 mg (lemon-lime); 200, 400 mg (cherry-banana) (phenylalanine); *Oral susp:* 125 mg/5 ml (banana), 250 mg/5 ml (75, 100, 150 ml) (orange); 200, 400 mg/5 ml (50, 75, 100 ml) (orange) (phenylalanine)

Augmentin ES-600 <3 months: not recommended; ≥3 months, <40 kg: 90 mg/kg/day divided q 12 hours x 10 days; *see page* 591 *for dose by weight table;* ≥40 kg: not recommended
Oral susp: 600 mg/5 ml (50, 75, 100, 125, 150, 200 ml) (strawberry cream) (phenylalanine)

Augmentin XR <16 years: use other forms; ≥16 years: 2 tabs q 12 hours x 7-10 days
Tab: 1000*mg 8-16 mg/kg/day in 3-4 divided doses x 10 days; *see page* 590 *for dose by weight table;* administer with TMP-SMX; ≥12 years: 300 mg qid x 10 days; administer with fluoroquinolone

▻ ***clindamycin***

Cleocin (G) *Cap:* 75 (tartrazine), 150 (tartrazine), 300 mg
Cleocin Pediatric Granules (G) *Oral susp:* 75 mg/5 ml (100 ml) (cherry)

▶ *doxycycline* (D)(G) <8 years: not recommended; ≥8 years, ≤100 lb: 2 mg/lb on first day in 2 divided doses, followed by 1 mg/lb/day in 1-2 divided doses x 5-10 days; ≥8 years, >100 lb: 100 mg bid x 5-10 days; *see page* 605 *for dose by weight table*

Acticlate *Tab:* 75, 150**mg
Adoxa *Tab:* 50, 75, 100, 150 mg ent-coat
Doryx *Tab:* 50, 75, 100, 150, 200 mg del-rel
Doxteric *Tab:* 50 mg del-rel
Monodox *Cap:* 50, 75, 100 mg
Oracea *Cap:* 40 mg del-rel
Vibramycin *Tab:* 100 mg; *Cap:* 50, 100 mg; *Syr:* 50 mg/5 ml (raspberry-apple) (sulfites); *Oral susp:* 25 mg/5 ml (raspberry)
Vibra-Tab *Tab:* 100 mg film-coat

Comment: ***doxycycline*** is contraindicated <8 years-of-age, in pregnancy, and lactation (discolors developing tooth enamel). A side effect may be photosensitivity (photophobia). Do not take with antacids, calcium supplements, milk or other dairy, or within 2 hours of taking another drug.

▶ *penicillin v potassium* (B)(G) <12 years: 50 mg/kg/day in 4 divided doses x 3 days; see *page* 616 *for dose by weight table;* ≥12 years: 500 mg PO qid x 3 days

Pen-VK *Tab:* 250, 500 mg; *Oral soln:* 125 mg/5 ml (100, 200 ml); 250 mg/5 ml (100, 150, 200 ml)

BITE: HUMAN

TETANUS PROPHYLAXIS

▶ *tetanus toxoid* vaccine (C) 0.5 ml IM x 1 dose if previously immunized

Vial: 5 Lf units/0.5 ml (0.5, 5 ml)
Prefilled syringe: 5 Lf units/0.5 ml (0.5 ml)
see ***Tetanus*** *page* 445 for patients not previously immunized

ANTI-INFECTIVES

▶ *amoxicillin+clavulanate* (B)(G)

Augmentin <40 kg: 40-45 mg/kg/day divided tid x 10 days or 90 mg/kg/day divided bid x 10 days; *see page* 590 *for dose by weight table;* ≥40 kg: 500 mg tid or 875 mg bid x 10 days

Tab: 250, 500, 875 mg; *Chew tab:* 125, 250 mg (lemon-lime); 200, 400 mg (cherry-banana) (phenylalanine); *Oral susp:* 125 mg/5 ml (banana), 250 mg/5 ml (75, 100, 150 ml) (orange); 200, 400 mg/5 ml (50, 75, 100 ml) (orange) (phenylalanine)

Augmentin ES-600 <3 months: not recommended; ≥3 months, <40 kg: 90 mg/kg/day divided q 12 hours x 10 days; *see page* 591 *for dose by weight table;* ≥40 kg: not recommended

Oral susp: 600 mg/5 ml (50, 75, 100, 125, 150, 200 ml) (strawberry cream) (phenylalanine)

Augmentin XR <16 years: use other forms; ≥16 years: 2 tabs q 12 hours x 7-10 days

Tab: 1000*mg ext-rel

▶ *cefoxitin* (B) <3 months: not recommended; ≥3 months: 80-160 mg/kg/day IM in 3-4 divided doses x 10 days; max 12 gm/day

Mefoxin Injectable *Vial:* 1, 2 gm

▶ *ciprofloxacin* (C) <18 years: not recommended; ≥18 years: 500 mg bid x 10 days; max 1.5 gm/day

Cipro (G) *Tab:* 250, 500, 750 mg; *Oral susp:* 250, 500 mg/5 ml (100 ml) (strawberry)
Cipro XR *Tab:* 500, 1000 mg ext-rel
ProQuin XR *Tab:* 500 mg ext-rel

Comment: ***ciprofloxacin*** is contraindicated <18 years-of-age, and during pregnancy and lactation. Risk of tendonitis or tendon rupture.

▶ ***erythromycin base*** **(B)(G)** <45 kg: 30-40 mg/kg/day in 4 divided doses x 10 days; ≥45 kg: 250 mg qid x 10 days
Ery-Tab *Tab:* 250, 333, 500 mg ent-coat
PCE *Tab:* 333, 500 mg

▶ ***erythromycin ethylsuccinate*** **(B)(G)** 30-50 mg/kg/day in 4 divided doses x 10 days; may double dose with severe infection; *see page* 607 *for dose by weight table;* max 100 mg/kg/day or 400 mg qid
EryPed *Oral susp:* 200 mg/5 ml (100, 200 ml) (fruit); 400 mg/5 ml (60, 100, 200 ml) (banana); *Oral drops:* 200, 400 mg/5 ml (50 ml) (fruit); *Chew tab:* 200 mg wafer (fruit)
E.E.S. *Oral susp:* 200, 400 mg/5 ml (100 ml) (fruit)
E.E.S. Granules *Oral susp:* 200 mg/5 ml (100, 200 ml) (cherry)
E.E.S. 400 Tablets *Tab:* 400 mg

▶ ***trimethoprim+sulfamethoxazole*** *[TMP-SMX]* **(D)(G)**
Bactrim, Septra <12 years: not recommended; ≥12 years: 2 tabs bid x 10 days
Tab: trim 80 mg+sulfa 400 mg*
Bactrim DS, Septra DS <12 years: not recommended; ≥12 years: 1 tab bid x 10 days
Tab: trim 160 mg+sulfa 800 mg*
Bactrim Pediatric Suspension, Septra Pediatric Suspension <2 months: not recommended; ≥2 months-12 years: 40 mg/kg/day of ***sulfamethoxazole*** in 2 doses bid; >12 years: use tabs
Oral susp: trim 40 mg+sulfa 200 mg per 5 ml (100 ml) (cherry) (alcohol 0.3%)

BLEPHARITIS

OPHTHALMIC AGENTS

▶ ***erythromycin*** ophthalmic ointment **(B)** apply 1/2 inch bid-qid x 14 days; then q HS x 10 days
Ilotycin *Oint:* 5 mg/gm (1/2 oz)

▶ ***polymyxin b+bacitracin*** ophthalmic ointment **(C)** apply 1/2 inch bid-qid x 14 days; then q HS
Polysporin *Oint: poly* b 10,000 U+baci 500 U (3.75 gm)

▶ ***polymyxin b+bacitracin+neomycin*** ophthalmic ointment **(C)** apply 1/2 inch bid-qid x 14 days; then q HS
Neosporin *Oint: poly* b 10,000 U+baci 400 U/*neo* 3.5 mg/gm (3.75 gm)

▶ ***sodium sulfacetamide*** **(C)**
Bleph-10 Ophthalmic Solution <2 years: not recommended; 2-12 years: years: 1-2 drops q 2-3 hours during the day x 7-14 days; >12 years: 2 drops q 4 hours x 7-14 days
Ophth soln: 10% (2.5, 5, 15 ml) (benzalkonium chloride)
Bleph-10 Ophthalmic Ointment <2 years: not recommended; ≥2 years: apply 1/2 inch qid and HS x 7-14 days
Ophth oint: 10% (3.5 gm) (phenylmercuric acetate)

SYSTEMIC AGENTS

▻ ***tetracycline*** **(D)(G)** <8 years: not recommended; ≥8 years, ≤100 lb: 25-50 mg/kg/day in 4 divided doses x 7-10 days; *see page* 618 *for dose by weight table*; >8 years, >100 lb: 250 mg qid x 7-10 days

Achromycin V *Cap:* 250, 500 mg

Sumycin *Tab:* 250, 500 mg; *Cap:* 250, 500 mg; *Oral susp:* 125 mg/5 ml (100, 200 ml) (fruit) (sulfites)

Comment: ***tetracycline*** is contraindicated <8 years-of-age, in pregnancy, and lactation (discolors developing tooth enamel). A side effect may be photosensitivity (photophobia). Do not give with antacids, calcium supplements, milk <u>or</u> other dairy, <u>or</u> within two hours of taking another drug.

BRONCHIOLITIS

Inhaled Beta2-Agonists (Bronchodilators) *see* ***Asthma*** *page* 29
Oral Beta-2 Agonists (Bronchodilators) *see* ***Asthma*** *page* 36
Inhaled Corticosteroids *see* ***Asthma*** *page* 31
Parenteral Corticosteroids *see page* 547
Oral Corticosteroids *see page* 546

BRONCHITIS: ACUTE & ACUTE EXACERBATION OF CHRONIC BRONCHITIS (AECB)

Comment: Antibiotics are seldom needed for treatment of acute bronchitis because the etiology is usually viral.
Inhaled Beta2-Agonists (Bronchodilators) *see* ***Asthma*** *page* 29
Oral Beta2-Agonists (Bronchodilators) *see* ***Asthma*** *page* 36

ANTI-INFECTIVES FOR SECONDARY BACTERIAL INFECTION

▻ ***amoxicillin*** **(B)(G)** <40 kg (88 lb): 20-40 mg/kg/day in 3 divided doses x 10 days <u>or</u> 25-45 mg/kg/day in 2 divided doses x 10 days; *see page* 588 *for dose by weight table;* ≥40 kg: 500-875 mg bid <u>or</u> 250-500 mg tid x 10 days

Amoxil *Cap:* 250, 500 mg; *Tab:* 875*mg; *Chew tab:* 125, 200, 250, 400 mg (cherry-banana-peppermint) (phenylalanine); *Oral susp:* 125, 250 mg/5 ml (80, 100, 150 ml) (strawberry); 200, 400 mg/5 ml (50, 75, 100 ml) (bubble gum); *Oral drops:* 50 mg/ml (30 ml) (bubble gum)

Moxatag *Tab:* 775 mg ext-rel

Trimox *Tab:* 125, 250 mg; *Cap:* 250, 500 mg; *Oral susp:* 125, 250 mg/5 ml (80, 100, 150 ml) (raspberry-strawberry)

▻ ***amoxicillin+clavulanate*** **(B)(G)**

Augmentin <40 kg: 40-45 mg/kg/day divided tid x 10 days <u>or</u> 90 mg/kg/day divided bid x 10 days; *see page* 590 *for dose by weight table;* ≥40 kg: 500 mg tid <u>or</u> 875 mg bid x 10 days

Tab: 250, 500, 875 mg; *Chew tab:* 125, 250 mg (lemon-lime); 200, 400 mg (cherry-banana) (phenylalanine); *Oral susp:* 125 mg/5 ml (banana), 250 mg/5 ml (75, 100, 150 ml) (orange); 200, 400 mg/5 ml (50, 75, 100 ml) (orange) (phenylalanine)

Augmentin ES-600 <3 months: not recommended; ≥3 months, <40 kg: 90 mg/kg/day divided q 12 hours x 10 days; *see page* 591 *for dose by weight table;* ≥40 kg: not recommended

Oral susp: 600 mg/5 ml (50, 75, 100, 125, 150, 200 ml) (strawberry cream) (phenylalanine)

Augmentin XR <16 years: use other forms; ≥16 years: 2 tabs q 12 hours x 7-10 days

Tab: 1000*mg ext-rel

➢ ***ampicillin*** **(B)** <12 years: not recommended for bronchitis in children; ≥12 years: 250-500 mg qid x 10 days

Omnipen, Principen *Cap:* 250, 500 mg; *Oral susp:* 125, 250 mg/5 ml (100, 150, 200 ml) (fruit)

➢ ***azithromycin*** **(B)(G)** <12 years: not recommended for bronchitis in children; ≥12 years: 500 mg x 1 dose on day 1, then 250 mg daily on days 2-5 or 500 mg once daily x 3 days or 2 gm in a single-dose

Zithromax *Tab:* 250, 500, 600 mg; *Oral susp:* 100 mg/5 ml (15 ml); 200 mg/5 ml(15, 22.5, 30 ml) (cherry); *Pkt:* 1 gm for reconstitution (cherry-banana)

Zithromax Tri-Pak *Tab:* 3 x 500 mg tabs/pck

Zithromax Z-Pak *Tab:* 6 x 250 mg tabs/pck

Zmax *Oral susp:* 2 gm ext-rel for reconstitution (cherry-banana) (148 mg Na^{+})

➢ ***cefaclor*** **(B)(G)** <16 years: not recommended; ≥16 years: 250-500 mg q 8 hours x 10 days; max 2 gm/day

Tab: 500 mg; *Cap:* 250, 500 mg; *Susp:* 125 mg/5 ml (75, 150 ml) (strawberry); 187 mg/5 ml (50, 100 ml) (strawberry); 250 mg/5 ml (75, 150 ml) (strawberry); 375 mg/5 ml (50, 100 ml) (strawberry)

Cefaclor Extended Release <16 years: not recommended; ≥16 years: 500 mg bid (clinically equivalent to 250 mg immed-rel caps tid); swallow whole; take with meals

Tab: 375, 500 mg ext-rel

➢ ***cefadroxil*** **(B)** <12 years: 30 mg/kg/day in 2 divided doses x 10 days; *see page* 595 *for dose by weight table;* ≥12 years: 1-2 gm in 1-2 divided doses x 10 days

Duricef *Tab:* 1 gm; *Cap:* 500 mg; *Oral susp:* 250 mg/5 ml (100 ml); 500 mg/5 ml (75, 100 ml) (orange-pineapple)

➢ ***cefdinir*** **(B)** <6 months: not recommended; 6 months-12 years: 14 mg/kg/day in 1-2 divided doses x 10 days; *see page* 596 *for dose by weight table;* >12 years: 300 mg bid x 10 days or 600 mg daily x 10 days

Omnicef *Cap:* 300 mg; *Oral susp:* 125 mg/5 ml (60, 100 ml) (strawberry)

➢ ***cefditoren pivoxil*** **(B)** <12 years: not recommended; ≥12 years: 400 mg bid x 10 days

Spectracef *Tab:* 200 mg

Comment: **Spectracef** is contraindicated with milk protein allergy or carnitine deficiency.

➢ ***cefixime*** **(B)(G)** <6 months: not recommended; 6 months-12 years, <50 kg: 8 mg/kg/day in 1-2 divided doses x 10 days; *see page* 597 *for dose by weight table;* >12 years, >50 kg: 400 mg once daily x 10 days

Suprax *Tab:* 400 mg; *Cap:* 400 mg; *Oral susp:* 100, 200, 500 mg/5 ml (50, 75, 100 ml) (strawberry)

➢ ***cefpodoxime proxetil*** **(B)** <2 months: not recommended; ≥2 months-12 years: 10 mg/kg/day (max 400 mg/dose) or 5 mg/kg/day bid (max 200 mg/dose) x 10 days; *see page* 598 *for dose by weight table;* >12 years: 200 mg bid x 10 days

Vantin *Tab:* 100, 200 mg; *Oral susp:* 50, 100 mg/5 ml (50, 75, 100 mg) (lemon creme)

➢ ***cefprozil*** **(B)** <2 years: not recommended; 2-12 years: 15 mg/kg bid x 10 days; *see page* 599 *for dose by weight table;* >12 years: 250-500 mg bid or 500 mg daily x 10 days

Cefzil *Tab:* 250, 500 mg; *Oral susp:* 125, 250 mg/5 ml (50, 75, 100 ml) (bubble gum) (phenylalanine)

- ▻ ***ceftibuten*** **(B)** <12 years: 9 mg/kg daily x 10 days; max 400 mg/day; *see page* 600 *for dose by weight table;* ≥12 years: 400 mg daily x 10 days
    - **Cedax** *Cap:* 400 mg; *Oral susp:* 90 mg/5 ml (30, 60, 90, 120 ml); 180 mg/5 ml (30, 60, 120 ml) (cherry)
- ▻ ***ceftriaxone*** **(B)(G)** <12 years: 50 mg/kg IM daily; continue 2 days after clinical stability; ≥12 years: 1-2 gm IM daily; continue 2 days after signs of infection have disappeared; max 4 gm/day
    - **Rocephin** *Vial:* 250, 500 mg; 1, 2 gm
- ▻ ***cephalexin*** **(B)(G)** <12 years: 25-50 mg/kg/day in 4 divided doses x 10 days; *see page* 601 *for dose by weight table;* ≥12 years: 250-500 mg qid x 10 days
    - **Keflex** *Cap:* 250, 333, 500, 750 mg; *Oral susp:* 125, 250 mg/5 ml (100, 200 ml) (strawberry)
- ▻ ***clarithromycin*** **(C)(G)** <6 months: not recommended; ≥6 months-12 years: 7.5 mg/kg bid x 7 days; *see page* 602 *for dose by weight table;* >12 years: 500 mg or 500 mg ext-rel once daily x 7 days
    - **Biaxin** *Tab:* 250, 500 mg
    - **Biaxin Oral Suspension** *Oral susp:* 125, 250 mg/5 ml (50, 100 ml) (fruit punch)
    - **Biaxin XL** *Tab:* 500 mg ext-rel

Comment: The FDA is advising caution before prescribing ***clarithromycin*** to patients with heart disease because of a potential increased risk of heart problems or death that can occur years later. This recommendation is based on a review of the results of a 10-year follow-up study of patients with coronary heart disease from a large clinical trial that first observed this safety issue. Consider risk benefit and the use of other antibiotics in such patients.

- ▻ ***dirithromycin*** **(C)(G)** <12 years: not recommended; ≥12 years: 500 mg daily x 7 days
    - **Dynabac** *Tab:* 250 mg
- ▻ ***doxycycline*** **(D)(G)** <8 years: not recommended; ≥8 years, ≤100 lb: 2 mg/lb on first day in 2 divided doses, followed by 1 mg/lb/day in 1-2 divided doses; ≥8 years, >100 lb: 40-100 mg bid; *see page* 605 *for dose by weight table*
    - **Acticlate** *Tab:* 75, 150**mg
    - **Adoxa** *Tab:* 50, 75, 100, 150 mg ent-coat
    - **Doryx** *Tab:* 50, 75, 100, 150, 200 mg del-rel
    - **Doxteric** *Tab:* 50 mg del-rel
    - **Monodox** *Cap:* 50, 75, 100 mg
    - **Oracea** *Cap:* 40 mg del-rel
    - **Vibramycin** *Tab:* 100 mg; *Cap:* 50, 100 mg; *Syr:* 50 mg/5 ml (raspberry-apple) (sulfites); *Oral susp:* 25 mg/5 ml (raspberry)
    - **Vibra-Tab** *Tab:* 100 mg film-coat

Comment: ***doxycycline*** is contraindicated <8 years-of-age, in pregnancy, and lactation (discolors developing tooth enamel). A side effect may be photosensitivity (photophobia). Do not give with antacids, calcium supplements, milk or other dairy, or within 2 hours of taking another drug.

- ▻ ***erythromycin ethylsuccinate*** **(B)(G)** 30-50 mg/kg/day in 4 divided doses x 7 days; may double dose with severe infection; max 100 mg/kg/day or 400 mg qid; *see page* 607 *for dose by weight table*
    - **EryPed** *Oral susp:* 200 mg/5 ml (100, 200 ml) (fruit); 400 mg/5 ml (60, 100, 200 ml) (banana); *Oral drops:* 200, 400 mg/5 ml (50 ml) (fruit); *Chew tab:* 200 mg wafer (fruit)
    - **E.E.S.** *Oral susp:* 200, 400 mg/5 ml (100 ml) (fruit)
    - **E.E.S. Granules** *Oral susp:* 200 mg/5 ml (100, 200 ml) (cherry)
    - **E.E.S. 400 Tablets** *Tab:* 400 mg

▶ ***gemifloxacin*** **(C)(G)** <18 years: not recommended; ≥18 years: 320 mg once daily x 5-7 days

Factive *Tab:* 320*mg

Comment: ***gemifloxacin*** is contraindicated <18 years-of-age, and during pregnancy and lactation. Risk of tendonitis or tendon rupture.

▶ ***levofloxacin*** **(C)** <18 years: not recommended; ≥18 years: *Uncomplicated:* 500 mg daily x 7 days; *Complicated:* 750 mg daily x 7 days

Levaquin *Tab:* 250, 500, 750 mg

Comment: ***levofloxacin*** is contraindicated <18 years-of-age, and during pregnancy and lactation. Risk of tendonitis or tendon rupture.

▶ ***loracarbef*** **(B)** <12 years: 15 mg/kg/day in 2 divided doses x 7 days; *see page* 614 *for dose by weight table*; ≥12 years: 200-400 mg bid x 7 days

Lorabid *Pulvule:* 200, 400 mg; *Oral susp:* 100 mg/5 ml (50, 100 ml); 200 mg/5 ml (50, 75, 100 ml) (strawberry bubble gum)

▶ ***moxifloxacin*** **(C)(G)** <18 years: not recommended; ≥18 years: 400 mg daily x 5 days

Avelox *Tab:* 400 mg; *Premixed* IV soln: 400 mg/250 ml (latex-free, preservative-free)

Comment: ***moxifloxacin*** is contraindicated <18 years-of-age and during pregnancy and lactation. Risk of tendonitis or tendon rupture.

▶ ***ofloxacin*** **(C)(G)** <18 years: not recommended; ≥18 years: 400 mg bid x 10 days

Floxin *Tab:* 200, 300, 400 mg

▶ ***telithromycin*** **(C)** <18 years: not recommended; ≥18 years: 2 x 400 mg tabs in a single-dose daily x 5 days

Ketek *Tab:* 400 mg

Comment: telithromycin is a ketolide indicated for the treatment of moderate-to-severe CAP).

▶ ***tetracycline*** **(D)(G)** <8 years: not recommended; ≥8 years, ≤100 lb: 25-50 mg/kg/day in 4 divided doses x 7 days; *see page* 618 *for dose by weight table* ; ≥8 years, >100 lb: 250-500 mg qid x 7 days

Achromycin V *Cap:* 250, 500 mg

Sumycin *Tab:* 250, 500 mg; *Cap:* 250, 500 mg; *Oral susp:* 125 mg/5 ml (100, 200 ml) (fruit) (sulfites)

Comment: ***tetracycline*** is contraindicated <8 years-of-age, in pregnancy, and lactation (discolors developing tooth enamel). A side effect may be photosensitivity (photophobia). Do not give with antacids, calcium supplements, milk or other dairy, or within two hours of taking another drug.

▶ ***trimethoprim+sulfamethoxazole [TMP-SMX]*** **(D)(G)**

Bactrim, Septra <12 years: not recommended; ≥12 years: 2 tabs bid x 10 days

Tab: trim 80 mg+*sulfa* 400 mg*

Bactrim DS, Septra DS <12 years: not recommended; ≥12 years: 1 tab bid x 10 days

Tab: trim 160 mg+*sulfa* 800 mg*

Bactrim Pediatric Suspension, Septra Pediatric Suspension <2 months: not recommended; ≥2 months-12 years: 40 mg/kg/day of ***sulfamethoxazole*** in 2 doses bid; >12 years: use tabs

Oral susp: trim 40 mg+*sulfa* 200 mg per 5 ml (100 ml) (cherry) (alcohol 0.3%)

BULIMIA NERVOSA

SELECTIVE SEROTONIN REUPTAKE INHIBITOR (SSRI)

▶ ***fluoxetine*** (C)(G)

Prozac <8 years: not recommended; 8-17 years: initially 10 mg/day; may increase after 1 week to 20 mg/day; range 20-60 mg/day; range for lower weight children, 20-30 mg/day; >17 years: initially 20 mg daily; may increase after 1 week; doses >20 mg/day should be divided into AM and noon doses; max 80 mg/day

Cap: 10, 20, 40 mg; *Tab:* 30*, 60*mg; *Oral soln:* 20 mg/5 ml (4 oz) (mint)

Prozac Weekly <12 years: not recommended; ≥12 years: following daily ***fluoxetine*** therapy at 20 mg/day for 13 weeks, may initiate **Prozac Weekly** 7 days after the last 20 mg ***fluoxetine*** dose

Cap: 90 mg ent-coat del-rel pellets

BURN: MINOR

▷ ***silver sulfadiazine*** (B)(G) <12 years: not established; ≥12 years: apply bid

Silvadene *Crm:* 1% (20 gm tube; 20, 50, 85, 400, 1,000 gm jar)

Comment: ***silver sulfadiazine*** is contradicted in sulfa allergy, late pregnancy, within the first 2 months after birth, premature infants.

TOPICAL & TRANSDERMAL ANESTHETICS

Comment: ***lidocaine*** gel, cream, lotion, or patch is not recommended <12 years-of-age and should not be applied to non-intact skin

▷ ***lidocaine*** burn gel (B)(G)

▷ ***lidocaine*** cream (B)(G)

LidaMantle *Crm:* 3% (1, 2 oz)

Lidoderm *Crm:* 3% (85 gm)

▷ ***lidocaine*** lotion (B)(G)

LidaMantle *Lotn:* 3% (177 ml)

▷ ***lidocaine*** 5% patch (B)(G) <12 years: not established; ≥12 years: apply up to 3 patches at one time for up to 12 hours/24 hour period (12 hours on/12 hours off); patches may be cut into smaller sizes before removal of the release liner; do not reuse

Lidoderm *Patch:* 5% (10 x 14 cm; 30/carton)

▷ ***lidocaine*** 2.5%+***prilocaine*** 2.5% <12 years: not established; ≥12 years: apply sparingly to the burn bid-tid prn

Emla Cream (B) (5, 30 gm)

BURSITIS

Acetaminophen for IV Infusion *see **Pain** page* 322
NSAIDs *see page* 539
Other Oral Analgesics *see **Pain** page* 324
Topical & Transdermal NSAIDs *see **Pain** page* 323
Parenteral Corticosteroids *see page* 547
Oral Corticosteroids *see page* 546

CANDIDIASIS: ABDOMEN, BLADDER, ESOPHAGUS, KIDNEY

▷ ***voriconazole*** (D)(G) <12 years: not recommended; ≥12 years: *PO:* <40 kg: 100 mg q 12 hours; may increase to150 mg q 12 hours if inadequate response; ≥40 kg: 200 mg q 12 hours; may increase to 300 mg q 12 hours if inadequate; *IV*: 6 mg/kg q 12 hours x 2 doses; then 4 mg/kg q 12 hour; max rate 3 mg/kg/hour over 1-2 hours

Vfend *Tab:* 50, 200 mg

Vfend I.V. for Injection *Vial:* 200 mg pwdr for reconstitution (preservative-free)

Vfend *Oral susp:* 40 mg/ml pwdr for reconstitution (75 ml) (orange)

CANDIDIASIS: ORAL (THRUSH)

ORAL ANTIFUNGALS

▶ ***clotrimazole*** (C) <3 years: not recommended; ≥3 years: *Prophylaxis:* 1 troche dissolved in mouth tid; *Treatment:* 1 troche dissolved in mouth 5 x/day x 10-14 days
Mycelex Troches *Troches:* 10 mg

▶ ***fluconazole*** (C) <2 weeks: not recommended; 2 weeks-12 years: 6 mg/kg x 1 day; then 3 mg/kg/day for at least 3 weeks; *see page* 610 *for dose by weight table;* >12 years: 200 mg x 1 dose first day; then 100 mg once daily x 13 days
Diflucan *Tab:* 50, 100, 150, 200 mg; *Oral susp:* 10, 40 mg/ml (35 ml) (orange) (sucrose)

▶ ***gentian violet*** (G) apply to oral mucosa with a cotton swab tid x 3 days

▶ ***itraconazole*** (C) <12 years: 5 mg/kg daily x 7-14 days; max 200 mg/day; *see page* 613 *for dose by weight table;* ≥12 years: 200 mg daily x 7-14 days
Sporanox *Oral soln:* 10 mg/ml (150 ml) (cherry-caramel); *Pulse Pack:* 100 mg caps (7/pck)

▶ ***miconazole*** (C) <16 years: not recommended; ≥16 years: 1 buccal tab once daily x 14 days; apply to upper gum region; hold place 30 seconds; do not crush, chew, or swallow
Oravig *Buccal tab:* 50 mg (14/pck)

▶ ***nystatin*** (C)(G)
Mycostatin 1-2 pastilles dissolved slowly in mouth 4-5 x/day x 10-14 days; max 14 days
Pastille: 200,000 units/pastille (30 pastilles/pck)
Mycostatin Suspension *Infants:* 1 ml in each cheek qid after feedings; *Older children:* 4-6 ml qid swish and swallow
Oral susp: 100,000 units/ml (60 ml w. dropper)

INVASIVE INFECTION

▶ ***posaconazole*** (D) <13 years: not recommended; ≥13 years: take with food; 100 mg bid on day one; then 100 mg once daily x 13 days; refractory, 400 mg bid
Noxafil *Oral susp:* 40 mg/ml (105 ml) (cherry)
Comment: **Noxafil** is indicated as prophylaxis for invasive aspergillus and candida infections in patients >13 years old who are at high risk due to being severely compromised.

CANDIDIASIS: SKIN

TOPICAL ANTIFUNGALS

▶ ***butenafine*** (B)(G) <12 years: not recommended; ≥12 years: apply bid x 1 week or once daily x 4 weeks
Lotrimin Ultra (C)(OTC) *Crm:* 1% (12, 24 gm)
Mentax *Crm:* 1% (15, 30 gm)
Comment: ***butenafine*** is a benzylamine, not an azole. Fungicidal activity continues for at least 5 weeks after the last application.

▶ ***ciclopirox*** (B)
Loprox Cream <10 years: not recommended; ≥10 years: apply bid; max 4 weeks
Crm: 0.77% (15, 30, 90 gm)
Loprox Lotion <10 years: not recommended; ≥10 years: apply bid; max 4 weeks
Lotn: 0.77% (30, 60 ml)
Loprox Gel <16 years: not recommended; ≥16 years: apply bid; max 4 weeks
Gel: 0.77% (30, 45 gm)

➢ *clotrimazole* (B) <12 years: not recommended; ≥12 years: apply bid x 7 days
  Lotrimin *Crm:* 1% (15, 30, 45 gm)
  Lotrimin AF (OTC) *Crm:* 1% (12 gm); *Lotn:* 1% (10 ml); *Soln:* 1% (10 ml)

➢ *econazole* (C) Pediatric: <12 years: not recommended; ≥12 years: apply bid x 14 days
  Spectazole *Crm:* 1% (15, 30, 85 gm)

➢ *ketoconazole* (C) <12 years: not recommended; ≥12 years: apply once daily x 14 days
  Nizoral Cream *Crm:* 2% (15, 30, 60 gm)

➢ *miconazole* 2% (C) <12 years: not recommended; ≥12 years: apply once daily x 2 weeks
  Lotrimin AF Spray Liquid (OTC) *Spray liq:* 2% (113 gm) (alcohol 17%)
  Lotrimin AF Spray Powder (OTC) *Spray pwdr:* 2% (90 gm) (alcohol 10%)
  Monistat-Derm *Crm:* 2% (1, 3 oz); *Spray liq:* 2% (3.5 oz); *Spray pwdr:* 2%(3 oz)

➢ *nystatin* (C) dust affected skin freely bid-tid
  Nystop Powder *Pwdr:* 100,000 U/gm (15 gm)

ORAL ANTIFUNGALS

➢ *amphotericin b* (B)
  Fungizone *Oral susp:* 100 mg/ml (24 ml w. dropper)

➢ *ketoconazole* (C)(G) <2 years: not recommended; ≥2 years-12 years: 3.3-6.6 mg/kg once daily x 4 weeks; >12 years: initially 200 mg once daily; max 400 mg/day x 4 weeks
  Nizoral *Tab:* 200 mg

Comment: Caution with ***ketoconazole*** due to potential for hepatotoxicity.

INVASIVE INFECTION

➢ *posaconazole* (D) <13 years: not recommended; ≥13 years: take with food; 100 mg bid on day one; then 100 mg once daily x 13 days; refractory, 400 mg bid x 13 days
  Noxafil *Oral susp:* 40 mg/ml (105 ml) (cherry)
  Comment: **Noxafil** is indicated as prophylaxis for invasive aspergillus and candida infections in patients >13 years old who are at high risk due to being severely compromised.

CANDIDIASIS: VULVOVAGINAL (MONILIASIS)

PROPHYLAXIS

➢ *acetic acid+oxyquinolone* (C) <12 years: not recommended; ≥12 years: one full applicator intravaginally bid for up to 30 days
  Relagard *Gel:* acetic acid 0.9%+oxyquin 0.025% (50 gm tube w. applicator)

Comment: The following treatment regimens for vulvovaginal candidiasis (VVC) are published in the **2015 CDC Sexually Transmitted Diseases Treatment Guidelines.** Treatment regimens are presented by generic drug name first, followed by information about brands and dose forms. Complicated VVC (recurrent, severe, non-albicans, or females with uncontrolled diabetes, debilitation, or immunosuppression) may require more intensive treatment and/or longer duration of treatment. VVC frequently occurs during pregnancy. Only topical azole therapies, applied for 7 days, are recommended during pregnancy.

ORAL RX AGENT

➢ *fluconazole* 150 mg in a single dose; complicated VVC, 150 mg x 3 doses on days 1, 4, 7 or weekly x 6 months

RX INTRAVAGINAL AGENTS

Regimen 1

- *butoconazole* 2% cream (bioadhesive product) 5 gm intravaginally in a single dose

Regimen 2

- *nystatin* 100,000-unit vaginal tablet once daily x 14 days

Regimen 3

- *terconazole* 0.4% cream 5 gm intravaginally once daily x 7 days

Regimen 4

- *terconazole* 0.8% cream 5 gm intravaginally once daily x 3 days

Regimen 5

- *terconazole* 80 mg vaginal suppository intravaginally once daily x 3 days

OTC INTRAVAGINAL AGENTS

Regimen 1

- *butoconazole* 2% cream 5 gm intravaginally once daily x 3 days

Regimen 2

- *clotrimazole* 1% cream intravaginally once daily x 7-14 days

Regimen 3

- *clotrimazole* 2% cream intravaginally once daily x 3 days

Regimen 4

- *miconazole* 2% cream intravaginally once daily x 7 days

Regimen 5

- *miconazole* 4% cream intravaginally once daily x 3 days

Regimen 6

- *miconazole* 100 mg vaginal suppository intravaginally once daily x 7 days

Regimen 7

- *miconazole* 200 mg vaginal suppository intravaginally once daily x 3 days

Regimen 8

- *miconazole* 1,200 mg vaginal suppository intravaginally in a single application

Regimen 9

- *tioconazole* 6.5% ointment 5 gm intravaginally in a single application

DRUG BRANDS AND DOSE FORMS

- *butoconazole* cream 2% (C)
  Gynazole-12% Vaginal Cream *Prefilled vag applicator:* 5 gm
  Femstat-3 Vaginal Cream (OTC) *Vag crm:* 2% (20 gm w. 3 applicators); *Prefilled vag applicator:* 5 gm (3/pck)

- *clotrimazole* (B)(OTC)
  - **Gyne-Lotrimin Vaginal Cream (OTC)** *Vag crm:* 1% (45 gm w. applicator)
  - **Gyne-Lotrimin Vaginal Suppository (OTC)** *Vag supp:* 100 mg (7/pck)
  - **Gyne-Lotrimin 3 Vaginal Suppository (OTC)** *Vag supp:* 200 mg (3/pck)
  - **Gyne-Lotrimin Combination Pack (OTC)** *Combination pck:* 7-100 mg supp with 7 gm 1% cream
  - **Gyne-Lotrimin 3 Combination Pack (OTC)** *Combination pck:* 200 mg supp (7/pck) plus 1% cream (7 gm)
  - **Mycelex-G Vaginal Cream** *Vag crm:* 1% (45, 90 gm w. applicator)
  - **Mycelex-G Vaginal Tab** 1 *Tab:* 500 mg (1/pck)
  - **Mycelex Twin Pack** *Twin pck:* 500 mg tab (7/pck) with 1% crm (7 gm)
  - **Mycelex-7 Vaginal Cream (OTC)** *Vag crm:* 1% (45 gm w. applicator)
  - **Mycelex-7 Vaginal Inserts (OTC)** *Vag insert:* 100 mg insert (7/pck)
  - **Mycelex-7 Combination Pack (OTC)** *Combination pck:* 100 mg inserts (7/pck) plus 1% crm (7 gm)
- *fluconazole* (C)
  - **Diflucan** *Tab:* 50, 100, 150, 200 mg; *Oral susp:* 10, 40 mg/ml (35 ml) (orange) (sucrose)
- *miconazole* (B)
  - **Monistat-3 Combination Pack (OTC)** *Combination pck:* 200 mg supp (3/pck) plus 2% crm (9 gm)
  - **Monistat-7 Combination Pack (OTC)** *Combination pck:* 100 mg supp (7/pck) plus 2% crm (9 gm)
  - **Monistat-7 Vaginal Cream (OTC)** *Vag crm:* 2% (45 gm w. applicator)
  - **Monistat-7 Vaginal Suppositories (OTC)** *Vag supp:* 100 mg (7/pck)
  - **Monistat-3 Vaginal Suppositories (OTC)** *Vag supp:* 200 mg (3/pck)
- *nystatin* (C)
  - **Mycostatin** *Vag tab:* 100,000 U (1/pck)
- *terconazole* (C)
  - **Terazol-3 Vaginal Cream** *Vag crm:* 0.8% (20 gm w. applicator)
  - **Terazol-3 Vaginal Suppositories** *Vag supp:* 80 mg supp (3/pck)
  - **Terazol-7 Vaginal Cream** *Vag crm:* 0.4% (45 gm w. applicator)
- *tioconazole* (C)
  - **1-Day (OTC)** *Vag oint:* 6.5% (prefilled applicator x 1)
  - **Monistat 1 Vaginal Ointment (OTC)** *Vag oint:* 6.5% (prefilled applicator x 1)
  - **Vagistat-1 Vaginal Ointment (OTC)** *Vag oint:* 6.5% (prefilled applicator x 1)

INVASIVE INFECTION

- *posaconazole* (D) <13 years: not recommended; ≥13 years: take with food; 100 mg bid on day 1; then 100 mg once daily x 13 days; refractory, 400 mg bid
  - **Noxafil** *Oral susp:* 40 mg/ml (105 ml) (cherry)
  - Comment: **Noxafil** is indicated as prophylaxis for invasive aspergillus and candida infections in patients ≥13 years old who are at high risk due to being severely compromised.

CANNABINOID HYPEREMESIS SYNDROME (CHS)

Comment: cannabinoid hyperemesis syndrome (CHS) is indicated by recurrent episodes of refractory nausea and vomiting with vague diffuse abdominal pain (accompanied by compulsive, frequent, hot baths or showers for relief of abdominal pain; these behaviors are thought to be learned through their cyclical periods of emesis) in the setting of chronic cannabis use (at least weekly for >2 years. The nausea and vomiting typically do not respond to antiemetic medications. 5HT3 (e.g., ***ondansetron***), D2 (e.g., ***prochlorperazine***), H1 (e.g., ***promethazine***), or neurokinin-1 receptor antagonists (e.g., ***aprepitant***) can be tried, but these therapies often are ineffective. The recovery phase can last weeks to months despite continued cannabis use prior to returning to the hyperemetic phase. Symptoms that are worse in the morning, with normal bowel habits, and negative evaluation, including laboratory, radiography, and endoscopy. Resolution requires cannabis cessation from 1 to 3 months. Returning to cannabis use often results in the returning of CHS.

REFERENCE

Fleming, JE, & Lockwood, S. (2017). Cannabinoid hyperemesis syndrome. *Fed Pract, 34*(10), 33–36.

PHENOTHIAZINES

▶ ***chlorpromazine*** **(C)(G)** 12-18 years: 0.25 mg/lb orally q 4-6 hours prn or 0.5 mg/lb rectally q 6-8 hours prn; >18 years: 10-25 mg PO q 4 hours prn or 50-100 mg rectally q 6-8 hours prn

Thorazine *Tab:* 10, 25, 50, 100, 200 mg; *Spansule:* 30, 75, 150 mg sust-rel; *Syr:* 10 mg/5 ml (4 oz; orange custard); *Conc:* 30 mg/ml (4 oz); 100 mg/ml (2, 8 oz); *Supp:* 25, 100 mg

▶ ***perphenazine*** **(C)** <12 years: not recommended; ≥12 years: 5 mg IM (may repeat in 6 hours) or 8-16 mg/day PO in divided doses; max 15 mg/day IM; max 24 mg/day PO

Trilafon *Tab:* 2, 4, 8, 16 mg; *Oral conc:* 16 mg/5 ml (118 ml); *Amp:* 5 mg/ml (1 ml)

▶ ***prochlorperazine*** **(C)(G)**

Compazine 20-29 lb: 2.5 mg daily bid prn; max 7.5 mg/day; 30-39 lb: 2.5 mg bid-tid prn; max 10 mg/day; 40-85 lb: 2.5 mg tid or 5 mg bid prn; max 15 mg/day; >85 lb: 5-10 mg tid-qid prn; usual max 40 mg/day

Tab: 5, 10 mg; *Syr:* 5 mg/5 ml (4 oz) (fruit)

Compazine Suppository 20-29 lb: 2.5 mg daily-bid prn; max 7.5; mg/day; 30-39 lb: 2.5 mg bid-tid prn; max 10 mg/day; 40-85 lb: 2.5 mg tid or 5 mg bid prn; max 15 mg/day; >85 lb: 25 mg rectally bid prn; usual max 50 mg/day

Rectal supp: 2.5, 5, 25 mg

Compazine Injectable ≥20 lb: 0.06 mg/kg x 1 dose; >12 years: 5-10 mg tid or qid prn

Vial: 5 mg/ml (2, 10 ml)

Compazine Spansule <12 years: not recommended; ≥12 years: 15 mg q AM prn or 10 mg q 12 hours prn usual max 40 mg/day

Spansule: 10, 15 mg sust-rel

▶ ***promethazine*** **(C)(G)** <2 years: not recommended; ≥2 years: 0.5 mg/lb or 6.25-25 mg q 4-6 hours prn; >12 years: 25 mg PO or rectally q 4-6 hours prn

Phenergan *Tab:* 12.5*, 25*, 50 mg; *Plain syr:* 6.25 mg/5 ml; *Fortis syr:* 25 mg/5 ml; *Rectal supp:* 12.5, 25, 50 mg

SUBSTANCE P/NEUROKININ 1 RECEPTOR ANTAGONIST

▶ ***aprepitant*** **(B)(G)** <6 years: not recommended; ≥6 years: use oral suspension (see mfr pkg insert for dose by weight; administer with 5HT-3 receptor antagonist; *Day 1:* 125 mg x 1 dose; *Starting Day 2:* 80 mg once daily in the morning

Emend *Cap:* 40, 80, 125 mg (2 x 80 mg bi-fold pck; 1 x 25 mg/2 x 80 mg tri-fold pck); *Oral susp:* 125 mg pwdr for oral suspension, single-dose pouch w. dispenser; *Vial:* 150 mg pwdr for reconstitution and IV infusion

SEROTONIN (5HT-3) RECEPTOR ANTAGONISTS

- *dolasetron* (B) <2 years: not recommended; 2-16 years: 1.8 mg/kg; >16 years: administer 100 mg IV over 30 seconds; max 100 mg/dose
  Anzemet *Tab:* 50, 100 mg; *Amp:* 12.5 mg/0.625 ml; *Prefilled carpuject syringe:* 12.5 mg (0.625 ml); *Vial:* 100 mg/5 ml (single-use); *Vial:* 500 mg/25 ml (multi-dose)
- *granisetron*
  Kytril (B) <2 years: not recommended; ≥2 years: 10 mcg/kg; administer IV over 30 seconds; max 1 dose/week
  Tab: 1 mg; *Oral soln:* 2 mg/10 ml (30 ml) (orange); *Vial:* 1 mg/ml (1 ml single-dose) (preservative-free); 1 mg/ml (4 ml multi-dose) (benzyl alcohol)
  Sancuso (B) apply 1 patch; remove 24 hours (minimum) to 7 days (maximum)
  Transdermal patch: 3.1 mg/day
- **Sustol** <18 years: not established; ≥18 years: administer SC over 20-30 seconds (due to drug viscosity) and not more frequently than once every 7 days; *CrCl 30-59 mL/min:* repeat dose no more than every 14th day; *CrCl <30 mL/min:* not recommended
  Syringe: 10 mg/0.4 ml ext-rel; prefilled single-dose/kit
  Comment: At least 60 minutes prior to administration, remove the **Sustol** kit from refrigeration; activate a warming pouch and wrap the syringe in the warming pouch for 5-6 minutes to warm it to room temperature.
- *ondansetron* (C)(G) <4 years: not recommended; 4-11 years: 4 mg q 4 hours x 3 doses; then 4 mg q 8 hours; >11 years: Oral Forms: 8 mg q 8 hours x 2 doses; then 8 mg q 12 hours
  Zofran *Tab:* 4, 8, 24 mg
  Zofran ODT *ODT:* 4, 8 mg (strawberry) (phenylalanine)
  Zofran Oral Solution *Oral soln:* 4 mg/5 ml (50 ml) (strawberry) (phenylalanine); *Parenteral form:* see mfr pkg insert
  Zofran Injection *Vial:* 2 mg/ml (2 ml single-dose); 2 mg/ml (20 ml muti-dose); 32 mg/50 ml (50 ml multi-dose); *Prefilled syringe:* 4 mg/2 ml, single-use (24/ carton)
  Zuplenz Oral Soluble Film: 4, 8 mg orally-disint (10/carton) (peppermint)
- *palonosetron* (B)(G) 6-17 years: 20 mcg/kg; max 1.5 mg/single dose; >17 years: administer 0.25 mg IV over 30 seconds; max 1 dose/week infuse over 15 minutes
  Aloxi *Vial (single-use):* 0.075 mg/1.5 ml; 0.25 mg/5 ml (mannitol)

CARCINOID SYNDROME DIARRHEA (CSD)

TRYPTOPHAN HYDROXYLASE

- *telotristat* <18 years: not established; ≥18 years: take with food; 250 mg tid
  Xermelo *Tab:* 250 mg (4 x 7 daily dose packs/carton)
  Comment: Take **Xermelo** in combination with somatostatin analog (SSA) therapy to treat patients inadequately controlled by SSA therapy. Breastfeeding females should monitor the infant for constipation.

CARPAL TUNNEL SYNDROME (CTS)

Acetaminophen for IV Infusion *see **Pain** page* 322
NSAIDs *see page* 539
Other Oral Analgesics *see **Pain** page* 324
Topical & Transdermal NSAIDs *see **Pain** page* 323
Parenteral Corticosteroids *see page* 547
Oral Corticosteroids *see page* 546

CAT SCRATCH FEVER (*BARTONELLA* INFECTION)

Comment: Cat scratch fever is usually self-limited. Treatment should be limited to severe or debilitating cases.

ANTI-INFECTIVES

- ***azithromycin*** **(B)(G)** <12 years: 12 mg/kg/day x 5 days; *see page* 593 *for dose by weight table*; max 500 mg/day; ≥12 years: 500 mg x 1 dose on day 1, then 250 mg daily on days 2-5 or 500 mg daily x 3 days or **Zmax** 2 gm in a single dose
  - **Zithromax** *Tab:* 250, 500, 600 mg; *Oral susp:* 100 mg/5 ml (15 ml); 200 mg/5 ml (15, 22.5, 30 ml) (cherry); *Pkt:* 1 gm for reconstitution (cherry-banana)
  - **Zithromax Tri-pak** *Tab:* 3 x 500 mg tabs/pck
  - **Zithromax Z-pak** *Tab:* 6 x 250 mg tabs/pck
  - **Zmax** *Oral susp:* 2 gm ext-rel for reconstitution (cherry-banana) (148 mg Na^+)
- ***doxycycline*** **(D)(G)** <8 years: not recommended; ≥8 years, ≤100 lb: 2 mg/lb on first day in 2 divided doses, followed by 1 mg/lb/day in 1-2 divided doses; ≥8 years, >100 lb: 100 mg bid; *see page* 605 *for dose by weight table*
  - **Acticlate** *Tab:* 75, 150**mg
  - **Adoxa** *Tab:* 50, 75, 100, 150 mg ent-coat
  - **Doryx** *Tab:* 50, 75, 100, 150, 200 mg del-rel
  - **Doxteric** *Tab:* 50 mg del-rel
  - **Monodox** *Cap:* 50, 75, 100 mg
  - **Oracea** *Cap:* 40 mg del-rel
  - **Vibramycin** *Tab:* 100 mg; *Cap:* 50, 100 mg; *Syr:* 50 mg/5 ml (raspberry-apple) (sulfites); *Oral susp:* 25 mg/5 ml (raspberry)
  - **Vibra-Tab** *Tab:* 100 mg film-coat

  Comment: ***doxycycline*** is contraindicated <8 years-of-age, in pregnancy, and lactation (discolors developing tooth enamel). A side effect may be photosensitivity (photophobia). Do not give with antacids, calcium supplements, milk or other dairy, or within 2 hours of taking another drug.
- ***erythromycin base*** **(B)(G)** 45 kg: 30-50 mg in 2-4 divided doses x 4 weeks; ≥45 kg: 500-1000 mg qid x 4 weeks
  - **Ery-Tab** *Tab:* 250, 333, 500 mg ent-coat
  - **PCE** *Tab:* 333, 500 mg
- ***erythromycin ethylsuccinate*** **(B)(G)** 30-50 mg/kg/day in 4 divided doses x 4 weeks; may double dose with severe infection; max 100 mg/kg/day or 400 mg qid; *see page* 607 *for dose by weight table*
  - **EryPed** *Oral susp:* 200 mg/5 ml (100, 200 ml) (fruit); 400 mg/5 ml (60, 100, 200 ml) (banana); *Oral drops:* 200, 400 mg/5 ml (50 ml) (fruit); Chew tab: 200 mg wafer (fruit)
  - **E.E.S.** *Oral susp:* 200, 400 mg/5 ml (100 ml) (fruit)
  - **E.E.S. Granules** *Oral susp:* 200 mg/5 ml (100, 200 ml) (cherry)
  - **E.E.S. 400 Tablets** *Tab:* 400 mg
- ***trimethoprim+sulfamethoxazole [TMP-SMX]*** **(D)(G)**
  - **Bactrim, Septra** <12 years: not recommended; ≥12 years: 2 tabs bid x 10 days
    Tab: trim 80 mg+sulfa 400 mg*
  - **Bactrim DS, Septra DS** <12 years: not recommended; ≥12 years: 1 tab bid x 10 days
    Tab: trim 160 mg+sulfa 800 mg*
  - **Bactrim Pediatric Suspension, Septra Pediatric Suspension** <2 months: not recommended; ≥2 months-12 years: 40 mg/kg/day of ***sulfamethoxazole*** in 2 doses bid; >12 years: use tabs
    Oral susp: trim 40 mg+sulfa 200 mg per 5 ml (100 ml) (cherry) (alcohol 0.3%)

CELLULITIS

Comment: Duration of treatment should be 10-30 days. Obtain culture from site. Consider blood cultures.

ANTI-INFECTIVES

▶ ***amoxicillin*** **(B)(G)** <40 kg (88 lb): 20-40 mg/kg/day in 3 divided doses x 10 days <u>or</u> 25-45 mg/kg/day in 2 divided doses x 10 days; *see page* 588 *for dose by weight table;* ≥40 kg: 500-875 mg bid <u>or</u> 250-500 mg tid x 10 days

Amoxil *Cap:* 250, 500 mg; *Tab:* 875*mg; *Chew tab:* 125, 200, 250, 400 mg (cherry-banana-peppermint) (phenylalanine); *Oral susp:* 125, 250 mg/5 ml (80, 100, 150 ml) (strawberry); 200, 400 mg/5 ml (50, 75, 100 ml) (bubble gum); *Oral drops:* 50 mg/ml (30 ml) (bubble gum)

Moxatag *Tab:* 775 mg ext-rel

Trimox *Tab:* 125, 250 mg; *Cap:* 250, 500 mg; *Oral susp:* 125, 250 mg/5 ml (80, 100, 150 ml) (raspberry-strawberry)

▶ ***amoxicillin+clavulanate*** **(B)(G)**

Augmentin <40 kg: 40-45 mg/kg/day divided tid x 10 days <u>or</u> 90 mg/kg/day divided bid x 10 days; *see page* 590 *for dose by weight table;* ≥40 kg: 500 mg tid <u>or</u> 875 mg bid x 10 days

Tab: 250, 500, 875 mg; *Chew tab:* 125, 250 mg (lemon-lime); 200, 400 mg (cherry-banana) (phenylalanine); *Oral susp:* 125 mg/5 ml (banana), 250 mg/5 ml (75, 100, 150 ml) (orange); 200, 400 mg/5 ml (50, 75, 100 ml) (orange) (phenylalanine)

Augmentin ES-600 <3 months: not recommended; ≥3 months, <40 kg: 90 mg/kg/day divided q 12 hours x 10 days; *see page* 591 *for dose by weight table;* ≥40 kg: not recommended

Oral susp: 600 mg/5 ml (50, 75, 100, 125, 150, 200 ml) (strawberry cream) (phenylalanine)

Augmentin XR <16 years: use other forms; ≥16 years: 2 tabs q 12 hours x 7-10 days

Tab: 1000*mg ext-rel

▶ ***azithromycin*** **(B)(G)** <12 years: 12 mg/kg/day x 5 days; *see page* 593 *for dose by weight table*; max 500 mg/day; ≥12 years: 500 mg x 1 dose on day 1, then 250 mg daily on days 2-5 <u>or</u> 500 mg daily x 3 days **oarsman** 2 gm in a single dose

Zithromax *Tab:* 250, 500, 600 mg; *Oral susp:* 100 mg/5 ml (15 ml); 200 mg/5 ml (15, 22.5, 30 ml) (cherry); *Pkt:* 1 gm for reconstitution (cherry-banana)

Zithromax Tri-pak *Tab:* 3 x 500 mg tabs/pck

Zithromax Z-pak *Tab:* 6 x 250 mg tabs/pck

Zmax *Oral susp:* 2 gm ext-rel for reconstitution (cherry-banana) (148 mg Na^+)

▶ ***cefaclor*** **(B)(G)** <1 month: not recommended; 1 month-12 years: 20-40 mg/kg in 2 <u>or</u> 3 divided doses x 10 days; *see page* 594 *for dose by weight table;* max 1 gm/day; >12 years: 375 mg q 12 hours x 10 days; max 2 gm/day

Tab: 500 mg; *Cap:* 250, 500 mg; *Susp:* 125 mg/5 ml (75, 150 ml) (strawberry); 187 mg/5 ml (50, 100 ml) (strawberry); 250 mg/5 ml (75, 150 ml) (strawberry); 375 mg/5 ml (50, 100 ml) (strawberry)

Cefaclor Extended Release <16 years: not recommended; ≥16 years: 500 mg bid x 10 days (clinically equivalent to 250 mg immed-rel caps tid); swallow whole; take with food

Tab: 375, 500 mg ext-rel

▶ ***cefpodoxime proxetil*** **(B)(G)** <2 months: not recommended; ≥2 months-12 years: 10 mg/kg/day (max 400 mg/dose) <u>or</u> 5 mg/kg/day bid (max 200 mg/dose) x 7-14 days; *see page* 598 *for dose by weight table;* >12 years: 400 mg bid x 7-14 days

Vantin *Tab:* 100, 200 mg; *Oral susp:* 50, 100 mg/5 ml (50, 75, 100 mg) (lemon creme)

- ***cefprozil*** **(B)** <2 years: not recommended; 2-12 years: 15 mg/kg bid x 10 days; *see page* 599 *for dose by weight table;* >12 years: 250-500 mg bid or 500 mg daily x 10 days

  Cefzil *Tab:* 250, 500 mg; *Oral susp:* 125, 250 mg/5 ml (50, 75, 100 ml) (bubble gum) (phenylalanine)

- ***ceftaroline fosamil*** **(B)** <18 years: not established: ≥18 years: administer 600 mg once every 12 hours, by IV infusion over 5-60 minutes, x 5-14 days

  Teflaro *Vial:* 400, 600 mg pwdr for reconstitution, single use (10/carton)

  Comment: **Teflaro** is indicated for the treatment of acute bacterial skin and skin structures infection (ABSSSI).

- ***ceftriaxone*** **(B)(G)** <12 years: 50-75 mg/kg IM in 1-2 divided doses x 5-14 days; max 2 gm/day; ≥12 years: 1-2 gm IM daily x 5-14 days; max 4 gm daily

  Rocephin *Vial:* 250, 500 mg; 1, 2 gm

- ***cephalexin*** **(B)(G)** <12 years: 25-50 mg/kg/day in 4 divided doses x 10 days; *see page* 601 *for dose by weight table;* ≥12 years: 500 mg bid x 10 days

  Keflex *Cap:* 250, 333, 500, 750 mg; *Oral susp:* 125, 250 mg/5 ml (100, 200 ml) (strawberry)

- ***clarithromycin*** **(C)(G)** <6 months: not recommended; ≥6 months-12 years: 7.5 mg/kg bid x 10 days; *see page* 602 *for dose by weight table;* >12 years: 500 mg q 12 hours or 500 mg ext-rel once daily x 10 days

  Biaxin *Tab:* 250, 500 mg

  Biaxin Oral Suspension *Oral susp:* 125, 250 mg/5 ml (50, 100 ml) (fruit punch)

  Biaxin XL *Tab:* 500 mg ext-rel

Comment: The FDA is advising caution before prescribing ***clarithromycin*** to patients with heart disease because of a potential increased risk of heart problems or death that can occur years later. This recommendation is based on a review of the results of a 10-year follow-up study of patients with coronary heart disease from a large clinical trial that first observed this safety issue. Consider risk benefit and the use of other antibiotics in such patients.

- ***dalbavancin*** **(C)** <18 years: not established; ≥18 years: 1,000 mg administered once as a single dose via IV infusion over 30 minutes or initially 1,000 mg once, followed by 500 mg 1 week later; infuse over 30 minutes; *CrCl <30 mL/min, not receiving dialysis:* initially 750 mg, followed by 375 mg 1 week later

  Dalvance *Vial:* 500 mg pwdr for reconstitution, single use (preservative-free)

  Comment: **Dalvance** is indicated for the treatment of acute bacterial skin and skin structures infection (ABSSSI) caused by gram positive bacteria.

- ***delafloxacin*** *IV infusion:* <18 years: not recommended; ≥18 years: administer 300 mg every 12 hours over 60 minutes x 5-14 days; *Tablet:* 450 mg every 12 hours x 5-14 days; dosage for patients with renal impairment is based on eGFR (see mfr pkg insert)

  Baxdela *Tab:* 450 mg; *Vial:* 300 mg pwdr for reconstitution and IV infusion

  Comment: **Baxdela**, a fluoroquinolone, is indicated for the treatment of acute bacterial skin and skin structure infections (ABSSSI) caused by designated susceptible bacteria. Fluoroquinolones have been associated with disabling and potentially irreversible serious adverse reactions that have occurred together, including tendinitis and tendon rupture, peripheral neuropathy, and central nervous system effects. Discontinue **Baxdela** immediately and avoid the use of fluoroquinolones, including **Baxdela**, in patients who experience any of these serious adverse reactions. Fluoroquinolones may exacerbate muscle weakness in patients with myasthenia gravis. Therefore, avoid **Baxdela** in patients with known history of myasthenia gravis. Most common adverse reactions are nausea, diarrhea, headache, transaminase elevations and vomiting. Closely monitor SCr in patients with severe renal impairment (eGFR 15-29 mL/min/1.73 m2) receiving intravenous ***delafloxacin***. If SCr level increases occur, consider changing to oral ***delafloxacin***. Discontinue **Baxdela** if eGFR decreases to <15 mL/min/1.73 m2. The limited available data with **Baxdela** use in pregnant females are insufficient to inform a drug-associated risk of major birth defects and miscarriages. There are no data available on the presence of ***delafloxacin*** in human milk or the effects on the breastfed infant. To report suspected adverse reactions, contact Melinta Therapeutics at 1-844-635-4682 or FDA at 1-800-FDA-1088 or visit www.fda.gov/medwatch

▶ ***dicloxacillin*** **(B)(G)** <12 years: 12.5-25 mg/kg/day in 4 divided doses x 10 days; *see page 604 for dose by weight table;* ≥12 years: 500 mg q 6 hours x 10 days
Dynapen *Cap:* 125, 250, 500 mg; *Oral susp:* 62.5 mg/5 ml (80, 100, 200 ml)

▶ ***dirithromycin*** **(C)(G)** <12 years: not recommended; ≥12 years: 500 mg once daily x 7-10 days
Dynabac *Tab:* 250 mg

▶ ***erythromycin base*** **(B)(G)** <45 kg: 30-50 mg in 2-4 divided doses x 7-10 days; ≥45 kg: 250 mg qid or 333 mg tid or 500 mg bid x 7-10 days; then taper to lowest effective dose
Ery-Tab *Tab:* 250, 333, 500 mg ent-coat
PCE *Tab:* 333, 500 mg

▶ ***erythromycin ethylsuccinate*** **(B)(G)** 30-50 mg/kg/day in 4 divided doses x 7-10 days; may double dose with severe infection; max 100 mg/kg/day or 400 mg qid; *see page 607 for dose by weight table*
EryPed *Oral susp:* 200 mg/5 ml (100, 200 ml) (fruit); 400 mg/5 ml (60, 100, 200 ml) (banana); *Oral drops:* 200, 400 mg/5 ml (50 ml) (fruit); *Chew tab:* 200 mg wafer (fruit)
E.E.S. *Oral susp:* 200, 400 mg/5 ml (100 ml) (fruit)
E.E.S. Granules *Oral susp:* 200 mg/5 ml (100, 200 ml) (cherry)
E.E.S. 400 Tablets *Tab:* 400 mg

▶ ***linezolid*** **(C)(G)** <5 years: 10 mg/kg q 8 hours x 10-14 days; 5-11 years: 10 mg/kg q 12 hours x 10-14 days; >11 years: 400-600 mg q 12 hours x 10-14 days
Zyvox *Tab:* 400, 600 mg; *Oral susp:* 100 mg/5 ml (150 ml) (orange) (phenylalanine)

Comment: ***linezolid*** is indicated to treat susceptible ***vancomycin***-resistant *E. faecium* infections of skin and skin structures, including diabetic foot without osteomyelitis.

▶ ***loracarbef*** **(B)** <12 years: 15 mg/kg/day in 2 divided doses x 10 days; *see page 614 for dose by weight table*; ≥12 years: 200 mg bid x 10 days
Lorabid *Pulvule:* 200, 400 mg; *Oral susp:* 100 mg/5 ml (50, 100 ml); 200 mg/5 ml (50, 75, 100 ml) (strawberry bubble gum)

▶ ***moxifloxacin*** **(C)(G)** <18 years: not recommended; ≥18 years: 400 mg daily x 5 days
Avelox *Tab:* 400 mg; *Premixed* IV soln: 400 mg/250 mg (latex-free, preservative-free)

Comment: ***moxifloxacin*** is contraindicated <18 years-of-age and during pregnancy and lactation. Risk of tendonitis or tendon rupture.

▶ ***oritavancin*** **(C)** <18 years: not established; ≥18 years: administer 1,200 mg as a single dose by IV infusion over 3 hours
Orbactiv *Vial:* 400 mg pwdr for reconstitution, single use (10/carton) (mannitol; preservative-free)
Comment: **Orbactiv** is indicated for the treatment of acute bacterial skin and skin structures infection (ABSSSI).

▶ ***penicillin v potassium*** **(B)** <12 years: 25-75 mg/kg day divided q 6-8 hours x 5-7 days; *see page 616 for dose by weight table;* ≥12 years: 250-500 mg q 6 hours x 5-7 days
Pen-VK *Tab:* 250, 500 mg; *Oral soln:* 125 mg/5 ml (100, 200 ml); 250 mg/5 ml (100, 150, 200 ml)

- ▶ ***tedizolid phosphate*** **(C)** <18 years: not established; ≥18 years: administer 200 mg once daily x 6 days, via PO or IV infusion over 1 hour

  Sivextro *Tab:* 200 mg (6/blister pck)

  Comment: **Sivextro** is indicated for the treatment of acute bacterial skin and skin structures infection (ABSSSI).
- ▶ ***tigecycline*** **(D)(G)** <18 years: not recommended; ≥18 years: 100 mg as a single dose; then 50 mg q 12 hours x 5-14 days; with severe hepatic impairment (Child-Pugh Class C), 100 mg as a single dose; then 25 mg q 12 hours

  Tygacil *Vial:* 50 mg pwdr for reconstitution and IV infusion (preservative-free)

  Comment: **Tygacil** is contraindicated in pregnancy, and lactation (discolors developing tooth enamel). A side effect may be photosensitivity (photo-phobia). Do not give with antacids, calcium supplements, milk or other dairy, or within two hours of taking another drug.

CERUMEN IMPACTION

OTIC ANALGESIC

- ▶ ***antipyrine+benzocaine+zinc acetate dihydrate*** otic **(C)** fill ear canal with solution; then moisten cotton plug with solution and insert into meatus; may repeat every 1-2 hours prn

  Otozin *Otic soln:* antipyr 5.4%+benz 1%+zinc 1% per ml (10 ml w. dropper)

CERUMINOLYTICS

- ▶ ***triethanolamine*** **(OTC)(G)** fill ear canal and insert cotton plug for 15-30 minutes before irrigating with warm water

  Cerumenex *Soln:* 10% (6, 12 ml)
- ▶ ***carbamide peroxide*** **(OTC)(G)** instill 5-10 drops in ear canal; keep drops in ear several minutes; then irrigate with warm water; repeat bid for up to 4 days

  Debrox *Soln:* 15, 30 ml squeeze bottle w. applicator

CHAGAS DISEASE (AMERICAN TRYPANOSOMIASIS)

Comment: Chagas disease is a protozoal parasite (*Trypanosoma cruzi*) infection with increasing prevalence in the US attributed to immigration from *T. cruzi*-endemic areas of South and Central Latin America. Approximately 300,000 persons in the US have chronic Chagas disease and up to 30% of them will develop clinically evident cardiovascular and/or gastrointestinal disease. Chagas Disease is one of the five neglected parasitic infections (NPIs) targeted by CDC for public health action. Transmitted by the bite of the triatomine bug ("kissing bug") which feeds on human blood, maternal-fetus vertical transmission, blood transfusion, consumption of contaminated food, and organ donation. A clinical marker is Romaña sign (periorbital swelling), chagoma (skin nodule), Schizotrypanides (nonpruritic morbilliform rash). Only two antiparasitic drugs, ***benznidazole*** and ***nifurtimox***, have demonstrated effectiveness altering the progression of this chronic disease. These drugs are not FDA approved and are available only from CDC under investigational protocols. Treatment is indicated for all cases of acute or reactivated Chagas disease and for chronic *Trypanosoma cruzi* infection in children ≤18. Congenital infections are considered acute disease. Treatment is strongly recommended up to 50 years old with chronic infection who do not already have advanced Chagas cardiomyopathy. For adults older than 50 years with chronic *T. cruzi* infection, the decision to treat with antiparasitic drugs should be individualized, weighing the potential benefits and risks for the patient.

Patients taking either of these drugs should have a CBC and CMP at the start of treatment and then bi-monthly for the duration of treatment to monitor for rare bone marrow suppression. Contraindications for treatment include severe hepatic and/or renal disease. As safety for infants exposed through breastfeeding has not been documented, withholding treatment while breastfeeding is also recommended. For emergencies (for example, acute Chagas disease with severe manifestations, Chagas disease in a newborn, or Chagas disease in an immunocompromised person) outside of regular business hours, call the CDC Emergency Operations Center (770-488-7100) and ask for the person on call for Parasitic Diseases. For more detailed information about screening, assessment, and treatment of this public health threat, see McDonald, J, & Mattingly, J. (November, 2016). Chagas disease: Creeping into family practice in the United States, *Clinician Reviews*, pp. 38-45, or call 404-718-4745 or e-mail questions to chagas@cdc.gov.

ANTI-PARASITIC AGENTS

- ***benznidazole*** (G) take with a meal to avoid GI upset; <12 years: 5-7.5 mg/kg/day divided bid x 60 days; ≥12 years: 5-7 mg/kg/day divided bid x 60 days
  Comment: Common side effects of ***benznidazole*** are allergic dermatitis, peripheral neuropathy, insomnia, anorexia with weight loss.
- ***nifurtimox*** (G) take with a meal to avoid GI upset; ≤10 years: 15-20 mg/kg/day divided tid-qid x 90 days; 11-16 years: 12.5-15 mg/kg/day divided tid-qid x 90 days; ≥17 years: 8-10 mg/kg/day divided tid-qid x 90 days
  Comment: Common side effects of ***nifurtimox*** are anorexia and weight loss, nausea, vomiting, polyneuropathy, headache, dizziness or vertigo.

CHANCROID

ANTI-INFECTIVES

- ***azithromycin*** (B)(G) <12 years: 12 mg/kg/day x 5 days; *see page* 593 *for dose by weight table*; max 500 mg/day; ≥12 years: 500 mg x 1 dose on day 1, then 250 mg daily on days 2-5 or 500 mg daily x 3 days **oarsman** 2 gm in a single dose
  - **Zithromax** *Tab:* 250, 500, 600 mg; *Oral susp:* 100 mg/5 ml (15 ml); 200 mg/5 ml (15, 22.5, 30 ml) (cherry); *Pkt:* 1 gm for reconstitution (cherry-banana)
  - **Zithromax Tri-pak** *Tab:* 3 x 500 mg tabs/pck
  - **Zithromax Z-pak** *Tab:* 6 x 250 mg tabs/pck
  - **Zmax** *Oral susp:* 2 gm ext-rel for reconstitution (cherry-banana) (148 mg reconstitution (cherry-banana))
- ***ceftriaxone*** (B)(G) <45 kg: 125 mg IM in a single dose; ≥45 kg: 250 mg IM in a single dose
  - **Rocephin** *Vial:* 250, 500 mg; 1, 2 gm
- ***ciprofloxacin*** (C) <18 years: not recommended; ≥18 years: 500 mg bid x 10 days; max 1.5 gm/day
  - **Cipro (G)** *Tab:* 250, 500, 750 mg; *Oral susp:* 250, 500 mg/5 ml (100 ml) (strawberry)
  - **Cipro XR** *Tab:* 500, 1,000 mg ext-rel
  - **ProQuin XR** *Tab:* 500 mg ext-rel

  Comment: ***ciprofloxacin*** is contraindicated <18 years-of-age, and during pregnancy and lactation. Risk of tendonitis or tendon rupture.
- ***erythromycin base*** (B)(G) <45 kg: 30-50 mg/kg/day divided bid-qid; max 100 mg/kg/day; >45 kg: 500 mg qid x 7 days
  - **Ery-Tab** *Tab:* 250, 333, 500 mg ent-coat
  - **PCE** *Tab:* 333, 500 mg

- ***erythromycin ethylsuccinate*** **(B)(G)** 30-50 mg/kg/day in 4 divided doses x 7 days; may double dose with severe infection; max 100 mg/kg/day or 400 mg qid; *see page 607 for dose by weight table*
  - **EryPed** *Oral susp:* 200 mg/5 ml (100, 200 ml) (fruit); 400 mg/5 ml (60, 100, 200 ml) (banana); *Oral drops:* 200, 400 mg/5 ml (50 ml) (fruit); *Chew tab:* 200 mg wafer (fruit)
  - **E.E.S.** *Oral susp:* 200, 400 mg/5 ml (100 ml) (fruit)
  - **E.E.S. Granules** *Oral susp:* 200 mg/5 ml (100, 200 ml) (cherry)
  - **E.E.S. 400 Tablets** *Tab:* 400 mg

CHEMOTHERAPY-RELATED NAUSEA/VOMITING

PHENOTHIAZINES

- ***chlorpromazine*** **(C)(G)** <6 months: not recommended; ≥6 months-12 years: 0.25 mg/lb orally q 4-6 hours prn or 0.5 mg/lb rectally q 6-8 hours prn; >12 years: 10-25 mg PO q 4 hours prn or 50-100 mg rectally q 6-8 hours prn
  - **Thorazine** *Tab:* 10, 25, 50, 100, 200 mg; *Spansule:* 30, 75, 150 mg sust-rel; *Syr:* 10 mg/5 ml (4 oz; orange custard); *Conc:* 30 mg/ml (4 oz); 100 mg/ml (2, 8 oz); *Supp:* 25, 100 mg
- ***perphenazine*** **(C)** <12 years: not recommended; ≥12 years: 5 mg IM (may repeat in 6 hours) or 8-16 mg/day PO in divided doses; max 15 mg/day IM; max 24 mg/day PO
  - **Trilafon** *Tab:* 2, 4, 8, 16 mg; *Oral conc:* 16 mg/5 ml (118 ml); *Amp:* 5 mg/ml (1 ml)
- ***prochlorperazine*** **(C)(G)**
  - **Compazine** <2 years or <20 lb: not recommended; 20-29 lb: 2.5 mg daily bid prn; max 7.5 mg/day; 30-39 lb: 2.5 mg bid-tid prn; max 10 mg/ day; 40-85 lb: 2.5 mg tid or 5 mg bid prn; max 15 mg/day; >85 lb: 5-10 mg tid-qid prn; usual max 40 mg/day
    - *Tab:* 5, 10 mg; *Syr:* 5 mg/5 ml (4 oz) (fruit)
  - **Compazine Suppository** 25 mg rectally bid prn; usual max 50 mg/day
    Pediatric: <2 years or <20 lb: not recommended; 20-29 lb: 2.5 mg daily-bid prn; max 7.5; mg/day; 30-39 lb: 2.5 mg bid-tid prn; max 10 mg/day; 40-85 lb: 2.5 mg tid or 5 mg bid prn; max 15 mg/day; >85 lb: 25 mg rectally bid prn; usual max 50 mg/day
    - *Rectal supp:* 2.5, 5, 25 mg
  - **Compazine Injectable** <2 years or <20 lb: not recommended; ≥2 years or ≥20 lb: 0.06 mg/kg x 1 dose; ≥12 years: 5-10 mg tid or qid prn
    - *Vial:* 5 mg/ml (2, 10 ml)
  - **Compazine Spansule** <12 years: not recommended; ≥12 years: 15 mg q AM prn or 10 mg q 12 hours prn usual max 40 mg/day
    - *Spansule:* 10, 15 mg sust-rel
- ***promethazine*** **(C)(G)** <2 years: not recommended; 2-12 years: 0.5 mg/lb or 6.25-25 mg q 4-6 hours prn; >12 years: 25 mg PO or rectally q 4-6 hours prn
  - **Phenergan** *Tab:* 12.5*, 25*, 50 mg; *Plain syr:* 6.25 mg/5 ml; *Fortis syr:* 25 mg/5 ml; *Rectal supp:* 12.5, 25, 50 mg

SUBSTANCE P/NEUROKININ 1 RECEPTOR ANTAGONIST

- ***aprepitant*** **(B)(G)** <6 months: years: not recommended; ≥6 months: use oral suspension (see mfr pkg insert for dose by weight; >12 years: administer with corticosteroid and 5HT-3 receptor antagonist; *Day 1 of chemotherapy cycle:* 125 mg 1 hour prior to chemotherapy *Day 2 & 3:* 80 mg in the morning
  - **Emend** *Cap:* 40, 80, 125 mg (2 x 80 mg bi-fold pck; 1 x 25 mg/2 x 80 mg tri-fold pck); *Oral susp:* 125 mg pwdr for oral suspension, single-dose pouch w. dispenser; *Vial:* 150 mg pwdr for reconstitution and IV infusion

5HT-3 RECEPTOR ANTAGONISTS

Comment: The selective 5HT-3 receptor antagonists indicated for prevention of nausea and vomiting associated with moderately to highly emetogenic chemotherapy.

▶ ***dolasetron*** **(B)** <2 years: not recommended; 2-16 years: 1.8 mg/kg; >16 years: administer 100 mg IV over 30 seconds, 30 min prior to administration of chemotherapy or 2 hours before surgery; max 100 mg/dose

Anzemet *Tab:* 50, 100 mg; *Amp:* 12.5 mg/0.625 ml; *Prefilled carpuject syringe:* 12.5 mg (0.625 ml); *Vial:* 100 mg/5 ml (single-use); *Vial:* 500 mg/25 ml (multi-dose)

▶ ***granisetron*** <2 years: not recommended; ≥2 years: 10 mcg/kg

Kytril (B) administer IV over 30 seconds, 30 min prior to administration of chemotherapy; max 1 dose/week

Tab: 1 mg; *Oral soln:* 2 mg/10 ml (30 ml; orange); *Vial:* 1 mg/ml (1 ml single-dose) (preservative-free); 1 mg/ml (4 ml multi-dose) (benzyl alcohol)

Sancuso (B) apply 1 patch 24-48 hours before chemo; remove 24 hours (minimum) to 7 days (maximum) after completion of treatment

Transdermal patch: 3.1 mg/day

▶ ***granisetron extended release injection*** <18 years: not recommended; ≥18 years: administer SC over 20-30 seconds (due to drug viscosity) on Day 1 of chemotherapy and not more frequently than once every 7 days; *CrCl 30-59 mL/min:* repeat dose no more than every 14th day; *CrCl <30 mL/min:* not recommended; for patients receiving MEC, the recommended ***dexamethasone*** dosage is 8 mg IV on Day 1; for patients receiving AC combination chemotherapy regimens, the recommended ***dexamethasone*** dosage is 20 mg IV on Day 1, followed by 8 mg PO bid on Days 2, 3 and 4; if **Sustol** is administered with an NK_1 receptor antagonist, see that drug's mfr pkg insert for the recommended ***dexamethasone*** dosing

Sustol *Syringe:* 10 mg/0.4 ml ext-rel; prefilled single-dose/kit

Comment: At least 60 minutes prior to administration, remove the **Sustol** kit from refrigeration; activate a warming pouch and wrap the syringe in the warming pouch for 5-6 minutes to warm it to room temperature.

▶ ***ondansetron*** **(C)(G)** <4 years: not recommended; 4-11 years: *Moderately emetogenic chemotherapy:* 4 mg q 4 hours x 3 doses beginning 30 min prior to start; then 4 mg q 8 hours x 1-2 days following; >11 years: Oral Forms: *Highly emetogenic chemotherapy:* 24 mg x 1 dose 30 min prior to start of single-day chemotherapy; *Moderately emetogenic chemotherapy:* 8 mg q 8 hours x 2 doses beginning 30 minutes prior to start of chemotherapy; then 8 mg q 12 hours x 1-2 days following

Zofran *Tab:* 4, 8, 24 mg

Zofran ODT *ODT:* 4, 8 mg (strawberry) (phenylalanine)

Zofran Oral Solution *Oral soln:* 4 mg/5 ml (50 ml) (strawberry) (phenylalanine); *Parenteral form:* see mfr pkg insert

Zofran Injection *Vial:* 2 mg/ml (2 ml single-dose); 2 mg/ml (20 ml multi-dose); 32 mg/50 ml (50 ml multi-dose); *Prefilled syringe:* 4 mg/2 ml, single-use (24/carton)

Zuplenz Oral Soluble Film: 4, 8 mg orally-disint (10/carton) (peppermint)

▶ ***palonosetron*** **(B)(G)** 1 month: not recommended; 1 month-17 years: 20 mcg/kg; max 1.5 mg single dose; infuse over 15 minutes beginning 30 minutes prior to administration of chemo; >17 years: *Chemotherapy:* administer 0.25 mg IV over 30 seconds, 30 min prior to administration of chemo; max 1 dose/week or 1 cap 1 hour before chemo; *Post-op:* administer 0.075 mg IV over 10 seconds immediately before induction of anesthesia

Aloxi *Vial (single-use):* 0.075 mg/1.5 ml; 0.25 mg/5 ml (mannitol)

CANNABINOIDS

- *dronabinol* **(C)(III)** <18 years: not recommended; ≥18 years: initially 5 mg/m^2 1-3 hours before chemotherapy; then q 2-4 hours prn; max 4-6 doses/day, 15 mg/m^2
  Marinol *Cap:* 2.5, 5, 10 mg (sesame seed oil)
- *nabilone* **(C)(II)** <18 years: not recommended; ≥18 years: 1-2 mg bid; max 6 mg/day in 3 divided doses; initially 1-3 hours before chemotherapy; may give 1-2 mg the night before chemo; may continue 48 hours after each chemo cycle
  Cesamet *Cap:* 1 mg (sesame seed oil)

CHICKENPOX (VARICELLA)

PROPHYLAXIS

- *Varicella virus* vaccine, live, attenuated **(C)**
  Varivax <12 months: not recommended; 12 months-12 years: 1 dose of 0.5 ml SC; repeat 4-6 weeks later; >12 years: 0.5 ml SC; repeat 4-8 weeks later
  Vial: 1350 PFU/0.5 ml single-dose w. diluent (preservative-free)

Comment: Administer **Varivax** SC in the deltoid for all ages.

TREATMENT

Antipyretics *see Fever page* 149

ORAL ANTIPRURITICS

- *diphenhydramine* **(B)(G)** <2 years: not recommended; 2-6 years: 6.25 mg q 4-6 hours; max 37.5 mg/day; >6-12 years: 12.5-25 mg q 4-6 hours; max 150 mg/day; >12 years: 25-50 mg q 6-8 hours; max 100 mg/day
  Benadryl (OTC) *Chew tab:* 12.5 mg (grape) (phenylalanine); *Liq:* 12.5 mg/5 ml (4, 8 oz); *Cap:* 25 mg; *Tab:* 25 mg; *Dye-free soft gel:* 25 mg; *Dye-free liq:* 12.5 mg/5 ml (4, 8 oz)
- *hydroxyzine* **(C)(G)** <6 years: 50 mg/day divided qid; 6-12 years: 50-100 mg/day divided qid; >12 years: 50-100 mg qid; max 600 mg/day
  Atarax *Tab:* 10, 25, 50, 100 mg; *Syr:* 10 mg/5 ml (alcohol 0.5%)
  Vistaril *Cap:* 25, 50, 100 mg; *Oral susp:* 25 mg/5 ml (4 oz) (lemon)

Comment: ***hydroxyzine*** is contraindicated in early pregnancy and in patients with a prolonged QT interval. It is not known whether this drug is excreted in human milk; therefore, ***hydroxyzine*** should not be given to nursing mothers.

PARENTERALRAL ANTIPRURITIC

- *diphenhydramine* injectable **(B)(G)** <12 years: *See mfr pkg insert:* 1.25 mg/kg up to 25 mg IM x 1 dose; then q 6 hours prn; ≥12 years: 25-50 mg IM immediately; then q 6 hours prn
  Benadryl Injectable *Vial:* 50 mg/ml (1 ml single use); 50 mg/ml (10 ml multi-dose); *Amp:* 10 mg/ml (1 ml); *Prefilled syringe:* 50 mg/ml (1 ml)

ANTIVIRALS

- *acyclovir* **(B)(G)** <2 years: not recommended; ≥2 years, <40 kg: 20 mg/kg qid x 5 days;≥2 years, >40 kg: 800 mg qid x 5 days; *see page* 586 *for dose by weight table*
  Zovirax *Cap:* 200 mg; *Tab:* 400, 800 mg
  Zovirax Oral Suspension *Oral susp:* 200 mg/5 ml (banana)

CHIKUNGUNYA VIRUS & CHIKUNGUNYA-RELATED ARTHRITIS

Comment: Acute infection with chikungunya virus is associated with fever, rash, headache, and muscle and joint pain, with outbreaks having been reported in Africa, Asia, the Indian and Pacific Ocean islands, and Europe. In 2013 for the first time the virus was first detected in the Caribbean region, and more than 1.2 million peoples in the Americas have now been infected. After transmission by an *Aedes aegypti* or *Aedes albopictus* mosquito bite, chikungunya virus undergoes local replication and then dissemination to lymphoid tissue," the researchers explained. Viremia is detectable for only 5 to 12 days, but animal studies have indicated that the virus can be found in lymphoid organs, joints, and muscles for several months and that viral RNA can be detected in muscle, liver, and spleen for long periods. But it is not known whether the remnants of the virus actually persist in humans and, if so, whether this can be causatively linked with chronic arthritis, which has implications for treatment. With no evidence of viral persistence, potential mechanisms for arthritis included epigenetic changes to host DNA, as has been observed with Epstein Barr virus infection, modification of macrophages, and molecular mimicry. There is currently no standard treatment for acute chikungunya virus infection or chikungunya-related arthritis, but various immunosuppressants such as ***methotrexate*** and ***hydroxychloroquine*** and biologics such as ***adalimumab*** (**Humira**) and ***etanercept*** (**Enbrel**) have been tried, despite concerns of renewed viral replication in the synovium and relapse of systemic viral infection. However, no relapses have been reported, and the lack of evidence of viral persistence in the joint seen in this analysis may provide some reassurance that treatment with immunosuppressant anti-rheumatic medications 2 years after infection is a viable option.

REFERENCES

Chang, AY, Martins, KAO, Encinales, L, *et al.* (2017). A cross-sectional analysis of chikungunya arthritis patients 22-months post-infection demonstrate no detectable viral persistence in synovial fluid. *Arthritis & Rheumatology*. doi:10.1002/art.40383

Chang, AY, Encinales, L, Porras, A, *et al.* (2017). Frequency of chronic joint pain following chikungunya infection: a colombian cohort study. *Arthritis & Rheumatology*. doi:10.1002/art.40384

CHLAMYDIA TRACHOMATIS

Comment: The following treatment regimens for *C. trachomatis* are published in the **2015 CDC Sexually Transmitted Diseases Treatment Guidelines**. Treatment regimens are presented by generic drug name first, followed by information about brands and dose forms. Treat all sexual contacts. Patients who are HIV-positive should receive the same treatment as those who are HIV-negative. Sexual abuse must be considered a cause of chlamydial infection in preadolescent children, although perinatally transmitted *C. trachomatis* infections of the nasopharynx, urogenital tract, and rectum may persist for >1 year.

RECOMMENDED REGIMENS: ADOLESCENT AND ≥18 YEARS, NON-PREGNANT

Regimen 1

- *azithromycin* 1 gm in a single dose

Regimen 2

- *doxycycline* 100 mg bid x 7 days

ALTERNATIVE REGIMENS: ADOLESCENT AND ≥18 YEARS, NON-PREGNANT

Regimen 1

- ***erythromycin base*** 500 mg qid x 7 days

Regimen 2

- ***erythromycin ethylsuccinate*** 800 mg qid x 7 days

Regimen 3

- ***levofloxacin*** 500 mg once daily x 7 days

Regimen 4

- ***ofloxacin*** 300 mg bid x 7 days

RECOMMENDED REGIMENS: PREGNANCY

Regimen 1

- ***azithromycin*** 1 gm in a single dose

Regimen 2

- ***amoxicillin*** (B)(G) <40 kg (88 lb): 20-40 mg/kg/day in 3 divided doses x 10 days or 25-45 mg/kg/day in 2 divided doses x 10 days; *see page* 588 *for dose by weight table;* ≥40 kg: 500 mg tid x 7 days

ALTERNATE REGIMENS: PREGNANCY

Regimen 1

- ***erythromycin base*** 500 mg qid x 7 days

Regimen 2

- ***erythromycin base*** 250 mg qid x 14 days

Regimen 3

- ***erythromycin ethylsuccinate*** 800 mg qid x 7 days

Regimen 4

- ***erythromycin ethylsuccinate*** 400 mg qid x 14 days

ALTERNATE REGIMENS: CHILDREN ≤8 YEARS

Regimen 1

- ***azithromycin*** 1 gm in a single dose

Regimen 2

- ***doxycycline*** 100 mg bid x 7 days

ALTERNATE REGIMEN: CHILDREN >45 KG; <8 YEARS

Regimen 1

- ***azithromycin*** 1 gm in a single dose

ALTERNATE REGIMENS: INFANTS

Regimen 1

▶ ***erythromycin base*** 50 mg/kg/day in divided doses qid x 14 days

Regimen 2

▶ ***erythromycin ethylsuccinate*** 50 mg/kg/day divided qid x 14 days

DRUG BRANDS AND DOSE FORMS

▶ ***azithromycin*** (B)(G) <12 years: 12 mg/kg/day x 5 days; *see page* 593 *for dose by weight table*; max 500 mg/day; ≥12 years: 500 mg x 1 dose on day 1, then 250 mg daily on days 2-5 or 500 mg daily x 3 days or **Zmax** 2 gm in a single dose

Zithromax *Tab:* 250, 500, 600 mg; *Oral susp:* 100 mg/5 ml (15 ml); 200 mg/5 ml (15, 22.5, 30 ml) (cherry); *Pkt:* 1 gm for reconstitution (cherry-banana)
Zithromax Tri-pak *Tab:* 3 x 500 mg tabs/pck
Zithromax Z-pak *Tab:* 6 x 250 mg tabs/pck
Zmax *Oral susp:* 2 gm ext-rel for reconstitution (cherry-banana) (148 mg Na^+)

▶ ***doxycycline*** (D)(G) <8 years: not recommended; ≥8 years, ≤100 lb: 2 mg/lb on first day in 2 divided doses, followed by 1 mg/lb/day in 1-2 divided doses; ≥8 years, >100 lb: 100 mg bid; *see page* 605 *for dose by weight table*

Acticlate *Tab:* 75, 150**mg
Adoxa *Tab:* 50, 75, 100, 150 mg ent-coat
Doryx *Tab:* 50, 75, 100, 150, 200 mg del-rel
Doxteric *Tab:* 50 mg del-rel
Monodox *Cap:* 50, 75, 100 mg
Oracea *Cap:* 40 mg del-rel
Vibramycin *Tab:* 100 mg; *Cap:* 50, 100 mg; *Syr:* 50 mg/5 ml (raspberry-apple) (sulfites); *Oral susp:* 25 mg/5 ml (raspberry)
Vibra-Tab *Tab:* 100 mg film-coat

Comment: ***doxycycline*** is contraindicated <8 years-of-age, in pregnancy, and lactation (discolors developing tooth enamel). A side effect may be photosensitivity (photophobia). Do not take with antacids, calcium supplements, milk or other dairy, or within 2 hours of taking another drug.

▶ ***erythromycin base*** (B)(G)

Ery-Tab *Tab:* 250, 333, 500 mg ent-coat
PCE *Tab:* 333, 500 mg

▶ ***erythromycin ethylsuccinate*** (B)(G)

EryPed *Oral susp:* 200 mg/5 ml (100, 200 ml) (fruit); 400 mg/5 ml (60, 100, 200 ml) (banana); *Oral drops:* 200, 400 mg/5 ml (50 ml) (fruit); *Chew tab:* 200 gaffer (fruit)
E.E.S. *Oral susp:* 200, 400 mg/5 ml (100 ml) (fruit)
E.E.S. Granules *Oral susp:* 200 mg/5 ml (100, 200 ml) (cherry)
E.E.S. 400 Tablets *Tab:* 400 mg

▶ ***levofloxacin*** (C)

Levaquin *Tab:* 250, 500, 750 mg

Comment: ***levofloxacin*** is contraindicated; <18 years-of-age, and during pregnancy and lactation. Risk of tendonitis or tendon rupture.

▶ ***ofloxacin*** (C)(G)

Floxin *Tab:* 200, 300, 400 mg

Comment: ***ofloxacin*** is contraindicated <18 years-of-age, and during pregnancy and lactation. Risk of tendonitis or tendon rupture.

CHOLANGITIS, PRIMARY BILIARY (PBC)

Comment: Monitor intensity of pruritis and administer antihistamines as appropriate for dermal pruritis. **Ocaliva (*obeticholic acid*)**, a farnesoid X receptor (FXR) agonist, is indicated for the treatment of primary biliary cholangitis (PBC) in combination with ***ursodeoxycholic acid*** (UDCA), in adults with an inadequate response to UDCA, or as monotherapy in adults unable to tolerate UDCA. This indication is approved under accelerated approval based on a reduction in alkaline phosphatase (ALP). An improvement in survival or disease-related symptoms has not been established. Continued approval for this indication may be contingent upon verification and description of clinical benefit in confirmatory trials.

FARNESOID X RECEPTOR (FXR) AGONIST

- ***obeticholic acid*** <18 years: not recommended; ≥18 years: initially 5 mg once daily (this lower starting dose is recommended to reduce pruritis); then after 3 months of treatment, if an adequate reduction in ALP and/or total bilirubin is not achieved, and if the patient is tolerating the drug, increase the dose to 10 mg once daily; take with or without food

  Ocaliva *Tab:* 5, 10 mg

  Comment: **Ocalvia** is contraindicated in patients with complete biliary obstruction. If this complication develops, discontinue **Ocaliva.**

Comment: Because PBC management strategies include bile acid binding resin (e.g., ***cholestyramine***, ***colestipol***, or ***colesevelam***), concurrent use with ***obeticholic acid*** should be separated by at least 4 hours. Concurrent use of ***obeticholic acid*** and ***warfarin*** may reduce the international normalized ratio (INR), monitor INR and adjust the ***warfarin*** dose as necessary. Monitor concentrations of CYP1A2 substrates with a narrow therapeutic index (e.g., ***theophylline*** and ***tizanidine***) as ***obeticholic acid*** a CYP1A2 inhibitor). Reduce the dose of **Ocaliva** in patients with moderate or severe hepatic impairment, and monitor LFTs and lipid levels (especially reduction in HDL).

URSODEOXYCHOLIC ACID (UDCA)

- ***ursodeoxycholic acid*** (UDCA) (G) in the first 3 months of treatment, the total daily dose should be divided tid (morning, midday, evening); as liver function values improve, the total daily dose may be taken once a day at bedtime; (see mfr pkg insert for dose table based on kilograms weight); monitor hepatic function every 4 weeks for the first 3 months; then, monitor hepatic function once every 3 months

  Ursofalk *Tab:* 500 mg film-coat; *Cap:* 250 mg, *Oral susp:* 250 mg/5 ml

Comment: ***ursodeoxycholic acid*** **(UDCA)** is indicated for the dissolution of cholesterol gall stones that are radioluscent (not visible on plain x-ray), ≤15 mm, and the gall bladder must still be functioning despite the gall stones.

BILE ACID BINDING RESINS

Comment: This drug class may produce or severely worsen pre-existing constipation. The dosage should be increased gradually in patients to minimize the risk of developing fecal impaction. Increased fluid and fiber intake should be encouraged to alleviate constipation and a stool softener may occasionally be indicated. If the initial dose is well tolerated, the dose may be increased as needed by one dose/day (at monthly intervals) with periodic monitoring of serum lipoproteins. If constipation worsens or the desired therapeutic response is not achieved at one to six doses/day, combination therapy or alternate therapy should be considered. Bile acid sequestrants may decrease absorption of fat-soluble vitamins. Use caution in patients susceptible to fat-soluble vitamin deficiencies.

▶ *cholestyramine* (C)(G) <12 years: 240 mg/kg/day of anhydrous cholestyramine resin in 2 to 3 divided doses, normally not to exceed 8 gm/day with dose titration based on response and tolerance; ≥12 years: starting dose: 1 packet or 1 scoopful of powder once daily for 5 to 7 days; then, increase to twice daily with monitoring of constipation and of serum lipoproteins, at least twice, 4 to 6 weeks apart; empty one packet into a glass or cup; add 1/2 to 1 cup (4 to 8 ounces) of water, fruit juice, or diet soft drink; stir well and drink immediately; do not swallow dry form; take with meals

Prevalite *Pwdr:* 4 gm/pkt, 4 gm/scoopful (1 level tsp) for oral suspension

▶ *colestipol* (C)(G) <12 years: not established; ≥12 years: Starting dose tabs: 2 gm once or twice daily; then, increases should occur at one or two month intervals; usual dose is 2 to 16 gm/day given once daily or in divided doses

Starting dose granules: 1 packet or 1 scoopful (1 level tsp) of granules once daily for 5 to 7 days, increasing to twice daily with monitoring of constipation and of serum lipoproteins, at least twice, 4 to 6 weeks apart; empty one packet or one scoopful (1 level tsp) of granules into a glass or cup; add 1/2 to 1 cup (4 to 8 ounces) of water, fruit juice, or diet soft drink; stir well and drink immediately; do not swallow dry form; take with meals

Colestid *Tab:* 1 gm; *Granules:* 5 gm/pkt, 5 gm/scoopful (1 level tsp) for oral suspension

Flavored Colestid *Granules:* 5 gm/pkt, 5 gm/scoopful (1 level tsp) for oral suspension (orange)

▶ *colesevelam* (C)(G)

Welchol <12 years: not established; ≥12 years: recommended dose is 6 tablets once daily or 3 tablets twice daily; take with a meal and liquid

Tab: 625 mg

Welchol for Oral Suspension <12 years: not established; ≥12 years: recommended dose is one 3.75 gm packet once daily or one 1.875 gm packet twice daily; empty one packet into a glass or cup; add 1/2 to 1 cup (4 to 8 ounces) of water, fruit juice, or diet soft drink; stir well and drink immediately; do not swallow dry form; take with meals

Pwdr: 3.75 gm/pkt (30 pkt/carton), 1.875 gm/pkt (60 pkt/carton) for oral suspension

CHOLELITHIASIS

▶ ***ursodeoxycholic acid*** (UDCA) **(G)** in the first 3 months of treatment, the total daily dose should be divided tid (morning, midday, evening); as liver function values improve, the total daily dose may be taken once a day at bedtime; (see mfr pkg insert for dose table based on kilograms weight); monitor hepatic function every 4 weeks for the first 3 months; then, monitor hepatic function once every 3 months

Ursofalk *Tab:* 500 mg film-coat; *Cap:* 250 mg, *Oral susp:* 250 mg/5 ml

Comment: ***ursodeoxycholic*** **(UDCA)** is indicated for the dissolution of cholesterol gall stones that are radioluscent (not visible on plain x-ray), ≤15 mm, and the gall bladder must still be functioning despite the gall stones

▶ ***ursodiol*** **(B)** <12 years: not recommended; ≥12 years: 8-10 mg/kg/day in 2-3 divided doses

Actigall *Cap:* 300 mg

Comment: **Actigall** is indicated for the dissolution of radiolucent, noncalciferous, gallstones <20 mm in diameter and for prevention of gallstones during rapid weight loss.

BILE ACID BINDING RESINS

Comment: This drug class may produce or severely worsen pre-existing constipation. The dosage should be increased gradually in patients to minimize the risk of developing fecal impaction. Increased fluid and fiber intake should be encouraged to alleviate constipation and a stool softener may occasionally be indicated. If the initial dose is well tolerated, the dose may be increased as needed by one dose/day (at monthly intervals) with periodic monitoring of serum lipoproteins. If constipation worsens or the desired therapeutic response is not achieved at one to six doses/day, combination therapy or alternate therapy should be considered. Bile acid sequestrants may decrease absorption of fat-soluble vitamins. Use caution in patients susceptible to fat-soluble vitamin deficiencies.

▶ ***cholestyramine*** (C)(G) <12 years: 240 mg/kg/day of anhydrous cholestyramine resin in 2 to 3 divided doses, normally not to exceed 8 gm/day with dose titration based on response and tolerance; ≥12 years: starting dose: 1 packet or 1 scoopful of powder once daily for 5 to 7 days; then, increase to twice daily with monitoring of constipation and of serum lipoproteins, at least twice, 4 to 6 weeks apart; empty one packet into a glass or cup; add 1/2 to 1 cup (4 to 8 ounces) of water, fruit juice, or diet soft drink; stir well and drink immediately; do not swallow dry form; take with meals

Prevalite *Pwdr:* 4 gm/pkt, 4 gm/scoopful (1 level tsp) for oral suspension

▶ ***colestipol*** (C)(G) <12 years: not established; ≥12 years: Starting dose tabs: 2 grams once or twice daily; then, increases should occur at one or two month intervals; usual dose is 2 to 16 grams/day given once daily or in divided doses

Starting dose granules: 1 packet or 1 scoopful (1 level tsp) of granules once daily for 5 to 7 days, increasing to twice daily with monitoring of constipation and of serum lipoproteins, at least twice, 4 to 6 weeks apart; empty one packet or one scoopful (1 level tsp) of granules into a glass or cup; add 1/2 to 1 cup (4 to 8 ounces) of water, fruit juice, or diet soft drink; stir well and drink immediately; do not swallow dry form; take with meals

Colestid *Tab:* 1 gm; *Granules:* 5 gm/pkt, 5 gm/scoopful (1 level tsp) for oral suspension

Flavored Colestid *Granules:* 5 gm/pkt, 5 gm/scoopful (1 level tsp) for oral suspension (orange)

▶ ***colesevelam*** (C)(G) <12 years: not recommended; ≥12 years: *s*

Welchol recommended dose is 6 tablets once daily or 3 tablets twice daily; take with a meal and liquid

Tab: 625 mg

Welchol for Oral Suspension <12 years: not established; ≥12 years: recommended dose is one 3.75 gm packet once daily or one 1.875 gm packet twice daily; empty one packet into a glass or cup; add 1/2 to 1 cup (4 to 8 ounces) of water, fruit juice, or diet soft drink; stir well and drink immediately; do not swallow dry form; take with meals

Pwdr: 3.75 gm/pkt (30 pkt/carton), 1.875 gm/pkt (60 pkt/carton) for oral suspension

CHOLERA (*VIBRIO CHOLERAE*)

Comment: June 10, 2016, the FDA approved the first vaccine for the prevention of cholera caused by serogroup O1 (the most predominant cause of cholera globally [WHO]) in patients aged 18-64 years traveling to cholera-affected areas (https://www.drugs.com/newdrugs/fda-approves-vaxchora-cholera-vaccine-live-oral-prevent-cholera-travelers-4396.html). **Vaxchora** (R) is the only FDA-approved vaccine for the prevention of cholera. The bacterium *Vibrio cholerae* is acquired by ingesting contaminated water or food and causes nausea, vomiting, and watery diarrhea that may be mild to severe. Profuse fluid loss may cause life-threatening dehydration if antibiotics and fluid replacement are not initiated promptly.

VACCINE PROPHYLAXIS

▶ ***Vibrio cholerae*** vaccine

Vaxchora reconstitute the buffer component in 100 ml purified bottled water; then add the active component (lyophilized *V. cholerae* CVD 103-HgR); total dose after reconstitution is 100 ml; instruct the patient to avoid eating or drinking fluids for 60 minutes before and after ingestion of the dose

Comment: **Vaxchora** is a live, attenuated vaccine that is taken as a single oral dose at least 10 days before travel to a cholera-affected area and at least 10 days before starting antimalarial prophylaxis. Diminished immune response occurs when taken concomitantly with ***chloroquine***. Avoid concomitant administration with systemic antibiotics since these agents may be active against the vaccine strain. Do not administer to patients who have received an oral or parental antibiotic within 14 days prior to vaccination. **Vaxchora** may be shed in the stool of recipients for at least 7 days. There is potential for transmission of the vaccine strain to non-vaccinated and immunocompromised close contacts. The Centers for Disease Control and Prevention and several health professional organizations state that vaccines given to a nursing mother do not affect the safety of breastfeeding for mothers or infants and that breastfeeding is not a contraindication to cholera vaccine. **Vaxchora** is not absorbed systemically, and maternal use is not expected to result in fetal exposure to the drug. The **Vaxchora** pregnancy exposure registry for reporting adverse events is 1-800-533-5899. There are 0 disease interactions, but at least 165 drug-drug interactions with **Vaxchora** (see mfr pkg insert).

TREATMENT

Comment: The first-line treatment for *V. cholerae* is oral rehydration therapy (ORT) and intravenous fluid replacement as indicated. Antibiotic therapy may shorten the duration and severity of symptoms, but is optional in other than severe cases. Although ***doxycycline*** is contraindicated in pregnancy and in children <8 years-of-age, the benefits may outweigh the risks (WHO, CDC, UNICEF). Although ***ciprofloxacin*** is contraindicated in children <18 years-of-age, the benefits may outweigh the risks (WHO, CDC, UNICEF). Cholera is not transmitted from person to person, but rather the fecal-oral route. Therefore, chemoprophylaxis is not usually required with strict hand hygiene and sanitation measures, and avoidance of contaminated food and water. Drugs and dosages for chemoprophylaxis are the same as for treatment.

NON-PREGNANT FEMALES ≤15 YEARS-OF-AGE

Regimen 1

▶ ***doxycycline*** (D)(G) 300 mg in a single dose

Acticlate *Tab:* 75, 150**mg
Adoxa *Tab:* 50, 75, 100, 150 mg ent-coat
Doryx *Tab:* 50, 75, 100, 150, 200 mg del-rel
Doxteric *Tab:* 50 mg del-rel
Monodox *Cap:* 50, 75, 100 mg
Oracea *Cap:* 40 mg del-rel
Vibramycin *Tab:* 100 mg; *Cap:* 50, 100 mg; *Syr:* 50 mg/5 ml (raspberry-apple) (sulfites); *Oral susp:* 25 mg/5 ml (raspberry)
Vibra-Tab *Tab:* 100 mg film-coat

Comment: ***doxycycline*** is contraindicated <8 years-of-age, in pregnancy, and lactation (discolors developing tooth enamel). A side effect may be photosensitivity (photophobia). Do not take with antacids, calcium supplements, milk or other dairy, or within 2 hours of taking another drug.

Regimen 2

▶ ***azithromycin*** (B) 1000 mg in a single dose
  Zithromax *Tab:* 250, 500, 600 mg
  Zmax *Oral susp:* 2 gm ext-rel for reconstitution (cherry-banana) (148 mg Na^+)
  or
▶ ***ciprofloxacin*** (C) 1000 mg in a single dose
  Cipro (G) *Tab:* 250, 500, 750 mg; *Oral susp:* 250, 500 mg/5 ml (100 ml) (strawberry)
  Cipro XR *Tab:* 500, 1000 mg ext-rel
  ProQuin XR *Tab:* 500 mg ext-rel

PREGNANT FEMALES ≥15 YEARS-OF-AGE

▶ ***azithromycin*** (B) 1,000 mg in a single dose
  Zithromax *Tab:* 250, 500, 600 mg
  Zmax *Oral susp:* 2 gm ext-rel for reconstitution (cherry-banana) (148 mg Na^+)
  or
▶ ***erythromycin*** (B)(G) 500 mg q 6 hours x 3 days
  E.E.S. 400 Tablets *Tab:* 400 mg
  Ery-Tab *Tab:* 250, 333, 500 mg ent-coat
  PCE *Tab:* 333, 500 mg

CHILDREN 3-15 YEARS-OF-AGE WHO CAN SWALLOW TABLETS

Regimen 1

▶ ***erythromycin*** (B)(G) 12.5 mg/kg q 6 hours x 3 days
  E.E.S. 400 Tablets *Tab:* 400 mg
  Ery-Tab *Tab:* 250, 333, 500 mg ent-coat
  PCE *Tab:* 333, 500 mg
  or
▶ ***azithromycin*** (B) 20 mg/kg in a single dose; max 1 gm
  Zithromax *Tab:* 250, 500, 600 mg; *Oral susp:* 100 mg/5 ml (15 ml); 200 mg/5 ml (15, 22.5, 30 ml) (cherry)
  Zmax *Oral susp:* 2 gm ext-rel for reconstitution (cherry-banana) (148 mg Na^+)

Regimen 2

▶ ***ciprofloxacin*** (D) <18 years usually not recommended; ***erythromycin*** or ***azithromycin*** preferred; consider risk benefit; 20 mg/kg in a single dose
  Cipro (G) *Tab:* 250, 500, 750 mg; *Oral susp:* 250, 500 mg/5 ml (100 ml) (strawberry)
  Cipro XR *Tab:* 500, 1000 mg ext-rel
  ProQuin XR *Tab:* 500 mg ext-rel
  or
▶ ***doxycycline*** (D)(G) <8 years usually not recommended; ***erythromycin*** or ***azithromycin*** preferred; consider risk benefit; >8 years: 2-4 mg/kg in a single dose
  Acticlate *Tab:* 75, 150**mg
  Adoxa *Tab:* 50, 75, 100, 150 mg ent-coat
  Doryx *Tab:* 50, 75, 100, 150, 200 mg del-rel

Doxteric *Tab:* 50 mg del-rel
Monodox *Cap:* 50, 75, 100 mg
Oracea *Cap:* 40 mg del-rel
Vibramycin *Tab:* 100 mg; *Cap:* 50, 100 mg; *Syr:* 50 mg/5 ml (raspberry-apple) (sulfites); *Oral susp:* 25 mg/5 ml (raspberry)
Vibra-Tab *Tab:* 100 mg film-coat

CHILDREN <3 YEARS-OF-AGE

Regimen 1

▶ ***erythromycin ethylsuccinate*** (B)(G) 12.5 mg/kg q 6 hours x 3 days; use suspension
E.E.S. *Oral susp:* 200, 400 mg/5 ml (100 ml) (fruit)
E.E.S. Granules *Oral susp:* 200 mg/5 ml (100, 200 ml) (cherry, fruit); *Chew tab* 200 mg wafer (fruit)
EryPed *Oral susp:* 200 mg/5 ml (100, 200 ml) (fruit); 400 mg/5 ml (60, 100, 200 ml) (banana); *Oral drops:* 200, 400 mg/5 ml (50 ml) (fruit); *Chew tab:* 200 mg wafer (fruit)

or

▶ ***azithromycin*** (B)(G) 20 mg/kg in a single dose; max 1 gm; use suspension
Zithromax *Tab:* 250, 500, 600 mg; *Oral susp:* 100 mg/5 ml (15 ml); 200 mg/5 ml(15, 22.5, 30 ml) (cherry)
Zmax *Oral susp:* 2 gm ext-rel for reconstitution (cherry-banana) (148 mg Na^+)

Regimen 2

▶ ***ciprofloxacin*** (C) <18 years usually not recommended; ***erythromycin*** or ***azithromycin*** preferred; consider risk benefit; 20 mg/kg in a single dose; use suspension
Cipro (G) *Oral susp:* 250, 500 mg/5 ml (100 ml) (strawberry)

or

▶ ***doxycycline*** (D)(G) <18 years usually not recommended; ***erythromycin*** or ***azithromycin*** preferred; consider risk/benefit; 2-4 mg/kg in a single dose; use suspension or syrup
Vibramycin *Syr:* 50 mg/5 ml (raspberry-apple) (sulfites); *Oral susp:* 25 mg/5 ml (raspberry)

☐ *CLOSTRIDIUM DIFFICILE*

Comment: Acid-suppressing drugs including proton pump inhibitors (PPIs), third- and fourth-generation cephalosporins, carbapenems, and ***piperacillin-tazobactam*** significantly increase the risk of hospital-onset *C. difficile* infection (CDI), according to the results of a recent study. Patients who received tetracyclines, macrolides, or ***clindamycin*** had lower risk of developing hospital-onset CDI.

REFERENCE

Watson, T, Hickok, J, Fraker, S, *et al.* (2017). Evaluating the risk factors for hospital-onset Clostridium difficile infections in a large healthcare system. *Clinical Infectious Diseases.* doi:10.1093/cid/cix1112

HUMAN IGG1 MONOCLONAL ANTIBODY

Comment: ***bezlotoxumab*** is a human IgG1 monoclonal antibody that inhibits the binding of *C. difficile* toxin B, preventing its effects on mammalian cells. ***bezlotoxumab*** does not bind to *C. difficile* toxin A. ***bezlotoxumab*** is indicated to reduce the recurrence of CDI in patients who are receiving antibacterial drug treatment of CDI and are at high risk for CDI recurrence. CDI recurrence is defined as a new episode of diarrhea associated with a positive stool test for toxigenic *C. difficile* following a clinical cure of the presenting CDI episode. It is not indicated for the primary treatment of CDI infection. It is to be used only in conjunction with appropriate primary drug treatment of CDI. Patients at high risk for CDI recurrence, studied in clinical trials establishing efficacy, include those ≥65 years-of-age, with a history of CDI in the previous 6 months, immunocompromised state, severe CDI at presentation, and *C. difficile* ribotype 027.

▶ ***bezlotoxumab*** (C) <18 years: not established; ≥18 years: administer a single dose of 10 mg/kg via IV infusion over 60 minutes
  Zinplava *Vial:* 40 ml single-use solution

GLYCOPEPTIDE ANTIBACTERIAL AGENT

Comment: **Firvanq** (***vancomycin*** oral solution) is a glycopeptide antibacterial agent FDA approved to treat *C. difficile*-associated diarrhea (CDAD) and entercolitis caused by *Staphylococcus aureus*, including methicillin-resistant strains (MRSA). **Firvanq** should be used only to treat or prevent infections that are proven or strongly suspected to be caused by susceptible bacteria. Orally administered ***vancomycin hcl*** is not effective for treatment of other types of infections. Prescribing **Firvanq** in the absence of a proven or strongly suspected bacterial infection is unlikely to provide benefit to the patient and increases the risk of the development of drug-resistant bacteria.

▶ ***vancomycin hcl oral solution*** see mfr pkg insert for preparation and important administration information; <18 years: CDAD and *Staphylococcal enterocolitis:* 40 mg/kg orally in 3 or 4 divided doses x 7-10 days; total daily dosage max 2 gm; ≥18 years: *CDAD* 125 mg orally 4 x/day x 10 days; *Staphylococcal enterocolitis:* 500 mg to 2 gm orally in 3 or 4 divided doses x 7-10 days
  Firvanq *Kit w. pwdr for oral soln:* 25, 50 mg/ml (150, 300 ml) equivalent to 3.75, 7.5, 10.5, or 15 gm ***vancomycin hcl***, and grape-flavored diluent
  Comment: Nephrotoxicity has occurred following oral ***vancomycin hcl*** therapy and can occur either during or after completion of therapy. The risk is increased in geriatric patients. Monitor renal function. Ototoxicity has occurred in patients receiving ***vancomycin hcl***. Assessment of auditory function may be appropriate in some instances. The most common adverse reactions (≥10%) have been nausea (17%), abdominal pain (15%) and hypokalemia (13%). There are no available data on **Firvanq** use in pregnant women to inform a drug associated risk of major birth defects or miscarriage. Available published data on vancomycin use in pregnancy during the second and third trimesters have not shown an association with adverse pregnancy related outcomes. There are insufficient data to inform the levels of ***vancomycin hcl*** in human milk. However, systemic absorption of ***vancomycin hcl*** following oral administration is expected to be minimal. There are no data on the effects of **Firvanq** on the breastfed infant.

COLIC: INFANTILE

▶ ***hyoscyamine*** (C)(G) 3-4 kg: 4 drops q 4 hours prn; max 24 drops/day; 5 kg: 5 drops q 4 hours prn; max 30 drops/day; 7 kg: 6 drops q 4 hours prn; max 36 drops/day; 10 kg: 8 drops q 4 hours prn; max 40 drops/day
  Levsin Drops *Oral drops:* 0.125 mg/ml (15 ml) (orange) (alcohol 5%)

▶ ***simethicone*** (C) 0.3 ml qid pc and HS
  Mylicon Drops (OTC) *Oral drops:* 40 mg/0.6 ml (30 ml)

COLONOSCOPY PREP/COLON CLEANSE

▶ ***sodium picosulfate+magnesium oxide+citric acid*** <18 years: not recommended; ≥18 years: reconstitute pwdr with cold water right before use; two dosing regimen options—each requires two separate dosing times; *Split Dose Method* (preferred): 1st dose during evening before the colonoscopy and 2nd dose the next day during the morning prior to the colonoscopy; *Day Before Method* (alternative, if split dose is not appropriate): 1st dose during afternoon or early evening before the colonoscopy and 2nd dose 6 hours later during evening before colonoscopy; additional clear liquids (no solid food or milk) must be consumed after every dose in both dosing regimens

Pediatric: <18 years: not recommended; ≥18 years: same as adult

Prepopik *Pwdr:* sod picos 10 mg+mag oxide 3.5 gm+anhy cit acid 12 gm/pkt pwdr for oral solution (2 pkts)

Comment: **Prepopik** is a combination of sodium picosulfate, a stimulant laxative, and magnesium oxide and anhydrous citric acid which form magnesium citrate, an osmotic laxative, indicated for cleansing of the colon as a preparation for colonoscopy in adults. Rule out diagnosis of suspected GI obstruction or perforation diagnosis before administration. **Prepopik** should be used during pregnancy only if clearly needed. **Prepopik** is contraindicated with severely reduced renal function (CrCl< 30 mL/min), GI obstruction or ileus, bowel perforation, toxic colitis or toxic megacolon, and gastric retention for any reason.

COMMON COLD (VIRAL UPPER RESPIRATORY INFECTION [URI])

Drugs for the Management of Allergy, Cough, and Cold *see page* 570
Oral Antipyretic-Analgesics *see **Fever** page* 149

NASAL SALINE DROPS & SPRAYS

▶ ***saline*** nasal spray (G)

Afrin Saline Mist w. Eucalyptol and Menthol (OTC) 1 month-2 years: 1-2 sprays in each nostril prn; >2-12 years: 1-4 sprays in each nostril prn; >12 years: 2-6 sprays in each nostril

Squeeze bottle: 45 ml

Afrin Moisturizing Saline Mist (OTC) 1 month-2 years: 1-2 sprays in each nostril prn; >2-12 years: 1-4 sprays in each nostril prn; >12 years: 2-6 sprays in each nostril prn

Squeeze bottle: 45 ml

Ocean Mist (OTC) 1 month-2 years: 1-2 sprays in each nostril prn; >2-12 years: 1-4 sprays in each nostril prn; >12 years: 2-6 sprays in each nostril prn

Squeeze bottle: saline 0.65% (45 ml) (alcohol-free)

Pediamist (OTC) 1 month-2 years: 1-2 sprays in each nostril prn; >2-12 years: 1-4 sprays in each nostril prn; >12 years: 2-6 sprays in each nostril prn

Squeeze bottle: saline 0.5% (15 ml) (alcohol-free)

NASAL SYMPATHOMIMETICS

▶ ***oxymetazoline*** (C)(OTC) <6 years: not recommended; 6-12 years: use 4-hour formulation; 2-3 drops or sprays q 4 hours prn; max duration 5 days; >12 years: may use 12-hour formulation; 2-3 drops or sprays in each nostril q 10-12 hours prn; max 2 doses/day; max duration 5 days

Afrin 12-Hour Extra Moisturizing Nasal Spray
Afrin 12-Hour Nasal spray Pump Mist

Afrin 12-Hour Original Nasal spray
Afrin 12-Hour Original Nose Drops
Afrin 12-Hour Severe Congestion Nasal Spray
Afrin 12-Hour Sinus Nasal Spray
Nasal spray: 0.05% (45 ml); *Nasal drops:* 0.05% (45 ml)
Afrin 4-Hour Nasal Spray
Neo-Synephrine 12 Hour Nasal Spray
Neo-Synephrine 12 Hour Extra Moisturizing Nasal Spray
Nasal spray: 0.05% (15 ml)

➢ ***phenylephrine*** (C)
Afrin Allergy Nasal Spray (OTC) <12 years: not recommended; ≥12 years: 2-3 sprays in each nostril q 4 hours prn; max duration 5 days
Nasal spray: 0.5% (15 ml)
Afrin Nasal Decongestant Children's Pump Mist (OTC) <6 years: not recommended; ≥6 years: 2-3 sprays in each nostril q 4 hours prn; max duration 5 days
Nasal spray: 0.25% (15 ml)
Neo-Synephrine Extra Strength (OTC) <12 years: not recommended; ≥12 years: 2-3 sprays or drops in each nostril q 4 hours prn; max duration 5 days
Nasal spray: 0.1% (15 ml); *Nasal drops:* 0.1% (15 ml)
Neo-Synephrine Mild Formula (OTC) <6 years: not recommended; ≥6 years: 2-3 sprays or drops in each nostril q 4 hours prn; max duration 5 days
Nasal spray: 0.25% (15 ml)
Neo-Synephrine Regular Strength (OTC) <12 years: not recommended; ≥12 years: 2-3 sprays or drops in each nostril q 4 hours prn; max duration 5 days
Nasal spray: 0.5% (15 ml); *Nasal drops:* 0.5% (15 ml)

➢ ***tetrahydrozoline*** (C)
Tyzine <6 years: not recommended; ≥6 years: 2-4 drops or 3-4 sprays in each nostril q 3-8 hours prn; max duration 5 days
Nasal spray: 0.1% (15 ml); *Nasal drops:* 0.1% (30 ml)
Tyzine Pediatric Nasal Drops 2-3 sprays or drops in each nostril q 3-6 hours prn
Nasal drops: 0.05% (15 ml)

CONJUNCTIVITIS: ALLERGIC

Oral Antihistamines *see* **Drugs for the Management of Allergy, Cough, and Cold Symptoms** *page* 570

OPHTHALMIC CORTICOSTEROIDS

Comment: Concomitant contact lens wear is contraindicated during therapy. Ophthalmic steroids are contraindicated with ocular, fungal, mycobacterial, viral (except herpes zoster), and untreated bacterial infection. Ophthalmic steroids may mask or exacerbate infection, and may increase intraocular pressure, optic nerve damage, cataract formation, or corneal perforation. Limit ophthalmic steroid use to 2-3 days if possible; usual max 2 weeks. With prolonged or frequent use, there is risk of corneal and scleral thinning and cataract formation.

➢ ***dexamethasone*** (C) <12 years: not recommended; ≥12 years: initially 1-2 drops hourly during the day and q 2 hours at night; then prolong dosing interval to 4-6 hours as condition improves
Maxidex *Ophth susp:* 0.1% (5, 15 ml) (benzalkonium chloride)

▶ ***dexamethasone phosphate*** (C) <12 years: not recommended; ≥12 years: initially 1-2 drops hourly during the day and q 2 hours at night; then 1 drop q 4-8 hours or more as condition improves

Decadron *Ophth soln:* 0.1% (5 ml) (sulfites)

▶ ***fluorometholone*** (C) <12 years: not recommended; ≥12 years: 1 drop bid-qid or 1/2 inch of ointment once daily-tid; may increase dose frequency during initial 24-48 hours

FML *Ophth susp:* 0.1% (5, 10, 15 ml) (benzalkonium chloride)
FML Forte *Ophth susp:* 0.25% (5, 10, 15 ml) (benzalkonium chloride)
FML S.O.P. Ointment *Ophth oint:* 0.1% (3.5 gm)

▶ ***fluorometholone acetate*** (C) <12 years: not recommended; ≥12 years: initially 2 drops q 2 hours during the first 24-48 hours; then 1-2 drops qid as condition improves

Flarex *Ophth susp:* 0.1% (2.5, 5 10 ml) (benzalkonium chloride)

▶ ***loteprednol etabonate*** (C)

Alrex <12 years: not recommended; ≥12 years: 1 drop qid
Ophth susp: 0.2% (5, 10 ml) (benzalkonium chloride)
Lotemax <12 years: not recommended; ≥12 years: 1-2 drops qid
Ophth susp: 0.5% (5, 10, 15 ml) (benzalkonium chloride)

▶ ***medrysone*** (C) <12 years: not recommended; ≥12 years: 1 drop up to q 4 hours

HMS *Ophth susp:* 1% (5, 10 ml) (benzalkonium chloride)

▶ ***rimexolone*** (C) <12 years: not recommended; ≥12 years: initially 1-2 drops hourly while awake x 1 week; then 1 drop q 2 hours while awake x 1 week; then taper as condition improves

Vexol *Ophth susp:* 0.1% (5, 10 ml) (benzalkonium chloride)

▶ ***prednisolone acetate*** (C)(G)

Econopred <12 years: not recommended; ≥12 years: 2 drops qid
Ophth susp: 0.125% (5, 10 ml)
Econopred Plus <12 years: not recommended; ≥12 years: 2 drops qid
Ophth susp: 1% (5, 10 ml)
Pred Forte <12 years: not recommended; ≥12 years: initially 2 drops hourly x 24-48 hours; then 1-2 drops bid-qid
Ophth susp: 1% (1, 5, 10, 15 ml) (benzalkonium chloride, sulfites)
Pred Mild <12 years: not recommended; ≥12 years: initially 2 drops hourly x 24-48 hours; then 1-2 drops bid-qid
Ophth susp: 0.12% (5, 10 ml) (benzalkonium chloride)

▶ ***prednisolone sodium phosphate*** (C) <12 years: not recommended; ≥12 years: initially 1-2 drops hourly during the day and q 2 hours at night; then 1 drop q 4 hours; then 1 drop tid-qid as condition improves

Inflamase Forte *Ophth soln:* 1% (5, 10, 15 ml) (benzalkonium chloride)
Inflamase Mild *Ophth soln:* 1/8% (5, 10 ml) (benzalkonium chloride)

OPHTHALMIC H1 ANTAGONISTS (ANTIHISTAMINES)

Comment: May insert contact lens 10 minutes after administration of ophthalmic antihistamine.

▶ ***emedastine*** (C) <3 years: not recommended; ≥3 years: 1 drop qid prn

Emadine *Ophth soln:* 0.05% (5 ml) (benzalkonium chloride)

▶ ***levocabastine*** (C) <12 years: not recommended; ≥12 years: 1 drop qid prn

Livostin *Ophth susp:* 0.05% (2.5, 5, 10 ml) (benzalkonium chloride)

▶ ***cetirizine*** (C) <2 years: not established; ≥2 years: 1 drop bid prn

Zerviate Ophthalmic *Ophth soln:* 0.24%/ml (5 ml [7.5 ml bottle]; 7.5 ml [10 ml bottle])

OPHTHALMIC MAST CELL STABILIZERS

Comment: Concomitant contact lens wear is contraindicated during treatment.

- ***cromolyn sodium*** **(B)** <4 years: not recommended; ≥4 years: 1-2 drops 4-6 x/day at regular intervals
  - **Crolom** *Ophth soln:* 4% (10 ml) (benzalkonium chloride)
- ***lodoxamide tromethamine*** **(B)** <2 years: not recommended; ≥2 years: 1-2 drops qid up to 3 months
  - **Alomide** *Ophth soln:* 1% (10 ml) (benzalkonium chloride)
- ***nedocromil*** **(B)** <3 years: not recommended; ≥3 years: 1-2 drops bid
  - **Alocril** *Ophth soln:* 2% (5 ml) (benzalkonium chloride)
- ***pemirolast potassium*** **(C)** 3 years: not recommended; ≥3 years: 1-2 drops qid
  - **Alamast** *Ophth soln:* 0.1% (10 ml) (lauralkonium chloride)

OPHTHALMIC ANTIHISTAMINE+MAST CELL STABILIZER COMBINATIONS

- ***alcaftadine*** **(B)** <2 years: not recommended; ≥2 years: 1 drop each eye daily
  - **Lastacaft** *Ophth soln:* 0.25% (6 ml) (benzalkonium chloride)

  Comment: May insert contact lens 10 minutes after ophthalmic administration.
- ***azelastine*** **(C)** <3 years: not recommended; ≥3 years: 1 drop each eye bid
  - **Optivar** *Ophth soln:* 0.05% (6 ml) (benzalkonium chloride)

  Comment: May insert contact lens 10 minutes after ophthalmic administration.
- ***bepotastine besilate*** **(C)** <2 years: not recommended; ≥2 years: 1 drop each eye bid
  - **Bepreve** *Ophth soln:* 1.5% (10 ml) (benzalkonium chloride)

  Comment: May insert contact lens 10 minutes after ophthalmic administration.
- ***epinastine*** **(C)(G)** <3 years: not recommended; ≥3 years: 1 drop each eye bid
  - **Elestat** *Ophth soln:* 0.05% (5 ml) (benzalkonium chloride)
- ***ketotifen fumarate*** **(C)** <3 years: not recommended; ≥3 years: 1 drop each eye q 8-12 hours
  - **Alaway (OTC)** *Ophth soln:* 0.025% (10 ml) (benzalkonium chloride)
  - **Claritin Eye (OTC)** *Ophth soln:* 0.025% (5 ml) (benzalkonium chloride)
  - **Refresh Eye Itch Relief (OTC)** *Ophth soln:* 0.025% (5 ml) (benzalkonium chloride)
  - **Zaditor (OTC)** *Ophth soln:* 0.025% (5 ml) (benzalkonium chloride)
  - **Zyrtec Itchy Eye (OTC)** *Ophth soln:* 0.025% (5 ml) (benzalkonium chloride)
- ***olopatadine*** **(C)** <3 years: not recommended; ≥3 years: 1 drop each eye bid
  - **Pataday (G)** *Ophth soln:* 0.2% (2.5 ml) (benzalkonium chloride)
  - **Patanol (G)** *Ophth soln:* 0.1% (5 ml) (benzalkonium chloride)
  - **Pazeo** *Ophth soln:* 0.7% (2.5 ml) (benzalkonium chloride)

  Comment: May insert contact lens 10 minutes after administration.

OPHTHALMIC VASOCONSTRICTORS

Comment: Concomitant contact lens wear is contraindicated during treatment.

- ***naphazoline*** **(C)** <12 years: not recommended; ≥12 years: 1-2 drops each eye qid prn
  - **Vasocon-A** *Ophth soln:* 0.1% (15 ml) (benzalkonium chloride)
- ***oxymetazoline*** **(OTC)** <6 years: not recommended; ≥6 years: 1-2 drops each eye qid prn
  - **Visine L-R** *Ophth soln:* 0.025% (15, 30 ml)
- ***tetrahydrozoline*** **(OTC)(G)** <6 years: not recommended; ≥6 years: 1-2 drops each eye qid prn
  - **Visine** *Ophth soln:* 0.05% (15, 22.5, 30 ml)

OPHTHALMIC VASOCONSTRICTOR+MOISTURIZER COMBINATION

Comment: Concomitant contact lens wear is contraindicated during treatment.

▶ ***tetrahydrozoline+polyethylene glycol 400+povidone+dextran 70*** (OTC) <6 years: not recommended; ≥6 years: 1-2 drops each eye qid prn

Advanced Relief Visine *Ophth soln:* tetra 0.025%+poly 1%+pov 1%+dex 0.1% (15, 30 ml)

OPHTHALMIC VASOCONSTRICTOR+ASTRINGENT COMBINATION

Comment: Concomitant contact lens wear is contraindicated during treatment.

▶ ***tetrahydrozoline+zinc sulfate*** (OTC) <6 years: not recommended; ≥6 years: 1-2 drops each eye qid prn

Visine AC *Ophth soln:* tetra 0.025%+zinc 0.05% (15, 30 ml)

OPHTHALMIC VASOCONSTRICTOR+ANTIHISTAMINE COMBINATIONS

Comment: Concomitant contact lens wear is contraindicated during treatment.

▶ ***naphazoline+pheniramine*** (C) <6 years: not recommended; ≥6 years: 1-2 drops each eye qid

Naphcon-A (OTC) *Ophth soln:* naph 0.025%+phen 0.3% (15 ml) (benzalkonium chloride)

OPHTHALMIC NSAIDs

Comment: Concomitant contact lens wear is contraindicated during treatment.

▶ ***bromfenac*** (C)(G) 1 drop affected eye(s) bid

Bromday Ophthalmic Solution *Ophth soln:* 0.09% (2.5 ml in 7.5 ml dropper bottle; 7.5 ml in 10 ml dropper bottle,)

Xibrom Ophthalmic Solution *Ophth soln:* 0.09% (2.5 ml in 7.5 ml dropper bottle; 7.5 ml in 10 ml dropper bottle)

▶ ***diclofenac sodium*** (B) <12 years: not recommended; ≥12 years: 1 drop affected eye(s) qid

Voltaren Ophthalmic Solution *Ophth soln:* 0.1% (2.5, 5 ml)

▶ ***ketorolac tromethamine*** (C) <3 years: not recommended; ≥3 years: 1 drop affected eye(s) qid; max x 4 days

Acular *Ophth soln:* 0.5% (3, 5, 10 ml) (benzalkonium chloride)

Acular LS *Ophth soln:* 0.4% (5 ml) (benzalkonium chloride)

Acular PF *Ophth soln:* 0.5% (0.4 ml; 12 single-use vials/carton) (preservative-free)

▶ ***nepafenac*** (C) <10 years: not recommended; ≥10 years: 1 drop affected eye(s) tid

Nevanac Ophthalmic Suspension *Ophth susp:* 0.1% (3 ml) (benzalkonium chloride)

CONJUNCTIVITIS & BLEPHAROCONJUNCTIVITIS: BACTERIAL

OPHTHALMIC ANTI-INFECTIVES

▶ ***azithromycin*** ophthalmic solution (B)(G) <1 year: not recommended; ≥1 year: 1 drop to affected eye(s) bid x 2 days; then 1 drop once daily for the next 5 days

AzaSite Ophthalmic Solution *Ophth susp:* 1% (2.5 ml) (benzalkonium chloride)

▶ ***bacitracin*** ophthalmic ointment (C)(G) apply 1/2 inch ribbon to the lower conjunctival sac of affected eye(s) 1-3 x daily x 7 days

Bacitracin Ophthalmic Ointment *Ophth oint:* 500 units/gm (3.5 gm)

▶ ***besifloxacin*** ophthalmic solution (C) <1 year: not recommended; ≥1 year: 1 drop to affected eye(s) tid x 7 days

Besivance Ophthalmic Solution *Ophth susp:* 0.6% (5 ml) (benzalkonium chloride)

▶ ***ciprofloxacin*** ophthalmic ointment **(C)** <2 years: not recommended; ≥2 years: apply 1/2 inch ribbon to the lower conjunctival sac of affected eye(s) tid x 2 days; then bid x 5 days

Ciloxan Ophthalmic Ointment *Ophth oint:* 0.3% (3.5 gm)

▶ ***ciprofloxacin*** ophthalmic solution **(C)** <1 years: not recommended; ≥1 year: 1-2 drops to affected eye(s) q 2 hours while awake x 2 days; then, q 4 hours while awake x 5 days

Ciloxan Ophthalmic Solution *Ophth soln:* 0.3% (2.5, 5, 10 ml) (benzalkonium chloride)

▶ ***erythromycin*** ophthalmic ointment **(B)** apply 1/2 inch ribbon to the lower conjunctival sac of affected eye(s) up to 6 x/day

Ilotycin Ophthalmic Ointment *Ophth oint:* 5 mg/gm (1/8 oz)

▶ ***gatifloxacin*** ophthalmic solution **(C)**

Zymar Ophthalmic Solution <1 year: not recommended; ≥1 year: initially 1 drop to affected eye(s) q 2 hours while awake up to 8 x/day for 2 days; then 1 drop qid while awake x 5 more days

Ophth soln: 0.3% (5 ml) (benzalkonium chloride)

Zymaxid Ophthalmic Solution(G) <1 year: not recommended; ≥1 year: initially 1 drop to affected eye(s) q 2 hours while awake up to 8 x/day on day 1; then 1 drop bid-qid while awake on days 2-7

Ophth soln: 0.5% (2.5 ml) (benzalkonium chloride)

▶ ***gentamicin sulfate*** ophthalmic ointment **(C)(G)** apply 1/2 inch ribbon to the lower conjunctival sac of affected eye(s) bid-tid

Garamycin Ophthalmic Ointment *Ophth oint:* 3 mg/gm (3.5 gm) (preservative-free formulation available)

Genoptic Ophthalmic Ointment *Ophth oint:* 3 mg/gm (3.5 gm)

Gentacidin Ophthalmic Ointment *Ophth oint:* 3 mg/gm (3.5 gm)

▶ ***gentamicin sulfate*** ophthalmic solution **(C)(G)** 1-2 drops to affected eye(s) q 4 hours x 7-14 days; max 2 drops q 1 h

Garamycin Ophthalmic Solution *Ophth soln:* 0.3% (5 ml) (benzalkonium chloride)

Genoptic Ophthalmic Solution *Ophth soln:* 0.3% (3, 5 ml)

▶ ***levofloxacin*** ophthalmic solution **(C)(G)** <1 year: not recommended; ≥1 years: 1-2 drops to affected eye(s) q 2 hours while awake on days 1 and 2 (max 8 x/day); then 1-2 drops q 4 hours while awake on days 3-7; max 4 x/day

Quixin Ophthalmic Solution *Ophth soln:* 0.5% (2.5, 5 ml) (benzalkonium chloride)

▶ ***moxifloxacin*** ophthalmic solution **(C)(G)** <1 year: not recommended; ≥1 year: 1 drop to affected eye(s) tid x 7 days

Moxeza Ophthalmic Solution (G) *Ophth soln:* 0.5% (3 ml)

Vigamox Ophthalmic Solution *Ophth soln:* 0.5% (3 ml)

▶ ***ofloxacin*** ophthalmic solution **(C)** <1 year: not recommended; ≥1 year: 1-2 drops to affected eye(s) q 2-4 hours x 2 days; then qid x 5 days

Ocuflox Ophthalmic Solution *Ophth soln:* 0.3% (5, 10 ml) (benzalkonium chloride)

▶ ***sulfacetamide*** ophthalmic solution and ointment **(C)**

Bleph-10 Ophthalmic Solution 1-2 drops to affected eye(s) q 2-3 hours during the day x 7-10 days

Ophth soln: 10% (2.5, 5, 15 ml) (benzalkonium chloride)

Bleph-10 Ophthalmic Ointment <2 years: not recommended; ≥2 years: apply 1/2 inch ribbon to the lower conjunctival sac of affected eye(s) q 3-4 hours and HS x 7-10 days

Ophth oint: 10% (3.5 gm) (phenylmercuric acetate)

Cetamide Ophthalmic Solution <2 years: not recommended; ≥2 years: initially 1-2 drops to affected eye(s) q 2-3 hours; then increase dosing interval as condition improves

Ophth soln: 15% (5, 15 ml)

Isopto Cetamide Ophthalmic Ointment <2 years: not recommended; ≥2 years: initially 1/2 inch ribbon in lower conjunctival sac of affected eye(s) q 3-4 hours; then increase dosing interval as condition improves

Ophth oint: 10% (3.5 gm)

Isopto Cetamide Ophthalmic Solution <2 years: not recommended; ≥2 years: initially 1-2 drops to affected eye(s)q 2-3 hours; then increase dosing interval as condition improves

Ophth soln: 15% (5, 15 ml)

▶ ***tobramycin*** **(B)**

Tobrex Ophthalmic Solution 1-2 drops to affected eye(s) q 4 hours

Ophth soln: 0.3% (5 ml) (benzalkonium chloride)

Tobrex Ophthalmic Ointment apply 1/2 inch ribbon to the lower conjunctiva sac of affected eye(s) bid-tid

Ophth oint: 0.3% (3.5 gm) (chlorobutanol)

OPHTHALMIC ANTI-INFECTIVE COMBINATIONS

▶ ***polymyxin b sulfate+bacitracin*** ophthalmic ointment **(C)** apply 1/2 inch ribbon to the lower conjunctival sac of affected eye(s) q 3-4 hours x 7-10 days

Polysporin Ophthalmic Ointment *Ophth oint:* poly b 10,000 U+bac 500 U (3.75 gm)

▶ ***polymyxin b sulfate+bacitracin zinc+neomycin sulfate*** ophthalmic ointment **(C)** apply 1/2 inch ribbon to the lower conjunctival sac of affected eye(s) q 3-4 hours x 7-10 days

Neosporin Ophthalmic Ointment *Ophth oint:* poly b 10,000 U+bac 400 U+neo 3.5 mg/gm (3.75 gm)

▶ ***polymyxin b sulfate+gramicidin+neomycin*** ophthalmic solution **(C)** <12 years: not recommended; ≥12 years: 1-2 drops to affected eye(s) q 1 hour x 2-3 doses; then 1-2 drops bid-qid x 7-10 days

Neosporin Ophthalmic Solution *Ophth soln:* poly b 10,000 U+gram 0.025 mg +neo 1.7 mg/gm (10 ml)

▶ ***trimethoprim+polymyxin b sulfate*** <2 years: not recommended; ≥2 years: ophthalmic solution **(C)** 1 drop to affected eye(s)q 3 hours x 7-10 days; max 6 doses/day

Polytrim *Ophth soln:* trim 1 mg+poly b 10,000 U/ml (10 ml) (benzalkonium chloride)

OPHTHALMIC ANTI-INFECTIVE+STEROID COMBINATIONS

Comment: Ophthalmic corticosteroids are contraindicated after removal of a corneal foreign body, epithelial herpes simplex keratitis, *varicella*, other viral infections of the cornea or conjunctiva, fungal ocular infections, and mycobacterial ocular infections. Limit ophthalmic steroid use to 2-3 days if possible; usual max 2 weeks. With prolonged or frequent use, there is risk of corneal and scleral thinning and cataract formation.

▶ ***gentamicin sulfate+prednisolone acetate*** ophthalmic suspension **(C)**

Pred-G Ophthalmic Suspension <12 years: not recommended; ≥12 years: 1 drop to affected eye(s) bid-qid; max 20 ml/therapeutic course

Ophth susp: gent 0.3%+pred 1%/ml (2, 5, 10 ml) (benzalkonium chloride)

Pred-G Ophthalmic Ointment <12 years: not recommended; ≥12 years: apply 1/2 inch ribbon to the lower conjunctiva sac of affected eye(s) once daily-tid; max 8 gm/therapeutic course

Ophth oint: gent 0.3%+pred 0.6%/gm (3.5 gm)

▶ ***neomycin sulfate+polymyxin b sulfate+dexamethasone*** ophthalmic suspension **(C)**

Maxitrol Ophthalmic Suspension <12 years: not recommended; ≥12 years: 1-2 drops to affected eye(s) q 1 hour (severe infection) or qid (mild to moderate infection)

Ophth susp: neo 0.35%+poly b 10,000 U+dexa 1%/ml (5 ml) (benzalkonium chloride)

Maxitrol Ophthalmic Ointment <12 years: not recommended; ≥12 years: apply 1/2 inch ribbon to the lower conjunctiva sac of affected eye(s) q 1 hour (severe infection) or qid (mild to moderate infection)

Ophth oint: neo 0.35%+poly b 10,000 U+dexa 0.1%/gm (3.5 gm)

▶ ***neomycin sulfate+polymyxin b sulfate+prednisolone acetate ophthalmic suspension*** **(C)** <12 years: not recommended; ≥12 years: 1-2 drops to affected eye(s) q 3-4 hours; more often as necessary; max 20 ml/therapeutic course

Poly-Pred Ophthalmic Suspension *Ophth susp:* neo 0.35%+poly b 10,000 U+pred 0.5%/ml (10 ml)

▶ ***polymyxin b sulfate+neomycin sulfate+hydrocortisone*** ophthalmic suspension **(C)** <12 years: not recommended; ≥12 years: 1-2 drops to affected eye(s) tid-qid; more often if necessary; max 20 ml/therapeutic course

Cortisporin Ophthalmic Suspension *Ophth susp:* poly b 10,000 U+neo 0.35%+hydro 1%/ml (7.5 ml) (thimerosal)

▶ ***polymyxin b sulfate+neomycin sulfate+bacitracin zinc+hydrocortisone*** ophthalmic ointment **(C)** <12 years: not recommended; ≥12 years: apply 1/2 inch ribbon to the lower conjunctival sac of affected eye(s) tid-qid; more often if necessary; max 8 gm/therapeutic course

Cortisporin Ophthalmic Ointment *Ophth oint:* poly b 10,000 U+neo 0.35%+bac 400 U+hydro 1%/gm (3.5 gm)

▶ ***sulfacetamide sodium+fluorometholone*** suspension **(C)** <12 years: not recommended; ≥12 years: 1 drop to affected eye(s) qid; max 20 ml/therapeutic course

FML-S *Ophth susp:* sulfa 10%+fluoro 0.1%/ml (5, 10, 15 ml) (benzalkonium chloride)

▶ ***sulfacetamide sodium+prednisolone acetate*** ophthalmic suspension and ointment **(C)**

Blephamide Liquifilm <6 years: not recommended; ≥6 years: 2 drops to affected eye(s) qid and HS

Ophth susp: sulfa 10%+pred 0.2%/ml (5, 10 ml) (benzalkonium chloride)

Blephamide S.O.P. Ophthalmic Ointment <6 years: not recommended; ≥6 years: apply 1/2 inch ribbon to the lower conjunctival sac of affected eye(s) tid-qid

Ophth oint: sulfa 10%+pred 0.2%/gm (3.5 gm) (benzalkonium chloride)

▶ ***sulfacetamide sodium+prednisolone sodium phosphate*** ophthalmic solution **(C)** <6 years: not recommended; ≥6 years: 2 drops to affected eye(s) q 4 hours

Vasocidin Ophthalmic Solution *Ophth soln:* sulfa 10%+pred 0.25%/ml (5, 10 ml)

▶ ***tobramycin+dexamethasone*** ophthalmic solution and ointment **(C)**

TobraDex Ophthalmic Solution <2 years: not recommended; ≥2 years: 1-2 drops q 4-6 hours; may start with 1-2 drops q 2 hours first 1-2 days; then 1-2 drops to affected eye(s) q 2-6 hours x 24-48 hours; then 4-6 hours; reduce frequency of dose as condition improves; max 20 ml per therapeutic course

Ophth susp: tobra 0.3%+dexa 0.1%/ml (2.5, 5 ml) (benzalkonium chloride)

TobraDex Ophthalmic Ointment <2 years: not recommended; ≥2 years: apply 1/2 inch ribbon to the lower conjunctival sac of affected eye(s) tid-qid; may use at HS in conjunction with daytime drops; max 8 gm/therapeutic course

Ophth oint: tobra 0.3%+dexa 0.1%/gm (3.5 gm) (chlorobutanol chloride)

TobraDex ST <12 years: not recommended; ≥12 years: 1-2 drops to affected eye(s) q 2-6 hours x 24-48 hours; then 4-6 hours; reduce frequency of dose as condition improves; max 20 ml per therapeutic course

Ophth susp: tobra 0.3%+dexa 0.05%/ml (2.5, 5, 10 ml) (benzalkonium chloride)

- ***tobramycin+loteprednol etabonate*** ophthalmic suspension **(C)** <12 years: not recommended; ≥12 years: 1-2 drops to affected eye(s) q 1-2 hours first 24-48 hours; reduce frequency of dose to q 4-6 hours as condition improves; max 20 ml per therapeutic course

  Zylet

  Ophth susp: tobra 0.3%+lote etab 0.5%/ml (2.5, 5, 10 ml) (benzalkonium chloride)

CONJUNCTIVITIS: CHLAMYDIAL

Comment: A chlamydial etiology should be considered for all infants aged ≤30 days that have conjunctivitis, especially if the mother has a history of chlamydia infection. Topical antibiotic therapy alone is inadequate for treatment for *ophthalmia neonatorum* caused by chlamydia and is unnecessary when systemic treatment is administered.

RECOMMENDED FIRST LINE REGIMEN

- ***erythromycin base*** (B)(G) <45 kg: 50 mg/kg/day in 4 divided doses x 14 days; ≥45 kg: 250 mg qid x 14 days <u>or</u> 500 mg qid x 7 days

  Ery-Tab *Tab:* 250, 333, 500 mg ent-coat

  PCE *Tab:* 333, 500 mg

- ***erythromycin ethylsuccinate*** (B)(G) 50 mg/kg/day in 4 divided doses x 14 days; max 100 mg/kg/day <u>or</u> 400 mg qid; *see page 607 for dose by weight table*

  EryPed *Oral susp:* 200 mg/5 ml (100, 200 ml) (fruit); 400 mg/5 ml (60, 100, 200 ml) (banana); Oral drops: 200, 400 mg/5 ml (50 ml) (fruit); *Chew tab:* 200 mg wafer (fruit)

  E.E.S. *Oral susp:* 200, 400 mg/5 ml (100 ml) (fruit)

  E.E.S. Granules *Oral susp:* 200 mg/5 ml (100, 200 ml) (cherry)

  E.E.S. 400 Tablets *Tab:* 400 mg

ALTERNATE REGIMEN

- ***azithromycin*** (B)(G) <12 years: 12 mg/kg/day x 5 days; *see page 593 for dose by weight table*; max 500 mg/day; ≥12 years: 500 mg x 1 dose on day 1, then 250 mg daily on days 2-5 <u>or</u> 500 mg daily x 3 days <u>or</u> **Zmax** 2 gm in a single dose

  Zithromax *Tab:* 250, 500, 600 mg; *Oral susp:* 100 mg/5 ml (15 ml); 200 mg/5 ml (15, 22.5, 30 ml) (cherry); *Pkt:* 1 gm for reconstitution (cherry-banana)

  Zithromax Tri-pak *Tab:* 3 x 500 mg tabs/pck

  Zithromax Z-pak *Tab:* 6 x 250 mg tabs/pck

  Zmax *Oral susp:* 2 gm ext-rel for reconstitution (cherry-banana) (148 mg Na^+)

CONJUNCTIVITIS: FUNGAL

- ***natamycin*** ophthalmic suspension **(C)** <1 year: not recommended; ≥1 year: 1 drop q 1-2 hours x 3-4 days; then 1 drop every 6 hours; treat for 14-21 days; withdraw dose gradually at 4- to 7-day intervals

  Natacyn Ophthalmic Suspension *Ophth susp:* 0.5% (15 ml) (benzalkonium chloride)

CONJUNCTIVITIS: GONOCOCCAL

RECOMMENDED REGIMENS

Regimen 1

- ***ceftriaxone*** (B)(G) <45 kg: 50 mg/kg IM x 1 dose; max 125 mg IM; ≥45 kg: 250 mg IM x 1 dose
  Rocephin *Vial:* 250, 500 mg; 1, 2 gm

Regimen 2

- ***erythromycin base*** (B)(G) <45 kg: 50 mg/kg/day in 4 divided doses x 10-14 days; ≥45 kg: 250 mg qid x 10-14 days
  Ery-Tab *Tab:* 250, 333, 500 mg ent-coat
  PCE *Tab:* 333, 500 mg
- ***erythromycin ethylsuccinate*** (B)(G) 50 mg/kg/day in 4 divided doses x 7 days; max 100 mg/kg/day or 400 mg qid; *see page 607 for dose by weight table*
  EryPed *Oral susp:* 200 mg/5 ml (100, 200 ml) (fruit); 400 mg/5 ml (60, 100, 200 ml) (banana); *Oral drops:* 200, 400 mg/5 ml (50 ml) (fruit); *Chew tab:* 200 mg wafer (fruit)
  E.E.S. *Oral susp:* 200, 400 mg/5 ml (100 ml) (fruit)
  E.E.S. Granules *Oral susp:* 200 mg/5 ml (100, 200 ml) (cherry)
  E.E.S. 400 Tablets *Tab:* 400 mg

ALTERNATE REGIMEN

- ***azithromycin*** (B)(G) <12 years: not recommended for bronchitis in children; ≥12 years: 500 mg x 1 dose on day 1; then 250 mg once daily on days; 2-5 or 500 mg daily x 3 days or 2 gm in a single dose
  Zithromax *Tab:* 250, 500, 600 mg; *Oral susp:* 100 mg/5 ml (15 ml); 200 mg/5 ml (15, 22.5, 30 ml) (cherry); Pkt: 1 gm for reconstitution (cherry-banana)
  Zithromax Tri-pak *Tab:* 3 x 500 mg tabs/pck
  Zithromax Z-pak *Tab:* 6 x 250 mg tabs/pck
  Zmax *Oral susp:* 2 gm ext-rel for reconstitution (cherry-banana) (148 mg Na^+)

CONJUNCTIVITIS: VIRAL

Comment: For prevention of secondary bacterial infection, see agents listed under bacterial conjunctivitis. Ophthalmic corticosteroids are contraindicated with herpes simplex, keratitis, *Varicella*, and other viral infections of the cornea.

- ***trifluridine*** ophthalmic suspension (C) <6 years: not recommended; ≥6 years: 1 drop q 2 hours while awake; max 9 drops/day; after re-epithelialization, 1 drop q 4 h x 7 days (at least 5 drops/day); max 21 days of therapy
  Viroptic Ophthalmic Solution *Ophth soln:* 1% (7.5 ml) (thimerosal)

CONSTIPATION: OCCASIONAL, INTERMITTENT

BULK-FORMING AGENTS

- ***calcium polycarbophil*** (C) <6 years: not recommended; 6-12 years: 1 tab daily to qid; >12 years: 2 tabs once daily-qid
  FiberCon (OTC) *Cplt:* 625 mg
  Konsyl Fiber Tablets (OTC) *Tab:* 625 mg

▶ ***methylcellulose***

Citrucel <6 years: not recommended; 6-12 years: 1/2 heaping tbsp in 4 oz cold water; >12 years: 1 heaping tbsp in 8 oz cold water tid

Oral pwdr: 16, 24, 30 oz and single-dose pkts (orange)

Citrucel Sugar-Free <6 years: not recommended; 6-12 years: 1 level tbsp in 4 oz cold water; >12 years: 1 heaping tbsp in 8 oz cold water tid

Oral pwdr: 16, 24, 30 oz and single-dose pkts (orange) (sugar-free, phenylalanine)

▶ ***psyllium husk*** **(B)** <6 years: not recommended; 6-12 years: 1/2 wafer, cap, or pkt in 8 oz liquid tid; >12 years: wafer or cap or 1 pkt or 1 rounded tsp (1 rounded tbsp for sugar-containing form) in 8 oz liquid tid

Metamucil (OTC)

Cap: psyllium husk 5.2 gm (100, 150/carton); Wafer: *psyllium husk* 3.4 gm/rounded tsp (24/carton) (apple crisp, cinnamon spice); *Plain and flavored pwdr:* 3.4 gm/rounded tsp (15, 20, 24, 29, 30, 36, 44, 48 oz); *Efferv sugar-free flav pkts:* 3.4 gm/pkt (30/pkt) (phenylalanine)

▶ ***psyllium*** hydrophilic mucilloid **(B)** <6 years: not recommended; 6-12 years: 1 rounded tsp in 8 oz liquid tid; >12 years: 2 rounded tsp in 8 oz water qid

Konsyl (OTC) *Pwdr:* 6 gm/rounded tsp (10.6, 15.9 oz); *Pwdr pkt:* 6 gm/rounded tsp (30/carton)

Konsyl-D (OTC) *Pwdr:* 3.4 gm/rounded tsp (11.5, 17.59 oz); *Pwdr pkt:* 3.4 gm/rounded tsp (30/carton)

Konsyl Easy Mix Formula (OTC) *Pwdr:* 3.4 gm/rounded tsp (8 oz) (sugar-free, low sodium)

Konsyl Orange (OTC) *Pwdr:* 3.4 gm/rounded tsp (19 oz); *Pwdr pkt:* 3.4 gm/rounded tsp (30/carton)

Konsyl Orange SF (OTC) *Pwdr:* 3.5 gm/rounded tsp (15 oz) (phenylalanine); *Pwdr pkt:* 3.5 gm/rounded tsp (30/carton) (phenylalanine)

STOOL SOFTENERS

▶ ***docusate sodium*** **(OTC)** <3 years: 10-40 mg/day; 3-6 years: 20-60 mg/day; >6-12 years: 40-120 mg/day; >12 years: 50-200 mg/day

Cap: 50, 100 mg; *Liq:* 10 mg/ml (30 ml w. dropper); *Syr:* 20 mg/5 ml (8 oz) (alcohol ≤1%)

Dialose 6 years: not recommended; ≥6 years: 1 tab q HS

Tab: 100 mg

Surfak (OTC) 12 years: not recommended; ≥12 years: 240 mg/day

Cap: 240 mg

OSMOTIC LAXATIVES

▶ ***lactulose*** **(B)(G)** 6 years: not recommended; ≥6 years: take 10-20 gm dissolved in 4 oz water once daily prn; max 40 gm/day

Kristalose *Crystals for oral soln:* 10, 20 gm single-dose pkts (30/carton)

▶ ***magnesium citrate*** **(B)(G)** <2 years: not recommended; 2-6 years: 4-12 ml once daily prn; ≥6-12 years: 50-100 ml once daily prn; >12 years: 1 full bottle (120-300 ml) once daily prn

Citrate of Magnesia (OTC) *Oral soln:* 300 ml

▶ ***magnesium hydroxide*** **(B)** <2 years: not recommended; 2-5 years: 5-15 ml/day in a single or divided doses; 6-11 years: 15-30 ml/day in a single or divided doses; >11 years: 30-60 ml/day in a single or divided doses prn

Milk of Magnesia *Liq:* 390 mg/5 ml (10, 15, 20, 30, 100, 120, 180, 360, 720 ml)

▶ ***polyethylene glycol (PEG)*** (C)(OTC)(G) ≤17: not recommended; >17 years: 1 tbsp (17 gm) dissolved in 4-8 oz water per day for up to max 7 days; may need 2-4 days for results

GlycoLax Powder for Oral Solution *Oral pwdr:* 7, 14, 30, and 45 dose bottles w. 17 gm dosing cup (gluten-free, sugar-free); 17 gm single-dose pkts (20/carton)

MiraLAX Powder for Oral Solution *Oral pwdr:* 7, 14, 30, and 45 dose bottles w. 17 gm dosing cup (gluten-free, sugar-free)

Polyethylene Glycol 3350 Powder for Oral Solution (G) *Oral pwdr:* 3350 gm w. dosing cup; 17 gm/scoop

Comment: *PEG* is an osmotic indicated for occasional constipation without affecting glucose and electrolyte levels. Contraindicated with suspected or known bowel obstruction.

STIMULANTS

▶ ***bisacodyl*** (B)(OTC) 2-3 tabs or 1 suppository bid prn

Dulcolax, Gentlax <12 years: 1/2 suppository once daily prn; 6-12 years: 1 tablet or 1/2 suppository once daily prn; >12 years: 1 tab or 1 rectal suppository

Tab: 5 mg; *Rectal supp:* 10 mg

Senokot <2 years: not recommended; 2-6 years: 1/4 tab or 1/2 tsp once daily prn; max 1 tab or 1/2 tsp bid; 6-12 years: 1 tab or 1/2 tsp once daily prn; max 2 tabs or 1 tsp once daily; >12 years: initially 2-4 tabs or 1 level tsp at HS prn; max 4 tabs or 2 tsp bid

Tab: 8.6*mg; *Granules:* 15 mg/tsp (2, 6, 12 oz) (cocoa)

Senokot Syrup <12 years: use Children's Syrup; ≥12 years: initially 10-15 ml at HS prn; max 15 ml bid

Syr: 8.8 mg/5 ml (2, 8 oz) (chocolate) (alcohol-free)

Senokot Children's Syrup (OTC) <2 years: not recommended; 2-6 years: 2.5-3.75 ml once daily prn; max 3.75 ml bid prn; ≥6-12 years: 5-7.5 ml once daily prn; max 7.5 ml bid

Syr: 8.8 mg/5 ml (2.5 oz) (chocolate) (alcohol-free)

Senokot Xtra (OTC) <2 years: not recommended; 2-6 years: use Children's Syrup; 6-12 years: 1/2 tab once daily at HS; max 1 tab bid; >12 years: 1 tab at HS prn; max 2 tabs bid

Tab: 17*mg

BULK-FORMING AGENT+STIMULANT COMBINATIONS

▶ ***psyllium+senna*** (B)

Perdiem (OTC) <7 years: not recommended; 7-11 years: 1 rounded tsp swallowed with 8 oz cool liquid qd-bid; >11 years: 1-2 rounded tsp swallowed with 8 oz cool liquid daily bid

Canister: 8.8, 14 oz; *Individual pkt:* 6 gm (6/pck)

SennaPrompt (OTC) <12 years: not recommended; ≥12 years: initially 2-5 caps bid

Cap: psyl 500 mg+*senna* 9 mg

STOOL SOFTENER+STIMULANT COMBINATIONS

▶ ***docusate+casanthranol*** (C)

Doxidan (OTC) <2 years: not recommended; ≥2 years-12 years: 1 cap/day; >12 years: 1-3 caps/day; max 1 week

Cap: doc 60 mg+cas 30 mg

Peri-Colace (OTC) <12 years: 5-15 ml q HS; ≥12 years: 1-2 caps or 15-30 ml q HS; max 2 caps or 30 ml bid or 3 caps q HS

Cap: doc 100 mg+cas 30 mg; *Syr:* doc 60 mg+cas 30 mg per 15 ml (8, 16 oz)

▶ ***docusate+senna*** concentrate **(C)**

Senokot S (OTC) <2 years: not recommended; 2-6 years: 1/2 tab daily; max 1 tab bid; >6-12 years: 1 tab daily; max 2 tabs bid; >12 years: 2 tabs q HS; max 4 tabs bid

Tab: doc 50 mg+senna 8.6 mg

ENEMAS AND OTHER AGENTS

▶ ***sodium biphosphate+sodium phosphate*** enema **(C)(OTC)**

Fleets Adult <2 years: not recommended; 2-12 years: 59 ml rectally; >12 years: 59-118 ml rectally

Enema: sod biphos 19 gm+sod phos 7 gm (59, 118 ml w. applicator)

Fleets Pediatric <12 years: 59 ml rectally; ≥12 years: use **Fleets Adult**

Enema: sod biphos 19 gm+sod phos 7 gm (59 ml w. applicator)

▶ ***glycerin*** suppositories **(C)(OTC)** <6 years: 1 pediatric suppository; ≥6 years: 1 adult suppository

CONSTIPATION: CHRONIC IDIOPATHIC (CIC)

GUANYLATE CYCLASE-C AGONISTS

Comment: Guanylate cyclase-c agonists increase intestinal fluid and intestinal transit time may induce diarrhea and bloating and therefore, are contraindicated with known or suspected mechanical GI obstruction.

▶ ***linaclotide*** **(C)** ≤18 years: not established (<6 years: contraindicated; 6-18 years: avoid); >18 years: 145 mcg orally once daily or 72 mcg orally once daily based on individual presentation or tolerability; take on an empty stomach at least 30 minutes before the first meal of the day; swallow whole, do not crush or chew cap or cap contents; may open cap and administer with applesauce or water (e.g., NGT, PEG tube)

Linzess *Cap:* 72, 145, 290 mcg

Comment: ***linaclotide*** and its active metabolite are negligibly absorbed systemically following oral administration and maternal use is not expected to result in fetal exposure to the drug. There is no information regarding the presence of ***plecanatide*** in human milk or its effects on the breastfed infant.

▶ ***plecanatide*** ≤18 years: not established (<6 years: contraindicated; 6-18 years: avoid); >18 years: take one tab once daily; if necessary, may crush and administer with applesauce or water (e.g., NGT, PEG tube)

Trulance *Tab:* 3 mg

Comment: Suspend ***plecanatide*** dosing and rehydrate if severe diarrhea occurs. Most common adverse reactions in CIC are sinusitis, URI, diarrhea, abdominal distension and tenderness, flatulence, increased liver enzymes. ***plecanatide*** and its active metabolite are negligibly absorbed systemically following oral administration and maternal use is not expected to result in fetal exposure to the drug. There is no information regarding the presence of ***plecanatide*** in human milk or its effects on the breastfed infant.

CHLORIDE CHANNEL ACTIVATOR

▶ ***lubiprostone*** **(C)** **<18 years:** not recommended; >18 years: **one** 24 mcg cap bid with food; swallow whole, do not break apart or chew

Amitiza *Cap:* 8, 24 mcg

Comment: **Amitiza** increases intestinal fluid and intestinal transit time. Suspend dosing and rehydrate if severe diarrhea occurs. **Amitiza** is contraindicated with known or suspected mechanical GI obstruction. Most common adverse reactions in CIC are nausea, diarrhea, headache, abdominal pain, abdominal distension, and flatulence.

CORNEAL EDEMA

▶ ***sodium chloride*** (G)

Various (OTC) 1-2 drops or 1 inch ribbon q 3-4 hours prn; reduce frequency as edema subsides

Ophth soln: 2, 5% (15, 30 ml); *Ophth oint:* 5% (3.5 gm)

CORNEAL ULCERATION

ANTIBACTERIAL OPHTHALMIC SOLUTION/OINTMENT

*See **Conjunctivitis & Blepharoconjunctivitis: Bacterial** page* 89

COSTOCHONDRITIS (CHEST WALL SYNDROME)

Acetaminophen for IV Infusion *see **Pain** page* 322
NSAIDs *see page* 539
Other Oral Analgesics *see **Pain** page* 324
Topical & Transdermal NSAIDs *see **Pain** page* 323
Parenteral Corticosteroids *see page* 547
Oral Corticosteroids *see page* 546

COXSACKIEVIRUS (HAND, FOOT, & MOUTH DISEASE)

NSAIDs *see page* 539
Other Oral Analgesics *see **Pain** page* 324
OTC throat Lozenges
OTC Cough Drops and Cough Syrup

Comment: Hand, foot, and mouth disease occurs most commonly in children ≤10 years-of-age. Although adults are susceptible, most have built up natural immunity. The causative organism, *Coxsackievirus*, is transmitted via droplet spread (coughing and/ or sneezing) and contact with contaminated objects and surfaces (same as influenza). Clinical signs and symptoms are typically relatively mild and include fever, sore throat, feeling generally unwell, malaise, headache, and poor appetite. Red spots, some painful blister-like lesions, most often appear on the tongue and roof of the mouth, palms of the hands, and soles of the feet (but not necessarily all three), and are often faint or sparse. Lesions, which are not pruritic, may also be noted on the dorsal surfaces of the hands/fingers and feet/ toes. Medical treatment, per se, is not required. Treatment in the home with age/ weight-dosed ibuprofen or acetaminophen for relief of sore throat, lesion pain, and fever. Other comfort measures include salt water gargles, throat lozenges, cough drops or cough syrup, and fluids. The disease typically resolves in 7 to 10 days.

CRAMPS: ABDOMINAL, INTESTINAL

ANTISPASMODIC-ANTICHOLINERGIC AGENTS

▶ ***dicyclomine*** (B)(G) <12 years: not recommended; ≥12 years: initially 20 mg bid-qid; may increase to 40 mg qid PO; usual IM dose 80 mg/day divided qid; do not use IM route for more than 1-2 days

Bentyl *Tab:* 20 mg; *Cap:* 10 mg; *Syr:* 10 mg/5 ml (16 oz); *Vial:* 10 mg/ml (10 ml); *Amp:* 10 mg/ml (2 ml)

▶ ***methscopolamine bromide*** **(B)** <12 years: not recommended; ≥12 years: 1 tab q 6 hours prn

Pamine *Tab:* 2.5 mg

Pamine Forte *Tab:* 5 mg

ANTICHOLINERGICS

▶ ***hyoscyamine*** **(C)(G)**

Anaspaz <2 years: not recommended; 2-12 years: 0.0625-0.125 mg q 4 hours prn; max 0.75 mg/day; >12 years: 1-2 tabs q 4 hours prn; max 12 tabs/day

Tab: 0.125*mg

Levbid <12 years: not recommended; ≥12 years: 1-2 tabs q 12 hours prn; max 4 tabs/day

Tab: 0.375*mg ext-rel

Levsin <6 years: not recommended; ≥6-12 years: 1 tab q 4 hours prn; >12 years: 1-2 tabs q 4 hours prn; max 12 tabs/day

Tab: 0.125*mg

Levsinex SL <2 years: not recommended; 2-12 years: 1 tab SL or PO q 4 hours; max 6 tabs/day; >12 years: 1-2 tabs q 4 hours SL or PO; max 12 tabs/day

Tab: 0.125 mg sublingual

Levsinex Timecaps <2 years: not recommended; 2-12 years: 1 cap q 12 hours; max 2 caps/day; >12 years; 1-2 caps q 12 hours; may adjust to 1 cap q 8 hours

Cap: 0.375 mg time-rel

NuLev <2 years: not recommended; 2-12 years: dissolve 1 tab on tongue, with or without water, q 4 hours prn; max 6 tabs/day; >12 years: dissolve 1-2 tabs on tongue, with or without water, q 4 hours prn; max 12 tabs/day

ODT: 0.125 mg (mint) (phenylalanine)

▶ ***simethicone*** **(C)(G)** 0.3 ml qid pc and HS

Mylicon Drops (OTC) *Oral drops:* 40 mg/0.6 ml (30 ml)

▶ ***phenobarbital+hyoscyamine+atropine+scopolamine*** **(C)(IV)(G)**

Donnatal <12 years: not recommended; ≥12 years: 1-2 tabs ac and HS

Tab: pheno 16.2 mg+hyo 0.1037 mg+atro 0.0194 mg+scop 0.0065 mg

Donnatal Elixir 20 lb: 1 ml q 4 hours or 1.5 ml q 6 hours; 30 lb: 1.5 ml q 4 hours or 2 ml q 6 hours; 50 lb: 1/2 tsp q 4 hours or 3/4 tsp q 6 hours; 75 lb: 3/4 tsp q 4 hours or 1 tsp q 6 hours; 100 lb: 1 tsp q 4 hours or 1 tsp q 6 hours; ≥12 years: 1-2 tsp ac and HS

Elix: pheno 16.2 mg+hyo 0.1037 mg+atro 0.0194 mg+scop 0.0065 mg per 5 ml (4, 16 oz)

Donnatal Extentabs <12 years: not recommended; ≥12 years: 1 tab q 12 hours

Tab: pheno 48.6 mg+hyo 0.3111 mg+atro 0.0582 mg+scop 0.0195 mg ext-rel

ANTICHOLINERGIC+SEDATIVE COMBINATION

▶ ***chlordiazepoxide+clidinium*** **(D)(IV)** <12 years: not recommended; ≥12 years: 1-2 caps ac and HS; max 8 caps/day

Librax *Cap:* chlor 5 mg+clid 2.5 mg

CROHN'S DISEASE

Parenteral Corticosteroids *see page* 547

Oral Corticosteroids *see page* 546

Comment: Standard treatment regimen for active disease (flare) is: antibiotic, antispasmodic, and bowel rest; progress to clear liquids; then progress to high-fiber diet. Long term management of chronic disease includes salicylates, immune modulators, and tumor necrosis factor (TNF) blockers.

ORAL ANTI-INFECTIVES

▶ ***metronidazole*** **(not for use in 1st; B in 2nd, 3rd)(G)** <12 years: 35-50 mg/kg/day in 3 divided doses x 10 days; ≥12 years: 500 mg tid or 750 mg bid; max 8 weeks

Flagyl *Tab:* 250*, 500*mg

Flagyl 375 *Cap:* 375 mg

Flagyl ER *Tab:* 750 mg ext-rel

Comment: Alcohol is contraindicated during treatment with oral ***metronidazole*** and for 72 hours after therapy due to a possible ***disulfiram***-like reaction (nausea, vomiting, flushing, headache).

SALICYLATES

▶ ***mesalamine*** (B)(G)

Asacol <12 years: not recommended; ≥12 years: 800 mg tid x 6 weeks; maintenance 1.6 gm/day in divided doses; swallow whole, do not crush or chew

Tab: 400 mg del-rel

Comment: 2 **Asacol** 400 mg tabs are not bioequivalent to 1 **Asacol HD** 800 mg tab.

Asacol HD <12 years: not recommended; ≥12 years: 1,600 mg tid x 6 weeks; swallow whole, do not crush or chew

Tab: 800 mg del-rel

Comment: 1 **Asacol HD** 800 mg tab is not bioequivalent to 2 **Asacol** 400 mg tabs

Canasa <12 years: not established; ≥12 years: 1 gm qid for up to 8 weeks

Rectal supp: 1 gm del-rel (30, 42/pck)

Delzicol <5 years: not established; >5 years: *Treatment:* 800 mg tid x 6 weeks; maintenance 1.6 gm/day in 2-4 divided doses daily; swallow whole; do not crush or chew

Cap: 400 mg del-rel

Comment: 2 **Delzicol** 400 mg caps are not bioequivalent to 1 ***mesalamine*** 800 mg del-rel tab

Lialda <18 years: not established; ≥18 years: 2.4-4.8 gm daily in a single dose for up to 8 weeks; swallow whole, do not crush or chew

Tab: 1.2 gm del-rel

Pentasa <12 years: not established; ≥12 years: 1 gm qid for up to 8 weeks; swallow whole, do not crush or chew

Cap: 250 mg cont-rel

Rowasa Enema <12 years: not established; ≥12 years: 4 gm rectally by enema q HS; retain for 8 hours x 3-6 weeks

Enema: 4 gm/60 ml (7, 14, 28/pck; kit, 7, 14, 28/pck w. wipes)

Rowasa Suppository <12 years: not established; ≥12 years: 1 suppository rectally bid x 3-6 weeks; retain for 1-3 hours or longer

Rectal supp: 500 mg

Sulfite-Free Rowasa Rectal Suspension <12 years: not established; ≥12 years: 4 gm rectally by enema q HS; retain for 8 hours x 3-6 weeks

Enema: 4 gm/60 ml (7, 14, 28/pck; kit, 7, 14, 28/pck w. wipes)

▶ ***olsalazine*** (C)

Dipentum <12 years: not established; ≥12 years: 1 gm/day in 2 divided doses; max 2 gm/day

Cap: 250 mg

Comment: Indicated in persons who cannot tolerate ***sulfasalazine***.

▶ ***sulfasalazine*** (B)(G)

Azulfidine <2 years: not recommended; 2-16 years: initially 40-60 mg/kg/day in 3-6 divided doses; max 2 gm/day; >16 years: initially 1-2 gm/day; increase to 3-4 gm/day in divided doses pc until clinical symptoms controlled; maintenance 2 gm/day; max 4 gm/day

Tab: 500*mg

Azulfidine EN <2 years: not recommended; 2-16 years: initially 40-60 mg/kg/day in 3-6 divided doses; max 2 gm/day; >16 years: initially 500 mg in the PM x 7 days; then 500 mg bid x 7 days; then 500 mg in the AM and 1 gm in the PM x 7 days; then 1 gm bid; max 4 gm/day

Tab: 500 mg ent-coat

▶ ***budesonide micronized*** **(C)(G)** <12 years: not established; ≥12 years: *Treatment* 9 mg once daily in the AM for up to 8 weeks; may repeat an 8-week course; *Maintenance of remission*: 6 mg once daily for up to 3 months

Entocort EC *Cap:* 3 mg ent-coat ext-rel granules

Comment: Taper other systemic steroids when transferring to **Entocort EC**. When corticosteroids are used chronically, systemic effects such as hypercorticism and adrenal suppression may occur. Corticosteroids can reduce the response of the hypothalamus-pituitary-adrenal (HPA) axis to stress. In situations where patients are subject to surgery or other stress situations, supplementation with a systemic corticosteroid is recommended. General precautions concerning corticosteroids should be followed.

PURINE ANTIMETABOLITE IMMUNOSUPPRESSANT

▶ ***azathioprine*** (D)(G)

Imuran *Tab:* 50*mg; *Injectable:* 100 mg

Comment: **Imuran** is usually administered on a daily basis. The initial dose should be approximately 1.0 mg/kg (50 to 100 mg) as a single dose or divided bid. Dose may be increased beginning at 6-8 weeks, and thereafter at 4-week intervals, if there are no serious toxicities and if initial response is unsatisfactory. Dose increments should be 0.5 mg/kg/day, up to max 2.5 mg/kg per day. Therapeutic response usually occurs after 6-8 weeks of treatment. An adequate trial should be a minimum of 12 weeks. Patients not improved after 12 weeks can be considered refractory. **Imuran** may be continued long-term in patients with clinical response, but patients should be monitored carefully, and gradual dosage reduction should be attempted to reduce risk of toxicities. Maintenance therapy should be at the lowest effective dose, and the dose given can be lowered decrementally with changes of 0.5 mg/kg or approximately 25 mg daily every 4 weeks while other therapy is kept constant. The optimum duration of maintenance **Imuran** has not been determined. **Imuran** can be discontinued abruptly, but delayed effects are possible.

TUMOR NECROSIS FACTOR (TNF) BLOCKERS

▶ ***adalimumab*** (B) <2 years, <10 kg: not recommended; 10-<15 kg: 10 mg every other week; 15-<30 kg: 20 mg every other week; ≥30 kg: 40 mg every other week; 2-17 years, supervise first dose; ≥12 years: 40 mg SC once every other week; may increase to once weekly without MTX; administer in abdomen or thigh; rotate sites

Humira *Prefilled syringe:* 20 mg/0.4 ml; 40 mg/0.8 ml single-dose (2/pck; 2, 6/starter pck) (preservative-free)

Comment: May use with ***methotrexate*** **(MTX)**, DMARDs, corticosteroids, salicylates, NSAIDs, or analgesics.

▶ ***adalimumab-adbm*** **(B)** <18 years: not recommended; ≥18 years: *First dose (Day 1):* 160 mg SC (4 x 40 mg injections in one day or 2 x 40 mg injections per day for two consecutive days); *Second dose two weeks later (Day 15):* 80 mg SC; *Two weeks later (Day 29):* begin a maintenance dose of 40 mg SC every other week

Cyltezo *Prefilled syringe:* 40 mg/0.8 ml single-dose (preservative-free)

Comment: **Cyltezo** is biosimilar to **Humira** ***(adalimumab)***.

➢ ***certolizumab*** **(B)** <12 years: not established; ≥12 years: 400 mg SC (2 x 200 mg inj at two different sites on day 1); then, 400 mg SC at weeks 2 and 4; maintenance 400 mg SC every 4 weeks; administer in abdomen or thigh; rotate sites

Cimzia *Vial:* 200 mg (2/pck); *Prefilled syringe:* 200 mg/ml single-dose (2/pck; 2, 6/starter pck) (preservative-free)

➢ ***infliximab*** *(tumor necrosis factor-alpha blocker)* ***infliximab*** *(tumor necrosis factor-alpha blocker)* <6 years: not recommended; ≥6 years: administer 5 mg/kg at 0, 2 and 6 weeks, then every 8 weeks; administer dose intravenously over a period of not less than 2 hours; must be refrigerated at 2°C to 8°C (36°F to 46°F); do not use beyond the expiration date as this product contains no preservative

Remicade *Vial:* 100 mg for reconstitution to 10 ml administration volume, single-dose (preservative-free)

Comment: **Remicade** is indicated to reduce signs and symptoms, and induce and maintain clinical remission, in adults and children ≥6 years-of-age with moderately to severely active disease who have had an inadequate response to conventional therapy and reduce the number of draining enterocutaneous and rectovaginal fistulas, and maintain fistula closure, in adults with fistulizing disease. Common adverse effects associated with **Rremicade** included abdominal pain, headache, pharyngitis, sinusitis, and upper respiratory infections. In addition, **Remicade** might increase the risk for serious infections, including tuberculosis, bacterial sepsis, and invasive fungal infections. Available data from published literature on the use of ***infliximab*** products during pregnancy have not reported a clear association with ***infliximab*** products and adverse pregnancy outcomes. ***infliximab*** products cross the placenta and infants exposed *in utero* should not be administered live vaccines for at least 6 months after birth. Otherwise, the infant may be at increased risk of infection, including disseminated infection which can become fatal. Available information is insufficient to inform the amount of ***infliximab*** products present in human milk or effects on the breastfed infant. To report suspected adverse reactions, contact Merck Sharp & Dohme Corp., a subsidiary of Merck & Co. at 1-877-888-4231 or FDA at 1-800-FDA-1088 or visit www.fda.gov/medwatch

➢ ***infliximab-abda*** *(tumor necrosis factor-alpha blocker)* **(B)**

Renflexis: see *infliximab* **(Remicade)** above for full prescribing information

Comment: **Renflexis** is a biosimilar to **Remicade** for the treatment of immune-disorders including Crohn's disease, ulcerative colitis, rheumatoid arthritis, ankylosing spondylitis, psoriatic arthritis and plaque psoriasis. **Renflexis** was approved under the FDA category for biosimilars and demonstrated no clinically meaningful differences for use, dosing regimens, strengths, dosage forms, and routes of administration from the FDA-approved biological product **Remicade.**

Inflectra: see ***infliximab*** **(Remicade)** above for full prescribing information

Comment: **Inflectra** is a biosimilar to **Remicade** for the treatment of immune-disorders including Crohn's disease, ulcerative colitis, rheumatoid arthritis, ankylosing spondylitis, psoriatic arthritis and plaque psoriasis. **Inflectra** was approved under the FDA category for biosimilars and demonstrated no clinically meaningful differences for use, dosing regimens, strengths, dosage forms, and routes of administration from the FDA-approved biological product **Remicade.**

➢ ***infliximab-qbtx*** *(tumor necrosis factor-alpha blocker)* **(B)**

Ifixi: see ***infliximab*** **(Remicade)** above for full prescribing information

Comment: **Ifixi** is a biosimilar to **Remicade** for the treatment of immune disorders including Crohn's disease, ulcerative colitis, rheumatoid arthritis, ankylosing spondylitis, psoriatic arthritis and plaque psoriasis. **Ifixi** was approved under the FDA category for biosimilars and demonstrated no clinically meaningful differences for use, dosing regimens, strengths, dosage forms, and routes of administration from the FDA-approved biological product **Remicade.**

INTEGRIN RECEPTOR ANTAGONIST (IMMUNOMODULATOR)

▶ ***natalizumab*** (C) <18 years: not established; ≥18 years: administer by IV infusion over 1 hour; monitor during and for 1 hour post infusion; 300 mg every 4 weeks; discontinue after 12 weeks if no therapeutic response, or if unable to taper off chronic concomitant steroids within 6 months; may continue aminosalicylates

Tysabri *Vial:* 300 mg single-dose, soln after dilution for IV infusion (preservative-free)

Comment: To report suspected adverse reactions, contact Biogen at 1-800-456-2255 or at FDA at 1-800-FDA-1088 or visit www.fda.gov/medwatch.

▶ ***vedolizumab*** (B) <18 years: not established; ≥18 years: administer by IV infusion over 30 minutes; 300 mg at weeks 0, 2, 6; then once every 8 weeks

Entyvio

Vial: 300 mg (20 ml) single-dose, pwdr for IV infusion after reconstitution (preservative-free)

Comment: To report suspected adverse reactions, contact Takeda Pharmaceuticals at 1-877-TAKEDA-7 (1-877-825-3327) or FDA at 1-800-FDA-1088 or visit www.fda.gov/medwatch

CRYPTOSPORIDIUM PARVUM

▶ ***nitazoxanide*** (B) <12 months: not recommended; 12-47 months: 5 ml q 12 hours x 3 days; 4-11 years: 10 ml q 12 hours x 3 days; ≥12 years: 500 mg by mouth q 12 hours x 3 days

Alinia *Oral susp:* 100 mg/5 ml (60 ml)

Comment: **Alinia** is an antiprotozoal for the treatment of diarrhea due to *G. lamblia* or *C. parvum.*

CYCLOSPORIASIS (*CYCLOSPORA CAYETANENSIS*)

Comment: The US Centers for Disease Control and Prevention (CDC), state and local health departments, and the US Food and Drug Administration have issued a Health Alert Network advisory after an increase in reported cases of cyclosporiasis, an intestinal illness caused by the parasite *Cyclospora cayetanensis.* Clinicians should consider a diagnosis of cyclosporiasis in patients who experience prolonged or remitting-relapsing diarrhea. Since May 1, 2017, 206 cases have been identified, more than twice the 88 cases reported from May 1 to August 3, 2016. Most laboratories in the United States do not routinely test for *Cyclospora*, even when a stool sample has been tested for parasites, so providers must specifically order the test. Several stool specimens may be required because *Cyclospora* oocysts may be shed intermittently and at low levels, even in persons with profuse diarrhea. Symptoms include watery diarrhea, which can be profuse, anorexia, fatigue, weight loss, nausea, flatulence, stomach cramps, myalgia, vomiting, and low-grade fever. Symptoms begin from 2 days to more than 2 weeks (average 7 days) after ingestion of the parasite. *Cyclospora* is food- and water-bone; it is not transmitted directly from person to person. The recommended treatment is ***trimethoprim+sulfamethoxazole*** (TMP/SMX). There are no effective alternatives for people who are allergic to or who cannot tolerate TMP/SMX; observation and symptomatic care is recommended for those patients. If untreated, illness may last for a few days to a month or longer.

▶ ***trimethoprim+sulfamethoxazole [TMP-SMX]*** (C)(G)

Bactrim, Septra <12 years: not recommended; ≥12 years: 2 tabs bid x 10 days

Tab: trim 80 mg+sulfa 400 mg*

Bactrim DS, Septra DS <12 years: not recommended; ≥12 years: 1 tab bid x 10 days

Tab: trim 160 mg+sulfa 800 mg*

Bactrim Pediatric Suspension, Septra Pediatric Suspension <2 months: not recommended; ≥2 months-12 years: 40 mg/kg/day of **sulfamethoxazole** in 2 doses bid; >12 years: use tabs

Oral susp: trim 40 mg+sulfa 200 mg per 5 ml (100 ml) (cherry) (alcohol 0.3%)

CYSTIC FIBROSIS

▶ ***acetylcysteine*** (B)(G) administer via face mask, mouth piece, tracheostomy T-piece, mist tent, or croupette; routine tracheostomy care, 1 to 2 ml of a 10% to 20% solution may be administered by direct instillation into the tracheostomy every 1 to 4 hours

Mucomyst *Vial:* 10, 20% (4, 10, 30 ml) soln for inhalation

Comment: **Mucomyst** is a mucolytic. For inhalation, the 10% concentration may be used undiluted; the 20% concentration should be diluted with sterile water or normal saline (either for injection or inhalation).

CYSTIC FIBROSIS TRANSMEMBRANE CONDUCTANCE REGULATOR (CFTR) POTENTIATOR

▶ ***ivacaftor*** (B) <2 years: not established; 2-6 years, <14 kg: one 50 mg packet mixed with 1 tsp (5 ml) soft food or liquid every 12 hours with fat-containing food; 2-6 years, ≥14 kg: one 75 mg packet mixed with 1 tsp (5 ml) soft food or liquid every 12 hours with fat-containing food; >6 years: 150 mg every 12 hours; administer with fat-containing food (e.g., eggs, butter, peanut butter, cheese pizza); avoid food and juices containing grapefruit or Seville oranges.

Kalydeco *Tab:* 150 mg film-coat; *Oral granules:* 50, 75 mg unit dose pkts (56 pkt/carton)

Comment: **Kalydeco** is indicated for the treatment of CF in patients who have a *G551D* co-mutation in the *CFTR* gene. If the patient's genotype is unknown, an FDA-cleared CF mutation test should be used to detect the presence of the *G551D* mutation. **Kalydeco** is not effective in patients with CF who are homozygous for the *F508del* mutation in the *CFTR* gene. Transaminases (ALT and AST) should be assessed prior to initiating **Kalydeco**, every 3 months during the first year of treatment, and annually thereafter. Patients who develop increased transaminase levels should be closely monitored until the abnormalities resolve. Dosing should be interrupted in patients with ALT or AST greater than 5 times the upper limit of normal (ULN). Following resolution of transaminase elevations, consider the benefits and risks of resuming **Kalydeco** dosing. Concomitant use with strong CYP3A inducers (e.g., ***rifampin***, St. John's Wort) substantially decreases exposure of **Kalydeco** (which may diminish effectiveness); therefore, co-administration is not recommended. Reduce dose to 150 mg twice weekly when co-administered with strong CYP3A inhibitors (e.g., ***ketoconazole***). Reduce dose to 150 mg once daily when co-administered with moderate CYP3A inhibitors. Caution is recommended in patients with severe renal impairment (CrCl <30 mL/min) or ESRD. No dose adjustment is necessary for patients with mild hepatic impairment (Child-Pugh Class A). A reduced dose of 150 mg once daily is recommended in patients with moderate hepatic impairment (Child-Pugh Class B). No studies have been conducted in patients with severe hepatic impairment (Child-Pugh Class C). The most commonly reported adverse reactions are headache, sore throat, nasopharyngitis, URI, nasal congestion, abdominal pain, nausea, diarrhea, dizziness, and rash. Excretion of **Kalydeco** into human milk is probable. To report suspected adverse reactions, contact Vertex Pharmaceuticals at 1-877-752-5933 or FDA at 1-800-FDA-1088 or visit www.fda.gov/medwatch.

(CFTR) POTENTIATOR COMBINATIONS

▶ ***lumacaftor+ivacaftor*** (B) <6years: not recommended; 6-11 years: 2 x 100/125 tabs q 12 hours; ≥12 years: 2 x 200/125 tabs q 12 hours

Orkambi *Tab:* luma 100 mg+iva 125 mg; luma 200 mg+iva 125 mg film-coat

Comment: **Orkambi** is indicated for the treatment of CF in patients age ≥6 years-of-age who are homozygous for the F508del mutation in the CFTR gene. The efficacy and safety of **Orkambi** have not been established in patients with CF other than those homozygous for the F508del mutation. If the patient's genotype is unknown, an FDA-cleared CF mutation test should be used to detect the presence of the F508del mutation on both alleles of the CFTR gene. Reduce the dose of **Orkambi** in patients with moderate-to severe-hepatic impairment. In patients with advanced liver disease, with caution and only if the benefits are expected to outweigh the risks. When initiating **Orkambi** in patients taking strong CYP3A inhibitors, reduce the dose of **Orkambi** for the first week of treatment. There are limited and incomplete human data from clinical trials and postmarketing reports on use of **Orkambi** or its individual components in pregnacy to inform a drug-associated risk. There is no information regarding the presence of ***lumacaftor*** or ***ivacaftor*** in human milk or effects on the breastfed infant. To report suspected adverse reactions, contact Vertex Pharmaceuticals at 1-877-634-8789 or FDA at 1-800-FDA-1088 or visit www.fda.gov/medwatch

▶ ***tezacaftor+ivacaftor plus ivacaftor*** (B) <12 years: not established; ≥12 years: 1 x fixed dose100/150 tab in the morning and 1 x 150 mg ***ivacaflor*** tab in the evening, approx 12 hours later. Take with fat-containing food. Avoid grapefruit and Seville oranges.

Symdeko *Tab:* teza 100 mg+iva 150 mg, fixed-dose combination *plus Tab:* iva 150 mg (4-week supply/carton)

Comment: **Symdeko** is indicated for the treatment of the underlying cause of CF in patients ≥12 years-of-age who have two copies of the F508del mutation in the CFTR gene or who have ≥1 mutation that is responsive to ***tevacaftor+ivacaftor***. If the patient's genotype is unknown, an FDA-cleared CF mutation test should be used to detect the presence of a CFTR mutation followed by verification with bi-directional sequencing when recommended by the mutation test instructions for use. Reduce dose with moderate to severe hepatic impairment. Reduce dose when co-administered with drugs that are moderate or strong CYP3A inhibitors. There are limited and incomplete human data from clinical trials and post-marketing reports on the use of **Symdeko** in pregnancy to inform a drug-associated risk. There is no information regarding the presence of ***tezacaftor*** or ***ivacaftor*** in human milk or effects on the breastfed infant. To report suspected adverse reactions, contact Vertex Pharmaceuticals at 1-877-634-8789 or FDA at 1-800-FDA-1088 or visit www.fda.gov/medwatch

URSODEOXYCHOLIC ACID (UDCA)

Comment: Indicated for liver disease associated with cystic fibrosis in children 6-18 years-of-age.

▶ ***ursodeoxycholic acid*** (UDCA) **(G)** in the first 3 months of treatment, the total daily dose should be divided tid (morning, midday, evening); as liver function values improve, the total daily dose may be taken once a day at bedtime; (see mfr pkg insert for dose table based on kilograms weight); monitor hepatic function every 4 weeks for the first 3 months; then, monitor hepatic function once every 3 months

Ursofalk *Tab:* 500 mg film-coat; *Cap:* 250 mg, *Oral susp:* 250 mg/5 ml

Comment: **ursodeoxycholic (UDCA)** is indicated for the dissolution of cholesterol gall stones that are radioluscent (not visible on plain x-ray), <15 mm, and the gall bladder must still be functioning despite the gall stones.

ANTI-INFECTIVE

▶ ***ciprofloxacin*** (C) <18 years: 20-40 mg/kg/day divided q 12 hours; ≥18 years: 500 mg bid x 7-10 days; max 1.5 gm/day

Cipro (G) *Tab:* 250, 500, 750 mg; *Oral susp:* 250, 500 mg/5 ml (100 ml) (strawberry)

Cipro XR *Tab:* 500, 1000 mg ext-rel

ProQuin XR *Tab:* 500 mg ext-rel

DEEP VEIN THROMBOSIS (DVT) PROPHYLAXIS

Anticoagulation Therapy *see page* 565

DEHYDRATION

ORAL REHYDRATION AND ELECTROLYTE REPLACEMENT THERAPY

▶ ***oral electrolyte replacement*** (OTC)(G)

KaoLectrolyte <12 years: not indicated; ≥12 years: 1 pkt dissolved in 8 oz water q 3-4 hours

Pkt: sodium 12 mEq+potassium 5 mEq+chloride 10 mEq+citrate 7 mEq+dextrose 5 gm+calories 22 per 6.2 gm

Pedialyte <2 years: as desired and as tolerated; ≥2 years: 1-2 liters/day

Oral soln: dextrose 20 gm+fructose 5 gm+sodium 25 mEq+potassium 20 mEq+chloride 35 mEq+citrate 30 mEq+calories 100 per liter (8 oz, 1 L)

Pedialyte Freezer Pops as desired and as tolerated

Pops: dextrose 1.6 gm+sodium 2.8 mEq+potassium 1.25 mEq+chloride 2.2 mEq+citrate 1.88 mEq+calories 6.25 per 62.5 ml (2.1 fl oz) pop

DENGUE FEVER

Dengue is the most common arthropod-borne viral (arboviral) illness in humans. The Centers for Disease Control and Prevention reports that cases of dengue in returning US travelers have increased steadily during the past 20 years, and dengue has become the leading cause of acute febrile illness in US travelers returning from the Caribbean, South America, and Asia. Dengue is transmitted by mosquitoes of the genus *Aedes*, which are widely distributed in subtropical and tropical areas of the world. A small percentage of persons who have previously been infected by one dengue serotype develop bleeding and endothelial leak upon infection with another dengue serotype. This syndrome is termed "dengue hemorrhagic fever." Dengue fever is typically a self-limited disease, with a mortality rate of less than 1%. When treated, dengue hemorrhagic fever has a mortality rate of 2%-5%, but when left untreated, the mortality rate is as high as 50%. Dengue fever is usually a self-limited illness. Supportive care with analgesics, fluid replacement, and bed rest is usually sufficient. Acetaminophen may be used to treat fever and relieve other symptoms. Aspirin, nonsteroidal anti-inflammatory drugs (NSAIDs), and corticosteroids should be avoided. Management of severe dengue requires careful attention to fluid management and proactive treatment of hemorrhage. Single dose methylprednisolone showed no mortality benefit in the treatment of dengue shock syndrome in a prospective, randomized, double-blind, placebo-controlled trial. **There is no specific antiviral treatment currently available for dengue fever. No vaccine is currently approved <u>or</u> in drug trials for the prevention of dengue infection.** Because lack of immunity to a single dengue strain is the major risk factor for dengue hemorrhagic fever and dengue shock syndrome, a vaccine must provide high levels of immunity to all 4 dengue strains to be clinically useful.

A live attenuated tetravalent vaccine against dengue was effective against all four serotypes of the virus and well-tolerated among children, according to researchers. Interim results from a phase II study showed that children at four study sites in dengue-endemic areas of Asia and Latin America who received the vaccine all had significantly higher levels of antibody titers 18 months later. The vaccine (TAK-003 or TDV) is comprised of a molecularly cloned attenuated strain of dengue serotype 2 (DENV-2), and engineered strains of dengue serotypes 1, 3 and 4 (DENV-1, DENV-3 and DENV-4). Prior phase I and phase II data found the vaccine was well-tolerated and immunogenic against all four dengue serotypes. The trial will take 48 months to complete. The trial is ongoing at three sites in the Dominican Republic (n=535), Panama (n=935), and the Philippines (n=330). Participants are "healthy" children, ages 2 to 17 years, randomized into three groups plus a placebo group. A phase III efficacy trial for the vaccine, entitled Tetravalent Immunization against Dengue Efficacy Study (TIDES) is currently being conducted in eight dengue-endemic countries, with data available in late 2018.

REFERENCES

Sáez-Llorens, X, Tricou, V, Yu, D, *et al.* (2018). Immunogenicity and safety of one versus two doses of tetravalent dengue vaccine in healthy children aged 2–17 years in Asia and Latin America: 18-month interim data from a phase 2, randomised, placebo-controlled study. *The Lancet Infectious Diseases, 18*(2), 162–170. doi:10.1016/s1473-3099(17)30632-1

Tricou, V, *et al. Progress in development of Takeda's tetravelent dengue vaccine ASTMH 2017*. Paper presented at the 2017 American Society of Tropical Medicine & Hygiene.

Yoon, I.-K, & Thomas, SJ. (2018). Encouraging results but questions remain for dengue vaccine. *The Lancet Infectious Diseases, 18*(2), 125–126. doi:10.1016/s1473-3099(17)30634-5

DENTAL ABSCESS

▶ ***amoxicillin+clavulanate*** **(B)(G)**

Augmentin <40 kg: 40-45 mg/kg/day divided tid x 10 days or 90 mg/kg/day divided bid x 10 days; *see page* 590 *for dose by weight table;* ≥40 kg: 500 mg tid or 875 mg bid x 10 days

Tab: 250, 500, 875 mg; *Chew tab:* 125, 250 mg (lemon-lime); 200, 400 mg (cherry-banana) (phenylalanine); *Oral susp:* 125 mg/5 ml (banana), 250 mg/5 ml (75, 100, 150 ml) (orange); 200, 400 mg/5 ml (50, 75, 100 ml) (orange) (phenylalanine)

Augmentin ES-600 <3 months: not recommended; ≥3 months, <40 kg: 90 mg/kg/day divided q 12 hours x 10 days; *see page* 591 *for dose by weight table;* ≥40 kg: not recommended

Oral susp: 600 mg/5 ml (50, 75, 100, 125, 150, 200 ml) (strawberry cream) (phenylalanine)

Augmentin XR <16 years: use other forms; ≥16 years: 2 tabs q 12 hours x 7-10 days

Tab: 1000*mg ext-rel

▶ ***clindamycin*****(B)(G)** <12 years: 8-16 mg/kg/day in 3-4 divided doses x 10 days; *see page* 603 *for dose by weight table;* administer with TMP-SMX; ≥12 years: 300 mg qid x 10 days; administer with fluoroquinolone

Cleocin *Cap:* 75 (tartrazine), 150 (tartrazine), 300 mg

Cleocin Pediatric Granules *Oral susp:* 75 mg/5 ml (100 ml) (cherry)

▶ ***erythromycin base*** **(B)(G)** <45 kg: 50 mg/kg/day in 4 divided doses x 10-14 days; ≥45 kg: 500 mg q 6 hours x 10 days

Ery-Tab *Tab:* 250, 333, 500 mg ent-coat

PCE *Tab:* 333, 500 mg

▶ ***erythromycin ethylsuccinate*** **(B)(G)** 30-50 mg/kg/day in 4 divided doses x 7 days; may double dose with severe infection; max 100 mg/kg/day or 400 mg qid; *see page* 607 *for dose by weight table*

EryPed *Oral susp:* 200 mg/5 ml (100, 200 ml) (fruit); 400 mg/5 ml (60, 100, 200 ml) (banana); *Oral drops:* 200, 400 mg/5 ml (50 ml) (fruit); *Chew tab:* 200 mg wafer (fruit)

E.E.S. *Oral susp:* 200, 400 mg/5 ml (100 ml) (fruit)

E.E.S. Granules *Oral susp:* 200 mg/5 ml (100, 200 ml) (cherry)

E.E.S. 400 Tablets *Tab:* 400 mg

▶ ***penicillin V potassium*** **(B)** <12 years: 25-75 mg/kg day divided q 6-8 hours x 5-7 days; *see page 616 for dose by weight table;* ≥12 years: 250-500 mg q 6 hours x 5-7 days

Pen-VK *Tab:* 250, 500 mg; *Oral soln:* 125 mg/5 ml (100, 200 ml); 250 mg/5 ml(100, 150, 200 ml)

DEPRESSION/MAJOR DEPRESSIVE DISORDER (MDD)

Comment: Abrupt withdrawal or interruption of treatment with an antidepressant medication is sometimes associated with an *antidepressant discontinuation syndrome* which may be mediated by gradually tapering the drug over a period of two weeks or longer, depending on the dose strength and length of treatment. Common symptoms of antidepressant withdrawal include flu-like symptoms, insomnia, nausea, imbalance, sensory disturbances, and hyperarousal. These medications include SSRIs, TCAs, MAOIs, and atypical agents such as ***venlafaxine*** **(Effexor)**, ***mirtazapine*** **(Remeron)**, ***trazodone*** **(Desyrel)**, and ***duloxetine*** **(Cymbalta)**. Common symptoms of the *serotonin discontinuation syndrome* include flu-like symptoms (nausea, vomiting, diarrhea, headaches, sweating), sleep disturbances (insomnia, nightmares, constant sleepiness), mood disturbances (dysphoria, anxiety, agitation), cognitive disturbances (mental confusion, hyperarousal), sensory and movement disturbances (imbalance, tremors, vertigo, dizziness, electric-shock-like sensations in the brain, often described by sufferers as "brain zaps").

SELECTIVE SEROTONIN REUPTAKE INHIBITORS (SSRIs)

Comment: Co-administration of SSRIs with TCAs requires extreme caution. Concomitant use of MAOIs and SSRIs is absolutely contraindicated. Avoid St. John's wort and other serotonergic agents. A potentially fatal adverse event is *serotonin syndrome*, caused by serotonin excess. Milder symptoms require HCP intervention to avert severe symptoms that can be rapidly fatal without urgent/emergent medical care. Symptoms include restlessness, agitation, confusion, tachycardia, hypertension, dilated pupils, muscle twitching, muscle rigidity, loss of muscle coordination, diaphoresis, diarrhea, headache, shivering, piloerection, hyperpyrexia, cardiac arrhythmias, seizures, loss of consciousness, coma, death. Common symptoms of the *serotonin discontinuation syndrome* include flu-like symptoms (nausea, vomiting, diarrhea, headaches, sweating), sleep disturbances (insomnia, nightmares, constant sleepiness), mood disturbances (dysphoria, anxiety, agitation), cognitive disturbances (mental confusion, hyperarousal, hallucinations), sensory and movement disturbances (imbalance, tremors, vertigo, dizziness, electric-shock-like sensations in the brain, often described by sufferers as "brain zaps").

▶ ***citalopram*** **(C)(G)** <12 years: not recommended; ≥12 years: initially 20 mg once daily; may increase after one week to 40 mg once daily; max 40 mg

Celexa *Tab:* 10, 20, 40 mg; *Oral soln:* 10 mg/5 ml (120 ml) (pepper mint) (sugar-free, alcohol-free, parabens)

▶ ***escitalopram*** **(C)(G)** <12 years: not recommended; 12-17 years: initially 10 mg daily; may increase to 20 mg daily after 3 weeks; >17 years: initially 10 mg daily; may increase to 20 mg daily after 1 week; *Hepatic impairment:* 10 mg once daily

Lexapro *Tab:* 5, 10*, 20*mg

Lexapro Oral Solution *Oral soln:* 1 mg/ml (240 ml) (peppermint) (parabens)

▶ *fluoxetine* (C)(G)

Prozac <8 years: not recommended; 8-17 years: initially 10 mg/day; may increase after 1 week to 20 mg/day; range 20-60 mg/day; range for lower weight children, 20-30 mg/day; >17 years: initially 20 mg daily; may increase after 1 week; doses >20 mg/day should be divided into AM and noon doses; max 80 mg/day

Cap: 10, 20, 40 mg; *Tab:* 30*, 60*mg; *Oral soln:* 20 mg/5 ml (4 oz) (mint)

Prozac Weekly <12 years: not recommended; ≥12 years: following daily ***fluoxetine*** therapy at 20 mg/day for 13 weeks, may initiate **Prozac Weekly** 7 days after the last 20 mg ***fluoxetine*** dose

Cap: 90 mg ent-coat del-rel pellets

▶ ***levomilnacipran*** (C) <12 years: not recommended; ≥12 years: swallow whole; initially 20 mg once daily for 2 days; then increase to 40 mg once daily; may increase dose in 40 mg increments at intervals of ≥2 days; max 120 mg once daily; *CrCl 30-59 mL/min:* max 80 mg oWnce daily; *CrCl 15-29 mL/min:* max 40 mg once daily

Fetzima *Cap:* 20, 40, 80, 120 mg ext-rel

▶ ***paroxetine maleate*** (D)(G)

Paxil <12 years: not recommended; ≥12 years: initially 20 mg daily in AM; may increase by 10 mg/day at weekly intervals as needed; max 60 mg/day

Tab: 10*, 20*, 30, 40 mg

Paxil CR <12 years: not recommended; ≥12 years: initially 25 mg daily in AM; may increase by 12.5 mg at weekly intervals as needed; max 62.5 mg/day

Tab: 12.5, 25, 37.5 mg cont-rel ent-coat

Paxil Suspension <12 years: not recommended; ≥12 years: initially 20 mg daily in AM; may increase by 10 mg/day at weekly intervals as needed; max 60 mg/day

Oral susp: 10 mg/5 ml (250 ml) (orange)

▶ ***paroxetine mesylate*** (D)(G) <12 years: not recommended; ≥12 years: initially 7.5 mg daily in AM; may increase by 10 mg/day at weekly intervals as needed; max 60 mg/day

Brisdelle *Cap:* 7.5 mg

▶ ***sertraline*** (C)(G) <6 years: not recommended; 6-<12 years: initially 25 mg daily; max 200 mg/day; 12-17 years: initially 50 mg daily; max 200 mg/day; >17 years: initially 50 mg daily; increase at 1 week intervals if needed; max 200 mg daily; dilute oral concentrate immediately prior to administration in 4 oz water, ginger ale, lemon lime soda, lemonade, <u>or</u> orange juice

Zoloft *Tab:* 25*, 50*, 100*mg; *Oral conc:* 20 mg per ml (60 ml) (alcohol 12%)

SEROTONIN-NOREPINEPHRINE REUPTAKE INHIBITORS (SNRIs)

▶ ***desvenlafaxine*** (C)(G) <18 years: not recommended; ≥18 years: swallow whole; initially 50 mg once daily; max 120 mg/day

Pristiq *Tab:* 50, 100 mg ext-rel

▶ ***duloxetine*** (C)(G) <12 years: not recommended; ≥12 years: swallow whole; initially 30 mg once daily x 1 week; then, increase to 60 mg once daily; max 120 mg/day

Cymbalta *Cap:* 20, 30, 40, 60 mg del-rel

▶ ***venlafaxine*** (C)(G)

Effexor initially <18 years: not recommended; ≥18 years: 75 mg/day in 2-3 divided doses; may increase at 4 day intervals in 75 mg increments to 150 mg/day; max 225 mg/day

Tab: 37.5, 75, 150, 225 mg

Effexor XR <18 years: not recommended; ≥18 years: initially 75 mg q AM; may start at 37.5 mg daily x 4-7 days, then increase by increments of up to 75 mg/day at intervals of at least 4 days; usual max 375 mg/day

Tab/Cap: 37.5, 75, 150 mg ext-rel

- *vortioxetine* (C) <18 years: not established; ≥18 years: initially 10 mg once daily; max 30 mg/day
  Brintellix *Tab:* 5, 10, 15, 20 mg

SELECTIVE SEROTONIN REUPTAKE INHIBITOR (SSRI) + 5HT-14 RECEPTOR PARTIAL AGONIST COMBINATION

- *vilazodone* (C) <18 years: not established; ≥18 years: take with food; initially 10 mg once daily x 7 days; then, 20 mg once daily x 7 days; then, 40 mg once daily
  Viibryd *Tab:* 10, 20, 40 mg

THIENOBENZODIAZEPINE+SSRI COMBINATION

- *olanzapine+fluoxetine* (C) <10 years: not established; ≥10 years: initially one 6/25 cap in the PM; titrate; max one 18/75 cap once daily in the PM
  Symbyax
  Cap: **Symbyax 3/25** olan 3 mg+fluo 25 mg
  Symbyax 6/25 olan 6 mg+fluo 25 mg
  Symbyax 6/50 olan 6 mg+fluo 50 mg
  Symbyax 12/25 olan 12 mg+fluo 25 mg
  Symbyax 12/50 olan 12 mg+fluo 50 mg
  Comment: **Symbyax** is a thienobenzodiazepine-SSRI indicated for the treatment of depressive episodes associated with bipolar depression disorder and treatment resistant depression (TRD).

TRICYCLIC ANTIDEPRESSANTS (TCAs)

Comment: Co-administration of SSRIs and TCAs requires extreme caution.

- *amitriptyline* (C)(G) <12 years: not recommended; ≥12 years: 10-20 mg q HS
  Tab: 10, 25, 50, 75, 100, 150 mg
- *amoxapine* (C) <12 years: not recommended; ≥12 years: initially 50 mg bid-tid; after 1 week may increase to 100 mg bid-tid; usual effective dose 200-300 mg/day; if total dose exceeds 300 mg/day, give in divided doses (max 400 mg/day); may give as a single bedtime dose (max 300 mg q HS)
  Tab: 25, 50, 100, 150 mg
- *clomipramine* (C)(G) <10 years: not recommended; 10-<16 years: initially 25 mg daily in divided doses; gradually increase; max 3 mg/kg or 100 mg, whichever is smaller; >16 years: initially 25 mg daily in divided doses; gradually increase to 100 mg during first 2 weeks; max 250 mg/day; total maintenance dose may be given at HS
  Anafranil *Cap:* 25, 50, 75 mg
- *desipramine* (C)(G) <12 years: not recommended; ≥12 years: 100-200 mg/day in single or divided doses; max 300 mg/day
  Norpramin *Tab:* 10, 25, 50, 75, 100, 150 mg
- *doxepin* (C)(G) <12 years: not recommended; ≥12 years: 75 mg/day; max 150 mg/day
  Cap: 10, 25, 50, 75, 100, 150 mg; Oral conc: 10 mg/ml (4 oz w. dropper)
- *imipramine* (C)(G) <12 years: not recommended; ≥12 years:
  Tofranil initially 75 mg daily (max 200 mg); adolescents initially 30-40 mg daily (max 100 mg/day); if maintenance dose exceeds 75 mg daily, may switch to **Tofranil PM** for divided or bedtime dose
  Tab: 10, 25, 50 mg
  Tofranil PM initially 75 mg daily 1 hour before HS; max 200 mg
  Cap: 75, 100, 125, 150 mg
- *nortriptyline* (D)(G) <12 years: not recommended; ≥12 years: initially 25 mg tid-qid; max 150 mg/day
  Pamelor *Cap:* 10, 25, 50, 75 mg; *Oral soln:* 10 mg/5 ml (16 oz)

▶ ***protriptyline*** (C) <12 years: not recommended; ≥12 years: initially 5 mg tid; usual dose 15-40 mg/day in 3-4 divided doses; max 60 mg/day

Vivactil *Tab:* 5, 10 mg

▶ ***trimipramine*** (C) <12 years: not recommended; ≥12 years: initially 75 mg/day in divided doses; max 200 mg/day

Surmontil *Cap:* 25, 50, 100 mg

AMINOKETONES

▶ ***bupropion HBr*** (C)(G)

Comment: Safety and effectiveness in the pediatric population have not been established. When considering the use of ***bupropion*** in a child or adolescent, balance the potential risks with the clinical need

Aplenzin <18 years: not recommended; ≥18 years: initially 100 mg bid for at least 3 days; may increase to 375 or 400 mg/day after several weeks; then after at least 3 more days, 450 mg in 4 divided doses; max 450 mg/day, 174 mg/single-dose

Tab: 174, 348, 522 mg

▶ ***bupropion HCl*** (C)(G)

Comment: Safety and effectiveness in the pediatric population have not been established. When considering the use of ***bupropion*** in a child or adolescent, balance the potential risks with the clinical need

Forfivo XL <18 years: not recommended; ≥18 years: do not use for initial treatment; use immediate-release bupropion forms for initial titration; switch to **Forfivo XL** 450 mg once daily when total dose/day reaches 450 mg; may switch to **Forfivo XL** when total dose/day reaches 300 mg for 2 weeks and patient needs 450 mg/day to reach therapeutic target; swallow whole, do not crush or chew

Tab: 450 mg ext-rel

Wellbutrin <18 years: not recommended; ≥18 years: initially 100 mg bid for at least 3 days; may increase to 375 or 400 mg/day after several weeks; then after at least 3 more days, 450 mg in 4 divided doses; max 450 mg/day, 150 mg/single-dose

Tab: 75, 100 mg

Wellbutrin SR <18 years: not recommended; ≥18 years: initially 150 mg in AM for at least 3 days; increase to 150 mg bid if well tolerated; usual dose 300 mg/day; max 400 mg/day

Tab: 100, 150 mg sust-rel

Wellbutrin XL <18 years: not recommended; ≥18 years: initially 150 mg in AM for at least 3 days; increase to 150 mg bid if well tolerated; usual dose 300 mg/day; max 450 mg/day

Tab: 150, 300 mg sust-rel

MONOAMINE OXIDASE INHIBITORS (MAOIs)

Comment: Many drug and food interactions with this class of drugs; use cautiously. Should be reserved for refractory depression that has not responded to other classes of antidepressants. Concomitant use of MAOIs and SSRIs is an absolute contraindication. See mfr pkg insert for drug and food interactions.

▶ ***isocarboxazid*** (C)(G) <16 years: not recommended; ≥16 years: initially 10 mg bid; increase by 10 mg every 2-4 days up to 40 mg/day; may increase by 20 mg/week to max 60 mg/day divided bid-qid

Marplan *Tab:* 10 mg

▶ ***phenelzine*** (C)(G) <16 years: not recommended; ≥16 years: initially 15 mg tid; max 90 mg/day

Nardil *Tab:* 15 mg

▻ *selegiline* (C) initially 10 mg tid; max 60 mg/day

Emsam *Transdermal patch:* 6 mg/24 Hr, 9 mg/24 Hr, 12 mg/24 Hr

Comment: With the **Emsam** transdermal patch 6 mg/24 Hr dose, the dietary restrictions commonly required when using non-selective MAOIs are not necessary.

▻ *tranylcypromine* (C) initially 10 mg tid; may increase in 10 mg/day every 1-3 weeks; max 60 mg/day

Parnate *Tab:* 10 mg

TETRACYCLICS

▻ *maprotiline* (B)(G) <18 years: not recommended; ≥18 years: initially 75 mg/day for 2 weeks then change gradually as needed in 25 mg increments; max 225 mg/day

Ludiomil *Tab:* 25, 50, 75 mg

▻ *mirtazapine* (C) <12 years: not recommended; ≥12 years: initially 15 mg q HS; increase at intervals of 1-2 weeks; usual range 15-45 mg/day; max 45 mg/day

Remeron *Tab:* 15*, 30*, 45*mg

Remeron SolTab *ODT:* 15, 30, 45 mg (orange) (phenylalanine)

▻ *chlordiazepoxide+amitriptyline* (C)(IV)

Limbitrol <12 years: not recommended; ≥12 years: 3-4 tabs in divided doses

Tab: chlor 5 mg+amit 12.5 mg

Limbitrol DS <18 years: not recommended; ≥18 years: 3-4 tabs in divided doses; max 6 tabs/day

Tab: chlor 10 mg+amit 25 mg

▻ *trazodone* (C)(G) <18 years: not recommended; ≥18 years: initially 150 mg/day in divided doses with food; increase by 50 mg/day q 3-4 days; max 400 mg/day in divided doses or 50-400 mg at HS

ATYPICAL ANTIPSYCHOTICS

▻ *aripiprazole* (C)(G) <10 years: not recommended; 10-17 years: initially 2 mg/day for 2 days; then, increase to 5 mg/day for 2 days; then, increase to target dose of 10 mg/day; may increase by 5 mg/day at 1 week intervals as needed to max 30 mg/day; >17 years: initially 15 mg daily; may increase to max 30 mg/day

Abilify *Tab:* 2, 5, 10, 15, 20, 30 mg

Abilify Discmelt *Tab:* 15 mg orally disintegrating (vanilla) (phenylalanine)

Abilify Maintena *Vial:* 300, 400 mg ext-rel pwdr for IM injection after reconstitution; 300, 400 mg single-dose prefilled dual-chamber syringes w. supplies

Comment: **Abilify** is indicated for acute and maintenance treatment of manic or mixed episodes in bipolar I disorder, as monotherapy or as an adjunct to ***lithium*** or ***valproate***, as adjunct to antidepressants for major depressive disorder (MDD), and for irritability associated with autistic disorder.

▻ *brexpiprazole* (C) <12 years: not recommended; ≥12 years: initially 0.5 or 1 mg once daily; titrate weekly up to target 2 mg/day; max 3 mg/day; *Moderate-severe hepatic impairment, renal impairment, or ESRD:* max 2 mg/day

Rexulti *Tab:* 0.25, 0.5, 1, 2, 3, 4 mg

DERMATITIS: ATOPIC (ECZEMA)

Parenteral Corticosteroids *see page* 547
Oral Corticosteroids *see page* 546
Topical Corticosteroids *see page* 542

PHOSPHODIESTERASE 4 INHIBITOR

▻ ***crisaborole 2%*** (C) apply sparingly bid; max 4 weeks
Pediatric: <2 years: not recommended; ≥2 years: same as adult
Eucrisa *Oint:* 2% (60 gm)

MOISTURIZING AGENTS

Aquaphor Healing Ointment (OTC) *Oint:* 1.75, 3.5, 14 oz (alcohol)
Eucerin Daily Sun Defense (OTC) *Lotn:* 6 oz (fragrance-free)
Comment: **Eucerin Daily Sun Defense** is a moisturizer with SPF-15 sunscreen.
Eucerin Facial Lotion (OTC) *Lotn:* 4 oz
Eucerin Light Lotion (OTC) *Lotn:* 8 oz
Eucerin Lotion (OTC) *Lotn:* 8, 16 oz
Eucerin Original Creme (OTC) *Crm:* 2, 4, 16 oz (alcohol)
Eucerin Plus Creme (OTC) *Crm:* 4 oz
Eucerin Plus Lotion (OTC) *Lotn:* 6, 12 oz
Eucerin Protective Lotion (OTC) *Lotn:* 4 oz (alcohol)
Comment: **Eucerin Protective Lotion** is a moisturizer with SPF-25 sunscreen.
Lac-Hydrin Cream (OTC) *Crm:* 280, 385 gm
Lac-Hydrin Lotion (OTC) *Lotn:* 25, 400 gm
Lubriderm Dry Skin Scented (OTC) *Lotn:* 6, 10, 16, 32 oz
Lubriderm Dry Skin Unscented (OTC) *Lotn:* 3.3, 6, 10, 16 oz (fragrance-free)
Lubriderm Sensitive Skin Lotion (OTC) *Lotn:* 3.3, 6, 10, 16 oz (lanolin-free)
Lubriderm Dry Skin (OTC) *Lotn (scented)*: 2.5, 6, 10, 16 oz;
Lotn (fragrance-free): 1, 2.5, 6, 10, 16 oz
Lubriderm Bath 1-2 capfuls in bath or rub onto wet skin as needed, then rinse
Oil: 8 oz
Moisturel apply as needed
Crm: 4, 16 oz; *Lotn:* 8, 12 oz; *Clnsr:* 8.75 oz

OATMEAL COLLOIDS

Aveeno (OTC) add to bath as needed
Regular: 1.5 oz (8/pck); *Moisturizing:* 0.75 oz (8/pck)
Aveeno Oil (OTC) add to bath as needed
Oil: 8 oz
Aveeno Moisturizing (OTC) apply as needed
Lotn: 2.5, 8, 12 oz; *Crm:* 4 oz
Aveeno Cleansing Bar (OTC) *Bar:* 3 oz
Aveeno Gentle Skin Cleanser (OTC) *Liq clnsr:* 6 oz

TOPICAL OIL

▻ ***fluocinolone acetamide*** 0.01% topical oil (C)
Derma-Smoothe/FS Topical Oil <6 years: not recommended; 6-12 years: apply sparingly bid for up to 4 weeks; >12 years: apply sparingly tid
Topical oil: 0.01% (4 oz) (peanut oil)

TOPICAL STEROIDS

(For other topical steroids, *see* **Topical Corticosteroids** *page* 542)
Comment: Topical steroids should be applied sparingly and for the shortest time necessary. Do not use in the diaper area. Do not use an occlusive dressing. Systemic

absorption of topical corticosteroids can induce reversible hypothalamic-pituitary-adrenal (HPA) axis suppression with the potential for clinical corticosteroid insufficiency.

▶ ***desonide*** 0.05% topical gel **(C)** apply sparingly bid-tid; max 4 weeks
Pediatric: <3 months: not recommended; ≥3 months: same as adult
Desonate *Gel:* 0.05% (60 gm) (89% purified water; fragrance-free, surfactant-free, alcohol-free)

SECOND GENERATION ORAL ANTIHISTAMINES

Comment: Second generation antihistamines are sedating, but much less so than the first generation antihistamines. All antihistamines are excreted into breast milk.

▶ ***cetirizine*** (C)(OTC)(G) <6 years: not recommended; ≥6-<65 years: initially 5-10 mg once daily; ≥65 years: 5 mg once daily
Children's Zyrtec Chewable *Chew tab:* 5, 10 mg (grape)
Children's Zyrtec Allergy Syrup *Syr:* 1 mg/ml (4 oz) (grape, bubble gum) (sugar-free, dye-free)
Zyrtec *Tab:* 10 mg
Zyrtec Hives Relief *Tab:* 10 mg
Zyrtec Liquid Gels *Liq gel:* 10 mg

▶ ***desloratadine*** (C)
Clarinex <6 years: not recommended; ≥6 years: 1/2-1 tab once daily
Tab: 5 mg
Clarinex RediTabs <6 years: not recommended; 6-12 years: 2.5 mg once daily; ≥12 years: 5 mg once daily
ODT: 2.5, 5 mg (tutti-frutti) (phenylalanine)
Clarinex Syrup <6 months: not recommended; 6-11 months: 1 mg (2 ml) once daily; 1-5 years: 1.25 mg (2.5 ml) once daily; 6-11 years: 2.5 mg (5 ml) once aily; ≥12 years: 5 mg (10 ml) once daily
Tab: 0.5 mg per ml (4 oz) (tutti-frutti) (phenylalanine)
Desloratadine ODT

▶ ***fexofenadine*** (C)(OTC)(G) 6 months-2 years: 15 mg bid; *CrCl ≤90 mL/min:* 15 mg once daily; 2-11 years: 30 mg bid; *CrCl ≤90 mL/min:* 30 mg once daily ≥12 years and older: ≥12 years: 60 mg once daily-bid or 180 mg once daily; *CrCl <90 mL/min:* 60 mg once daily **Allegra** *Tab:* 30, 60, 180 mg film-coat
Allegra Allergy *Tab:* 60, 180 mg film-coat
Allegra ODT *ODT:* 30 mg (phenylalanine)
Allegra Oral Suspension *Oral susp:* 30 mg/5 ml (6 mg/ml) (4 oz)

▶ ***levocetirizine*** (B)(OTC) administer dose in the PM; *Seasonal Allergic Rhinitis:* <2 years: not recommended; may start at ≥2 years; *Chronic Spontaneous/Idiopathic Urticaria (CSU/CIU), Perennial Allergic Rhinitis:* <6 months: not recommended; may start at ≥6 months; *Dosing by Age:* 6 months-5 years: max 1.25 mg once daily; 6-11 years: max 2.5 mg once daily; ≥12 years: 2.5-5 mg once daily; *Renal Dysfunction <12 years:* contraindicated; *Renal Dysfunction ≥12 years: CrCl 50-80 mL/min:* 2.5 mg once daily; *CrCl 30-50 mL/min:* 2.5 mg every other day; *CrCl: 10-30 mL/min:* 2.5 mg twice weekly (every 3-4 days); *CrCl <10 mL/min, ESRD or hemodialysis:* contraindicated
Children's Xyzal Allergy 24HR *Oral Soln:* 0.5 mg/ml (150 ml)
Xyzal Allergy 24HR *Tab:* 5*mg

▶ ***loratadine*** (C)(OTC)(G) <2 years: not recommended; 2-5 years: 5 mg once daily; ≥6 years: 5 mg bid or 10 mg once daily; *Hepatic or Renal Insufficiency:* (see mfr pkg insert)

Children's Claritin Chewables *Chew tab:* 5 mg (grape) (phenylalanine)
Children's Claritin Syrup 1 mg/ml (4 oz) (fruit) (sugar-free, alcohol-free, dye-free; sodium 6 mg/5 ml)
Claritin *Tab:* 10 mg
Claritin Hives Relief *Tab:* 10 mg
Claritin Liqui-Gels *Liq gel:* 10 mg
Claritin RediTabs 12 Hours *ODT:* 5 mg (mint)
Claritin RediTabs 24 Hours *ODT:* 10 mg (mint)

FIRST GENERATION ANTIHISTAMINES

▶ ***diphenhydramine*** **(B)(G)** <2 years: not recommended; 2-6 years: 6.25 mg q 4-6 hours; max 37.5 mg/day; >6-12 years: 12.5-25 mg q 4-6 hours; max 150 mg/day; >12 years: 25-50 mg q 6-8 hours; max 100 mg/day
Benadryl (OTC) *Chew tab:* 12.5 mg (grape) (phenylalanine); *Liq:* 12.5 mg/5 ml (4, 8 oz); *Cap:* 25 mg; *Tab:* 25 mg; *Dye-free soft gel:* 25 mg; *Dye-free liq:* 12.5 mg/5 ml (4, 8 oz)

▶ ***diphenhydramine injectable*** **(B)(G)** <12 years: *See mfr pkg insert:* 1.25 mg/kg up to 25 mg IM x 1 dose; then q 6 hours prn; ≥12 years: 25-50 mg IM immediately; then q 6 hours prn
Benadryl Injectable *Vial:* 50 mg/ml (1 ml single-use); 50 mg/ml (10 ml multi-dose);
Amp: 10 mg/ml (1 ml); *Prefilled syringe:* 50 mg/ml (1 ml)

▶ ***hydroxyzine*** **(C)(G)** <6 years: 50 mg/day divided qid prn; ≥6 years: 50-100 mg/day divided qid prn; max 600 mg/day; 25 mg tid prn; max 600 mg/day
AtaraxR *Tab:* 10, 25, 50, 100 mg; *Syr:* 10 mg/5 ml (alcohol 0.5%)
Vistaril *Cap:* 25, 50, 100 mg; *Oral susp:* 25 mg/5 ml (4 oz) (lemon)
Comment: hydroxyzine is contraindicated in early pregnancy and in patients with a prolonged QT interval. It is not known whether this drug is excreted in human milk; therefore, hydroxyzine should not be given to nursing mothers.

TOPICAL ANALGESICS

▶ ***capsaicin*** cream **(B)(G)** <2 years: not recommended; 2-12 years: apply sparingly to intact skin bid prn; >12 years: apply tid-qid prn
Axsain *Crm:* 0.075% (1, 2 oz)
Capsin (OTC) *Lotn:* 0.025, 0,075% (59 ml)
Capzasin-P (OTC) *Crm:* 0.025% (1.5 oz); *Lotn:* 0.025% (2 oz)
Capzasin-HP (OTC) *Crm:* 0.075% (1.5 oz); *Lotn:* 0.075% (2 oz)
Dolorac *Crm:* 0.025% (28 gm)
Double Cap (OTC) *Crm:* 0.05% (2 oz)
R-Gel *Gel:* 0.025% (15, 30 gm)
Zostrix (OTC) *Crm:* 0.025% (0.7, 1.5, 3 oz)
Zostrix HP (OTC) *Emol crm:* 0.075% (1, 2 oz)
Comment: Provides some relief by 1-2 weeks; optimal benefit may take 4-6 weeks. Avoid contact with mucous membranes.

▶ ***doxepin*** cream **(B)** <12 years: not recommended; ≥12 years: apply to affected area qid at intervals of at least 3-4 hours; max 8 days
Prudoxin *Crm:* 5% (45 gm)
Zonalon *Crm:* 5% (30, 45 gm)

▶ ***pimecrolimus*** 1% cream **(C)** <2 years: not recommended; ≥2 years: apply to affected area bid; do not occlude
Elidel *Crm:* 1% (30, 60, 100 gm)

Comment: ***pimecrolimus*** is indicated for short-term and intermittent long-term use. Discontinue use when resolution occurs. Contraindicated if the patient is immunosuppressed. Change to the 0.1% preparation or if secondary bacterial infection is present.

▶ ***tacrolimus*** **(C)** <2 years: not recommended; 2-15 years: use 0.03% strength; apply to affected area bid; continue for 1 week after clearing; >15 years: apply to affected area bid; do not occlude or apply to wet skin; continue for 1 week after clearing

Protopic *Oint:* 0.03, 0.1% (30, 60, 100 gm)

▶ ***trolamine salicylate*** <2 years: not recommended; ≥2 years: apply tid-qid prn to intact skin

Mobisyl *Crm:* 10%

Comment: Provides some relief by 1-2 weeks; optimal benefit may take 4-6 weeks.

TOPICAL ANESTHETIC

▶ ***lidocaine*** **(B)** reduce dosage commensurate with age, body weight, and physical condition (see pkg insert); apply to affected area bid-tid prn

Lidoderm *Crm:* 3% (85 gm)

INTERLEUKIN-4 RECEPTOR ALPHA ANTAGONIST

▶ ***dupilumab*** <18 years: not recommended; ≥18 years: administer SC into the upper arm, abdomen, or thigh; rotate sites; initially 600 mg (2 x 300 mg injections at different sites) followed by 300 mg SC once every other week; may use with or without topical corticosteroids; may use with calcineurin inhibitors, but reserve only for problem areas (e.g., face, neck, intertriginous, and genital areas); avoid live vaccines.

Dupixent Prefill syr: 300 mg/2 ml (2/pck without needle) (preservative-free)

Comment: ***dupilumab*** is a human monoclonal IgG4 antibody that inhibits interleukin-4 (IL-4) and interleukin-13 (IL-13) signaling by specifically binding to the IL4Rα subunit shared by the IL-4 and IL-13 receptor complexes, thereby inhibiting the release of pro-inflammatory cytokines, chemokines, and IgE. ***dupilumab*** is indicated for moderate-to-severe atopic dermatitis in patients who are not adequately controlled with topical prescription therapies or when they are not advisable.

DERMATITIS: CONTACT

Topical Corticosteroids *see page* 542
Parenteral Corticosteroids *see page* 547
Oral Corticosteroids *see page* 546

PROPHYLAXIS

▶ ***bentoquatam*** <6 years: not recommended; ≥6 years: apply as a wet film to exposed skin at least 15 minutes prior to possible contact; reapply at least q 4 hours; remove with soap and water

IvyBlock (OTC) *Soln:* 120 ml

Comment: Provides protection against genus rhus (poison ivy, oak, and sumac).

TREATMENT

Oatmeal Colloids

Aveeno (OTC) add to bath as needed

Regular: 1.5 oz (8/pck); *Moisturizing*: 0.75 oz (8/pck)

Aveeno Oil (OTC) add to bath as needed
Oil: 8 oz
Aveeno Moisturizing (OTC) apply as needed
Lotn: 2.5, 8, 12 oz; *Crm:* 4 oz
Aveeno Cleansing Bar (OTC) *Bar:* 3 oz
Aveeno Gentle Skin Cleanser (OTC) *Liq clnsr:* 6 oz

SECOND GENERATION ORAL ANTIHISTAMINES

Comment: The following drugs are second generation antihistamines. As such they minimally sedating, much less so than the first generation antihistamines. All antihistamines are excreted into breast milk.

▶ ***cetirizine*** (C)(OTC)(G) <6 years: not recommended; ≥6-<65 years: initially 5-10 mg once daily; ≥65 years: 5 mg once daily
Children's Zyrtec Chewable *Chew tab:* 5, 10 mg (grape)
Children's Zyrtec Allergy Syrup *Syr:* 1 mg/ml (4 oz) (grape, bubble gum) (sugar-free, dye-free)
Zyrtec *Tab:* 10 mg
Zyrtec Hives Relief *Tab:* 10 mg
Zyrtec Liquid Gels *Liq gel:* 10 mg

▶ ***desloratadine*** (C)
Clarinex <6 years: not recommended; ≥6 years: 1/2-1 tab once daily
Tab: 5 mg
Clarinex RediTabs <6 years: not recommended; 6-12 years: 2.5 mg once daily; ≥12 years: 5 mg once daily
ODT: 2.5, 5 mg (tutti-frutti) (phenylalanine)
Clarinex Syrup <6 months: not recommended; 6-11 months: 1 mg (2 ml) once daily; 1-5 years: 1.25 mg (2.5 ml) once daily; 6-11 years: 2.5 mg (5 ml) once daily; ≥12 years: 5 mg (10 ml) once daily
Tab: 0.5 mg per ml (4 oz) (tutti-frutti) (phenylalanine)
Desloratadine ODT <6 years: not recommended; 6-11 years: ½ tab once daily; ≥12 years: 1 tab once daily
ODT: 5 mg

▶ ***fexofenadine*** (C)(OTC)(G) <6 months: not recommended; 6 months-<2 years: 15 mg bid; *CrCl ≤90 mL/min:* 15 mg once daily; 2-11 years: 30 mg bid; *CrCl ≤90 mL/min:* 30 mg once daily; ≥12 years: 60 mg once daily-bid or 180 mg once daily; *CrCl <90 mL/min:* 60 mg once daily **Allegra** *Tab:* 30, 60, 180 mg film-coat
Allegra Allergy *Tab:* 60, 180 mg film-coat
Allegra ODT *ODT:* 30 mg (phenylalanine)
Allegra Oral Suspension *Oral susp:* 30 mg/5 ml (6 mg/ml) (4 oz)

▶ ***levocetirizine*** (B)(OTC) administer dose in the PM; *Seasonal Allergic Rhinitis:* <2 years: not recommended; may start at ≥2 years; *Chronic Spontaneous/Idiopathic Urticaria (CSU/CIU), Perennial Allergic Rhinitis:* <6 months: not recommended; may start at ≥ 6 months; *Dosing by Age:* 6 months-5 years: max 1.25 mg once daily; 6-11 years: max 2.5 mg once daily; ≥12 years: 2.5-5 mg once daily; *Renal Dysfunction <12 years:* contraindicated; *Renal Dysfunction ≥12 years: CrCl 50-80 mL/min:* 2.5 mg once daily; *CrCl 30-50 mL/min:* 2.5 mg every other day; *CrCl: 10-30 mL/min:* 2.5 mg twice weekly (every 3-4 days); *CrCl <10 mL/min, ESRD or hemodialysis:* contraindicated;
Children's Xyzal Allergy 24HR *Oral Soln:* 0.5 mg/ml (150 ml)
Xyzal Allergy 24HR *Tab:* 5*mg

▶ ***loratadine*** (C)(OTC)(G) <2 years: not recommended; 2-5 years: 5 mg once daily; ≥6 years: 5 mg bid or 10 mg once daily; *Hepatic or Renal Insufficiency:* (see mfr pkg insert)

Children's Claritin Chewables *Chew tab:* 5 mg (grape) (phenylalanine)
Children's Claritin Syrup 1 mg/ml (4 oz) (fruit) (sugar-free, alcohol-free, dye-free; sodium 6 mg/5 ml)
Claritin *Tab:* 10 mg
Claritin Hives Relief *Tab:* 10 mg
Claritin Liqui-Gels *Liq gel:* 10 mg
Claritin RediTabs 12 Hours *ODT:* 5 mg (mint)
Claritin RediTabs 24 Hours *ODT:* 10 mg (mint)

FIRST GENERATION ORAL ANTIHISTAMINES

➢ ***diphenhydramine*** **(B)(G)** <2 years: not recommended; 2-6 years: 6.25 mg q 4-6 hours; max 37.5 mg/day; >6-12 years: 12.5-25 mg q 4-6 hours; max 150 mg/day; >12 years: 25-50 mg q 6-8 hours; max 100 mg/day
Benadryl (OTC) *Chew tab:* 12.5 mg (grape) (phenylalanine); *Liq:* 12.5 mg/5 ml (4, 8 oz); *Cap:* 25 mg; *Tab:* 25 mg; *Dye-free soft gel:* 25 mg; *Dye-free liq:* 12.5 mg/5 ml (4, 8 oz)

➢ ***hydroxyzine*** **(C)(G)** <6 years: 50 mg/day divided qid prn; ≥6 years: 50-100 mg/day divided qid prn
Atarax *Tab:* 10, 25, 50, 100 mg; *Syr:* 10 mg/5 ml (alcohol 0.5%)
Vistaril *Cap:* 25, 50, 100 mg; *Oral susp:* 25 mg/5 ml (4 oz) (lemon)

Comment: ***hydroxyzine*** is contraindicated in early pregnancy and in patients with a prolonged QT interval. It is not known whether this drug is excreted in human milk; therefore, ***hydroxyzine*** should not be given to nursing mothers.

FIRST GENERATION PARENTERAL ANTIHISTAMINE

➢ ***diphenhydramine*** injectable **(B)(G)** <12 years: *See mfr pkg insert:* 1.25 mg/kg up to 25 mg IM x 1 dose; then q 6 hours prn; ≥12 years: 25-50 mg IM immediately; then q 6 hours prn
Benadryl Injectable *Vial:* 50 mg/ml (1 ml single use); 50 mg/ml (10 ml multi-dose); *Amp:* 10 mg/ml (1 ml); *Prefilled syringe:* 50 mg/ml (1 ml)

☐ DERMATITIS: GENUS RHUS (POISON OAK, POISON IVY, POISON SUMAC)

Topical Corticosteroids *see page* 542
Parenteral Corticosteroids *see page* 547
Oral Corticosteroids *see page* 546
OTC Calamine Lotion
OTC diphenhydramine cream

PROPHYLAXIS

➢ ***bentoquatam*** <6 years: not recommended; ≥6 years: apply as a wet film to exposed skin at least 15 minutes prior to possible contact; reapply at least q 4 hours; remove with soap and water
IvyBlock (OTC) *Soln:* 120 ml

Comment: Provides protection against genus rhus (poison oak, poison ivy, and poison sumac).

TREATMENT

Oatmeal Colloids

Aveeno (OTC) add to bath as needed
Regular: 1.5 oz (8/pck); *Moisturizing:* 0.75 oz (8/pck)

Aveeno Oil (OTC) add to bath as needed
Oil: 8 oz
Aveeno Moisturizing (OTC) apply as needed
Lotn: 2.5, 8, 12 oz; *Crm:* 4 oz
Aveeno Cleansing Bar (OTC) *Bar:* 3 oz
Aveeno Gentle Skin Cleanser (OTC) *Liq clnsr:* 6 oz

SECOND GENERATION ORAL ANTIHISTAMINES

Comment: The following drugs are second generation antihistamines. As such they minimally sedating, much less so than the first generation antihistamines. All antihistamines are excreted into breast milk.

▶ ***cetirizine*** (C)(OTC)(G) <6 years: not recommended; ≥6-<65 years: initially 5-10 mg once daily; ≥65 years: 5 mg once daily
Children's Zyrtec Chewable *Chew tab:* 5, 10 mg (grape)
Children's Zyrtec Allergy Syrup *Syr:* 1 mg/ml (4 oz) (grape, bubble gum) (sugar-free, dye-free)
Zyrtec *Tab:* 10 mg
Zyrtec Hives Relief *Tab:* 10 mg
Zyrtec Liquid Gels *Liq gel:* 10 mg

▶ ***desloratadine*** (C)
Clarinex <6 years: not recommended; ≥6 years: 1/2-1 tab once daily
Tab: 5 mg
Clarinex RediTabs <6 years: not recommended; 6-12 years: 2.5 mg once daily; ≥12 years: 5 mg once daily
ODT: 2.5, 5 mg (tutti-frutti) (phenylalanine)
Clarinex Syrup <6 months: not recommended; 6-11 months: 1 mg (2 ml) once daily; 1-5 years: 1.25 mg (2.5 ml) once daily; 6-11 years: 2.5 mg (5 ml) once daily; ≥12 years: 5 mg (10 ml) once daily
Tab: 0.5 mg per ml (4 oz) (tutti-frutti) (phenylalanine)
Desloratadine ODT <6 years: not recommended; 6-11 years: ½ tab once daily; ≥12 years: 1 tab once daily
ODT: 5 mg

▶ ***fexofenadine*** (C)(OTC)(G) <6 months: not recommended; 6 months-<2 years: 15 mg bid; *CrCl ≤90 mL/min:* 15 mg once daily; 2-11 years: 30 mg bid; *CrCl ≤90 mL/min:* 30 mg once daily; ≥12 years: 60 mg once daily-bid or 180 mg once daily; *CrCl <90 mL/min:* 60 mg once daily **Allegra** *Tab:* 30, 60, 180 mg film-coat
Allegra Allergy *Tab:* 60, 180 mg film-coat
Allegra ODT *ODT:* 30 mg (phenylalanine)
Allegra Oral Suspension *Oral susp:* 30 mg/5 ml (6 mg/ml) (4 oz)

▶ ***levocetirizine*** (B)(OTC) administer dose in the PM; *Seasonal Allergic Rhinitis:* <2 years: not recommended; may start at ≥2 years; *Chronic Spontaneous/Idiopathic Urticaria (CSU/CIU), Perennial Allergic Rhinitis:* <6 months: not recommended; may start at ≥ 6 months; *Dosing by Age:* 6 months-5 years: max 1.25 mg once daily; 6-11 years: max 2.5 mg once daily; ≥12 years: 2.5-5 mg once daily; *Renal Dysfunction <12 years:* contraindicated; *Renal Dysfunction ≥12 years: CrCl 50-80 mL/min:* 2.5 mg once daily; *CrCl 30-50 mL/min:* 2.5 mg every other day; *CrCl: 10-30 mL/min:* 2.5 mg twice weekly (every 3-4 days); *CrCl <10 mL/min, ESRD or hemodialysis:* contraindicated
Children's Xyzal Allergy 24HR *Oral Soln:* 0.5 mg/ml (150 ml)
Xyzal Allergy 24HR *Tab:* 5*mg

▶ ***loratadine*** (C)(OTC)(G) <2 years: not recommended; 2-5 years: 5 mg once daily; ≥6 years: 5 mg bid or 10 mg once daily; *Hepatic or Renal Insufficiency:* (see mfr pkg insert)

Children's Claritin Chewables *Chew tab:* 5 mg (grape) (phenylalanine)
Children's Claritin Syrup 1 mg/ml (4 oz) (fruit) (sugar-free, alcohol-free, dye-free; sodium 6 mg/5 ml)
Claritin *Tab:* 10 mg
Claritin Hives Relief *Tab:* 10 mg
Claritin Liqui-Gels *Liq gel:* 10 mg
Claritin RediTabs 12 Hours *ODT:* 5 mg (mint)
Claritin RediTabs 24 Hours *ODT:* 10 mg (mint)

FIRST GENERATION ORAL ANTIHISTAMINES

▶ ***diphenhydramine*** **(B)(G)** <2 years: not recommended; 2-6 years: 6.25 mg q 4-6 hours; max 37.5 mg/day; >6-12 years: 12.5-25 mg q 4-6 hours; max 150 mg/day; >12 years: 25-50 mg q 6-8 hours; max 100 mg/day
Benadryl (OTC) *Chew tab:* 12.5 mg (grape) (phenylalanine); *Liq:* 12.5 mg/5 ml (4, 8 oz); *Cap:* 25 mg; *Tab:* 25 mg; *Dye-free soft gel:* 25 mg; *Dye-free liq:* 12.5 mg/5 ml (4, 8 oz)

▶ ***hydroxyzine*** **(C)(G)** <6 years: 50 mg/day divided qid prn; ≥6 years: 50-100 mg/day divided qid prn
Atarax *Tab:* 10, 25, 50, 100 mg; *Syr:* 10 mg/5 ml (alcohol 0.5%)
Vistaril *Cap:* 25, 50, 100 mg; *Oral susp:* 25 mg/5 ml (4 oz) (lemon)

Comment: ***hydroxyzine*** is contraindicated in early pregnancy and in patients with a prolonged QT interval. It is not known whether this drug is excreted in human milk; therefore, ***hydroxyzine*** should not be given to nursing mothers.

FIRST GENERATION PARENTERAL ANTIHISTAMINE

▶ ***diphenhydramine*** injectable **(B)(G)** <12 years: *See mfr pkg insert:* 1.25 mg/kg up to 25 mg IM x 1 dose; then q 6 hours prn; ≥12 years: 25-50 mg IM immediately; then q 6 hours prn
Benadryl Injectable *Vial:* 50 mg/ml (1 ml single use); 50 mg/ml (10 ml multi-dose); *Amp:* 10 mg/ml (1 ml); *Prefilled syringe:* 50 mg/ml (1 ml)

DERMATITIS: SEBORRHEIC

ANTIFUNGAL SHAMPOOS AND TOPICAL AGENTS

▶ ***chloroxine*** shampoo **(C)** <12 years: not recommended; ≥12 years: massage onto wet scalp; wait 3 minutes, rinse, repeat, and rinse thoroughly; use twice weekly
Capitrol Shampoo *Shampoo:* 2% (4 oz)

▶ ***ciclopirox*** **(B)** apply gel once daily or apply cream or lotion twice daily, x 4 weeks or shampoo twice weekly; massage shampoo onto wet scalp; wait 3 minutes, rinse, repeat, and rinse thoroughly; shampoo twice weekly
Loprox Cream <10 years: not recommended
Crm: 0.77% (15, 30, 90 gm)
Loprox Gel <16 years: not recommended
Gel: 0.77% (30, 45 gm)
Loprox Lotion <10 years: not recommended
Lotn: 0.77% (30, 60 ml)
Loprox Shampoo *Shampoo:* 1% (120 ml)

▶ ***coal tar*** **(C)(G)**
Scytera (OTC) apply once daily-qid; use lowest effective dose
Foam: 2%

T/Gel Shampoo Extra Strength (OTC) use every other day; max 4 x/week; massage into wet scalp for 5 minutes; rinse; repeat
Shampoo: 1%
T/Gel Shampoo Original Formula (OTC) use every other day; max 7 x/week; massage into wet scalp for 5 minutes; rinse; repeat
Shampoo: 0.5%
T/Gel Shampoo Stubborn Itch Control (OTC) use every other day; max 7 x/week; massage into wet scalp for 5 minutes; rinse; repeat
Shampoo: 0.5%

▶ ***fluocinolone acetamide*** **(C)**
Derma-Smoothe/FS Shampoo <12 years: not recommended; ≥12 years: apply up to 1 oz to scalp daily, lather, and leave on x 5 minutes, then rinse twice
Shampoo: 0.01% (4 oz)
Derma-Smoothe/FS Topical Oil ***fluocinolone acetamide*** 0.01% topical oil **(C)** <6 years: not recommended; ≥6-12 years: apply sparingly bid for up to 4 weeks; >12 years: apply sparingly tid; for scalp psoriasis wet or dampen hair or scalp, then apply a thin film, massage well, cover with a shower cap and leave on for at least 4 hours or overnight, then wash hair with regular shampoo and rinse
Topical oil: 0.01% (4 oz) (peanut oil)

▶ ***ketoconazole*** **(C)** <12 years: not recommended; ≥12 years: apply cream or gel once daily x 4 week or apply up to 1 oz shampoo to scalp daily, lather, leave on x 5 minutes, then rinse twice
Nizoral Cream *Crm:* 2% (15, 30, 60 gm)
Nizoral Shampoo *Shampoo:* 2% (4 oz)
Xolegel *Gel:* 2% (45 gm)
Xolegel Duo *Kit:* **Xolegel** *Gel:* 2% (45 gm)
Xolex *Shampoo*: 2% (4 oz)

▶ ***selenium sulfide*** **(C)** <12 years: not recommended; ≥12 years: massage cream into scalp twice weekly x 2 weeks or massage into wet scalp, wait 2-3 minutes, rinse; repeat twice weekly x 2 weeks; may continue treatment with lotion of shampoo 1-2 x weekly as needed
Exsel Shampoo *Shampoo:* 2.5% (4 oz)
Selsun Rx *Lotn:* 2.5% (4 oz)
Selsun Shampoo *Shampoo:* 1% (120, 210, 240, 330 ml); 2.5% (120 ml)

▶ ***sodium sulfacetamide+sulfur*** **(C)**
Clenia Emollient Cream apply daily tid
Emol crm: sod sulfa 10%+sulfur 5% (10 oz) (alcohol-free)
Clenia Foaming Wash wash 1-2 x/daily
Wash: sod sulfa 10%+sulfur 5% (6, 12 oz) (alcohol-free)
Rosula Gel apply daily tid
Gel: sod sulfa 10%+sulfur 4.5% (45 ml)
Rosula Lotion apply daily tid
Lotn: sod sulfa 10%+sulfur 4.5% (45 ml) (alcohol-free)
Rosula Wash wash bid
Clnsr: sod sulfa 10%+sulfur 4.5% (12 oz) (alcohol-free)

TOPICAL STEROID

▶ ***betamethasone valerate*** 0.12% foam **(C)(G)** <12 years: not recommended; ≥12 years: apply twice daily in AM and PM; invert can and dispense a small amount of foam onto a clean saucer or another cool surface (do not apply directly to hand) and massage a small amount into affected area until foam disappears
Luxiq *Foam:* 100 gm
Other Topical Corticosteroids *see page* 542

DIABETIC PERIPHERAL NEUROPATHY (DPN)

NUTRITIONAL SUPPLEMENT

▶ ***L-methylfolate calcium(as metafolin)+pyridoxal 5-phosphate/methylcobalamin*** <12 years: not recommended; ≥12 years: 1 cap twice daily or 2 caps once daily

Metanx *Cap:* meta 3 mg+pyr 35 mg+methyl 2 mg

Comment: **Metanx** is indicated as adjunct treatment for patients with endothelial cell dysfunction, who have loss of protective sensation and neuropathic pain associated with diabetic peripheral neuropathy.

ORAL ANALGESICS

▶ ***acetaminophen*** (B)(G) *see* ***Fever*** *page* 149

▶ ***aspirin*** (D)(G) *see* ***Fever*** *page* 150

Comment: ***aspirin***-containing medications are contraindicated with history of allergic-type reaction to ***aspirin***, children and adolescents with *Varicella* or other viral illness, and 3rd trimester of pregnancy.

▶ ***tramadol*** (C)(IV)(G)

Comment: ***tramadol*** is known to be excreted in breast milk. The FDA and the European Medicines Agency (EMA) are investigating the safety of using ***tramadol***-containing medications to treat pain in children 12-18 years because of the potential for serious side effects, including slowed or difficult breathing.

Rybix ODT <12 years: contraindicated; 12-<18: use extreme caution; not recommended for children and adolescents with obesity, asthma, obstructive sleep apnea, or other chronic breathing problem, or for post-tonsillectomy/adenoidectomy pain; ≥18 years: initially 100 mg once daily; may increase by 100 mg every 5 days; max 300 mg/day; *CrCl <30 mL/min* or *severe hepatic impairment:* not recommended; *Cirrhosis:* max 50 mg q 12 hours

ODT: 50 mg (mint) (phenylalanine)

Ryzolt <12 years: contraindicated; 12-<18: use extreme caution; not recommended for children and adolescents with obesity, asthma, obstructive sleep apnea, or other chronic breathing problem, or for post-tonsillectomy/adenoidectomy pain; ≥18 years: initially 100 mg once daily; may increase by 100 mg every 5 days; max 300 mg/day; *CrCl <30 mL/min* or *severe hepatic impairment:* not recommended

Tab: 100, 200, 300 mg ext-rel

Ultram <12 years: contraindicated; 12-<18: use extreme caution; not recommended for children and adolescents with obesity, asthma, obstructive sleep apnea, or other chronic breathing problem, or for post-tonsillectomy/adenoidectomy pain; ≥18 years: 50-100 mg q 4-6 hours prn; max 400 mg/day; *CrCl <30 mL/min:* max 100 mg q 12 hours; *Cirrhosis:* max 50 mg q 12 hours

Tab: 50*mg

Ultram ER <12 years: contraindicated; 12-<18: use extreme caution; not recommended for children and adolescents with obesity, asthma, obstructive sleep apnea, or other chronic breathing problem, or for post-tonsillectomy/adenoidectomy pain; ≥18 years: initially 100 mg once daily; may increase by 100 mg every 5 days; max 300 mg/day; *CrCl <30 mL/min:* or *severe hepatic impairment:* not recommended

Tab: 100, 200, 300 mg ext-rel

▶ ***tramadol+acetaminophen*** (C)(IV)(G) <12 years: contraindicated; 12-<18: use extreme caution; not recommended for children and adolescents with obesity, asthma, obstructive sleep apnea, or other chronic breathing problem, or for post-tonsillectomy/adenoidectomy pain; ≥18 years: 2 tabs q 4-6 hours; max 8 tabs/day; 5 days; *CrCl <30 mL/min:* max 2 tabs q 12 hours; max 4 tabs/day x 5 days

Ultracet *Tab:* tram 37.5+acet 325 mg

Comment: ***tramadol*** is known to be excreted in breast milk. The FDA and the European Medicines Agency (EMA) are investigating the safety of using ***tramadol***-containing medications to treat pain in children 12-18 years because of the potential for serious side effects, including slowed or difficult breathing.

TOPICAL ANALGESICS

▶ ***capsaicin*** cream **(B)(G)** <2 years: not recommended; 2-12 years: apply sparingly to intact skin bid prn; >12 years: apply tid-qid prn

Axsain *Crm:* 0.075% (1, 2 oz)
Capsin (OTC) *Lotn:* 0.025, 0,075% (59 ml)
Capzasin-P (OTC) *Crm:* 0.025% (1.5 oz); *Lotn:* 0.025% (2 oz)
Capzasin-HP (OTC) *Crm:* 0.075% (1.5 oz); *Lotn:* 0.075% (2 oz)
Dolorac *Crm:* 0.025% (28 gm)
Double Cap (OTC) *Crm:* 0.05% (2 oz)
R-Gel *Gel:* 0.025% (15, 30 gm)
Zostrix (OTC) *Crm:* 0.025% (0.7, 1.5, 3 oz)
Zostrix HP (OTC) *Emol crm:* 0.075% (1, 2 oz)

Comment: Provides some relief by 1-2 weeks; optimal benefit may take 4-6 weeks. Avoid contact with mucous membranes.

▶ ***capsaicin*** 8% patch **(B)** <18 years: not recommended; ≥18 years: apply up to 4 patches for one 60-minute application to clean dry skin; may prep area with topical anesthetic; wear non-latex gloves; patches may be cut to size/shape; treatment may be repeated every 3 months

Qutenza *Patch:* 8% 1640 mcg/cm (179 mg) (1 or 2 patches w. 1-50 gm tube cleansing gel/carton)

▶ ***lidocaine*** 5% patch **(B)(G)** <12 years: not recommended; ≥12 years: apply up to 3 patches at one time for up to 12 hours/24-hour period (12 hours on/12 hours off); patches may be cut into smaller sizes before removal of the release liner; do not reuse

Lidoderm *Patch:* 5% 10 x 14 cm (30 patches/carton)

ANTICONVULSANTS

Gamma Aminobutyric Acid Analog

▶ ***gabapentin*** **(C)** <3 years: not recommended; 3-12 years: initially 10-15 mg/kg/day in 3 divided doses; max 12 hours between doses; titrate over 3 days; 3-4 years: titrate to 40 mg/kg/day; 5-12 years: titrate to 25-35 mg/kg/day; max 50 mg/kg/day; >12 years: initially 300 mg on Day 1; then 600 mg on Day 2; then 900 mg on Days 3-6; then 1,200 mg on Days 7-10; then 1,500 mg on Days 11-14; titrate up to 1,800 mg on Day 15; take entire dose once daily with the evening meal; do not crush, split, or chew

Gralise (C) *Tab:* 300, 600 mg
Neurontin (G) *Tab:* 600*, 800*mg; *Cap:* 100, 300, 400 mg; *Oral soln:* 250 mg/5 ml (480 ml) (strawberry-anise)

▶ ***gabapentin enacarbil*** **(C)** <18 years: not recommended; ≥18 years: 600 mg once daily at about 5:00 PM; if dose not taken at recommended time, next dose should be taken the following day; swallow whole; take with food; *CrCl 30-59 mL/min*: 600 mg on Day 1, Day 3, and every day thereafter; *CrCl <30 mL/min*: or hemodialysis: not recommended

Horizant *Tab:* 300, 600 mg ext-rel

Comment: Avoid abrupt cessation of ***gabapentin enacarbil.*** To discontinue, withdraw gradually over 1 week or longer.

▻ ***pregabalin (GABA analog)*** (C)(V) <18 years: not recommended; ≥18 years:
Lyrica initially 50 mg tid; may titrate to 100 mg tid within one week; max 600 mg divided tid; discontinue over 1 week
Cap: 25, 50, 75, 100, 150, 200, 225, 300 mg; *Oral soln:* 20 mg/ml
Lyrica CR *Tab:* usual dose: 165 mg once daily; may increase to 330 mg/day within 1 week; max 660 mg/day; discontinue over 1 week
Tab: 82.5, 165, 330 mg ext-rel

TRICYCLIC ANTIDEPRESSANTS (TCAs)

Comment: Co-administration of SSRIs and TCAs requires extreme caution.

▻ ***amitriptyline*** (C)(G) <12 years: not recommended; ≥12 years: 10-20 mg q HS *Tab:* 10, 25, 50, 75, 100, 150 mg

▻ ***amoxapine*** (C) <12 years: not recommended; ≥12 years: initially 50 mg bid-tid; after 1 week may increase to 100 mg bid-tid; usual effective dose 200-300 mg/day; if total dose exceeds 300 mg/day, give in divided doses (max 400 mg/day); may give as a single bedtime dose (max 300 mg q HS)
Tab: 25, 50, 100, 150 mg

▻ ***clomipramine*** (C)(G) <10 years: not recommended; 10-<16 years: initially 25 mg daily in divided doses; gradually increase; max 3 mg/kg or 100 mg, whichever is smaller; >16 years: initially 25 mg daily in divided doses; gradually increase to 100 mg during first 2 weeks; max 250 mg/day; total maintenance dose may be given at HS
Anafranil *Cap:* 25, 50, 75 mg

▻ ***desipramine*** (C)(G) <12 years: not recommended; ≥12 years: 100-200 mg/day in single or divided doses; max 300 mg/day
Norpramin *Tab:* 10, 25, 50, 75, 100, 150 mg

▻ ***doxepin*** (C)(G) <12 years: not recommended; ≥12 years: 75 mg/day; max 150 mg/day
Cap: 10, 25, 50, 75, 100, 150 mg; Oral conc: 10 mg/ml (4 oz w. dropper)

▻ ***imipramine*** (C)(G) <12 years: not recommended; ≥12 years:
Tofranil initially 75 mg daily (max 200 mg); adolescents initially 30-40 mg daily (max 100 mg/day); if maintenance dose exceeds 75 mg daily, may switch to **Tofranil PM** for divided or bedtime dose
Tab: 10, 25, 50 mg
Tofranil PM initially 75 mg daily 1 hour before HS; max 200 mg
Cap: 75, 100, 125, 150 mg

▻ ***nortriptyline*** (D)(G) <12 years: not recommended; ≥12 years: initially 25 mg tid-qid; max 150 mg/day
Pamelor *Cap:* 10, 25, 50, 75 mg; *Oral soln:* 10 mg/5 ml (16 oz)

▻ ***protriptyline*** (C) <12 years: not recommended; ≥12 years: initially 5 mg tid; usual dose 15-40 mg/day in 3-4 divided doses; max 60 mg/day
Vivactil *Tab:* 5, 10 mg

▻ ***trimipramine*** (C) <12 years: not recommended; ≥12 years: initially 75 mg/day in divided doses; max 200 mg/day
Surmontil *Cap:* 25, 50, 100 mg

DIABETIC RETINOPATHY, MACULAR EDEMA, MACULAR DEGENERATION

VASCULAR ENDOTHELIAL GROWTH FACTOR (VEGF) INHIBITOR

Comment: Diabetic retinopathy is the leading cause of blindness among working-age adults in the US. **Lucentis *(ranibizumab)*** is only one FDA-approved drug for the treatment of diabetic retinopathy. Additional labeled indications include treatment of diabetic macular edema (DME), treatment of neovascular (wet) age-related macular degeneration (AMD), treatment of macular edema following retinal vein occlusion (RVO), and treatment of myopic choroidal neovascularization (mCNV).

▶ ***ranibizumab*** **(D)** <18 years: not established; ≥18 years:

Neovascular (wet) Age-related Macular Degeneration (AMD): Intravitreal: 0.5 mg once a month (approximately every 28 days). Frequency may be reduced (e.g., 4 to 5 injections over 9 months) after the first 3 injections or may be reduced after the first 4 injections to once every 3 months if monthly injections are not feasible. *Note:* A regimen averaging 4 to 5 doses over 9 months is expected to maintain visual acuity and an every 3-month dosing regimen has reportedly resulted in a ~5 letter (1 line) loss of visual acuity over 9 months, as compared to monthly dosing which may result in an additional ~1 to 2 letter gain

Diabetic macular edema (DME): Intravitreal: 0.3 mg once a month (approximately every 28 days); in clinical trials, monthly doses of 0.5 mg were also studied

Diabetic retinopathy (DR): Intravitreal: 0.3 mg once a month (approximately every 28 days)

Macular edema following retinal vein occlusion (RVO): Intravitreal: 0.5 mg once a month (approximately every 28 days)

Myopic choroidal neovascularization (mCNV): Intravitreal: 0.5 mg once a month (approximately every 28 days) for up to 3 months; may re-treat if necessary

Lucentis *Prefilled syringe:* 10 mg/ml solution (0.5 mg/0.05 ml single-dose); 6 mg/ml (0.3 mg/0.05 ml single-dose) for intra-vitreal injection (preservative-free); *Vial:* 10 mg/ml (**Lucentis** 0.5 mg/0.05 ml single-dose); 6 mg/ml solution (**Lucentis** 0.3 mg/0.05 ml single-dose) for intra-vitreal injection (preservative-free); a 5-micron sterile filter needle (19 gauge x 1-1/2 inch) is required for preparation, but not included; keep refrigerated; do not freeze; protect vial from light; see mfr pkg insert

Comment: **Lucentis** is a recombinant humanized monoclonal antibody fragment which binds to and inhibits human vascular endothelial growth factor A (VEGF-A). **Lucentis** inhibits VEGF from binding to its receptors and thereby suppressing neovascularization and slowing vision loss. Contraindications include ocular or periocular infection, and active intraocular inflammation. For ophthalmic intravitreal injection only. Each vial or prefilled syringe should only be used for the treatment of a single eye. If the contralateral eye requires treatment, a new vial or prefilled syringe should be used and the sterile field, syringe, gloves, drapes, eyelid speculum, filter, and injection needles should be changed before **Lucentis** is administered to the other eye. Adequate anesthesia and a topical broad-spectrum antimicrobial agent should be administered prior to the procedure. Refer to manufacturer labeling for additional detailed information. Based on its mechanism of action, adverse effects on pregnancy would be expected. Information related to use in pregnancy is limited. The intravitreal injection procedure should be carried out under controlled aseptic conditions, which include the use of sterile gloves, a sterile drape, and a sterile eyelid speculum (or equivalent). Adequate anesthesia and a broad-spectrum microbicide should be given prior to the injection. Prior to and 30 minutes following the intravitreal injection, patients should be monitored for elevation in intraocular pressure using tonometry. Each prefilled syringe or vial should only be used for the treatment of a single eye. If the contralateral eye requires treatment, a new prefilled syringe or vial should be used and the sterile field, syringe, gloves, drapes, eyelid speculum, filter needle (vial only), and injection needles should be changed. Solomon, SD, Chew, E, Duh, EJ, *et al*. Diabetic retinopathy: A position statement by the American Diabetes Association [published online February 21, 2017]. *ADA*.

DIAPER RASH

Topical Corticosteroids *see page* 542

Comment: Low to intermediate potency topical corticosteroids are indicated if inflammation is present.

PROTECTIVE BARRIERS

▶ ***aloe+vitamin e+zinc oxide*** ointment apply at each diaper change after thoroughly cleansing skin

Balmex *Oint:* 2, 4 oz tube; 16 oz jar

▶ ***vitamin a*** & ***d*** (G) ointment apply at each diaper change after thoroughly cleansing skin

A&D Ointment *Oint:* 1.5, 4 oz

▶ ***zinc oxide*** (G) cream and ointment apply at each diaper change after thoroughly cleansing the skin

A&D Ointment with Zinc Oxide *Oint:* 10% (1.5, 4 oz)
Desitin *Oint:* 40% (1, 2, 4, 9 oz)
Desitin Cream *Crm:* 10% (2, 4 oz)

TOPICAL ANTIFUNGALS

Comment: Use if caused by *Candida albicans*.

▶ ***butenafine*** (B)(G) <12 years: not recommended; ≥12 years: apply bid x 1 week <u>or</u> once daily x 4 weeks

Lotrimin Ultra (C)(OTC) *Crm:* 1% (12, 24 gm)
Mentax *Crm:* 1% (15, 30 gm)

Comment: ***butenafine*** is a benzylamine, not an azole. Fungicidal activity continues for at least 5 weeks after last application.

▶ ***clotrimazole*** (B) apply to affected area bid x 7 days

Lotrimin (OTC) *Crm:* 1% (15, 30, 45 gm)
Lotrimin AF (OTC) *Crm:* 1% (12 gm); *Lotn:* 1% (10 ml); *Soln:* 1% (10 ml)

▶ ***econazole*** (C) apply bid x 7 days

Spectazole *Crm:* 1% (15, 30, 85 gm)

▶ ***ketoconazole*** (C) apply to affected area bid x 7 days

Nizoral Cream *Crm:* 2% (15, 30, 60 gm)

▶ ***nystatin*** (C)(G) apply bid x 7 days

Mycostatin *Crm:* 100,000 U/gm (15, 30 gm)

COMBINATION AGENT

▶ ***clotrimazole+betamethasone*** cream (C)(G) apply bid x 7 days

Lotrisone *Crm:* 15, 45 gm

DIARRHEA: ACUTE

▶ ***attapulgite*** (C)

Donnagel (OTC) <3 years: not recommended; 3-6 years: 7.5 ml; >6-12 years: 15 ml; >12 years: 30 ml after each loose stool; max 7 doses/day x 2 days

Liq: 600 mg/15 ml (120, 240 ml)

Donnagel Chewable Tab (OTC) <3 years: not recommended; 3-6 years: 1/2 tab after each loose stool; max 7 doses/day; >6-12 years: 1 tab after each loose stool; max tabs/day; >12 years: 2 tabs after each loose stool; max 14 tabs/day

Chew tab: 600 mg

Kaopectate (OTC) <3 years: not recommended; 3-6 years: 7.5 ml after each loose stool; >6-12 years: 15 ml after each loose stool; >12 years: 30 ml after each loose stool; max 7 doses/day x 2 days

Liq: 600 mg/15 ml (120, 240 ml)

▶ ***bismuth subsalicylate*** **(C; D in 3rd)(G)**

Pepto-Bismol (OTC) <3 years (14-18 lb): 2.5 ml q 4 hours; max 6 doses/day; <3 years(18-28 lb): 5 ml q 4 hours; max 6 doses/day; 3-6 years: 1/3 tab or 5 ml q 30-60 minutes; max 8 doses/day; >6-9 years: 2/3 tab or 10 ml q 30-60 minutes; max 8 doses/day; >9-12 years: 1 tab or 15 ml q 30-60 minutes; max 8 doses/day; >12 years: 2 tabs or 30 ml q 30-60 minutes as needed; max 8 doses/day

Chew tab: 262 mg; *Liq:* 262 mg/15 ml (4, 8, 12, 16 oz)

Pepto-Bismol Maximum Strength **(OTC)** <3 years: not recommended; 3-6 years: 5 ml q 60 minutes; max 4 doses/day; >6-9 years: 10 ml q 60 minutes; max 4 doses/day; >9-12 years: 15 ml q 60 minutes; max 4 doses/day; >12 years: 30 ml q 60 minutes; max 4 doses/day

Liq: 525 mg/15 ml (4, 8, 12, 16 oz)

Comment: ***aspirin***-containing medications are contraindicated with history of allergic type reaction to ***aspirin***, children and adolescents with *Varicella* or other viral illness, and 3rd trimester pregnancy.

▶ ***calcium polycarbophil*** **(C)** <6 years: not recommended; 6-12 years: 1 tab daily qid; >12 years: 2 tabs daily qid

Fibercon (OTC) *Cplt:* 625 mg

▶ ***crofelemer*** **(C)** <12 years: not recommended; ≥12 years: 2 tabs once daily; swallow whole with or without food; do not crush or chew

Mytesi *Tab:* 125 mg del-rel

Comment: ***crofelemer*** is indicated for the symptomatic relief of non-infectious diarrhea in patients ≥18 years with HIV/AIDS on antiretroviral therapy.

▶ ***difenoxin+atropine*** **(C)** <2 years: not recommended; ≥2 years: 2 tabs, then 1 tab after each loose stool or 1 tab q 3-4 hours as needed; max 8 tab/day x 2 days

Motofen *Tab:* dif 1 mg+atro 0.025 mg

▶ ***diphenoxylate+atropine*** **(C)(V)(G)** <2 years: not recommended; 2-12 years: initially 0.3-0.4 mg/kg/day in 4 divided doses; >12 years: 2 tabs or 10 ml qid until diarrhea is controlled

Lomotil *Tab:* diphen 2.5 mg+atrop 0.025 mg; *Liq:* diphen 2.5 mg+atrop 0.025 mg per 5 ml (2 oz)

▶ ***loperamide*** **(B)(OTC)(G)**

Imodium <5 years: not recommended; ≥5 years: 4 mg initially, then 2 mg after each loose stool; max 16 mg/day x 2 days

Cap: 2 mg

Imodium A-D <2 years: not recommended; 2-5 years (24-47 lb): 1 mg up to tid x 2 days; 6-8 years (48-59 lb): 2 mg initially, then 1 mg after each loose stool; max 4 mg/day x 2 days; 9-11 years (60-95 lb): 2 mg initially, then 1 after each loose stool; max 6 mg/day x 2 days; >11 years: 4 mg initially, then 2 mg after each loose stool; usual max 8 mg/day x 2 days

Cplt: 2 mg; *Liq:* 1 mg/5 ml (2, 4 oz) (cherry-mint) (alcohol 0.5%)

▶ ***loperamide+simethicone*** **(B)(OTC)(G)**

Imodium Advanced <6 years: not recommended; 6-8 years: chew 1 tab after loose stool, then chew 1/2 tab after next loose stool; ≥8-11 years: chew 1 tab after loose stool, then chew 1/2 tab after next loose stool; max 3 tabs/day; >11 years: 2 tabs chewed after loose stool, then 1 after the next loose stool; max 4 tabs/day

Chew tab: loper 2 mg+simeth 125 mg (vanilla-mint)

ORAL REHYDRATION AND ELECTROLYTE REPLACEMENT THERAPY

▶ *oral electrolyte replacement* (OTC)

CeraLyte 50 <4 years: not indicated; ≥4 years: dissolve in 8 oz water

Pkt: sodium 50 mEq+potassium 20 mEq+chloride 40 mEq+citrate 30 mEq+rice syrup solids 40 gm+calories 190 per liter (mixed berry) (gluten-free)

CeraLyte 70 <4 years: not indicated; ≥4 years: dissolve in 8 oz water

Pkt: sodium 70 mEq+potassium 20 mEq+chloride 60 mEq+citrate 30 mEq+rice syrup solids 40 gm+calories 165 per liter (natural, lemon) (gluten-free)

KaoLectrolyte <2 years: not indicated; ≥2 years: 1 pkt dissolved in 8 oz water q 3-4 hours

Pkt: sodium 12 mEq+potassium 5 mEq+chloride 10 mEq+citrate 7 mEq+dextrose 5 gm+calories 22 per 6.2 gm

Pedialyte <2 years: as desired and as tolerated; ≥2 years: 1-2 L/day

Oral soln: dextrose 20 gm+fructose 5 gm+sodium 25 mEq+potassium 20 mEq+chloride 35 mEq+citrate 30 mEq+calories 100 per liter (8 oz, 1 L)

Pedialyte Freezer Pops as desired and as tolerated

Pops: dextrose 1.6 gm+sodium 2.8 mEq+potassium 1.25 mEq+chloride 2.2 mEq+citrate 1.88 mEq+calories 6.25 per 6.25 ml pop (8 oz, 1 L)

DIARRHEA: CARCINOID SYNDROME (CSD)

TRYPTOPHAN HYDROXYLASE

▶ ***telotristat*** <18 years: not established; ≥18 years: take with food; 250 mg tid

Xermelo *Tab:* 250 mg (4 x 7 daily dose pcks/carton

Comment: Take **Xermelo** in combination with somatostatin analog (SSA) therapy to treat patients inadequately controlled by SSA therapy. Breastfeeding females should monitor the infant for constipation. ESRD requiring dialysis not studied.

DIARRHEA: CHRONIC

▶ ***cholestyramine*** (C)

Questran Powder for Oral Suspension initially 1 pkt or scoop daily; usual maintenance 2-4 pkts or scoops daily in 2 doses; max 6 pkts or scoops daily

Oral pwdr: 9 gm pkts; 9 gm equals 4 gm *anhydrous cholestyramine resin* (60/pck); *Bulk can:* 378 gm w. scoop

Questran Light initially 1 pkt or scoop daily; usual maintenance 2-4 pkts or scoops daily in 2 doses

Light: 5 gm pkts; 5 gm equals 4 gm *anhydrous cholestyramine resin* (60/pck); *Bulk can:* 210 gm w. scoop

Comment: Use ***cholestyramine*** only if diarrhea is due to bile salt malabsorption.

▶ ***crofelemer*** (C) not established; <12 years: not recommended; ≥12 years: 2 tabs daily; swallow whole with or without food; do not crush or chew

Mytesi *Tab:* 125 mg del-rel

Comment: ***crofelemer*** is indicated for the symptomatic relief of non-infectious diarrhea in patients ≥18 years with HIV/AIDS on antiretroviral therapy.

▶ ***difenoxin+atropine*** (C)

Motofen <2 years: not recommended; ≥2 years: 2 tabs, then 1 tab after each loose stool or 1 tab q 3-4 hours prn; max 8 tab/day x 2 days

Tab: dif 1 mg+atrop 0.025 mg

▶ ***diphenoxylate+atropine*** **(B)(V)(G)**

Lomotil <2 years: not recommended; 2-12 years: initially 0.3-0.4 mg/kg/day in 4 divided doses; >12 years: 5-20 mg/day in divided doses

Tab: diphen 2.5 mg+atrop 0.025 mg; *Liq:* diphen 2.5 mg+atrop 0.025 mg per 5 ml (2 oz w. dropper)

▶ ***attapulgite*** (C)(G)

Donnagel (OTC) <2 years: not recommended; 2-6 years: 7.5 ml after each loose stool; >6 years: 30 ml after each loose stool; max 7 doses/day

Liq: 600 mg/15 ml (120, 240 ml)

Donnagel Chewable Tab <3 years: not recommended; 3-6 years: 1/2 tab after each stool; max 7 doses/day; >6-12 years: 1 tab after each loose stool; max 7 tabs/day; >12 years: 2 tabs after each loose stool; max 14 tabs/day

▶ ***loperamide*** **(B)(OTC)(G)**

Imodium (OTC) <5 years: not recommended; ≥5 years: 4-16 mg/day in divided doses

Cap: 2 mg

Imodium A-D (OTC) <2 years: not recommended; 2-5 years (24-47 lb): 1 mg up to tid x 2 days; >5-8 years (48-59 lb): 2 mg initially, then 1 mg after each loose stool; max 4 mg/day x 2 days; >8-11 years (60-95 lb): 2 mg initially, then 1 mg after each loose stool; max 6 mg/day x 2 days; >11 years: 4-16 mg/day in divided doses

Cplt: 2 mg; *Liq:* 1 mg/5 ml (2, 4 oz)

▶ ***loperamide+simethicone*** (B)(OTC)(G)

Imodium Advanced <6 years: not recommended; 6-8 years: chew 1 tab after loose stool, then chew 1/2 tab after next loose stool; 9-11 years: chew 1 tab after loose stool, then chew 1/2 tab after next loose stool; max 3 tabs/day; >11 years: 2 tabs chewed after loose stool, then 1 after the next loose stool; max 4 tabs/day

Chew tab: loper 2 mg+simeth 125 mg

DIARRHEA: TRAVELERS

▶ ***ciprofloxacin*** (C) <18 years: not recommended; ≥18 years: 500 mg bid x 3 days; max 1.5 gm/day

Cipro (G) *Tab:* 250, 500, 750 mg; *Oral susp:* 250, 500 mg/5 ml (100 ml) (strawberry)

Cipro XR *Tab:* 500, 1000 mg ext-rel

ProQuin XR *Tab:* 500 mg ext-rel

Comment: ***ciprofloxacin*** is contraindicated <18 years-of-age, and during pregnancy, and lactation. Risk of tendonitis or tendon rupture.

▶ ***rifaximin*** (C) <12 years: not recommended; ≥12 years: 200 mg tid x 3 days; discontinue if diarrhea worsens or persists more than 24 hours; not for use if diarrhea is accompanied by fever or blood in the stool or if causative organism other than *E. coli* is suspected.

Xifaxan *Tab:* 200 mg

▶ ***trimethoprim+sulfamethoxazole [TMP-SMX]*** (C)(G)

Bactrim, Septra <12 years: not recommended; ≥12 years: 2 tabs bid x 10 days

Tab: trim 80 mg+sulfa 400 mg*

Bactrim DS, Septra DS <12 years: not recommended; ≥12 years: 1 tab bid x 10 days

Tab: trim 160 mg+sulfa 800 mg*

Bactrim Pediatric Suspension, Septra Pediatric Suspension <2 months: not recommended; ≥2 months-12 years: 40 mg/kg/day of ***sulfamethoxazole*** in 2 doses bid; >12 years: use tabs

Oral susp: trim 40 mg+sulfa 200 mg per 5 ml (100 ml) (cherry) (alcohol 0.3%)

DIGITALIS TOXICITY

Comment: The digitalis therapeutic index is narrow, 0.8-1.2 ng/mL. Whether acute or chronic toxicity, the patient should be treated in the emergency department and/or admitted to in-patient service for continued monitoring and care. Signs and symptoms of digitalis toxicity include: loss of appetite, nausea, vomiting, abdominal pain, diarrhea, visual disturbances (diplopia, blurred, or yellow vision, yellow-green halos around lights and other visual images, spots, blind spots), decreased urine output, generalized edema, orthopnea, confusion, delirium, decreased consciousness, potentially lethal cardiac arrhythmias (ranging from ventricular tachycardia (VT) and ventricular fibrillation (VF) to sino-atrial heart block AVB). Treatment measures include repeated doses of charcoal via NG tube administered after gastric lavage for acute ingestion (methods to induce vomiting are usually discouraged because vomiting can worsen bradyarrhythmias), digitalis binders. Monitoring includes: serial ECGs, serum digitalis level, chemistries, potassium (hyperkalemia), magnesium (hypomagnesemia), BUN and creatinine.

DIGOXIN BINDER

➢ ***digoxin (immune fab [ovine])*** (B) contents of one vial of **Digibind** or **Digifab** neutralizes 0.5 mg ***digoxin***; dose based on amount of ***digoxin*** or ***digitoxin*** to be neutralized; see mfr pkg insert
  Digibind *Vial:* 38 mg
  Digifab *Vial:* 40 mg for IV injection after reconstitution (preservative-free)

DIPHTHERIA

Prophylaxis *see* ***Childhood Immunizations*** *page* 525

POST-EXPOSURE PROPHYLAXIS FOR NON-IMMUNIZED PERSONS

➢ ***erythromycin base*** (B)(G) 45 kg: 50 mg/kg/day in 4 divided doses x 14 days; ≥45 kg: 500 mg qid x 14 days
  Ery-Tab *Tab:* 250, 333, 500 mg ent-coat
  PCE *Tab:* 333, 500 mg

➢ ***erythromycin ethylsuccinate*** (B)(G) 30-50 mg/kg/day in 4 divided doses x 14 days; may double dose with severe infection; max 100 mg/kg/day or 400 mg qid; *see page* 607 *for dose by weight table*
  EryPed *Oral susp:* 200 mg/5 ml (100, 200 ml) (fruit); 400 mg/5 ml (60, 100, 200 ml) (banana); *Oral drops:* 200, 400 mg/5 ml (50 ml) (fruit); *Chew tab:* 200 mg wafer (fruit)
  E.E.S. *Oral susp:* 200, 400 mg/5 ml (100 ml) (fruit)
  E.E.S. Granules *Oral susp:* 200 mg/5 ml (100, 200 ml) (cherry)
  E.E.S. 400 Tablets *Tab:* 400 mg

➢ ***Immunization Series***
  See ***Childhood Immunizations*** *page* 525

POST-EXPOSURE PROPHYLAXIS FOR IMMUNIZED PERSONS

➢ ***Diphtheria*** immunization booster

DIVERTICULITIS

➢ ***amoxicillin*** (B)(G) <40 kg (88 lb): 20-40 mg/kg/day in 3 divided doses x 10 days or 25-45 mg/kg/day in 2 divided doses x 10 days; *see page* 588 *for dose by weight table;* ≥40 kg: 500-875 mg bid or 250-500 mg tid x 10 days

Amoxil *Cap:* 250, 500 mg; *Tab:* 875*mg; *Chew tab:* 125, 200, 250, 400 mg(cherry-banana-peppermint) (phenylalanine); *Oral susp:* 125, 250 mg/5 ml(80, 100, 150 ml) (strawberry); 200, 400 mg/5 ml (50, 75, 100 ml) (bubble gum); *Oral drops:* 50 mg/ml (30 ml) (bubble gum)

Moxatag *Tab:* 775 mg ext-rel

Trimox *Tab:* 125, 250 mg; *Cap:* 250, 500 mg; *Oral susp:* 125, 250 mg/5 ml (80, 100, 150 ml) (raspberry-strawberry)

▶ ***amoxicillin+clavulanate*** **(B)(G)**

Augmentin <40 kg: 40-45 mg/kg/day divided tid x 10 days <u>or</u> 90 mg/kg/day divided bid x 10 days; *see page* 590 *for dose by weight table;* ≥40 kg: 500 mg tid <u>or</u> 875 mg bid x 10 days

Tab: 250, 500, 875 mg; *Chew tab:* 125, 250 mg (lemon-lime); 200, 400 mg (cherry-banana) (phenylalanine); *Oral susp:* 125 mg/5 ml (banana), 250 mg/5 ml (75, 100, 150 ml) (orange); 200, 400 mg/5 ml (50, 75, 100 ml) (orange) (phenylalanine)

Augmentin ES-600 <3 months: not recommended; ≥3 months, <40 kg: 90 mg/kg/day divided q 12 hours x 10 days; *see page* 591 *for dose by weight table;* ≥40 kg: not recommended

Oral susp: 600 mg/5 ml (50, 75, 100, 125, 150, 200 ml) (strawberry cream) (phenylalanine)

Augmentin XR <16 years: use other forms; ≥16 years: 2 tabs q 12 hours x 7-10 days

Tab: 1000*mg ext-rel

▶ ***ciprofloxacin*** **(C)** <18 years: not recommended; ≥18 years: 500 mg bid x 7 days; max 1.5 gm/day

Cipro (G) *Tab:* 250, 500, 750 mg; *Oral susp:* 250, 500 mg/5 ml (100 ml) (strawberry)

Cipro XR *Tab:* 500, 1000 mg ext-rel

ProQuin XR *Tab:* 500 mg ext-rel

Comment: ***ciprofloxacin*** is contraindicated <18 years-of-age, and during pregnancy, and lactation. Risk of tendonitis <u>or</u> tendon rupture.

▶ ***metronidazole*** **(not for use in 1st; B in 2nd, 3rd)(G)** 250-500 mg q 8 hours <u>or</u> 750 mg q 12 hours x 7 days

Flagyl *Tab:* 250*, 500*mg

Flagyl 375 *Cap:* 375 mg

Flagyl ER *Tab:* 750 mg ext-rel

Comment: Alcohol is contraindicated during treatment with oral ***metronidazole*** and for 72 hours after therapy due to a possible ***disulfiram***-like reaction (nausea, vomiting, flushing, headache).

▶ ***trimethoprim+sulfamethoxazole [TMP-SMX]*** **(D)(G)**

Bactrim, Septra <12 years: not recommended; ≥12 years: 2 tabs bid x 10 days

Tab: trim 80 mg+sulfa 400 mg*

Bactrim DS, Septra DS <12 years: not recommended; ≥12 years: 1 tab bid x 10 days

Tab: trim 160 mg+sulfa 800 mg*

Bactrim Pediatric Suspension, Septra Pediatric Suspension <2 months: not recommended; ≥2 months-12 years: 40 mg/kg/day of ***sulfamethoxazole*** in 2 doses bid; >12 years: use tabs

Oral susp: trim 40 mg+sulfa 200 mg per 5 ml (100 ml) (cherry) (alcohol 0.3%)

DIVERTICULOSIS

BULK-PRODUCING AGENTS

see ***Constipation*** *page* 94

DRY EYE SYNDROME

OPHTHALMIC IMMUNOMODULATOR/ANTI-INFLAMMATORY

▶ ***cyclosporine*** (C) <16 years: not recommended; ≥16 years: 1 drop q 12 hours
Restasis *Ophth emul:* 0.05% (0.4 ml) (preservative-free)
Comment: Ophthalmic immunomodulators are contraindicated with active ocular infection. Allow at least 15 minutes between doses of artificial tears. May reinsert contact lenses 15 minutes after treatment.

OCULAR LUBRICANTS

Comment: Remove contact lens prior to using an ocular lubricant.
▶ ***dextran 70+hypromellose*** 1-2 drops prn
Bion Tears (OTC) *Ophth soln:* single-use containers (28/pck) (preservative-free)
▶ ***hydroxypropyl cellulose*** apply 1/2 inch ribbon <u>or</u> 1 insert in each inferior cul-de-sac 1-2 x/day prn
Lacrisert *Ophth inserts:* 5 mg (60/pck) (preservative-free)
Hypotears Ophthalmic Ointment (OTC) *Ophth oint:* 1% (3.5 gm) (preservative-free)
Comment: Place insert in the inferior cul-de-sac of the eye, beneath the base of the tarsus, not in opposition to the cornea nor beneath the eyelid at the level of the tarsal plate.
▶ ***hydroxypropyl methylcellulose*** 1-2 drops prn
GenTeal Mild, GenTeal Moderate (OTC) *Ophth soln:* (15 ml) (perborate)
GenTeal Severe (OTC) *Ophth soln:* (15 ml) (carbopol 980, perborate)
▶ ***petrolatum+mineral oil*** apply 1/2 inch ribbon prn
Hypotears Ophthalmic Ointment (OTC) *Ophth oint:* 1% (3.5 gm) (benzalkonium chloride, alcohol 1%)
Hypotears PF Ophthalmic Ointment (OTC) *Ophth oint:* 1% (3.5 gm) (preservative-free, alcohol 1%)
Lacri-Lube (OTC) *Ophth oint:* 1% (3.5, 7 gm)
Lacri-Lube NP (OTC) *Ophth oint:* 1% (0.7 gm, 24/pck) (preservative-free)
▶ ***petrolatum+lanolin+mineral oil*** apply 1/4 inch ribbon prn
Duratears Naturale (OTC) *Ophth oint:* 3.5 gm (preservative-free)
▶ ***polyethylene glycol+glycerin+hydroxypropyl methylcellulose*** 1-2 drops prn
Visine Tears (OTC) *Ophth soln:* 1% (15, 30 ml)
▶ ***polyethylene glycol 400 0.4%+propylene glycol 0.3%*** 1-2 drops prn
Systane (OTC) *Ophth soln:* (15, 30, 40 ml) (polyquaternium-1, zinc chloride); *Vial:* 0.01 oz (28) (preservative-free)
Systane Ultra (OTC) *Ophth soln:* (10, 20 ml) (aminomethylpropanol, polyquaternium-1, sorbitol (zinc chloride); *Vial:* 0.01 oz (24) (preservative-free)
▶ ***polyvinyl alcohol*** 1-2 drops prn
Hypotears (OTC) *Ophth soln:* 1% (15, 30 ml)
Hypotears PF (OTC) 1-2 drops q 3-4 hours prn
Ophth soln: 1% (0.02 oz single-use containers, 30/pck) (preservative-free)
▶ ***propylene glycol*** 0.6% 1-2 drops prn
Systane Balance (OTC) *Ophth soln:* (10 ml) (polyquaternium-1)

DUCHENNE MUSCULAR DYSTROPHY (DMD)

▶ ***deflazacort*** (B) <5 years: not established; ≥ 5 years: 0.9 mg/kg/day administered once daily; take with <u>or</u> without food; may crush and mix with applesauce (then take immediately)
Emflaza *Tab:* 6, 18, 30, 36 mg; *Oral susp:* 22.75 mg/ml (13 ml)

Comment: **Emflaza** is the first FDA-approved corticosteroid indicated for this condition to decrease inflammation and reduce the activity of the immune system. The side effects caused by **Emflaza** are similar to those experienced with other corticosteroids. The most common side effects include facial puffiness (cushingoid appearance), weight gain, increased appetite, upper respiratory tract infection, cough, extraordinary daytime urinary frequency (pollakiuria), hirsutism, and central obesity. Other side effects that are less common include problems with endocrine function, increased susceptibility to infection, elevation in blood pressure, risk of gastrointestinal perforation, serious skin rashes, behavioral and mood changes, decrease in the density of the bones and vision problems such as cataracts. Patients receiving immunosuppressive doses of corticosteroids should not be given live or live attenuated vaccines (LAVs). Moderate or strong CYP3A4 inhibitors, give one third of the recommended dosage of **Emflaza**. Avoid use of moderate or strong CYP3A4 inducers with **Emflaza**, as they may reduce efficacy. Dosage must be decreased gradually if the drug has been administered for more than a few days. Use only the oral dispenser provided with the product. After withdrawing the appropriate dose into the oral dispenser, slowly add the oral suspension into 3 to 4 ounces of juice or milk and mix well. The dose should then be administered immediately. Do not administer with grapefruit. Discard any unused **Emflaza Oral Suspension** remaining after 1 month of first opening the bottle.

REFERENCE

FDA News Release: FDA approves drug to treat Duchenne muscular dystrophy (2/9/17) https:/www.fda.gov/NewsEvents/Newsroom/PressAnnouncements/ucm540945.htm

▶ ***eteplirsen*** 30 mg/kg via IV infusion over 35-60 minutes once weekly
Exondys *Vial:* 100 mg/2 ml (50 mg/ml), 500 mg/10 ml

Comment: **Exondys** is indicated for patients who have a confirmed mutation of the dystrophin gene amenable to exon 51 skipping (which affects about 13% of patients with DMD).

DYSHIDROSIS

Topical Corticosteroids *see page* 542

Comment: Intermediate to high potency ophthalmic steroid treatment is indicated for dyshidrosis.

DYSFUNCTIONAL UTERINE BLEEDING (DUB)

Oral Prescription NSAIDs *see page* 539
Other Oral Analgesics *see* ***Pain*** *page* 324

▶ ***medroxyprogesterone acetate*** (X) 10 mg daily x 10-13 days
Provera *Tab:* 2.5, 5, 10 mg
See **Oral and Injectable Progesterone-only Contraceptives** *page* 537

▶ ***combined oral contraceptives*** (X) with 35 mcg ***estrogen***-equivalent
see **Combined Oral Contraceptives** *page* 528

DYSLIPIDEMIA (HYPERCHOLESTEROLEMIA, HYPERLIPIDEMIA, MIXED DYSLIPIDEMIA)

Comment: As recommended by the American Heart, Lung, and Blood Institute, children and adolescents should be screened for dyslipidemia once between 9 and 11 years and once between 17 and 21 years.

OMEGA 3-FATTY ACID ETHYL ESTERS

Comment: ***Vascepa, Lovaza,*** and ***Epanova*** are indicated for the treatment of TG ≥500 mg/dL.

- ***icosapent ethyl (omega 3-fatty acid ethyl ester of EPA)*** **(C)** <18 years: not recommended; ≥18 years: 2 caps bid with food; max 4 g/day; swallow whole, do not crush or chew
  - **Vascepa sgc:** 0.5, 1 gm (α-tocopherol 4 mg/cap)
- ***omega 3-acid ethyl esters*** **(C)(G)**
  - **Lovaza** <18 years: not recommended; ≥18 years: 2 gm bid or 4 gm once daily
    - *Soft gel cap:* 1 gm (α-tocopherol 4 mg/cap)
  - **Epanova** <18 years: not recommended; ≥18 years: 2 gm bid or 4 gm once daily; swallow whole, do not crush or chew
    - *Gelcap:* 1 gm

MICROSOMAL TRIGLYCERIDE-TRANSFER PROTEIN (MTP) INHIBITOR

- ***lomitapide mesylate*** **(X)** <12 years: not recommended; ≥12 years: 10 mg daily
  - **Juxtapid** *Cap:* 5, 10, 20 mg
  - Comment: **Juxtapid** is an adjunct to low-fat diet and other lipid-lowering treatments, including LDL apheresis where available, to reduce LDL-C, total cholesterol, apo-B, and non-HDL-C in patients with homozygous familial hypercholesterolemia (HoFH); not for patients with hypercholesterolemia who do not have HoFH.

OLIGONUCLEOTIDE INHIBITOR OF APO B-100 SYNTHESIS

- ***mipomersen*** **(B)** <12 years: not established; ≥12 years: administer 200 mg SC once weekly, on the same day, in the upper arm, abdomen, or thigh; administer 1st injection under appropriate professional supervision
  - **Kynamro** *Vial, Prefilled syringe:* 200 mg mg/ml soln for SC inj single-use vial (preservative-free)
  - Comment: **Kynamro** is an adjunct to low-fat diet and other lipid-lowering treatments, to reduce LDL-C, apo-B, total cholesterol (TC), non-HDL-C in patients with homozygous familial hypercholesterolemia (HoFH).

CHOLESTEROL ABSORPTION INHIBITOR

- ***ezetimibe*** **(C)(G)** <10 years: not recommended; ≥10 years: 10 mg daily
  - **Zetia** *Tab:* 10 mg

Comment: ***ezetimibe*** is contraindicated with concomitant statins in liver disease, persistent elevations in serum transaminase, pregnancy, and nursing mothers. Concomitant fibrates are not recommended. Potentiated by ***fenofibrate, gemfibrozil,*** and possibly ***cyclosporine***. Separate dosing of bile acid sequestrants is required; take ***ezetimibe*** at least 2 hours before or 4 hours after.

PROPROTEIN CONVERTASE SUBTILISIN KEXIN TYPE 9 (PCSK9) INHIBITOR

Comment: PCSK9 inhibitors are an adjunct to maximally tolerated statin therapy in persons who require additional lowering of LDL-C.

- ***alirocumab*** <18 years: not established; ≥18 years: administer SC in the upper outer arm, abdomen, or thigh; initially 75 mg SC once every 2 weeks; measure LDL 4-8 weeks after initiation or titration; if inadequate response, may increase to 150 mg SC every 2 weeks or 300 mg SC once monthly
  - **Praluent**

Soln for SC inj: 75, 150 mg/ml (1 ml) single-use prefilled syringe (preservative-free)

Comment: The FDA has approved a new once-monthly 300 mg dosing option for **Praluent** injection, for the treatment of patients with high low-density lipoprotein (LDL) cholesterol. The drug is indicated as an adjunct to diet and statin therapy for patients with heterozygous familial hypercholesterolemia (HeFH) or clinical atherosclerotic cardiovascular disease (ASCVD) who require additional LDL lowering. The most common side effects of **Praluent** include injection site reactions, symptoms of the common cold, and flu-like symptoms. Each 150 mg pen delivers the dose over 20 seconds. A 300 mg once monthly dose = administration of 2 x 150 mg pens. **Praluent** is contraindicated in the 2nd and 3rd trimester of pregnancy.

▻ ***evolocumab***

Repatha <12 years: HeFH, primary hyperlipidemia: not established; HoFH: <13 years: not established; >13 years: administer SC in the upper outer arm, elbow, or thigh; measure LDL 4-8 weeks after initiation; *HeFH* or *primary hyperlipidemia:* 140 mg SC once every 2 weeks or 420 mg once monthly; *HoFH:* 420 mg once monthly

Soln for SC inj: single-use prefilled syringe; 140 mg/syringe; single-use prefilled SureClick Autoinjector (140 mg/syringe preservative-free)

Comment: To administer 420 mg of **Repatha**, administer 150 mg SC x 3 within 30 minutes. Although **Repatha** does not have an assigned pregnancy category, it is contraindicated in pregnancy.

HMG-COA REDUCTASE INHIBITORS (STATINS)

Comment: The statins decrease total cholesterol, LDL-C, TG, and apo-B, and increase HDL-C. Before initiating and at 4-6 weeks, 3 months, and 6 months of therapy, check fasting lipid profile and LFTs. Side effects include myopathy and increased liver enzymes. Relative contraindications include concomitant use of cyclosporine, a macrolide antibiotic, various oral antifungal agents, and CYP-450 inhibitors. An absolute contraindication is active or chronic liver disease.

▻ ***atorvastatin*** **(X)(G)** <10 years: not recommended; ≥10 years (female post-menarche): initially 10 mg daily; usual range 10-80 mg/day

Lipitor *Tab:* 10, 20, 40, 80 mg

▻ ***fluvastatin*** **(X)(G)** <18 years: not recommended; ≥18 years; initially 20-40 mg q HS; usual range 20-80 mg/day

Lescol *Cap:* 20, 40 mg

Lescol XL *Tab:* 80 mg ext-rel

▻ ***lovastatin*** **(X)**

Mevacor <10 years: not recommended; 10-17 years: initially 10-20 mg daily at evening meal; may increase at 4-week intervals; max 40 mg daily; >17 years: initially 20 mg daily at evening meal; may increase at 4-week intervals; max 80 mg/day in single or divided doses; if concomitant fibrates, niacin, or *CrCl <30 mL/min*, usual max 20 mg/day

Tab: 10, 20, 40 mg

Altoprev <20 years: not recommended; ≥20 years: initially 20 mg daily at evening meal; may increase at 4-week intervals; max 60 mg/day; if concomitant fibrates, or ***niacin***; >1 gm/day, usual max 40 mg/day; if concomitant cyclosporine, ***amiodarone***, or ***verapamil***, or *CrCl <30 mL/min*, usual max 20 mg/day

Tab: 10, 20, 40, 60 mg ext-rel

- ***pitavastatin*** **(X)(G)** <12 years: not established; initially 2 mg q HS; may increase to 4 mg after 4 weeks; max 4 mg/day; if concomitant ***erythromycin*** *or CrCl <60 mL/min;* 1 mg/day with usual max 2 mg/day; if concomitant ***rifampin***, max 2 mg once daily
  - **Livalo** *Tab:* 1, 2, 4 mg
  - **Nikita** *Tab:* 1, 2, 4 mg
- ***pravastatin*** **(X)** <8 years: not recommended; 8-13 years: 20 mg daily; >13-18 years: 40 mg daily; >18 years: initially 10-20 mg q HS; usual range 10-40 mg/day; may start at 40 mg/day
  - **Pravachol** *Tab:* 10, 20, 40, 80 mg
- ***rosuvastatin*** **(X)(G)** <10 years: not recommended; 10-17 years: 5-20 mg/day; max 20 mg/day; >17 years: initially 10-20 mg q HS; usual range 5-40 mg/day; adjust at 4-week intervals
  - **Crestor** *Tab:* 5, 10, 20, 40 mg
- ***simvastatin*** **(X)** <10 years: not recommended; ≥10 years (female post menarche): initially 20 mg q PM; usual range 5-80 mg/day; adjust at 4-week intervals
  - **Zocor** *Tab:* 5, 10, 20, 40, 80 mg

CHOLESTEROL ABSORPTION INHIBITOR+HMG-COA REDUCTASE INHIBITOR COMBINATION

- ***ezetimibe+atorvastatin*** **(X)(G)** Take once daily in the PM; may start at 10/40; swallow whole, do not cut, crush, or chew
  Pediatric: <17 years: not recommended; ≥17 years: same as adult
  - *Tab:* **Liptruzet 10/10** ezet 10 mg+atorva 10 mg
  - **Liptruzet 10/20** ezet 10 mg+atorva 20 mg
  - **Liptruzet 10/40** ezet 10 mg+atorva 40 mg
  - **Liptruzet 10/80** ezet 10 mg+atorva 80 mg
- ***ezetimibe+simvastatin*** **(X)(G)** <17 years: not recommended; ≥17 years: take once daily in the PM; may start at **10/40**; swallow whole
  - **Vytorin**
  - *Tab:* **Vytorin 10/10** ezet 10 mg+simva 10 mg
  - **Vytorin 10/20** ezet 10 mg+simva 20 mg
  - **Vytorin 10/40** ezet 10 mg+simva 40 mg
  - **Vytorin 10/80** ezet 10 mg+simva 80 mg

ISOBUTYRIC ACID DERIVATIVES AND FIBRATE

Comment: These agents decrease total cholesterol, LDL-C, and TG; increase HDL-C. They are indicated when the primary problem is very high TG level. Side effects include epigastric discomfort, dyspepsia, abdominal pain, cholelithiasis, myopathy, and neutropenia. Before initiating, and at 4-6 weeks, 3 months, and 6 months of therapy, check fasting CBC, lipid profile, LFT, and serum creatinine. Absolute contraindications include severe renal disease and severe hepatic disease.

ISOBUTYRIC ACID DERIVATIVES

- ***gemfibrozil*** (C)(G) <12 years: not recommended; ≥12 years: 600 mg bid 30 minutes before AM and PM meal
  - **Lopid** *Tab:* 600*mg

FIBRATES (FIBRIC ACID DERIVATIVES)

- ***fenofibrate*** (C)(G) <12 years: not recommended; ≥12 years: take with meals; adjust at 4- to 8-week intervals; discontinue if inadequate response after 2 months; lowest dose or contraindicated with renal impairment

Antara 43-130 mg daily; max 130 mg/day
Cap: 43, 87, 130 mg
Fenoglide 40-120 mg daily; max 120 mg/day
Tab: 40, 120 mg
FibriCor 30-105 mg daily; max 105 mg/day
Tab: 30, 105 mg
TriCor 48-145 mg daily; max 145 mg/day
Tab: 48, 145 mg
TriLipix 45-135 mg daily; max 135 mg/day
Cap: 45, 135 mg del-rel
Lipofen 50-150 mg daily; max 150 mg/day
Cap: 50, 150 mg
Lofibra 67-200 mg daily; max 200 mg/day
Tab: 67, 134, 200 mg

NICOTINIC ACID DERIVATIVES

Comment: Nicotinic acid derivatives decrease total cholesterol, LDL-C, and TG; increase HDL-C. Before initiating and at 4-6 weeks, 3 months, and 6 months of therapy, check fasting lipid profile, LFT, glucose, and uric acid. Side effects include hyperglycemia, upper GI distress, hyperuricemia, hepatotoxicity, and significant transient skin flushing. Take with food and take ***aspirin*** 325 mg 30 minutes before niacin dose to decrease flushing. Relative contraindications include diabetes, hyperuricemia (gout), and PUD and absolute contraindications include severe gout and chronic liver disease.

▶ ***niacin*** (C)
Niaspan (G) <21 years: not recommended; 375 mg daily for 1st week, then 500 mg daily for 2nd week, then 750 mg daily for 3rd week, then 1 gm daily for weeks 4-7; may increase by 500 mg q 4 weeks; usual range 1-2 gm/day; max 2 gm/day
Tab: 500, 750, 1000 mg ext-rel
Slo-Niacin <12 years: not recommended; ≥12 years: one 250 or 500 mg tab q AM or HS or one-half 750 mg tab q AM or HS
Tab: 250, 500, 750 mg cont-rel

BILE ACID SEQUESTRANTS

Comment: Bile acid sequestrants decrease total cholesterol, LDL-C, and increase HDL-C, but have no effect on triglycerides. A relative contraindication is TG ≥200 mg/dL and an absolute contraindication is TG ≥400 mg/dL. Before initiating and at 4-6 weeks, 3 months, and 6 months of therapy, check fasting lipid profile. Side effects include sandy taste in mouth, abdominal gas, abdominal cramping, and constipation. These agents decrease the absorption of many other drugs.

▶ ***cholestyramine*** (C)
Questran Powder for Oral Suspension <12 years: see mfr pkg insert; ≥12 years: initially 1 pkt or scoop daily; usual maintenance 2-4 pkts or scoops daily in 2 divided doses; max 6 pkts or scoops daily
Pwdr: 9 gm pkts; 9 gm equals 4 gm anhydrous ***cholestyramine*** resin for reconstitution (60/pck); *Bulk can:* 378 gm w. scoop
Questran Light <12 years: see mfr pkg insert; ≥12 years: initially 1 pkt or scoop daily; usual maintenance 2-4 pkts or scoops daily in 2 doses
Light: 5 gm pkts; 5 gm equals 4 gm anhydrous ***cholestyramine*** resin (60/pck): *Bulk can:* 210 gm w. scoop

▶ ***colesevelam*** (B)
Monotherapy: <12 years: not recommended; ≥12 years: 3 tabs bid or 6 tabs once daily or one 1.875 gm pkt bid or one 3.75 gm pkt once daily

WelChol *Tab:* 625 mg; *Pwdr for oral susp:* 1.875 gm pwdr pkts (60/carton); 3.75 gm pwdr pkts (30/carton) (citrus) (phenylalanine)

Comment: **WelChol** is indicated as adjunctive therapy to improve glycemic control in patients >18 years with type 2 diabetes. It can be added to ***metformin***, sulfonylureas, or ***insulin*** alone or in combination with other antidiabetic agents

▶ ***colestipol*** (C)

Comment: ***colestipol*** lowers LDL and total cholesterol.

Colestid <12 years: not recommended; ≥12 years: 2-16 gm daily in a single or divided doses; granules: 5-30 gm daily in a single or divided dose

Tab: 1 gm (120); *Granules:* unflavored: 5 gm pkt (30, 90/carton); unflavored bulk: 300, 500 gm w. scoop; orange-flavored: 7.5 gm pkt (60/carton) (aspartame, phenylalanine); orange-flavored bulk: 450 gm w. scoop (aspartame); flavored: 7.5 gm pkt

Colestid Tab initially 2 gm bid; increase by 2 gm bid at 1-2-month intervals; usual maintenance 2-16 gm/day

Tab: 1 gm

ANTILIPID COMBINATIONS

Nicotinic Acid Derivative+HMG-CoA Reductase Inhibitor Combinations

▶ ***niacin+lovastatin*** (X)

Advicor <18 years: not recommended; ≥18 years: swallow whole at bedtime with a low-fat snack; may pretreat with aspirin; start at lowest niacin dose; may titrate niacin by no more than 500 mg/day every 4 weeks; max 2000/40 daily

Tab: **Advicor 500/20** nia 500 mg ext-rel+lova 20 mg
Advicor 750/20 nia 750 mg ext-rel+lova 20 mg
Advicor 1000/20 nia 1000 mg ext-rel+lova 20 mg
Advicor 1000/40 nia 1000 mg ext-rel+lova 40 mg

▶ ***niacin+simvastatin*** (X)

Simcor <18 years: not recommended; ≥18 years: swallow whole at bedtime with a low-fat snack; may pretreat with ***aspirin***; start at lowest ***niacin*** dose; may titrate ***niacin*** by no more than 500 mg/day every 4 weeks; max 2000/40 daily; take aspirin 325 mg 30 minutes before dose to decrease niacin flushing.

Tab: **Simcor 500/20** nia 500 mg ext-rel+simva 20 mg
Simcor 750/20 nia 750 mg ext-rel+simva 20 mg
Simcor 1000/20 nia 1000 mg ext-rel+simva 20 mg
Simcor 500/40 nia 500 mg ext-rel+simva 40 mg
Simcor 1000/40 nia 1000 mg ext-rel+simva 40 mg

ANTIHYPERTENSIVE+ANTILIPID COMBINATIONS

Calcium Channel Blocker+HMG-CoA Reductase Inhibitor (Statin) Combinations

▶ ***amlodipine+atorvastatin*** (X)(G)

Caduet <10 years: not recommended; ≥10 years (female, post-menarche):select according to blood pressure and lipid values; titrate amlodipine over 7-14 days; titrate atorvastatin according to monitored lipid values; max amlodipine 10 mg/day and max atorvastatin 80 mg/day; for contraindications and precautions for CCB and statin therapy, see to mfr pkg insert

Tab: **Caduet 5/10** amlo 5 mg+ator 10 mg
Caduet 5/20 amlo 5 mg+ator 20 mg

Caduet 5/40 amlo 5 mg+ator 40 mg
Caduet 5/80 amlo 5 mg+ator 80 mg
Caduet 10/10 amlo 10 mg+ator 10 mg
Caduet 10/20 amlo 10 mg+ator 20 mg
Caduet 10/40 amlo 10 mg+ator 40 mg
Caduet 10/80 amlo 10 mg+ator 80 mg

DYSMENORRHEA: PRIMARY

NSAIDs *see page* 539
Other Oral Analgesics *see* ***Pain*** *page* 324
Combined Oral Contraceptives *see page* 528

BENZENEACETIC ACID DERIVATIVE

▷ ***diclofenac*** (C) <14 years: not recommended; ≥14 years: 50-100 mg once; then 50 tid
Cataflam *Tab:* 50 mg
Voltaren *Tab:* 25, 50, 75 mg ent-coat
Voltaren-XR *Tab:* 100 mg ext-rel
Comment: ***diclofenac*** is contraindicated with ***aspirin*** allergy and late (≥30 weeks) pregnancy.

FENAMATE

Comment: Avoid ***aspirin*** with a fenamate.
▷ ***mefenamic acid*** (C) <14 years: not recommended; >14 years: 500 mg once; then 250 mg q 6 hours for up to 2-3 days; take with food
Ponstel *Cap:* 250 mg

COX-2 INHIBITORS

Comment: Cox-2 inhibitors are contraindicated with history of asthma, urticaria, and allergic-type reactions to ***aspirin***, other NSAIDs, and sulfonamides, 3rd trimester of pregnancy, and coronary artery bypass graft (CABG) surgery.
▷ ***celecoxib*** (C)(G) <18 years: not recommended; ≥18 years: 100-400 mg bid; max 800 mg/day
Celebrex *Cap:* 50, 100, 200, 400 mg
▷ ***meloxicam*** (C)(G)
Mobic <2 years, <60 kg: not recommended; ≥2, ≥60 kg: 0.125 mg/kg; max 7.5 mg once daily; ≥18 years: initially 7.5 mg once daily; max 15 mg once daily; *Hemodialysis:* max 7.5 mg/day
Tab: 7.5, 15 mg; *Oral susp:* 7.5 mg/5 ml (100 ml) (raspberry)
Vivlodex <18 years: not established; ≥18 years: initially 5 mg qd; may increase to max 10 mg/day; *Hemodialysis:* max 5 mg/day
Cap: 5, 10 mg

EDEMA

THIAZIDE DIURETICS

▷ ***chlorthalidone*** (B)(G) initially 30-60 mg daily <u>or</u> 60 mg on alternate days; max 90-120 mg/day
Thalitone *Tab:* 15 mg

- ▶ ***chlorothiazide*** **(B)(G)** <6 months: up to 15 mg/lb/day in 2 divided doses; ≥6 months-12 years: 10 mg/lb/day in 2 divided doses; max 375 mg/day; >12 years: 0.5-1 gm/day in a single or divided doses; max 2 gm/day
  - **Diuril** *Tab:* 250*, 500*mg; *Oral susp:* 250 mg/5 ml (237 ml)
- ▶ ***hydrochlorothiazide*** **(B)(G)** <12 years: not recommended; ≥12 years:
  - **Esidrix** 25-200 mg daily
    - *Tab:* 25, 50, 100 mg
  - **Microzide** 12.5 mg daily; usual max 50 mg/day
    - *Cap:* 12.5 mg
- ▶ ***hydroflumethiazide*** **(B)** <2 years: not recommended; ≥2 years: 50-200 mg/day in a single or 2 divided doses
  - **Saluron** *Tab:* 50 mg
- ▶ ***polythiazide*** **(C)** <2 years: not recommended; ≥2 years: 1-4 mg daily
  - **Renese** *Tab:* 1, 2, 4 mg

POTASSIUM-SPARING DIURETICS

- ▶ ***amiloride*** **(B)(G)** <12 years: not recommended; ≥12 years: initially 5 mg; may increase to 10 mg; max 20 mg
  - *Tab:* 5 mg
- ▶ ***spironolactone*** **(D)** <12 years: not recommended; ≥12 years: initially 25-200 mg in a single or divided doses; titrate at 2-week intervals
  - **Aldactone (G)** *Tab:* 25, 50*, 100*mg
  - **CaroSpir** *Oral susp:* 25 mg/5 ml (118, 473 ml) (banana)
- ▶ ***triamterene*** **(B)** <12 years: not recommended; ≥12 years: 100 mg bid; max 300 mg
  - **Dyrenium** *Cap:* 50, 100 mg

LOOP DIURETICS

- ▶ ***bumetanide*** **(C)(G)** <18 years: not recommended; ≥18 years: 0.5-2 mg daily; may repeat at 4-5 hour intervals; max 10 mg/day
  - *Tab:* 1*mg

  Comment: ***bumetanide*** is contraindicated with sulfa drug allergy.
- ▶ ***ethacrynic acid*** **(B)(G)** ≤1 month: not recommended; >1 month-12 years: initially 25 mg/day; then adjust dose in 25 mg increments; >12 years: max 50-200 mg once daily
  - **Edecrin** *Tab:* 25, 50 mg
- ▶ ***ethacrynate sodium*** *for IV injection* **(B)(G)** <1 month: not recommended; ≥1 month-12 years: use the smallest effective dose; initially 25 mg; then careful stepwise increments in dosage of 25 mg to achieve effective maintenance; ≥12 years: administer smallest dose required to produce gradual weight loss (about 1-2 pounds per day); onset of diuresis usually occurs at 50-100 mg in children ≥12 years; after diuresis has been achieved, the minimally effective dose (usually 50-200 mg/day) may be administered on a continuous or intermittent dosage schedule; dose titrations are usually in 25-50 mg increments to avoid derangement electrolyte and water excretion; the patient should be weighed under standard conditions before and during administration of ***ethacrynate sodium;*** the following schedule may be helpful in determining the lowest effective dose: *Day 1:* 50 mg once daily after a meal; *Day 2:* 50 mg bid after meals, if necessary; *Day 3:* 100 mg in the morning and 50-100 mg following the afternoon or evening meal, depending upon response to the morning dose; a few patients may require initial and maintenance doses as high as 200 mg bid; these higher doses, which should be achieved gradually, are most often required in patients with severe, refractory edema
  - **Sodium Edecrin** *Vial:* 50 mg single-dose

    Comment: **Sodium Edecrin** is more potent than more commonly used loop and thiazide diuretics. Treatment of the edema associated with congestive heart failure, cirrhosis of the liver, and renal disease, including the nephrotic syndrome, short-term management of ascites due to malignancy, idiopathic edema, and lymphedema, short-term management of hospitalized pediatric patients, other than infants, with congenital heart disease or the nephrotic syndrome. IV **Sodium Edecrin** is indicated when a rapid onset of diuresis is desired, e.g., in acute pulmonary edema or when gastrointestinal absorption is impaired or oral medication is not practical.

- ***furosemide*** (C)(G) <12 years: not recommended; ≥12 years: initially 20-80 mg as a single dose
  - **Lasix** *Tab:* 20, 40*, 80 mg; *Oral soln:* 10 mg/ml (2, 4 oz w. dropper)

Comment: ***furosemide*** is contraindicated with sulfa drug allergy.

- ***torsemide*** (B) <12 years: not recommended; ≥12 years: 5 mg daily; may increase to 10 mg daily
  - **Demadex** *Tab:* 5*, 10*, 20*, 100*mg

OTHER DIURETICS

- ***indapamide*** (B) <12 years: not recommended; ≥12 years: initially 1.25 mg daily; may titrate every 4 weeks if needed; max 5 mg/day
  - **Lozol** *Tab:* 1.25, 2.5 mg

Comment: ***indapamide*** is contraindicated with sulfa drug allergy.

- ***metolazone*** (B)
  - **Mykrox** <12 years: not recommended; ≥12 years: initially 0.5 mg q AM; max 1 mg/day
    - *Tab:* 0.5 mg
  - **Zaroxolyn** <12 years: not recommended; ≥12 years: 2.5-5 mg once daily
    - *Tab:* 2.5, 5, 10 mg

Comment: ***metolazone*** is contraindicated with sulfa drug allergy.

DIURETIC COMBINATIONS

- ***amiloride+hydrochlorothiazide*** (B)(G) <12 years: not recommended; ≥12 years: initially 1 tab daily; may increase to 2 tabs/day in a single or divided doses
  - **Moduretic** *Tab:* amil 5 mg+hydro 50 mg*
- ***spironolactone+hydrochlorothiazide*** (D)(G) <12 years: not recommended; ≥12 years: usual maintenance is 100 mg each of spironolactone and hydrochlorothiazide daily, in a single dose or in divided doses; range 25-200 mg of each component daily depending on the response to the initial titration
  - **Aldactazide 25** *Tab:* spiro 25 mg+hydro 25 mg
  - **Aldactazide 50** *Tab:* spiro 50 mg+hydro 50 mg
- ***triamterene+hydrochlorothiazide*** (C)(G) <12 years: not recommended; ≥12 years:
  - **Dyazide** 1-2 caps once daily
    - *Cap:* triam 37.5 mg+hydro 25 mg
  - **Maxzide** 1 tab once daily
    - *Tab:* triam 75 mg+hydro 50 mg*
  - **Maxzide-25** 1-2 tabs once daily
    - *Tab:* triam 37.5 mg+hydro 25 mg*

ENCOPRESIS

INITIAL BOWEL EVACUATION

- ***mineral oil*** (C) 1 oz x 1 day

Comment: Mineral oil can inhibit absorption of fat-soluble vitamins (A, D, E, and K).

- *bisacodyl* (B) <12 years: 1/2 suppository daily prn; ≥12 years: 1 suppository daily prn
  - **Dulcolax** *Rectal supp:* 10 mg
- *glycerin* suppository <6 years: 1 pediatric suppository; ≥6 years: 1 adult suppository

MAINTENANCE

- *mineral oil* (C) 5-15 ml once daily
- *multivitamin* (A) 1 daily

ENDOMETRIOSIS

Comment: Endometriosis can begin in teens as early as the first menstrual period. Treatment options for adolescents and adults are the same. Acetaminophen and (NSAIDs) can help relieve the pain, but they do not affect the endometriosis itself. Combination contraceptives reduce the amount of menstrual flow can often reduce the pain associated with endometriosis symptoms while producing shorter and lighter menstrual cycles.

Acetaminophen for IV Infusion *see* ***Pain*** *page* 322
NSAIDs *see page* 539
Other Oral Analgesics *see* ***Pain*** *page* 324
Contraceptives *see page* 527

MEDICAL MARIJUANA FOR ENDOMETRIOSIS PAIN

Comment: The functioning of the uterus is related to the body's internal cannabinoid system, which has led researchers to explore medical marijuana as a pain management option. A 2010 study examined the effects of cannabinoids on controlling endometriosis growth and pain in rats. The researchers found the results promising.

PROGESTERONE-ONLY CONTRACEPTIVES

- *medroxyprogesterone* (X) 30 mg daily
  - **Provera** *Tab:* 2.5, 5, 10 mg
- *medroxyprogesterone acetate* injectable (X) 100-400 mg IM monthly
  - **Depo-Provera** Injectable: 300 mg/ml (2.5, 10 ml)
- *norethindrone acetate* (X) initially 5 mg daily x 2 weeks; then increase by 2.5 mg/day every 2 weeks up to 15 mg/day maintenance dose; then continue for 6 to 9 months unless breakthrough bleeding is intolerable
  - **Aygestin** *Tab:* 5*mg

GONADOTROPIN-RELEASING HORMONE ANALOGS (GnRDa)

Comment: These agonists can have unpleasant side effects (e.g., hot flashes, vaginal dryness, bone loss, changes in mood).

- *goserelin (GnRH analog)* implant (X) implant SC into upper abdominal wall; 1 SC implant q 28 days for up to 6 months; re-treatment not recommended
  Pediatric: <18 years: not recommended; >18 years: same as adult
  - **Zoladex** SC implant in syringe: 3.6 mg
- *leuprolide acetate (GnRH analog)* (X)
  Pediatric: <18 years: not recommended; >18 years: same as adult
  - **Lupron Depot 3.75 mg** 3.75 mg SC monthly for up to 6 months; may repeat one 6-month cycle
    - *Syringe:* 3.75 mg (single-dose depo susp for SC injection)

Lupron Depot-3 Month 22.5 mg SC q 3 months (84 days); max 2 injections
Syringe: 22.5 mg (single-dose depo susp for IM injection)

Comment: Do not split doses.

▶ ***nafarelin acetate*** **(X)** 1 spray (200 mcg) into one nostril q AM, then 1 spray (200 mcg) into the other nostril q PM x 6 months; if no response after 2 months, may increase to 2 sprays (400 mcg) bid
Pediatric: <18 years: not recommended; >18 years: same as adult
Synarel *Nasal spray:* 2 mg/ml (10 ml)

Comment: Start ***nafarelin acetate*** (**Synarel**) on the 3rd or 4th day of the menstrual period or after a negative pregnancy test.

SYNTHETIC STEROID DERIVED FROM ETHISTERONE

▶ ***danazol*** **(X)** start on 3rd or 4th day of menstrual period or after a negative pregnancy test; initially 400 mg bid; gradual downward titration of dosage may be considered dependent upon patient response; mild cases may respond to 100-200 mg bid
Pediatric: <18 years: not recommended; >18 years: same as adult
Danocrine *Cap:* 50, 100, 200 mg

Comment: ***danazol*** is a synthetic steroid derived from ethisterone. It suppresses the pituitary-ovarian axis. This suppression is probably a combination of depressed hypothalamic-pituitary response to lowered ***estrogen*** production, the alteration of sex steroid metabolism, and interaction of ***danazol*** with sex hormone receptors. The only other demonstrable hormonal effects are weak androgenic activity and depression of both follicle-stimulating hormone (FSH) andmluteinizing hormone (LH) output. Recent evidence suggests a direct inhibitory effect at gonadal sites and a binding of **Danocrine** to receptors of gonadal steroids at target organs. In addition, **Danocrine** has been shown to significantly decrease IgG, IgM and IgA levels, as well as phospholipid and IgG isotope autoantibodies in patients with endometriosis and associated elevations of autoantibodies, suggesting this could be another mechanism by which it facilitates regression of endometrial lesions. **Danocrine** alters the normal and ectopic endometrial tissue so that it becomes inactive and atrophic. Complete resolution of endometrial lesions occurs in the majority of cases. Changes in the menstrual pattern may occur. Generally, the pituitary-suppressive action of **Danocrine** is reversible. Ovulation and cyclic bleeding usually return within 60 to 90 days when therapy with **Danocrine** is discontinued. **Danocrine** is also used to treat fibrocystic breast disease (reduces breast tissue nodularity and breast pain) and hereditary angioedema (to prevent attacks). Contraindications include pregnancy, breastfeeding, active or history of thromboembolic disease/event, porphyria, undiagnosed abnormal genital bleeding, androgen-dependent tumor, and markedly impaired hepatic, renal, or cardiac function.

☐ ENURESIS: PRIMARY, NOCTURNAL

VASOPRESSIN

▶ ***desmopressin acetate*** **(B)**
DDAVP <6 years: not recommended; ≥6 years: usual dose 0.2 mg before bedtime
Tab: 0.1*, 0.2*mg
DDAVP Rhinal Tube <6 years: not recommended; ≥6 years: 10 mcg or 0.1 ml of soln each nostril (20 mcg total dose) before bedtime
Nasal spray: 10 mcg/actuation (5 ml, 50 sprays); *Rhinal tube*: 0.1 mg/ml (2.5 ml)

TRICYCLIC ANTIDEPRESSANTS (TCAs)

Comment: Co-administration of SSRIs and TCAs requires extreme caution.

- *amitriptyline* (C)(G) <12 years: not recommended; ≥12 years: initially 10 mg before bedtime; use lowest effective dose
  - *Tab:* 10, 25, 50, 75, 100, 150 mg
- *amoxapine* (C) <12 years: not recommended; ≥12 years: initially 25 mg before bedtime; use lowest effective dose
  - *Tab:* 25, 50, 100, 150 mg
- *clomipramine* (C)(G) <10 years: not recommended; ≥10 years: initially 25 mg before bedtime; use lowest effective dose
  - **Anafranil** *Cap:* 25, 50, 75 mg
- *desipramine* (C)(G) <12 years: not recommended; ≥12 years: initially 25 mg before bedtime; use lowest effective dose
  - **Norpramin** *Tab:* 10, 25, 50, 75, 100, 150 mg
- *doxepin* (C)(G) <12 years: not recommended; ≥12 years: initially 10 mg before bedtime; use lowest effective dose
  - *Cap:* 10, 25, 50, 75, 100, 150 mg; Oral conc: 10 mg/ml (4 oz w. dropper)
- *imipramine* (C)(G) <12 years: not recommended; ≥12 years:
  - **Tofranil** initially 10 mg at bedtime; use lowest effective dose; if bedtime dose exceeds 75 mg daily, may switch to **Tofranil PM**
    - *Tab:* 10, 25, 50 mg
  - **Tofranil PM** initially 75 mg before bedtime; use lowest effective dose
    - *Cap:* 75, 100, 125, 150 mg
- *nortriptyline* (D)(G) <12 years: not recommended; ≥12 years: initially 10 mg before bedtime; use lowest effective dose
  - **Pamelor** *Cap:* 10, 25, 50, 75 mg; *Oral soln:* 10 mg/5 ml (16 oz)
- *protriptyline* (C) <12 years: not recommended; ≥12 years: initially 5 mg before bedtime; use lowest effective dose
  - **Vivactil** *Tab:* 5, 10 mg
- *trimipramine* (C) <12 years: not recommended; ≥12 years: initially 25 mg before bedtime; use lowest effective dose
  - **Surmontil** *Cap:* 25, 50, 100 mg

EOSINOPHILIC GRANULOMATOSIS WITH POLYANGIITIS (FORMERLY, CHURG-STRAUSS SYNDROME)

Comment: Eosinophilic granulomatosis with polyangiitis (EGPA) is a rare autoimmune disease that causes vasculitis, an inflammation in the wall of blood vessels of the body. EGPA is a characterized by asthma, high levels of eosinophils, and inflammation of small- to medium-sized blood vessels affecting organ systems including the lungs, GI tract, skin, heart, and nervous system. **Nucala *(mepolizumab)*** is the first FDA-approved therapy specifically to treat EGPA. This expanded indication of **Nucala** meets a critical, unmet need for EGPA patients. It's notable that patients taking **Nucala** in clinical trials reported a significant improvement in their symptoms. The FDA granted this application Priority Review and Orphan Drug designations. Orphan Drug designation provides incentives to assist and encourage the development of drugs for rare diseases.

REFERENCE

https:/www.fda.gov/NewsEvents/Newsroom/PressAnnouncements/ucm588594.htm

HUMANIZED INTERLEUKIN-5 ANTAGONIST MONOCLONAL ANTIBODY

▶ ***mepolizumab*** <12 years: not recommended; ≥12 years: 100 mg SC once every 4 weeks in upper arm, abdomen, or thigh

Nucala *Vial:* 100 mg pwdr for reconstitution, single-use (preservative-free)

Comment: **Nucala** is an add-on maintenance treatment for severe asthma. There is a pregnancy exposure registry that monitors pregnancy outcomes in women exposed to **Nucala** during pregnancy. Healthcare providers can enroll patients or encourage patients to enroll themselves by calling 1-877-311-8972 <u>or</u> visiting www.mothertobaby.org/asthma.

EPICONDYLITIS

Acetaminophen for IV Infusion *see* ***Pain*** *page* 322
NSAIDs *see page* 539
Other Oral Analgesics *see* ***Pain*** *page* 324
Topical & Transdermal NSAIDs *see* ***Pain*** *page* 323
Parenteral Corticosteroids *see page* 547
Oral Corticosteroids *see page* 546

EPIDIDYMITIS

Comment: The following treatment regimens for epididymitis are published in the **2015 CDC Transmitted Diseases Treatment Guidelines**. Treatment regimens are presented by generic drug name first, followed by information about brands and dose forms. Empiric treatment requires concomitant treatment of chlamydia. Treat all sexual contacts. Patients who are HIV-positive should receive the same treatment as those who are HIV-negative.

RECOMMENDED REGIMEN

Regimen 1

▶ ***ceftriaxone*** (B)(G) 250 mg IM in a single dose

<u>plus</u>

▶ ***doxycycline*** (D)(G) 100 mg bid x 10 days

RECOMMENDED REGIMENS: LIKELY CAUSED BY ENTERIC ORGANISMS

Regimen 1

▶ ***levofloxacin*** (C) 500 mg daily x 10 days

Regimen 2

▶ ***ofloxacin*** (C)(G) 300 mg bid x 10 day

DRUG BRANDS AND DOSE FORMS

▶ ***ceftriaxone*** (B)(G)

Rocephin *Vial:* 250, 500 mg; 1, 2 gm

▶ ***doxycycline*** (D)(G)

Acticlate *Tab:* 75, 150**mg

Adoxa *Tab:* 50, 75, 100, 150 mg ent-coat

Doryx *Tab:* 50, 75, 100, 150, 200 mg del-rel
Doxteric *Tab:* 50 mg del-rel
Monodox *Cap:* 50, 75, 100 mg
Oracea *Cap:* 40 mg del-rel
Vibramycin *Tab:* 100 mg; *Cap:* 50, 100 mg; *Syr:* 50 mg/5 ml (raspberry-apple) (sulfites); *Oral susp:* 25 mg/5 ml (raspberry)
Vibra-Tab *Tab:* 100 mg film-coat

Comment: ***doxycycline*** is contraindicated <8 years-of-age, in pregnancy, and lactation (discolors developing tooth enamel). A side effect may be photosensitivity (photophobia). Do not take with antacids, calcium supplements, milk or other dairy, or within 2 hours of taking another drug.

- ***levofloxacin*** **(C)**
  Levaquin *Tab:* 250, 500, 750 mg; *Oral soln:* 25 mg/ml (480 ml) (benzyl alcohol)

Comment: ***levofloxacin*** is contraindicated <18 years-of-age, and during pregnancy, and lactation. Risk of tendonitis or tendon rupture.

- ***ofloxacin*** **(C)(G)**
  Floxin *Tab:* 200, 300, 400 mg

Comment: ***ofloxacin*** is contraindicated <18 years-of-age, and during pregnancy and lactation. Risk of tendonitis or tendon rupture.

ERYSIPELAS

Comment: Erysipelas is most commonly due to GABHS (Group A beta-hemolytic Strept).

TREATMENT OF CHOICE

- ***penicillin v potassium*** **(B)** <12 years: 25-75 mg/kg day divided q 6-8 hours x 10 days; *see page 616 for dose by weight table;* ≥12 years: 250-500 mg q 6 hours x 10 days
  Pen-VK *Tab:* 250, 500 mg; *Oral soln:* 125 mg/5 ml (100, 200 ml); 250 mg/5 ml (100, 150, 200 ml)

TREATMENT IF PENICILLIN ALLERGIC

- ***erythromycin base*** **(B)(G)** <40 kg: 30-40 mg/kg/day divided q 6 hours x 10 days; ≥40 kg: 250 mg q 6 hours x 10 days
  Ery-Tab *Tab:* 250, 333, 500 mg ent-coat
  PCE *Tab:* 333, 500 mg

Comment: ***erythromycin*** may increase INR with concomitant ***warfarin***, as well as increase serum level of ***digoxin***, benzodiazepines and statins.

- ***erythromycin ethylsuccinate*** **(B)(G)** 30-50 mg/kg/day in 4 divided doses x 7 days; may double dose with severe infection; max 100 mg/kg/day or 400 mg qid; *see page 607 for dose by weight table*
  EryPed *Oral susp:* 200 mg/5 ml (100, 200 ml) (fruit); 400 mg/5 ml (60, 100, 200 ml) (banana); *Oral drops:* 200, 400 mg/5 ml (50 ml) (fruit); *Chew tab:* 200 mg wafer (fruit)
  E.E.S. *Oral susp:* 200, 400 mg/5 ml (100 ml) (fruit)
  E.E.S. Granules *Oral susp:* 200 mg/5 ml (100, 200 ml) (cherry)
  E.E.S. 400 Tablets *Tab:* 400 mg

Comment: ***erythromycin*** may increase INR with concomitant ***warfarin***, as well as increase serum level of ***digoxin***, benzodiazepines and statins.

EXOCRINE PANCREAS INSUFFICIENCY (EPI)/PANCREATIC ENZYME DEFICIENCY

Comment: Seen in chronic pancreatitis, post-pancreatectomy, cystic fibrosis, post-GI tract bypass surgery, and ductal obstruction from neoplasia. May sprinkle cap; however, do not crush or chew cap or tab. May mix with applesauce or other acidic food; follow with water or juice. Do not let any drug remain in mouth. Take dose with (not before or after) each meal and snack (half dose with snacks). Base dose on lipase units; adjust per diet and clinical response (i.e., steatorrhea). Pancrelipase products are interchangeable. Contraindicated with pork protein hypersensitivity.

PANCRELIPASE PRODUCTS

▶ *pancreatic enzymes* (C)

Creon <12 months: 2,000-4,000 units per 120 ml formula or per breastfeeding (do not mix directly into formula or breast milk; 12 months-4 years: 1,000 units/kg per meal; max 2,500 units/kg per meal <10,000 units/kg per day; >4 years: 500 units/kg per meal; max 2,500 units/kg per meal or <10,000 units/kg per day or <4,000 units/gm fat ingested per day

Cap: **Creon 3000** *lip* 3,000 units+*pro* 9,500 units+*amyl* 15,000 units del-rel
Creon 6000 *lip* 6,000 units+*pro* 19,000 units+*amyl* 30,000 units del-rel
Creon 12000 *lip* 12,000 units+*pro* 38,000 units+amyl 60,000 units del-rel
Creon 24000 *lip* 24,000 units+pro 76,000 units+*amyl* 120,000 units del-rel
Creon 36000 *lip* 36,000 units+*pro* 114,000 units+*amyl* 180,000 units del-rel

Cotazym <12 years: not recommended; ≥12 years: 1-3 tabs just prior to each meal or snack

Tab: **Cotazym** *lip* 1,000 units+*pro* 12,500 units+*amyl* 12,500 units del-rel
Cotazym-S *lip* 5,000 units+*pro* 20,000 units+*amyl* 20,000 units del-rel

Donnazyme <12 years: not recommended; ≥12 years: 1-3 caps just prior to each meal or snack

Cap: **Donnazyme** *lip* 5,000 units+*pro* 20,000 units+*amyl* 20,000 units del-rel

Ku-Zyme 1-2 caps just prior to each meal or snack

Cap: **Ku-Zyme:** *lip* 12,000 units+*pro* 15,000 units+*amyl* 15,000 units del-rel

Kutrase <12 years: not recommended; ≥12 years: 1-2 caps just prior to each meal or snack

Cap: **Kutrase:** *lip* 12,000 units+*pro* 30,000 units+*amyl* 30,000 units del-rel

Pancreaze <12 months: 2,000-4,000 lipase units per 120 ml formula or per breastfeeding; ≥12 months-<4 years: 1,000 lipase units/kg per meal; 4-12 years: 500 lipase units/kg per meal; >12 years: 2,500 lipase units/kg per meal or <10,000 lipase units/kg per day or <4,000 lipase units/gm fat ingested per day

Cap: **Pancreaze 4200** *lip* 4,200 units+*pro* 10,000 units+*amyl* 17,500 units ec-microtabs
Pancreaze 10500 *lip* 10,500 units+*pro* 25,000 units+*amyl* 43,750 units ec microtabs
Pancreaze 16800 *lip* 16,800 units+*pro* 40,000 units+*amyl* 70,000 units ec-microtabs
Pancreaze 21000 *lip* 21,000 units+*pro* 37,000 units+*amyl* 61,000 units ec-microtabs

Pertyze 12 months-4 years and ≥8 kg: initially 1,000 lipase units/kg per meal; ≥4 years and ≥16 kg: initially 500 lipase units/kg per meal; *Both:* 2,500 lipase units/kg per meal or <10,000 units/kg per day or <4,000 lipase units/gm fat ingested per day

Cap: **Pertyze 8000** *lip* 8,000 units+*pro* 28,750 units+*amyl* 30,250 units del-rel

Pertyze 16000 *lip* 16,000 units+*pro* 57,500 units+*amyl* 65,000 units del-rel

Ultrase 1-3 tabs just prior to each meal or snack

Cap: **Ultrase** *lip* 4,500 units+*pro* 20,000 units+*amyl* 25,000 units del-rel

Ultrase MT *lip* 12,000 units+*pro* 39,000 units+*amyl* 39,000 units del-rel

Ultrase MT 18 *lip* 18,000 units+*pro* 58,500 units+*amyl* 58,500 units del-rel

Ultrase MT 20 *lip* 20,000 units+*pro* 65,000 units+*amyl* 65,000 units del-rel

Viokace <12 years: not established; ≥12 years: initially 500 lip units/kg per meal; max 2,500 lipase units/kg per meal, or <10,000 lipase units/kg per meal, or <4,000 units/gm fat ingested per day

Tab: **Viokace 8** *lip* 8,000 units+*pro* 30,000 units+*amyl* 30,000 units

Viokace 16 *lip* 16,000 units+*pro* 60,000 units+*amyl* 60,000 units

Viokace 10440 *lip* 10,440 units+*pro* 39,150 units+*amyl* 39,150 units

Viokace 20880 *lip* 20,880 units+*pro* 78,300 units+*amyl* 78,300 units

Comment: **Viokace 10440** and **Viokace 20880** should be taken with a daily proton pump inhibitor.

Viokace Powder 1/4 tsp (0.7 gm) with meals

Viokace Powder *lip* 16,800 units+*pro* 70,000 units+*amyl* 70,000 units 1/4 (8 oz)

Zenpep <12 months: 2,000-4,000 units per 120 ml formula or per breast feeding (do not mix directly into formula or breast milk); 12 months-4 years: 1,000 units/kg per meal; max 2,500 units/kg per meal <10,000 units/kg per day; >4 years: 500 units/kg per meal; max 2,500 units/kg per meal or <10,000 units/kg per day or <4,000 units/gm fat ingested per day

Cap: **Zenpep 5000** *lip* 5,000 units+pro 17,000 units+*amyl* 27,000 units del-rel

Zenpep 10000 *lip* 10,000 units+*pro* 34,000 units+*amyl* 55,000 units del-rel

Zenpep 15000 *lip* 15,000 units+*pro* 51,000 units+*amyl* 82,000 units del-rel

Zenpep 20000 *lip* 20,000 units+*pro* 68,000 units+*amyl* 109,000 units del-rel

Zymase <12 years: not recommended; ≥12 years: 1-3 caps just prior to each meal or snack

Cap: **Zymase** *lip* 12,000 units+*pro* 24,000 units+*amyl* 24,000 units del-rel

EYE PAIN

Acetaminophen for IV Infusion *see* ***Pain*** *page* 322

OPHTHALMIC NSAIDs

Comment: Concomitant contact lens wear is contraindicated during therapy. Etiology of eye pain must be known prior to use of these agents

- ***diclofenac*** **(B)** <12 years: not recommended; ≥12 years: 1 drop affected eye qid
  Voltaren Ophthalmic Solution *Ophth soln:* 0.1% (2.5, 5 ml)
- ***ketorolac tromethamine*** **(C)** <3 years: not recommended; ≥3 years: 1 drop affected eye qid for up to 4 days
  Acular *Ophth soln:* 0.5% (3, 5, 10 ml; benzalkonium chloride)
  Acular LS *Ophth soln:* 0.4% (5 ml; benzalkonium chloride)
  Acular PF *Ophth soln:* 0.5% (0.4 ml; 12 single-use vials/carton) (preservative-free)
- ***nepafenac*** **(C)** <10 years: not recommended; ≥10 years: 1 drop affected eye tid
  Nevanac Ophthalmic Suspension *Ophth susp:* 0.1% (3 ml) (benzalkonium chloride)

OPHTHALMIC STEROIDS

Comment: Contraindications: ocular fungal, viral, or mycobacterial infections. Effectiveness of treatment should be assessed after 2 days. The corticosteroid should be tapered and treatment concluded within 14 days if possible due to risk of corneal and/or scleral thinning with prolonged use.

▶ ***difluprednate*** **(C)** <12 years: not recommended; ≥12 years: 1 drop affected eye qid; *Post-op pain:* beginning 24 hours after surgery, 1 drop affected eye qid; continue for 2 weeks post-op; then bid x 1 week; then taper until resolved
  Durezol Ophthalmic Solution *Ophth emul:* 0.05% (5 ml)

▶ ***etabonate*** **(C)** <12 years: not recommended; ≥12 years: 1 drop affected eye qid
  Alrex Ophthalmic Solution *Ophth emul:* 0.2% (5 ml) (benzalkonium chloride)

FACIAL HAIR: EXCESSIVE/UNWANTED

TOPICAL HAIR GROWTH RETARDANT

▶ ***eflornithine*** 13.9% cream (C) <12 years: not recommended; ≥12 years: apply a thin layer to affected areas of face and under the chin bid at least 8 hours apart; rub in thoroughly; do not wash treated area for at least 4 hours following application
  Vaniqa *Crm:* 13.9% (30, 60 gm)
  Comment: After **Vaniqa** dries, may apply cosmetics or sunscreen. Hair removal techniques may be continued as needed.

FECAL ODOR

▶ ***bismuth subgallate powder*** **(B)(OTC)** 1-2 tabs tid with meals
  Devrom *Chew tab:* 200 mg; *Cap:* 200 mg
  Comment: **Devrom** is an internal (oral) deodorant for control of odors from ileostomy or colostomy drainage or fecal incontinence.

FEVER (PYREXIA)

ACETAMINOPHEN FOR IV INFUSION

▶ ***acetaminophen*** injectable **(B)(G)** <2 years: not recommended; 2-13 years <50 kg: 15 mg/kg q 6 hours prn or 12.5 mg/kg q 4 hours prn; max 750 mg single-dose; max 75 mg/kg per day; >13 years: administer by IV infusion over 15 minutes; 1,000 mg q 6 hours prn or 650 mg q 4 hours prn; max 4,000 mg/day
  Ofirmev *Vial:* 10 mg/ml (100 ml) (preservative-free)
  Comment: The **Ofirmev** vial is intended for single use. If any portion is withdrawn from the vial, use within 6 hours. Discard the unused portion. For pediatric patients, withdraw the intended dose and administer via syringe pump. Do not admix **Ofirmev** with any other drugs. **Ofirmev** is physically incompatible with ***diazepam*** and ***chlorpromazine hydrochloride***.

▶ ***acetaminophen*** **(B)(G)**
  Children's Tylenol (OTC) 10-20 mg/kg q 4-6 hours prn
    Oral susp: 80 mg/tsp
      4-11 months (12-17 lb): 1/2 tsp q 4 hours prn; 12-23 months (18-23 lb): 3/4 tsp q 4 hours prn; 2-3 years (24-35 lb): 1 tsp q 4 hours prn; 4-5 years(36-47 lb): 1 tsp q 4 hours prn; 6-8 years (48-59 lb): 2 tsp q 4 hours prn; 9-10 years (60-71 lb): 2 tsp q 4 hours prn; 11 years (72-95 lb): 3 tsp q 4 hours prn; All: max 5 doses/day

Elix: 160 mg/5 ml (2, 4 oz)

Chew tab: 80 mg

2-3 years (24-35 lb): 2 tabs q 4 hours prn; 4-5 years (36-47 lb): 3 tabs q 4 hours prn; 6-8 years (48-59 lb): 4 tabs q 4 hours prn; 9-10 years (60-71 lb): 5 tabs q 4 hours prn; 11 years (72-95 lb): 6 tabs q 4 hours prn; All: max 5 doses/day

Junior Strength:

6-8 years: 2 tabs q 4 hours prn; 9-10 years: 2 tabs q 4 hours prn; 11 years: 3 tabs q 4 hours prn; 12 years: 4 tabs q 4 hours prn; All: max 5 doses/day

Chew tab: 160 mg

Junior cplt: 160 mg

Infant's Drops and Suspension: 80 mg/0.8 ml (1/2, 1 oz)

<3 months: 0.4 ml q 4 hours prn; 4-11 months: 0.8 ml q 4 hours prn; 12-23 months: 1.2 ml q 4 hours prn; 2-3 years (24-35 lb): 1.6 ml q 4 hours prn; 4-5 years (36-47 lb): 2.4 ml q 4 hours prn; All: max 5 doses/day

Extra Strength Tylenol (G)(OTC) <12 years: not recommended; ≥12 years: 500-1000 mg q 4-6 hours prn; max 4 gm/day

Tab/Cplt/Gel tab/Gel cap: 500 mg; *Liq:* 500 mg/15 ml (8 oz)

FeverAll Extra Strength Tylenol (OTC) <3 months: not recommended; 3-36 months: 80 mg q 4 hours prn; 3-6 years: 120 mg q 4 hours prn; ≥6 years: 325 mg q 4 hours prn; *Rectal supp:* 80, 120, 325 mg (6/carton)

Maximum Strength Tylenol Sore Throat (OTC) <12 years: not recommended; ≥12 years: 500-1000 mg q 4-6 hours prn

Liq: 1000 mg/30 ml (8 oz)

Tylenol (OTC) <6 years: not recommended; 6-11 years: 325 mg q 4-6 hours prn; max 1.625 gm/day; ≥12 years: 650 mg q 4-6 hours; max 4 gm/day

▻ ***aspirin*** **(D)(G)**

Bayer (OTC) <6 years: not recommended; 6-11 years: 325 mg q 4-6 hours prn; max 1.625 gm/day; >11 years: 325-650 mg q 4 hours prn; max: 5 doses/day

Tab/Cplt: 325 mg ext-rel

Extra Strength Bayer (OTC) <6 years: not recommended; 6-11 years: 325 mg q 4-6 hours prn; max 1.625 gm/day; ≥12 years: 500-1000 mg q 4-6 hours prn; max 4 gm/day

Cplt: 500 mg

Extended-Release Bayer 8 Hour (OTC) <12 years: not recommended; ≥12 years: 650-1300 mg q 8 hours prn

Cplt: 650 mg ext-rel

Comment: ***aspirin***-containing medications are contraindicated with history of allergic-type reaction to ***aspirin***, children and adolescents with *Varicella* or other viral illness, and 3rd trimester of pregnancy.

▻ ***aspirin+caffeine*** **(D)(G)**

Anacin (OTC) <6 years: not recommended; 6-12 years: 400 mg q 4 hours prn; max 2 gm/day; ≥12 years: 800 mg q 4 hours prn; max 4 gm/day

Tab/Cplt: 400 mg

Anacin Maximum Strength (OTC) <12 years: not recommended; ≥12 years: 1 gm tid-qid

Tab: 500 mg

Comment: ***aspirin***-containing medications are contraindicated with history of allergic-type reaction to ***aspirin***, children and adolescents with *Varicella* or other viral illness, and 3rd trimester of pregnancy.

▻ ***aspirin+antacid*** **(D)(G)**

Extra Strength Bayer Plus (OTC) <12 years: not recommended; ≥12 years: 500 mg-1 gm q 4-6 hours prn; usual max 4 gm/day

Cplt: 500 mg aspirin + calcium carbonate

Bufferin (OTC) <12 years: not recommended; ≥12 years: 650 mg q 4 hours; max 3.9 mg/day

Tab: 325 mg aspirin+calcium carbonate+magnesium carbonate+magnesium oxide

Comment: ***aspirin***-containing medications are contraindicated with history of allergic-type reaction to ***aspirin***, children and adolescents with *Varicella* or other viral illness, and 3rd trimester of pregnancy.

➢ ***ibuprofen* (B; not for use in 3rd)(G)**

Comment: *ibuprofen* is contraindicated in children <6 months-of-age.

Children's Advil (OTC), ElixSure IB (OTC), Motrin (OTC), PediaCare (OTC), PediaProfen (OTC)5-10 mg/kg q 6-8 hours; max 40 mg/kg/day; <24 lb (<2 years):individualize; 24-35 lb (2-3 years): 5 ml q 6-8 hours prn; 36-47 lb (4-5 years): 7.5 ml q 6-8 hours prn; 48-59 lb (6-8 years): 10 ml or 2 tabs q 6-8 hours prn; 60-71 lb (9-10 years): 12.5 ml or 2 tabs q 6-8 hours prn; 72-95 lb (11 years): 15 ml or 3 tabs q 6-8 hours prn

Oral susp: 100 mg/5 ml (2, 4 oz) (berry); *Junior tabs:* 100 mg

Children's Motrin Drops (OTC), PediaCare Drops (OTC) n <24 lb (<2 years): individualize; 24-35 lb (2-3 years): 2.5 ml q 6-8 hours prn; *Oral drops:* 50 mg/1.25 ml (15 ml; berry)

Children's Motrin Chewables and Caplets (OTC) 48-59 lb (6-8 years): 200 mg q 6-8 hours prn; 60-71 lb (9-10 years): 250 mg q 6-8 hours prn; 72-95 lb (11 years): 300 mg q 6-8 hours prn; ≥12 years: 400 mg q 4 hours prn

Chew tab: 100*mg (citrus; phenylalanine)

Cplt: 100 mg

Motrin (OTC) <6 months: not recommended; >6 months, fever <102.5: 5 mg/kg q6-8 hours prn; >6 months, fever >102.5: 10 mg/kg q 6-8 hours prn; *All:* max 40 mg/kg/day; ≥12 years: 400 mg q 6 hours prn

Tab: 400 mg; *Cplt:* 100*mg; *Chew tab:* 50*, 100*mg (citrus; phenylalanine); *Oral susp:* 100 mg/5 ml (4, 16 oz) (berry); *Oral drops:* 40 mg/ml (15 ml) (berry)

Advil (OTC), Motrin IB (OTC), Nuprin (OTC) <12 years: not recommended; ≥12 years: 200-400 mg q 4-6 hours; max 1.2 gm/day

Tab/Cplt/Gel cap: 200 mg

➢ ***naproxen* (B)(G)**

Aleve (OTC) <2 years: not recommended; ≥2 years-6 years: 2.5-5 mg/kg bid-tid; max: 15 mg/kg/day; 400 mg x 1 dose; then 200 mg q 8-12 hours prn; max 10 days

Tab/Cplt/Gel cap: 200 mg

Anaprox <12 years: not recommended; ≥12 years: 550 mg x 1 dose; then 550 mg q 12 hours or 275 mg q 6-8 hours prn; max 1.375 gm first day and 1.1 gm/day thereafter

Tab: 275 mg

Anaprox DS <12 years: not recommended; ≥12 years: 1 tab bid

Tab: 550 mg

EC-Naprosyn <12 years: not recommended; ≥12 years: 375 or 500 mg bid prn; may increase dose up to max 1500 mg/day as tolerated

Tab: 375, 500 mg del-rel

Naprelan <12 years: not recommended; ≥12 years: 1 gm daily or 1.5 gm daily for limited time; max 1 gm/day thereafter

Tab: 375, 500 mg

Naprosyn <12 years: not recommended; ≥12 years: initially 500 mg, then 500 mg q 12 hours or 250 mg q 6-8 hours prn; max 1.25 gm first day and 1 gm/day thereafter

Tab: 250, 375, 500 mg; *Oral susp:* 125 mg/5 ml (473 ml) (pineapple-orange)

FIBROCYSTIC BREAST DISEASE

Contraceptives *see page* 527

- ***spironolactone*** **(D)**10 mg bid premenstrually
  - **Aldactone (G)** *Tab:* 25, 50*, 100*mg
  - **CaroSpir** *Oral susp:* 25 mg/5 ml (118, 473 ml) (banana)
- ***vitamin E*** **(A)** 400-600 IU daily
- ***vitamin B6*** **(A)** 50-100 mg daily
- ***danazol*** **(X)** <18 years: not recommended; ≥18 years: start on 3rd or 4th day of menstrual period or after a negative pregnancy test; 50-200 mg bid x 2-6 months
  - **Danocrine** *Cap:* 50, 100, 200 mg

Comment: ***danazol*** is a synthetic steroid derived from ethisterone. It suppresses the pituitary-ovarian axis. This suppression is probably a combination of depressed hypothalamic-pituitary response to lowered ***estrogen*** production, the alteration of sex steroid metabolism, and interaction of ***danazol*** with sex hormone receptors. The only other demonstrable hormonal effects are weak androgenic activity and depression of both follicle-stimulating hormone (FSH) and luteinizing hormone (LH) output. Recent evidence suggests a direct inhibitory effect at gonadal sites and a binding of **Danocrine** to receptors of gonadal steroids at target organs. In addition, **Danocrine** has been shown to significantly decrease IgG, IgM and IgA levels, as well as phospholipid and IgG isotope autoantibodies in patients with endometriosis and associated elevations of autoantibodies, suggesting this could be another mechanism by which it facilitates regression of fibrocystic breast disease. **Danocrine** usually produces partial to complete disappearance of breast tissue nodularity and complete relief of pain and tenderness. Changes in the menstrual pattern may occur. Generally, the pituitary-suppressive action of **Danocrine** is reversible. Ovulation and cyclic bleeding usually return within 60 to 90 days when therapy with **Danocrine** is discontinued. **Danocrine** is also used to treat endometriosis (to relieve associated abdominal pain) and hereditary angioedema (to prevent attacks). Contraindications include pregnancy, breastfeeding, active or history of thromboembolic disease/event, porphyria, undiagnosed abnormal genital bleeding, androgen-dependent tumor, and markedly impaired hepatic, renal, or cardiac function.

FIBROMYALGIA

Acetaminophen for IV Infusion *see* ***Pain*** *page* 322
NSAIDs *see page* 539
Other Oral Analgesics *see* ***Pain*** *page* 324
Topical & Transdermal NSAIDs *see* ***Pain*** *page* 323
Parenteral Corticosteroids *see page* 547
Oral Corticosteroids *see page* 546

SEROTONIN-NOREPINEPHRINE REUPTAKE INHIBITORS (SNRIs)

- ***duloxetine*** **(C)(G)** <12 years: not recommended; ≥12 years: swallow whole; initially 30 mg once daily x 1 week; then increase to 60 mg once daily; max 120 mg/day
  - **Cymbalta** *Cap:* 20, 30, 60 mg ent-coat pellets
- ***milnacipran*** **(C)(G)** <17 years: not recommended; ≥17 years: *Day 1:* 12.5 mg once; *Days 2-3:* 12.5 mg bid; *Days 4-7:* 25 mg bid; max 100 mg bid
  - **Savella** *Tab:* 12.5, 25, 50, 100 mg

GAMMA-AMINOBUTYRIC ACID ANALOG

▶ *gabapentin* (C) <3 years: not recommended; 3-12 years: initially 10-15 mg/kg/day in 3 divided doses; max 12 hours between doses; titrate over 3 days; 3-4 years: titrate to 40 mg/kg/day; 5-12 years: titrate to 25-35 mg/kg/day; max 50 mg/kg/day; >12 years: initially 300 mg on Day 1; then 600 mg on Day 2; then 900 mg on Days 3-6; then 1200 mg on Days 7-10; then 1500 mg on Days 11-14; titrate up to 1800 mg on Day 15; take entire dose once daily with the evening meal; do not crush, split, or chew

Gralise *Tab:* 300, 600 mg

Neurontin (G) *Tab:* 600*, 800*mg; *Cap:* 100, 300, 400 mg; *Oral soln:* 250 mg/5 ml (480 ml) (strawberry-anise)

Comment: Avoid abrupt cessation of ***gabapentin***. To discontinue, withdraw gradually over 1 week or longer.

▶ ***gabapentin enacarbil*** (C) <12 years: not recommended: ≥12 years: 600 mg once daily at about 5: 00 PM; if dose not taken at recommended time, next dose should be taken the following day; swallow whole; take with food; *CrCl 30-59 mL/min:* 600 mg on Day 1, Day 3, and every day thereafter; *CrCl <30 mL/min:* or on hemodialysis: not recommended

Horizant *Tab:* 300, 600 mg ext-rel

Comment: Avoid abrupt cessation of ***gabapentin*** and ***gabapentin enacarbil***. To discontinue, withdraw gradually over 1 week or longer.

ALPHA-2 DELTA LIGAND

▶ ***pregabalin (GABA analog)*** (C)(V) <18 years: not recommended; ≥18 years:

Lyrica initially 50 mg tid; may titrate to 100 mg tid within one week; max 600 mg divided tid; discontinue over 1 week

Cap: 25, 50, 75, 100, 150, 200, 225, 300 mg; *Oral soln:* 20 mg/ml

Lyrica CR *Tab:* usual dose: 165 mg once daily; may increase to 330 mg/day within 1 week; max 660 mg/day; discontinue over 1 week

Tab: 82.5, 165, 330 mg ext-rel

OTHER AGENTS

▶ ***amitriptyline*** (C)(G) <12 years: not recommended; ≥12 years: 20 mg q HS; may increase gradually to max 50 mg q HS

Tab: 10, 25, 50, 75, 100, 150 mg

▶ ***cyclobenzaprine*** (B)(G) <15 years: not recommended; ≥15 years: 10 mg tid; usual range 20-40 mg/day in divided doses; max 60 mg/day x 2-3 weeks or 15 mg ext-rel once daily; max 30 mg ext-rel/day x 2-3 weeks

Amrix *Cap:* 15, 30 mg ext-rel

Fexmid *Tab:* 7.5 mg

Flexeril *Tab:* 5, 10 mg

▶ ***eszopiclone*** (pyrrolopyrazine) (C)(IV)(G) <18 years: not recommended; ≥18 years: 1-3 mg; max 3 mg/day x 1 month; do not take if unable to sleep for at least 8 hours before required to be active again; delayed effect if taken with a meal

Lunesta *Tab:* 1, 2, 3 mg

▶ ***flurazepam*** (X)(IV)(G) <18 years: not recommended; ≥18 years: 15 mg q HS; may increase to 30 mg q HS

Dalmane *Cap:* 15, 30 mg

▶ ***trazodone*** (C)(G) <18 years: not recommended; ≥18 years: 50 mg q HS

Desyrel *Tab:* 50, 100, 150, 300 mg

▶ ***triazolam*** (X)(IV)(G) <18 years: not recommended; ≥18 years: 0.125 mg q HS, may increase gradually to 0.5 mg

Halcion *Tab:* 0.125, 0.25*mg

- ***zaleplon*** (imidazopyridine) **(C)(IV)** <12 years: not recommended; ≥12 years: 5-10 mg at HS or after going to bed if unable to sleep; do not take if unable to sleep for at least 4 hours before required to be active again; max 20 mg/day x 1 month; delayed effect if taken with a meal

    Sonata *Cap:* 5, 10 mg (tartrazine)

    Comment: **Sonata** is indicated for the treatment of insomnia when a middle-of-the-night awakening is followed by difficulty returning to sleep.

- ***zolpidem*** oral solution spray (imidazopyridine hypnotic) **(C)(IV)** <18 years: not recommended; ≥18 years: 2 actuations (10 mg) immediately before bedtime; *Debilitated, or hepatic impairment:* 2 actuations (5 mg); max 2 actuations (10 mg)

    ZolpiMist *Oral soln spray*: 5 mg/actuation (60 metered actuations) (cherry)

  Comment: The lowest dose of ***zolpidem*** in all forms is recommended for females as drug elimination is slower than in men.

- ***zolpidem*** tabs (pyrazolopyrimidine hypnotic) **(B)(IV)(G)** <18 years: not recommended; ≥18 years: 5-10 mg or 6.25-12.5 ext-rel q HS prn; max 12.5 mg/day x 1 month; do not take if unable to sleep for at least 8 hours before required to be active again; delayed effect if taken with a meal

    Ambien *Tab:* 5, 10 mg

    Ambien CR *Tab:* 6.25, 12.5 mg ext-rel

  Comment: The lowest dose of ***zolpidem*** in all forms is recommended for females as drug elimination is slower than in males.

- ***zolpidem*** sublingual tabs (imidazopyridine hypnotic) **(C)(IV)(G)** <18 years: not recommended; ≥18 years: dissolve 1 tab under the tongue; allow to disintegrate completely before swallowing; take only once per night and only if at least 4 hours of bedtime remain before planned time for awakening

    Edluar *SL Tab:* 5, 10 mg

    Intermezzo *SL Tab:* 1.75, 3.5 mg

    Comment: **Intermezzo** is indicated for the treatment of insomnia when a middle-of-the-night awakening is followed by difficulty returning to sleep.

Comment: The lowest dose of ***zolpidem*** in all forms is recommended for females as drug elimination is slower than in males.

FIFTH DISEASE (ERYTHEMA INFECTIOSUM)

Antipyretics *see* ***Fever*** *page* 149

FLATULENCE

- ***simethicone*** (C)(G)

    Gas-X (OTC) 2-4 tabs pc and HS prn

      Tab: 40, 80, 125 mg; *Cap:* 125 mg

    Mylicon (OTC) 2-4 tabs pc and HS prn

      Tab: 40, 80, 125 mg; *Cap:* 125 mg

    Phazyme-95 1-2 tabs with each meal and HS prn

      Tab: 95 mg

    Phazyme Infant Oral Drops <2 years: 0.3 ml qid pc and HS prn; 2-12 years: 0.6 ml qid pc and HS prn; >12 years: 1.2 ml qid pc and HS prn; *Oral drops:* 40 mg/0.6 ml (15, 30 ml w. calibrated dropper) (orange) (alcohol-free)

    Maximum Strength Phazyme 1-2 caps with each meal and HS prn

      Cap: 125 mg

FLUORIDATION, WATER, <0.6 PPM

▶ ***fluoride*** (G)

Luride *Water fluoridation 0.3-0.6 ppm:* <3 years: use drops; 6 months-3 years: 0.125 mg daily; 4-6 years: 0.25 mg daily; 7-16 years: 0.5 mg daily; *Water fluoridation <0.3 ppm:* <3 years: use drops; 6 months-3 years: 0.25 mg daily; 3-6 years: 0.5 mg daily; >6-16 years: 1 mg daily

Chew tab: 0.25, 0.5, 1 mg (sugar-free)

Luride Drops *Water fluoridation 0.3-0.6 ppm:* 6 months-3 years: 0.25 ml once daily; 4-6 years: 0.5 ml once daily; 7-16 years: 1 ml once daily; *Water fluoridation <0.3 ppm:* 6 months-3 years: 0.5 ml once daily; 4-6 years: 1 ml once daily; 7-16 years: 2 ml daily

Oral drops: 0.5 mg/ml (50 ml) (sugar-free)

COMBINATION AGENTS

▶ ***fluoride+vitamin a+vitamin d+vitamin c*** (G) *Water fluoridation 0.3-0.6 ppm:* <3 years: not recommended; 3-6 years: 0.25 mg fluoride/day; 7-16 years: 0.5 mg fluoride/day; *Water fluoridation <0.3 ppm:* <6 months: not recommended; 6 months-3 years: 0.25 mg fluoride/day; 4-6 years: 0.5 mg fluoride/day; 7-16 years: 1 mg fluoride/day

Tri-Vi-Flor Drops

Oral drops: fluor 0.25 mg+vit a 1500 u+vit d 400 u+vit c 35 mg per ml (50 ml)

Oral drops: fluor 0.5 mg+vit a 1500 u+vit d 400 u+vit c 35 mg per ml (50 ml)

▶ ***fluoride+vitamin a+vitamin d+vitamin c+iron*** *Water fluoridation 0.3-0.6 ppm:* <3 years: not recommended; 3-6 years: 0.25 mg fluoride/day; 7-16 years: 0.5 mg fluoride/day; *Water fluoridation <0.3 ppm:* <6 months: not recommended; 6 months-3 years: 0.25 mg fluoride/day; 4-6 years: 0.5 mg fluoride/day; 7-16 years: 1 mg fluoride/day

Tri-Vi-Flor w. Iron Drops

Oral drops: fluor 0.25 mg+vit a 1500 u+vit d 400 u+vit c 35 mg+iron 10 mg per ml (50 ml)

FOLLICULITIS BARBAE

Topical Corticosteroids *page 542*

TOPICAL AGENTS

▶ ***benzoyl peroxide*** (B) apply after shaving; may discolor clothing and linens.

Benzac-W initially apply to affected area once daily; increase to bid-tid as tolerated

Gel: 2.5, 5, 10% (60 gm)

Benzac-W Wash wash affected area bid

Wash: 5% (4, 8 oz); 10% (8 oz)

Benzagel apply to affected area one or more x/day

Gel: 5, 10% (1.5, 3 oz) (alcohol 14%)

Benzagel Wash wash affected area bid

Gel: 10% (6 oz)

Desquam X_5 wash affected area bid

Wash: 5% (5 oz)

Desquam X_{10} wash affected area bid

Wash: 10% (5 oz)

Triaz apply to affected area daily bid

Lotn: 3, 6, 9% (bottle), 3% (tube); *Pads:* 3, 6, 9% (jar)

ZoDerm apply once or twice daily

Gel: 4.5, 6.5, 8.5% (125 ml); *Crm:* 4.5, 6.5, 8.5% (125 ml); *Clnsr:* 4.5, 6.5, 8.5% (400 ml)

▶ ***clindamycin*** topical **(B)** apply bid

Cleocin T *Pad:* 1% (60/pck; alcohol 50%); *Lotn:* 1% (60 ml); *Gel:* 1% (30, 60 gm);*Soln w. applicator:* 1% (30, 60 ml) (alcohol 50%)

Clindagel *Gel:* 1% (42, 77 gm)

Clindets *Pad:* 1% (60/pck)

Evoclin *Foam:* 1% (50, 100 gm) (alcohol)

▶ ***clindamycin+benzoyl peroxide*** topical **(C)** ***benzoyl peroxide*** may discolor clothing and linens; <12 years: not recommended; ≥12 years:

Acanya (G) apply qd-bid

Gel: clin 1.2%+benz 2.5% (50 gm)

BenzaClin apply bid

Gel: clin 1%+benz 5% (25, 50 gm)

Duac apply daily in the evening

Gel: clin 1%+benz 5% (45 gm)

Onexton Gel apply once daily

Gel: clin 1.2%+benz 3.75% (50 gm pump) (alcohol-free) (preservative-free)

▶ ***dapsone*** topical **(C)(G)** <12 years: not recommended; ≥12 years: apply bid

Aczone *Gel:* 5% (30 gm)

▶ ***tazarotene*** **(X)(G)** <12 years: not recommended; ≥12 years: apply daily at HS

Avage Cream *Crm:* 0.1% (30 gm)

Tazorac Cream *Crm:* 0.05, 0.1% (15, 30, 60 gm)

Tazorac Gel *Gel:* 0.05, 0.1% (30, 100 gm)

▶ ***tretinoin*** **(C)** <12 years: not recommended; ≥12 years: apply q HS

Atralin Gel *Gel:* 0.05% (45 gm)

Avita *Crm:* 0.025% (20, 45 gm); *Gel:* 0.025% (20, 45 gm)

Renova *Crm:* 0.02% (40 gm); 0.05% (40, 60 gm)

Retin-A Cream *Crm:* 0.025, 0.05, 0.1% (20, 45 gm)

Retin-A Gel *Gel:* 0.01, 0.025% (15, 45 gm) (alcohol 90%)

Retin-A Liquid *Liq:* 0.05% (28 ml) (alcohol 55%)

Retin-A Micro *Microspheres:* 0.04, 0.1% (20, 45 gm)

Tretin-X Cream *Crm:* 0.075% (35 gm) (parabens-free, alcohol-free, propylene glycol-free)

Retin-A Micro *Microspheres:* 0.04, 0.1% (20, 45 gm)

FOREIGN BODY: ESOPHAGUS

▶ ***glucagon*** **(B)** 0.02 mg/kg IV or IM with serial x-rays; max 1 mg

Glucagon (rDNA origin or beef/pork derived)

Vial: 1 mg/ml w. diluent

Comment: ***glucagon*** facilitates passage of foreign body from esophagus into stomach.

FOREIGN BODY: EYE

▶ ***proparacaine*** 1-2 drops to anesthetize surface of eye; then flush with normal saline

Ophthaine *Ophth soln:* 0.5% (15 ml)

Comment: *proparacaine* facilitates the search, location, and removal of foreign body and examination of the cornea.

GASTRITIS/DYSPEPSIA

Antacids *see GERD page* 158
H_2 Antagonists *see GERD page* 159

GASTRITIS-RELATED NAUSEA/VOMITING

OTC ANTI-EMETIC

▶ ***phosphorylated carbohydrate*** solution **(C)(G)** 1-2 tbsp q 15 minutes until nausea subsides; max 5 doses/day
Emetrol (OTC) *Soln:* dextrose 1.87 gm+fructose 1.87 gm+phosphoric acid 21.5 mg per 5 ml (4, 8, 16 oz)

Rx ANTI-EMETICS

▶ ***ondansetron*** (C)(G) 8 mg q 8 hours x 2 doses; then 8 mg q 12 hours
Pediatric: <4 years: not recommended; 4-11 years: 4 mg q 4 hours x 3 doses; then 4 mg q 8 hours
Zofran *Tab:* 4, 8, 24 mg
Zofran ODT *ODT:* 4, 8 mg (strawberry) (phenylalanine)
Zofran Oral Solution *Oral soln:* 4 mg/5 ml (50 ml) (strawberry) (phenylalanine); *Parenteral form:* see mfr pkg insert
Zofran Injection *Vial:* 2 mg/ml (2 ml single-dose); 2 mg/ml (20 ml multi-dose); 32 mg/50 ml (50 ml multi-dose); *Prefilled syringe:* 4 mg/2 ml, single-use (24/carton)
Zuplenz Oral Soluble Film: 4, 8 mg oral-dis (10/carton) (peppermint)

▶ ***phosphorylated carbohydrate*** solution **(C)(G)** <10 years: 1-2 tbsp q 15 minutes until nausea subsides; max 5 doses/day; ≥10 years: 1-2 tsp q 15 minutes until nausea subsides; max 5 doses/day
Emetrol (OTC) *Soln:* dextrose 1.87 gm+fructose 1.87 gm+phosphoric acid 21.5 mg per 5 ml (4, 8, 16 oz)

▶ ***promethazine*** (C) <2 years: not recommended; 2-12 years: 0.5 mg/lb or 6.25-25 mg q 4-6 hours PO or rectally; >12 years: 12.5-25 q 4-6 hours PO or rectally
Phenergan *Tab:* 12.5*, 25*, 50 mg; *Plain syr:* 6.25 mg/5 ml; *Fortis syr:* 25 mg/5 ml; *Rectal supp:* 12.5, 25, 50 mg; *Amp:* 25, 50 mg/ml (1 ml)

Comment: ***promethazine*** is contraindicated in children with uncomplicated nausea, dehydration, Reye's syndrome, history of sleep apnea, asthma, and lower respiratory disorders in children. ***Promethazine*** lowers the seizure threshold in children, may cause cholestatic jaundice, anticholinergic effects, extrapyramidal effects, and potentially fatal respiratory depression.

▶ ***ondansetron*** (C)(G) <4 years: not recommended; 4-11 years: 4-8 mg bid prn; >11 years: 8 mg q 8 hours prn
Zofran *Tab:* 4, 8, 24 mg
Zofran Injection *Vial:* 2 mg/ml (2 ml) single-dose; 2 mg/ml (20 ml) multidose) for IV or IM administration
Zofran ODT *ODT:* 4, 8 mg (strawberry) (phenylalanine)
Zofran Oral Solution *Oral soln:* 4 mg/5 ml (50 ml) (strawberry)
Zuplenz Oral Soluble Film: 4, 8 mg orally-disint (10/carton) (peppermint)

GASTROESOPHAGEAL REFLUX (GER), GASTROESOPHAGEAL REFLUX DISEASE (GERD), AND IDIOPATHIC GASTRIC ACID HYPERSECRETION (IGAH)

Comment: Precipitators of gastric reflux include narcotics, benzodiazepines, calcium antagonists, alcohol, nicotine, chocolate, and peppermint. Issues associated with H2 secretion and gastrointestinal health (e.g., chronic remitting gastritis, Barrett's esophagitis, peptic ulcer disease [PUD)]), other organ system impairments (e.g., CVD, metabolic syndrome, hepatitis, autoimmune and immunodeficiency disorders, renal insufficiency, iatrogenic consequences of treatments (e.g., steroids, NSAIDs, immune modulators), (advanced age,) and lifestyle (dietary habits and general nutritional health). Risk/benefit discussions with patients can be challenging, but are necessary for informed decision-making and prudent prescribing.

ANTACIDS

Comment: Antacids with ***aluminum hydroxide*** may potentiate constipation. Antacids with ***magnesium hydroxide*** may potentiate diarrhea.

▶ ***aluminum hydroxide*** **(C)** <12 years: not recommended; ≥12 years:

ALTernaGEL (OTC) 5-10 ml between meals and HS prn; max 90 ml/day

Liq: 500 mg/5 ml (5, 12 oz)

Amphojel (OTC) 10 ml 5-6 x/day between meals and HS prn; max 60 ml/day

Oral susp: 320 mg/5 ml (12 oz)

Amphojel Tab (OTC) 600 mg 5-6 x/day between meals and HS prn; max 3.6 gm/day

Tab: 300, 600 mg

▶ ***aluminum hydroxide+magnesium carbonate*** **(C)(OTC)(G)** <12 years: not recommended; ≥12 years:

Maalox HRF 10-20 ml qid pc and HS prn

Oral susp: alum 280 mg+mag 350 mg per 10 ml (10 oz)

▶ ***aluminum hydroxide+magnesium hydroxide*** **(C)(OTC)(G)** <12 years: not recommended; ≥12 years:

Maalox 10-20 ml qid and HS prn

Oral susp: 200 mg per 5 ml (5, 12, 26 oz) (mint, lemon, cherry)

Maalox Therapeutic Concentrate 10-20 ml qid pc and HS prn

Oral susp: alum 600 mg+mag 300 mg per 5 ml (12 oz) (mint)

▶ ***aluminum hydroxide+magnesium hydroxide+simethicone*** **(C)(OTC)(G)** <12 years: not recommended; ≥12 years:

Maalox Plus 10-20 ml qid pc and HS prn

Tab: alum 200 mg+mag 200 mg+sim 25 mg

Extra Strength Maalox Plus 10-20 ml qid pc and HS prn

Tab: alum 350 mg+mag 350 mg+sim 30 mg

Oral susp: alum 500 mg+mag 450 mg+sim 40 mg per 5 ml (5, 12, 26 oz)

Extra Strength Maalox Plus Tab 1-3 tabs qid pc and HS prn

Tab: alum 350 mg+mag 350 mg+sim 30 mg

Mylanta 10-20 ml between meals and HS prn

Liq: alum 200 mg+mag 200 mg+sim 20 mg per 5 ml (5, 12, 24 oz)

Mylanta Double Strength 10-20 ml between meals and HS prn

Liq: alum 700 mg+mag 400 mg+sim 40 mg per 5 ml (5, 12, 24 oz)

▶ ***aluminum hydroxide+magnesium trisilicate*** **(C)(G)** <12 years: not recommended; ≥12 years:

Gaviscon chew 2-4 tabs qid pc and HS prn

Tab: alum 80 mg+mag 20 mg

Gaviscon Liquid 15-30 ml qid pc and HS prn
Liq: alum 95 mg+mag 359 mg per 15 ml (6, 12 oz)
Gaviscon Extra Strength 2-4 tabs qid pc and HS prn
Tab: alum 160 mg+mag 105 mg
Gaviscon Extra Strength Liquid 10-20 ml qid prn
Liq: alum 508 mg+mag 475 mg per 10 ml (12 oz)

▶ ***aluminum hydroxide+magnesium hydroxide+simethicone*** (C)(OTC)(G) <12 years: not recommended; ≥12 years:
Maalox Maximum Strength 10-20 ml qid prn; max 60 ml/day
Oral susp: alum 500 mg+mag 450 mg+sim 40 mg per 5 ml (5, 12, 26 oz) (mint, cherry)

▶ ***calcium carbonate*** (C)(OTC)(G)
Children's Mylanta Tab <2 years: not recommended; 2-5 years (24-47 lb): 1 tab as needed up to tid; 6-11 years (48-95 lb): 2 tabs as needed up to tid
Tab: 400 mg
Children's Mylanta <2 years: not recommended; 2-5 years (24-47 lb): 1 tab as needed up to tid; 6-11 years (48-95 lb): 2 tabs as needed up to tid; >11 years: 2-4 tabs as needed
Liq: 400 mg/5 ml (4 oz)
Maalox Tab <12 years: not recommended; ≥12 years: chew 2-4 tabs prn; max 12 tabs/day
Chew tab: 600 mg (wild berry, lemon, wintergreen) (phenylalanine)
Maalox Maximum Strength Tab <12 years: not recommended; ≥12 years: 1-2 tabs prn; max 8 tabs/day
Tab: 1 gm (wild berry, lemon, wintergreen; phenylalanine)
Rolaids Extra Strength <12 years: not recommended; ≥12 years: 1-2 tabs dissolved in mouth or chewed q 1 hour prn; max 8 tabs/day
Tab: 1000 mg
Tums <12 years: not recommended; ≥12 years: 1-2 tabs dissolved in mouth or chewed q 1 hour prn; max 16 tabs/day
Tab: 500 mg
Tums E-X <12 years: not recommended; ≥12 years: 1-2 tabs dissolved in mouth or chewed q 1 hour prn; max 16 tabs/day
Tab: 750 mg

▶ ***calcium carbonate+magnesium carbonate*** (C)
Mylanta Gel Caps (OTC) <12 years: not recommended; ≥12 years: 2-4 caps prn
Gel cap: calib 550 mg+mag 125 mg

▶ ***calcium carbonate+magnesium hydroxide*** (C) <12 years: not recommended; ≥12 years:
Mylanta Tab 2-4 tabs between meals and HS prn
Tab: calib 350 mg+mag 150 mg
Mylanta DS Tab 2-4 tabs between meals and HS prn
Tab: calib 700 mg+mag 300 mg
Rolaids Sodium-Free 1-2 tabs dissolved in mouth or chewed q 1 hour as needed
Tab: calib 317 mg+mag 64 mg

▶ ***dihydroxyaluminum***
Rolaids (OTC) 1-2 tabs dissolved in mouth or chewed q 1 hour prn; max 24 tabs/day
Tab: 334 mg

H2 ANTAGONISTS

▶ ***cimetidine*** (B)(OTC)(G) <16 years: not recommended; ≥16 years: 800 mg bid or 400 mg qid; max 12 weeks
Tagamet 800 mg bid or 400 mg qid; max 12 weeks
Tab: 200, 300, 400*, 800*mg

Tagamet HB *Prophylaxis:* 1 tab ac; *Treatment:* 1 tab bid
Tab: 200 mg
Tagamet HB Oral Suspension *Prophylaxis:* 1-3 tsp ac; *Treatment:* 1 tsp bid
Oral susp: 200 mg/20 ml (12 oz)
Tagamet Liquid *Liq:* 300 mg/5 ml (mint-peach) (alcohol 2.8%)

▶ ***famotidine*** **(B)(OTC)(G)**0.5 mg/kg/day q HS prn or in 2 divided doses; max 40 mg/day
Maximum Strength Pepcid AC 1 tab ac
Tab: 20 mg
Pepcid 20-40 mg bid; max 6 weeks
Tab: 20 mg; *Tab*: 40 mg; Oral susp: 40 mg/5 ml (50 ml)
Pepcid AC 1 tab ac; max 2 doses/day
Tab/Rapid dissolving tab: 10 mg
Pepcid Complete (OTC) 1 tab ac; max 2 doses/day
Tab: fam 10 mg+$CaCO_2$ 800 mg+mag hydroxide 165 mg
Pepcid RPD *Tab:* 20, 40 mg rapid dissolv

▶ ***nizatidine*** **(B)(OTC)(G)** <12 years: not recommended; ≥12 years: 150 mg bid or 300 mg once daily
Axid *Cap:* 150, 300 mg; *Oral soln:* 15 mg/ml (480 ml) (bubble gum)

▶ ***ranitidine*** **(B)(OTC)(G)** <1 month: not recommended; 1 month-16 years: 2-4 mg/kg/day in 2 divided doses; max 300 mg/day; *Duodenal/Gastric Ulcer:* 2-4 mg/kg/day divided bid; max 300 mg/day; *Erosive Esophagitis:* 5-10 mg/kg/day divided bid; max 300 mg/day; 20 lb, 9 kg: 0.6 ml; 30 lb, 13.6 kg: 0.9 ml; 40 lb, 18.2 kg: 1.2 ml; 50 lb, 22.7 kg: 1.5 ml; 60 lb, 27.3 kg: 1.8 ml; 70 lb, 31.8 kg: 2.1 ml
Zantac 150 mg bid or 300 mg q HS
Tab: 150, 300 mg
Zantac 75 1 tab ac
Tab: 75 mg
Zantac EFFERdose dissolve 25 mg tab in 5 ml water and dissolve 150 mg tab in 6-8 oz water
Efferdose: 25, 150 mg effervescent
Zantac Syrup *Syr:* 15 mg/ml (peppermint) (alcohol 7.5%)

▶ ***ranitidine*** **(B)(OTC)(G)** <1 month: not recommended; 1 month-16 years: 2-4 mg/kg/day in 2 divided doses; max 300 mg/day; *Duodenal/Gastric Ulcer:* 2-4 mg/kg/day divided bid; max 300 mg/day; *Erosive Esophagitis:* 5-10 mg/kg/day divided bid; max 300 mg/day; 20 lb, 9 kg: 0.6 ml; 30 lb, 13.6 kg: 0.9 ml; 40 lb, 18.2 kg: 1.2 ml; 50 lb, 22.7 kg: 1.5 ml; 60 lb, 27.3 kg: 1.8 ml; 70 lb, 31.8 kg: 2.1 ml
Zantac 150 mg bid or 300 mg q HS
Tab: 150, 300 mg
Zantac 75 1 tab ac
Tab: 75 mg
Zantac EFFERdose dissolve 25 mg tab in 5 ml water and dissolve 150 mg tab in 6-8 oz water
Efferdose: 25, 150 mg effervescent
Zantac Syrup *Syr:* 15 mg/ml (peppermint) (alcohol 7.5%)

▶ ***ranitidine bismuth citrate*** **(C)** <12 years: not recommended; ≥12 years: 400 mg bid
Tritec *Tab:* 400 mg

PROTON PUMP INHIBITORS (PPIs)

Comment: A recent study of 144,032 incident users of acid suppression therapy, including 125,596 PPI users and 18,436 histamine H_2 receptor antagonist users were followed over 5 years. The researchers reported PPI users had an increased risk of having an eGFR <60 mL/min/$1.73m^2$, incident CKD, eGFR decline over 30%, and ESRD or eGFR decline over 50%, as compared to those taking H2 blockers. They concluded, "reliance on antecedent acute kidney injury (AKI) as a warning sign to guard against the risk of chronic kidney disease (CKD) among PPI users is not sufficient as a sole mitigation strategy." Further, timely PPI discontinuation is warranted if there is a first AKI to avoid progression to CKD.

REFERENCE

Xie, Y, Bowe, B, Li, T, *et al.* (2017). Long-term kidney outcomes among users of proton pump inhibitors without intervening acute kidney injury. *Kidney International, 91*(6), 1482–1494. doi:10.1016/j.kint.2016.12.021

Comment: Practice guidelines from the American Gastroenterological Association (AGA) address risks and recommendations for prescribing PPI therapy based on an extensive review of the literature. PPI use may increase the risk for fracture, vitamin B12 deficiency, hypomagnesemia, iron-deficiency anemia, small intestinal bacterial overgrowth (SIBO), *C. difficile* infection, kidney disease, cardiovascular disease (CVD), pneumonias, and dementia. Healthcare providers are advised to discuss the risks/benefits of PPI therapy with respect to each individual patient's situation.

REFERENCE

Freedberg, DE, Kim, LS, & Yang, Y-X. (2017). The risks and benefits of long-term use of proton pump inhibitors: expert review and best practice advice from the american gastroenterological association. *Gastroenterology, 152*(4), 706–715. doi:10.1053/j.gastro.2017.01.031

▶ ***dexlansoprazole*** **(B)(G)** <18 years: not recommended; ≥18 years: 30-60 mg daily for up to 4 weeks

  Dexilant *Cap:* 30, 60 mg ent-coat del-rel granules; may open and sprinkle on applesauce; do not crush or chew granules

  Dexilant SoluTab *Tab:* 30 mg del-rel orally-disint

▶ ***esomeprazole*** **(B)(OTC)(G)** <1 month: not established; 1 month-<1 year, 3-5 kg: 2.5 mg; 5-7.5 kg: 5 mg; >7.5-12 kg: 10 mg; 1-11 years, <20 kg: 10 mg; ≥20 kg: 10-20 mg; 12-17 years: 20 mg; max 8 weeks; >17 years: 20-40 mg once daily; max 8 weeks; take 1 hour before food; swallow whole or mix granules with food or juice and take immediately; do not crush or chew granules

  Nexium *Cap:* 20, 40 mg ent-coat del-rel pellets

  Nexium for Oral Suspension *Oral susp:* 10, 20, 40 mg ent-coat del-rel granules/pkt; mix in 2 tbsp water and drink immediately; 30 pkt/carton

▶ ***lansoprazole*** **(B)(OTC)(G)** <1 year: not recommended; ≥1 year: 15-30 mg daily for up to 8 weeks; may repeat course; take before eating

  Prevacid *Cap:* 15, 30 mg ent-coat del-rel granules; swallow whole or mix granules with food or juice and take immediately; do not crush or chew granules; follow with water

  Prevacid for Oral Suspension *Oral susp:* 15, 30 mg ent-coat del-rel granules/pkt; mix in 2 tbsp water and drink immediately; 30 pkt/carton (strawberry)

  Prevacid SoluTab *ODT:* 15, 30 mg (strawberry) (phenylalanine)

  Prevacid 24HR 15 mg ent-coat del-rel granules; swallow whole or mix granules with food or juice and take immediately; do not crush or chew granules; follow with water

▶ ***omeprazole*** **(C)(OTC)(G)**

  Prilosec <1 year: not recommended; ≥1 year: 5-<10 kg: 5 mg daily; 10-<20 kg: 10 mg daily; ≥20 kg: 20-40 mg daily for 14 days; may repeat course in 4 months; take before eating; swallow whole or mix granules with applesauce and take immediately; do not crush or chew granules; follow with water

    Cap: 10, 20, 40 mg ent-coat del-rel granules

Prilosec OTC <18 years: not recommended; >18 years:
Tab: 20 mg del-rel (regular, wild berry)

➢ ***pantoprazole*** **(B)(G)** <12 years: not recommended; ≥12 years: 40 mg daily
Tab: 40 mg ent-coat del-rel
Protonix for Oral Suspension
Oral susp: 40 mg ent-coat del-rel granules/pkt; mix in 1 tsp apple juice for 5 seconds or sprinkle on 1 tsp applesauce, and swallow immediately; do not mix in water or any other liquid or food; take approximately 30 minutes prior to a meal; 30 pkt/carton

➢ ***rabeprazole*** **(B)(OTC)(G)** <1 year: not recommended; 1-11 years, <15 kg: 5 mg once daily for up to 12 weeks; >11 years, ≥15 kg: 20 mg daily after breakfast; may open cap and sprinkle contents on a small amount of soft food or liquid
AcipHex *Tab:* 20 mg ent-coat del-rel
AcipHex Sprinkle *Cap:* 5, 10 mg del-rel

PROTON PUMP INHIBITOR+SODIUM BICARBONATE COMBINATION

➢ ***omeprazole+sodium bicarbonate*** **(B)(G)** <18 years: not recommended; ≥18 years: 20 mg daily; do not crush or chew; max 8 weeks
Zegerid *Cap:* omep 20 mg+sod bicarb 1100 mg; omep 40 mg+sod bicarb 1100 mg
Zegerid OTC (OTC) *Cap:* omep 20 mg+sod bicarb 1100 mg
Zegerid for Oral Suspension *Pwdr for oral susp:* omep 20 mg+sod bicarb 1680 mg; omep 40 mg+sod bicarb 1680 mg (30 pkt/carton)

PROMOTILITY AGENT

➢ ***metoclopramide*** **(B)(G)** <18 years: not recommended; ≥18 years: 10-15 mg qid 30 minutes ac and HS prn; up to 20 mg prior to provoking situation; max 12 weeks per therapeutic course
Metozolv ODT *ODT:* 5, 10 mg (mint)
Reglan *Tab:* 5*, 10 mg; *Syr:* 5 mg/5 ml
Reglan ODT *ODT:* 5, 10 mg (orange)

Comment: metoclopramide is contraindicated when stimulation of GI motility may be dangerous. Observe for tardive dyskinesia and Parkinsonism. Avoid concomitant drugs that may cause an extrapyramidal reaction (e.g., phenothiazines, ***haloperidol***).

GIARDIASIS (*GIARDIA LAMBLIA*)

➢ ***metronidazole*** **(not for use in 1st; B in 2nd, 3rd)(G)** <12 years: 35-50 mg/kg/day in 3 divided doses x 10 days; ≥12 years: 250 mg tid x 5-10 days
Flagyl *Tab:* 250*, 500*mg
Flagyl 375 *Cap:* 375 mg
Flagyl ER *Tab:* 750 mg ext-rel

Comment: Alcohol is contraindicated during treatment with oral ***metronidazole*** and for 72 hours after therapy due to a possible ***disulfiram***-like reaction (nausea, vomiting, flushing, headache).

➢ ***nitazoxanide*** **(B)** <1 year: not recommended; 1-3 years; 100 mg q 12 hours x 3 days; >3-11 years: 200 mg q 12 hours x 3 days; ≥11 years: 500 mg q 12 hours x 3 days; take with food
Alinia *Tab:* 500 mg; *Oral susp:* 100 mg/5 ml (60 ml)
Comment: **Alinia** is an antiprotozoal for the treatment of diarrhea due to *G. lamblia* or *C. parvum.*

- ▶ *tinidazole* **(not for use in 1st; B in 2nd, 3rd)** <3 years: not recommended; 3-12 years: 50 mg/kg once daily x 3-5 days; take with food; max 2 gm/day; >12 years: 2 gm once daily x 3-5 days; take with food
  Tindamax *Tab:* 250*, 500*mg

GINGIVITIS/PERIODONTITIS

ANTI-INFECTIVE ORAL RINSES

Comment: Oral treatments should be preceded by brushing and flossing the teeth. Avoid foods and liquids for 2-3 hours after a treatment.

- ▶ *chlorhexidine gluconate* **(B)(G)** swish 15 ml undiluted for 30 seconds bid; do not swallow; do not rinse mouth after treatment.
  Peridex, PerioGard *Oral soln:* 0.12% (480 ml)

GLAUCOMA: OPEN ANGLE/OCULAR HYPERTENSION

Comment: Other ophthalmic medications should not be administered within 5-10 minutes of administering an ophthalmic antiglaucoma medication. Contact lenses should be removed prior to instillation of antiglaucoma medications and may be replaced 15 minutes later. Interactions with ophthalmic antiglaucoma agents include MAOIs, CNS depressants, beta-blockers, tricyclic antidepressants, and hypoglycemics. Choices for medical treatment in progressive cases include *betaxolol* eye drops which have a beneficial effect on optic nerve blood flow in addition to intraocular pressure IOP reduction. Other beta blockers and adrenergic drugs (such as dipivefrine) should better be avoided because of the probability of nocturnal systemic hypotension and optic nerve hypoperfusion (e.g., in patients with untreated obstructive sleep apnea). Prostaglandin derivatives tend to have greater IOP-lowering effect which may be of overriding consideration. *dorzolamide-timolol* fixed combination is a safe and effective IOP-lowering agent in patients with normal tension glaucoma (NTG). *brimonidine* significantly improved retinal vascular autoregulation in NTG patients.

OPHTHALMIC ALPHA-2A AGONISTS

Comment: Ophthalmic $alpha_{2a}$-agonists are contraindicated with concomitant MAOI use. Cautious use with CNS depressants, beta-blockers (ocular and systemic), antihypertensives, cardiac glycosides, and tricyclic antidepressants.

- ▶ *apraclonidine* ophthalmic solution **(C)** <12 years: not recommended; ≥12 years: 1-2 drops affected eye tid
  Iopidine *Ophth soln:* 0.5% (5 ml) (benzalkonium chloride)
- ▶ ***brimonidine tartrate*** ophthalmic solution **(B)** <2 years: not recommended; ≥2 years: 1 drop affected eye q 8 hours
  Alphagan P *Ophth soln:* 0.1, 0.15% (5, 10, 15 ml) (purite)

OPHTHALMIC CARBONIC ANHYDRASE INHIBITORS

Comment: Ophthalmic carbonic anhydrase inhibitors are contraindicated in patients with sulfa allergy.

- ▶ *brinzolamide* ophthalmic suspension **(C)** <12 years: not recommended; ≥12 years: 1 drop affected eye tid
  Azopt *Ophth susp:* 1% (2.5, 5, 10, 15 ml) (benzalkonium chloride)
- ▶ *dorzolamide* ophthalmic solution **(C)(G)** <12 years: not recommended; ≥12 years: 1 drop affected eye tid
  Trusopt *Ophth soln:* 2% (10 ml) (benzalkonium chloride)

OPHTHALMIC ALPHA-2 ADRENERGIC RECEPTOR AGONIST+CARBONIC ANHYDRASE INHIBITOR

▶ ***brimonidine+brinzolamide*** **(C)** <12 years: not recommended; ≥12 years: 1 drop affected eye tid

Simbrinza *Ophth soln:* brim 1% mg+brinz 0.2% per ml (10 ml)

OPHTHALMIC CHOLINERGICS (MIOTICS)

▶ ***carbachol+hydroxypropyl methylcellulose*** ophthalmic solution **(C)** <12 years: not recommended; ≥12 years: 2 drops affected eye tid

Isopto Carbachol *Ophth soln:* carb 0.75% or 2.25%+hydroxy 1% (15 ml); carb 1.5% or 3%+hydroxy 1% (15, 30 ml) (benzalkonium chloride)

▶ ***pilocarpine*** **(C)(G)** <12 years: not recommended; ≥12 years:

Isopto Carpine 2 drops affected eye tid-qid
Ophth soln: 1, 2, 4% (15 ml) (benzalkonium chloride)

Ocusert Pilo change ophthalmic insert once weekly
Ophth inserts: 20 mcg/Hr (8/pck)

Pilocar Ophthalmic Solution 1-2 drops affected eye 1-6 x/day
Ophth soln: 0.5, 1, 2, 3, 4, 6, 8% (15 ml)

Pilopine HS apply 1/2 inch ribbon in lower conjunctival sac q HS
Ophth gel: 4% (4 gm)

OPHTHALMIC CHOLINESTERASE INHIBITORS

▶ ***demecarium bromide*** ophthalmic solution **(X)** <12 years: not recommended; ≥12 years: 1-2 drops affected eye q 12-48 hours

Humorsol Ocumeter *Ophth soln:* 0.125, 0.25% (5 ml)

▶ ***echothiophate iodide*** ophthalmic solution **(C)** <12 years: not recommended; ≥12 years: initially 1 drop of 0.03% affected eye bid; then increase strength as needed

Phospholine Iodide *Ophth soln:* 0.03, 0.06, 0.125, 0.25% (5 ml)

OPHTHALMIC CARDIOSELECTIVE BETA-BLOCKERS

Comment: Ophthalmic beta-blockers are generally contraindicated in severe COPD, history of or current bronchial asthma, sinus bradycardia, 2nd or 3rd degree AV block.

▶ ***betaxolol*** ophthalmic solution **(C)(G)** <12 years: not recommended; ≥12 years: 1-2 drops affected eye bid

Betoptic *Ophth soln:* 0.5% (5, 10, 15 ml) (benzalkonium chloride)

Betoptic S *Ophth soln:* 0.25% (2.5, 5, 10, 15 ml) (benzalkonium chloride)

OPHTHALMIC BETA-BLOCKERS (NON-CARDIOSELECTIVE)

Comment: Ophthalmic beta-blockers are generally contraindicated in severe COPD, history of or current bronchial asthma, sinus bradycardia, 2nd or 3rd degree AV block.

▶ ***carteolol*** ophthalmic solution **(C)(G)** <12 years: not recommended; ≥12 years: 1 drop affected eye bid

Ocupress *Ophth soln:* 1% (5, 10, 15 ml) (benzalkonium chloride)

▶ ***levobunolol*** ophthalmic solution **(C)** <12 years: not recommended; ≥12 years: 1-2 drops affected eye bid

Betagan *Ophth soln:* 0.5% (5, 10, 15 ml) (benzalkonium chloride)

▶ ***metipranolol*** ophthalmic solution **(C)(G)** <12 years: not recommended; ≥12 years: 1 drop affected eye bid

OptiPranolol *Ophth soln:* 0.3% (5, 10 ml) (benzalkonium chloride)

▶ ***timolol*** ophthalmic solution and gel **(C)(G)** <12 years: not recommended; ≥12 years:

Betimol 1 drop affected eye bid

Ophth soln: 0.25, 0.5% (5, 10, 15 ml) (benzalkonium chloride)

Istalol 1 drop affected eye daily

Ophth soln: 0.5% (2.5, 5 ml) (preservative-free)

Timoptic 1 drop affected eye bid

Ophth soln: 0.25, 0.5% (5, 10, 15 ml) (benzalkonium chloride)

Timoptic Ocudose 1 drop bid

Ophth soln: 0.25, 0.5% (0.2 ml/dose, 60 dose) (preservative-free)

Timoptic-XE 1 drop affected eye bid

Ophth gel: 0.25, 0.5% (2.5, 5 ml) (preservative-free)

OPHTHALMIC ALPHA-2A AGONIST+ NON-CARDIOSELECTIVE BETA-BLOCKER COMBINATION

Comment: Generally contraindicated in severe COPD, history of or current bronchial asthma, sinus bradycardia, 2nd or 3rd degree AV block.

▶ ***brimonidine tartrate+timolol*** ophthalmic solution **(C)**: <2 years: not recommended; ≥2 years: 1 drop affected eye bid

Combigan *Ophth soln:* brimo 0.2%+timo 0.5% (5, 10, 15 ml) (benzalkonium chloride)

OPHTHALMIC PROSTAMIDE ANALOGS

▶ ***bimatoprost*** ophthalmic solution **(C)(G)** <16 years: not recommended; ≥16 years: 1 drop q affected eye HS

Lumigan *Ophth soln:* 0.01, 0.03% (2.5, 5, 7.5 ml) (benzalkonium chloride)

▶ ***latanoprost*** ophthalmic solution **(C)** <12 years: not recommended; ≥12 years: 1 drop affected eye q HS

Xalatan *Ophth soln:* 0.005% (2.5 ml) (benzalkonium chloride)

▶ ***tafluprost*** ophthalmic solution **(C)** <12 years: not recommended; ≥12 years: 1 drop affected eye q HS

Zioptan *Ophth soln:* 0.0015% (0.3 ml single use, 30-60/carton) (preservative-free)

▶ ***travoprost*** ophthalmic solution **(C)(G)** <16 years: not recommended; ≥16 years: 1 drop affected eye q HS

Travatan *Ophth soln:* 0.004% (2.5, 5 ml) (benzalkonium chloride)

Travatan Z *Ophth soln:* 0.004% (2.5, 5 ml) (boric acid, propylene glycol, sorbitol, zinc chloride)

PROSTAGLANDIN ANALOG (WITH NITRIC OXIDE METABOLITE)

▶ ***latanoprostene bunod*** ophthalmic solution **(C)** ≤16 years: not recommended (because of potential safety concerns related to increased pigmentation following long-term chronic use); >16 years:1 drop affected eye once daily

Vyzulta *Ophth soln:* 0.024% (5 ml) (benzalkonium chloride)

Comment: **Vyzulta** is a prostaglandin analog with nitric oxide as one of its metabolites. **Vyzulta** exerts a dual mechanism of action through latanoprost acid and butanediol mononitrate, working in the uveoscleral pathway and Schlemm's canal. Most common ocular adverse reactions with incidence ≥ 2% are conjunctival hyperemia (6%), eye irritation (4%), eye pain (3%), and instillation site pain (2%). There may be increased pigmentation of the iris and periorbital tissue. Iris pigmentation is likely to be permanent. There may be gradual changes to eyelashes including increased length, increased thickness and number of eyelashes, that is usually reversible upon discontinuation of treatment. There are no available human data for the use of **Vyzulta** during pregnancy to inform any drug associated risks. There are no data on the presence of **Vyzulta** in human milk or effects on the breastfed infant.

OPHTHALMIC SYMPATHOMIMETICS

Comment: Contraindicated in narrow-angle glaucoma. Use with caution in cardiovascular disease, hypertension, hyperthyroidism, diabetes, and asthma.

▶ ***dipivefrin*** ophthalmic solution **(B)** <12 years: not recommended; ≥12 years: 1 drop affected eye q 12 hours

Propine *Ophth soln:* 0.1% (5, 10, 15 ml) (benzalkonium chloride)

OPHTHALMIC CARBONIC ANHYDRASE INHIBITOR+NON-CARDIOSELECTIVE BETA-BLOCKER

▶ ***dorzolamide+timolol*** ophthalmic solution **(C)** <12 years: not recommended; ≥12 years: 1 drop affected eye bid

Cosopt *Ophth soln:* dorz 2%+tim 0.5% (10 ml) (benzalkonium chloride)

Cosopt PF *Ophth soln:* dorz 2%+tim 0.5% (10 ml) (preservative-free)

OPHTHALMIC SYNTHETIC DOCOSANOID

▶ ***unoprostone isopropyl*** ophthalmic solution **(C)** <12 years: not recommended; ≥12 years: 1 drop affected eye bid

Rescula *Ophth soln:* 0.15% (5 ml) (benzalkonium chloride)

OPHTHALMIC RHO KINASE INHIBITOR

▶ ***netarsudil*** ophthalmic solution **(C)** <18 years: not established; ≥18 years: 1 drop affected eye once daily in the PM

Rhopressa *Ophth soln:* 0.02% (0.2 mg/ml, 2.5 ml) (benzalkonium chloride)

ORAL CARBONIC ANHYDRASE INHIBITORS

▶ ***acetazolamide*** **(C)** <12 years: not recommended; ≥12 years: 250-1000 mg/day in divided doses or 500 mg bid sust-rel tabs; max 1 gm/day

Diamox *Tab:* 125*, 250*mg

Diamox Sequels *Tab:* 500 mg sust-rel

▶ ***methazolamide*** (C)(G) <12 years: not recommended; ≥12 years: 50-100 mg bid-tid times daily

Neptazane *Tab:* 25, 50 mg

Comment: Administer ophthalmic osmotic and miotic agents concomitantly.

GONORRHEA (*NEISSERIA GONORRHOEAE*)

Comment: The following treatment regimens for *N. gonorrhoeae* are published in the **2015 CDC Transmitted Diseases Treatment Guidelines**. Treatment regimens are presented by generic drug name first, followed by information about brands and dose forms. Empiric treatment requires concomitant treatment of chlamydia. Treat all sexual contacts. Patients who are HIV-positive should receive the same treatment as those who are HIV-negative. Sexual abuse must be considered a cause of gonococcal infection in preadolescent children.

RECOMMENDED REGIMENS, ≥12 YEARS: UNCOMPLICATED INFECTIONS OF THE CERVIX, URETHRA, AND RECTUM

Regimen 1

- *ceftriaxone* 250 mg IM in a single dose
  plus
- *azithromycin* 1 gm in a single dose

Regimen 2

- *ceftriaxone* 250 mg IM in a single dose
  plus
- *doxycycline* 100 mg bid x 7 days

RECOMMENDED REGIMENS, ≥12 YEARS: UNCOMPLICATED INFECTIONS OF THE PHARYNX

Regimen 1

- *ceftriaxone* 250 mg IM in a single dose
  plus
- *azithromycin* 1 gm in a single dose

Regimen 2

- *ceftriaxone* 250 mg IM in a single dose
  plus
- *doxycycline* 100 mg bid x 7 days

RECOMMENDED REGIMENS, CHILDREN ≥45 KG, ≥8 YEARS: UNCOMPLICATED INFECTIONS OF THE CERVIX, URETHRA, AND RECTUM

Regimen 1

- *ceftriaxone* 250 mg IM in a single dose
  plus
- *azithromycin* 1 gm in a single dose

RECOMMENDED REGIMEN: CHILDREN ≥45 KG

Regimen 1

- *ceftriaxone* 250 mg IM in a single dose

RECOMMENDED REGIMEN: CHILDREN >45 KG WHO HAVE GONOCOCCAL BACTEREMIA OR GONOCOCCAL ARTHRITIS

Regimen 1

- *ceftriaxone* 50 mg/kg IM or IV in a single dose daily x 7 days

RECOMMENDED REGIMENS, CHILDREN <45 KG, <8 YEARS: UNCOMPLICATED GONOCOCCAL VULVOVAGINITIS, CERVICITIS, URETHRITIS, PHARYNGITIS, OR PROCTITIS

Regimen 1

- *ceftriaxone* 250 mg IM in a single dose

RECOMMENDED REGIMEN, CHILDREN <45 KG, <8 YEARS: GONOCOCCAL BACTEREMIA OR ARTHRITIS

Regimen 1

- *ceftriaxone* 50 mg/kg (max dose 1 gm) IM or IV in a single dose daily x 7 days

DRUG BRANDS AND DOSE FORMS

- *azithromycin* (B)(G)
  - **Zithromax** *Tab:* 250, 500, 600 mg; *Oral susp:* 100 mg/5 ml (15 ml); 200 mg/5 ml (15, 22.5, 30 ml) (cherry); *Pkt:* 1 gm for reconstitution (cherry-banana)
  - **Zithromax Tri-pak** *Tab:* 3 x 500 mg tabs/pck
  - **Zithromax Z-pak** *Tab:* 6 x 250 mg tabs/pck
  - **Zmax** *Oral susp:* 2 gm ext-rel for reconstitution (cherry-banana) (148 mg Na^+)
- *ceftriaxone* (B)(G)
  - **Rocephin** *Vial:* 250, 500 mg; 1, 2 gm
- *doxycycline* (D)(G) <8 years: not recommended
  - **Acticlate** *Tab:* 75, 150**mg
  - **Adoxa** *Tab:* 50, 75, 100, 150 mg ent-coat
  - **Doryx** *Tab:* 50, 75, 100, 150, 200 mg del-rel
  - **Doxteric** *Tab:* 50 mg del-rel
  - **Monodox** *Cap:* 50, 75, 100 mg
  - **Oracea** *Cap:* 40 mg del-rel
  - **Vibramycin** *Tab:* 100 mg; *Cap:* 50, 100 mg; *Syr:* 50 mg/5 ml (raspberry-apple) (sulfites); *Oral susp:* 25 mg/5 ml (raspberry)
  - **Vibra-Tab** *Tab:* 100 mg film-coat

ALTERNATIVE THERAPY

- *azithromycin* (B) <12 years: not recommended; ≥12 years: 2 gm x 1 dose
  - **Zithromax** *Tab:* 250, 500, 600 mg; *Oral susp:* 100 mg/5 ml (15 ml); 200 mg/5 ml (15, 22.5, 30 ml) (cherry); *Pkt:* 1 gm for reconstitution (cherry-banana)
  - **Zithromax Tri-pak** *Tab:* 3 x 500 mg tabs/pck
  - **Zithromax Z-pak** *Tab:* 6 x 250 mg tabs/pck
  - **Zmax** *Oral susp:* 2 gm ext-rel for reconstitution (cherry-banana) (148 mg Na^+)
- *cefotaxime* 500 mg IM x 1 dose
  - **Claforan** *Vial:* 500 mg; 1, 2 gm
- *cefotetan* <12 years: not recommended; ≥12 years: 1 gm IM x 1 dose
  - **Cefotan** *Vial:* 1, 2 gm
- *cefoxitin* (B) <3 months: not recommended; ≥3 months: 2 gm IM x 1 dose
  - **Mefoxin** *Vial:* 1, 2 gm

    plus
- *probenecid* (B)(G)
  - **Benemid** <2 years: not recommended; 2-14 years: 25 mg/kg 30 minutes before *cefoxitin*; >14 years: 1 gm 30 minutes before *cefoxitin*
    - *Tab:* 500*mg; *Cap:* 500 mg
- *cefpodoxime proxetil* (B) <2 months: not recommended; 2 months-12 years: 10 mg/kg/day (max 400 mg/dose) or 5 mg/kg/day bid (max 200 mg/dose); ≥12 years: 200 mg x 1 dose
  - **Vantin** *Tab:* 100, 200 mg; *Oral susp:* 50, 100 mg/5 ml (50, 75, 100 mg) (lemon creme)
- *ceftizoxime* (B) <6 months: not recommended; ≥6 months: 1 gm IM x 1 dose
  - **Cefizox** *Vial:* 500 mg; 1, 2, 10 g

▶ *demeclocycline* (X) <8 years: not recommended; ≥8 years: initially 600 mg, followed by 300 mg q 12 hours x 4 days (total 3 gm)
  Declomycin *Tab:* 300 mg
 Comment: ***demeclocycline*** is contraindicated <8 years-of-age, in pregnancy, and lactation (discolors developing tooth enamel). A side effect may be photosensitivity (photophobia). Do not give with antacids, calcium supplements, or other dairy, or within two hours of taking another drug.

▶ ***enoxacin*** (C) <18 years: not recommended; ≥18 years: 400 mg x 1 dose
  Penetrex *Tab:* 200, 400 mg

▶ ***lomefloxacin*** (C) <18 years: not recommended; ≥18 years: 400 mg x 1 dose
  Maxaquin *Tab:* 400 mg

▶ ***norfloxacin*** (C) <18 years: not recommended; ≥18 years: 800 mg x 1 dose
  Noroxin *Tab:* 400 mg

▶ ***spectinomycin*** (B) <12 years: 40 mg/kg IM x 1 dose; ≥12 years: 2 gm IM x 1 dose
  Trobicin *Vial:* 2 gm

GOUT (HYPERURICEMIA)

Acetaminophen for IV Infusion *see page* 322
NSAIDs *see page* 539
Other Oral Analgesics *see* ***Pain*** *page* 324
Topical & Transdermal NSAIDs *see* ***Pain*** *page* 323
Parenteral Corticosteroids *see page* 547
Oral Corticosteroids *see page* 546
Pseudogout *see page* 382

XANTHINE OXIDASE INHIBITORS (PROPHYLAXIS)

▶ *allopurinol* (C)(G) **6 years: max 150 mg/day; 6-10 years: max 400 mg/day; >10 years:** 200-300 mg in 1-3 doses; max 800 mg/day; max single dose 300 mg
  Zyloprim *Tab:* 100*, 300*mg

▶ ***potassium citrate*** (C)(G) <12 years: not recommended; ≥12 years: 30 mEq qid
  Urocit-K *Tab:* 5, 10, 15 mEq ext-rel
 Comment: ***potassium citrate*** is contraindicated in hyperkalemia. Encourage patients to limit salt intake and maintain liberal hydration (urine volume should be at least 2 liters/day). Target urine pH is 6.0-7.0 and urine citrate at least 320 mg/day and close to the normal mean of 640 mg/day. Take with food.

ACUTE ATTACK

▶ *colchicine* (C)(G) <12 years: not recommended; ≥12 years: 0.6-1.2 mg at first sign of attack; then 0.6 mg every hour or 1.2 mg every 2 hours until pain relief; then consider 0.6 mg/day or every other day for maintenance
  Colcrys *Tab:* 0.6 mg
  Mitigare *Cap:* 0.6 mg
 Comment: Do not take ***colchicine*** concurrently with ***allopurinol***.

▶ *febuxostat* (C)(G) <18 years: not recommended; ≥18 years: initially 40 mg daily; after 2 weeks, may increase to 80 mg daily.
  Uloric *Tab:* 40, 80 mg
 Comment: Gout flare prophylaxis with ***colchicine*** or NSAID is recommended on initiation of ***febuxostat*** and up to 6 months.

PEGYLATED URIC ACID SPECIFIC ENZYME

▶ ***pegloticase*** (C) <18 years: not recommended; ≥18 years: pre-medicate with antihistamine and corticosteroid; 8 mg once every 2 weeks; administer IV infusion after dilution over at least 2 hours; observe at least 1 hour post-infusion

Krystexxa *Vial:* 8 mg/ml (1 ml) single-use pwdr for IV infusion after dilution

Comment: Slow rate, or stop and restart at lower rate, if infusion reaction occurs (e.g., **Krystexxa** is contraindicated with G6PD deficiency; screen patients of African or Mediterranean descent). **Krystexxa** is not for the treatment of asymptomatic hyperuricemia.

URICOSURIC AGENT

▶ ***probenecid*** (C)(G) <18 years: not recommended; ≥18 years: 250 mg bid x 1 week; maintenance 500 mg bid

Tab: 500*mg; *Cap:* 500 mg

Comment: Avoid concomitant use of ***probenecid*** and salicylates.

URICOSURIC+ANTI-INFLAMMATORY COMBINATIONS

▶ ***probenecid+colchicine*** (G) <18 years: not recommended; ≥18 years: 1 tab once daily x 1 week; then, 1 tab bid thereafter

Tab: prob 500 mg+colch 0.5 mg

Comment: ***probenecid+colchicine*** is contraindicated in the treatment of acute gout attack, patients with blood dyscrasias, and patients with uric acid kidney stones. Concomitant salicylates antagonize the uricosuric effects.

▶ ***sulfinpyrazone*** (C) <18 years: not recommended; ≥18 years: initially 200-400 mg bid; may gradually increase to 800 mg bid

Anturane *Cap:* 100, 200 mg

Comment: Goal is serum uric acid <6.5 mg/dL.

XANTHINE OXIDASE INHIBITOR

▶ ***febuxostat*** (C) <18 years: not established; ≥18 years: 40 mg once daily x 2 weeks; if serum uric acid is not <6 mg/dL, may increase to 80 mg once daily

Uloric *Tab:* 40, 80 mg

SELECTIVE URIC ACID REABSORPTION INHIBITOR (SURI)

▶ ***lesinurad*** (C) <18 years: not established; ≥18 years: 200 mg once daily in combination with a xanthine oxidase inhibitor (XOI)

Zurampic *Tab:* 200 mg

Comment: **Zurampic** inhibits URATI, a urate transporter, which is responsible for the majority of renal absorption of uric acid and (OAT) 4, organic anion transporter, a uric acid transporter involved in diuretic-induced hyperuricemia. Do not use as monotherapy. Use in combination with an XOI, such as ***allopurinol*** or ***febuxostat***, (to reduce the production of uric acid). Do not initiate if CrCl <45 mL/min, ESRD, dialysis, or kidney transplant.

XANTHINE OXIDASE INHIBITOR+URATI INHIBITOR COMBINATION

▶ ***allopurinol+lesinurad*** <18 years: not established; ≥18 years: take 1 tab once daily

Duzallo *Tab:* 200/200, 300/200 mg

Comment: The US Food and Drug Administration recently approved **Duzallo** for the treatment of hyperuricemia associated with gout in patients who have not achieved target serum uric acid (sUA) levels with ***allopurinol*** alone. **Duzallo** is the first drug to combine ***allopurinol***, the current standard of care for hyperuricemia associated with gout, and ***lesinurad***, the most recent FDA-approved treatment for this condition. The fixed-dose combination addresses the overproduction and underexcretion of serum uric acid. Patients with asymptomatic hyperuricemia are not recommended to receive **Duzallo**. Common adverse reactions associated with **Duzallo** include headache, influenza, higher levels of blood creatinine, and heart burn. In addition, **Duzallo** has a boxed warning for the risk of acute renal failure associated with ***lesinurad***. There are no available human data on use of **Duzallo** or ***lesinurad*** in pregnancy to inform a drug-associated risk of adverse developmental outcomes. Limited published data on ***allopurinol*** use in pregnancy do not demonstrate a clear pattern or increase in frequency of adverse development outcomes. There is no information regarding the presence of **Duzallo** or ***lesinurad*** in human milk or the effects on the breastfed infant. Based on information from a single case report, ***allopurinol*** and its active metabolite, ***oxypurinol***, were detected in the milk of a mother at five weeks postpartum. The effect of ***allopurinol*** on the breastfed infant is unknown. CrCl 45-< 60 mL/min: adjust the allopurinol to a medically appropriate dose (200 mg). CrCl <45, ***allopurinol*** not recommended. Max ***lesinurad*** 200 mg/day. In clinical trials evaluating the safety and efficacy of this combined therapy among adult patients with gout who failed to achieve target sUA levels on ***allopurinol*** alone, **Duzallo** was found to nearly double the number of patients who achieved target sUA at 6 months, mean sUA was reduced to less than 6 mg/dL by 1 month, and this level was maintained through 12 months.

GOUTY ARTHRITIS

Acetaminophen for IV Infusion *see **Pain** page* 322
NSAIDs *see page* 539
Other Oral Analgesics *see **Pain** page* 324
Topical & Transdermal NSAIDs *see **Pain** page* 323
Parenteral Corticosteroids *see page* 547
Oral Corticosteroids *see page* 546

TOPICAL ANALGESICS

▶ ***capsaicin*** (B)(G) <2 years: not recommended; ≥2 years: apply tid-qid prn to intact skin

- **Axsain** *Crm:* 0.075% (1, 2 oz)
- **Capsin** *Lotn:* 0.025, 0.075% (59 ml)
- **Capzasin-P (OTC)** *Crm:* 0.025% (1.5 oz); *Lotn:* 0.025% (2 oz)
- **Dolorac** *Crm:* 0.025% (28 gm)
- **Double Cap (OTC)** *Crm:* 0.05% (2 oz)
- **R-Gel** *Gel:* 0.025% (15, 30 gm)
- **Zostrix (OTC)** *Crm:* 0.025% (0.7, 1.5, 3 oz)
- **Zostrix HP (OTC)** *Emol crm:* 0.075% (1, 2 oz)

Comment: Provides some relief by 1-2 weeks; optimal benefit may take 4-6 weeks.

ORAL SALICYLATE

▶ ***indomethacin*** (C) <14 years: usually not recommended; <2-14 years, if risk warranted: 1-2 mg/kg/day in divided doses; max 3-4 mg/kg/day (or 150-200 mg/day, whichever is less); ≤14 years: ER cap not recommended; >14 years: initially 25 mg bid-tid; increase as needed at weekly intervals by 25-50 mg/day; max 200 mg/day

Cap: 25, 50 mg; *Susp:* 25 mg/5 ml (pineapple-coconut, mint; alcohol 1%); *Supp:* 50 mg; *ER Cap:* 75 mg ext-rel

Comment: ***indomethacin*** is indicated only for acute painful flares. Administer with food and/or antacids. Use lowest effective dose for shortest duration.

NSAID PLUS PPI

- *esomeprazole+naproxen* **(C; not for use in 3rd)(G)** <18 years: not recommended; ≥18 years: 1 tab bid; use lowest effective dose for the shortest duration; swallow whole; take at least 30 minutes before a meal
  - **Vimovo** *Tab:* nap 375 mg+eso 20 mg ext-rel; nap 500 mg+eso 20 mg ext-rel

COX-2 INHIBITORS

Comment: Cox-2 inhibitors are contraindicated with history of asthma, urticaria, and allergic-type reactions to ***aspirin***, other NSAIDs, and sulfonamides, 3rd trimester of pregnancy, and coronary artery bypass graft (CABG) surgery.

- ***celecoxib*** **(C)(G)** <18 years: not recommended; ≥18 years: 100-400 mg bid; max 800 mg/day
  - **Celebrex** *Cap:* 50, 100, 200, 400 mg
- ***meloxicam*** **(C)(G)**
  - **Mobic** <2 years, <60 kg: not recommended; ≥2 years, ≥60 kg-12 years: 0.125 mg/kg; max 7.5 mg once daily; ≥12 years: initially 7.5 mg once daily; max 15 mg once daily; Hemodialysis: max 7.5 mg/day
    - *Tab:* 7.5, 15 mg; *Oral susp:* 7.5 mg/5 ml (100 ml) (raspberry)
  - **Vivlodex** <18 years: not established; ≥18 years: initially 5 mg qd; may increase to max 10 mg/day; Hemodialysis: max 5 mg/day
    - *Cap:* 5, 10 mg

GRANULOMA INGUINALE (DONOVANOSIS)

Comment: The following treatment regimens are published in the **2015 CDC Sexually Transmitted Diseases Treatment Guidelines.** Treatment regimens are for patients ≥18 years only; consult a specialist for treatment of patients less than 18 years-of-age. Treatment regimens are presented by generic drug name first, followed by information about brands and dose forms. Persons who have sexual contact with a patient who has had granuloma inguinale within the past 60 days before onset of the patient's symptoms should be examined and offered therapy. Patients who are HIV-positive should receive the same treatment as those who are HIV-negative; however, the addition of a parenteral aminoglycoside (e.g., ***gentamicin***) can also be considered.

RECOMMENDED REGIMEN

- ***doxycycline*** 100 mg bid x at least 3 weeks and until all lesions have completely healed

ALTERNATE REGIMENS

- ***azithromycin*** (B)(G)1 gm once weekly for at least 3 weeks and until all lesions have completely healed
- ***ciprofloxacin*** (C) 750 mg bid x at least 3 weeks and until all lesions have completely healed; max 1.5 gm/day
- ***erythromycin base*** 500 mg qid x 14 days or ***erythromycin ethylsuccinate*** 400 mg qid x 14 days
- ***trimethoprim+sulfamethoxazole*** 1 double-strength (160/800) dose bid x at least 3 weeks and until all lesions have completely healed

DRUG BRANDS AND DOSE FORMS

- ***azithromycin*** (B)(G)
  - **Zithromax** *Tab:* 250, 500, 600 mg; *Oral susp:* 100 mg/5 ml (15 ml); 200 mg/5 ml (15, 22.5, 30 ml) (cherry); *Pkt:* 1 gm for reconstitution (cherry-banana)

Zithromax Tri-pak *Tab:* 3 x 500 mg tabs/pck
Zithromax Z-pak *Tab:* 6 x 250 mg tabs/pck
Zmax *Oral susp:* 2 gm ext-rel for reconstitution (cherry-banana) (148 mg Na^+)

▶ ***ciprofloxacin*** **(C)**
Cipro (G) *Tab:* 250, 500, 750 mg; *Oral susp:* 250, 500 mg/5 ml (100 ml) (strawberry)
Cipro XR *Tab:* 500, 1000 mg ext-rel
ProQuin XR *Tab:* 500 mg ext-rel

Comment: ***ciprofloxacin*** is contraindicated <18 years-of-age, and during pregnancy, and lactation. Risk of tendonitis or tendon rupture.

▶ ***doxycycline*** **(D)(G)** <8 years: not recommended; ≥8 years, <100 lb: 2 mg/lb on first day in 2 divided doses, followed by 1 mg/lb/day in 1-2 divided doses; ≥8 years, ≥100 lb: 40-100 mg bid; *see page* 605 *for dose by weight table*
Acticlate *Tab:* 75, 150**mg
Adoxa *Tab:* 50, 75, 100, 150 mg ent-coat
Doryx *Tab:* 50, 75, 100, 150, 200 mg del-rel
Doxteric *Tab:* 50 mg del-rel
Monodox *Cap:* 50, 75, 100 mg
Oracea *Cap:* 40 mg del-rel
Vibramycin *Tab:* 100 mg; *Cap:* 50, 100 mg; *Syr:* 50 mg/5 ml (raspberry-apple) (sulfites); *Oral susp:* 25 mg/5 ml (raspberry)
Vibra-Tab *Tab:* 100 mg film-coat

Comment: ***doxycycline*** is contraindicated <8 years-of-age, in pregnancy, and lactation (discolors developing tooth enamel). A side effect may be photosensitivity (photophobia). Do not give with antacids, calcium supplements, milk or other dairy, or within 2 hours of taking another drug.

▶ ***erythromycin base*** **(B)(G)**
Ery-Tab *Tab:* 250, 333, 500 mg ent-coat
PCE *Tab:* 333, 500 mg

▶ ***erythromycin ethylsuccinate*** **(B)(G)**
EryPed *Oral susp:* 200 mg/5 ml (100, 200 ml) (fruit); 400 mg/5 ml (60, 100, 200 ml) (banana); *Oral drops:* 200, 400 mg/5 ml (50 ml) (fruit); *Chew tab:* 200 mg wafer (fruit)
E.E.S. *Oral susp:* 200, 400 mg/5 ml (100 ml) (fruit)
E.E.S. Granules *Oral susp:* 200 mg/5 ml (100, 200 ml) (cherry)
E.E.S. 400 Tablets *Tab:* 400 mg

▶ ***trimethoprim+sulfamethoxazole [TMP-SMX]*** **(C)(G)**
Bactrim, Septra <12 years: not recommended; ≥12 years: 2 tabs bid x 10 days
Tab: trim 80 mg+sulfa 400 mg*
Bactrim DS, Septra DS <12 years: not recommended; ≥12 years: 1 tab bid x 10 days
Tab: trim 160 mg+sulfa 800 mg*
Bactrim Pediatric Suspension, Septra Pediatric Suspension <2 months: not recommended; ≥2 months-12 years: 40 mg/kg/day of ***sulfamethoxazole*** in 2 doses bid; >12 years: use tabs
Oral susp: trim 40 mg+sulfa 200 mg per 5 ml (100 ml) (cherry) (alcohol 0.3%)

GROWTH FAILURE

Comment: Administer growth hormones by SC injection into thigh, buttocks, or abdomen. Rotate sites with each dose. Contraindicated in children with fused epiphyses or evidence of neoplasia.

▶ ***mecasermin (recombinant human insulin-like growth factor-1 [rhIGF-1])***

Increlex (B) see mfr pkg insert

Vial: 10 mg/ml (benzyl alcohol)

Comment: **Increlex** is indicated for growth failure in children with severe primary IGF-1 deficiency (primary IGFD) or in those with growth hormone (GH) gene deletion who have developed neutralizing antibodies to GH.

▶ ***somatropin*** (rDNA origin)

Genotropin (B) <12 years: usually 0.16-0.024 mg/kg/week divided into 6-7 doses; ≥12 years: initially not more than 0.04 mg/kg/week divided into 6-7 doses; may increase at 4-8 week intervals; max 0.08 mg/kg/week divided into 6-7 doses

Intra-Mix Device: 1.5 mg (1.3 mg/ml after reconstitution), 5.8 mg (5 mg/ml after reconstitution) (two-chamber cartridge w. diluent); *Pen* or *Intra-Mix Device:* 5.8 mg (5 mg/ml after reconstitution), 13.8 mg (512 mg/ml after reconstitution) (two-chamber cartridge w. diluent)

Genotropin Miniquick (B) <12 years: usually 0.16-0.024 mg/kg/week divided into 6-7 doses; ≥12 years: initially not more than 0.04 mg/kg/week divided into 6-7 doses; may increase at 4-8-week intervals; max 0.08 mg/kg/week divided into 6-7 doses

MiniQuick: 0.2, 0.4, 0.6, 0.8, 1, 1.2, 1.4, 1.6, 1.8, 2 mg/0.25 ml (pwdr for SC injection after reconstitution) (two-chamber cartridge w. diluent)

Humatrope (C) <12 years: initially 0.18 mg/kg/week IM or SC divided into equal doses give neither on 3 alternate days or 6 x/week; max 0.3 mg/kg/week

Vial: 5 mg w. 5 ml diluent

Norditropin (C) <12 years: 0.024-0.034 mg/kg 6-7 x/week SC

Vial: 4 mg (12 IU), 8 mg (24 IU); *Cartridge for inj:* 5, 10, 15 mg/1.5 ml; *Flex-Pro prefilled pen:* 5, 10, 15 mg/1.5 ml; *NordiFlex prefilled pen:* 5, 10, 15 mg/1.5 ml; 30 mg/3 ml

Nutropin (C) <12 years: 0.7 mg/kg/week SC in divided daily doses

Vial: 5, 10 mg/vial w. diluent

Nutropin AQ (C) <12 years: *Prepubertal:* up to 0.043 mg/kg SC daily; *Pubertal:* up to 0.1 mg/kg SC daily; *Turner Syndrome:* up to 0.0375 mg/kg/week divided into equal doses 3-7 x/week; ≥12 years: initially not more than 0.006 mg/kg SC daily; may increase to max 0.025 mg/kg SC daily

Vial: 5 mg/ml (2 ml)

Nutropin Depot (C) 1.5 mg/kg SC monthly on same day each month; max 22.5 mg/inj; divide injection if >22.5 mg

Vial: 13.5, 18, 22.5 mg/vial (pwdr for injection after reconstitution; single use w. diluent and needle)

Omnitrope (B) 0.16-0.24 mg/kg/week SC divided 3-7 x/week

Vial: 5.8 mg

Omnitrope Pen 5 (B) 0.16-0.24 mg/kg/week SC divided 3-7 x/week

Cartridge for inj: 5 mg/1.5 ml

Omnitrope Pen 10 (B) 0.16-0.24 mg/kg/week SC divided 3-7 x/week

Cartridge for inj: 10 mg/1.5 ml

Saizen (B)(G) 0.18 mg/kg/week IM or SC divided 3-7 x/week

Vial: 5 mg (pwdr for SC injection w. diluent)

Serostim (B) 0.1 mg/kg SC once daily at HS; max 6 mg

Vial: 5, 4, 6, 8.8 mg (pwdr for SC injection w. diluent) (benzyl alcohol)

HEADACHE: MIGRAINE & CLUSTER

ERGOTAMINE AGENTS

Comment: Do not use an ergotamine-type drug within 24 hours of any triptan or other 5-HT agonist.

▶ ***dihydroergotamine mesylate*** (X) <12 years: not recommended; ≥12 years: **DHE 45** 1 mg SC, IM, or IV; may repeat at 1 hour intervals; max 3 mg/day SC or IM/day; max 2 mg IV/day; max 6 mg/week

Amp: 1 mg/ml (1 ml)

Migranal 1 spray in each nostril; may repeat 15 minutes later; max 6 sprays/day and 8 sprays/week

Nasal spray: 4 mg/ml; 0.5 mg/spray (caffeine)

▶ ***ergotamine*** (X)(G) <12 years: not recommended; ≥12 years: 1 tab SL at onset of attack; then q 30 minutes as needed; max 3 tabs/day and 5 tabs/week

Tab: 2 mg

▶ ***ergotamine+caffeine*** (X)(G) <12 years: not recommended; ≥12 years:

Cafergot 2 tabs at onset of attack; then 1 tab every 1/2 hour if needed; max 6 tabs/attack and 10 tabs/week

Tab: ergot 1 mg+caf 100 mg

Cafergot Suppository 1 suppository rectally at onset of headache; may repeat x 1 after 1 hour; max 2/attack, 5/week

Rectal supp: ergot 2 mg+caf 100 mg

5-HT RECEPTOR AGONISTS

Comment: Contraindications to 5-HT receptor agonists include cardiovascular disease, ischemic heart disease, cerebral vascular syndromes, peripheral vascular disease, uncontrolled hypertension, hemiplegic or basilar migraine. Do not use any triptan within 24 hours of ergot-type drugs or other 5-HT1A agonists, or within 2 weeks of taking an MAOI.

▶ ***almotriptan*** (C)(G) <12 years: not recommended; ≥12 years: 6.25 or 12.5 mg; may repeat once after 2 hours; max 2 doses/day

Axert *Tab:* 6.25 mg (6/card), 12.5 mg (12/card)

Comment: ***almotriptan*** is indicated for patients 12-17 years-of-age with PMHx migraine headache lasting ≥4 hours untreated.

▶ ***eletriptan*** (C)(G) <18 years: not recommended; ≥18 years: 20 or 40 mg; may repeat once after 2 hours; max 80 mg/day

Relpax *Tab:* 20, 40 mg

▶ ***frovatriptan*** (C)(G) <18 years: not recommended; ≥18 years: 2.5 mg with fluids; may repeat once after 2 hours; max 7.5 mg/day

Frova *Tab:* 2.5 mg

▶ ***naratriptan*** (C) <18 years: not recommended; ≥18 years: 1 or 2.5 mg with fluids; may repeat once after 4 hours; max 5 mg/day

Amerge *Tab:* 1, 2.5 mg

▶ ***rizatriptan*** (C) <18 years: not recommended; ≥18 years: initially 5 or 10 mg; may repeat in 2 hours if needed; max 30 mg/day

Maxalt *Tab:* 5, 10 mg

Maxalt-MLT *ODT:* 5, 10 mg (peppermint) (phenylalanine)

▶ ***sumatriptan*** (C)(G) <18 years: not recommended; ≥18 years:

Alsuma 6 mg SC to the upper arm or lateral thigh only; may repeat after 1 hour if needed; max 2 doses/day

Prefilled syringe: 6 mg/0.5 ml (2/pck with autoinjector)

Imitrex Injectable 4-6 mg SC; may repeat after 1 hour if needed; max 2 doses/day

Prefilled syringe: 4, 6 mg/0.5 ml (2/pck with or without autoinjector)

Imitrex Nasal Spray (G) 5-20 mg intranasally; may repeat once after 2 hours if needed; max 40 mg/day

Nasal spray: 5, 20 mg/spray (single-dose)

Imitrex Tab 25-200 mg x 1 dose; may be repeated at intervals of at least 2 hours if needed; max 200 mg/day

Tab: 25, 50, 100 mg rapid-rel

Imitrex STATdose Pen 6 mg/0.5 mg SC; may repeat once after 2 hours if needed; max 2 doses/day

Prefilled needle-free autoinjector delivery system: 6 mg/0.5 ml (6/pck)

Onzetra Xsail each disposable white nosepiece contains half a dose of medication (11 mg of sumatriptan); a full dose is 22 mg; do not use more than 2 nosepieces per dose; attach the mouthpiece and one nasal piece; then press the white button on the delivery device to pierce the capsule in the nasal piece, then insert the nasal piece into one nostril and blow into the mouth piece to deliver the nasal powder in the contents of one capsule (11 mg); repeat in the opposite nostril for a total single 22 mg dose

Cap: 11 mg nasal pwdr; *Kit:* nosepieces (2), capsules (2), reusable breath powered delivery device (1)

Sumavel DosePro 6 mg SC to the upper arm or lateral thigh only; may repeat after 1 hour if needed; max 2 doses/day

Prefilled needle-free delivery system: 6 mg/0.5 ml (6/pck)

Zembrace SymTouch administer 3 mg SC at onset of headache; may repeat hourly; max 12 mg/24 hours

Autoinjector: 3 mg/0.5 ml (prefilled single-dose disposable autoinjector)

➢ ***zolmitriptan*** **(C)(G)** <18 years: not recommended; ≥18 years: initially 2.5 mg; may repeat after 2 hours if needed; max 10 mg/day

Zomig *Tab:* 2.5*, 5 mg

Zomig Nasal Spray *Nasal spray:* 5 mg/spray (6 single-dose/carton)

Zomig-ZMT *ODT:* 2.5 mg (6 tabs), 5*mg (3 tabs) (orange) (phenylalanine)

5-HT RECEPTOR AGONIST+NSAID COMBINATION

➢ ***sumatriptan+naproxen*** **(C; D in 3rd)** <18 years: not recommended; ≥18 years:

Treximet initially 1 tab; may repeat after 2 hours; max 2 doses/day

Tab: suma 85 mg+naprox 500 mg (9/blister card)

Comment: Do not use ***sumatriptan*** within 24 hours of ergot-type drugs or other 5-HT agonists, or within 2 weeks of taking an MAOI.

OTHER ANALGESICS

➢ ***acetaminophen+aspirin+caffeine*** **(D)(G)**

Comment: ***aspirin***-containing medications are contraindicated with history of allergic-type reaction to ***aspirin***, children and adolescents with *Varicella* or other viral illness, and 3rd trimester of pregnancy.

Excedrin Migraine (OTC) <12 years: not recommended; ≥12 years: 2 tabs q 6 hours prn; max 8 tabs/day x 2 days

Tab: acet 250 mg+asp 250 mg+caf 65 mg

➢ ***diclofenac potassium powder for oral solution*** **(C; D ≥30 weeks)(G)** <18 years: not established; ≥18 years: empty the contents of one pkt into a cup containing 1-2 oz or 2-4 tbsp (30-60 ml) of water, mix well, and drink immediately; water only, no other liquids; take on an empty stomach; use the lowest effective dose for the shortest duration of time; safety and effectiveness of a 2nd dose has not been established

Cambia *Pwdr for oral soln:* 50 mg/pkt (3 pkts/set, conjoined with a perforated border

Comment: **Cambia** is not indicated for migraine prophylaxis. May not be bioequivalent with other ***diclofenac*** forms (e.g., ***diclofenac sodium*** ent-coat tabs, ***diclofenac sodium*** ext-rel tabs, ***diclofenac potassium*** immed-rel tabs) even of the mg strength is the same, therefore, it's not possible to convert dosing from any other diclofenac formulation to **Cambia**. **Cambia** is contraindicated in the setting of coronary artery bypass graft. Use of **Cambia** should not be considered with hepatic impairment, gastric/duodenal ulcer, starting at 30 weeks gestation (risk of premature closure of the ductus arteriosus in the fetus), concomitant NSAIDs, SSRIs, anticoagulants/antiplatelets, any risk factor for potential bleeding.

▶ ***isometheptene mucate+dichloralphenazone+acetaminophen*** (C)(IV)
  Midrin <12 years: not recommended; ≥12 years: 2 caps initially; then 1 cap q 1 hour until relieved; max 5 caps/12 hours
    Cap: iso 65 mg+dichlor 100 mg+acet 325 mg

PROPHYLAXIS

▶ ***topiramate*** (D)(G) <12 years: not recommended; ≥12 years: initially 25 mg daily in the PM and titrate up daily as tolerated; then 25 mg bid; then, 25 mg in the AM and 50 mg in the PM; then, 50 mg bid
  Topamax *Tab:* 25, 50, 100, 200 mg
  Topamax Sprinkle Caps *Cap:* 15, 25 mg
  Trokendi XR *Cap:* 25, 50, 100, 200 mg ext-rel
  Qudexy XR *Cap:* 25, 50, 100, 150, 200 mg ext-rel

BETA-BLOCKERS

▶ ***atenolol*** (D)(G) <12 years: not recommended; ≥12 years: initially 25 mg bid; max 150 mg/day in divided doses
  Tenormin *Tab:* 25, 50, 100 mg

▶ ***metoprolol succinate*** (C)(G) <12 years: not recommended; ≥12 years: initially 12.5-25 mg in a single dose daily; increase weekly if needed; reduce if symptomatic bradycardia occurs; max 400 mg/day
  Toprol-XL *Tab:* 25*, 50*, 100*, 200*mg ext-rel

▶ ***metoprolol tartrate*** (C)(G) <12 years: not recommended; ≥12 years: initially 25-50 mg bid; increase weekly if needed; max 400 mg/day
  Lopressor *Tab:* 25, 37.5, 50, 75, 100 mg

▶ ***nadolol*** (C)(G) <12 years: not recommended; ≥12 years: initially 20 mg daily; max 240 mg/day in divided doses
  Corgard *Tab:* 20*, 40*, 80*, 120*, 160*mg

▶ ***propranolol*** (C)(G)
  Inderal <12 years: not recommended; ≥12 years: initially 10 mg bid; usual range 160-320 mg/day in divided doses
    Tab: 10*, 20*, 40*, 60*, 80*mg
  Inderal LA <12 years: not recommended; ≥12 years: initially 80 mg daily in a single dose; increase q 3-7 days; usual range 120-160 mg/day; max 320 mg/day in a single dose
    Cap: 60, 80, 120, 160 mg sust-rel
  InnoPran XL <12 years: not recommended; ≥12 years: initially 80 mg q HS; max 120 mg/day
    Cap: 80, 120 mg ext-rel

▶ ***timolol*** (C)(G) <12 years: not recommended; ≥12 years: initially 10 mg bid; increase weekly if needed; usual maintenance 20-40 mg/day; max 60 mg/day in 2 divided doses
  Blocadren *Tab:* 5, 10*, 20*mg

CALCIUM ANTAGONISTS

▶ ***diltiazem*** (C)(G) <12 years: not recommended; ≥12 years:
  Cardizem initially 30 mg qid; may increase gradually every 1-2 days; max 360 mg/day in divided doses
    Tab: 30, 60, 90, 120 mg

Cardizem CD initially 120-180 mg once daily; adjust at 1- to 2-week intervals; max 480 mg/day
Cap: 120, 180, 240, 300, 360 mg ext-rel
Cardizem LA initially 180-240 mg once daily; titrate at 2-week intervals; max 540 mg/day
Tab: 120, 180, 240, 300, 360, 420 mg ext-rel
Cardizem SR initially 60-120 mg bid; adjust at 2-week intervals; max 360 mg/day
Cap: 60, 90, 120 mg sust-rel

➢ ***nifedipine*** **(C)(G)** <12 years: not recommended; ≥12 years:
Adalat initially 10 mg tid; usual range 10-20 mg tid; max 180 mg/day
Cap: 10, 20 mg
Procardia initially 10 mg tid; titrate over 7-14 days: max 30 mg/dose and 180 mg/day in divided doses
Cap: 10, 20 mg
Procardia XL initially 30-60 mg daily; titrate over 7-14 days; max 90 mg/day in divided doses

➢ ***verapamil*** **(C)(G)** <12 years: not recommended; ≥12 years:
Calan 80-120 mg tid; increase daily or weekly if needed
Tab: 40, 80*, 120*mg
Covera HS initially 180 mg q HS; titrate in steps to 240 mg; then to 360 mg; then to 480 mg if needed
Tab: 180, 240 mg ext-rel
Isoptin initially 80-120 mg tid
Tab: 40, 80, 120 mg
Isoptin SR initially 120-180 mg in the AM; may increase to 240 mg in the AM; then, 180 mg q 12 hours or 240 mg in the AM and 120 mg in the PM; then, 240 mg q 12 hours
Tab: 120, 180*, 240*mg sust-rel

TRICYCLIC ANTIDEPRESSANTS (TCAs)

Comment: Co-administration of SSRIs and TCAs requires extreme caution.

➢ ***amitriptyline*** **(C)(G)** <12 years: not recommended; ≥12 years: 10-20 mg q HS *Tab:* 10, 25, 50, 75, 100, 150 mg

➢ ***amoxapine*** **(C)** <12 years: not recommended; ≥12 years: initially 50 mg bid-tid; after 1 week may increase to 100 mg bid-tid; usual effective dose 200-300 mg/day; if total dose exceeds 300 mg/day, give in divided doses (max 400 mg/day); may give as a single bedtime dose (max 300 mg q HS)
Tab: 25, 50, 100, 150 mg

➢ ***clomipramine*** **(C)(G)** <10 years: not recommended; 10-<16 years: initially 25 mg daily in divided doses; gradually increase; max 3 mg/kg or 100 mg, whichever is smaller; >16 years: initially 25 mg daily in divided doses; gradually increase to 100 mg during first 2 weeks; max 250 mg/day; total maintenance dose may be given at HS
Anafranil *Cap:* 25, 50, 75 mg

➢ ***desipramine*** **(C)(G)** <12 years: not recommended; ≥12 years: 100-200 mg/day in single or divided doses; max 300 mg/day
Norpramin *Tab:* 10, 25, 50, 75, 100, 150 mg

➢ ***doxepin*** **(C)(G)** <12 years: not recommended; ≥12 years: 75 mg/day; max 150 mg/day
Cap: 10, 25, 50, 75, 100, 150 mg; Oral conc: 10 mg/ml (4 oz w. dropper)

➢ ***imipramine*** **(C)(G)** <12 years: not recommended; ≥12 years:
Tofranil initially 75 mg daily (max 200 mg); adolescents initially 30-40 mg daily (max 100 mg/day); if maintenance dose exceeds 75 mg daily, may switch to **Tofranil PM** for divided or bedtime dose
Tab: 10, 25, 50 mg

Tofranil PM initially 75 mg daily 1 hour before HS; max 200 mg
Cap: 75, 100, 125, 150 mg

▶ ***nortriptyline*** **(D)(G)** <12 years: not recommended; ≥12 years: initially 25 mg tid-qid; max 150 mg/day
Pamelor *Cap:* 10, 25, 50, 75 mg; *Oral soln:* 10 mg/5 ml (16 oz)

▶ ***protriptyline*** **(C)** <12 years: not recommended; ≥12 years: initially 5 mg tid; usual dose 15-40 mg/day in 3-4 divided doses; max 60 mg/day
Vivactil *Tab:* 5, 10 mg

▶ ***trimipramine*** **(C)** <12 years: not recommended; ≥12 years: initially 75 mg/day in divided doses; max 200 mg/day
Surmontil *Cap:* 25, 50, 100 mg

SSRI ANTIDEPRESSANTS

Comment: Co-administration of SSRIs with TCAs requires extreme caution. Concomitant use of MAOIs and SSRIs is absolutely contraindicated. Avoid other serotonergic drugs. A potentially fatal adverse event is *serotonin syndrome*, caused by serotonin excess. Milder symptoms require HCP intervention to avert severe symptoms that can be rapidly fatal without urgent/emergent medical care. Symptoms include restlessness, agitation, confusion, hallucinations, tachycardia, hypertension, dilated pupils, muscle twitching, muscle rigidity, loss of muscle coordination, diaphoresis, diarrhea, headache, shivering, piloerection, hyperpyrexia, cardiac arrhythmias, seizures, loss of consciousness, coma, death. Abrupt withdrawal or interruption of treatment with an antidepressant medication is sometimes associated with an *antidepressant discontinuation syndrome*, which may be mediated by gradually tapering the drug over a period of two weeks or longer, depending on the dose strength and length of treatment. Common symptoms of the *serotonin discontinuation syndrome* include flu-like symptoms (nausea, vomiting, diarrhea, headaches, sweating), sleep disturbances (insomnia, nightmares, constant sleepiness), mood disturbances (dysphoria, anxiety, agitation), cognitive disturbances (mental confusion, hyperarousal), sensory and movement disturbances (imbalance, tremors, vertigo, dizziness, electric-shock-like sensations in the brain, often described by sufferers as "brain zaps").

▶ ***fluoxetine*** **(C)(G)**
Prozac <8 years: not recommended; 8-17 years: initially 10-20 mg/day; start lower weight children at 10 mg/day; if starting at 10 mg daily, may increase after 1 week to 20 mg once daily; >17 years: initially 20 mg daily; may increase after 1 week; doses >20 mg/day may be divided into AM and noon doses; max 80 mg/day
Cap: 10, 20, 40 mg; *Tab:* 30*, 60*mg; *Oral soln:* 20 mg/5 ml (4 oz) (mint)
Prozac Weekly <12 years: not recommended; ≥12 years: following daily ***fluoxetine*** therapy at 20 mg/day for 13 weeks, may initiate **Prozac Weekly** 7 days after the last 20 mg ***fluoxetine*** dose; 1 90 mg cap once weekly on the same day
Cap: 90 mg ent-coat del-rel pellets

ANTICONVULSANTS

▶ ***divalproex sodium*** **(D)** <10 years: not recommended; ≥10 years: *Delayed-release*: initially 250 mg bid; titrate weekly to usual max 500 mg bid; *Extended-release*: initially 500 mg once daily; may increase after one week to 1 gm once daily
Depakene *Cap:* 250 mg del-rel; syr: 250 mg/5 ml (16 oz)
Depakote *Tab:* 125, 250, 500 mg del-rel
Depakote ER *Tab:* 250, 500 mg ext-rel
Depakote Sprinkle *Cap:* 125 mg del-rel

CALCITONIN GENE-RELATED PEPTIDE RECEPTOR ANTAGONIST

Comment: **Aimovig** ***(erenumab-aooe)*** is a preventive treatment for patients >18 years-of-age with migraine, self-administered as a once-monthly SC injection, from a new class of drugs that block the activity of calcitonin gene-related peptide, which is involved in migraine attacks.

▶ ***erenumab-aooe*** <18 years: not recommended; ≥18 years: administer by SC injection only in the abdomen, thigh, or upper arm; recommended dose is 70 mg SC once monthly; some patients may benefit from a dosage of 140 mg SC once monthly (i.e., two consecutive injections of 70 mg each); the needle shield within the white cap of the prefilled autoinjector and the gray needle cap of the prefilled syringe contain dry natural rubber (a derivative of latex), which may cause allergic reactions in individuals sensitive to latex

Aimovig *Autoinjector:* 70 mg/ml (1 ml), prefilled single-dose, SureClick

Comment: The most common adverse side effects are injection site reaction and constipation. There are no adequate data on the developmental risk associated with the use of **Aimovig** in pregnant females. There are no data on the presence of ***erenumab-aooe*** in human milk or effects on the breastfed infant. Safety and effectiveness in pediatric patients have not been established.

OTHER AGENT

▶ ***methysergide*** (C) <18 years: not recommended; ≥18 years: 4-8 mg daily in divided doses with food; max 8 mg/day; max 6 month treatment course; wean off over last 2-3 weeks of treatment course; separate treatment courses by 3-4 week drug-free intervals

Sansert *Tab:* 2 mg

Comment: ***methysergide maleate*** is indicated for the prevention or reduction of intensity and frequency of vascular headaches. It is contraindicated in pregnancy due to its oxytocic actions. ***methysergide maleate*** is a semi-synthetic compound structurally related to ergotamine, and thus it may appear in breast milk. Ergot alkaloids have been reported to cause nausea, vomiting, diarrhea and weakness in the nursing infant and suppression of prolactin secretion and lactation in the mother.

MAGNESIUM SUPPLEMENTS

▶ ***magnesium*** (B) monitor serum magnesium level

Slow-Mag <12 years: not recommended; ≥12 years: 2 tabs daily

Tab: 64 mg (as chloride)+110 mg (as carbonate)

▶ ***magnesium oxide*** (B) monitor serum magnesium level

Mag-Ox 400 <12 years: not recommended; ≥12 years: 1-2 tabs daily

Tab: 400 mg

HEADACHE: TENSION, MUSCLE CONTRACTION

Acetaminophen for IV Infusion *see* ***Pain*** *page* 322
NSAIDs *see page* 539
Other Oral Analgesics *see* ***Pain*** *page* 324
Topical & Transdermal NSAIDs *see* ***Pain*** *page* 323
Parenteral Corticosteroids *see page* 547
Oral Corticosteroids *see page* 546

ORAL ANALGESIC COMBINATIONS

▶ ***butalbital+acetaminophen*** (C)(G) <12 years: not recommended; ≥12 years:

Phrenilin 1-2 tabs q 4 hours prn; max 6 tabs/day

Tab: but 50 mg+acet 325 mg

Phrenilin Forte 1 tab or cap q 4 hours prn; max 6 caps/day
Cap/Tab: but 50 mg+acet 650 mg

▶ ***butalbital+acetaminophen+caffeine*** (C)(G) <12 years: not recommended; ≥12 years:
Fioricet 1-2 tabs q 4 hours prn; max 6/day
Tab: but 50 mg+acet 325 mg+caf 40 mg
Zebutal 1 cap q 4 hours prn; max 5/day
Cap: but 50 mg+acet 500 mg+caf 40 mg

▶ ***butalbital+acetaminophen+codeine+caffeine*** (C)(III)(G) <18 years: not recommended; ≥18 years:
Fioricet with Codeine 1-2 tabs at onset q 4 hours prn; max 6 tabs/day
Tab: but 50 mg+acet 325 mg+cod 30 mg+caf 40 mg

Comment: ***Codeine*** is known to be excreted in breast milk. <12 years: not recommended; 12-<18: use extreme caution; not recommended for children and adolescents with asthma or other chronic breathing problem. The FDA and the European Medicines Agency (EMA) are investigating the safety of using ***codeine*** containing medications to treat pain, cough and colds, in children 12-<18 years because of the potential for serious side effects, including slowed or difficult breathing.

▶ ***butalbital+aspirin+caffeine*** (C)(III)(G) <18 years: not recommended; ≥18 years:
Fiorinal 1-2 tabs or caps q 4 hours prn; max 6 caps/tabs/day
Tab/Cap: but 50 mg+*asp* 325 mg+caf 40 mg

▶ ***butalbital+aspirin+codeine+caffeine*** (C)(III)(G) <18 years: not recommended; ≥18 years:
Fiorinal with Codeine 1-2 caps q 4 hours prn; max 6 caps/day
Cap: but 50 mg+asp 325 mg+cod 30 mg+caf 40 mg

Comment: ***Codeine*** is known to be excreted in breast milk. <12 years: not recommended; 12-<18: use extreme caution; not recommended for children and adolescents with asthma or other chronic breathing problem. The FDA and the European Medicines Agency (EMA) are investigating the safety of using ***codeine*** containing medications to treat pain, cough and colds, in children 12-<18 years because of the potential for serious side effects, including slowed or difficult breathing. ***aspirin***-containing medications are contraindicated with history of allergic-type reaction to ***aspirin***, children and adolescents with *Varicella* or other viral illness, and 3rd trimester of pregnancy.

▶ ***butorphanol tartrate***(C)(IV)(G) <18 years: not recommended; ≥18 years: initially 1 spray (1 mg) in one nostril and may repeat after 60-90 minutes (*Elderly* 90-120 minutes) in opposite nostril if needed or 1 spray in each nostril and may repeat q 3-4 hours prn
Butorphanol Nasal Spray *Nasal spray:* 1 mg/actuation (10 mg/ml, 2.5 ml)
Stadol Nasal Spray *Nasal spray:* 1 mg/actuation (10 mg/ml, 2.5 ml)

▶ ***tramadol*** (C)(IV)(G) <18 years: not recommended; ≥18 years:

Comment: ***tramadol*** is known to be excreted in breast milk. The FDA and the European Medicines Agency (EMA) are investigating the safety of using ***tramadol***-containing medications to treat pain in children 12-18 years because of the potential for serious side effects, including slowed or difficult breathing.

Rybix ODT <18 years: not recommended; ≥18 years: initially 100 mg once daily; may increase by 100 mg every 5 days; max 300 mg/day; *CrCl <30 mL/min or severe hepatic impairment:* not recommended; *Cirrhosis:* max 50 mg q 12 hours
ODT: 50 mg (mint) (phenylalanine)

Ryzolt <18 years: not recommended; ≥18 years: initially 100 mg once daily; may increase by 100 mg every 5 days; max 300 mg/day; *CrCl <30 mL/min or severe hepatic impairment:* not recommended
Tab: 100, 200, 300 mg ext-rel

Ultram <18 years: not recommended; ≥18 years: 50-100 mg q 4-6 hours prn; max 400 mg/day; *CrCl <30 mL/min:* max 100 mg q 12 hours; *Cirrhosis:* max 50 mg q 12 hours

Tab: 50*mg

Ultram ER <18 years: not recommended; ≥18 years: initially 100 mg once daily; may increase by 100 mg every 5 days; max 300 mg/day; *CrCl <30 mL/min. or severe hepatic impairment:* not recommended

Tab: 100, 200, 300 mg ext-rel

▶ ***tramadol+acetaminophen*** (C)(IV)(G) <18 years: not recommended; ≥18 years: 2 tabs q 4-6 hours; max 8 tabs/day; 5 days; *CrCl <30 mL/min:* max 2 tabs q 12 hours; max 4 tabs/day x 5 days

Ultracet *Tab:* tram 37.5+acet 325 mg

Comment: ***tramadol*** is known to be excreted in breast milk. The FDA and the European Medicines Agency (EMA) are investigating the safety of using ***tramadol***-containing medications to treat pain in children 12-18 years because of the potential for serious side effects, including slowed or difficult breathing.

TRICYCLIC ANTIDEPRESSANTS (TCAs)

Comment: Co-administration of SSRIs and TCAs requires extreme caution.

▶ ***amitriptyline*** (C)(G) <12 years: not recommended; ≥12 years: 10-20 mg q HS *Tab:* 10, 25, 50, 75, 100, 150 mg

▶ ***amoxapine*** (C) <12 years: not recommended; ≥12 years: initially 50 mg bid-tid; after 1 week may increase to 100 mg bid-tid; usual effective dose 200-300 mg/day; if total dose exceeds 300 mg/day, give in divided doses (max 400 mg/day); may give as a single bedtime dose (max 300 mg q HS)

Tab: 25, 50, 100, 150 mg

▶ ***clomipramine*** (C)(G) <10 years: not recommended; 10-<16 years: initially 25 mg daily in divided doses; gradually increase; max 3 mg/kg or 100 mg, whichever is smaller; >16 years: initially 25 mg daily in divided doses; gradually increase to 100 mg during first 2 weeks; max 250 mg/day; total maintenance dose may be given at HS

Anafranil *Cap:* 25, 50, 75 mg

▶ ***desipramine*** (C)(G) <12 years: not recommended; ≥12 years: 100-200 mg/day in single or divided doses; max 300 mg/day

Norpramin *Tab:* 10, 25, 50, 75, 100, 150 mg

▶ ***doxepin*** (C)(G) <12 years: not recommended; ≥12 years: 75 mg/day; max 150 mg/day

Cap: 10, 25, 50, 75, 100, 150 mg; Oral conc: 10 mg/ml (4 oz w. dropper)

▶ ***imipramine*** (C)(G) <12 years: not recommended; ≥12 years:

Tofranil initially 75 mg daily (max 200 mg); adolescents initially 30-40 mg daily (max 100 mg/day); if maintenance dose exceeds 75 mg daily, may switch to **Tofranil PM** for divided or bedtime dose

Tab: 10, 25, 50 mg

Tofranil PM initially 75 mg daily 1 hour before HS; max 200 mg

Cap: 75, 100, 125, 150 mg

▶ ***nortriptyline*** (D)(G) <12 years: not recommended; ≥12 years: initially 25 mg tid-qid; max 150 mg/day

Pamelor *Cap:* 10, 25, 50, 75 mg; *Oral soln:* 10 mg/5 ml (16 oz)

▶ ***protriptyline*** (C) <12 years: not recommended; ≥12 years: initially 5 mg tid; usual dose 15-40 mg/day in 3-4 divided doses; max 60 mg/day

Vivactil *Tab:* 5, 10 mg

▶ ***trimipramine*** (C) <12 years: not recommended; ≥12 years: initially 75 mg/day in divided doses; max 200 mg/day

Surmontil *Cap:* 25, 50, 100 mg

MAGNESIUM SUPPLEMENTS

▶ *magnesium* (B)
  Slow-Mag 2 tabs daily
    Tab: 64 mg (as chloride)+110 mg (as carbonate)

▶ *magnesium oxide* (B)
  Mag-Ox 400 1-2 tabs daily
    Tab: 400 mg

HEART FAILURE (HF)

HEART FAILURE AND DIABETES

Comment: Heart failure (HF) in the presence of type 2 diabetes (**T2DM**) has a 5-year survival rate on par with some of the worst diseases, such as lung cancer, because diabetes makes the pathophysiology of heart failure worse. Diabetes amplifies the neurohormonal response to heart failure, so it drives progressive heart failure and increases the risk for sudden death. As left ventricular function decreases, patients with diabetes have heightened activation of the renin angiotensin system (RAS). They have increased left ventricular hypertrophy, and they have increased sympathetic nervous system activation. A "four Ds" framework that clinicians can use to improve prognosis in these patients: (1) ***Loop diuretics*** to get the patient out of congestive cardiac syndrome as quickly as possible; (2) ***Disease modification*** with beta-blockers (ββs) and ACE inhibitors, to the maximal dose tolerated, the mainstays of treatment for patients with heart failure (ACEI's protect these patients against cardiac myocyte cell death and vasoconstriction and ββs protect against the activation of the sympathetic nervous system [SNS]); (3) Consider ***device therapy*** (including defibrillators and resynchronization therapy); and (4) ***Optimize diabetes management***.

REFERENCE

Reported by Mark Kearney, MD, Director of the Leeds Institute of Cardiovascular & Metabolic Medicine at Leeds (England) University at the World Congress on Insulin Resistance, Diabetes & Cardiovascular Disease [published online January 28, 2018]. https:/www.mdedge.com/clinicalendocrinologynews/article/157198/diabetes/learn-four-ds-approach-heart-failure-diabetes

ACE INHIBITORS (ACEIs)

▶ *captopril* (**C; D in 2nd, 3rd**)(**G**) <12 years: not recommended; ≥12 years: initially 25 mg tid; after 1-2 weeks may increase to 50 mg tid; max 450 mg/day
  Capoten *Tab:* 12.5*, 25*, 50*, 100*mg

▶ *enalapril* (**D**) <12 years: not recommended; ≥12 years: initially 5 mg daily; usual dosage range 10-40 mg/day; max 40 mg/day
  Epaned Oral Solution *Oral soln:* 1 mg/ml (150 ml) (mixed berry)
  Vasotec (**G**) *Tab:* 2.5*, 5*, 10, 20 mg

▶ *fosinopril* (**C; D in 2nd, 3rd**) <6 years, <50 kg: not recommended; 6-12 years, ≥50 kg: 5-10 mg daily; ≥12 years: initially 10 mg daily, usual maintenance 20-40 mg/day in a single or divided doses
  Monopril *Tab:* 10*, 20, 40 mg

▶ *lisinopril* (**D**)
  Prinivil <12 years: not recommended; ≥12 years: initially 10 mg daily; usual range 20-40 mg/day
    Tab: 5*, 10*, 20*, 40 mg

Qbrelis Oral Solution administer as a single dose once daily; <6 years, *GFR <30 mL/min:* not recommended; ≥6 years, *GFR >30 mL/min:* initially 0.07 mg/kg, max 5 mg; adjust according to BP up to a max 0.61 mg/kg (40 mg) once daily
Oral soln: 1 mg/ml (150 ml)
Zestril <12 years: not recommended; ≥12 years: initially 10 mg daily; usual range 20-40 mg/day
Tab: 2.5, 5*, 10, 20, 30, 40 mg

▶ ***quinapril*** **(C; D in 2nd, 3rd)** <12 years: not recommended; ≥12 years: initially 5 mg bid; increase weekly to 10-20 mg bid
Accupril *Tab:* 5*, 10, 20, 40 mg

▶ ***ramipril*** **(C; D in 2nd, 3rd)** <12 years: not recommended; ≥12 years: initially 2.5 mg bid; usual maintenance 5 mg bid
Altace *Tab/Cap:* 1.25, 2.5, 5, 10 mg

▶ ***trandolapril*** **(C; D in 2nd, 3rd)** <12 years: not recommended; ≥12 years: initially 1 mg daily; titrate to dose of 4 mg daily as tolerated
Mavik *Tab:* 1*, 2, 4 mg

BETA-BLOCKERS (CARDIOSELECTIVE)

▶ ***carvedilol*** (C)
Coreg <18 years: not recommended; ≥18 years: initially 3.125 mg bid; may increase at 1-2 week intervals to 12.5 mg bid; usual max 50 mg bid
Tab: 3.125, 6.25, 12.5, 25 mg
Coreg CR <18 years: not recommended; ≥18 years: initially 10 mg once daily x 2 weeks; may double dose at 2 week intervals; max 80 mg once daily; may open caps and sprinkle on food
Cap: 10, 20, 40, 80 mg cont-rel

▶ ***metoprolol succinate*** (C)(G) <12 years: not recommended; ≥12 years: initially 12.5-25 mg in a single dose daily; increase weekly if needed; reduce if symptomatic bradycardia occurs; max 400 mg/day
Toprol-XL *Tab:* 25*, 50*, 100*, 200*mg ext-rel

▶ ***metoprolol tartrate*** (C)(G) <12 years: not recommended; ≥12 years: initially 25-50 mg bid; increase weekly if needed; max 400 mg/day
Lopressor *Tab:* 25, 37.5, 50, 75, 100 mg

ANGIOTENSIN II RECEPTOR BLOCKERS (ARBs)

▶ ***valsartan*** **(C; D in 2nd, 3rd)** <6 years: not recommended; ≥6-16 years: initially 0.65 mg/kg bid; max 40 mg/day; dose range 0.65-1.35 mg/kg bid; max 40-160 mg/day; ≥17 years: initially 40-80 mg bid; *Target maintenance dose:* increase dose as tolerated or after 2-4 weeks to 160 mg bid
Diovan *Tab:* 40*, 80, 160, 320 mg
Prexxartan *Oral soln:* 20mg/5 ml; 80/20 ml; 120, 473 ml; 20 ml unit-dose cup

Comment: ***Post-Myocardial Infarction:*** <6 years: not recommended; ≥6-16 years: initially 0.65 mg/kg bid; max 20 mg/day; dose range 0.65-1.35 mg/kg bid; max 40-160 mg/day; ≥17 years: initially 40-80 mg bid; *Target maintenance dose:* increase dose as tolerated or after 2-4 weeks to 160 mg bid

NEPRILYSIN INHIBITOR+ARB COMBINATION

▶ ***sacubitril+valsartan*** (D) <12 years: not established; ≥12 years: initially 49/51 bid; double dose after 2-4 weeks; maintenance 97/103 bid; *GFR <30 mL/min* or *moderate hepatic impairment:* initially 24/26 bid; double dose every 2-4 weeks to target maintenance 97/103 bid

Entresto
Tab: **Entresto 24/26** sacu 24 mg+val 26 mg
Entresto 49/51 sacu 49 mg+val 51 mg
Entresto 97/103 sacu 97 mg+val 103 mg

ALDOSTERONE RECEPTOR BLOCKER

▶ ***eplerenone*** **(B)** <12 years: not recommended; ≥12 years: initially 25 mg once daily; titrate within 4 weeks to 50 mg once daily; adjust dose based on serum K^+

Inspra *Tab:* 25, 50 mg

Comment: **Inspra** is contraindicated with concomitant potent CYP3A4 inhibitors. Risk of hyperkalemia with concomitant ACEI or ARB. Monitor serum potassium at baseline, 1 week, and 1 month. Caution with serum *Cr >2 mg/dL* (male) or >1.8 mg/dL (female) and/or *CrCl <50 mL/min*, and DM with proteinuria.

THIAZIDE DIURETICS

Comment: Monitor hydration status, blood pressure, urine output, serum K^+.

▶ ***chlorothiazide*** **(C)(G)** <6 months: up to 15 mg/lb/day in 2 divided doses; ≥6 months-12 years: 10 mg/lb/day in 2 divided doses; >12 years: 0.5-1 gm/day in single or divided doses; max 2 gm/day

Diuril *Tab:* 250*, 500*mg; *Oral susp:* 250 mg/5 ml (237 ml)

▶ ***hydrochlorothiazide*** **(B)(G)**

Esidrix <12 years: not recommended; ≥12 years: 25-100 mg once daily
Tab: 25, 50, 100 mg

Microzide <12 years: not recommended; ≥12 years: 12.5 mg daily; usual max 50 mg/day
Cap: 12.5 mg

▶ ***polythiazide*** **(C)** <12 years: not recommended; ≥12 years: 2-4 mg once daily

Renese *Tab:* 1, 2, 4 mg

POTASSIUM-SPARING DIURETICS

Comment: Monitor hydration status, blood pressure, urine output, serum K^+.

▶ ***amiloride*** **(B)** <12 years: not recommended; ≥12 years: initially 5 mg once daily; may increase to 10 mg; max 20 mg

Midamor *Tab:* 5 mg

▶ ***spironolactone*** **(D)** <12 years: not established; ≥12 years: initially 50-100 mg in a single or divided doses; titrate at 2 week intervals

Aldactone (G) *Tab:* 25, 50*, 100*mg
CaroSpir *Oral susp:* 25 mg/5 ml (118, 473 ml) (banana)

LOOP DIURETICS

Comment: Monitor hydration status, blood pressure, urine output, serum K^+

▶ ***bumetanide*** **(C)(G)** <18 years: not recommended; ≥18 years: 0.5-2 mg as a single dose; may repeat at 4-5 hour intervals; max 10 mg/day

Bumex *Tab:* 0.5*, 1*, 2*mg

Comment: ***bumetanide*** is contraindicated with sulfa drug allergy.

▶ ***ethacrynic acid*** **(B)(G)** ≤1 month: not recommended; >1 month-12 years: initially 25 mg/day; then adjust dose in 25 mg increments; >12 years: max 50-200 mg once daily

Edecrin *Tab:* 25, 50 mg

- ▶ ***ethacrynate sodium*** **(B)(G)** <1 month: not recommended; ≥1 month-12 years: **use the smallest effective dose;** initially 25 mg; then careful stepwise increments in dosage of 25 mg to achieve effective maintenance; ≥12 years: administer smallest dose required to produce gradual weight loss (about 1-2 pounds per day); onset of diuresis usually occurs at 50-100 mg in children ≥12 years; after diuresis has been achieved, the minimally effective dose (usually 50-200 mg/day) may be administered on a continuous or intermittent dosage schedule; dose titrations are usually in 25-50 mg increments to avoid derangement electrolyte and water excretion; the patient should be weighed under standard conditions before and during administration of ***ethacrynate sodium;*** the following schedule may be helpful in determining the lowest effective dose: *Day 1:* 50 mg once daily after a meal; *Day 2:* 50 mg bid after meals, if necessary; *Day 3:* 100 mg in the morning and 50-100 mg following the afternoon or evening meal, depending upon response to the morning dose; a few patients may require initial and maintenance doses as high as 200 mg bid; these higher doses, which should be achieved gradually, are most often required in patients with severe, refractory edema

    Sodium Edecrin *Vial:* 50 mg single-dose

    Comment: **Sodium Edecrin** is more potent than more commonly used loop and thiazide diuretics. Treatment of the edema associated with congestive heart failure, cirrhosis of the liver, and renal disease, including the nephrotic syndrome, short-term management of ascites due to malignancy, idiopathic edema, and lymphedema, short-term management of hospitalized pediatric patients, other than infants, with congenital heart disease or the nephrotic syndrome. IV **Sodium Edecrin** is indicated when a rapid onset of diuresis is desired, e.g., in acute pulmonary edema or when gastrointestinal absorption is impaired or oral medication is not practical.

- ▶ ***furosemide*** **(C)(G)** <12 years: not established; ≥12 years: initially 40 mg bid

    Lasix *Tab:* 20, 40*, 80 mg; *Oral soln:* 10 mg/ml (2, 4 oz w. dropper)

  Comment: ***furosemide*** is contraindicated with sulfa drug allergy.

- ▶ ***torsemide*** **(B)** <12 years: not established; ≥12 years: 5 mg once daily; may increase to 10 mg daily

    Demadex *Tab:* 5*, 10*, 20*, 100*mg

OTHER DIURETICS

Comment: Monitor hydration status, blood pressure, urine output, serum K^+.

- ▶ ***indapamide*** (B) <12 years: not established; ≥12 years: initially 1.25 mg once daily; may titrate dosage upward every 4 weeks if needed; max 5 mg/day

    Lozol *Tab:* 1.25, 2.5 mg

  Comment: ***indapamide*** is contraindicated with sulfa drug allergy.

- ▶ ***metolazone*** **(B)** <12 years: not established; ≥12 years: 2.5-5 mg once daily

  Comment: ***metolazone*** is contraindicated with sulfa drug allergy.

DIURETIC COMBINATIONS

Comment: Monitor hydration status, blood pressure, urine output, serum K^+.

- ▶ ***amiloride+hydrochlorothiazide*** **(B)(G)** <12 years: not established; ≥12 years: initially 1 tab once daily; may increase to 2 tabs/day in a single or divided doses

    Moduretic *Tab:* amil 5 mg+hctz 50 mg*

- ▶ ***spironolactone+hydrochlorothiazide*** **(D)(G)**

    Aldactazide <12 years: not established; ≥12 years: **25** usual maintenance 50-100 mg in a single or divided doses

      Tab: spiro 25 mg+hctz 25 mg

Aldactazide 50 <12 years: not established; ≥12 years: usual maintenance 50-100 mg in a single or divided doses

Tab: spiro 50 mg+hctz 50 mg

▶ ***triamterene+hydrochlorothiazide*** (C)(G)

Dyazide <12 years: not established; ≥12 years: 1-2 caps daily

Cap: triam 37.5 mg+hctz 25 mg

Maxzide <12 years: not established; ≥12 years: 1 tab once daily

Tab: triam 75 mg+hctz 50 mg*

Maxzide-25 <12 years: not established; ≥12 years: 1-2 tabs once daily

Tab: triam 37.5 mg+hctz 25 mg*

NITRATE+PERIPHERAL VASODILATOR COMBINATION

▶ ***isosorbide dinitrate+hydralazine*** (C) <12 years: not established; ≥12 years: initially 1 tab tid; may reduce to 1/2 tab tid if not tolerated; titrate as tolerated after 3-5 days; max 2 tabs tid

BiDil *Tab:* isosor 20 mg+hydral 37.5 mg

Comment: **BiDil** is an adjunct to standard therapy in self-identified Black persons to improve survival, to prolong time to hospitalization for heart failure, and to improve patient-reported functional status.

CARDIAC GLYCOSIDES

Comment: Therapeutic serum level of is 0.8-2 mcg/ml.

▶ ***digoxin*** (C)(G) *Total oral digitalizing dose (in 24 hours)*: <2 years: 40-50 mcg/kg; 2-10 years: 30-40 mcg/kg; >10 years: 0.75-1.5 mg; *Daily oral maintenance dose (single dose)*: <2 years: 10-12 mcg/kg; 2-10 years: 8-10 mcg/kg; >10 years: 0.125–0.5 mg; 1-1.5 mg IM, IV, or PO in divided doses over 1-3 days as a loading dose; usual maintenance 0.125-0.5 mg/day

Comment: For more information on the use of ***digoxin*** in heart failure, see Jain, S, & Vaidyanathan, B. (2009). Digoxin in management of heart failure in children: Should it be continued or relegated to the history books? *Annals of Pediatric Cardiology, 2*(2), 149–152.

Lanoxicaps <10 years: use elixir or parenteral form

Cap: 0.05, 0.1, 0.2 mg soln-filled (alcohol)

Lanoxin <10 years: use elixir or parenteral form

Tab: 0.0625, 0.125*, 0.1875, 0.25*mg; *Elix:* 0.05 mg/ml (2 oz w. dropper) (lime) (alcohol 10%)

Lanoxin Injection *Amp:* 0.25 mg/ml (2 ml)

Lanoxin Injection Pediatric *Amp:* 0.1 mg/ml (1 ml)

OTHER

▶ ***ivabradine*** (D) <18 years: not established; ≥18 years: initially 5 mg bid with food; assess after 2 weeks and adjust dose to achieve a resting heart rate 50-60 bpm; thereafter, adjust dose as needed based on resting heart rate and tolerability; max 7.5 mg bid; in patients with a history of conduction defects, or for whom bradycardia could lead to hemodynamic compromise, initiate at 2.5 mg bid before increasing the dose based on heart rate

Corlanor *Tab:* 5, 7.5 mg

Comment: **Corlanor** is indicated to reduce the risk of hospitalization for worsening heart failure in patients with stable, symptomatic, chronic heart failure with left ventricular ejection fraction (LVEF) ≤35%, who are in sinus rhythm with resting heart rate ≤70 bpm and either are on maximally tolerated doses of beta-blockers or have a contraindication to beta-blocker use. **Corlanor** is contraindicated with acute decompensated heart failure, BP <90/50, sick sinus syndrome (SSS), sino-atrial block, and 3rd degree AV block (unless patient has a functioning demand pacemaker). **Corlanor** may cause fetal toxicity when administered to pregnant females based on embryo-fetal toxicity and cardiac teratogenic effects observed in animal studies. Therefore, females should to use effective contraception when taking this drug.

HELICOBACTER PYLORI (H. PYLORI) INFECTION

ERADICATION REGIMENS

Comment: There are many H2 receptor blocker-based and PPI-based treatment regimens suggested in the professional literature for the eradication of the *H. pylori* organism and subsequent ulcer healing. Generally, regimens range from 10-14 days for eradication and 2-6 more weeks of continued gastric acid suppression. A three- or four-antibiotic combination may increase treatment effectiveness and decrease the likelihood of resistant strain emergence. Empirical treatment is not recommended. Diagnosis should be confirmed before treatment is started. Antibiotic choices include ***doxycycline***, ***tetracycline***, ***amoxicillin***, ***amoxicillin+clavulanate***, ***clarithromycin***, ***clindamycin***, and ***metronidazole***. Follow-up visits are recommended at 2 and 6 weeks to evaluate treatment outcomes.

- **Regimen 1: Helidac Therapy (D)** ***bismuth subsalicylate*** <12 years: not recommended; ≥12 years: 525 mg qid + ***tetracycline*** 500 mg qid + ***metronidazole*** 250 mg qid x 14 days; *Pack: bismuth subsalicylate chew tab:* 262.4 mg (112/pck); ***tetracycline*** *cap:* 500 mg (56/pck); *metronidazole Tab:* 250 mg (56/pck)
- **Regimen 2: PrevPac (D)(G)** <12 years: not recommended; ≥12 years: ***amoxicillin*** 500 mg 2 caps bid + ***lansoprazole*** 30 mg bid + ***clarithromycin*** 500 mg bid x 14 days (one card per day); *Kit:* ***lansoprazole*** *cap:* 30 mg (2/card); ***amoxicillin*** *cap:* 500 mg (4/card); ***clarithromycin*** *tab:* 500 mg (2/card) (14 daily cards/carton)
- **Regimen 3: Pylera (D)** <12 years: not recommended; ≥12 years: take 3 caps qid after meals and at bedtime x 10 days; take with 8 oz water plus ***omeprazole*** 20 mg bid, with breakfast and dinner, for 10 days

  Cap: ***bismuth subsalicylate*** 140 mg + ***tetracycline*** 125 mg + ***metronidazole*** 125 mg (120 caps)

  Comment: ***omeprazole*** not included with **Pylera**.
- **Regimen 4: Omeclamox-Pak (C)** <12 years: not recommended; ≥12 years: ***omeprazole*** 20 mg bid + ***amoxicillin*** 1000 bid + ***clarithromycin*** 500 mg bid x 10 days

  Kit: ***omeprazole*** *cap:* 20 mg (2/pck); ***amoxicillin*** *cap:* 500 mg (4/pck); ***clarithromycin*** *tab:* 500 mg (2/pck) (10 pcks/carton)
- **Regimen 5: (C)** <12 years: not recommended; ≥12 years: ***omeprazole*** 40 mg daily + ***clarithromycin*** 500 mg tid x 2 weeks; then continue ***omeprazole*** 10-40 mg daily x 6 more weeks
- **Regimen 6: (B)** <12 years: not recommended; ≥12 years: ***lansoprazole*** 30 mg tid + ***amoxicillin*** 1 gm tid x 10 days; then continue ***lansoprazole*** 15-30 mg daily x 6 more weeks
- **Regimen 7: (C)** <12 years: not recommended; ≥12 years: ***omeprazole*** 40 mg daily + ***amoxicillin*** 1 gm bid + ***clarithromycin*** 500 mg bid x 10 days; then continue ***omeprazole*** 10-40 mg daily x 6 more weeks
- **Regimen 8: (D)** <12 years: not recommended; ≥12 years: ***bismuth subsalicylate*** 525 mg qid + ***metronidazole*** 250 mg qid + ***tetracycline*** 500 mg qid + H2 receptor agonist x 2 weeks; then continue H2 receptor agonist x 6 more weeks
- **Regimen 9: (not for use in 1st; B in 2nd, 3rd)** <12 years: not recommended; ≥12 years: ***bismuth subsalicylate*** 525 mg qid + ***metronidazole*** 250 mg qid + ***amoxicillin***

500 mg qid + H2 receptor agonist x 2 weeks; then continue H2 receptor agonist x 6 more weeks

- **Regimen 10: (C)** <12 years: not recommended; ≥12 years: ***ranitidine bismuth citrate*** 400 mg bid + ***clarithromycin*** 500 mg bid x 2 weeks; then continue ***ranitidine bismuth citrate*** 400 mg bid x 2 more weeks
- **Regimen 11: (D)** <12 years: not recommended; ≥12 years: ***omeprazole*** 20 mg or ***lansoprazole*** 30 mg q AM + ***bismuth subsalicylate*** 524 mg qid + ***metronidazole*** 500 mg tid + ***tetracycline*** 500 mg qid x 2 weeks; then continue ***omeprazole*** 20 mg or ***lansoprazole*** 30 mg q AM for 6 more weeks

HEMOPHILIA A (CONGENITAL FACTOR VIII DEFICIENCY) WITH FACTOR VIII INHIBITORS

- ***emicizumab-kxwh*** initially 3 mg/kg by SC injection once weekly for the first 4 weeks; followed by 1.5 mg/kg once weekly

  Hemlibra *Vial:* 30 mg/ml (single-dose); 60 mg/0.4 ml (single-dose); 105 mg 0.7 ml (single-dose); 150 mg/ml (single-dose)

Comment: **Hemlibra** is a bispecific factor IXa- and factor X-directed antibody indicated for routine prophylaxis to prevent or reduce the frequency of bleeding episodes in adult and pediatric patients with hemophilia A (congenital factor VIII deficiency) with factor VIII inhibitors. Laboratory *Coagulation Test Interference*: **Hemlira** interferes with activated clotting time (ACT), activated partial thrombo-plastin time (aPTT), and coagulation laboratory tests based on aPTT, including one stage aPTT-based single-factor assays, aPTT-based Activated Protein C
Resistance (APC-R), and Bethesda assays (clotting-based) for factor VIII (FVIII) inhibitor titers. Intrinsic pathway clotting-based laboratory tests should not be used. Black Box Warning (BBW): Cases of thrombotic microangiopathy and thrombotic events were reported when on average a cumulative amount of >100 U/kg/24 hours of activated prothrombin complex concentrate (aPCC) was administered for 24 hours or more to patients receiving Hemlibra prophylaxis. Monitor for the development of thrombotic microangiopathy and thrombotic events if aPCC is administered. Discontinue aPCC and suspend dosing of **Hemlibra** if symptoms occur. Most common adverse reactions (incidence are injection site reactions, headache, and arthralgia. There are no available data on **Hemlibra** use in pregnant women to inform a drug-associated risk of major birth defects and miscarriage. Women of childbearing potential should use contraception while receiving **Hemlibra** and **Hemlibra** should be used during pregnancy only if the potential benefit for the mother outweighs the risk to the fetus. There is no information regarding the presence of ***emicizumab-kxwh*** in human milk or effects on the breastfed child. To report suspected adverse reactions, contact Genentech at 1-888-835-2555 or FDA at 1-800-FDA-1088 or visit www.fda.gov/medwatch

HEMORRHOIDS

- ***dibucaine*** (C)(OTC)(G) <12 years: not recommended; ≥12 years: 1 applicatorful or suppository bid and after each stool; max 6/day

  Nupercainal (OTC) *Rectal oint:* 1% (30, 60 gm); *Rectal supp:* 1% (12, 14/pck)
- ***hydrocortisone*** (C)(OTC)(G)

  Anusol-HC 1 <12 years: not recommended; ≥12 years: suppository rectally bid-tid or 2 suppositories bid x 2 weeks

  Rectal supp: 25 mg (12, 24/pck)

  Anusol-HC Cream <12 years: not recommended; ≥12 years: 2.5% apply bid-qid prn

  Rectal crm: 2.5% (30 gm)

Anusol HC-1 <12 years: not recommended; ≥12 years: apply tid-qid prn; max 7 days
Rectal crm: 1% (0.7 oz)
Hydrocortisone Rectal Cream <12 years: not recommended; ≥12 years: apply tid-qid prn; max 7 days
Rectal crm: 1, 2.5% (30 gm)
Nupercainal <12 years: not recommended; ≥12 years: apply tid-qid prn
Rectal crm: 1% (30 gm)
Proctocort <12 years: not recommended; ≥12 years: 1 suppository rectally bid-tid prn or 2 suppositories bid x 2 weeks
Rectal supp: 30 mg (12/pck)
Proctocream HC 2.5% <12 years: not recommended; ≥12 years: apply rectally bid-qid prn
Rectal crm: 2.5% (30 gm)
Proctofoam HC 1% <12 years: not recommended; ≥12 years: apply rectally tid-qid prn
Rectal foam: 1% (14 applications/10 gm)

➢ ***hydrocortisone+pramoxine*** **(C)** <12 years: not recommended; ≥12 years: 1 applicatorful tid-qid and after each stool; max 2 weeks
Procort *Rectal crm:* hydro 1.85%+pramox 1.15% (30 gm)

➢ ***hydrocortisone+lidocaine*** **(B)** <12 years: not recommended; ≥12 years: apply bid-tid prn
AnaMantle HC *Crm/Lotn:* hydrocort 5%+lido 3% (1 oz)
LidaMantle HC *Crm/Lotn:* hydrocort 5%+lido 3% (1 oz)

➢ ***petrolatum+mineral oil+shark liver oil+phenylephrine*** **(C)(OTC)(G)**
Preparation H Ointment <12 years: not recommended; ≥12 years: apply up to qid prn
Rectal oint: 1, 2 oz

➢ ***petrolatum+glycerin+shark liver oil+phenylephrine*** **(C)(OTC)(G)**
Preparation H Cream <12 years: not recommended; ≥12 years: apply up to qid prn
Rectal crm: 0.9, 1.8 oz

➢ ***phenylephrine+cocoa butter+shark liver oil*** **(C)(OTC)(G)**
Preparation H Suppositories <12 years: not recommended; ≥12 years: 1 suppository or 1 application of rectal ointment or cream, up to qid
Rectal supp: phenyle 0.25%+cocoa 85.5%+shark 3% (12, 24, 45/pck); *Rectal oint:* phenyle 0.25%+petro 1.9%+mineral oil 14%+shark liv 3% (1, 2 oz); Rectal crm: phenyle 0.25%+petro 18%+gly 12%+shark liv 3% (0.9, 1.8 oz)

➢ ***witch hazel*** *Topical solution/gel* **(OTC)**
Tucks <12 years: not recommended; ≥12 years: apply up to 6 x/day; leave on x 5-15 minutes
Pad: 12, 40, 100/pck; *Gel:* 19.8 gm

➢ ***lidocaine*** 3% cream **(B)** <12 years: reduce dosage commensurate with age, body weight, and physical condition; ≥12 years: apply bid-tid prn
LidaMantle *Crm:* 3% (1 oz)

Bulk-forming Agents, Stool Softeners, and Stimulant Laxatives *see* ***Constipation*** *page* 94

HEPATITIS A (HAV)

Comment: Administer a 2-dose series. Schedule first immunization at least 2 weeks before expected exposure. Booster dose recommended 6-12 months later. Under 1 year-of-age administer in the vastus lateralis; over 1 year-of-age administer in deltoid.

PROPHYLAXIS (HEPATITIS A)

▶ ***hepatitis a vaccine, inactivated*** (C)

Havrix 1,440 El.U IM <2 years: not recommended; 2-18 years: 0.5 ml IM; repeat in 6-18 months; >18 years: repeat in 6-12 months

Vial: 25 U/ml single-dose (preservative-free); *Prefilled syringe:* 25 U/ml (0.5, 1 ml) single-dose

Vaqta 25 U (1 ml) IM; <2 years: not recommended; 2-18 years: 0.5 ml IM; repeat in 6-18 months; >18 years: repeat in 6 months

Vial: 25 U/ml single-dose (preservative-free); *Prefilled syringe:* 25 U/ml, (0.5, 1 ml) (single-dose)

PROPHYLAXIS (HEPATITIS A AND B COMBINATION)

▶ ***hepatitis a inactivated+hepatitis b surface antigen (recombinant vaccine)*** (C)

Twinrix <18 years: not recommended; ≥18 years: 1 ml IM in deltoid; repeat in 1 month and 6 months

Vial (soln): hepatitis a inactivated 720 IU+*hepatitis b* surface antigen (recombinant) 20 mcg/ml (1, 10 ml); *Prefilled syringe:* hepatitis a inactivated 720 IU+hepatitis b surface antigen (recombinant) 20 mcg/ml

HEPATITIS B (HBV)

PROPHYLAXIS (HEPATITIS B)

Comment: Administer IM; under 1 year-of-age, administer in vastus lateralis. Over 1 year-of-age, administer in the deltoid. Administer a 3-dose series; *First dose:* newborn (or now); *Second dose:* 1-2 months after first dose; *Third dose:* 6 months after first dose.

▶ ***hepatitis b recombinant vaccine*** (C)

Engerix-B Adult infant-19 years: 10 mcg (1/2 ml) IM; repeat in 1 and 6 month; >19 years: 20 mcg (1 ml) IM; repeat in 1 and 6 months

Vial: 20 mcg/ml single-dose (preservative-free, thimerosal); *Prefilled syringe:* 20 mcg/ml

Engerix-B Pediatric/Adolescent infant-19 years: 10 mcg IM; repeat in 1 and 6 months

Vial: 10 mcg/0.5 ml single-dose (preservative-free, thimerosal)

Prefilled syringe: 10 mcg/0.5 ml

Recombivax HB Adult >19 years: 10 mcg (1 ml) IM in deltoid; repeat in 1 and 6 months

Vial: 10 mcg/ml single-dose; *Vial:* 10 mcg/3 ml multidose

Recombivax HB Pediatric/Adolescent birth-19 years: 5 mcg (0.5 ml) IM; repeat in 1 and 6 months; >19 years: use adult formulation or 10 mcg (1 ml) pediatric/adolescent formulation; <19 years: 5 mcg (0.5 ml) IM; repeat in 1 and 6 months

Vial: 5 mcg/0.5 ml single-dose

PROPHYLAXIS (HEPATITIS A AND B COMBINATION)

Comment: Administer IM; under 1 year-of-age, administer in vastus lateralis. Over 1 year-of-age, administer in the deltoid. Administer a 3-dose series; *First dose:* newborn (or now); *Second dose:* 1-2 months after first dose; *Third dose:* 6 months after first dose.

▶ ***hepatitis a inactivated+hepatitis b surface antigen (recombinant) vaccine*** (C)

Twinrix 1 ml IM in deltoid; repeat in 1 and 6 months

Vial (soln): hepatitis a inactivated 720 IU+hepatitis b surface antigen (recombinant) 20 mcg/ml (1, 10 ml); *Prefilled syringe:* hepatitis a inactivated 720 IU+hepatitis b surface antigen (recombinant) 20 mcg/ml

CHRONIC HBV INFECTION TREATMENT

Nucleoside Analogs (Reverse Transcriptase Inhibitors and HBV Polymerase Inhibitors)

Comment: Nucleoside analogs are indicated for chronic hepatitis infection with viral replication and either elevated ALT/AST or histologically active disease.

- ***adefovir dipivoxil*** (C)(G) <12 years: not recommended; ≥12 years: 10 mg daily; *CrCl 20-49 mL/min*: 10 mg q 48 hours; *CrCl 10-19 mL/min*: 10 mg q 72 hours
  Hepsera *Tab:* 10 mg
- ***entecavir*** (C)(G) take on an empty stomach; <16 years: not recommended; ≥16 years:
  Nucleoside naïve: 0.5 mg daily; *Nucleoside naïve, CrCl 30-49 mL/min:* 0.25 mg daily; *Nucleoside naïve, CrCl 10-29 mL/min:* 0.15 mg daily; *Nucleoside naïve, CrCl <10 mL/min:* 0.05 mg daily; ***lamivudine**-refractory:* 1 mg daily; ***lamivudine**-refractory, renal impairment:* see mfr pkg insert
  Baraclude *Tab:* 0.5, 1 mg; *Oral Soln:* 0.05 mg/ml (orange; parabens)
- ***lamivudine*** (C)(G) <2 years: not recommended; 2-17 years: 3 mg/kg (max 100 mg) once daily; >17 years: 100 mg daily; *CrCl <5 mL/min:* 35 mg for 1st dose, then 10 mg once daily; *CrCl 5-14 mL/min:* 35 mg for 1st dose, then 15 mg once daily; *CrCl 15-29 mL/min:* 100 mg for 1st dose, then 25 mg once daily; *CrCl 30-49 mL/min:* 100 mg for 1st dose, then 50 mg once daily
  Epivir-HBV *Tab:* 100 mg
  Epivir-HBV Oral Solution *Oral Soln:* 5 mg/ml (240 ml) (strawberry-banana)
- ***telbivudine*** (C) <2 years: not recommended; 2-17 years: 3 mg/kg (max 100 mg) once daily; >17 years: 600 mg daily; *CrCl <40 mL/min:* 600 mg q 72 hours; *CrCl 30-49 mL/min:* 600 mg q 48 hours
  Tyzeka *Tab:* 600 mg
- ***tenofovir alafenamide (TAF)*** (C) <18 years: not established; take with food; ≥18 years: take 1 tab once daily with concomitant carbamazepine 2 tablets
  Vemlidy *Tab:* 25 mg

  Comment: No dosage adjustment of **Vemlidy** is required in patients with mild hepatic impairment (Child-Pugh Class A). The safety and efficacy of **Vemlidy** in patients with decompensated cirrhosis (Child-Pugh B or C) have not been established; therefore **Vemlidy** is not recommended in patients with decompensated (Child-Pugh Class B or C) hepatic impairment, Healthcare providers are encouraged to register patients by calling the Antiretroviral Pregnancy Registry (APR) at 1-800-258-4263.

Interferon Alpha

- ***interferon alfa-2b*** (C) <1 year: not recommended; >1 year-12 years: 3 million IU/m^2 2-3 x/week x 1 week; then increase to 6 million IU/m^2 3 x/week to 16-24 weeks; max 10 million IU/dose; reduce dose by half or interrupt dose if WBCs, granulocyte count, or platelet count decreases; >12 years: 5 million IU SC or IM daily or 10 million IU SC or IM 3 x/week x 16 weeks; reduce dose by half or interrupt dose if WBCs, granulocyte count, or platelet count decreases
  Intron A *Vial (pwdr):* 5, 10, 18, 25, 50 million IU/vial (pwdr + diluent; single-dose) (benzoyl alcohol); *Vial (soln):* 3, 5, 10 million IU/vial (single-dose); *Multi-dose vials (soln):* 18, 25 million IU/vial soln; *Multi-dose pens (soln):* 3, 5, 10 million IU/0.2 ml (6 doses/pen)

HEPATITIS C (HCV)

CHRONIC HCV INFECTION TREATMENT

Nucleoside Analogs (Reverse Transcriptase Inhibitors)

Comment: Nucleoside analogs are indicated for patients with compensated liver disease previously untreated with ***alpha interferon*** or who have relapsed after ***alpha interferon*** therapy. Primary toxicity is hemolytic anemia. Contraindicated in male partners of pregnant females; use 2 forms of contraception during therapy and for 6 months after discontinuation.

- ***ribavirin*** (X)(G) <5 years: not established; >5-<18 years: 23-33 kg: 400 mg/day; 34-46 kg: 600 mg/day; 47-59 kg: 800 mg/day; 60-75 kg: 1 gm/day; 1.2 gm/day; >75 kg: *Genotype 2, 3:* treat for 24 weeks; *Genotype 1, 4:* treat for 48 weeks; reduce dose or discontinue if hematologic abnormalities occur; >18 years: take with food in 2 divided doses; *Genotype 2, 3:* 800 mg/day x 24 weeks; *Genotype 1, 4, <75 kg:* 1 gm/day x 48 weeks; >75 km 1.2 gm/day x 48 weeks; *HIV co-infection:* 800 mg/day x 48 weeks; *CrCl 30-50 mL/min:* alternate 200 mg and 400 mg every other day; *CrCl <30 mL/min or hemodialysis:* reduce dose or discontinue if hematologic abnormalities occur
  - **Copegus** *Tab:* 200 mg
  - **Rebetol** *Cap:* 200 mg
  - **Rebetol Oral Solution** *Oral soln:* 40 mg/ml (120 ml) (bubble gum)
  - **Ribasphere RibaPak 600 mg** *Tab:* 600 mg (14/pck)
  - **Virazole** *Vial:* 6 gm for inhalation

Interferon Alpha

- ***interferon alfacon-1*** (C)
  - **Infergen** <18 years: not recommended; ≥18 years: 9 mcg SC 3 x/week x 24 weeks, then 15 mcg SC 3 x/week x 6 months; allow at least 48 hours between doses
    - *Vial (soln):* 9, 15 mcg/vial soln (6 single-dose/pck) (preservative-free)
- ***interferon alfa-2b*** (C)
  - **Intron A** <18 years: not recommended; ≥18 years:
    - *Vial (pwdr):* 5, 10, 18, 25, 50 million IU/vial (pwdr w. diluent; single-dose) (benzoyl alcohol); *Vial (soln):* 3, 5, 10 million IU/vial (single-dose); *Multi-dose vials (soln):* 18, 25 million IU/vial; *Multi-dose pens (soln):* 3, 5, 10 million IU/0.2 ml (6 doses/pen)
- ***peginterferon alfa-2a*** (C) administer 180 mcg SC once weekly (on the same day of the week); treat for 48 weeks; consider discontinuing if adequate response after 12-24 weeks
  - **PEGasys** *Vial:* 180 mcg/ml (single-dose); *Monthly pck (vials):* 180 mcg/ml (1 ml, 4/pck)
- ***peginterferon alfa-2b*** (C) <18 years: not recommended; ≥18 years: administer SC once weekly (on the same day of the week); treat for 1 year; consider discontinuing if inadequate response after 24 weeks; 37-45 kg: 40 mcg (100 mg/ml, 0.4 ml); 46-56 kg: 50 mcg (100 mg/ml, 0.5 ml); 57-72 kg: 64 mcg (160 mg/ml, 0.4 ml); 73-88 kg: 80 mcg (160 mg/ml, 0.5 ml); 89-106 kg: 96 mcg (240 mg/ml, 0.4 ml); 107-136 kg: 120 mcg (240 mg/ml, 0.5 ml); 137-160 kg: 150 mcg (300 mg/ml, 0.5 ml)
  - **PEG-Intron** *Vial:* 50, 80, 120, 150 mcg/ml (single-dose)
  - **PEG-Intron Redipen** *Pen:* 50, 80, 120, 150 mcg/ml (disposable pens)

HCV NS5A Inhibitor

➢ ***daclatasvir*** **(X)** <18 years: not recommended; ≥18 years: 60 mg once daily for 12 weeks (with ***sofosbuvir***); if ***sofosbuvir*** is discontinued, ***daclatasvir*** should also be discontinued; with concomitant CY3P inhibitors, reduce dose to 30 mg once daily; with concomitant CY3P inducers, increase dose to 90 mg once daily

Daklinza *Tab:* 30, 60 mg

Comment: **Daklinza** is indicated in combination with ***sofosbuvir*** with or without ***ribavirin***, for the treatment of HCV genotypes 1 and 3, and in patients with comorbid HIV-1 infection, advanced cirrhosis, or post-liver transplant recurrence of HCV.

HCV NS5B Polymerase Inhibitor

➢ ***sofosbuvir*** **(B)** <12 years: not established; ≥12-17 years, ≥35 kg (77 lb): take with or without food; taken only as a component on a combination antiviral treatment regimen; *Genotype 2:* 400 mg once daily plus ***ribavirin*** x 12 weeks without cirrhosis or with compensated cirrhosis; *Genotype 3:* 400 mg once daily plus ***ribavirin*** x 24 weeks without cirrhosis or with compensated cirrhosis; ≥18 years: *Genotype 1:* 400 mg once daily plus ***simeprevir*** x12 weeks or x 24 weeks; *Alternate:* 400 mg once daily with ***daclatasvir*** x12 weeks; *Genotype 2:* 400 mg once daily plus ***daclatasvir*** x12 weeks or x 16-24 weeks (duration depends on cirrhosis status--refer to AASLD/IDSA hepatitis C guidelines; *Genotype 3:* 400 mg once daily plus ***daclatasvir*** x12 weeks; *Genotype 4:* 400 mg once daily plus ***daclatasvir*** x 12 weeks; *Hepatocellular Cancer Awaiting Transplant:* 400 mg once daily plus ***ribavirin***

Sovaldi *Tab:* 400 mg film-coat

Comment: *CrCl ≥30:* no adjustment; *CrCl <30:* not defined; *Hemodialysis:* not defined; *Hepatic Impairment:* no adjustment; *Decompensated Hepatic Disease:* not defined. Refer to AASLD/IDSA hepatitis C guidelines for more information. Because **Sovaldi** is used in combination with other antiviral drugs for treatment of HCV infection, consult the prescribing information for these drugs used in combination with **Sovaldi**. Warnings and precautions related to these drugs also apply to their use in **Sovaldi** combination treatment. Hepatitis B virus (HBV) reactivation has been reported in HCV/HBV co-infected patients who were undergoing or had completed treatment with HCV direct acting antivirals, and who were not receiving HBV antiviral therapy. Some cases have resulted in fulminant hepatitis, hepatic failure, and death. Cases have been reported in patients who are HBsAg positive and also in patients with serologic evidence of resolved HBV infection (i.e., HBsAg negative and anti-HBc positive). HBV reactivation has also been reported in patients receiving certain immunosuppressant or chemotherapeutic agents; the risk of HBV reactivation associated with treatment with HCV direct-acting antivirals may be increased in these patients. HBV reactivation is characterized as an abrupt increase in HBV replication manifesting as a rapid increase in serum HBV DNA level. In patients with resolved HBV infection, reappearance of HBsAg can occur. Reactivation of HBV replication may be accompanied by hepatitis, i.e., increases in aminotransferase levels and, in severe cases, increases in bilirubin levels, liver failure, and death can occur. P-gp inducers (e.g., ***rifampin***, St. John's wort) in the intestine may significantly decrease ***sofosbuvir*** plasma concentrations and may lead to a reduced therapeutic effect of **Sovaldi**: therefore, the use of ***rifampin*** and St. John's wort with **Sovaldi** is not recommended. Serious risk of symptomatic bradycardia when co-administered with ***amiodarone*** and another HCV direct-acting antiviral (DAA).

HCV NS5A Inhibitor+HCV NS3/4A Protease Inhibitor Combinations

➢ ***elbasvir+grazoprevir*** <18 years: not recommended; ≥18 years: 1 tab as a single dose once daily; see mfr pkg insert for length of treatment

Zepatier *Tab:* elba 50 mg+grazo 100 mg

Comment: **Zepatier** is contraindicated with moderate <u>or</u> severe hepatic impairment, concomitant ***atazanavir***, ***carbamazepine***, ***cyclosporine***, ***darunavir***, ***efavirenz***, ***lopinavir***, ***phenytoin***, ***rifampin***, ***saquinavir***, St. John's wort, ***tipranavir***. When co-administered with ***ribavirin***, pregnancy category **X.**

➢ ***glecaprevir+pibrentasvir*** <18 years: not recommended; ≥18 years: take 3 tablets (total daily dose: ***glecaprevir*** 300 mg and ***pibrentasvir*** 120 mg) once daily with food.

Mavyret *Tab:* gleca 100 mg+pibre 40 mg

Comment: **Mavyret** is a drug for the treatment of adults who have chronic Hepatitis C virus genotypes 1, 2, 3, 4, 5 <u>or</u> 6 infection and who do not have cirrhosis <u>or</u> who have early stage cirrhosis. **Mavyret** may cause serious liver problems including liver failure and death in patients who had hepatitis B virus infection. This is because the hepatitis B virus could become active again (i.e., reactivated) during <u>or</u> after treatment with **Mavyret**. Test all patients for HBV infection by measuring HBsAg and anti-HBc prior to initiating therapy with **Mavyret.** The most common side effects of **Mavyret** are headache and tiredness. See mfr insert for table of recommended duration of treatment based on patient characteristics. No adequate human data are available to establish whether <u>or</u> not **Mavyret** poses a risk to pregnancy outcomes. It is not known whether the components of **Mavyret** are excreted in human breast milk <u>or</u> have effects on the breastfed infant.

HCV NS5A Inhibitor+HCV NS3/4A Protease Inhibitor+CYP3A Inhibitor Combinations

➢ ***ombitasvir+paritaprevir+ritonavir*** **(B)** <18 years: not recommended; ≥18 years: 2 tabs once daily in the AM x 12 weeks

Technivie *Tab:* omvi 25 mg+pari 75 mg+rito 50 mg (4 x 7 daily dose pcks/carton)

Comment: **Technivie** is indicated for use in chronic HCV genotype 4 without cirrhosis. **Technivie** is not for use with moderate hepatic impairment.

HCV NS3/4A+Protease Inhibitor Combinations

➢ ***simeprevir*** **(C)** <18 years: not recommended; ≥18 years: 150 mg once daily; swallow whole; take with food, not for monotherapy; do not reduce dose <u>or</u> interrupt therapy; if discontinued, do not reinitiate; discontinue if HCV-RNA levels indicate futility; discontinue if ***peginterferon***, ***ribavirin***, <u>or</u> ***sofosbuvir*** is permanently discontinued; *Treatment-naïve, treatment relapses, with <u>or</u> without cirrhosis:* treat x 12 weeks (***simeprevir*** + ***peginterferon*** + ***ribavirin***) followed by additional 12 weeks ***peginterferon*** + ***ribavirin*** (total = 24 weeks). *Partial and non-responders, with <u>or</u> without cirrhosis:* treat x 12 weeks (***simeprevir*** + ***peginterferon*** + ***ribavirin***) followed by additional 36 weeks ***peginterferon*** + ***ribavirin*** (total = 48 weeks); *Treatment-naïve <u>or</u> treatment-experienced without cirrhosis:* treat x 12 weeks (***simeprevir*** + ***sofosbuvir***); *Treatment-naïve <u>or</u> treatment-experienced with cirrhosis:* treat x 24 weeks (***simeprevir*** + ***sofosbuvir***)

Olysio *Cap:* 150 mg

HCV NS5A Inhibitor+HCV NS5B Polymerase Inhibitor Combinations

➢ ***ledipasvir+sofosbuvir*** <12 years: not recommended; ≥12 years: *Treatment-naïve, without cirrhosis, with pretreatment HCV RNA <6 million IU/ml:* 1 tab daily x 8 weeks; *Treatment-naïve with <u>or</u> without cirrhosis <u>or</u> treatment-experienced without cirrhosis:* 1 tab daily x 12 weeks; *Treatment-experienced with cirrhosis:* 1 tab daily x 24 weeks; *In combination with **ribavirin**:* 1 tab daily x 12 weeks

Harvoni *Tab:* ledi 90 mg+sofo 400 mg

Comment: **Harvoni** is indicated for patients with advanced liver disease, genotype 1, 4, 5, <u>or</u> 6 infection: chronic HCV genotype 1- <u>or</u> 4-infected liver transplant recipients with <u>or</u> without cirrhosis <u>or</u> with compensated cirrhosis (Child-Pugh Class A), and for HCV genotype 1-infected patients with decompensated cirrhosis (Child-Pugh Class B/C), including those who have undergone liver transplantation. No adequate human data are available to establish whether or not **Harvoni** poses a risk to pregnancy outcomes; the background risk of major birth defects and miscarriage for the indicated population is unknown. If **Harvoni** is administered with ***ribavirin***, the combination regimen is contraindicated **(X)** in pregnant females and in males whose female partners are pregnant. It is not known whether **Harvoni** and its metabolites are present in human breast milk, affect human milk production, or have effects on the breastfed infant. If **Harvoni** is administered with ***ribavirin***, the nursing mother's information for ***ribavirin*** also applies to this combination regimen.

- ***sofosbuvir+velpatasvir*** <18 years: not established; ≥18 years: *Without cirrhosis or compensated cirrhosis (Child-Pugh Class A):* 1 tablet daily x 12 weeks; *Decompensated cirrhosis (Child-Pugh B or C):* 1 tablet daily plus ***ribavirin*** (RBV)

  Epclusa *Tab:* sofo 400 mg+velpa 100 mg

  Comment: **Epclusa** is indicated for patients with chronic HCV with genotype 12, 3, 4, 5, or 6 infection.

HCV NS5A Inhibitor+HCV NS3/4A Protease Inhibitor+CYP3A Inhibitor Combination

- ***sofosbuvir+velpatasvir*** **(B)** <12 years: not established; ≥12 years: 1 tab daily

  Viekira XR *Tab:* dasa 200 mg+omvi 8.33 mg+pari 50 mg+rito 33.33 mg ext-rel (4 weekly cartons, each containing 7 daily dose packs/carton)

  Comment: **Viekira XR** is indicated for HCV genotype 1 with mild liver dysfunction (Child-Pugh Class A). **Viekira XR** is contraindicated for moderate (Child-Pugh Class B) to severe (Child-Pugh Class C) liver dysfunction. No adjustment is recommended with mild, moderate, or severe renal dysfunction.

HCV NS5A Inhibitor+HCV NS3/4A Protease Inhibitor+CYP3A Inhibitor PLUS HCV NS5B Polymerase Inhibitor Combination

- ***ombitasvir+paritaprevir+ritonavir*** plus ***dasabuvir*** **(B)** <12 years: not established; ≥12 years: 2 combination tablets orally once a day (in the morning); ***dasabuvir***: 250 mg orally twice a day (morning and evening)

  Viekira Pak *Tab:* omvi 12.5 mg+pari 75 mg+rito 50 mg plus *Tab:* dasa 250 mg (28 day supply/pck)

  Comment: **Viekira Pak** is indicated for mild liver dysfunction (Child-Pugh Class A). **Viekira Pak** is contraindicated for moderate (Child-Pugh Class B) to severe (Child-Pugh C) liver dysfunction. No adjustment is recommended with mild, moderate, or severe renal dysfunction.

HCV NS5B Polymerase Inhibitor+HCV NS5A Inhibitor+HCV NS3/4A Protease Inhibitor Combination

- ***sofosbuvir+velpatasvir+voxilaprevir***: <12 years: not established; ≥12 years: 1 tablet once daily with food x 12 weeks; pre-test for HBV infection by measuring HBsAg and anti-HBc prior to the initiation of therapy

  Vosevi *Tab:* sofo 400 mg+velpa 100 mg+voxil 100 mg fixed-dose combination

  Comment: **Vosevi** is not recommended in patients with moderate or severe hepatic impairment (Child-Pugh Class B or C). A dosage recommendation cannot be made for patients with severe renal impairment or end stage renal disease. **Vosevi** is contraindicated while taking any medicines containing ***rifampin*** (**Rifater, Rifamate,**

Rimactane, Rifadin). **Vosevi** is indicated for the treatment of adult pa-tients with chronic HCV infection without cirrhosis or with compensated cirrhosis (Child-Pugh Class A) who have: (1) genotype 1, 2, 3, 4, 5, or 6 infection and have previously been treated with an HCV regimen containing an NS5A inhibitor or (2) genotype 1a or 3 infection and have previously been treated with an HCV regimen containing ***sofosbuvir*** without an NS5A inhibitor. Duration of treatment is 12 weeks. Additional benefit of **Vosevi** over ***sofosbuvir+velpatasvir*** has not been demonstrated with genotype 1b, 2, 4, 5, or 6 infection previously treated with ***sofosbuvir*** without an NS5A inhibitor. Because there is risk of Hepatitis B virus reactivation, test all patients for evidence of current or prior HBV infection before initiation of HCV treatment. Monitor HCV/HBV co-infected patients for HBV reactivation and hepatitis flare during HCV treatment and post-treatment follow-up. Initiate appropriate patient management for HBV infection as clinically indicated. The most common adverse reactions are headache, fatigue, diarrhea, and nausea. To report a suspected adverse reaction, contact Gilead Sciences at 1-800-GILEAD-5 or FDA at 1-800-FDA-1088 or visit www.fda.gov/medwatch

TRIPLE TREATMENT REGIMEN

Sovaldi+Harvoni+Ribavirin Combination Treatment Regimen

Comment: For this FDA-approved triple therapy regimen, follow the recommended regimen for each individual drug. Patients who are co-infected with hepatitis B are at risk for HBV reactivation during or after treatment with HCV direct-acting retrovirals. Therefore, patients should be screened for current or past HBV infection before starting this triple therapy regimen.

HEREDITARY ANGIOEDEMA (HAE), C1 ESTERASE INHIBITOR DEFICIENCY

Comment: Agents administered for the treatment of hereditary angioedema carry a risk of hypersensitivity reactions, which are similar to HAE attacks, and the patient should be monitored closely for signs and symptoms accordingly (e.g., hives, urticaria, tightness of the chest, wheezing, hypotension and/or anaphylaxis).

HAE PROPHYLAXIS

- ***danazol*** (X) <18 years: not recommended; ≥18 years: *Females:* start on 3rd or 4th day of menstrual period or after a negative pregnancy test; *Males/Females:* dosage requirements for continuous treatment of hereditary angioedema should be adjusted based on individual clinical response; initially 200 mg bid-tid; after a favorable initial response is achieved (prevention of episodes of edematous attacks), continuing dosage should be determined by decreasing the dosage by 50% or less at intervals of 1 to 3 months or longer if frequency of attacks prior to treatment dictates; if an attack occurs, daily dosage may be increased by up to 200 mg. During the dose adjusting phase, close monitoring of the patient's response is indicated, particularly if the patient has a history of airway involvement.

  Danocrine *Cap:* 50, 100, 200 mg

Comment: ***danazol*** is a synthetic steroid derived from ethisterone. It suppresses the pituitary-ovarian axis. This suppression is probably a combination of depressed hypothalamic-pituitary response to lowered ***estrogen*** production, the alteration of sex steroid metabolism, and interaction of ***danazol*** with sex hormone receptors. The only other demonstrable hormonal effects are weak androgenic activity and depression of both follicle-stimulating hormone (FSH) and luteinizing hormone (LH) output. Recent evidence suggests a direct inhibitory effect at gonadal sites and a binding of

Danocrine to receptors of gonadal steroids at target organs. In addition, **Danocrine** has been shown to significantly decrease IgG, IgM and IgA levels, as well as phospholipid and IgG isotope autoantibodies in patients with endometriosis and associated elevations of autoantibodies, suggesting this could be another mechanism by which it facilitates regression of fibrocystic breast disease. Changes in the menstrual pattern may occur. Generally, the pituitary-suppressive action of **Danocrine** is reversible. Ovulation and cyclic bleeding usually return within 60 to 90 days when therapy with **Danocrine** is discontinued. In the treatment of hereditary angioedema, **Danocrine** at effective doses prevents attacks of the disease characterized by episodic edema of the abdominal viscera, extremities, face, and airway which may be disabling and, if the airway is involved, fatal. In addition, **Danocrine** corrects partially or completely the primary biochemical abnormality of hereditary angioedema by increasing the levels of the deficient C1 esterase inhibitor (C1EI). As a result of this action the serum levels of the C4 component of the complement system are also increased. **Danocrine** is also used to treat endometriosis (to relieve associated abdominal pain) and fibrocystic breast disease (to reduce breast tissue nodularity and breast pain/ tenderness. Contraindications include pregnancy, breastfeeding, active or history of thromboembolic disease/ event, porphyria, undiagnosed abnormal genital bleeding, androgen-dependent tumor, and markedly impaired hepatic, renal, or cardiac function.

C1 ESTERASE INHIBITOR [HUMAN]

▶ ***C1 esterase inhibitor (human)*** <12 years: not established; ≥12 years: administer 60 International Units per kg body weight SC in the abdomen twicem weekly (every 3 or 4 days); administer at room temperature within 8 hours after reconstitution; use a silicone-free syringe for reconstitution and administration; use either the Mix2Vial transfer set provided with **Haegarda** or a commercially available 566 double-ended needle and vented filter spike

Haegarda *Vial:* 2000, 3000 IU C1 INH pwdr for reconstitution, single-use

Comment: **Haegarda is** a plasma-derived concentrate of C1 esterase inhibitor [human], a serine proteinase inhibitor. Iindicated for routine prophylaxis to prevent HAE attacks in adults and adolescents. It is not indicated for treating acute attacks of HAE. **Haegarda** is the first C1 esterase inhibitor (human) SC injection approved for self-administration by the patient or caregiver after healthcare provider instruction. An international consensus panel states that human plasma-derived C1 esterase inhibitor is considered to be the therapy of choice for both treatment and prophylaxis of maternal hereditary angioedema during lactation. There are no prospective clinical data from **Haegarda** use in pregnant women. C1-INH is a normal component of human plasma. There is no information regarding the excretion of **Haegarda** in human milk or effect the breastfed infant. The developmental and health benefits of breastfeeding should be considered along with the mother's clinical need for **Haegarda** and any potential adverse effects on the breastfed infant from **Haegarda** or from the underlying maternal condition.

HAE ACUTE ATTACK

C1 ESTERASE INHIBITOR [HUMAN]

▶ ***C1 esterase inhibitor [human]*** (C) <12 years: not established; ≥12 years: reconstitute pwdr using the sterile water provided; administer 20 IU/kg body weight via IVP injection at approximately 4 ml/min, at room temperature within 8 hours of reconstitution; store the vial at room temperature in the original carton to protect from light; appropriately trained patients may self-administer upon recognition of an HAE attack; hypersensitivity reactions may occur, therefore, have epinephrine immediately available for treatment of acute severe hypersensitivity reaction

Berinert *Vial:* 500 Units/10 ml vial, single-use, pwdr for reconstitution with the 10 ml sterile water diluent (provided)

Comment: To report suspected adverse reactions, contact the CSL Behring Pharmacovigilance Department at 1-866-915-6958 or to the FDA at 1-800-FDA-1088 or visit www.fda.gov/medwatch

▶ ***C1 esterase inhibitor [human]*** (C) <16 years: not established; ≥16 years: administer 1,000 Units (2 x 500 U vials) via IVP injection, after reconstitution with 5 ml sterile H2O/vial; reconstitute 1,000 U pwdr in a 10 ml syringe with 10 ml sterile water; administer over 10 minutes (1 ml/min) at room temperature within 3 hours of reconstitution; each 1,000 Unit treatment is administered every 3-4 days; hypersensitivity reactions may occur, therefore, have epinephrine immediately available for treatment of acute severe hypersensitivity reaction

Cinryze *Vial:* 500 Units/8 ml vial pwdr for reconstitution (sterile water diluent not provided)

Comment: No adequate and well-controlled studies have been conducted in pregnant women. It is not known whether **Cinryze** can cause fetal harm when administered to a pregnant woman or can affect reproduction capacity. **Cinryze** should be administered to a pregnant woman only if clearly needed. It is not known whether **Cinryze** is excreted in human milk. **Cinryze** is made from human plasma and may contain infectious agents (e.g. viruses and, theoretically, the Creutzfeldt-Jakob disease agent). To report suspected adverse reactions, contact ViroPharma Medical Information at 1-866-331-5637 or FDA at 1-800-FDA-1088 or visit www.fda.gov/medwatch

C1 ESTERASE INHIBITOR [RECOMBINANT]

▶ ***C1 esterase inhibitor [recombinant]*** (B) <13 years: not established; ≥13 years: reconstitute 2.100 IU pwdr (1 vial) with 14 ml sterile H2O; administer reconstituted solution at room temperature, slow IVP injection over approximately 5 minutes; appropriately trained patients may self-administer upon recognition of HAE attack; Weight-based dose: <84 kg: 50 IU /kg [wt in kg ÷ 3 = vol (ml) reconst soln for administration]; ≥84 kg: 4,200 IU (28 ml, 2 vials); if the attack symptoms persist, an additional (second) dose can be administered at the recommended dose level; do not exceed 4200 IU per dose; max two doses within a 24 hour period; hypersensitivity reactions may occur, therefore, have epinephrine immediately available for treatment of acute severe hypersensitivity reaction

Ruconest *Vial:* 2,100 IU, pwdr, single-use for IVP injection after reconstitution (sterile water diluent not provided)

Comment: To report **Ruconest** suspected adverse reactions, contact Salix Pharmaceuticals, Inc. at 1-800-508-0024 or FDA at 1-800-FDA-1088 or visit www.fda.gov/medwatch

BRADYKINEN B2 RECEPTOR ANTAGONIST

▶ ***icatibant*** (C) <18 years: not established; ≥18 years: administer 30 mg SC injection in the abdominal area; if response is inadequate or symptoms recur, additional injections of 30 mg may be administered at intervals of at least 6 hours; max 3 injections/24 hours; patients may self-administer upon recognition of an HAE attack

Firazyr *Prefilled syringe:* 10 mg/ml (3 ml) single-dose w. 25 gauge luer lock needle (1/carton, 3 cartons/pck)

Comment: **Firazyr**, as a bradykinin B2 receptor antagonist, may attenuate the antihypertensive effect of ACE inhibitors. The most commonly reported adverse reaction is injection site reaction (97% in clinical trials). To report suspected adverse reactions, contact Shire Human Genetic Therapies OnePath at 1-800-828-2088 or FDA at 1-800-FDA-1088 or visit www.fda.gov/medwatch

PLASMA KALLIKREIN INHIBITOR

▶ ***ecallantide*** (C) <12 years: not established; ≥12 years: administer 30 mg (3 ml) SC in three 10 mg (I ml) injections; if an attack persists, an additional dose of 30 mg may be administered within a 24 hour period; should only be administered by a healthcare professional with appropriate medical support to manage anaphylaxis and hereditary angioedema

Kalbitor *Vial:* 10 mg/ml (1/carton, 3 vials/pkg) single-use

Comment: Anaphylaxis has occurred in 3.9% of patients treated with **Kalbitor**. Therefore, **Kakbitor** should only be administered in a setting equipped to manage anaphylaxis and hereditary angioedema. Given the similarity in hypersensitivity symptoms and acute HAE symptoms, monitor patients closely for hypersensitivity reactions. To report suspected adverse reactions, contact Dyax Corp at 1-888-452-5248 or FDA at 1-800-FDA-1088 or www.fda.gov/medwatch

HERPANGINA

ANALGESICS

▶ ***acetaminophen*** (B) *see* ***Fever*** *page* 149

▶ ***tramadol*** (C)(IV)(G)

Comment: ***tramadol*** is known to be excreted in breast milk. The FDA and the European Medicines Agency (EMA) are investigating the safety of using ***tramadol***-containing medications to treat pain in children 12-18 years because of the potential for serious side effects, including slowed or difficult breathing.

Rybix ODT <18 years: not recommended; ≥18 years: initially 100 mg once daily; may increase by 100 mg every 5 days; max 300 mg/day; *CrCl <30 mL/min or severe hepatic impairment:* not recommended; *Cirrhosis:* max 50 mg q 12 hours

ODT: 50 mg (mint) (phenylalanine)

Ryzolt <18 years: not recommended; ≥18 years: initially 100 mg once daily; may increase by 100 mg every 5 days; max 300 mg/day; *CrCl <30 mL/min or severe hepatic impairment:* not recommended

Tab: 100, 200, 300 mg ext-rel

Ultram <18 years: not recommended; ≥18 years: 50-100 mg q 4-6 hours prn; max 400 mg/day; *CrCl <30 mL/min:* max 100 mg q 12 hours; *Cirrhosis:* max 50 mg q 12 hours

Tab: 50*mg

Ultram ER <18 years: not recommended; ≥18 years: initially 100 mg once daily; may increase by 100 mg every 5 days; max 300 mg/day; *CrCl <30 mL/min: or severe hepatic impairment:* not recommended

Tab: 100, 200, 300 mg ext-rel

▶ ***tramadol+acetaminophen*** (C)(IV)(G) <12 years: contraindicated; 12-<18: use extreme caution; not recommended for children and adolescents with obesity, asthma, obstructive sleep apnea, or other chronic breathing problem, or for post-tonsillectomy/adenoidectomy pain; ≥18 years: 2 tabs q 4-6 hours; max 8 tabs/day; 5 days; *CrCl <30 mL/min:* max 2 tabs q 12 hours; max 4 tabs/day x 5 days

Ultracet *Tab:* tram 37.5+acet 325 mg

Comment: ***tramadol*** is known to be excreted in breast milk. The FDA and the European Medicines Agency (EMA) are investigating the safety of using ***tramadol***-containing medications to treat pain in children 12-18 years because of the potential for serious side effects, including slowed or difficult breathing.

TOPICAL ANESTHETICS

▶ ***lidocaine*** viscous soln (**B**) <4 years: apply 1.25 ml to affected area with cotton-tipped applicator; may repeat after 3 hours; max 8 doses/day; ≥4 years, able to gargle or rinse/spit: 15 ml gargle or rinse/spit; repeat after 3 hours; max 8 doses/day

Xylocaine 2% Viscous Solution *Viscous soln:* 2% (20, 100, 450 ml)

Antipyretics *see* ***Fever*** *page* 149

HERPES GENITALIS (HSV TYPE II)

Comment: The following treatment regimens are published in the **2015 CDC Sexually Transmitted Diseases Treatment Guidelines**. Treatment regimens are for patients 18 years-of-age or older only; consult a specialist for treatment of patients less than 18 years-of-age. Treatment regimens are presented in alphabetical order by generic drug name, followed by a listing of brands with dose forms.

RECOMMENDED REGIMENS: FIRST CLINICAL EPISODE

Regimen 1

▶ ***acyclovir*** <18 years: not established; ≥18 years: 400 mg tid x 7-10 days or 200 mg 5 x/day x 10 days or until clinically resolved

Regimen 2

▶ ***acyclovir*** cream <18 years: not established; ≥18 years: apply q 3 hours 6 x/day x 7 days

Regimen 3

▶ ***famciclovir*** <18 years: not established; ≥18 years: 250 mg tid x 7-10 days or until clinically resolved

Regimen 4

▶ ***valacyclovir*** <18 years: not established; ≥18 years: 1 gm bid x 10 days or until clinically resolved

RECOMMENDED RECURRENT/EPISODIC REGIMENS

Comment: Initiate treatment of recurrent episodes within 1 day of onset of lesions.

Regimen 1

▶ ***acyclovir*** <18 years: not established; ≥18 years: 200 mg 5 x/day x 5 days

Regimen 2

▶ ***famciclovir*** <18 years: not established; ≥18 years: 125 mg bid x 5 days

Regimen 3

▶ ***valacyclovir*** <18 years: not established; ≥18 years: 500 mg bid x 3-5 days or until clinically resolved

SUPPRESSION THERAPY REGIMENS

Regimen 1

- *acyclovir* <18 years: not established; ≥18 years: 400 mg bid x 1 year

Regimen 2

- *famciclovir* <18 years: not established; ≥18 years: 250 mg bid x 1 year

Regimen 3

- *valacyclovir* <18 years: not established; ≥18 years: 500 mg daily x 1 year (for ≤9 recurrences/year) or 1 gm daily x 1 year (for ≥10 recurrences/year)

DAILY SUPPRESSIVE REGIMENS FOR PERSONS WITH HIV

Regimen 1

- *acyclovir* <18 years: not established; ≥18 years: 400-800 mg bid-tid

Regimen 2

- *famciclovir* <18 years: not established; ≥18 years: 500 mg bid

Regimen 3

- *valacyclovir* <18 years: not established; ≥18 years: 500 mg bid

RECURRENT/EPISODIC REGIMENS FOR PERSONS WITH HIV

Regimen 1

- *acyclovir* <18 years: not established; ≥18 years: 400 mg tid x 5-10 days

Regimen 2

- *famciclovir* <18 years: not established; ≥18 years: 500 mg bid x 5-10 days

Regimen 3

- *valacyclovir* <18 years: not established; ≥18 years: 1 gm bid x 5-10 days

DRUG BRANDS AND DOSE FORMS

- *acyclovir* (B)(G)
  - **Zovirax** *Cap:* 200 mg; *Tab:* 400, 800 mg
  - **Zovirax Oral Suspension** *Oral susp:* 200 mg/5 ml (banana)
  - **Zovirax Cream** *Crm:* 5% (3, 15 gm); *Oint:* 5% (3, 15 gm)
- *famciclovir* (B)(G)
  - **Famvir** *Tab:* 125, 250, 500 mg
- *valacyclovir* (B)(G)
  - **Valtrex** *Cplt:* 500, 1,000 mg

☐ HERPES LABIALIS/HERPES FACIALIS (HERPES SIMPLEX VIRUS TYPE I, COLD SORE, FEVER BLISTER)

PRIMARY INFECTION

- *acyclovir* (B)(G) <12 years: *see page 586 for dose by weight table*; ≥12 years: do not chew, crush, or swallow the buccal tab; apply within 1 hour of symptom onset and before appearance of lesion; apply a single buccal tab to the upper gum region on the affected side and hold in place for 30 seconds

Sitavig *Buccal tab:* 50 mg

Comment: **Sitavig** is contraindicated with allergy to milk protein concentrate.

- *valacyclovir* (B) <12 years: not recommended; >12 years: 2 gm q 12 hours x 1 day

  Valtrex *Cplt:* 500, 1,000 mg

SUPPRESSION THERAPY (FOR ≥6 OUTBREAKS/YEAR)

- *acyclovir* (B)(G) <2 years: not recommended; ≥2 years, <40 kg: 20 mg/kg 2-5 x/day x 1 year; >2 years, >40 kg: 200 mg 2-5 x/day x 1 year; *see page* 586 *for dose by weight table;*

  Zovirax *Cap:* 200 mg; *Tab:* 400, 800 mg

  Zovirax Oral Suspension *Oral susp:* 200 mg/5 ml (banana)

TOPICAL ANTIVIRAL THERAPY

- *acyclovir* (B)(G) <2 years: not recommended; ≥2 years: apply q 3 hours 6 x/day x 7 days

  Zovirax Cream *Crm:* 5% (3, 15 gm); *Oint:* 5% (3, 15 gm)

- *docosanol* (B) <12 years: not recommended; ≥12 years: apply and gently rub in 5 times daily until healed

  Abreva (OTC) *Crm:* 10% (2 gm)

- *penciclovir* (B) <12 years: not recommended; ≥12 years: apply q 2 hours while awake x 4 days

  Denavir *Crm:* 1% (2 gm)

TOPICAL ANTIVIRAL+CORTICOSTEROID THERAPY

- *acyclovir+hydrocortisone* (B)(G) <12 years: not recommended; ≥12 years: cream apply to affected area 5 x/day x 5 days

  Crm: 1% (2, 5 gm)

HERPES ZOSTER (HZ, SHINGLES)

Postherpetic Neuralgia *see page* 366

PROPHYLAXIS VACCINE

Comment: Herpes zoster (shingles) vaccine is indicated for adults >50 years-of-age (<50 years: not recommended). The vaccine is not for preventing primary infection (chickenpox).

- ***zoster vaccine recombinant, adjuvanted*** administer one 0.5 mL dose at month 0 followed by second dose anytime between 2–6 months later; administer immediately upon reconstitution or store refrigerated and use within 6 hours.

  Pediatric: <18 years: not established

  Shingrix *Vial:* 0.5 ml single-dose susp for IM injection after reconstitution with diluent (10/carton) (preservative-free)

ORAL ANTIVIRALS

- *famciclovir* (B) <18 years: not recommended; ≥18 years: 500 mg tid x 7 days

  Famvir *Tab:* 125, 250, 500 mg

▶ ***valacyclovir*** (B) <12 years: not recommended; ≥12 years: 1 gm tid x 7 days
  Valtrex *Cplt:* 500, 1,000 mg

▶ ***acyclovir*** (B)(G) <2 years: not recommended; ≥2 years, <40 kg: 20 mg/kg 5 x/day x 7-10 days; >2 years, >40 kg: 800 mg 5 x/day x 7-10 days; *see page* 586 *for dose by weight table;* ≥12 years: 800 mg 5 x/day x 7-10 days
  Zovirax *Cap:* 200 mg; *Tab:* 400, 800 mg
  Zovirax Oral Suspension *Oral susp:* 200 mg/5 ml (banana)

PROPHYLAXIS AGAINST SECONDARY INFECTION

▶ ***silver sulfadiazine*** (B)(G) <12 years: not established; ≥12 years: apply bid-qid
  Silvadene *Crm:* 1% (20 gm tube; 20, 50, 85, 400, 1,000 gm jar)

Comment: ***silver sulfadiazine*** is contradicted in sulfa allergy, late pregnancy, within the first 2 months after birth, premature infants.

ORAL ANALGESICS

Other Oral Analgesics *see* ***Pain*** *page* 324

▶ ***acetaminophen*** **(B)** *see* ***Fever*** *page* 149

▶ ***aspirin*** **(D)** *see* ***Fever*** *page* 150

Comment: ***aspirin***-containing medications are contraindicated with history of allergic-type reaction to ***aspirin***, children and adolescents with *varicella* or other viral illness, and 3rd trimester of pregnancy.

▶ ***tramadol*** (C)(IV)(G)

Comment: ***tramadol*** is known to be excreted in breast milk. The FDA and the European Medicines Agency (EMA) are investigating the safety of using ***tramadol***-containing medications to treat pain in children 12-18 years because of the potential for serious side effects, including slowed or difficult breathing.

  Rybix ODT <18 years: not recommended; ≥18 years: initially 100 mg once daily; may increase by 100 mg every 5 days; max 300 mg/day; *CrCl <30 mL/min or severe hepatic impairment:* not recommended; *Cirrhosis:* max 50 mg q 12 hours *ODT:* 50 mg (mint) (phenylalanine)

  Ryzolt <18 years: not recommended; ≥18 years: initially 100 mg once daily; may increase by 100 mg every 5 days; max 300 mg/day; *CrCl <30 mL/min or severe hepatic impairment:* not recommended
    Tab: 100, 200, 300 mg ext-rel

  Ultram <18 years: not recommended; ≥18 years: 50-100 mg q 4-6 hours prn; max 400 mg/day; *CrCl <30 mL/min:* max 100 mg q 12 hours; *Cirrhosis:* max 50 mg q 12 hours
    Tab: 50*mg

  Ultram ER <18 years: not recommended; ≥18 years: initially 100 mg once daily; may increase by 100 mg every 5 days; max 300 mg/day; *CrCl <30 mL/min: or severe hepatic impairment:* not recommended
    Tab: 100, 200, 300 mg ext-rel

▶ ***tramadol+acetaminophen*** (C)(IV)(G) <12 years: contraindicated; 12-<18: use extreme caution; not recommended for children and adolescents with obesity, asthma, obstructive sleep apnea, or other chronic breathing problem, or for post-tonsillectomy/adenoidectomy pain; ≥18 years: 2 tabs q 4-6 hours; max 8 tabs/day; 5 days; *CrCl <30 mL/min:* max 2 tabs q 12 hours; max 4 tabs/day x 5 days
  Ultracet *Tab:* tram 37.5+acet 325 mg

Comment: ***tramadol*** is known to be excreted in breast milk. The FDA and the European Medicines Agency (EMA) are investigating the safety of using ***tramadol***-containing medications to treat pain in children 12-18 years because of the potential for serious side effects, including slowed or difficult breathing.

SECONDARY INFECTION PROPHYLAXIS

▶ *silver sulfadiazine* (B)(G) <12 years: not established; ≥12 years: apply bid-qid
Silvadene *Crm:* 1% (20 gm tube; 20, 50, 85, 400, 1,000 gm jar)

Comment: ***silver sulfadiazine*** is contradicted in sulfa allergy, late pregnancy, within the first 2 months after birth, premature infants.

HERPES ZOSTER OPHTHALMICUS (HZO)

Comment: Herpes Zoster ophthalmicus (HZO) is an ophthalmologic emergency. Standard therapy involves initiating systemic (oral or intravenous) antiviral therapy as soon as possible. Pharmacotherapy options include ***acyclovir***, ***valacyclovir***, and ***famciclovir***. IV acyclovir is recommended for immunocompromised persons. Duration of treatment is 7-10 or 14 days, depending on severity. Ocular complications include conjunctivitis with or without superimposed bacterial infections, episcleritis, scleritis, keratitis, and uveitis, involvement of the 3rd, 4th, and 5th cranial nerves, acute optic neuritis, and necrotizing retinopathy (that often leads to permanent vision loss). Corticosteroids reduce the duration of pain during the acute phase, however, they have not been shown to decrease the incidence of postherpetic neuralgia and can exacerbate some ocular complications. Ophthalmology consultation is mandatory before initiating corticosteroid therapy.

REFERENCES

Anderson, E, Fantus, RJ, & Haddadin, RI. (2017). Diagnosis and management of herpes zoster ophthalmicus. *Disease-a-month*, *63*(2), 38–44.

Vrcek, I, Choudhury, E, Durairaj, V. (2017). Herpes zoster ophthalmicus: A review for the internist. *The American Journal of Medicine*, *130*(1), 21–26.

Parenteral Corticosteroids *see page* 547
Oral Corticosteroids *see page* 546

ORAL ANTIVIRALS

▶ *acyclovir* (B)(G) <2 years: not recommended; 2 years, <40 kg: 20 mg/kg 5 x/day x 7-10 days; 2 years, >40 kg: 800 mg 5 x/day x 7-10 days; *see page* 586 *for dose by weight* 800 mg 5 x/day x 7-10 days; >12 years: 800 mg 5 x/day x 7-10 days
Zovirax *Cap:* 200 mg; *Tab:* 400, 800 mg; *IVF bag:* 500 mg, 1 gm pre-mixed in 0.9% NS
Zovirax Oral Suspension *Oral susp:* 200 mg/5 ml (banana)

▶ *famciclovir* (B) <18 years: not recommended; >18 years: 500 mg tid x 7-10 days
Famvir *Tab:* 125, 250, 500 mg

▶ *valacyclovir* (B) <12 years: not recommended; >12 years: 1 gm tid x 7-10 days
Valtrex *Cplt:* 500, 1 gm

HICCUPS: INTRACTABLE

▶ *chlorpromazine* (C) <6 months: not recommended; ≥6 months: 0.25 mg/lb orally q 4-6 hours prn <u>or</u> 0.5 mg/lb rectally q 6-8 hours prn; ≥12 years: 25-50 mg tid-qid
Thorazine *Tab:* 10, 25, 50, 100, 200 mg; *Spansule:* 30, 75, 150 mg sust-rel; *Syr:* 10 mg/5 ml (4 oz; orange custard); *Oral conc:* 30 mg/ml (4 oz); 100 mg/ml (2, 8 oz); *Supp:* 25, 100 mg

HIDRADENITIS SUPPURATIVA

ORAL ANTI-INFECTIVES

▶ ***doxycycline*** **(D)(G)** <8 years: not recommended; ≥8 years, <100 lb: 2 mg/lb on first day in 2 divided doses, followed by 1 mg/lb/day in 1-2 divided x 7-14 days; ≥8 years, ≥100 lb: 100 mg bid x 7-14 days; *see page 605 for dose by weight table*

Acticlate *Tab:* 75, 150**mg
Adoxa *Tab:* 50, 75, 100, 150 mg ent-coat
Doryx *Tab:* 50, 75, 100, 150, 200 mg del-rel
Doxteric *Tab:* 50 mg del-rel
Monodox *Cap:* 50, 75, 100 mg
Oracea *Cap:* 40 mg del-rel
Vibramycin *Tab:* 100 mg; *Cap:* 50, 100 mg; *Syr:* 50 mg/5 ml (raspberry-apple) (sulfites); *Oral susp:* 25 mg/5 ml (raspberry)
Vibra-Tab *Tab:* 100 mg film-coat

Comment: ***doxycycline*** is contraindicated <8 years-of-age, in pregnancy, and lactation (discolors developing tooth enamel). A side effect may be photosensitivity (photophobia). Do not take with antacids, calcium supplements, milk or other dairy, or within 2 hours of taking another drug.

▶ ***erythromycin base*** **(B)(G)** <45 kg: 30-50 mg in 2-4 divided doses x 7-14 days; ≥45 kg: 1-1.5 gm divided qid x 7-14 days

Ery-Tab *Tab:* 250, 333, 500 mg ent-coat
PCE *Tab:* 333, 500 mg

▶ ***erythromycin ethylsuccinate*** **(B)(G)** 30-50 mg/kg/day in 4 divided doses x 7-14 days; may double dose with severe infection; max 100 mg/kg/day; *see page 607 for dose by weight table*

EryPed *Oral susp:* 200 mg/5 ml (100, 200 ml) (fruit); 400 mg/5 ml (60, 100, 200 ml) (banana); *Oral drops:* 200, 400 mg/5 ml (50 ml) (fruit); *Chew tab:* 200 mg wafer (fruit)
E.E.S. *Oral susp:* 200, 400 mg/5 ml (100 ml) (fruit)
E.E.S. Granules *Oral susp:* 200 mg/5 ml (100, 200 ml) (cherry)
E.E.S. 400 Tablets *Tab:* 400 mg

▶ ***minocycline*** **(D)(G)** <8 years: not recommended, ≥8 years: 100 mg bid x 7-14 days

Dynacin *Cap:* 50, 100 mg
Minocin *Cap:* 50, 75, 100 mg; *Oral susp:* 50 mg/5 ml (60 ml) (custard) (sulfites, alcohol 5%)

Comment: ***minocycline*** is contraindicated <8 years-of-age, in pregnancy, and lactation (discolors developing tooth enamel). A side effect may be photosensitivity (photophobia). Do not give with antacids, calcium supplements, milk or other dairy, or within two hours of taking another drug.

▶ ***tetracycline*** **(D)(G)** <8 years: not recommended; ≥8 years, <100 lb: 25-50 mg/kg/day in 4 divided doses x 7-14 days; *see page 618 for dose by weight table*; ≥8 years, ≥100 lb: 250 mg qid or 500 mg tid x 7-14 days

Achromycin V *Cap:* 250, 500 mg
Sumycin *Tab:* 250, 500 mg; *Cap:* 250, 500 mg; *Oral susp:* 125 mg/5 ml (100, 200 ml) (fruit) (sulfites)

Comment: ***tetracycline*** is contraindicated <8 years-of-age, in pregnancy, and lactation (discolors developing tooth enamel). A side effect may be photosensitivity (photophobia). Do not give with antacids, calcium supplements, milk or other dairy, or within two hours of taking another drug.

TOPICAL ANTI-INFECTIVES

▶ *clindamycin* (B)(G) apply bid x 7-14 days
 Cleocin T *Pad:* 1% (60/pck; alcohol 50%); *Lotn:* 1% (60 ml); *Gel:* 1% (30, 60 gm); *Soln w. applicator:* 1% (30, 60 ml; alcohol 50%)

HOOKWORM (UNCINARIASIS, CUTANEOUS LARVAE MIGRANS)

ANTHELMINTICS

Comment: Oral bioavailability of anthelmintics is enhanced when administered with a fatty meal (estimated fat content 40 gm).

▶ ***albendazole*** (C) take with a meal; may crush and mix with food; may repeat in 3 weeks if needed; <2 years: 200 mg bid x 7 days; 2-12 years: 400 mg once daily x 7 days; >12 years: 400 mg bid x 7 days
 Albenza *Tab:* 200 mg

Comment: ***albendazole*** is a broad-spectrum benzimidazole carbamate anthelmintic.

▶ ***ivermectin*** (C) take with water; chew or crush and mix with food; may repeat in 3 months if needed; <15 kg: not recommended; ≥15 kg: 200 mcg/kg as a single dose
 Stromectol *Tab:* 3, 6*mg

▶ ***mebendazole*** (C)(G) take with a meal; chew or crush and mix with food; may repeat in 3 weeks if needed; <2 years: not recommended; ≥2 years: 100 mg bid x 3 days
 Emverm *Chew tab:* 100 mg
 Vermox *Chew tab:* 100 mg

▶ ***pyrantel pamoate*** (C) take with a meal; may open capsule and sprinkle or mix with food; treat x 3 days; may repeat in 2-3 weeks if needed; treat x 3 days; 11 mg/kg/dose; max 1 gm/dose; <25 lb: not recommended; 25-37 lb: 1/2 tsp/dose; 38-62 lb: 1 tsp/dose; 63-87 lb: 1 tsp/dose; 88-112 lb: 2 tsp/dose; 113-137 lb: 2 tsp/dose; 138-162 lb: 3 tsp/dose; 163-187 lb: 3 tsp/dose; >187 lb: 4 tsp/dose
 Antiminth *Cap:* 180 mg; *Liq:* 50 mg/ml (30 ml); 144 mg/ml (30 ml); *Oral susp:* 50 mg/ml (60 ml)
 Pin-X (OTC) *Cap:* 180 mg; *Liq:* 50 mg/ml (30 ml); 144 mg/ml (30 ml); *Oral susp:* 50 mg/ml (30 ml)

▶ ***thiabendazole*** (C) take with a meal; may crush and mix with food; treat x 7 days; <30 lb: consult mfr pkg insert; ≥30 lb: 25 mg/kg/dose bid with meals; 30-50 lb: 250 mg bid with meals; >50 lb: 10 mg/lb/dose bid with meals; max 1.5 gm/dose; max 3 gm/day
 Mintezol *Chew tab:* 500*mg (orange); *Oral susp:* 500 mg/5 ml (120 ml) (orange)

Comment: ***thiabendazole*** is not for prophylaxis. May impair mental alertness. May not be available in the US.

HUMAN IMMUNODEFICIENCY VIRUS (HIV) EXPOSURE & ANTIRETROVIRAL PrEP/nPrEP

Antiretroviral drug brand names and dose forms (*see* ***Anti-HIV Drugs*** *page* 562)

Antiretroviral prophylactic treatment regimens for occupational HIV exposure (PrEP) and non-occupational exposure (nPrEP) are referenced from the **2015 CDC Sexually Transmitted Diseases Treatment Guidelines, MMWR**, and **NIH** available at: https://www.cdc.gov/hiv/pdf/programresources/cdc-hiv-npep-guidelines.pdf

In this section, the 2015 CDC-recommended highly active antiretroviral treatment (HAART) regimens are followed by a listing of the single and combination drugs with dosing regimens and dose forms. **Appendix S** is an alphabetical listing of the HIV drugs and dose forms. For more information on the management of HIV infection in adolescents and ≥18 years, see ***Guidelines for the Use of Antiretroviral Agents in HIV-1-Infected Adults and Adolescents:*** https://aidsinfo.nih.gov/contentfiles/lvguidelines/adultandadolescentgl.pdf

For specific dosing information in the management of HIV infection in children, see ***Guidelines for Use of Antiretroviral Agents in Pediatric HIV Infection:*** https://www.aidsinfo.nih.gov/contentfiles/lvguidelines/pediatricguidelines.pdf
Providers should consult, and refer HIV-infected patients to, a specialist and/or specialty community services for age-appropriate dosing regimens and other specific pediatric considerations.
Initiation of PrEP/nPrEP with ART as soon as possible increases the likelihood of prophylactic benefit. Treatment regimens must be initiated ≥72 hours following exposure. A 28-day course of ART is recommended for persons with ***substantial risk for HIV exposure*** (i.e., exposure of vagina, rectum, eye, mouth, or other mucous membrane, non-intact skin, or percutaneous contact with blood, semen, vaginal secretions, breast milk, or any body fluid that is visibly contaminated with blood, when the source is known to be infected with HIV). ART is not recommended for persons with ***negligible risk for HIV exposure*** (i.e., exposure of vagina, rectum, eye, mouth, or other mucus membrane, intact or non-intact skin, or percutaneous contact with urine, nasal secretions, saliva, sweat, or tears, if not visibly contaminated with blood, regardless of the known or suspected HIV status of the source). There is no evidence indicating any specific antiretroviral medication, or combination of medications is optimal for suppressing local viral replication. There is no evidence to indicate that a 3-drug ART regimen is any more beneficial than a 2-drug regimen. When the source person is available for interview and testing, his or her history of retroviral medication use and most recent/current viral load measurement should be considered when selecting an ART treatment regimen (e.g., to help avoid prescribing an antiretroviral medication to which the source virus is likely to be resistant). Register pregnant patients exposed to antiretroviral agents to the Antiretroviral Pregnancy Registry (APR) at 1-800-258-4263. The Centers for Disease Control and Prevention recommend that HIV-infected mothers not breastfeed their infants to avoid risking postnatal transmission of HIV infection.

REGIMENS

Non-Nucleoside Reverse Transcriptase Inhibitor (NNRTI)-Based Regimen

- ***efavirenz*** plus (***lamivudine*** or ***emtricitabine***) plus (***zidovudine*** or ***tenofovir***)

Protease Inhibitor (PI)-Based Regimens

- ***lopinavir+ritonavir*** (co-formulated as **Kaletra**) plus (***lamivudine*** or ***emtricitabine***) plus ***zidovudine***
- ***darunavir+cobicistat*** (co-formulated as **Prezcobix**) plus other retroviral agents

ALTERNATIVE REGIMENS

NNRTI-Based Regimen

- ***efavirenz*** plus (***lamivudine*** or ***emtricitabine***) plus (***abacavir*** or ***didanosine*** or ***stavudine***)

  Comment: ***efavirenz*** should be avoided in pregnant females and females of childbearing potential.

Protease Inhibitor-Based Regimens

Regimen 1

- *atazanavir* plus (*lamivudine* or *emtricitabine*) plus (*zidovudine* or *stavudine* or *abacavir* or *didanosine*) or (*tenofovir* plus *ritonavir* (100 mg/day)

Regimen 2

- *fosamprenavir* plus (*lamivudine* or *emtricitabine*) plus (*zidovudine* or *stavudine*) or (*abacavir* or *tenofovir* or *didanosine*)

Regimen 3

- *fosamprenavir+ritonavir* plus (*lamivudine* or *emtricitabine*) plus (*zidovudine* or *stavudine* or *abacavir* or *tenofovir* or *didanosine*)

Regimen 4

- *indinavir+ritonavir* plus (*lamivudine* or *emtricitabine*) plus (*zidovudine* or *stavudine* or *abacavir* or *tenofovir* or *didanosine*)

  Comment: Using *ritonavir* with *indinavir* may increase risk for renal adverse events.

Regimen 5

- *lopinavir/ritonavir* (coformulated as **Kaletra**) plus (*lamivudine* or *emtricitabine*) plus (*stavudine* or *abacavir* or *tenofovir* or *didanosine*)

Regimen 6

- *nelfinavir* plus (*lamivudine* or *emtricitabine*) plus (*zidovudine* or *stavudine* or *abacavir* or *tenofovir* or *didanosine*)

Regimen 7

- *saquinavir+ritonavir* plus (*lamivudine* or *emtricitabine*) plus (*zidovudine* or *stavudine* or *abacavir* or *tenofovir* or *didanosine*)

Triple Nucleoside Reverse Transcriptase Inhibitor (NRTI)-Based Regimen

- *abacavir* plus *lamivudine* plus *zidovudine*

Comment: Triple NRTI therapy should be used only when an NNRTI- or PI-based regimen cannot or should not be used.

BRAND NAMES, DOSING, AND DOSE FORMS: SINGLE AGENTS

Integrase Strand Transfer Inhibitors (INSTIs)

- ***dolutegravir*** (C) <12 years, <40 kg: not established; ≥12 years, ≥40 kg: *Treatment-naïve or treatment-experienced but INSTI-naïve:* 50 mg once daily; *Treatment-naïve or treatment-experienced or and co-administered with* ***efavirenz****, FPV/r, TPV/r, or* ***rifampin****:* 50 mg bid; *INSTI-experienced with certain INSTI-associated resistance substitutions:* 50 mg bid

  Tivicay *Tab:* 10, 25, 50 mg
- ***raltegravir (as potassium)*** (C) <4 weeks: not recommended; ≥4 weeks, 3-11 kg [oral suspension] 3-<4 kg: 20 mg bid; 4-<6 kg: 30 mg bid; 6-<8 kg: 40 mg bid; 8-<11 kg: 60 mg bid; ≥11-<25 kg [oral suspension/chewable tab]; 6 mg/kg/dose bid; see mfr pkg insert for dose by weight table;≥25 kg and unable to swallow tablet use chewable tab; 25-<28 kg: 150 mg bid; 28-<40 kg: 200 mg bid; ≥40 kg: 300 mg bid; 6 years **25** kg, and

able to swallow tablets use film-coat tab; 400 mg bid; take with concomitant ***rifampin*** 800 mg bid; swallow film-coated tablets whole; do not crush or chew

Isentress *Tab:* 400 mg film-coat; *Chew tab:* 25, 100*mg (orange banana) (phenylalanine)

Isentress HD *Tab:* 600 mg film-coat

Isentress Oral Suspension *Oral susp:* 100 mg/pkt pwdr for oral susp (banana)

Comment: Oral suspension, chewable tablets and film-coated ***raltegravir*** tablets are not bioequivalent. Max dose for chewable tablets is 300 mg twice daily. Previously, the maximum dose for film-coated tablets was 400 mg twice daily. However, the US Food and Drug Administration has recently approved a new 1200 mg daily dosage of **Isentress HD** (***raltegravir***) for the treatment of HIV-1 infection in adults, and pediatric patients who weigh > 40 kg and are treatment-naïve or whose virus has been suppressed on an initial regimen of 400 mg twice-daily dose of **Isentress HD. Isentress HD** is administered as two 600 mg film-coated oral tablets in combination with other antiretroviral agents, and can be taken with or without food. Co-administration of **Isentress HD** can include a wide range of antiretroviral agents and non-antiretroviral agents, however aluminum and/or magnesium-containing antacids, calcium carbonate antacids, ***rifampin***, ***tipranavir+ritonavir***, ***etravirine***, and other strong inducers of drug metabolizing enzymes are not recommended to be combined with **Isentress HD**. Healthcare providers should consider the potential for drug-drug interactions prior to and during treatment with **Isentress HD** and any other recommended agents. Adverse effects associated with treatment included abdominal pain, diarrhea, vomiting and decreased appetite. In addition, severe, potentially life-threatening and fatal skin reactions can occur, including Stevens-Johnson syndrome, hypersensitivity reaction, and toxic epidermal necrolysis. Treatment should be immediately discontinued if severe hypersensitivity, severe rash, or rash with systemic symptoms or liver aminotransferase elevations develop.

Nucleoside Reverse Transcriptase Inhibitors (NRTIs)

▶ ***abacavir sulfate*** (C)(G) <3 months: not recommended; 3 months-16 years: [tablet/oral solution] 16 mg/kg qd or 8 mg/kg bid; max 300 mg bid; >14 kg: see mfr pkg insert for tablet dosing by weight table; *Mild hepatic impairment:* use oral solution for titration

Ziagen (as sulfate) *Tab:* 300*mg

Ziagen Oral Solution *Oral soln:* 20 mg/ml (240 ml) (strawberry-banana) (parabens, propylene glycol)

▶ ***didanosine*** (C)

Videx EC <20 kg: not recommended (use oral solution); 20-<25 kg: 200 mg; 25-<60 kg: 250 mg; ≥60 kg: 400 mg; *CrCl 30-59 mL/min:* <60 kg: 125 mg; ≥60 kg: 200 mg; *CrCl 10-29 mL/min:* 125 mg; *CrCl <10 mL/min or dialysis:* <60 kg: use oral solution ≥60 kg: 125 mg; take once daily on an empty stomach; swallow whole, do not crush or chew

Cap: 125, 200, 250, 400 mg ent-coat del-rel; *Chew tab:* 25, 50, 100, 150, 200 mg (mandarin orange) (buffered with calcium carbonate and magnesium hydroxide, phenylalanine)

Videx Pediatric Pwdr for Solution <2 weeks: not recommended; 2 weeks-8 months: 100 mg/m² bid; >8 months: 120 mg/m² bid; *Renal impairment:* consider reducing dose or increasing dosing interval; take on an empty stomach

Pwdr for oral soln: 2, 4 gm (120, 240 ml)

Comment: ***didanosine*** is contraindicated with concomitant ***allopurinol*** or ***ribavirin***.

▶ ***emtricitabine*** **(B)** <3 months: 3 mg/kg oral soln once daily; 3 months-17 years, 6 mg/kg once daily; ≤33 kg: use oral soln, max 240 mg (24 ml); >33 kg: 200 mg cap once daily; max 240 mg/day; ≥18 years: 200 mg once daily; *CrCl 30-49 mL/min:* 200 mg q 48 hours; *CrCl 5-29 mL/min:* 200 mg q 72 hours; *CrCl <15 mL/min* or *dialysis:* 200 mg q 96 hours

Emtriva *Cap:* 200 mg

Emtriva Oral Solution *Oral soln:* 10 mg/ml (170 ml) (cotton candy)

▶ ***lamivudine*** **(C)(G)** <3 months: not established; 3 months-16 years: 4 mg/kg oral soln or tab bid; [tab] 14-<20 kg: 150 mg once daily or 75 mg bid; ≥20-<25 kg: 225 mg once daily or 75 mg in the AM and 150 mg in the PM; ≥25 kg: 300 mg once daily or 150 mg bid; max 8 mg/kg once daily or 150 mg bid or 300 mg once daily; >16 years: *CrCl ≥50 mL/min:* 300 mg qd or 150 mg bid; *CrCl >30-50 ml/min:* 150 mg qd; *CrCl 15-29:* first dose 150 mg, then 100 mg once daily; *CrCl 5-14 ml/min:* first dose 150 mg, then 50 mg qd; *CrCl <5 mL/min:* first dose 50 mg, then 25 mg once daily; max 8 mg/kg once daily or 150 mg bid

Epivir *Tab:* 150*, 300 mg

Epivir Oral Solution *Oral soln:* 10 mg/ml (240 ml) (strawberry-banana) (sucrose 3 gm/15 ml)

Comment: With renal impairment reduce ***lamivudine*** dose or extend dosing interval.

▶ ***stavudine*** **(C)(G)** birth-13 days: [tablet/oral solution] 0.5 mg/kg q 12 hours; >14 days, <30 kg: [tablet/oral solution] 1 mg/kg q 12 hours; ≥30-<60 kg: 30 mg q 12 hours; ≥60 kg: 40 mg q 12 hours; ≤60 kg: 30 mg q 12 hours; *If peripheral neuropathy develops:* discontinue; *After resolution, ≥60 kg:* may restart at 20 mg q 12 hours; *After resolution, ≤60 kg:* may restart at 15 mg q 12 hours; *if neuropathy returns:* consider permanent discontinuation; *CrCl 10-50 mL/min, ≥60 kg:* 20 mg q 12 hours; *CrCl 10-50 mL/min, ≥60 kg:* 15 mg q 12 hours; *Hemodialysis, ≥60 kg:* 20 mg q 24 hours; *Hemodialysis, ≤60 kg:* 15 mg q 24 hours; administer at the same time of day; *Hemodialysis:* administer at the end of dialysis

Zerit *Cap:* 15, 20, 30, 40 mg

Zerit for Oral Solution *Oral soln:* 1 mg/ml pwdr for reconstitution (fruit) (dye-free)

▶ ***tenofovir disoproxil fumarate*** **(C)(G)** <2 years: not established; 2-12 years: 8 mg/kg once daily; >12 years, 35 kg: 300 mg once daily; mix oral pwdr with 2-4 oz soft food; max 300 mg once daily; *CrCl 30-49 mL/min:* max 300 mg q 48 hours; *CrCl 10-29:* max 300 mg q 72-96 hours; *Hemodialysis:* max 300 mg once every 7 days or after a total of 12 hours of dialysis; *CrCl <10 mL/min:* not recommended

Viread *Tab:* 150, 200, 250, 300 mg; *Oral pwdr:* 40 mg/gm (60 gm w. dosing scoop)

▶ ***zidovudine*** **(C)(G)** *Treatment of HIV-1 infection:* 4-<9 kg: 24 mg/kg/day divided bid or tid; ≥9-30 kg: 18 mg/kg/day divided bid or tid; ≥30 kg: 600 mg/day divided bid or tid; *Prevention of maternal-fetal neonatal transmission: <12 hours after birth until 6 weeks of age:* [Solution] 2 mg/kg q 6 hours until 6 weeks-of-age; [IV] 1.5 mg/kg infused over 30 minutes q 6 hours until 6 weeks-of-age; max 200 mg q 8 hours; *ESRD/dialysis:* max 100 mg q 6-8 hours; *Vertical transmission, severe anemia,* or *neutropenia:* see mfr pkg insert

Retrovir Tablets *Tab:* 300 mg

Retrovir Capsules *Cap:* 100 mg

Retrovir Syrup *Syrup:* 50 mg/5 ml (strawberry)

Retrovir IV *Vial:* 10 mg/ml after dilution (20 ml) (preservative-free)

Non-Nucleoside Reverse Transcriptase Inhibitors (NNRTIs)

▶ ***delavirdine mesylate*** **(C)** <16 years: not established; ≥16 years: 400 mg (4 x 100 mg or 2 x 200 mg) tablets tid in combination with other antiretroviral agents

Rescriptor *Tab:* 100, 200 mg

Comment: The 100 mg **Rescriptor** tablets may be dispersed in water prior to consumption. To prepare a dispersion, add four 100 mg Rescriptor tablets to at least 3 ounces of water, allow to stand for a few minutes, and then stir until a uniform dispersion occurs. The dispersion should be consumed promptly. The glass should be rinsed with water and the rinse swallowed to ensure the entire dose is consumed. The 200 mg tablets should be taken as intact tablets, because they are not readily dispersed in water.

- ***efavirenz*** **(D)(G)** ≤3 months: not established; >3 months, ≤3.5 kg: [tablet/capsule] 3.5-<5 kg: 100 mg once daily; 5-<7.5 kg: 150 mg once daily; 7.5-<15 kg: 200 mg once daily; 15-<20 kg: 250 mg once daily; 20-<25 kg: 300 mg once daily; 25-<32.5 kg: 350 once daily; 32.5-<40 kg: 400 mg once daily; >40 kg: 600 mg once daily; max 600 mg once daily

  Comment: For children who cannot swallow capsules, the capsule contents can be administered with a small amount of food (applesauce, grape jelly, yogurt) or 2 tsp room temperature infant formula using the capsule sprinkle method of administration. See mfr pkg insert for instructions. Tablets should not be crushed or chewed. Administer at bedtime to limit CNS effects. Consider pretreatment with antihistamine to minimize rash.

  Sustiva *Tab:* 75, 150, 600, 800 mg; *Cap:* 50, 200 mg

- ***etravirine*** **(B)** <3 years: not recommended; ≥3 years, >16 kg: 16-< 20 kg: 100 mg bid; 20-<25 kg: 125 mg bid; 25-<30 kg: 150 mg bid; ≥30 kg: 200 mg (1 x 200 mg tablet or 2 x 100 mg tablets) bid following a meal; max 200 mg bid; take following a meal

  Intelence *Tab:* 25*, 100, 200 mg

- ***nevirapine*** **(B)(G)** <6 years: not recommended; 6-<18 years: BSA 0.58-0.83 kg/m^2: 200 mg once daily; BSA 0.84-1.16 kg/m^2: 300 mg once daily; BSA ≥1.17 kg/m^2: 400 mg once daily; max 400 mg once daily; ≥18 years: initially one 200 mg tablet of immediate-release **Viramune** once daily for the first 14 days in combination with other antiretroviral agents; then one 400 mg tablet of **Viramune XR** once daily

  Comment: Children must initiate therapy with immediate-release **Viramune** for the first 14 days; ≥15 days: [oral suspension/tablet]: 150 mg/m^2 once daily for 14 days, then 150 mg/m^2 bid. The 14-day lead-in period has been found to lessen the frequency of rash.

  Viramune *Tab:* 200*mg

  Viramune Oral Suspension *Oral susp:* 50 mg/5 ml (240 ml)

  Viramune XR *Tab:* 100, 400 mg ext-rel

- ***rilpivirine*** **(D)** <12 years: not recommended; ≥12 years, >35 kg: 25 mg once daily; *If concomitant **rifabutin**:* 50 mg once daily: *If concomitant **rifabutin** stopped:* 25 mg once daily

  Edurant *Tab:* 25 mg

Nucleoside and Non-Nucleoside Reverse Transcriptase Inhibitor (NRTI/NNRTI) Combinations

- **Atripla (B)** ***efavirenz+emtricitabine+tenofovir disoproxil fumarate*** <12 years: not recommended; ≥12 years, 40 kg: 1 tab once daily preferably at HS; take on an empty stomach; *Concomitant **rifabutin**:* >50 kg: take additional ***efavirenz*** 200 mg/day

  Tab: efa 600 mg+emtri 200 mg+teno dis fum 300 mg

- **Complera (B)** ***emtricitabine+tenofovir disoproxil fumarate+rilpivirine*** *<12* years, <35 kg: not established; ≥12 years, ≥35 kg: 1 tab once daily; *CrCl <50 mL/min:* not recommended; *Concomitant **rifabutin**:* take additional ***ribavirin*** 25 mg qd

  Tab: emtri 200 mg+teno dis 300 mg+rilpiv 25 mg

Protease Inhibitors (PIs)

- ***atazanavir*** **(B)(G)** <3 months: not recommended; ≥3 mos, 5 kg: [oral powder] 5-<15 kg: 200 mg (4 packets) plus ***ritonavir*** 80 mg once daily; 15-<25 kg: 250 mg (5 packets) plus ***ritonavir*** 80 mg once daily; ≥**25** kg, unable to swallow capsules: 300 mg (6 packets) plus *ritonavir* once daily; 6 yrs, <15 kg: [capsule] 15-<20 kg: 150 mg plus ***ritonavir*** 100 mg once daily; 20-<40 kg: 200 mg plus ***ritonavir*** 100 mg once daily; ≥40 kg: 300 mg plus ***ritonavir*** 100 mg once daily; [capsule]15-<20 kg: 150 mg plus ***ritonavir*** 100 mg once daily; 20-<40 kg: 200 mg plus ***ritonavir*** 100 mg once daily; ≥40 kg: 300 mg plus ***ritonavir*** 100 mg once daily; max dose 400 mg once daily; *Treatment-naïve, ≥40 kg: Recommended regimen:* 300 mg plus ***ritonavir*** 100 mg once daily; *Unable to tolerate* ***ritonavir****:* 400 mg once daily; *In combination with* ***efavirenz****:* 400 mg plus ***ritonavir*** 100 mg once daily; *Treatment-experienced. ≥40 kg: Recommended regimen:* 300 mg plus ***ritonavir*** 100 mg once daily; *In combination with both an H_2-blocker* or *PPI and* ***tenofovir****:* 400 mg plus ***ritonavir*** 100 mg once daily; take with food

Reyataz *Cap:* 100, 150, 200, 300 mg; *Oral pwdr:* 50 mg/pkt (30/carton) (phenylalanine)

Comment: Administration of ***atazanavir*** with ***rotinavir*** is preferred. Dose for treatment-naïve children ≥13 years-of-age and ≥40 kg unable to tolerate ***rotinavir***, administer 400 mg once daily. See mfr pkg insert for special dosing considerations when combining ***atazanavir*** with other retrovirals.

▶ ***darunavir*** **(C)(G)** <3 years: nor recommended; ≥3 years, 10 kg [oral solution/tablet/capsule] *Treatment-naïve* or *experienced without* ***darunavir****-associated substitutions:* 10-<15 kg: 35 mg/kg once daily plus ***ritonavir*** 7 mg/kg once daily; 15-<30 kg: 600 mg plus ***ritonavir*** 100 mg once daily; 30-<40 kg: 675 mg plus ***ritonavir*** 100 mg once daily; ≥40 kg: 800 mg plus ***ritonavir*** 100 mg once daily; *Treatment-experienced with ≥1* ***darunavir****-associated substitution(s):* 10-15 kg: 20 mg/kg bid plus ***ritonavir*** 3 mg/kg bid; 15-<30 kg: 375 mg plus ***ritonavir*** 48 mg bid; 30-<40 kg: 450 mg plus ***ritonavir*** 60 mg bid; ≥40 kg: 600 mg plus ***ritonavir*** 100 mg bid

Prezista *Tab:* 75, 150, 600, 800 mg film-coat

Prezista Oral Suspension *Susp:* 100 mg/ml (strawberry cream)

Comment: **Prezista** is FDA approved for treatment of HIV-1-infected pregnant females and for the treatment of children >3 years-of-age in combination with ***ritonavir*** and other antiretrovirals.

Comment: **Prezista** is FDA approved for treatment of HIV-1-infected pregnant females and for the treatment of children >3 years-of-age in combination with ***ritonavir*** and other antiretrovirals.

▶ ***fosamprenavir*** **(C)(G)** <4 weeks: not recommended; *Protease inhibitor-naïve, ≥4 weeks-18 years* or *protease inhibitor-experienced:* ≥6 months, <11 kg: 45 mg/kg plus ***ritonavir*** 7 mg/kg bid; 11-<15 kg: 30 mg/kg plus ***ritonavir*** 3 mg/kg bid; 15 kg-<20 kg: 23 mg/kg plus ***ritonavir*** 3 mg/kg bid; ≥20 kg: 18 mg/kg plus ***ritonavir*** 3 mg/kg bid; *Protease inhibitor-naïve, ≥2 years:* 30 mg/kg bid without ***ritonavir****:* max dose 700 mg plus ***ritonavir*** 100 mg bid; *Max dosing: Treatment-naïve:* 1,400 mg bid or 1,400 mg once daily plus ***ritonavir*** 200 mg once daily or 1,400 mg once daily plus ***ritonavir*** 100 mg once daily or 700 mg bid plus ***ritonavir*** 100 mg bid; *Protease inhibitor-experienced:* 700 mg bid plus ***ritonavir*** 100 mg bid

Lexiva: *Tab: 700 mg film-coat*

Lexiva Oral Suspension *Oral susp:* 50 mg/ml (225 ml) (grape-bubble gum-peppermint)

Comment: ***fosamprenavir*** 1 ml is equivalent to approximately 43 mg of ***amprenavir*** 1 ml.

▶ ***indinavir sulfate*** **(C)** <18 years: not established (3-18 years, doses of 500 mg/m^2 every 8 hours have been used; see mfr pkg insert); ≥18 years: 800 mg q 8 hours; *Concomitant* ***rifabutin****:* 1 gm q 8 hours and reduce ***rifabutin*** dose by half; *Hepatic insufficiency* or *concomitant* **ketoconazole, itraconazole,** or ***delavirdine****:* 600 mg q 8 hours; take with water on an empty stomach or with a light meal

Crixivan *Cap:* 100, 200, 333, 400 mg

▶ ***nelfinavir mesylate*** **(B)** <2 years: not established; 2-13 years: 45-55 mg/kg bid or 25-35 mg/kg tid; take with a meal; max 2,500 mg/day; ≥13 years: 1250 mg (5 x 250 mg tablets or 2 x 625 mg tablets) bid or 750 mg (3 x 250 mg tablets) tid; take with a meal; may dissolve tablets in a small amount of water; max 2500 mg/day

Viracept *Tab:* 250, 625 mg

Viracept Oral Powder *Oral pwdr:* 50 mg/gm (144 gm) (phenylalanine)

Comment: The 250 mg **Viracept** tablets are interchangeable with oral powder, the 625 mg tablets are not.

▶ ***raltegravir (as potassium)*** **(B)** <4 weeks, <3 kg: not recommended; ≥4 weeks, 3-11 kg: [oral suspension] 3-<4 kg: 20 mg bid; 4-<6 kg: 30 mg bid; 6-<8 kg: 40 mg bid; 8-<11 kg: 60 mg bid; ≥11-<25 kg: [oral suspension/chewable tablet] 6 mg/kg/dose bid; see mfr pkg insert for dosage by weight;≥25 kg and unable to swallow tablet: [chewable tablet]25-<28 kg: 150 mg bid; 28-<40 kg: 200 mg bid; ≥40 kg: 300 mg bid; ≥6 years, ≥25 kg, able to swallow tablets: 400 mg film-coat tablet bid

Comment: Oral suspension, chewable tablets, and film-coated tablets are not bioequivalent. Chewable tablet max dose 300 mg bid. Film-coated tablets max dose 400 mg bid. Oral suspension max dose 100 mg bid.

Isentress *Tab:* 400 mg film-coat; *Chew tab:* 25, 100*mg (orange-banana) (phenylalanine)

Isentress Oral Suspension *Oral susp:* 100 mg/pkt pwdr for oral susp (banana)

▶ ***ritonavir*** **(B)(G)** <1 month: not recommended; ≥1 month: 350-400 mg/m^2 bid; initiate at 250 mg/m^2 bid and titrate upward every 2-3 days by 50 mg/m^2 bid; max dose 600 mg bid

Comment: Lower doses of ***ritonavir*** have been used to boost other protease inhibitors but the ***ritonavir*** doses used for boosting have not been specifically approved in children.

Norvir *Tab:* 100 mg film-coat; *Gel cap:* 100 mg (alcohol)

Norvir Oral Solution *Oral soln:* 80 mg/ml, 600 mg/7.5 ml (8 oz) (peppermint-caramel) (alcohol)

Comment: **Norvir** tablets should be swallowed whole. Take **Norvir** with meals. Patients may improve the taste of **Norvir Oral Solution** by mixing with chocolate milk, **Ensure**, or **Advera** within one hour of dosing. Dose reduction of **Norvir** is necessary when used with other protease inhibitors (***atazanavir***, ***darunavir***, ***fosamprenavir***, ***saquinavir***, and ***tipranavir***). Patients who take the 600 mg gel cap bid may experience more gastrointestinal side effects such as nausea, vomiting, abdominal pain, or diarrhea when switching from the gel cap to the tablet because of greater maximum plasma concentration (Cmax) achieved with the tablet. These adverse events (gastrointestinal or paresthesias) may diminish as treatment is continued.

▶ ***saquinavir mesylate*** **(B)** <16 years: not established; ≥16 years: 1 gm bid plus ***ritonavir*** 100 mg bid (take both at the same time); *Treatment-naïve or switching from a* ***delavirdine****- or* ***rilpivirine****-containing regimen:* initially 500 mg bid x 7 days, then increase to 1 gm bid plus ***ritonavir*** 100 mg bid; take within 2 hours after a meal

Fortovase *Tab/Cap:* 200 mg

Invirase *Tab:* 500 mg; *Cap:* 200 mg

▶ ***tipranavir*** **(C)** <2 years: not recommended; 2-18 yrs: [capsule/oral solution] 14 mg/kg plus ***ritonavir*** 6 mg/kg bid or 375 mg/m^2 plus ***ritonavir*** 150 mg/m^2 bid; max 500 mg plus ***ritonavir*** 200 mg bid

Aptivus *Gel cap:* 250 mg (alcohol)

Aptivus Oral Solution *Oral soln:* 100 mg/ml (buttermint-butter toffee) (Vit E 116 IU/ml)

Fusion Inhibitors—CCR5 Coreceptor Antagonists

- *enfuvirtide* (B) <6 years: not established; 6-16 years: administer 2 mg/kg SC bid; max 90 mg SC bid; rotate injection sites
  Fuzeon *Vial:* 90 mg/ml pwdr for SC inj after reconstitution (1 ml, 60 vials/kit) (preservative-free)
- *maraviroc* (B) <16 years: not established; ≥16 years: must be administered concomitant with other retrovirals; *Concomitant potent CYP3A inhibitors (with or without a potent CYP3A inducer) including protease inhibitors (except* ***tipranavir+ritonavir),*** ***delavirdine, ketoconazole, itraconazole, clarithromycin,*** *other potent CYP3A inhibitors (e.g.,* ***nefazodone, telithromycin****): CrCl ≥30 mL/min:* 150 mg bid; *CrCl <30 mL/min, dialysis:* not recommended; *Potent CYP3A inducers (without a potent CYP3A inhibitor) including* ***efavirenz, rifampin, etravirine, carbamazepine, phenobarbital,*** *and* ***phenytoin****:* 300 mg bid*; CrCl ≥30 mL/min:* 600 mg bid; *<30 mL/min:* not recommended; *other concomitant agents, including* ***tipranavir+ritonavir, nevirapine, raltegravir,*** *all NRTIs, and* ***enfuvirtide****:* 300 mg bid
  Selzentry *Tab:* 150, 300 mg film-coat

BRAND NAMES, DOSING, AND DOSE FORMS: COMBINATION AGENTS

- **Atripla (B)** ***efavirenz+emtricitabine+tenofovir disoproxil fumarate*** *<12* years: not established; ≥12 years, ≥40 kg: 1 tablet once daily on an empty stomach; bedtime dosing may improve the tolerability of nervous system symptoms; *CrCl <50 mL/min:* not recommended
  Tab: efa 600 mg+emtri 200 mg+teno dis fum 300 mg film-coat
- **Combivir (C)(G)** ***lamivudine+zidovudine*** *<12* years: not recommended; ≥12 years, ≥30 kg: 1 tablet bid with food
  Tab: lami 150 mg+zido 300 mg
- **Complera (B)** ***emtricitabine+tenofovir disoproxil fumarate+rilpivirine*** <12 years, <40 kg: not recommended; ≥12 years, ≥40 kg: 1 tablet once daily; *CrCl <50 mL/min:* not recommended
  Tab: emtri 200 mg+teno dis 300 mg+rilpiv 25 mg
- **Descovy (D)** ***emtricitabine+tenofovir alafenamide*** <12 years, <35 kg: not recommended; ≥12 years, ≥35 kg: 1 tablet once daily with or without food; *CrCl <30 mL/min:* not recommended
  Tab: emtri 200 mg+teno ala 25 mg
  Comment: Patients with HIV-1 should be tested for the presence of chronic hepatitis B virus (HBV) before initiating antiretroviral therapy. **Descovy** is not approved for the treatment of chronic HBV infection, and the safety and efficacy of **Descovy** have not been established in patients co-infected with HIV-1 and HBV.
- **Epzicom (B)** ***abacavir sulfate+lamivudine*** <25 kg: use individual components; ≥25 kg: one tablet once daily; *Mild hepatic impairment or CrCl <50 mL/min:* not recommended
  Tab: aba 600 mg+lami 300 mg
- **Evotaz (B)** ***atazanavir+cobicistat*** <18 years: not established; ≥18 years: 1 tab once daily
  Tab: ataz 600 mg+cobi 300 mg
- **Genvoya (B)** ***elvitegravir+cobicistat+emtricitabine+tenofovir alafenamide*** *<12* years: not established; ≥12 years, ≥35 kg: 1 tab once daily; *Severe hepatic impairment or CrCl <30 mL/min:* not recommended; take with food
  Tab: elvi 150 mg+cobi 150 mg+emtri 200 mg+teno 10 mg
- **Kaletra, Kaletra Oral Solution(C)(G)** ***lopinavir+ritonavir*** dose calculation is based on the ***lopinavir*** component; <14 days: not recommended; 14 days-6 months: 16 mg/kg

bid; ≥6 months-12 years: [tablet/capsule/solution] 7-<15 kg: 12 mg/kg bid (13 mg/kg plus ***nevirapine***); 15-40 kg: 10 mg/kg bid (11 mg/kg plus ***nevirapine)***, >40 kg, >12 years: ***lopinavir*** 400 mg bid (533 mg plus ***nevirapine***); max ***lopinavir*** 400 mg bid for patients who are not receiving ***nevirapine*** or ***efavirenz;*** **Kaletra** should not be used in combination with NNRTIs in children <6 months-of-age; see mfr pkg insert for BSA-based dosing; swallow whole, do not crush or chew; take with or without food

Tab: **Kaletra 100/25** lopin 100 mg+riton 25 mg
Kaletra 200/50 lopin 200 mg+riton 50 mg *Oral soln:* lopin 80 mg+riton 20 mg per ml, lopin 400 mg+riton 500 mg per 5 ml (160 ml) (cotton candy) (alcohol 42.4%)

▶ **Odefsey (D)** ***emtricitabine+rilpivirine+tenofovir alafenamide*** <12 years, <35 kg: not established; ≥12 years: 1 tab once daily with food; *CrCl <30 mL/min:* not recommended

Tab: emtri 200 mg+rilpi 25 mg+teno alafen 25 mg

▶ **Prezcobix (C)** ***darunavir+cobicistat*** <18 years: not recommended; ≥18 years: 1 tab once daily; *Treatment-naïve and treatment-experienced with no* ***darunavir*** *resistance-associated substitution:* 800 mg once daily plus ***ritonavir*** 100 mg once daily; *Treatment-experienced with at least one* ***darunavir*** *resistance associated substitution:* 600 mg bid plus ***ritonavir*** 100 mg bid; take with food; *CrCl <70 mL/min:* not recommended

Tab: darun 800 mg+cobi 150 mg

▶ **Stribild (B)(G)** ***elvitegravir+cobicistat+emtricitabine+tenofovir disoproxil fumarate*** <18 years: not established; ≥18 years: 1 tab once daily; *CrCl <70 mL/min:* not recommended; *if CrCl declines to <50 mL/min during treatment:* discontinue; *Severe hepatic impairment:* not recommended

Tab: elvi 150 mg+cobi 150 mg+emtri 200 mg+teno dis fum 300 mg

▶ **Triumeq (C)(G)** ***abacavir sulfate+dolutegravir+lamivudine*** <18 years: not established; ≥18 years: 1 tab once daily

Tab: aba 600 mg+dolu 50 mg+lami 300 mg

▶ **Trizivir (C)(G)** ***abacavir sulfate+lamivudine+zidovudine*** <40 kg: not recommended; ≥40 kg: 1 tab bid

Tab: aba 300 mg+lami 150 mg+zido 300 mg

▶ **Truvada (B)(G)** ***emtricitabine+tenofovir disoproxil fumarate*** <17 kg: not established; 17-<22 kg: 100/150 once daily; 22-<28 kg: 133/200 once daily; 28-35 kg: 167/250 once daily; ≥35 kg: 200/300 once daily

Tab: **Truvada 100/150** emt 100 mg+teno 150 mg
Truvada 133/200 emt 133 mg+teno 200 mg
Truvada 167/250 emt 167 mg+teno 250 mg
Truvada 200/300 emt 200 mg+teno 300 mg

Comment: **Truvada** is indicated for treatment of HIV-1 infection and pre-exposure prophylaxis (PrEP) to reduce the risk of sexually acquired HIV-1 in persons at high risk for exposure, ≥18 years-of-age, in combination with safe sex practices.

HUMAN PAPILLOMAVIRUS (HPV, VENEREAL WART)

TREATMENT

see ***Wart: Venereal*** *page* 504

PROPHYLAXIS

Comment: *Administer IM in deltoid. Administer a 3-dose series; First dose:* females (10-25 years-of-age) and males (9-15 years-of-age); *Second dose:* 1-2 months after first dose; *Third dose:* 6 months after first dose. HPV vaccination is indicated for the prevention of cervical, vulvar, vaginal, and anal cancers. Register pregnant patients exposed to **Gardasil** by calling 1-800-986-8999.

- ***bivalent human papillomavirus types 16 and 18 vaccine, aluminum adsorbed*** (B) <10 years: not applicable; ≥10 years: administer in the deltoid; 1st dose 0.5 ml IM on elected date; then, 2nd dose 0.5 ml IM 1 month later; then, 3rd dose 0.5 ml IM 6 months after the first dose (5 months after 2nd dose)
  Cervarix *Vial:* susp for IM inj (single-dose; prefilled syringe) (preservative-free)
- ***quadrivalent human papillomavirus types 6, 11, 16, and 18 vaccine, recombinant, aluminum adsorbed*** (B) <9 years: not applicable; ≥9 years: administer in the deltoid or upper thigh; 1st dose 0.5 ml IM on elected date; then, 2nd dose 0.5 ml IM 2 months later; then, 3rd dose 0.5 ml IM 6 months after the first dose (4 months after 2nd dose)
  Gardasil *Vial:* susp for IM inj (single-dose; prefilled syringe w. needles or tip caps) (preservative-free)
- ***quadrivalent human papillomavirus types 6, 11, 16, 18, 31, 33, 45, 52, and 58 vaccine, recombinant, aluminum adsorbed*** (B) <9 years: not applicable; 9-26 years-of-age: administer in the deltoid or thigh; 1st dose 0.5 ml IM on elected date; then, 2nd dose 0.5 ml IM 2 months later; then, 3rd dose 0.5 ml IM 6 months after the 1st dose (4 months after 2nd dose)
  Gardasil 9 *Vial:* susp for IM inj (0.5 ml single-dose; prefilled syringe w. needles or tip caps) (preservative-free)

HYPEREMESIS GRAVIDARUM: NAUSEA/VOMITING OF PREGNANCY

ANTIHISTAMINE+VITAMIN B ANALOG

- ***doxylamine succinate+pyridoxine hydrochloride*** <18 years: not established; ≥18 years: one tab at HS prn; if symptoms are not adequately controlled, the dose can be increased to max one tablet in the AM and one tab at HS
  Bonjesta *Tab:* doxy 20 mg+pyri 20 mg ext-rel

Comment: **Bonjesta** is indicated for nausea/vomiting of pregnancy in women who do not respond to conservative management. Somnolence (severe drowsiness) can occur when used in combination with alcohol or other sedating medications. Use with caution in patients with asthma, increased intraocular pressure, narrow angle glaucoma, stenosing peptic ulcer, pyloroduodenal obstruction and urinary bladder-neck obstruction.

HYPERHIDROSIS (PERSPIRATION, EXCESSIVE)

Comment: Hyperhidrosis is a common, self-limiting problem that affects 2% to3% of the US population. Patients may complain of localized sweating of the hands, feet, face, or axillae or more systemic, generalized sweating in multiple locations and report a significant impact on their quality of life.

REFERENCE

Varella, AY, Fukuda, JM, Telvelis, MP, *et al.* (2016). Translation and validation of Hyperhidrosis Disease Severity Scale. *Revista Da Associação Médica Brasileira, 62*(9), 843–847.

- ***aluminum chloride*** 20% solution apply q HS; wash treated area the following morning; after 1-2 treatments, may reduce frequency to 1-2 x/week
  Drysol *Soln:* 35, 60 ml (alcohol 93%) cont-rel

Comment: Apply to clean dry skin (e.g., underarms). Do not apply to broken, irritated, or recently shaved skin.

ANTICHOLINERGIC

Comment: ***oxybutynin***, a cholinergic antagonist commonly prescribed for overactive bladder, is the first oral agent to emerge as a treatment option for hyperhidrosis.

REFERENCES

Scholhammer, M, Brenaut, E, Menard-Andivot, N, *et al.* (2015). Oxybutynin as a treatment for generalized hyperhidrosis: a randomized, placebo-controlled trial. *British Journal of Dermatology, 173*(5), 1163–1168.

Wolosker, N, de Campos, JR, Kauffman, P, *et al.* (2012). A randomized placebo-controlled trial of oxybutynin for the initial treatment of palmar and axillary hyperhidrosis. *Journal of Vascular Surgery, 55*(6), 1696–1700.

▶ ***oxybutynin chloride*** **(B)**

Ditropan <5 years: not recommended; 5-12 years: 5 mg bid; max 15 mg/day; ≥16 years: 5 mg bid-tid; max 20 mg/day

Tab: 5*mg; *Syr:* 5 mg/5 ml

Ditropan XL <6 years: not recommended; ≥6-12 years: initially 5 mg once daily; may increase weekly in 5 mg increments as needed; max 20 mg/day; **>12 years:** initially 5 mg daily; may increase weekly in 5-mg increments as needed; max 30 mg/day

Tab: 5, 10, 15 mg ext-rel

GelniQUE 3 mg Pump *Pump:* <14 years: not recommended; ≥14 years: apply 3 pumps (84 mg) once daily to clean dry intact skin on the abdomen, upper arm, shoulders, or thighs; rotate sites; wash hands; avoid washing application site for 1 hour after application

Gel: 3% (92 gm, metered pump dispenser) (alcohol)

GelniQUE 1 gm Sachet apply 1 gm gel (1 sachet) once daily to dry intact skin on abdomen, upper arms/shoulders, or thighs; rotate sites; wash hands; avoid washing application site for 1 hour after application

Gel: 10%, 1 gm/sachet (30/carton) (alcohol)

Oxytrol Transdermal Patch (OTC) <14 years: not recommended; ≥14 years: apply patch to clean dry area of the abdomen, hip, or buttock; one patch twice weekly; rotate sites

Transdermal patch: 3.9 mg/day

HYPERHOMOCYSTEINEMIA

Comment: Elevated homocysteine is associated with cognitive impairment, vascular dementia, and dementia of the Alzheimer's type.

HOMOCYSTEINE-LOWERING NUTRITIONAL SUPPLEMENTS

▶ ***L-methylfolate calcium (as metafolin)+pyridoxyl 5-phosphate+methyl****cobalamin* <12 years: not recommended; ≥12 years: take 1 cap daily

Metanx *Cap:* metafo 3 mg+pyrid 35 mg+methyl 2 mg (gluten-free, yeast-free, lactose-free)

Comment: **Metanx** is indicated as adjunct treatment of endothelial dysfunction and/or hyperhomocysteinemia in patients who have lower extremity ulceration.

▶ ***L-methylfolate calcium (as metafolin)+methylcobalamin+n-acetylcysteine*** <12 years: not recommended; ≥12 years: take 1 cap daily

Cerefolin *Cap:* metafo 5.6 mg+methyl 2 mg+n-ace 600 mg (gluten-free, yeast-free, lactose-free)

Comment: **Cerefolin** is indicated in the dietary management of patients treated for early memory loss, with emphasis on those at risk for neurovascular oxidative stress, hyperhomocysteinemia, mild to moderate cognitive impairment with or without vitamin B12 deficiency, vascular dementia, or Alzheimer's disease.

HYPERKALEMIA

HYPERKALEMIA CATION EXCHANGE RESINS

Comment: Normal serum K^+ range is approximately 3.5-5.5 mEq/L. Hyperkalemia is associated with cardiac dysrhythmias and metabolic acidosis. Risk factors include kidney disease, heart failure, and drugs that inhibit the renin-angiotensin-aldosterone system (RAAS) including ACEIs, ARBs, direct renin inhibitors, and aldosterone antagonists. Cation exchange resins are not for emergency treatment of life-threatening hyperkalemia, severe constipation, bowel obstruction or impaction. May cause GI irritability, ulceration, necrosis, sodium retention, hypocalcemia, hypomagnesemia, fecal impaction, ischemic colitis. Avoid non-absorbable cation-donating antacids and laxatives (e.g., ***magnesium hydroxide, aluminum hydroxide***). Concomitant sorbitol should be avoided because it may cause intestinal necrosis.

▶ ***patiromer sorbitex calcium*** **(B)** <18 years: not established; ≥18 years: initially 8.4 gm once daily; adjust dosage as prescribed based on potassium concentration and target range; may increase dosage at 1-week (or longer) intervals in increments of 8.4 gm; max dose 25.2 gm once daily; prepare immediately prior to administration; do not take in dry form; administer or without food; measure 1/3 cup of water and pour half into a glass; then add **Veltassa** and stir; add the remaining water and stir well; the powder will not dissolve and the mixture will look cloudy; add more water as needed for desired consistency; do not heat or mix with heated food or fluids

Veltassa *Pkt:* 8, 4, 16.8, 25.2 gm pwdr for oral susp, 30 single-use pkts/carton

Comment: Take **Veltassa** at least 3 hours before or 3 hours after any other medicine taken by mouth. Store packets in the refrigerator. It stored at room temperature, product must be used within 3 months.

▶ ***sodium polystyrene sulfonate*** **(C)(G)** Use 1 gm/1 mEq of K^+ as basis of calculation; see mfr literature

Kayexalate *Susp:* 15 gm 1-4 times daily; *Rectal Enema:* 30-50 gm in 100 ml every 6 hours

HYPERPARATHYROIDISM

▶ ***calcifediol*** **(C)(G)** <18 years: not established; ≥18 years: 1 cap daily

Rayaldee *Cap:* 30 mcg ext-rel

Comment: **Rayaldee** is indicated for the prevention and treatment of secondary hyperparathyroidism associated with chronic kidney disease (CKD), stage 3 or 4 and serum total 25-hydroxyvitamin D levels <30 mg/ml.

▶ ***paricalcitol*** **(C)(G)** <18 years: not established; ≥18 years: administer 0.04-1 mcg/kg (2.8-7 mcg) IV bolus, during dialysis, no more than every other day; may be increased by 2-4 mcg every 2-4 weeks; monitor serum calcium and phosphorus during dose adjustment periods; if Ca x P >75, immediately reduce dose or discontinue until these levels normalize; discard unused portion of single-use vials immediately

Zemplar *Vial:* 2, 5 mcg/ml soln for inj

Comment: **Zemplar** is indicated for the prevention and treatment of secondary hyperparathyroidism associated with chronic kidney disease, stage 5.

HYPERPHOSPHATEMIA

PHOSPHATE BINDERS

Comment: Monitor for development of hypercalcemia. Normal serum PO_4^- is 2.5-4.5 mg/dL and normal serum calcium is 8.5-10.5 mg/dL.

- ***calcium acetate*** (C)(G) <12 years: not established; ≥12 years: initially 2 tabs or caps with each meal; then, titrate gradually to keep serum phosphate at <6 mg/dL; usual maintenance is 3-4 tabs or caps with each meal
  - **PhosLo** *Tab:* 667 mg; *Cap:* 667 mg
- ***lanthanum carbonate*** (C)(G) <12 years: not established; ≥12 years: initially 750 mg to 1.5 gm per day in divided doses; take with meals; titrate at 2-3-week intervals in increments of 750 mg/day based on serum phosphate; usual range 1.5-3 gm/day; usual max 3,750 mg/day
  - **Fosrenol** *Chew tab:* 250, 500, 750 mg; 1 g
- ***sevelamer*** (C)(G) <12 years: not recommended; ≥12 years: for patients not taking a phosphate binder, take tid with meals; swallow whole; titrate by 1 tab per meal at 1 week intervals to keep serum phosphorus 3.5-5.5 mg/dL; switching from calcium acetate to ***sevelamer***, see mfr pkg insert. *Serum phosphorus* >5.5 to >7.5 mg/dL: 800 mg tid; *Serum phosphorus* 7.5-9: 1.2-1.6 gm tid
  - **Renagel** *Tab:* 400, 800 mg
  - **Renvela** *Tab:* 800 mg

HYPERPIGMENTATION

Comment: De-pigmenting agents may be used for hyperpigmented skin conditions including chloasma, melasma, freckles, senile lentigines. Limit treatments to small areas at one time. Sunscreen ≥30 SPF recommended.

- ***hydroquinone*** (C)(G) apply sparingly to affected area and rub in bid
  - **Lustra** *Crm:* 4% (1, 2 oz) (sulfites)
  - **Lustra AF** *Crm:* 4% (1, 2 oz) (sunscreen, sulfites)
- ***monobenzone*** (C) apply sparingly to affected area and rub in bid-tid; depigmentation occurs in 1-4 months
  - **Benoquin** *Crm:* 20% (1.25 oz)
- ***tazarotene*** (X)(G) <12 years: not recommended; ≥12 years: apply daily at HS
  - **Avage Cream** *Crm:* 0.1% (30 gm)
  - **Tazorac Cream** *Crm:* 0.05, 0.1% (15, 30, 60 gm)
  - **Tazorac Gel** *Gel:* 0.05, 0.1% (30, 100 gm)
- ***tretinoin*** (C)(G) <12 years: not recommended; ≥12 years: apply daily at HS
  - **Atralin Gel** *Gel:* 0.05% (45 gm)
  - **Avita** *Crm:* 0.025% (20, 45 gm); *Gel:* 0.025% (20, 45 gm)
  - **Renova** *Crm:* 0.02% (40 gm); 0.05% (40, 60 gm)
  - **Renova** *Crm:* 0.02% (40 gm); 0.05% (40, 60 gm)
  - **Retin-A Cream** *Crm:* 0.025, 0.05, 0.1% (20, 45 gm)
  - **Retin-A Gel** *Gel:* 0.01, 0.025% (15, 45 gm) (alcohol 90%)
  - **Retin-A Liquid** *Soln:* 0.05% (alcohol 55%)
  - **Retin-A Micro Gel** *Gel:* 0.04, 0.08, 0.1% (20, 45 gm)
  - **Tretin-X Cream** *Crm:* 0.075% (35 gm) (parabens-free, alcohol-free, propylene glycol-free)
  - **Retin-A Micro** *Microspheres:* 0.04, 0.1% (20, 45 gm)

COMBINATION AGENTS

▶ ***hydroquinone+fluocinolone+tretinoin*** (C) <12 years: not recommended; ≥12 years: apply sparingly to affected area and rub in daily at HS

Tri-Luma *Crm:* hydro 4%+fluo 0.01%+tretin 0.05% (30 gm) (parabens, sulfites)

▶ ***hydroquinone+padimate o+oxybenzone+octyl methoxycinnamate*** (C) <12 years: not recommended; ≥12 years: apply sparingly to affected area and rub in bid

Glyquin *Crm:* 4% (1 oz jar)

▶ ***hydroquinone+ethyl dihydroxypropyl PABA+dioxybenzone+oxybenzone*** (C) <12 years: not recommended; ≥12 years: apply sparingly to affected area and rub in bid; max 2 months

Solaquin *Crm:* hydro 2%+PABA 5%+dioxy 3%+oxy 2% (1 oz) (sulfites)

▶ ***hydroquinone+padimate+dioxybenzone+oxybenzone*** (C) <12 years: not recommended; ≥12 years: apply sparingly to affected area and rub in bid; max 2 months

Solaquin Forte *Crm:* hydro 4%+pad 0.5%+dioxy 3%+oxy 2% (1 oz) (sunscreen, sulfites)

▶ ***hydroquinone+padimate+dioxybenzone*** (C) <12 years: not recommended; ≥12 years: apply sparingly to affected area and rub in bid; max 2 months

Solaquin Forte Gel: hydro 4%+pad 0.5%+dioxy 3% (1 oz) (alcohol, sulfites)

HYPERPROLACTINEMIA

DOPAMINE RECEPTOR AGONIST

▶ ***dostinex*** (B)(G) <12 years: not established; ≥12 years: initial therapy is 0.25 mg twice a week; may increase by 0.25 mg twice weekly up to 1 mg twice a week according to the patient's serum prolactin level; dose increases should not occur more than every 4 weeks; after a normal serum prolactin level has been maintained for 6 months, may be discontinued, with periodic monitoring of serum prolactin level to determine if/when treatment should be reinstituted

Cabergoline *Tab:* 0.5 mg

Comment: **Cabergoline** is indicated to treat hyperprolactinemia disorders due to idiopathic or pituitary adenoma.

HYPERTENSION: PRIMARY, ESSENTIAL

see JNC-8 Recommendations page 516

BETA-BLOCKERS (CARDIOSELECTIVE)

Comment: Cardioselective beta-blockers are less likely to cause bronchospasm, peripheral vasoconstriction, or hypoglycemia than non-cardioselective beta-blockers.

▶ ***acebutolol*** (B)(G) <12 years: not recommended; ≥12 years: initially 400 mg in 1-2 divided doses; usual range 200-800 mg/day; max 1.2 gm/day in 2 divided doses

Sectral *Cap:* 200, 400 mg

▶ ***atenolol*** (D)(G) <12 years: not recommended; ≥12 years: initially 50 mg daily; may increase after 1-2 weeks to 100 mg daily; max 100 mg/day

Tenormin *Tab:* 25, 50, 100 mg

▶ ***betaxolol*** (C) <12 years: not recommended; ≥12 years: initially 10 mg daily; may increase to 20 mg/day after 7-14 days; usual max 20 mg/day

Kerlone *Tab:* 10*, 20 mg

- ▶ ***bisoprolol*** (C) <12 years: not recommended; ≥12 years: 5 mg daily; max 20 mg daily
  - **Zebeta** *Tab:* 5*, 10 mg
- ▶ ***metoprolol succinate*** (C)(G) <12 years: not recommended; ≥12 years: initially 12.5-25 mg in a single dose daily; increase weekly if needed; reduce if symptomatic bradycardia occurs; max 400 mg/day
  - **Toprol-XL** *Tab:* 25*, 50*, 100*, 200*mg ext-rel
- ▶ ***metoprolol tartrate*** (C)(G) <12 years: not recommended; ≥12 years: initially 25-50 mg bid; increase weekly if needed; max 400 mg/day
  - **Lopressor** *Tab:* 25, 37.5, 50, 75, 100 mg
- ▶ ***nebivolol*** (C)(G) <12 years: not recommended; ≥12 years: initially 5 mg daily; may increase at 2 week intervals; max 40 mg/day
  - **Bystolic** *Tab:* 2.5, 5, 10, 20 mg

BETA-BLOCKERS (NON-CARDIOSELECTIVE)

Comment: Non-cardioselective beta-blockers are more likely to cause bronchospasm, peripheral vasoconstriction, <u>and/or</u> hypoglycemia than cardioselective beta-blockers.

- ▶ ***nadolol*** (C)(G) <12 years: not recommended; ≥12 years: initially 40 mg daily; usual maintenance 40-80 mg daily; max 320 mg/day
  - **Corgard** *Tab:* 20*, 40*, 80*, 120*, 160*mg
- ▶ ***penbutolol*** (C) <12 years: not recommended; ≥12 years: 20 mg once daily
  - **Levatol** *Tab:* 20*mg
- ▶ ***pindolol*** (B)(G) <12 years: not recommended; ≥12 years: initially 5 mg bid; may increase after 3-4 weeks in 10 mg increments; max 60 mg/day
  - **Pindolol** *Tab:* 5, 10 mg
  - **Visken** *Tab:* 5, 10 mg
- ▶ ***propranolol*** (C)(G)
  - **Inderal** <12 years: initially 1 mg/kg/day; usual range 2-4 mg/kg/day in 2 divided doses; max 16 mg/kg/day; ≥12 years: initially 40 mg bid; usual maintenance 120-240 mg/day; max 640 mg/day
    - *Tab:* 10*, 20*, 40*, 60*, 80*mg
  - **Inderal LA** <12 years: not recommended; ≥12 years: initially 80 mg daily in a single dose; increase q 3-7 days; usual range 120-160 mg/day; max 320 mg/day in a single dose
    - *Cap:* 60, 80, 120, 160 mg sust-rel
  - **InnoPran XL** <12 years: not recommended; ≥12 years: initially 80 mg q HS; max 120 mg/day
    - *Cap:* 80, 120 mg ext-rel
- ▶ ***timolol*** (C)(G) <12 years: not recommended; ≥12 years: initially 10 mg bid; increase weekly if needed; usual maintenance 20-40 mg/day; max 60 mg/day in 2 divided doses
  - **Blocadren** *Tab:* 5, 10*, 20*mg

BETA-BLOCKER (NON-CARDIOSELECTIVE)+ALPHA-1 BLOCKER COMBINATIONS

- ▶ ***carvedilol*** (C)
  - **Coreg** <1 years: not recommended; ≥1 years: initially 6.25 mg bid; may increase at 1-2-week intervals to 12.5 mg bid; max 25 mg bid
    - *Tab:* 3.125, 6.25, 12.5, 25 mg
  - **Coreg CR** <18 years: not recommended; ≥18 years: initially 20 mg once daily for 2 weeks; may increase at 1-2-week intervals; max 80 mg once daily
    - *Tab:* 10, 20, 40, 80 mg cont-rel

▶ *carteolol* (C) <12 years: not recommended; ≥12 years: initially 2.5 mg daily, gradually increase to 5 or 10 mg daily; usual maintenance 2.5-5 mg daily
Cartrol
Tab: 2.5, 5 mg
▶ *labetalol* (C)(G) <12 years: not recommended; ≥12 years: initially 100 mg bid; increase after 2-3 days if needed; usual maintenance 200-400 mg bid; max 2.4 gm/day
Normodyne *Tab:* 100*, 200*, 300 mg
Trandate *Tab:* 100*, 200*, 300*mg

DIURETICS

Thiazide Diuretics

▶ *chlorthalidone* (B)(G) <12 years: not established; ≥12 years: initially 15 mg daily; may increase to 30 mg once daily based on clinical response; max 45-60 mg/day
Chlorthalidone *Tab:* 25, 50 mg **Thalitone** *Tab:* 15 mg
▶ *chlorothiazide* (B)(G) <6 months: up to 15 mg/lb/day in 2 divided doses; ≥6 months-<12 years: 10 mg/lb/day in 2 divided doses; ≥12 0.5-1 gm/day in a single or divided doses; max 2 gm/day
Diuril *Tab:* 250*, 500*mg; *Oral susp:* 250 mg/5 ml (237 ml)
▶ *hydrochlorothiazide* (B)(G)
Esidrix <12 years: not recommended; ≥12 years: 25 mg once daily; usual max 100 mg/day 25-100 mg once daily
Tab: 25, 50, 100 mg
Hydrochlorothiazide <12 years: not recommended; ≥12 years: 12.5 mg once daily; usual max 50 mg/day
Tab: 25*, 50*mg
Microzide <12 years: not recommended; ≥12 years: 12.5 mg once daily; usual max 50 mg/day
Cap: 12.5 mg
▶ *polythiazide* (C) <12 years: not recommended; ≥12 years: 2-4 mg once daily
Renese *Tab:* 1, 2, 4 mg

Potassium-Sparing Diuretics

▶ *amiloride* (B)(C) <12 years: not recommended; ≥12 years: initially 5 mg; may increase to 10 mg; max 20 mg
Midamor *Tab:* 5 mg
▶ *spironolactone* (D) <12 years: not recommended; ≥12 years: initially 50-100 mg in a single or divided doses; titrate at 2-week intervals
Aldactone (G) *Tab:* 25, 50*, 100*mg
CaroSpir *Oral susp:* 25 mg/5 ml (118, 473 ml) (banana)
▶ *triamterene* (B) <12 years: not recommended; ≥12 years: 100 mg bid; max 300 mg
Dyrenium *Cap:* 50, 100 mg

Loop Diuretics

▶ *bumetanide* (C)(G) <18 years: not recommended; ≥18 years: 0.5-2 mg daily; may repeat at 4-5-hour intervals; max 10 mg/day
Bumex *Tab:* 0.5*, 1*, 2*mg
Comment: ***bumetanide*** is contraindicated with sulfa drug allergy.
▶ *ethacrynic acid* (B)(G) ≤1 month: not recommended; >1 month-12 years: initially 25 mg/day; then adjust dose in 25 mg increments; >12 years: max 50-200 mg once daily
Edecrin *Tab:* 25, 50 mg

- ***ethacrynate sodium*** **(B)(G)** <1 month: not recommended; ≥1 month-12 years: use the smallest effective dose; initially 25 mg; then careful stepwise increments in dosage of 25 mg to achieve effective maintenance; ≥12 years: administer smallest dose required to produce gradual weight loss (about 1-2 pounds per day); onset of diuresis usually occurs at 50-100 mg in children ≥12 years; after diuresis has been achieved, the minimally effective dose (usually 50-200 mg/day) may be administered on a continuous or intermittent dosage schedule; dose titrations are usually in 25-50 mg increments to avoid derangement electrolyte and water excretion; the patient should be weighed under standard conditions before and during administration of ***ethacrynate sodium;*** the following schedule may be helpful in determining the lowest effective dose; *Day 1:* 50 mg once daily after a meal; *Day 2:* 50 mg bid after meals, if necessary; *Day 3:* 100 mg in the morning and 50-100 mg following the afternoon or evening meal, depending upon response to the morning dose; a few patients may require initial and maintenance doses as high as 200 mg bid; these higher doses, which should be achieved gradually, are most often required in patients with severe, refractory edema

    Sodium Edecrin *Vial:* 50 mg single-dose

    Comment: **Sodium Edecrin** is more potent than more commonly used loop and thiazide diuretics. Treatment of the edema associated with congestive heart failure, cirrhosis of the liver, and renal disease, including the nephrotic syndrome, short-term management of ascites due to malignancy, idiopathic edema, and lymphedema, short-term management of hospitalized pediatric patients, other than infants, with congenital heart disease or the nephrotic syndrome. IV **Sodium Edecrin** is indicated when a rapid onset of diuresis is desired, for example, in acute pulmonary edema or when gastrointestinal absorption is impaired or oral medication is not practical.

- ***furosemide*** **(C)(G)** <12 years: not recommended; ≥12 years: initially 40 mg bid

    Lasix *Tab:* 20, 40*, 80 mg; *Oral Soln:* 10 mg/ml (2, 4 oz w. dropper)

  Comment: ***furosemide*** is contraindicated with sulfa drug allergy.

- ***torsemide*** **(B)** <12 years: not recommended; ≥12 years: 5 mg once daily; may increase to 10 mg once daily

    Demadex *Tab:* 5*, 10*, 20*, 100*mg

Other Diuretics

- ***indapamide*** **(B)** <12 years: not recommended; ≥12 years: initially 1.25 mg once daily; may titrate dosage upward q 4 weeks if needed; max 5 mg/day

    Lozol *Tab:* 1.25, 2.5 mg

  Comment: ***indapamide*** is contraindicated with sulfa drug allergy.

- ***metolazone*** **(B)** <12 years: not recommended; ≥12 years: 2.5-5 mg qd

    Zaroxolyn *Tab:* 2.5, 5, 10 mg

  Comment: ***metolazone*** is contraindicated with sulfa drug allergy.

DIURETIC COMBINATIONS

- ***amiloride+hydrochlorothiazide*** **(B)(G)** <12 years: not recommended; ≥12 years: initially 1 tab daily; may increase to 2 tabs/day in a single or divided doses

    Moduretic *Tab:* amil 5 mg+hctz 50 mg*

- ***spironolactone+hydrochlorothiazide*** **(D)(G)**

    Aldactazide 25 <12 years: not recommended; ≥12 years: usual maintenance 50-100 mg in a single or divided doses

        Tab: spiro 25 mg+hctz 25 mg

    Aldactazide 50 <12 years: not recommended; ≥12 years: usual maintenance 50-100 mg in a single or divided doses

        Tab: spiro 50 mg+hctz 50 mg

▶ ***triamterene+hydrochlorothiazide*** **(C)(G)**

Dyazide <12 years: not recommended; ≥12 years: 1-2 caps once daily

Cap: triam 37.5 mg+hctz 25 mg

Maxzide <12 years: not recommended; ≥12 years: 1 tab once daily

Tab: triam 75 mg+hctz 50 mg*

Maxzide-25 <12 years: not recommended; ≥12 years: 1-2 tabs once daily

Tab: triam 37.5 mg+hctz 25 mg*

ANGIOTENSIN CONVERTING ENZYME INHIBITORS (ACEIs)

Comment: Black patients receiving ACEI monotherapy have been reported to have a higher incidence of angioedema compared to non-Blacks. Non-Blacks have a greater decrease in BP when ACEIs are used compared to Black patients.

▶ ***benazepril*** **(D)(G)** <12 years: not recommended; ≥12 years: initially 10 mg daily; usual maintenance 20-40 mg/day in 1-2 divided doses; usual max 80 mg/day

Lotensin *Tab:* 5, 10, 20, 40 mg

▶ ***captopril*** **(D)(G)** <12 years: not recommended; ≥12 years: initially 25 mg bid-tid; after 1-2 weeks increase to 50 mg bid-tid

Capoten *Tab:* 12.5*, 25*, 50*, 100*mg

▶ ***enalapril*** **(D)** <12 years: not recommended; ≥12 years: initially 5 mg daily; usual dosage range 10-40 mg/day; max 40 mg/day

Epaned Oral Solution *Oral soln:* 1 mg/ml (150 ml) (mixed berry)

Vasotec (G) *Tab:* 2.5*, 5*, 10, 20 mg

▶ ***fosinopril*** **(D)** <6 years, <50 kg: not recommended; ≥6-12 years, >50 kg: 5-10 mg once daily; ≥12 years: initially 10 mg daily; usual maintenance 20-40 mg/day in a single <u>or</u> divided doses; max 80 mg/day

Monopril *Tab:* 10*, 20, 40 mg

▶ ***lisinopril*** **(D)**

Prinivil <6 years, <50 kg: not recommended; ≥6-12 years: initially 10 mg once daily; usual range 20-40 mg/day

Tab: 5*, 10*, 20*, 40 mg

Qbrelis Oral Solution <6 years, GFR <30 mL/min: not recommended; ≥6-12 years, GFR >30 mL/min: initially 0.07 mg/kg, max 5 mg; adjust according to BP up to a max 0.61 mg/kg (40 mg) once daily; administer as a single dose once daily

Oral soln: 1 mg/ml (150 ml)

Zestril <12 years: not recommended; ≥12 years: initially 10 mg daily; usual range 20-40 mg/day

Tab: 2.5, 5*, 10, 20, 30, 40 mg

▶ ***moexipril*** **(D)** <12 years: not recommended; ≥12 years: initially 7.5 mg daily; usual range 15-30 mg/day in 1-2 divided doses; max 30 mg/day

Univasc *Tab:* 7.5*, 15*mg

▶ ***perindopril*** **(D)** <12 years: not recommended; ≥12 years: 2-8 mg daily-bid; max 16 mg/day

Aceon *Tab:* 2*, 4*, 8*mg

▶ ***quinapril*** **(D)** <12 years: not recommended; ≥12 years: initially 10 mg once daily; usual maintenance 20-80 mg daily in 1-2 divided doses

Accupril *Tab:* 5*, 10, 20, 40 mg

▶ ***ramipril*** **(D)(G)** <12 years: not recommended; ≥12 years: initially 2.5 mg bid; usual maintenance 2.5-20 mg in 1-2 divided doses

Altace *Tab/Cap:* 1.25, 2.5, 5, 10 mg

▶ ***trandolapril*** **(C; D in 2nd, 3rd)** <12 years: not recommended; ≥12 years: initially 1-2 mg once daily; adjust at 1-week intervals; usual range 2-4 mg in 1-2 divided doses; max 8 mg/day

Mavik *Tab:* 1*, 2, 4 mg

ANGIOTENSIN II RECEPTOR BLOCKERS (ARBs)

- ***azilsartan medoxomil*** (D) <12 years: not recommended; ≥12 years: *Monotherapy, not volume depleted:* 80 mg once daily; *Volume-depleted (concomitant high-dose diuretic):* initially 40 mg once daily
- **Edarbi** *Tab:* 40, 80 mg***candesartan*** (D)(G) <12 years: not recommended; ≥12 years: initially 16 mg daily; range 8-32 mg in 1-2 divided doses
  Atacand *Tab:* 4, 8, 16, 32 mg
- ***eprosartan*** (D)(G) <12 years: not recommended; ≥12 years: initially 400 mg bid or 600 mg once daily; max 800 mg/day
  Teveten *Tab:* 400, 600 mg
- ***irbesartan*** (D)(G) <12 years: not recommended; ≥12 years: initially 150 mg daily; titrate up to 300 mg
  Avapro *Tab:* 75, 150, 300 mg
- ***losartan*** (D)(G) <12 years: not recommended; ≥12 years: initially 50 mg daily; max 100 mg/day
  Cozaar *Tab:* 25, 50, 100 mg
- ***olmesartan medoxomil*** (D)(G) <6 years: not recommended; ≥6-16 years: 20-35 kg: initially 10 mg once daily; after 2 weeks, may increase to max 20 mg once daily; ≥6-16 years: >35 kg: initially 20 mg once daily; after 2 weeks, may increase to max 40 mg once daily; ≥16 years: initially 20 mg once daily; after 2 weeks, may increase to 40 mg once daily
  Benicar *Tab:* 5, 20, 40 mg
- ***telmisartan*** (D)(G) <12 years: not recommended; ≥12 years: initially 40 mg once daily
  Micardis *Tab:* 20, 40, 80 mg
- ***valsartan*** (C; **D in 2nd, 3rd**) (G) <6 years: not recommended; ≥6-16 years: initially 0.65 mg/kg bid; max 40 mg/day; dose range 0.65-1.35 mg/kg bid; max 40-160 mg/day; ≥17 years: initially 40-80 mg bid; *Target maintenance dose:* increase dose as tolerated or after 2-4 weeks to 160 mg bid
  Diovan *Tab:* 40*, 80, 160, 320 mg
  Prexxartan *Oral soln:* **20mg/5 ml; 80/20 ml;** 120, 473 ml; 20 ml unit-dose cup
  Comment: ***Post-myocardial infarction:*** <6 years: not recommended; ≥6-16 years: initially 0.65 mg/kg bid; max 20 mg/day; dose range 0.65-1.35 mg/kg bid; max 40-160 mg/day; ≥17 years: initially 40-80 mg bid; *Target maintenance*

CALCIUM CHANNEL BLOCKERS (CCBs)

Benzothiazepines

- ***diltiazem*** (C)(G)
  Cardizem <12 years: not established; ≥12 years: initially 30 mg qid; may increase gradually every 1-2 days; max 360 mg/day in divided doses
  Tab: 30, 60, 90, 120 mg
  Cardizem CD <12 years: not established; ≥12 years: initially 120-180 mg daily; adjust at 1-2-week intervals; max 480 mg/day
  Cap: 120, 180, 240, 300, 360 mg ext-rel
  Cardizem LA <12 years: not established; ≥12 years: initially 180-240 mg daily; titrate at 2-week intervals; max 540 mg/day
  Tab: 120, 180, 240, 300, 360, 420 mg ext-rel
  Cardizem SR <12 years: not established; ≥12 years: initially 60-120 mg bid; adjust at 2-week intervals; max 360 mg/day
  Cap: 60, 90, 120 mg sust-rel
  Cartia XT <12 years: not established; ≥12 years: initially 180 or 240 mg once daily; max 540 mg once daily
  Cap: 120, 180, 240, 300 mg ext-rel

Dilacor XR <12 years: not established; ≥12 years: initially 180 or 240 mg in AM; usual range 180-480 mg/day; max 540 mg/day

Cap: 120, 180, 240 mg ext-rel

Tiazac (G) <12 years: not established; ≥12 years: initially 120-240 mg daily; adjust at 2-week intervals; usual max 540 mg/day

Cap: 120, 180, 240, 300, 360, 420 mg ext-rel

▶ ***diltiazem maleate*** **(C)** <12 years: not recommended; ≥12 years: initially 120-180 mg daily; adjust at 2-week intervals; usual range 120-480 mg daily

Tiamate *Cap:* 120, 180, 240 mg ext-rel

Dihydropyridines

▶ ***amlodipine*** **(C)** <12 years: not established; ≥12 years: initially 5 mg once daily; max 10 mg/day

Norvasc *Tab:* 2.5, 5, 10 mg

▶ ***clevidipine butyrate*** **(C)** <18 years: not recommended; ≥18 years: administer by IV infusion; initially 1-2 mg/hour; double dose at 90-second intervals until BP approaches goal; then titrate slower; adjust at 5-10-minute intervals; maintenance 4-6 mg/hour; usual max, 16-32 mg/hour; do not exceed 1,000 ml (21 mg/hour for 24 hours) due to lipid load

Cleviprex *Vial:* 0.5 mg/ml soln for IV infusion (single use, 50, 100 ml) (lipids)

Comment: **Cleviprex** is indicated to reduce blood pressure when oral therapy is not feasible or desirable. **Cleviprex** is contraindicated with egg or soy allergy.

▶ ***felodipine*** **(C)(G)** <12 years: not recommended; ≥12 years: initially 5 mg daily; usual range 2.5-10 mg daily; adjust at 2-week intervals; max 10 mg/day

Plendil *Tab:* 2.5, 5, 10 mg ext-rel

▶ ***isradipine*** **(C)**

DynaCirc <12 years: not recommended; ≥12 years: initially 2.5 mg bid; adjust in increments of 5 mg/day at 2-4-week intervals; max 20 mg/day

Cap: 2.5, 5 mg

DynaCirc CR <12 years: not recommended; ≥12 years: initially 5 mg daily; adjust in increments of 5 mg/day at 2-4-week intervals; max 20 mg/day

Tab: 5, 10 mg cont-rel

▶ ***nicardipine*** **(C)(G)**

Cardene <18 years: not recommended; ≥18 years: initially 20 mg tid; adjust at intervals of at least 3 days; max 120 mg/day

Cap: 20, 30 mg

Cardene SR <12 years: not recommended; ≥12 years: 30-60 mg bid

Cap: 30, 45, 60 mg sust-rel

▶ ***nifedipine*** **(C)(G)**

Adalat <12 years: not recommended; ≥12 years: initially 10 mg tid; usual range 10-20 mg tid; max 180 mg/day

Cap: 10, 20 mg

Adalat CC <12 years: not recommended; ≥12 years: initially 10 mg tid; usual range 10-20 mg tid; max 180 mg/day

Cap: 30, 60, 90 mg ext-rel

Afeditab CR <12 years: not recommended; ≥12 years: initially 30 mg once daily; titrate over 7-14 days; max 90 mg/day

Cap: 30, 60 mg ext-rel

Procardia <12 years: not recommended; ≥12 years: initially 10 mg tid; titrate over 7-14 days: max 30 mg/dose and 180 mg/day in divided doses

Cap: 10, 20 mg

Procardia XL <12 years: not recommended; ≥12 years: initially 30-60 mg daily; titrate over 7-14 days; max dose 90 mg/day

Tab: 30, 60, 90 mg ext-rel

▶ *nisoldipine* (C)

Sular <12 years: not recommended; ≥12 years: initially 20 mg daily; may increase by 10 mg weekly; usual maintenance 20-40 mg/day; max 60 mg/day

Tab: 10, 20, 30, 40 mg ext-rel

Diphenylalkylamines

▶ *verapamil* (C)(G)

Calan <12 years: not recommended; ≥12 years: 80-120 mg tid; may titrate up; usual max 360 mg in divided doses

Tab: 40, 80*, 120*mg

Calan SR <12 years: not recommended; ≥12 years: initially 120 mg in the AM; may titrate up; max 480 mg/day in divided doses

Cplt: 120, 180*, 240*mg sust-rel

Covera HS <12 years: not recommended; ≥12 years: initially 180 mg q HS; titrate to 240 mg; then to 360 mg; then to 480 mg if needed

Tab: 180, 240 mg ext-rel

Isoptin <12 years: not recommended; ≥12 years: initially 80-120 mg tid

Tab: 40, 80, 120 mg

Isoptin SR <12 years: not recommended; ≥12 years: initially 120-180 mg in the AM; may increase to 240 mg in the AM; then 180 mg q 12 hours or 240 mg in the AM and 120 mg in the PM; then 240 mg q 12 hours

Tab: 120, 180*, 240*mg sust-rel

Verelan <12 years: not recommended; ≥12 years: initially 240 mg once daily; adjust in 120 mg increments; max 480 mg/day

Cap: 120, 180, 240, 360 mg sust-rel

Verelan PM <12 years: not recommended; ≥12 years: initially 200 mg q HS; may titrate upward to 300 mg; then 400 mg if needed

Cap: 100, 200, 300 mg ext-rel

ALPHA-1 ANTAGONISTS

Comment: Educate the patient regarding potential side effects of hypotension when taking an alpha-1 antagonist, especially with first dose ("first dose effect"). Start at lowest dose and titrate upward.

▶ *doxazosin* (C)(G) <12 years: not recommended; ≥12 years: initially 1 mg once daily at HS; increase dose slowly every 2 weeks if needed; max 16 mg/day

Cardura *Tab:* 1*, 2*, 4*, 8*mg

Cardura XL *Tab:* 4, 8 mg

▶ *prazosin* (C)(G) <12 years: not recommended; ≥12 years: first dose at HS, 1 mg bid-tid; increase dose slowly; usual range 6-15 mg/day in divided doses; max 20-40 mg/day

Minipress *Cap:* 1, 2, 5 mg

▶ *terazosin* (C) <12 years: not recommended; ≥12 years: 1 mg q HS, then increase dose slowly; usual range 1-5 mg q HS; max 20 mg/day

Hytrin *Cap:* 1, 2, 5, 10 mg

CENTRAL ALPHA-AGONISTS

▶ *clonidine* (C)

Catapres <12 years: not recommended; ≥12 years: initially 0.1 mg bid; usual range 0.2-0.6 mg/day in divided doses; max 2.4 mg/day; *Tab:* 0.1*, 0.2*, 0.3*mg

Catapres-TTS <12 years: not recommended; ≥12 years: 0.1 mg patch weekly; increase after 1-2 weeks if needed; max 0.6 mg/day

Patch: 0.1, 0.2 mg/day (12/carton); 0.3 mg/day (4/carton)

Kapvay (G) <12 years: not recommended; ≥12 years: initially 0.1 mg bid; usual range 0.2-0.6 mg/day in divided doses; max 2.4 mg/day; *Tab:* 0.1, 0.2 mg
Nexiclon XR <12 years: not recommended; ≥12 years: initially 0.18 mg (2 ml) suspension or 0.17 mg tab once daily; usual max 0.52 mg (6 ml suspension) once daily
Tab: 0.17, 0.26 mg ext-rel; *Oral susp:* 0.09 mg/ml ext-rel (4 oz)

- ***guanabenz*** (C)(G) <12 years: not recommended; ≥12 years: initially 4 mg bid; may increase by 4-8 mg/day every 1-2 weeks; max 32 mg/day
  Tab: 4, 8 mg
- ***guanfacine*** (B)(G) <12 years: not recommended; ≥12 years: initially 1 mg/day q HS; may increase to 2 mg/day q HS; usual max 3 mg/day
  Tenex *Tab:* 1, 2 mg
- ***methyldopa*** (B)(G) <12 years: initially 10 mg/kg/day in 2-4 divided doses; max 65 mg/kg/day or 3 gm/day, whichever is less; ≥12 years: initially 250 mg bid-tid; titrate at 2-day intervals; usual maintenance 500 mg/day to 2 gm/day; max 3 gm/day
  Aldomet *Tab:* 125, 250, 500 mg; *Oral susp:* 250 mg/5 ml (473 ml)

ALDOSTERONE RECEPTOR BLOCKER

- ***eplerenone*** (B) <12 years: not recommended; ≥12 years: 25-50 mg daily; may increase to 50 mg bid; max 100 mg/day
  Inspra *Tab:* 25, 50 mg
  Comment: Contraindicated with concomitant potent CYP3A4 inhibitors. Risk of hyperkalemia with concomitant ACE-I or ARB. Monitor serum potassium at baseline, 1 week, and 1 month. Caution with serum Cr >2 mg/dL (male) or >1.8 mg/dL (female) and/or *CrCl <50 mL/min*, and DM with proteinuria.

PERIPHERAL ADRENERGIC BLOCKER

- ***guanethidine*** (C) <12 years: not recommended; ≥12 years: initially 10 mg daily; may adjust dose at 5-7 day intervals; usual range 25-50 mg/day
  Ismelin *Tab:* 10, 25 mg

DIRECT RENIN INHIBITOR

- ***aliskiren*** (D) <18 years: not recommended; ≥18 years: initially 150 mg once daily; max 300 mg/day
  Tekturna *Tab:* 150, 300 mg

PERIPHERAL VASODILATORS

- ***hydralazine*** (C)(G) <12 years: initially 0.75 mg/kg/day in 4 divided doses; increase gradually over 3-4 weeks; max 7.5 mg/kg/day or 2,000 mg/day; ≥12 years: initially 10 mg qid x 2-4 days; then increase to 25 mg qid for remainder of 1st week; then increase to 50 mg qid; max 300 mg/day
  Tab: 10, 25, 50, 100 mg
- ***minoxidil*** (C) <12 years: initially 0.2 mg/kg daily; may increase in 50%-100% increments every 3 days; usual range 0.25-1 gm/kg/day; max 50 mg/day; ≥12 years: initially 5 mg daily; may increase at 3-day intervals to 10 mg/day, then 20 mg/day, then 40 mg/day; usual range 10-40 mg/day; max 100 mg/day
  Loniten *Tab:* 2.5*, 10*mg

ACEI+DIURETIC COMBINATIONS

- ***benazepril+hydrochlorothiazide*** (D)
  Lotensin HCT <12 years: not recommended; ≥12 years: 1 tab once daily; titrate individual components

Tab: **Lotensin HCT 5/6.25** benaz 5 mg+hctz 6.25 mg*
Lotensin HCT 10/12.5 benaz 10 mg+hctz 12.5 mg*
Lotensin HCT 20/12.5 benaz 20 mg+hctz 12.5 mg*
Lotensin HCT 20/25 benaz 20 mg+hctz 25 mg*

▶ ***captopril+hydrochlorothiazide*** (D)(G)
Capozide <12 years: not recommended; ≥12 years: 1 tab once daily; titrate individual components
Tab: **Capozide 25/15** capt 25 mg+hctz 15 mg*
Capozide 25/25 capt 25 mg+hctz 25 mg*
Capozide 50/15 capt 50 mg+hctz 15 mg*
Capozide 50/25 capt 50 mg+hctz 25 mg*

▶ ***enalapril+hydrochlorothiazide*** (D)
Vaseretic <12 years: not recommended; ≥12 years: 1 tab once daily; titrate individual components
Tab: **Vaseretic 5/12.5** enal 5 mg+hctz 12.5 mg
Vaseretic 10/25 enal 10 mg+hctz 25 mg

▶ ***lisinopril+hydrochlorothiazide*** (D)
Prinzide <12 years: not recommended; ≥12 years: 1 tab once daily; titrate individual components
Tab: **Prinzide 10/12.5** lis 10 mg+hctz 12.5 mg
Prinzide 20/12.5 lis 20 mg+hctz 12.5 mg
Prinzide 20/25 lis 20 mg+hctz 25 mg
Zestoretic <12 years: not recommended; ≥12 years: 1 tab once daily; titrate individual components; *CrCl <40 mL/min:* not recommended
Tab: **Zestoretic 10/12.5** lis 10 mg+hctz 12.5 mg
Zestoretic 20/12.5 lis 20 mg+hctz 12.5 mg*
Zestoretic 20/25 lis 20 mg+hctz 25 mg

▶ ***moexipril+hydrochlorothiazide*** (D)
Uniretic <12 years: not recommended; ≥12 years: 1 tab once daily; titrate individual components
Tab: **Uniretic 7.5/12.5** moex 7.5 mg+hctz 12.5 mg*
Uniretic 15/12.5 moex 15 mg+hctz 12.5 mg*
Uniretic 15/25 moex 15 mg+hctz 25 mg*

▶ ***quinapril+hydrochlorothiazide*** (D)
Accuretic <12 years: not recommended; ≥12 years: 1 tab once daily; titrate individual components
Tab: **Accuretic 10/12.5** quin 10 mg+hctz 12.5 mg*
Accuretic 20/12.5 quin 20 mg+hctz 12.5 mg*
Accuretic 20/25 quin 20 mg+hctz 25 mg*

ARB+DIURETIC COMBINATIONS

▶ ***azilsartan+chlorthalidone*** (D)
Edarbyclor <18 years: not recommended; ≥18 years: 1 tab once daily; titrate individual components
Tab: **Edarbyclor 40/12.5** azil 40 mg+chlor 12.5 mg
Edarbyclor 40/25 azil 40 mg+chlor 25 mg

▶ ***candesartan+hydrochlorothiazide*** (D) <12 years: not recommended; ≥12 years: 1 tab once daily; titrate individual components
Atacand HCT
Tab: **Atacand HCT 16/12.5** cande 16 mg+hctz 12.5 mg
Atacand HCT 32/12.5 cande 32 mg+hctz 12.5 mg

➢ *eprosartan+hydrochlorothiazide* (D)
Teveten HCT <12 years: not recommended; ≥12 years: 1 tab once daily; titrate individual components
Tab: **Teveten HCT 600/12.5** epro 600 mg+hctz 12.5 mg
Teveten HCT 600/25 epro 600 mg+hctz 25 mg

➢ *irbesartan+hydrochlorothiazide* (D)
Avalide <12 years: not recommended; ≥12 years: 1 tab once daily; titrate individual components
Tab: **Avalide 150/12.5** irbes 150 mg+hctz 12.5 mg
Avalide 300/12.5 irbes 300 mg+hctz 12.5 mg

➢ *losartan+hydrochlorothiazide* (D)(G)
Hyzaar <12 years: not recommended; ≥12 years: 1 tab once daily; titrate individual components
Tab: **Hyzaar 50/12.5** losar 50 mg+hctz 12.5 mg
Hyzaar 100/12.5 losar 100 mg+hctz 12.5 mg
Hyzaar 100/25 losar 100 mg+hctz 25 mg

➢ *olmesartan medoxomil+hydrochlorothiazide* (D)(G)
Benicar HCT <12 years: not recommended; ≥12 years: 1 tab once daily; titrate individual components
Tab: **Benicar HCT 20/12.5** *olme* 20 mg+hctz 12.5 mg
Benicar HCT 40/12.5 *olme* 40 mg+hctz 12.5 mg
Benicar HCT 40/25 *olme* 40 mg+hctz 25 mg

➢ *telmisartan+hydrochlorothiazide* (D)(G)
Micardis HCT <12 years: not recommended; ≥12 years: 1 tab once daily; titrate individual components
Tab: **Micardis HCT 40/12.5** telmi 40 mg+hctz 12.5 mg
Micardis HCT 80/12.5 telmi 80 mg+hctz 12.5 mg
Micardis HCT 80/25 telmi 80 mg+hctz 25 mg

➢ *valsartan+hydrochlorothiazide* (D)
Diovan HCT <12 years: not recommended; ≥12 years: 1 tab once daily; titrate individual components
Tab: **Diovan HCT 80/12.5** vals 80 mg+hctz 12.5 mg
Diovan HCT 160/12.5 vals 160 mg+hctz 12.5 mg
Diovan HCT 160/25 vals 160 mg+hctz 25 mg
Diovan HCT 320/12.5 vals 320 mg+hctz 12.5 mg
Diovan HCT 320/25 vals 320 mg+hctz 25 mg

CENTRAL ALPHA-AGONIST+DIURETIC COMBINATIONS

➢ *clonidine+chlorthalidone* (C)
Combipres <12 years: not recommended; ≥12 years: 1 tab daily-bid
Tab: **Combipres 0.1** clon 0.1 mg+chlor 15 mg*
Combipres 0.2 clon 0.2 mg+chlor 15 mg*
Combipres 0.3 clon 0.3 mg+chlor 15 mg*

➢ *methyldopa+hydrochlorothiazide* (C)(G)
Aldoril <12 years: not recommended; ≥12 years: initially **Aldoril 15** bid-tid or **Aldoril 25** bid; titrate individual components
Tab: **Aldoril 15** meth 250 mg+hctz 15 mg
Aldoril 25 meth 250 mg+hctz 25 mg
Aldoril D30 meth 500 mg+hctz 30 mg
Aldoril D50 meth 500 mg+hctz 50 mg

BETA-BLOCKER (CARDIOSELECTIVE)+DIURETIC COMBINATIONS

▶ *atenolol+chlorthalidone* (D)(G)

Tenoretic <12 years: not recommended; ≥12 years: initially ***tenoretic*** 50 mg once daily; may increase to ***tenoretic*** 100 mg once daily

Tab: **Tenoretic 50/25** aten 50 mg+chlor 25 mg*
Tenoretic 100/25 aten 100 mg+chlor 25 mg*

▶ *bisoprolol+hydrochlorothiazide* (C)

Ziac <12 years: not recommended; ≥12 years: initially one 2.5/6.25 mg tab daily; adjust at 2 week intervals; max two 10/6.25 mg tabs daily

Tab: **Ziac 2.5** biso 2.5 mg+hctz 6.25 mg
Ziac 5 biso 5 mg+hctz 6.25 mg
Ziac 10 biso 10 mg+hctz 6.25 mg

▶ *metoprolol succinate+hydrochlorothiazide* (C)

Lopressor HCT <12 years: not recommended; ≥12 years: titrate individual components

Tab: **Lopressor HCT 50/25** meto succ 50 mg+hctz 25 mg*
Lopressor HCT 100/25 meto succ 100 mg+hctz 25 mg*
Lopressor HCT 100/50 meto succ 100 mg+hctz 50 mg*

▶ *metoprolol succinate+ext-rel hydrochlorothiazide* (C)

Dutoprol <12 years: not established; ≥12 years: titrate individual components; may titrate to max 200/25 mg once daily

Tab: **Dutoprol 25/12.5** meto succ 25 mg+ext-rel hctz 12.5 mg
Dutoprol 50/12.5 meto succ 50 mg+ext-rel hctz 12.5 mg
Dutoprol 100/12.5 meto succ 100 mg+ext-rel hctz 12.5 mg

BETA-BLOCKER (NON-CARDIOSELECTIVE)+DIURETIC COMBINATIONS

▶ *nadolol+bendroflumethiazide* (C)

Corzide <12 years: not recommended; ≥12 years: titrate individual components

Tab: **Corzide 40/5** nado 40 mg+bend 5 mg*
Corzide 80/5 nado 80 mg+bend 5 mg*

▶ *propranolol+hydrochlorothiazide* (C)(G)

Inderide <12 years: not recommended; ≥12 years: titrate individual components

Tab: **Inderide 40/25** prop 40 mg+hctz 25 mg*
Inderide 80/25 prop 80 mg+hctz 25 mg*
Inderide LA titrate individual components

Cap: **Inderide LA 80/50** prop 80 mg+hctz 50 mg sust-rel
Inderide LA 120/50 prop 120 mg+hctz 50 mg sust-rel
Inderide LA 160/50 prop 160 mg+hctz 50 mg sust-rel

▶ *timolol+hydrochlorothiazide* (C)

Timolide <12 years: not recommended; ≥12 years: usual maintenance 2 tabs/day in a single or 2 divided doses

Tab: timo 10 mg+hctz 25 mg

BETA-BLOCKER (CARDIOSELECTIVE)+ARB COMBINATION

▶ *nebivolol+valsartan* (X) <12 years: not recommended; ≥12 years: 1 tab daily; may initiate when inadequately controlled on ***nebivolol*** 10 mg or ***valsartan*** 80 mg

Byvalson *Tab:* nebi 5 mg+val 80 mg

ALPHA-1 ANTAGONIST+DIURETIC COMBINATIONS

▶ *prazosin+polythiazide* (C)
Minizide <12 years: not recommended; ≥12 years: titrate individual components
Cap: **Minizide 1** praz 1 mg+poly 0.5 mg
Minizide 2 praz 2 mg+poly 0.5 mg
Minizide 5 praz 5 mg+poly 0.5 mg

PERIPHERAL ADRENERGIC BLOCKER+HCTZ COMBINATIONS

▶ *guanethidine+hydrochlorothiazide* (C)
Esimil <12 years: not recommended; ≥12 years: titrate individual components
Tab: **Esimil 10/25** guan 1 mg+hctz 25 mg

ACEI+CCB COMBINATIONS

▶ *amlodipine+benazepril* (D) <12 years: not recommended; ≥12 years: titrate individual components
Lotrel
Cap: **Lotrel 2.5/10** amlo 2.5 mg+benaz 10 mg
Lotrel 5/10 amlo 5 mg+benaz 10 mg
Lotrel 5/20 amlo 5 mg+benaz 20 mg
Lotrel 10/20 amlo 10 mg+benaz 20 mg
Lotrel 5/40 amlo 5 mg+benaz 40 mg
Lotrel 10/40 amlo 10 mg+benaz 40 mg

▶ *amlodipine+perindopril* (D)
Prolastin <12 years: not recommended; ≥12 years: titrate individual components
Cap: **Prolastin 2.5/3.5** amlo 2.5 mg+peri 3.5 mg
Prolastin 5/7 amlo 5 mg+peri 7 mg
Prolastin 5/14 amlo 5 mg+peri 14 mg

▶ *enalapril+diltiazem* (D)
Teczem <12 years: not recommended; ≥12 years: titrate individual components
Tab: enal 5 mg+dil 180 mg ext-rel

▶ *enalapril+felodipine* (D)
Lexxel <12 years: not recommended; ≥12 years: initially 1 tab daily; after 1-2 weeks may increase to 2 tabs/day; titrate individual components
Tab: **Lexxel 5/2.5** enal 5 mg+felo 2.5 mg ext-rel
Lexxel 5/5 enal 5 mg+felo 5 mg ext-rel

▶ *perindopril+amlodipine* (D)
Prestalia <12 years: not recommended; ≥12 years: titrate individual components; max 14/10 once daily
Tab: **Prestalia 3.5/2.5** peri 3.5 mg+amlo 2.5 mg
Prestalia 7/5 peri 7 mg+amlo 5 mg
Prestalia 14/10 peri 14 mg+amlo 10 mg

▶ *trandolapril+verapamil* (D)
Tarka <12 years: not recommended; ≥12 years: titrate individual components
Tab: **Tarka 1/240** tran 1 mg+ver 240 mg ext-rel
Tarka 2/180 tran 2 mg+ver 180 mg ext-rel
Tarka 2/240 tran 2 mg+ver 240 mg ext-rel
Tarka 4/240 tran 4 mg+ver 240 mg ext-rel

DRI+HCTZ COMBINATIONS

▶ *aliskiren+hydrochlorothiazide* (D) <12 years: not recommended; ≥12 years: initially ***aliskiren*** 150 mg once daily; max ***aliskiren*** 300 mg/day

Tekturna HCT

Tab: **Tekturna HCT 150/12.5** alisk 150 mg+hctz 12.5 mg
Tekturna HCT 150/25 alisk 150 mg+hctz 25 mg
Tekturna HCT 300/12.5 alisk 300 mg+hctz 12.5 mg
Tekturna HCT 300/25 alisk 300 mg+hctz 25 mg

DRI+ARB COMBINATIONS

▶ *aliskiren+valsartan* (D)

Valturna <12 years: not recommended; ≥12 years: initially 150/160 once daily; may increase to max 300/320 once daily

Tab: **Valturna 150/160** alisk 150 mg+vals 160 mg
Valturna 300/320 alisk 300 mg+vals 320 mg

DRI+CCB COMBINATIONS

▶ *aliskiren+amlodipine* (D)

Tekamlo <12 years: not recommended; ≥12 years: initially 150/5 once daily; may increase to max 300/10 once daily

Tab: **Tekamlo 150/5** alisk 150 mg+amlo 5 mg
Tekamlo 150/10 alisk 150 mg+amlo 10 mg
Tekamlo 300/5 alisk 300 mg+amlo 5 mg
Tekamlo 300/10 alisk 300 mg+amlo 10 mg

DRI+CCB+HCTZ COMBINATIONS

▶ *aliskiren+amlodipine+hydrochlorothiazide* (D)

Amturnide <12 years: not recommended; ≥12 years: initially 150/5/12.5 once daily; may increase to max 300/10/25 once daily

Tab: **Amturnide 150/5/12.5** alisk 150 mg+amlo 5 mg+hctz 12.5 mg
Amturnide 300/5/12.5 alisk 300 mg+amlo 5 mg+hctz 12.5 mg
Amturnide 300/5/25 alisk 300 mg+amlo 5 mg+hctz 25 mg
Amturnide 300/10/25 alisk 300 mg+amlo 10 mg+hctz 25 mg

ARB+CCB COMBINATIONS

▶ *amlodipine+valsartan medoxomil* (D)(G)

Exforge <12 years: not recommended; ≥12 years: 1 tab daily; titrate individual components at 1-week intervals; max 10/320 daily

Tab: **Exforge 5/160** amlo 5 mg+vals 160 mg
Exforge 5/320 amlo 5 mg+vals 320 mg
Exforge 10/160 amlo 10 mg+vals 160 mg
Exforge 10/320 amlo 10 mg+vals 320 mg

▶ *amlodipine+olmesartan* (D)(G)

Azor <12 years: not recommended; ≥12 years: titrate individual components

Tab: **Azor 5/20** amlo 5 mg+olme 20 mg
Azor 10/20 amlo 10 mg+olme 20 mg
Azor 5/40 amlo 5 mg+olme 40 mg
Azor 10/40 amlo 10 mg+olme 40 mg

▶ *telmisartan+amlodipine* (D)

Twynsta <12 years: not recommended; ≥12 years: initially 40/5 once daily; titrate at 1 week intervals; max 80/10 once daily

Tab: **Twynsta 40/5** telmi 40 mg+amlo 5 mg
Twynsta 40/10 telmi 40 mg+amlo 10 mg
Twynsta 80/5 telmi 80 mg+amlo 5 mg
Twynsta 80/10 telmi 80 mg+amlo 10 mg

ARB+CCB+HCTZ COMBINATIONS

➢ ***amlodipine+valsartan medoxomil+hydrochlorothiazide*** (D)(G)

Exforge HCT: <12 years: not recommended; ≥12 years: initially 5/160/12.5 once daily; may titrate at 1-week intervals to max 10/320/25 once daily

Tab: **Exforge HCT 5/160/12.5** amlo 5 mg+vals 160 mg+hctz 12.5 mg
Exforge HCT 5/160/25 amlo 5 mg+vals 160 mg+hctz 25 mg
Exforge HCT 10/160/12.5 amlo 10 mg+vals 160 mg+hctz 12.5 mg
Exforge HCT 10/160/25 amlo 10 mg+vals 160 mg+hctz 25 mg
Exforge HCT 10/320/25 amlo 10 mg+vals 320 mg+hctz 25 mg

➢ ***olmesartan medoxomil+amlodipine+hydrochlorothiazide*** (D)(G)

Tribenzor: <12 years: not recommended; ≥12 years: initially 40/5/12.5 once daily; may titrate at 1-week intervals to max 40/10/25 daily

Tab: **Tribenzor 40/5/12.5** olme 40 mg+amlo 5 mg+hctz 12.5 mg
Tribenzor 40/5/25 olme 40 mg+amlo 5 mg+hctz 25 mg
Tribenzor 40/10/12.5 olme 40 mg+amlo 10 mg+hctz 12.5 mg
Tribenzor 40/10/25 olme 40 mg+amlo 10 mg+hctz 25 mg

OTHER COMBINATION AGENTS

➢ ***clonidine+chlorthalidone*** (C)

Clorpres <12 years: not recommended; ≥12 years: initially 0.1/15 once daily; may titrate to max 0.3/15 bid

Tab: **Clorpres 0.1/15** clon 0.1 mg+chlor 15 mg
Clorpres 0.2/15 clon 0.2 mg+chlor 15 mg
Clorpres 0.3/15 clon 0.3 mg+chlor 15 mg

➢ ***reserpine+hydroflumethiazide*** (C)

Salutensin <12 years: not recommended; ≥12 years: initially 1.25/25 once daily; may titrate to 1.25/25 bid or 1.25/50 once daily

Tab: **Salutensin 1.25/25** enal 1.25 mg+hydro flu 25 mg
Salutensin 1.25/50: enal 1.25 mg+hydro flu 50 mg

ANTIHYPERTENSION+ANTILIPID COMBINATIONS

CCB+Statin Combinations

➢ ***amlodipine+atorvastatin*** (X)

Caduet <10 years: not established; ≥10 years (female post menarche) select according to blood pressure and lipid values; titrate ***amlodipine*** over 7-14 days; titrate ***atorvastatin*** according to monitored lipid values; max ***amlodipine*** 10 mg/day and max ***atorvastatin*** 80 mg/day; refer to contraindications and precautions for CCB and statin therapy

Tab: **Caduet 2.5/10** amlo 2.5 mg+ator 10 mg
Caduet 2.5/20 amlo 2.5 mg+ator 20 mg
Caduet 5/10 amlo 5 mg+ator 10 mg
Caduet 5/20 amlo 5 mg+ator 20 mg
Caduet 5/40 amlo 5 mg+ator 40 mg
Caduet 5/80 amlo 5 mg+ator 80 mg
Caduet 10/10 amlo 10 mg+ator 10 mg
Caduet 10/20 amlo 10 mg+ator 20 mg
Caduet 10/40 amlo 10 mg+ator 40 mg
Caduet 10/80 amlo 10 mg+ator 80 mg

HYPERTHYROIDISM

- *methimazole* (D) <12 years: initially 0.4 mg/kg/day in 3 divided doses; maintenance 0.2 mg/kg/day <u>or</u> 1/2 initial dose; ≥12 years: initially 15-60 mg/day in 3 divided doses; maintenance 5-15 mg/day

  Tapazole *Tab:* 5*, 10*mg

  Comment: ***methimazole*** potentiates anticoagulants. Contraindicated in nursing mothers.

- *propylthiouracil (ptu)* (D)(G)

  Propyl-Thyracil <6 years: not recommended; ≥6-10 years: initially 50-150 mg/day <u>or</u> 5-7 mg/kg/day in 3 divided doses; >10 years: initially 150-300 mg/day <u>or</u> 5-7 mg/kg/day in 3 divided doses; *maintenance:* 0.2 mg/kg/day <u>or</u> 1/2-2/3 of initial dose; initially 100-900 mg/day in 3 divided doses; maintenance usually 50-600 mg/day in 2 divided doses

  Tab: 50*mg

  Comment: Preferred agent in pregnancy. Side effects include dermatitis, nausea, agranulocytosis, and hypothyroidism. Should be taken regularly for 2 years. Do not discontinue abruptly.

BETA-ADRENERGIC BLOCKER

- *propranolol* (C)(G)

  Inderal <12 years: not recommended; ≥12 years: 40-240 mg once daily

  Tab: 10*, 20*, 40*, 60*, 80*mg

  Inderal LA <12 years: not recommended; ≥12 years: initially 80 mg daily in a single dose; increase q 3-7 days; usual range 120-160 mg/day; max 320 mg/day in a single dose

  Cap: 60, 80, 120, 160 mg sust-rel

  InnoPran XL <12 years: not recommended; ≥12 years: initially 80 mg q HS; max 120 mg/day

  Cap: 80, 120 mg ext-rel

HYPERTRIGLYCERIDEMIA

OMEGA 3-FATTY ACID ETHYL ESTERS

Comment: ***Vascepa***, ***Lovaza***, and **Epanova** are indicated for the treatment of TG ≥500 mg/dL.

- ***icosapent ethyl (omega 3-fatty acid ethyl ester of EPA)*** **(C)** <18 years: not recommended; ≥18 years: 2 caps bid with food; max 4 gm/day; swallow whole, do not crush <u>or</u> chew

  Vascepa *sgc:* 1 gm (α-tocopherol 4 mg/cap)

- ***omega 3-fatty acid ethyl esters*** (C)(G) <18 years: not recommended; ≥18 years: 2 gm bid <u>or</u> 4 gm daily; swallow whole, do not crush <u>or</u> chew

  Lovaza *Gelcap:* 1 gm (α-tocopherol 4 mg/cap) **(C)** take 2-4 *gel caps* (2-4 gm) daily without regard to meals

  Epanova *Gelcap:* 1 gm

ISOBUTYRIC ACID DERIVATIVE

- *gemfibrozil* (C)(G) <12 years: not recommended; ≥12 years: 600 mg bid 30 minutes before AM and PM meals

  Lopid *Tab:* 600*mg

FIBRATES (FIBRIC ACID DERIVATIVES)

▻ ***fenofibrate*** **(C)** take with meals; adjust at 4-8-week intervals; discontinue if inadequate response after 2 months; lowest dose or contraindicated with renal impairment

Antara <12 years: not recommended; ≥12 years: 43-130 mg once daily; max 130 mg/day

Cap: 43, 87, 130 mg

FibriCor <12 years: not recommended; ≥12 years: 30-105 mg once daily; max 105 mg/day

Tab: 30, 105 mg

TriCor (G) <12 years: not recommended; ≥12 years: 48-145 mg once daily; max 145 mg/day

Tab: 48, 145 mg

TriLipix (G) <12 years: not recommended; ≥12 years: 45-135 mg once daily; max 135 mg/day

Cap: 45, 135 mg del-rel

Lipofen (G) <12 years: not recommended; ≥12 years: 50-150 mg once daily; max 150 mg/day

Cap: 50, 150 mg

Lofibra <12 years: not recommended; ≥12 years: 67-200 mg daily; max 200 mg/day

Tab: 67, 134, 200 mg

NICOTINIC ACID DERIVATIVES

Comment: Contraindicated in liver disease. Decrease total cholesterol, LDL-C, and TG; increase HDL-C. Before initiating and at 4-6 weeks, 3 months, and 6 months of therapy, check fasting lipid profile or as indicated by manufacturer, LFT, glucose, and uric acid. Significant side effect of transient skin flushing. Take with food and take ***aspirin*** 325 mg 30 minutes before dose to decrease flushing.

▻ ***niacin*** **(C)**

Niaspan <12 years: not recommended; ≥12 years: 375 mg daily for 1st week; then, 500 mg daily for 2nd week; then, 750 mg daily for 3rd week; then, 1 gm daily for weeks 4-7; may increase by 500 mg q 4 weeks; usual range 1-3 gm/day

Tab: 500, 750, 1,000 mg ext-rel

Slo-Niacin <12 years: not recommended; ≥12 years: 250 mg or 500 mg or 750 mg q AM or HS

Tab: 250, 500, 750 mg cont-rel

HMG-COA REDUCTASE INHIBITORS

▻ ***atorvastatin*** **(X)(G)** <10 years: not recommended; ≥10 years (female post menarche): initially 10 mg daily; usual range 10-80 mg daily

Lipitor *Tab:* 10, 20, 40, 80 mg

▻ ***fluvastatin*** **(X)(G)** <18 years: not recommended; ≥18 years: initially 20-40 mg q HS; usual range 20-80 mg/day

Lescol *Cap:* 20, 40 mg

Lescol XL *Tab:* 80 mg ext-rel

▻ ***lovastatin*** **(X)** <10 years: not recommended; 10-17 years: initially 10-20 mg daily at evening meal; may increase at 4 week intervals; max 40 mg daily; *Concomitant fibrates, niacin, or CrCl <40 mL/min:* usual max 20 mg/day initially 20 mg daily at evening meal; may increase at 4 week intervals; max 80 mg/day in a single or divided doses; *Concomitant fibrates,* ***niacin****, or CrCl <40 mL/min:* usual max 20 mg/day

Mevacor *Tab:* 10, 20, 40 mg

- *pravastatin* (X)(G) <8 years: not recommended; 8-13 years: 20 mg q HS; 14-17 years: 40 mg q HS; >17 years: initially 10-20 mg q HS; usual range 10-80 mg/day; may start at 40 mg/day
  Pravachol *Tab:* 10, 20, 40, 80 mg
- *rosuvastatin* (X)(G) <10 years: not recommended; 10-17 years: 5-20 mg q HS; >17 years: initially 20 mg q HS; usual range 5-40 mg/day; adjust at 4 week intervals; max 20 mg q HS
  Crestor *Tab:* 5, 10, 20, 40 mg
- *simvastatin* (X)(G) <10 years: not recommended; 10-17 years: initially 10 mg q HS; may increase at 4 week intervals; >17 years: initially 20 mg q HS; usual range 5-80 mg/day; adjust at 4 week intervals; max 40 mg q HS
  Zocor *Tab:* 5, 10, 20, 40, 80 mg

NICOTINIC ACID DERIVATIVE+HMG-COA REDUCTASE INHIBITOR COMBINATION

- *niacin+lovastatin* (X) **Advicor** <18 years: not recommended; ≥18 years: take 1 tab once daily
  Tab: **Advicor 500/20** niac 500 mg ext-rel+lova 20 mg
  Advicor 750/20 niac 750 mg ext-rel+lova 20 mg
  Advicor 1,000/20 niac 1,000 mg ext-rel+lova 20 mg

HYPOCALCEMIA

Comment: Hypocalcemia resulting in metabolic bone disease may be secondary to hyperparathyroidism, pseudoparathyroidism, and chronic renal disease. Normal serum Ca^{++} range is approximately 8.5-12 mg/dL. Signs and symptoms of hypocalcemia include confusion, increased neuromuscular excitability, muscle spasms, paresthesias, hyperphosphatemia, positive Chvostek's sign, and positive Trousseau's sign. Signs and symptoms of hypercalcemia include fatigue, lethargy, decreased concentration and attention span, frank psychosis, anorexia, nausea, vomiting, constipation, bradycardia, heart block, shortened QT interval. Foods high in calcium include almonds, broccoli, baked beans, salmon, sardines, buttermilk, turnip greens, collard greens, spinach, pumpkin, rhubarb, and bran. Recommended daily calcium intake: 1-3 years: 700 mg; 4-8 years: 1,000 mg; 9-18 years: 1,300 mg; >18 years: 1,000 mg; pregnancy or nursing: 1,000-1,300 mg. Recommended daily vitamin D intake: >1 year: 600 IU; The American Academy of Rheumatology (AAR) recommends the following daily doses for anyone on a chronic oral corticosteroid regimen: ***Calcium*** 1,200-1,500 mg/day and ***vitamin D*** 800-1,000 IU/day.

CALCIUM SUPPLEMENTS

Comment: Take ***calcium*** supplements after meals to avoid gastric upset. Dosages of ***calcium*** over 2,000 mg/day have not been shown to have any additional benefit. ***calcium*** decreases ***tetracycline*** absorption. ***calcium*** absorption is decreased by corticosteroids.

- *calcitonin-salmon* (C)
  Miacalcin 200 units (1 spray intranasally) once daily; alternate nostrils each day
  Nasal spray: 14 dose (2 ml)
  Miacalcin injection 100 units/day SC or IM
  Vial: 2 ml
- *calcium carbonate* (C)(OTC)(G)
  Rolaids chew 2 tabs bid; max 14 tabs/day
  Tab: calcium carbonate: 550 mg
  Rolaids Extra Strength chew 2 tabs bid; max 8 tabs/day
  Tab: 1,000 mg

Tums chew 2 tabs bid; max 16 tabs/day
Tab: 500 mg
Tums Extra Strength chew 2 tabs bid; max 10 tabs/day
Tab: 750 mg
Tums Ultra chew 2 tabs bid; max 8 tabs/day
Tab: 1,000 mg
Os-Cal 500 (OTC) 1-2 tab bid-tid
Tab: elemental calcium carbonate 500 mg

▶ ***calcium carbonate+vitamin d*** (C)(G)
Os-Cal 250/D (OTC) 1-2 tabs tid
Tab: elemental calcium carbonate 250 mg+vit d 125 IU
Os-Cal 500/D (OTC) 1-2 tabs bid-tid
Tab: elemental calcium carbonate 500 mg+vit d 125 IU
Viactiv (OTC) 1 tab tid
Chew tab: elemental calcium 500 mg/vit d 125 IU+vit a 100 IU+vit k 40 mEq

▶ ***calcium citrate***
Citracal (OTC) 1-2 tabs bid
Tab: elemental calcium citrate 200 mg

▶ ***calcium citrate+vitamin d*** (C)(G)
Citracal+D (OTC) 1-2 cplts bid
Cplt: elemental cal cit 315 mg+vit d 200 IU
Citracal 250+D (OTC) 1-2 tabs bid
Tab: elemental cal cit 250 mg+vit d 62.3 IU

VITAMIN D ANALOGS

Comment: Concurrent ***vitamin D*** supplementation is contraindicated for patients taking ***calcitriol*** or ***doxercalciferol*** due to the risk of ***vitamin D*** toxicity. Symptoms of hypervitaminosis D: hypercalcemia, hypercalciuria, elevated creatinine, erythema multiforme, hyperphosphatemia. Maintain adequate daily calcium and fluid intake. Keep serum calcium times phosphate (Ca x P) product below 70. Monitor serum calcium (esp. during dose titration), phosphorus, other lab values (see literature for frequency)

▶ **calcitriol** (C)(G) <12 years: *Predialysis:* <3 years: 10-15 ng/kg per day; ≥3 years: initially 0.25 mcg daily; may increase to 0.5 mcg daily; *Dialysis:* not recommended; *Hypoparathyroidism:* initially 0.25 mcg daily in the AM; may increase by 0.25 mcg day at 2-4 week intervals; usual maintenance: (1-5 years): 0.25-0.75 mcg daily; (≥6 years): 0.5-2 mcg daily; *Pseudohypoparathyroidism:* (<6 years): insufficient data, see mfr pkg insert; ≥12 years: *Predialysis:* initially 0.25 mcg daily; may increase to 0.5 mcg daily *Dialysis:* initially 0.25 mcg daily; may increase by 0.25 mcg daily at 4-8 week intervals; usual maintenance: 0.5-1 mcg daily. *Hypoparathyroidism:* initially 0.25 mcg q AM; may increase by 0.25 mcg/day at 4-8 week intervals; usual maintenance 0.5-2 mcg/day
Rocaltrol *Cap:* 0.25, 0.5 mcg
Rocaltrol Solution *Soln:* 1 mcg/ml (15 ml, single-use dispensers)

Comment: ***calcitriol*** is indicated for the treatment of secondary hyperparathyroidism and resultant metabolic bone disease in predialysis patients (CrCl 15-55 mL/min), hypocalcemia and resultant metabolic bone disease in patients on chronic renal dialysis, hypocalcemia in hypoparathyroidism, and pseudohypoparathyroidism.

▶ ***doxercalciferol*** (C)(G) <12 years: not established; ≥12 years: *Dialysis:* initially 10 mcg 3 x/week at dialysis; adjust to maintain intact parathyroid hormone (iPTH) between 150-300 pg/mL; if iPTH is not lowered by 50% and fails to reach target range, may increase by 2.5 mcg at 8-week intervals; max 20 mcg 3 x/week; if iPTH <100 pg/mL, suspend for 1 week, then resume at a dose that is at least 2.5 mcg lower; *Predialysis:* initially 1 mcg once daily; may increase by 0.5 mcg at 2 week intervals to target iPTH levels; max 3.5 mcg/day

Hectorol *Cap:* 0.25, 0.5, 1, 2.5 mcg

Comment: Oral **Hectorol** is indicated for the treatment of secondary hyperparathyroidism in patients with chronic kidney disease (CKD) on dialysis; *Predialysis stage 3 or 4 CKD:* use oral form only.

Hectoral Injection <12 years: not recommended; ≥12 years: 4 mcg 3 x weekly after dialysis; adjust dose to maintain intact parathyroid hormone (iPTH) between 150-300 pg/mL; if iPTH is not lowered by 50% and fails to reach target range, may increase by 1-2 mcg at 8 week intervals; max 18 mcg/week; if iPTH <100 pg/mL, suspend for 1 week, then resume at a dose that is at least 1 mcg lower

Vial: 2 mcg/ml (1, 2 ml single-dose; 2 ml multi-dose)

Comment: **Hectorol Injection** is indicated for the treatment of secondary hyperparathyroidism in patients with chronic kidney disease (CKD) on dialysis.

▶ ***paricalcitol*** (C)(G) <18 years: not established; ≥18 years: administer 0.04-1 mcg/kg (2.8-7 mcg) IV bolus, during dialysis, no more than every other day; may be increased by 2-4 mcg/dose every 2-4 weeks; monitor serum calcium and phosphorus during dose adjustment periods; if Ca x P >75, immediately reduce dose or discontinue until these levels normalize; discard unused portion of single-use vials immediately

Zemplar *Vial:* 2, 5 mcg/ml soln for inj

Comment: ***paricalcitol*** is indicated for the prevention and treatment of secondary hyperparathyroidism associated with chronic kidney disease (CKD) stage 5.

BIOENGINEERED REPLICA OF HUMAN PARATHYROID HORMONE

▶ ***bioengineered replica of human parathyroid hormone*** (C) before starting, confirm 25-hydroxyvitamin D stores are sufficient; if insufficient, replace to sufficient levels per standard of care; confirm serum calcium is above 7.5 mg/dL; the goal of treatment is to achieve serum calcium within the lower half of the normal range; administer SC into the thigh once daily; alternate thighs; initially, 50 mcg/day; when initiating, decrease dose of active vitamin D by 50%, if serum calcium is above 7.5 mg/dL; monitor serum calcium levels every 3 to 7 days after starting or adjusting dose and when adjusting either active vitamin D or calcium supplements dose. Abrupt interruption or discontinuation of **Natpara** can result in severe hypocalcemia. Resume treatment with, or increase the dose of, an active form of vitamin D and calcium supplements. Monitor for signs and symptoms of hypocalcemia and monitor serum calcium levels, In the case of a missed dose, the next **Natpara** dose should be administered as soon as reasonably feasible and additional exogenous calcium should be taken in the event of hypocalcemia.

Natpara *Soln for inj:* 25, 50, 75, 100 mcg (2/pkg) multiple dose, dual-chamber glass cartridge containing a sterile powder and diluent

Comment: **Natpara** is indicated as an adjunct to calcium and vitamin D in patients with hypoparathyroidism. Because of a potential risk of osteosarcoma, use **Natpara** only in patients who cannot be well-controlled on calcium and active forms of vitamin D alone and for whom the potential benefits are considered to outweigh the potential risk. Avoid use of **Natpara** in patients who are at increased baseline risk for osteosarcoma, such as patients with Paget's disease of bone or unexplained elevations of alkaline phosphatase, pediatric and patients ≥18 years with open epiphyses, patients with hereditary disorders predisposing to osteosarcoma or patients with a prior history of external beam or implant radiation therapy involving the skeleton. Because of the risk of osteosarcoma, **Natpara** is available only through a restricted program under a Risk Evaluation and Mitigation Strategy (REMS) at www.natparaREMS.com

HYPOKALEMIA

Comment: Normal serum K^+ range is approximately 3.5-5.5 mEq/L. Signs and symptoms of hypokalemia include neuromuscular weakness, muscle twitching and cramping, hyporeflexia, postural hypotension, anorexia, nausea and vomiting, depressed ST segments, flattened T waves, and cardiac tachyarrhythmias. Signs and symptoms of hyperkalemia include peaked T waves, elevated ST segment, and widened QRS complexes.

PROPHYLAXIS

Comment: Usual dose range is 8-10 mEq/day.

TREATMENT OF HYPOKALEMIA: NON-EMERGENCY (K^+<3.5 mEq/L)

Comment: Usual dose range 40-120 mEq/day in divided doses. Solutions are preferred; potentially serious GI side effects may occur with tablet formulations or when taken on an empty stomach.

POTASSIUM SUPPLEMENTS

Comment: Potassium supplements should be taken with food. Solutions are the preferred form. Extended-release and sustained-release forms should be swallowed whole; do not crush or chew. Potassium supplementation is indicated for hypokalemia including that caused by diuretic use, and digitalis intoxication without atrioventricular (AV) block.

▶ ***potassium*** **(C)(G)** <12 years: not established; ≥12 years:

KCL Solution Oral soln: 10% (30 ml unit dose, 50/case)
K-Dur (as chloride) *Tab:* 10, 20* mEq sust-rel
K-Lor for Oral Solution (as chloride) *Pkts* for reconstitution: 20 mEq/pkt (fruit)
Klor-Con/25 (as chloride) *Pkts* for reconstitution: 25 mEq/pkt
Klor-Con/EF 25 (as bicarbonate) *Pkts* for reconstitution: 25 mEq/pkt (effervescent) (fruit)
Klor-Con Extended-Release (as chloride) *Tab:* 8, 10 mEq ext-rel
Klor-Con M (as chloride) *Tab:* 10, 15*, 20* mEq ext-rel
Klor-Con Powder (as chloride) 20, 25 mEq *Pkts* for reconstitution: (30/carton) (fruit)
Klorvess (as bicarbonate and citrate) *Tab:* 20 mEq effervescent for solution; *Granules:* 20 mEq/pkt effervescent for solution; *Oral liq:* 20 mEq/15 ml (16 oz)
Klotrix (as chloride) *Tab:* 10 mEq sust-rel
K-Lyte (as bicarbonate and citrate) *Tab:* 25 mEq effervescent for solution (lime, orange)
K-Lyte/CL (as chloride) *Tab:* 25 mEq effervescent for solution (citrus, fruit)
K-Lyte/CL 50 (as chloride) *Tab:* 50 mEq effervescent for solution (citrus, fruit)
K-Lyte/DS (as bicarbonate and citrate) *Tab:* 50 mEq effervescent for solution (lime, orange)
K-Tab (as chloride) *Tab:* 10 mEq sust-rel
Micro-K (as chloride) *Cap:* 8, 10 mEq sust-rel
Potassium Chloride Extended Release Caps *Cap:* 8, 10 mEq ext-rel
Potassium Chloride Sust-Rel Tabs *Tab/Cap:* 10 mEq sust-rel
Potassium Chloride ER *Tab:* 8 mEq (600 mg), 10 mEq (750 mg)

HYPOMAGNESEMIA

Comment: Normal serum Mg^{++} range is approximately 1.2-2.6 mEq/L. Signs and symptoms of hypomagnesemia include confusion, disorientation, hallucinations, hyperreflexia, tetany, convulsions, tachyarrhythmia, positive Chvostek's sign, and positive Trousseau's sign. Signs and symptoms of hypermagnesemia include drowsiness, lethargy, muscle weakness, hypoactive reflexes, slurred speech, bradycardia, hypotension, convulsions, and cardiac arrhythmias.

MAGNESIUM SUPPLEMENTS

- ***magnesium*** (B) <12 years: not established; ≥12 years: 2 tabs daily
  Slow-Mag *Tab:* 64 mg (as chloride)+110 mg (as carbonate)
- ***magnesium oxide*** (B) <12 years: not established; ≥12 years: 1 tab daily
  Mag-Ox 400 *Tab:* 400 mg

HYPOPARATHYROIDISM

VITAMIN D ANALOGS

Comment: Concurrent vitamin D supplementation is contraindicated for patients taking ***calcitriol*** or ***doxercalciferol*** owing to the risk of vitamin D toxicity.

- ***calcitriol*** (C) <12 years: initially 0.25 mcg q AM; may increase by 0.25 mcg/day at 4 to 8 week intervals; usual maintenance 0.5-2 mcg/day; ≥12 years: initially 0.25 mcg daily; may increase by 0.25 mcg/day at 2-4-week intervals; usual maintenance (1-6 years) 0.25-0.75 mcg/day, (≥6 years) 0.5-2 mcg/day
  Rocaltrol *Cap:* 0.25, 0.5 mcg
  Rocaltrol Solution *Soln:* 1 mcg/ml (15 ml, single-use dispensers)
- ***doxercalciferol*** (C) <12 years: initially 0.25 mcg q AM; may increase by 0.25 mcg/day at 4-8-week intervals; usual maintenance 0.5-2 mcg/day; ≥12 years: initially 0.25 mcg daily; may increase by 0.25 mcg/day at 2-4-week intervals; usual maintenance (1-6 years) 0.25-0.75 mcg/day, (≥6 years) 0.5-2 mcg/day
  Hectorol *Cap:* 0.25, 0.5 mcg
- ***teriparatide*** (C) <12 years: not recommended; ≥12 years: 20 mcg SC daily in the thigh or abdomen; may treat for up to 2 years
  Forteo *Multidose pen:* 250 mcg/ml (3 ml)
  Comment: **Forteo** is indicated for the treatment of osteoporosis in females who are at high risk for fracture and to increase bone mass in males with primary or hypogonadal osteoporosis who are at high risk for fracture.

HUMAN PARATHYROID HORMONE RELATED PEPTIDE (PTHRP) ANALOG

- ***abaloparatide*** (C) Administer 80 mcg SC once daily into the periumbilical region of the abdomen; sit or lie down in case of orthostatic hypotension, especially for first dose; patients should receive supplemental calcium and vitamin D if dietary intake is inadequate
  Tymlos *Multi-dose pen:* 3120 mcg/1.56 ml (2000 mcg/ml, 30 daily doses) disposable

Comment: **Tymlos** is indicated for the treatment of postmenopausal osteoporosis in women who are at high risk for fracture (defined as a history of osteoporotic fracture, or multiple risk factors for fracture, or patients who have failed or are intolerant to other available osteoporosis therapy. **Tymlos** is not recommended in patients who are at risk for osteosarcoma (boxed warning). Cumulative use of **Tymlos** or other parathyroid analogs (e.g., ***teriparatide***) for >2 years during a patient's lifetime is not recommended (boxed warning). Avoid use in patients with pre-existing hypercalcemia and those known to have an underlying hypercalcemic disorder, such as primary hyperparathyroidism. Monitor urine calcium if preexisting hypercalciuria or active urolithiasis are suspected.

BIOENGINEERED REPLICA OF HUMAN PARATHYROID HORMONE

▶ ***bioengineered replica of human parathyroid hormone*** (C) <12 years: not established; ≥12 years: initially inject mg IM into the thigh once daily; when initiating, decrease dose of active vitamin D by 50% if serum calcium is above 7.5 mg/dL; monitor serum calcium levels every 3-7 days after starting or adjusting dose and when adjusting either active vitamin D or calcium supplements dose

Natpara *Soln for inj:* 25, 50, 75, 100 mcg (2/pkg) multiple dose, dual-chamber glass cartridge containing a sterile powder and diluent

Comment: **Natpara** is indicated as an adjunct to calcium and vitamin D in patients with parathyroidism.

HYPOPHOSPHATASIA (OSTEOMALACIA, RICKETS)

Comment: Hypophosphatasia (HPP) is an inborn error of metabolism marked by abnormally low serum alkaline phosphatase activity and phosphoethanolamine in the urine. It is manifested by osteomalacia in older adolescents and rickets in infants and children. It is most severe in infants under 6 months-of-age. With congenital absence of alkaline phosphatase, an enzyme essential to the calcification of bone tissue, complications include vomiting, growth retardation, and often death in infancy. Surviving children have numerous skeletal abnormalities and dwarfism.

▶ ***asfotase alfa*** 6 mg/kg/week SC, administered as 2 mg/kg or 1 mg/kg 6 x/week; max 9 mg/kg/week SC administered as 3 mg/kg 3 x/week

Strensiq *Vial:* 18 mg/0.45 ml, 28 mg/0.7 ml, 40 mg/ml, 80 mg/0.8 ml for SC inj, single use (1, 12/carton) (preservative-free)

Comment: **Strensiq** is the first FDA-approved (2015) treatment for perinatal, infantile, and juvenile onset HPP. Prior to the availability of **Strensiq**, there was no effective treatment and patient prognosis was very poor.

HYPOPHOSPHATEMIA: X-LINKED (XLH)

FIBROBLAST GROWTH FACTOR 23 (FGF23) BLOCKING ANTIBODY

Comment: **Crysvita** is a fibroblast growth factor 23 (FGF23) blocking antibody indicated for the treatment of X-linked hypophosphatemia (XLH) in adult and pediatric patients ≥1 year-of-age. For SC administration only.

▶ ***burosumab-twza*** (C) <1 year: not recommended; >1-17 years: starting dose 0.8 mg/kg rounded to the nearest 10 mg; min starting dose 10 mg; max dose 90 mg; administer SC every 2 weeks; dose may be increased up to approximately 2 mg/kg (max 90 mg), administered every two weeks to achieve normal serum phosphorus; ≥18 years: 1 mg/kg body weight rounded to the nearest 10 mg up to max dose of 90 mg administered every four weeks

Crysvita *Vial:* 10, 20, 30 mg/ml (1 ml) single-dose

Comment: **Crysvita** is contraindicated in patients with severe renal impairment or end stage renal disease (ESRD). The most common adverse side effects associated with **Crysvita** in pediatric XLH patients are headache, injection site reaction, vomiting, pyrexia, pain in extremity, and decreased serum vitamin D. The most common adverse side effects associated with **Crysvita** in patients with XLH ≥18 years-of-age are back pain, headache, tooth infection, restless leg syndrome, dizziness, constipation, decreased serum vitamin D, and increased serum phosphorus. There are no available data on ***burosumab-twza*** use to inform a drug-associated risk of adverse developmental outcomes in pregnancy. There are no data to inform the presence of ***burosumab-twza*** in human milk or effects on the breastfed infant. To report suspected adverse reactions, contact Ultragenyx at 1-888-756-8657 or FDA at 1-800-FDA-1088 or www.fda.gov/medwatch

HYPOTENSION: NEUROGENIC, ORTHOSTATIC

ALPHA-1 AGONIST

➢ ***midodrine*** (C)(G) <12 years: not recommended; ≥12 years: 10 mg tid at 3-4-hour intervals; take while upright; take last dose at least 4 hours before bedtime

ProAmatine *Tab:* 2.5*, 5*, 10*mg

SYNTHETIC AMINO ACID PRECURSOR OF NOREPINEPHRINE

➢ ***droxidopa*** (C) <12 years: not recommended; ≥12 years: initially 100 mg, taken 3 x/day, upon arising in the morning, at midday, and in the late afternoon at least 3 hours prior to bedtime (to reduce the potential for supine hypertension during sleep); administer with or without; swallow whole; titrate to symptomatic response, in increments of 100 mg tid every 24-48 hours; max 600 mg tid (max total 1,800 mg/day)

Northera *Cap:* 100, 200, 300 mg

Comment: **Northera** is indicated for the treatment of orthostatic dizziness, lightheadedness, or feeling about to black out in patients ≥18 years-of-age with symptomatic neurogenic orthostatic hypotension (NOH) caused by primary autonomic failure (Parkinson's disease [PD], multiple system atrophy [MSA], and pure autonomic failure), dopamine beta-hydroxylase deficiency, and non-diabetic autonomic neuropathy. Effectiveness beyond 2 weeks of treatment has not been established. The continued effectiveness of **Northera** should be assessed. Administering **Northera** in combination with other agents that increase blood pressure (e.g., norepinephrine, ephedrine, midodrine, triptans) would be expected to increase the risk for supine hypertension.

HYPOTHYROIDISM

Comment: Take thyroid replacement hormone in the morning on an empty stomach. Start thyroid hormone replacement at 25 mcg/day. Target TSH is 0.4-5.5 mIU/L; target T4 is 4.5-12.5 ng/L. Signs and symptoms of thyroid toxicity include tachycardia, palpitations, nervousness, chest pain, heat intolerance, and weight loss.

ORAL THYROID HORMONE SUPPLEMENTS

T3

➢ ***liothyronine*** (A) initially 5 mcg/day; may increase by 5 mcg/day every 3-4 days; *Cretinism:* maintenance dose: <1 year: 20 mcg/day; 1-3 years: 50 mcg/day; >3 years: initially 25 mcg daily; may increase by 25 mcg every 1-2 weeks as needed; usual maintenance 25-75 mcg/day

Cytomel *Tab:* 5, 25, 50 mcg

T4

➢ ***levothyroxine*** (A)(G)

Levoxyl <6 months: 8-10 mcg/kg/day; 6-12 months: 6-8 mcg/kg/day; >1-5 years: 5-6 mcg/kg/day; 6-12 years: 4-5 mcg/kg/day; >12 years: initially 25-100 mcg/day; increase by 25 mcg/day q 2-3 weeks as needed; maintenance 100-200 mcg/day

Tab: 25*, 50* (dye-free), 75*, 88*, 100*, 112*, 125*, 137*, 150*, 175*, 200*, 300*mcg

Synthroid <6 months: 8-10 mcg/kg/day; 6-12 months: 6-8 mcg/kg/day; >1-5 years: 5-6 mcg/kg/day; 6-12 years: 4-5 mcg/kg/day; >12 years: initially 50 mcg/day; increase by 25 mcg/day q 2-3 weeks as needed; max 300 mcg/day

Tab: 25*, 50* (dye-free), 75*, 88*, 100*, 112*, 125*, 137*, 150*, 175*, 200*, 300*mcg

Unithroid 0-3 months: 10-15 mcg/kg/day; 3-6 months: 8-10 mcg/kg/day; 6-12 months: 6-8 mcg/kg/day; 1-5 years: 5-6 mcg/kg/day; 6-12 years: 4-5 mcg/kg/day; >12 years: 2-3 mcg/kg/day; *Growth and puberty complete:* initially 50 mcg/day; increase by 25 mcg/day q 2-3 weeks as needed; max 300 mcg/day

Tab: 25*, 50* (dye-free), 75*, 88*, 100*, 112*, 125*, 150*, 175*, 200*, 300*mcg

T3+T4 COMBINATION

▷ ***liothyronine+levothyroxine*** (A) <6 months: 4.6-6 mcg/kg/day; 6-12 months: 3.6-4.8 mcg/kg/day; >1-5 years: 3-3.6 mcg/kg/day; 6-12 years: 2.4-3 mcg/kg/day; >12 years: 1.2-1.8 mcg/kg/day; *Growth and puberty complete:* initially 15-30 mg/day; increase by 15 mg/day q 2-3 weeks to target goal; usual maintenance 60-120 mg/day

Armour Thyroid Tab *Tab:* per grain: T3 9 mcg/T4 38 mcg: 1/4, 1/2, 1, 1, 2, 3*, 4*, 5* gr; 15, 30, 60, 90, 120, 180*, 240*, 300*mg

Thyrolar *Tab: per grain:* T3 12.5 mcg+T4 50 mcg: 1/4, 1/5, 1, 2, 3 gr

PARENTERAL THYROID HORMONE SUPPLEMENT

▷ ***levothyroxine sodium*** (A)(G) <12 years: not recommended; ≥12 years: 1/2 oral dose by IV or IM and titrate; *Myxedema Coma:* 200-500 mcg IV x 1 dose; may administer 100-300 mcg (or more) IV on second day if needed; then 50-100 mcg IV daily; switch to oral form as soon as possible

T4 *Vial:* 100, 200, 500 mcg (pwdr for IM or IV administration after reconstitution)

HYPOTRICHOSIS (THIN/SPARSE EYELASHES)

PROSTAGLANDIN ANALOG

▷ ***bimatoprost*** ophthalmic solution (C)(G) <16 years: not recommended; ≥16 years: apply one drop nightly directly to the skin of the upper eyelid margin at the base of the eyelashes using the accompanying applicators; blot any excess solution beyond the eyelid margin; dispose of the applicator after one use; repeat for the opposite eyelid margin using a new sterile applicator. Repeat treatment of the opposite eye using a new applicator

Latisse *Ophth soln:* 0.03% (3 ml in 5 ml bottle w. 70 disposable sterile applicators; 5 ml in 5 ml bottle w. 140 disposable sterile applicators)

Comment: **Latisse** is indicated to treat hypotrichosis of the eyelashes by increasing their growth including length, thickness and darkness. Ensure the face is clean, all makeup is removed, and contact lenses removed. Place one drop of **Latisse** on the disposable sterile applicator and brush cautiously along the skin of the upper eyelid margin at the base of the eyelashes. Do not to apply to the lower eyelash line. If eyelid skin darkening occurs, it may be reversible after discontinuation of **Latisse**. If any **Latisse** solution gets into the eye proper, it will not cause harm; the eye should not be rinsed. Any excess solution outside the upper eyelid margin should be blotted with a tissue or other absorbent material. Onset of effect is gradual but is not significant in the majority of patients until 2 months. The effect is not permanent and can be expected to gradually return to previous. Additional applications of **Latisse** will not increase the growth of eyelashes.

IDIOPATHIC PULMONARY FIBROSIS (IPF)

Comment: Idiopathic pulmonary fibrosis (IPF) is a chronic, progressive, interstitial lung disease of unknown etiology. There are few effective therapies and the mortality rate is high. New treatments for IPF are urgently needed. Antiinflammatory therapy with corticosteroids or immunosuppressants fails to significantly improve the survival time of patients with IPF. Other pharmacological interventions, which include *nintedanib, etanercept, warfarin, gleevec*, and *bosentan*, remain controversial. *pirfenidone* was approved by the European Medicines Agency in 2011. In a 2016 study, *N-Acetylcysteine* was found to have a significant effect only on decreases in percentage of predicted vital capacity and 6 minutes walking test distance. *N*-acetylcysteine showed no beneficial effect on changes in forced vital capacity, changes in predicted carbon monoxide diffusing capacity, rates of adverse events, <u>or</u> death rates.

REFERENCES

Canestaro, WJ, Forrester, SH, & Raghu, G, *et al.* (2016). Drug treatment of idiopathic pulmonary fibrosis: Systematic review and network meta-analysis. *Chest, 149*(3), 756–766.

Sun, T, Liu, J, & Zhao, DW. (2016). Efficacy of N-Acetylcysteine in idiopathic pulmonary fibrosis: A systematic review and meta-analysis. *Medicine, 95*(19), e3629.

➢ ***azathioprine*** **(D)** <12 years: not recommended; ≥12 years: 1 mg/kg/day in a single or divided doses; may increase by 0.5 mg/kg/day q 4 weeks; max 2.5 mg/kg/day; minimum trial to ascertain effectiveness is 12 weeks

  Azasan *Tab* 75*, 100*mg

  Imuran *Tab* 50*mg

➢ ***nintedanib*** **(D)** <12 years: not established; ≥12 years: 150 mg bid, 12 hours apart; max 300 mg/day; take with food at the same time each day

  Ofev *Cap:* 100, 150 mg

  Comment: Monitor liver enzymes. If elevated LFTs (3 < AST/ALT <5 x ULN) without severe liver damage, interrupt therapy <u>or</u> reduce dose to 100 mg bid. When liver enzymes return to baseline, restart at 100 mg bid and titrate up.

➢ ***pirfenidone*** **(C)** <12 years: not established; ≥12 years: *Days 1-7:* 1 cap tid; *Days 8-14:* 2 caps tid; *Days 15 and ongoing:* 3 caps tid; max 9 caps/day; take with food at the same time each day

  Esbriet *Gelcap:* 267 mg

IMMUNODEFICIENCY: PRIMARY, HUMORAL (PHI)

Comment: Primary Humoral Immunodeficiency (PHI) includes, but is not limited to, Congenital or X-linked Agammaglobulinemia, Common Variable Immunodeficiency, Wiskott-Aldrich Syndrome, Severe Combined Immuno- deficiencies. For chronic inflammatory demyelenating polyneuropathy (CIDP) *see page* 363

IMMUNE GLOBULIN, HUMAN

➢ ***immune globulin subcutaneous [human] 20% liquid*** <2 years: not recommended; ≥2 years: via SC infusion only; *Infusion sites:* abdomen, thigh, upper arm, <u>and/or</u> lateral hip; may use up to 8 injection sites simultaneously, with at least 2 inches between sites; *Infusion volume:* for the first infusion, up to 15 ml per injection site; may increase to 20 ml per site after the fourth infusion; max 25 ml per site as tolerated; *Infusion rate:* first infusion, up to 15 ml/hr per site; may increase, to max 25 ml/hr per site as tolerated; however, maximum flow rate is not to exceed a total of 50 ml/hr for all sites combined before switching to **Hizentra**, obtain the patient's serum IgG trough level to guide subsequent dose adjustments; adjust the dose based on clinical response and serum IgG trough levels; administer at regular intervals from daily up to every 2 week.

Weekly dosing: start **Hizentra** 1 week after last Immune Globulin Intravenous, Human (IGIV) infusion; initial weekly dose: [previous IGIV dose (in grams) x 1.37] divided by # of weeks between IGIV doses

Biweekly dosing (every 2 weeks): start **Hizentra** 1 or 2 weeks after the last IGIV infusion or 1 week after the last weekly IGSC infusion; administer twice the calculated weekly dose

Frequent dosing (2 to 7 times per week): start **Hizentra** 1 week after the last IGIV or IGSC infusion; divide the calculated weekly dose by the desired number of times per week

Hizentra *Vial:* 0.2 mg/ml (20%; 5, 10, 20, 50 ml)

Comment: IgA-deficient patients with anti-IgA antibodies are at greater risk of severe hypersensitivity and anaphylactic reactions. Thrombosis may occur following treatment with immune globulin products, including **Hizentra**. Aseptic meningitis syndrome has been reported with IGIV and IGSC, including **Hizentra**. Monitor renal function in patients at risk of acute renal failure (ARF). Monitor for clinical signs and symptoms of hemolysis. Monitor for pulmonary adverse reactions (transfusion-related acute lung injury [TRALI]). **Hizentra** is made from human blood and may contain infectious agents (e.g., viruses, the variant Creutzfeldt-Jakob disease (vCJD) agent and, theoretically, the Creutzfeldt-Jakob disease (CJD) agent). Monitor for clinical signs and symptoms of hemolysis. The most common adverse reactions observed in ≥5% of study subjects were local infusion site reactions, headache, diarrhea, fatigue, back pain, nausea, pain in extremity, cough, upper respiratory tract infection, rash, pruritus, vomiting, abdominal pain (upper), migraine, arthralgia, pain, fall and nasopharyngitis. No human or animal reproduction studies have not been conducted with **Hizentra**. It is not known whether **Hizentra** can cause fetal harm when administered during pregnancy. No human data are available to inform maternal use of **Hizentra** on the breastfed infant. Safety and effectiveness of weekly **Hizentra** administration have not been established in children <2 years of age. To report suspected adverse reactions, contact CSL Behring Pharmacovigilance at 1-866-915-6958 or FDA at 1-800-FDA-1088 or www.fda.gov/medwatch

☐ IMPETIGO CONTAGIOSA (INDIAN FIRE)

Comment: The most common infectious organisms are *Staphylococcus aureus* and *Streptococcus pyogenes*.

TOPICAL ANTI-INFECTIVES

▶ ***mupirocin*** **(B)(G)** apply to lesions bid; apply to walls of nares bid

Bactroban *Oint:* 2% (22 gm); *Crm:* 2% (15, 30 gm)

Centany *Oint:* 2% (15, 30 gm)

ORAL ANTI-INFECTIVES

▶ ***amoxicillin*** **(B)(G)** <40 kg (88 lb): 20-40 mg/kg/day in 3 divided doses x 10 days or 25-45 mg/kg/day in 2 divided doses x 10 days; *see page* 588 *for dose by weight table;* ≥40 kg: 500-875 mg bid or 250-500 mg tid x 10 days

Amoxil *Cap:* 250, 500 mg; *Tab:* 875*mg; *Chew tab:* 125, 200, 250, 400 mg (cherry-banana-peppermint) (phenylalanine); Oral susp: 125, 250 mg/5 ml (80, 100, 150 ml) (strawberry); 200, 400 mg/5 ml (50, 75, 100 ml) (bubble gum); Oral drops: 50 mg/ml (30 ml) (bubble gum)

Moxatag *Tab:* 775 mg ext-rel

Trimox *Tab:* 125, 250 mg; *Cap:* 250, 500 mg; *Oral susp:* 125, 250 mg/5 ml (80, 100, 150 ml) (raspberry-strawberry)

▶ ***amoxicillin+clavulanate*** **(B)(G)**

Augmentin <40 kg: 40-45 mg/kg/day divided tid x 10 days or 90 mg/kg/day divided bid x 10 days; *see page 590 for dose by weight table;* ≥40 kg: 500 mg tid or 875 mg bid x 10 days

Tab: 250, 500, 875 mg; *Chew tab:* 125, 250 mg (lemon-lime); 200, 400 mg (cherry-banana) (phenylalanine); *Oral susp:* 125 mg/5 ml (banana), 250 mg/5 ml (75, 100, 150 ml) (orange); 200, 400 mg/5 ml (50, 75, 100 ml) (orange) (phenylalanine)

Augmentin ES-600 <3 months: not recommended; ≥3 months, <40 kg: 90 mg/kg/day divided q 12 hours x 10 days; *see page 591 for dose by weight table;* ≥40 kg: not recommended

Oral susp: 600 mg/5 ml (50, 75, 100, 125, 150, 200 ml) (strawberry cream) (phenylalanine)

Augmentin XR <16 years: use other forms; ≥16 years: 2 tabs q 12 hours x 7-10 days

Tab: 1000*mg ext-rel

▶ ***azithromycin*** **(B)(G)** <12 years: 12 mg/kg/day x 5 days; *see page 593 for dose by weight table*; max 500 mg/day; ≥12 years: 500 mg x 1 dose on day 1, then 250 mg daily on days 2-5 or 500 mg daily x 3 days or **Zmax** 2 gm in a single dose

Zithromax *Tab:* 250, 500, 600 mg; *Oral susp:* 100 mg/5 ml (15 ml); 200 mg/5 ml (15, 22.5, 30 ml) (cherry); *Pkt:* 1 gm for reconstitution (cherry-banana)

Zithromax Tri-pak *Tab:* 3 x 500 mg tabs/pck

Zithromax Z-pak *Tab:* 6 x 250 mg tabs/pck

Zmax *Oral susp:* 2 gm ext-rel for reconstitution (cherry-banana) (148 mg Na^+)

▶ ***cefaclor*** **(B)(G)** <1 month: not recommended; 1 month-12 years: 20-40 mg/kg divided bid x 10 days; *see page 594 for dose by weight table;* max 1 gm/day; >12 years: 250-500 mg q 8 hours x 10 days; max 2 gm/day

Tab: 500 mg; *Cap:* 250, 500 mg; *Susp:* 125 mg/5 ml (75, 150 ml) (strawberry); 187 mg/5 ml (50, 100 ml) (strawberry); 250 mg/5 ml (75, 150 ml) (strawberry); 375 mg/5 ml (50, 100 ml) (strawberry)

Cefaclor Extended Release <16 years: not recommended; ≥16 years: 500 mg bid x 10 days (clinically equivalent to 250 mg immed-rel caps tid); swallow whole; take with meals

Tab: 375, 500 mg ext-rel

▶ ***cefadroxil*** <12 years: 30 mg/kg/day in 2 divided doses x 10 days; *see page 595 for dose by weight table;* ≥12 years: 1-2 gm in a single or 2 divided doses x 10 days

Duricef *Cap:* 500 mg; *Tab:* 1 gm; *Oral susp:* 250 mg/5 ml (100 ml); 500 mg/5 ml (75, 100 ml) (orange-pineapple)

▶ ***cefpodoxime proxetil*** **(B)** <2 months: not recommended; 2 months-12 years: 10 mg/kg/day (max 400 mg/dose) or 5 mg/kg/day bid (max 200 mg/dose) x 10 days; *see page 598 for dose by weight table;* >12 years: 200 mg bid x 10 days

Vantin *Tab:* 100, 200 mg; *Oral susp:* 50, 100 mg/5 ml (50, 75, 100 mg) (lemon creme)

▶ ***cefprozil*** **(B)** ≤6 months: not recommended; 6 months-12 years: 7.5 mg/kg bid x 10 days; *see page 599 for dose by weight table;* >12 years: 250-500 mg bid or 500 mg daily x 10 days 500 mg bid x 10 days

Cefzil *Tab:* 250, 500 mg; *Oral susp:* 125, 250 mg/5 ml (50, 75, 100 ml) (bubble gum) (phenylalanine)

▶ ***ceftaroline fosamil*** **(B)** administer by IV infusion after reconstitution every 12 hours x 5-14 days; *CrCl >50 mL/min:* 600 mg; *CrCl >30-<50 mL/min:* 400 mg; *CrCl >1 5-<30 mL/min:* 300 mg; ESRD: 200 mg

Teflaro *Vial:* 400, 600 mg

- ***cephalexin*** **(B)(G)** <12 years: 25-50 mg/kg/day in 4 divided doses x 10 days; *see page* 601 *for dose by weight table*; ≥12 years: 250-500 mg qid or 500 mg bid x 10 days
  - **Keflex** *Cap:* 250, 333, 500, 750 mg; *Oral susp:* 125, 250 mg/5 ml (100, 200 ml) (strawberry)
- ***clarithromycin*** **(C)(G)** <6 months: not recommended; ≥6 months-12 years: 7.5 mg/kg bid x 7 days; *see page* 602 *for dose by weight table;* >12 years: 500 mg or 500 mg ext-rel daily x 7 days
  - **Biaxin** *Tab:* 250, 500 mg
  - **Biaxin Oral Suspension** *Oral susp:* 125, 250 mg/5 ml (50, 100 ml) (fruit punch)
  - **Biaxin XL** *Tab:* 500 mg ext-rel

Comment: The FDA is advising caution before prescribing ***clarithromycin*** to patients with heart disease because of a potential increased risk of heart problems or death that can occur years later. This recommendation is based on a review of the results of a 10-year follow-up study of patients with coronary heart disease from a large clinical trial that first observed this safety issue. Consider risk benefit and the use of other antibiotics in such patients.

- ***dicloxacillin*** **(B)(G)** <12 years: 12.5-25 mg/kg/day in 4 divided doses x 10 days; *see page* 604 *for dose by weight table;* ≥12 years: 500 mg q 6 hours x 10 days
  - **Dynapen** *Cap:* 125, 250, 500 mg; *Oral susp:* 62.5 mg/5 ml (80, 100, 200 ml)
- ***erythromycin base*** **(B)(G)** <45 kg: 30-50 mg in 2-4 divided doses x 7-10 days; ≥45 kg: 250 mg qid, or 333 mg tid, or 500 mg bid x 7-10 days
  - **Ery-Tab** *Tab:* 250, 333, 500 mg ent-coat
  - **PCE** *Tab:* 333, 500 mg

Comment: ***erythromycin*** may increase INR with concomitant ***warfarin***, as well as increase serum level of ***digoxin***, benzodiazepines and statins.

- ***erythromycin ethylsuccinate*** **(B)(G)** 30-50 mg/kg/day in 4 divided doses x 7-10 days; may double dose with severe infection; max 100 mg/kg/day or 400 mg qid; *see page* 607 *for dose by weight table*
  - **EryPed** *Oral susp:* 200 mg/5 ml (100, 200 ml) (fruit); 400 mg/5 ml (60, 100, 200 ml) (banana); *Oral drops:* 200, 400 mg/5 ml (50 ml) (fruit); *Chew tab:* 200 mg wafer (fruit)
  - **E.E.S.** *Oral susp:* 200, 400 mg/5 ml (100 ml) (fruit)
  - **E.E.S. Granules** *Oral susp:* 200 mg/5 ml (100, 200 ml) (cherry)
  - **E.E.S. 400 Tablets** *Tab:* 400 mg

Comment: ***erythromycin*** may increase INR with concomitant ***warfarin***, as well as increase serum level of ***digoxin***, benzodiazepines and statins.

- ***loracarbef*** **(B)** <12 years: 15 mg/kg/day in 2 divided doses x 10 days; *see page 614 for dose by weight table*; ≥12 years: 200 mg bid x 10 days
  - **Lorabid** *Pulvule:* 200, 400 mg; *Oral susp:* 100 mg/5 ml (50, 100 ml); 200 mg/5 ml (50, 75, 100 ml) (strawberry bubble gum)
- ***penicillin g (benzathine)*** **(B)** <12 years: <60 lb: 300,000-600,000 units IM x 1 dose; ≥60 lb: 900,000 units x 1 dose; ≥12 years: 1.2 million units IM x 1 dose
  - **Bicillin L-A** *Cartridge-needle unit:* 600,000 units (1 ml); 1.2 million units (2 ml)
- ***penicillin g (benzathine+procaine)*** **(B)(G)** <30 lb: 600,000 units IM x 1 dose; 30-60 lb: 900,000-1.2 million units IM x 1 dose; ≥12 years: 2.4 million units IM x 1 dose
  - **Bicillin C-R** *Cartridge-needle unit:* 600,000 units (1 ml); 1.2 million units (2 ml); 2.4 million units (4 ml)
- ***penicillin v potassium*** **(B)** <12 years: 25-75 mg/kg day divided q 6-8 hours x 3 days; *see page* 616 *for dose by weight table;* ≥12 years: 250-500 mg q 6 hours x 10 days
  - **Pen-VK** *Tab:* 250, 500 mg; *Oral soln:* 125 mg/5 ml (100, 200 ml); 250 mg/5 ml (100, 150, 200 ml)

INCONTINENCE: FECAL

Comment: Treatment of fecal incontinence in patients who have failed conservative therapy (e.g., diet, fiber therapy, antimotility agents).

▶ ***dextranomer microspheres+sodium hyaluronate*** <18 years: not recommended; ≥18 years:
Pretreatment: bowel preparation using enema (required) and prophylactic antibiotics (recommended) prior to injection;
Treatment: inject slowly into the deep submucosal layer in the proximal part of the high pressure zone of the anal canal about 5 mm above the dentate line; 4 x 1 ml injections in the following order: posterior, left lateral, anterior, right lateral; keep needle in place 15-30 seconds to minimize leakage; use a new needle for each syringe and injection site;
Post-treatment: avoid hot baths and physical activity during first 24 hours; avoid antidiarrheal drugs, sexual intercourse, and strenuous activity for 1 week; avoid anal manipulation for 1 month;
Retreatment: may repeat if needed with max 4 ml, no sooner than 4 weeks after the first injection; point of injection should be made in between initial injection sites (i.e., shifted 1/8 of a turn)
Solesta dex micro 50 mg+sod hyal 15 mg per ml; *Syringe:* 1 ml (4 w. needles)

INCONTINENCE: URINARY (STRESS INCONTINENCE & OVERACTIVE BLADDER & ATONIC BLADDER)

See **Enuresis** *page* 143

▶ ***pseudoephedrine*** (C)(G) 30-60 mg tid
Sudafed (OTC) *Tab:* 30 mg; *Liq:* 15 mg/5 ml (1, 4 oz)

VASOPRESSIN

▶ ***desmopressin acetate (DDAVP)*** (B)(G)
DDAVP <6 years: not recommended; ≥6 years: 0.5 mg daily <u>or</u> q HS prn; ≥12 years: usual dosage 0.1-1.2 mg/day in 2-3 divided doses; 0.2 mg q HS prn for nocturnal enuresis
Tab: 0.1*, 0.2*mg
DDAVP Rhinal Tube <6 years: not recommended; ≥6 years: 10 mcg <u>or</u> 0.1 ml of soln each nostril (20 mcg total dose) q HS prn; max 40 mcg total dose
Rhinal tube: 0.1 mg/ml (2.5 ml)

BETA-3 ADRENERGIC AGONIST

▶ ***mirabegron*** (C) <12 years: not established; ≥12 years: initially 25 mg once daily; max 50 mg once daily; *Severe renal impairment:* 25 mg once daily
Myrbetriq *Tab:* 25, 50 mg ext-rel

Comment: **Myrbetriq** ***(mirabegron)*** is FDA-approved to be taken in combination with **VESIcare** ***(solifenacin succinate)*** for the treatment of overactive bladder (OAB) with symptoms of frequency, urgency, and urge urinary incontinence.

MUSCARINIC RECEPTOR ANTAGONISTS

▶ ***fesoterodine*** (C)(G) <12 years: not recommended; ≥12 years: 4 mg daily; max 8 mg/day
Toviaz *Tab:* 4, 8 mg ext-rel

▶ ***tolterodine tartrate*** **(C)(G)** <12 years: not established; ≥12 years: **Detrol** 2 mg bid; may decrease to 1 mg bid

Tab: 1, 2 mg

Detrol LA 2-4 mg once daily

Cap: 2, 4 mg ext-rel

ANTISPASMODIC/ANTICHOLINERGICS

▶ ***darifenacin*** **(C)(G)** <12 years: not recommended; ≥12 years: not recommended; ≥12 years: 7.5-15 mg daily with liquid; max 15 mg/day

Enablex *Tab:* 7.5, 15 mg ext-rel

▶ ***dicyclomine*** **(B)(G)** <12 years: not recommended; ≥12 years: 10-20 mg qid

Bentyl *Tab:* 20 mg; *Cap:* 10 mg; *Syr:* 10 mg/5 ml (16 oz)

▶ ***flavoxate*** **(B)** <12 years: not recommended; ≥12 years: 100-200 mg tid-qid

Urispas *Tab:* 100 mg

▶ ***hyoscyamine*** **(C)(G)**

Anaspaz <2 years: not recommended; 2-12 years: 0.0625-0.125 mg q 4 hours prn; max 0.75 mg/day; >12 years: 1-2 tabs q 4 hours prn; max 12 tabs/day

Tab: 0.125*

Levbid <12 years: not recommended; ≥12 years: 1-2 tabs q 12 hours prn; max 4 tabs/day

Tab: 0.375*mg ext-rel

Levsin <6 years: not recommended; 6-12 years: 1 tab q 4 hours prn; >12 years: 1-2 tabs q 4 hours prn; max 12 tabs/day

Tab: 0.125*mg;

Levsin Drops <12 years: 3.4 kg: 4 drops q 4 hours prn; max 24 drops/day; 5 kg: 5 drops q 4 hours prn; max 30 drops/day; 7 kg: 6 drops q 4 hours prn; max 36 drops/day; 10 kg: 8 drops q 4 hours prn; max 40 drops/day; ≥12 years: 1-2 ml q 4 hours prn; max 60 ml/day

Oral drops: 0.125 mg/ml (15 ml) (orange) (alcohol 5%)

Levsin Elixir <12 years: <10 kg: use drops; 10-19 kg: 1.25 ml q 4 hours prn; 20-39 kg: 2.5 ml q 4 hours prn; 40-49 kg: 3.75 ml q 4 hours prn; ≥50 kg: 5 ml q 4 hours prn; ≥12 years: 5-10 ml q 4 hours prn

Elix: 0.125 mg/5 ml (16 oz) (orange) (alcohol 20%)

Levsinex SL <2 years: not recommended; 2-12 years: 1 tab q 4 hours; max 6 tabs/day; >12 years:

Tab: 0.125 mg sublingual; ≥12 years: 1-2 tabs q 4 hours SL or PO; max 12 tabs/day

Levsinex Timecaps <2 years: not recommended; 2-12 years: 1 cap q 12 hours; max 2 caps/day; >12 years: 1-2 caps q 12 hours; may adjust to 1 cap q 8 hours

Cap: 0.375 mg time-rel

NuLev <2 years: not recommended; 2-12 years: dissolve 1 tab on tongue, with or without water, q 4 hours prn; max 6 tabs/day; >12 years: dissolve 1-2 tabs on tongue, with or without water, q 4 hours prn; max 12 tabs/day

ODT: 0.125 mg (mint; phenylalanine)

▶ ***oxybutynin chloride*** **(B)**

Ditropan <5 years: not recommended; 5-12 years: 5 mg bid; max 15 mg/day; >12 years: 5 mg bid-tid; max 20 mg/day

Tab: 5*mg; *Syr:* 5 mg/5 ml

Ditropan XL <6 years: not recommended; ≥6 years: initially 5 mg once daily; may increase weekly in 5 mg increments as needed; max 20 mg/day; ≥12 years: initially 5 mg daily; may increase weekly in 5 mg increments as needed; max 30 mg/day

Tab: 5, 10, 15 mg ext-rel

GelniQUE 3 mg Pump: <6 years: not recommended; ≥6 years: apply 3 pumps (84 mg) once daily to clean dry intact skin on the abdomen, upper arm, shoulders, or thighs; rotate sites; wash hands; avoid washing application site for 1 hour after application

Gel: 3% (92 gm, metered pump dispenser) (alcohol)

GelniQUE 1 gm Sachet: <6 years: not recommended; ≥6 years: apply 1 gm gel (1 sachet) once daily to dry intact skin on abdomen, upper arms/shoulders, or thighs; rotate sites; wash hands; avoid washing application site for 1 hour after application

Gel: 10% (1 gm/sachet, 30/carton) (alcohol)

Oxytrol Transdermal Patch (OTC) <12 years: not established; ≥12 years: apply patch to clean dry area of the abdomen, hip, or buttock; one patch twice weekly; rotate sites

Transdermal patch: 3.9 mg/day

▶ ***propantheline*** (C) <12 years: not recommended; ≥12 years: 15-30 mg tid

Pro-Banthine *Tab:* 7.5, 15 mg

▶ ***solifenacin*** (C)(G) <12 years: not recommended; ≥12 years: 5-10 mg daily

VESIcare *Tab:* 5, 10 mg

Comment: **Myrbetriq *(mirabegron)*** is FDA-approved to be taken in combination with **VESIcare *(solifenacin succinate)*** for the treatment of overactive bladder (OAB) with symptoms of frequency, urgency, and urge urinary incontinence.

▶ ***trospium chloride*** (C)(G)

Sanctura <6 years: not recommended; ≥6 years: 20 mg twice daily; ≥75 years: *CrCl ≤30 mL/min:* 20 mg once daily

Tab: 20 mg

Sanctura XR <6 years: not recommended; ≥6 years: 60 mg daily in the morning

Cap: 60 mg ext-rel

Comment: Take ***trospium chloride*** on an empty stomach.

OVERFLOW INCONTINENCE+ATONIC BLADDER

▶ ***bethanechol*** (C) <12 years: not recommended; ≥12 years: 10-30 mg tid

Urecholine *Tab:* 5, 10, 25, 50 mg

INFLUENZA (FLU)

Comment: Egg allergy affects as many as 2% of children in the US. New data have affirmed what the American College of Allergy, Asthma and Immunology said has been known for several years: there are no special precautions needed to dispense the influenza vaccine in people with egg allergy. Based on recommendations from the clinical immunization safety assessment hypersensitivity working group of the ACIP, the members voted during the meeting this week to recommend administration of trivalent inactivated influenza vaccine to patients with a history of egg allergy. The consensus of the working group: egg allergy of any severity, including anaphylaxis, should not be a contraindication of the administration of the influenza vaccine, but rather a precaution. Both the single-dose and two-dose methods are appropriate for administering influenza vaccine to those who are allergic to eggs. No special precautions beyond those recommended for providing any vaccine to any patient are necessary for administration of influenza vaccine to persons allergic to eggs. The recommendation will be included in the ACIP draft guidelines for use of influenza vaccines for the upcoming season.

REFERENCES

Greenhawt, M, Turner, PJ, & Kelso, JM. (2018). Administration of influenza vaccines to egg allergic recipients: a practice parameter update 2017. *Annals of Allergy, Asthma & Immunology, 120*(1), 49–52. doi:10.1016/j.anai.2017.10.020

Turner, PJ, Southern, J, Andrews, NJ, *et al.* (2015). Safety of live attenuated influenza vaccine in atopic children with egg allergy. *Journal of Allergy and Clinical Immunology, 136*(2), 376–381. doi:10.1016/j.jaci.2014.12.1925

Comment: Until official guidelines are available, provider discretion should be used with appropriate precautions with individual patient consideration and informed consent. Refer to mfr's pkg insert for product maker's recommendations and precautions. With the exception of **Flucelvax**, current flu vaccine mfr pkg inserts report that flu vaccine is contraindicated with allergy to egg or chicken proteins, or egg products, and all flu vaccines are contraindicated with allergy to latex, active infection, acute respiratory disease, active neurological disorder; history of Guillain-Barre syndrome. Have epinephrine 1:1,000 on hand. Flu vaccine is contraindicated for children under 18 years-of-age who are taking ***aspirin*** and/or an ***aspirin***-containing product due to the risk of developing Reye's syndrome. Under 1 year-of-age, administer flu vaccine in the vastus lateralis in two split doses one month apart. Over 1 year-of-age, administer flu vaccine in the deltoid. Flu vaccine formulations change annually. Administer flu vaccine 1 month before flu season. Flu vaccine delivered via nasal spray may be administered earlier.

PROPHYLAXIS (NASAL SPRAY)

▶ ***trivalent, live attenuated influenza vaccine, types a and b*** (C) ≤5 years: not recommended; ≥5 years: 1 spray each nostril

Never vaccinated with **FluMist**: 5-8 years: 2 divided doses 46-74 days apart.

Previously vaccinated with **FluMist**: 5-8 years: 1 spray each nostril

FluMist Nasal Spray 0.5 ml spray annually

Nasal spray: 0.5 ml (0.25 ml/spray) (10/carton) (preservative-free)

PROPHYLAXIS (INJECTABLE)

▶ ***quadrivalent inactivated influenza subvirion vaccine, types a and b*** (C) <3 years: not recommended; ≥3 years: 0.5 ml IM annually

Fluad 0.5 ml IM annually

Comment: **Fluad** is the first seasonal influenza vaccine with adjuvant, indicated for persona ≥65 years-of-age. Adjuvants are incorporated into some vaccine formulations to enhance or direct the immune response.

Fluarix Quadrivalent *Prefilled syringes:* 0.5 ml (10/carton; preservative-free, latex-free)

▶ ***trivalent inactivated influenza subvirion vaccine, types A and B***

Afluria (B) <5 years: not recommended; 5-8 years: 1-2 doses/season at least 4 weeks apart; >9 years: 1 dose/season

Comment: Contraindicated with allergy to egg or chicken protein, neomycin, polymyxin, or history of life-threatening reaction to any previous fly vaccine.

Fluarix (B) 0.5 ml IM annually; <3 years: not recommended; 3-9 years (previously unvaccinated or vaccinated for the first time last season with one dose of flu vaccine): 2 doses per season at least 1 month apart; 3-9 years (previously vaccinated with two doses of flu vaccine); and >9 years: 1 dose per season

Prefilled syringe: 0.5 ml single-dose (5/carton) (may contain trace amounts of hydrocortisone, gentamicin; preservative-free)

Comment: Contraindicated with allergy to egg protein.

Flublok <18 years: not recommended; ≥18 years: 0.5 ml IM in the deltoid annually
Vial: 0.5 ml single-dose (10/carton) (preservative-free, egg protein-free, antibiotic-free, latex-free)

Comment: **Flublok** is a cell culture-derived vaccine and, therefore, is an alternative to the traditional egg-based vaccines. Contains 3 times the amount of active ingredient in traditional flu vaccines

Flucelvax <18 years: not established; ≥18 years: 0.5 ml IM annually
Prefilled syringes: 0.5 ml (10/carton; preservative-free, latex-free)

Comment: **Flucelvax** is a cell culture-derived vaccine and, therefore, is an alternative to the traditional egg-based vaccines.

FluLaval (C) <3 years: not established; 3-8 years, *never received the vaccine:* 2 doses/season administered at least 4 weeks apart; 3-8 years, *vaccinated in a previous season:* 1-2 doses/season administered at least 4 weeks apart; ≥9 years: one dose/season; a single dose is 0.5 ml; all ages, administer IM in the deltoid
Vial: 5 ml multi-dose (10 doses)

Comment: Contraindicated with allergy to egg protein.

FluShield <6 months: not recommended; *Never vaccinated:* <9 years: 2 doses at least 4 weeks apart; 9-12 years: same as adult; *Previously vaccinated:* 6-35 months: 0.25 ml IM x 1 dose; 3-8 years: 0.5 ml IM annually

Fluzone 0.5 ml IM annually
Vial: 5 ml (thimerosal)

Comment: Contraindicated with allergy to egg protein, or history of life-threatening reaction to any previous flu vaccine.

Fluzone Preservative-Free: Adult Dose <6 months: not recommended; *Not previously vaccinated:* 6 months-8 years: 0.25 ml IM; repeat in 1 month; *Previously vaccinated:* 6-35 months: 0.25 ml IM x 1 dose; ≥3 years: 0.5 ml IM annually *Prefilled syringe*: 0.5 ml (10/carton) (preservative-free, trace thimerosal)

Fluzone Preservative-Free: Pediatric Dose <6 months: not recommended; *Not previously vaccinated:* 6 months-8 years: 0.25 ml IM; repeat in 1 month; *Previously vaccinated:* 6-35 months: 0.25 ml IM x 1 dose; ≥3 years: 0.5 ml IM (use **Fluzone for Adult**). All ages: administer in the deltoid
Prefilled syringe: 0.5 ml (10/carton; preservative-free; trace thimerosal)

Comment: Contraindicated with allergy to egg protein, or history of life-threatening reaction to any previous flu vaccine.

PROPHYLAXIS AND TREATMENT

Neuraminidase Inhibitors

Comment: Effective for influenza type A and B. Indicated for treatment of uncomplicated acute illness in patients who have been symptomatic for no more than 2 days; therefore, start within 2 days of symptom onset or exposure. Indicated for influenza prophylaxis in patients ≥3 months of age.

▶ ***oseltamivir phosphate*** (C)(G) *Prophylaxis:* <1 year: not recommended; 1-12 years: <15 kg: 30 mg once daily x 10 days; 16-23 kg: 45 mg once daily x 10 days; 24-40 kg: 60 mg once daily x 10 days; >40 kg: 75 mg daily for at least 7 days and up to 6 weeks for community outbreak; *Treatment:* <1 year: not recommended; 1-12 years: <15 kg: 30 mg bid x 5 days; 16-23 kg: 45 mg bid x 5 days; 24-40 kg: 60 mg bid x 5 days; >40 kg: 75 mg bid x 5 days; initiate treatment only if symptomatic <2 days

Tamiflu *Cap:* 30, 45, 75 mg; *Oral susp:* 6 mg/ml pwdr for reconstitution (60 ml w. oral dispenser) (tutti-frutti)

Comment: **Tamiflu** is effective for influenza type A and B.

▶ *zanamivir* (C) <7 years: not recommended; ≥7 years: 2 inhalations (10 mg) bid x 5 days
Relenza Inhaler *Inhaler:* 5 mg/inh blister (4 blisters/Rotadisk, 5 Rotadisks/carton w. 1 inhaler)
Comment: **Relenza Inhaler** is effective for influenza type A and B. Use caution with asthma.

INSECT BITE/STING

Topical Corticosteroids *see page* 542
Parenteral Corticosteroids *see page* 547
Oral Corticosteroids *see page 546*

TOPICAL ANESTHETIC

▶ *lidocaine* 3% cream **(B)** apply bid-tid prn; reduce dosage commensurate with age, body weight, and physical condition
LidaMantle *Crm:* 3% (1 oz)

EPINEPHRINE

▶ *epinephrine* (C)(G) <12 years: 0.01 ml/kg SC; ≥12 years: 1:1,000 0.3-0.5 ml

TETANUS PROPHYLAXIS

▶ *tetanus toxoid* vaccine **(C)(G)** 0.5 ml IM x 1 dose if previously immunized
Vial: 5 Lf units/0.5 ml (0.5, 5 ml); *Prefilled syringe:* 5 Lf units/0.5 ml (0.5 ml) (For patients not previously immunized *see* ***Tetanus*** *page* 445)

INSOMNIA

Tricyclic Antidepressants *see* ***Depression*** *page* 110

MELATONIN RECEPTOR AGONIST

▶ *ramelteon* (C)(IV) <12 years: not recommended; ≥12 years: 8 mg within 30 minutes of bedtime; delayed effect if taken with a meal
Rozerem *Tab:* 8 mg

NON-BENZODIAZEPINES

▶ *eszopiclone* (pyrrolopyrazine) **(C)(IV)(G)** <18 years: not recommended; ≥18 years: 1-3 mg; max 3 mg/day x 1 month; do not take if unable to sleep for at least 8 hours before required to be active again; delayed effect if taken with a meal
Lunesta *Tab:* 1, 2, 3 mg

▶ *zaleplon* (imidazopyridine) **(C)(IV)(G)** <12 years: not recommended; ≥12 years: 5-10 mg at HS or after going to bed if unable to sleep; do not take if unable to sleep for at least 4 hours before required to be active again; max 20 mg/day x 1 month; delayed effect if taken with a meal
Sonata *Cap:* 5, 10 mg (tartrazine)
Comment: **Sonata** is indicated for the treatment of insomnia when a middle-of-the-night awakening is followed by difficulty returning to sleep.

▶ *zolpidem* oral solution spray (imidazopyridine hypnotic) **(C)(IV)** <18 years: not recommended; ≥18 years: 2 actuations (10 mg) immediately before bedtime; *Debilitated,* or *hepatic impairment:* 2 actuations (5 mg); max 2 actuations (10 mg)
ZolpiMist *Oral soln spray*: 5 mg/actuation (60 metered actuations) (cherry)

Comment: The lowest dose of ***zolpidem*** in all forms is recommended for females as drug elimination is slower than in males.

▷ ***zolpidem*** tabs (pyrazolopyrimidine hypnotic) **(B)(IV)(G)** <18 years: not recommended; ≥18 years: 5-10 mg or 6.25-12.5 ext-rel q HS prn; max 12.5 mg/day x 1 month; do not take if unable to sleep for at least 8 hours before required to be active again; delayed effect if taken with a meal

Ambien *Tab:* 5, 10 mg

Ambien CR *Tab:* 6.25, 12.5 mg ext-rel

Comment: The lowest dose of ***zolpidem*** in all forms is recommended for females as drug elimination is slower than in men.

▷ ***zolpidem*** sublingual tabs (imidazopyridine hypnotic) **(C)(IV)(G)** <18 years: not recommended; ≥18 years: dissolve 1 tab under the tongue; allow to disintegrate completely before swallowing; take only once per night and only if at least 4 hours of bedtime remain before planned time for awakening

Edluar *SL Tab:* 5, 10 mg

Intermezzo *SL Tab:* 1.75, 3.5 mg

Comment: **Intermezzo** is indicated for the treatment of insomnia when a middle-of-the-night awakening is followed by difficulty returning to sleep. The lowest dose of ***zolpidem*** in all forms is recommended for females as drug elimination is slower than in males.

OREXIN RECEPTOR ANTAGONIST

▷ ***suvorexant*** **(C)(IV)** <12 years: not recommended; ≥12 years: use lowest effective dose; take 30 minutes before bedtime; do not take if unable to sleep for ≥7 hours, max 20 mg

Belsomra *Tab:* 5, 10, 15, 20 mg (30/blister pck)

BENZODIAZEPINES

▷ ***estazolam*** **(X)(IV)(G)** <18 years: not recommended; ≥18 years: initially 1 mg q HS prn; may increase to 2 mg q HS

ProSom *Tab:* 1*, 2*mg

▷ ***flurazepam*** **(X)(IV)(G)** <15 years: not recommended; ≥15 years: 30 mg q HS prn; *Debilitated:* 15 mg

Dalmane *Cap:* 15, 30 mg

▷ ***temazepam*** **(X)(IV)(G)** <18 years: not recommended; ≥18 years: 7.5-30 mg q HS prn; short term, 7-10 days; max 30 mg; max 1 month

Restoril *Cap:* 7.5, 15, 22.5, 30 mg

▷ ***triazolam*** **(X)(IV)** <18 years: not recommended; ≥18 years: 0.125-0.25 mg q HS prn; short term, 7-10 days; max 0.5 mg; max 1 month

Halcion *Tab:* 0.125, 0.25*mg

BARBITURATE

▷ ***pentobarbital*** **(D)(II)(G)**

Nembutal <12 years: not recommended; ≥12 years: 50 or 100 mg q HS prn

Cap: 50, 100 mg

Nembutal Suppository one supp q HS prn; <2 months: not recommended; 2-12 months (10-20 lb): 30 mg supp; >1 year-4 years (21-40 lb): 30 or 60 mg supp; 5-12 years (41-80 lb): 60 mg supp; >12-14 years (81-110 lb): 60 or 120 mg supp; >14 years: 120 or 200 mg supp q HS prn

Rectal supp: 30, 60, 120, 200 mg

ORAL H1 RECEPTOR AGONIST (FIRST GENERATION ANTIHISTAMINE)

▶ *doxepin* (C) <12 years: not recommended; ≥12 years: 3-6 mg q HS prn; *Hepatic impairment, tendency to urinary retention:* initially 3 mg
Silenor *Tab:* 3, 6 mg

ANALGESIC+FIRST GENERATION ANTIHISTAMINE COMBINATIONS

▶ *acetaminophen+diphenhydramine* (B) <12 years: not recommended; ≥12 years: 2 tabs q HS prn
Excedrin PM (OTC) *Tab/Gel tab:* acet 500 mg+diphen 38 mg
Tylenol PM (OTC) *Tab/Cap/Gel cap:* acet 500 mg+diphen 25 mg

INTERSTITIAL CYSTITIS

Acetaminophen for IV Infusion *see* ***Pain*** *page* 322
Oral Prescription NSAIDs *see page* 539
Comment: Avoid peppers and spicy food, citrus, vinegar, caffeine (e.g., coffee, tea, cola), alcohol, carbonated beverages, and other GU tract irritants.

MANAGEMENT OF PAIN AND URINARY URGENCY

Acetaminophen for IV Infusion *see* ***Pain*** *page* 322
Oral Prescription NSAIDs *see page* 539
▶ *phenazopyridine* (B)(G) <12 years: not recommended; ≥12 years: 95-200 mg q 6 hours prn; max 2 days
AZO Standard, Prodium, Uristat (OTC) *Tab:* 95 mg
AZO Standard Maximum Strength (OTC) *Tab:* 97.5 mg
Pyridium, Urogesic *Tab:* 100, 200 mg *phenazopyridine* (B)(G) 190-200 mg tid; max 2 days
Azo Standard (OTC) *Tab:* 95 mg
Azo Standard Maximum Strength (OTC) *Tab:* 97.5 mg
Pyridium *Tab:* 100, 200 mg ent-coat
Uristat (OTC) *Tab:* 95 mg
Urogesic *Tab:* 100, 200 mg
▶ *hyoscyamine* (C)(G)
Anaspaz <2 years: not recommended; 2-12 years: 0.0625-0.125 mg q 4 hours prn; max 0.75 mg/day; >12 years: 1-2 tabs q 4 hours prn; max 12 tabs/day
Tab: 0.125*mg
Levbid <12 years: not recommended; ≥12 years: 1-2 tabs q 12 hours prn; max 4 tabs/day
Tab: 0.375*mg ext-rel
Levsin <6 years: not recommended; 6-12 years: 1 tab q 4 hours prn; ≥12 years: 1-2 tabs q 4 hours prn; max 12 tabs/day
Tab: 0.125*mg
Levsin Drops <3 kg: not recommended: 3.4 kg: 4 drops q 4 hours prn; max 24 drops/day; 5 kg: 5 drops q 4 hours prn; max 30 drops/day; 7 kg: 6 drops q 4 hours prn; max 36 drops/day; 10 kg: 8 drops q 4 hours prn; max 40 drops/day; >10 kg: 1-2 ml q 4 hours prn; max 60 ml/day
Oral drops: 0.125 mg/ml (15 ml) (orange) (alcohol 5%)
Levsin Elixir <10 kg: use drops; 10-19 kg: 1.25 ml q 4 hours prn; 20-39 kg: 2.5 ml q 4 hours prn; 40-49 kg: 3.75 ml q 4 hours prn; ≥50 kg: 5 ml q 4 hours prn
Elix: 0.125 mg/5 ml (16 oz) (orange) (alcohol 20%)

Levsinex SL <2 years: not recommended; 2-12 years: 1 tab q 4 hours; max 6 tabs/day; >12 years: 1-2 tabs q 4 hours SL or PO; max 12 tabs/day
SL tab: 0.125 mg
Levsinex Timecaps <2 years: not recommended; 2-12 years: 1 cap q 12 hours; max 2 caps/day; >12 years: 1-2 caps q 12 hours; may adjust to 1 cap q 8 hours
Cap: 0.375 mg time-rel
NuLev <2 years: not recommended; 2-12 years: dissolve 1 tab on tongue, with or without water, q 4 hours prn; max 6 tabs/day; >12 years: dissolve 1-2 tabs on tongue, with or without water, q 4 hours prn; max 12 tabs/day
ODT: 0.125 mg (mint) (phenylalanine)

- ***methenamine+na phosphate monobasic+phenyl salicylate+methylene blue+hyoscyamine sulfate*** **(C)** <6 years: not recommended; ≥6 years: individualize dose (see mfr pkg insert)
Uribel *Cap:* meth 118 mg+sod phos 40.8 mg+phenyl sal 36 mg+methyl blue 10 mg+hyoscy 0.12 mg
- ***methenamine+phenyl salicylate+methylene blue+benzoic acid+atropine sulfate+hyoscyamine sulfate*** **(C)(G)** <6 years: not recommended; ≥6 years: 2 tabs qid
Urised *Tab:* meth 40.8 mg+phenyl sal 18.1 mg+methyl blue 5.4 mg+benz acid 4.5 mg+atro sul 0.03 mg+hyoscy 0.03 mg
Comment: **Urised** imparts a blue-green color to urine which may stain fabrics.
- ***oxybutynin chloride*** **(B)**
Ditropan <5 years: not recommended; 5-12 years: 5 mg bid; max 15 mg/day; ≥12 years: 5 mg bid-tid; max 20 mg/day
Tab: 5*mg; *Syr:* 5 mg/5 ml
Ditropan XL <12 years: not recommended; ≥12 years: initially 5 mg daily; may increase weekly in 5 mg increments as needed; max 30 mg/day
Tab: 5, 10, 15 mg ext-rel
- ***pentosan*** **(B)** <16 years: not recommended; ≥16 years: 100 mg tid; re-evaluate at 3 and 6 months
Elmiron *Cap:* 100 mg

URINARY TRACT ANALGESIA

- ***phenazopyridine*** **(B)(G)** <12 years: not recommended; ≥12 years: 95-200 mg q 6 hours prn; max 2 days
AZO Standard, Prodium, Uristat (OTC) *Tab:* 95 mg
AZO Standard Maximum Strength (OTC) *Tab:* 97.5 mg
Pyridium, Urogesic *Tab:* 100, 200 mg
Azo Standard (OTC) *Tab:* 95 mg
Azo Standard Maximum Strength (OTC) *Tab:* 97.5 mg
Pyridium *Tab:* 100, 200 mg ent-coat
Uristat (OTC) *Tab:* 95 mg
Urogesic *Tab:* 100, 200 mg
Comment: *Phenazopyridine* imparts an orange-red color to urine which may stain fabrics.
- ***propantheline*** **(C)** <12 years: not recommended; ≥12 years: 15-30 mg tid
Pro-Banthine *Tab:* 7.5, 15 mg
- ***tolterodine tartrate*** **(C)(G)**
Detrol <12 years: not recommended; ≥12 years: 2 mg bid; may decrease to 1 mg bid
Tab: 1, 2 mg
Detrol XL 2-4 mg daily
Cap: 2, 4 mg ext-rel

ANTICHOLINERGIC+SEDATIVE COMBINATION

- ***chlordiazepoxide+clidinium*** (D)(IV) <12 years: not recommended; ≥12 years: 1-2 caps ac and HS; max 8 caps/day
  Librax *Cap:* chlor 5 mg+clid 2.5 mg

TRICYCLIC ANTIDEPRESSANTS (TCAs)

Comment: Co-administration of SSRIs and TCAs requires extreme caution.

- ***amitriptyline*** (C)(G) <12 years: not recommended; ≥12 years: 10-20 mg q HS
  Tab: 10, 25, 50, 75, 100, 150 mg
- ***amoxapine*** (C) <12 years: not recommended; ≥12 years: initially 50 mg bid-tid; after 1 week may increase to 100 mg bid-tid; usual effective dose 200-300 mg/day; if total dose exceeds 300 mg/day, give in divided doses (max 400 mg/day); may give as a single bedtime dose (max 300 mg q HS)
  Tab: 25, 50, 100, 150 mg
- ***clomipramine*** (C)(G) <10 years: not recommended; 10-<16 years: initially 25 mg daily in divided doses; gradually increase; max 3 mg/kg or 100 mg, whichever is smaller;>16 years: initially 25 mg daily in divided doses; gradually increase to 100 mg during first 2 weeks; max 250 mg/day; total maintenance dose may be given at HS
  Anafranil *Cap:* 25, 50, 75 mg
- ***desipramine*** (C)(G) <12 years: not recommended; ≥12 years: 100-200 mg/day in single or divided doses; max 300 mg/day
  Norpramin *Tab:* 10, 25, 50, 75, 100, 150 mg
- ***doxepin*** (C)(G) <12 years: not recommended; ≥12 years: 75 mg/day; max 150 mg/day
  Cap: 10, 25, 50, 75, 100, 150 mg; Oral conc: 10 mg/ml (4 oz w. dropper)
- ***imipramine*** (C)(G) <12 years: not recommended; ≥12 years:
  Tofranil <12 years: not recommended; ≥12 years: adolescents initially 30-40 mg daily (max 100 mg/day); if maintenance dose exceeds 75 mg daily, may switch to **Tofranil PM** for divided or bedtime dose
    Tab: 10, 25, 50 mg
  Tofranil PM initially 75 mg daily 1 hour before HS; max 200 mg
    Cap: 75, 100, 125, 150 mg
- ***nortriptyline*** (D)(G) <12 years: not recommended; ≥12 years: initially 25 mg tid-qid; max 150 mg/day
  Pamelor *Cap:* 10, 25, 50, 75 mg; *Oral soln:* 10 mg/5 ml (16 oz)
- ***protriptyline*** (C) <12 years: not recommended; ≥12 years: initially 5 mg tid; usual dose 15-40 mg/day in 3-4 divided doses; max 60 mg/day
  Vivactil *Tab:* 5, 10 mg
- ***trimipramine*** (C) <12 years: not recommended; ≥12 years: initially 75 mg/day in divided doses; max 200 mg/day
  Surmontil *Cap:* 25, 50, 100 mg

INTERTRIGO

See Candidiasis: Skin *page* 60
Topical Antifungals *see* ***Tinea Corporis*** *page* 447
Topical Anti-infectives *see* ***Skin Infection: Bacterial*** *page* 427
Topical Corticosteroids *see page* 542
OTC hydrocortisone 1% paste or ointment
OTC Zinc Oxide paste or ointment
OTC A&D Ointment

Comment: Treatment is dependent on symptoms and presence of infection. Intertrigo is an irritant dermatitis in the intertriginous zones (skin creases and folds) characterized by inflammation and excoriation caused by skin-to-skin friction, moisture, and heat and may be itching, stinging, burning with a musty odor. Common areas at risk include breast folds, axillae, groin folds, buttocks folds, and the abdominal panniculus in obese persons, finger and toe webs. Treatment includes keeping the areas clean, moisture-free, application of a steroid cream and a protective lubricant barrier. Intertrigo may be complicated by a superimposed infection such as yeast (*Candida albicans*), dermatophytic fungi, or bacteria. Oral agents may be required based on severity of the skin breakdown and invasive infectious process. Apply appropriate topical anti-infective first and barrier product last. Non-medicated powders (e.g., corn starch) are contraindicated in the affected areas as they trap moisture. Exposure to light and air when possible and as appropriate facilitates integumentary healing.

IRITIS: ACUTE

- ***loteprednol etabonate*** **(C)** <12 years: not recommended; ≥12 years: 1-2 drops qid; may increase to 1 drop hourly as needed
  Lotemax Ophthalmic Solution *Ophth soln:* 0.3% (2.5, 5, 10, 15 ml)
- ***prednisone acetate*** (C) <12 years: not recommended; ≥12 years: 1 drop q 1 hour x 24-48 hours, then 1 drop q 2 hours while awake x 24-48 hours, then 1 drop bid-qid until resolved
  Pred Forte *Ophth soln:* 1% (1, 5, 10, 15 ml)

IRON OVERLOAD

IRON CHELATING AGENTS

- ***deferasirox (tridentate ligand)*** (C)(G) <2 years: not recommended; ≥2 years: initially 20 mg/kg/day; titrate; may increase 5-10 mg/kg q 3-6 months based on serum ferritin trends; max 30 mg/kg/day
  Exjade *Tab for oral soln:* 125, 250, 500 mg
  Jadenu *Tab:* 90, 180, 360 mg film-coat
  Jadenu Sprinkle *Sachet:* 90, 180, 360 mg (30/carton)
  Comment: ***deferasirox*** is an orally active chelator selective for iron. It is indicated for the treatment of chronic iron overload due to blood transfusions (transfusional hemosiderosis). Monitor serum ferritin monthly. Consider interrupting therapy if serum ferritin falls below 500 mcg/L. Take ***deferasirox*** **(Exjade, Jadenu, Jadenu Sprinkle)** on an empty stomach. Completely disperse tablet(s) for oral solution in 3.5 oz liquid if dose is ≤1 gm <u>or</u> 7 oz liquid if dose is ≥1 gm.
- ***succimer*** (C) <12 years: not recommended; ≥12 years: initially 10 mg/kg q 8 hours x 5 days; then, reduce frequency to every 12 hours x 14 more days; allow at least 14 days between courses unless blood lead levels indicate need for prompt treatment
  Chemet *Cap:* 100 mg
  Comment: **Chemet** *is* indicated for the treatment of lead poisoning when blood lead level 45 mcg/dL. Treatment for more than 3 consecutive weeks is not recommended. Monitor hydration, renal, and hepatic function.

IRRITABLE BOWEL SYNDROME WITH CONSTIPATION (IBS-C)

Bulk-Producing Agents, Laxatives, Stool Softeners *see **Constipation** page* 94

GUANYLATE CYCLASE-C AGONISTS

Comment: Guanylate cyclase-c agonists increase intestinal fluid and intestinal transit time may induce diarrhea and bloating and therefore, are contraindicated with known or suspected mechanical GI obstruction.

- *linaclotide* (C) <18 years: not established (<6 years: contraindicated; 6-18 years: avoid); >18 years: 290 mcg orally once daily; take on an empty stomach at least 30 minutes before the first meal of the day; swallow whole, do not crush or chew cap or cap contents; may open cap and administer with applesauce or water (e.g., NGT, PEG tube)

  Linzess *Cap:* 72, 145, 290 mcg

  Comment: *linaclotide* and its active metabolite are negligibly absorbed systemically following oral administration and maternal use is not expected to result in fetal exposure to the drug. There is no information regarding the presence of ***plecanatide*** in human milk or its effects on the breastfed infant.

CHLORIDE CHANNEL ACTIVATOR

- *lubiprostone* (C) <18 years: not recommended; >18 years: **one** 8 mcg cap bid with food and water; swallow whole, do not break apart or chew

  Amitiza *Cap:* 8, 24 mcg

  Comment: **Amitiza** increases intestinal fluid and intestinal transit time. Suspend dosing and rehydrate if severe diarrhea occurs. **Amitiza** is contraindicated with known or suspected mechanical GI obstruction. Most common adverse reactions in CIC are nausea, diarrhea, headache, abdominal pain, abdominal distension, and flatulence.

IRRITABLE BOWEL SYNDROME WITH DIARRHEA (IBS-D)

Bulk-Producing Agents *see* ***Constipation*** *page* 94

CONSTIPATING AGENTS

- *difenoxin+atropine* (C) <12 years: not recommended; ≥12 years: 2 tabs, then 1 tab after each loose stool or 1 tab q 3-4 hours as needed; max 8 tab/day x 2 days

  Motofen *Tab:* difen 1 mg+atro 0.025 mg

- *diphenoxylate+atropine* (C)(G) <2 years: not recommended; 2-12 years: initially 0.3-0.4 mg/kg/day in 4 divided doses; >12 years: 2 tabs or 10 ml qid

  Lomotil *Tab:* difen 2.5 mg+atro 0.025 mg; *Liq:* difen 2.5 mg+atro 0.025 mg per 5 ml (2 oz)

- *eluxadoline* (NA)(IV) <12 years: not established; ≥12 years: 100 mg bid; 75 mg bid if unable to tolerate 100 mg, or without a gall bladder, or mild-to-moderate hepatic impairment, or receiving concomitant OATP1B1 inhibitors

  Viberzi 4 mg initially, then 2 mg after each loose stool; max 16 mg/day

  Tab: 75, 100 mg film-coat

  Comment: *eluxadoline* is a mu-opioid receptor agonist. It is contraindicated with biliary obstruction, Sphincter of Oddi disease or dysfunction, alcohol abuse or addiction, pancreatitis, pancreatic duct obstruction, severe hepatic impairment, and mechanical GI obstruction.

- *loperamide* (B)(G)

  Imodium (OTC) <5 years: not recommended; ≥5 years: 4 mg initially, then 2 mg after each loose stool; max 16 mg/day

  Cap: 2 mg

Imodium A-D (OTC) <2 years: not recommended; 2-5 years (24-47 lb): 1 mg up to tid x 2 days; 6-8 years (48-59 lb): 2 mg initially, then 1 mg after each loose stool; max 4 mg/day x 2 days; 9-11 years (60-95 lb): 2 mg initially, then 1 mg after each loose stool; max 6 mg/day x 2 days; ≥12 years: 4 mg initially, then 2 mg after each loose stool; usual max 8 mg/day x 2 days

Cplt: 2 mg; *Liq:* 1 mg/5 ml (2, 4 oz)

➢ ***loperamide+simethicone*** (B)(G)

Imodium Advanced (OTC) <6 years: not recommended; 6-8 years: 1 tab chewed after loose stool, then 1/2 after next loose stool; max 2 tabs/day; 9-11 years: 1 tab chewed after loose stool, then 1/2 after next loose stool; max 3 tabs/day; ≥12 years: 2 tabs chewed after loose stool, then 1 after the next loose stool; max 4 tabs/day

Chew tab: lop 2 mg+sim 125 mg

SEROTONIN (5-HT3) RECEPTOR ANTAGONIST

➢ ***alosetron*** (B)(G) <12 years: not recommended; ≥12 years: initially 0.5 mg bid; may increase to 1 mg bid after 4 weeks if starting dose is tolerated but inadequate

Lotronex *Tab:* 0.5, 1 mg

ANTISPASMODIC+ANTICHOLINERGIC COMBINATIONS

➢ ***dicyclomine*** (B)(G) <12 years: not recommended; ≥12 years: initially 20 mg bid-qid; may increase to 40 mg qid PO; usual IM dose 80 mg/day divided qid; do not use IM route for more than 1-2 days

Bentyl *Tab:* 20 mg; *Cap:* 10 mg; *Syr:* 10 mg/5 ml (16 oz); *Vial:* 10 mg/ml (10 ml); *Amp:* 10 mg/ml (2 ml)

➢ ***methscopolamine bromide*** (B) <12 years: not recommended; ≥12 years: 1 tab q 6 hours prn

Pamine *Tab:* 2.5 mg

Pamine Forte *Tab:* 5 mg

ANTICHOLINERGICS

➢ ***hyoscyamine*** (C)(G)

Anaspaz <2 years: not recommended; 2-12 years: 0.0625-0.125 mg q 4 hours prn; max 0.75 mg/day; >12 years: 1-2 tabs q 4 hours prn; max 12 tabs/day

Tab: 0.125*mg

Levbid <12 years: not recommended; ≥12 years: 1-2 tabs q 12 hours prn; max 4 tabs/day

Tab: 0.375*mg ext-rel

Levsin <6 years: not recommended; 6-12 years: 1 tab q 4 hours prn; >12 years: 1-2 tabs q 4 hours prn; max 12 tabs/day

Tab: 0.125*mg

Levsinex SL <2 years: not recommended; 2-12 years: 1 tab q 4 hours; max 6 tabs/day; >12 years: 1-2 tabs q 4 hours SL or PO; max 12 tabs/day

Tab: 0.125 mg sublingual

Levsinex Timecaps <2 years: not recommended; 2-12 years: 1 cap q 12 hours; max 2 caps/day; >12 years: 1-2 caps q 12 hours; may adjust to 1 cap q 8 hours

Cap: 0.375 mg time-rel

NuLev <2 years: not recommended; 2-12 years: dissolve 1 tab on tongue, with or without water, q 4 hours prn; max 6 tabs/day; >12 years: dissolve 1-2 tabs on tongue, with or without water, q 4 hours prn; max 12 tabs/day

ODT: 0.125 mg (mint; phenylalanine)

➢ ***simethicone*** (C)(G) 0.3 ml qid pc and HS

Mylicon Drops (OTC) *Oral drops:* 40 mg/0.6 ml (30 ml)

▶ ***phenobarbital+hyoscyamine+atropine+scopolamine*** **(C)(IV)(G)**

Donnatal <12 years: not recommended; ≥12 years: 1-2 tabs ac and HS

Tab: pheno 16.2 mg+hyo 0.1037 mg+atro 0.0194 mg+scop 0.0065 mg

Donnatal Elixir <12 years: not recommended; ≥12 years: 1-2 tsp ac and HS 20 lb: 1 ml q 4 hours or 1.5 ml q 6 hours; 30 lb: 1.5 ml q 4 hours or 2 ml q 6 hours; 50 lb: 1/2 tsp q 4 hours or 3/4 tsp q 6 hours; 75 lb: 3/4 tsp q 4 hours or 1 tsp q 6 hours; 100 lb: 1 tsp q 4 hours or 1 tsp q 6 hours

Elix: pheno 16.2 mg+hyo 0.1037 mg+atro 0.0194 mg+scop 0.0065 mg per 5 ml (4, 16 oz)

Donnatal Extentabs <12 years: not recommended; ≥12 years: 1 tab q 12 hours

Tab: pheno 48.6 mg+hyo 0.3111 mg+atro 0.0582 mg+scop 0.0195 mg ext-rel

ANTICHOLINERGIC+SEDATIVE COMBINATION

▶ ***chlordiazepoxide+clidinium*** **(D)(IV)** <12 years: not recommended; ≥12 years: 1-2 caps ac and HS: max 8 caps/day

Librax *Cap:* chlor 5 mg+clid 2.5 mg

TRICYCLIC ANTIDEPRESSANTS (TCAs)

Comment: Co-administration of SSRIs and TCAs requires extreme caution.

▶ ***amitriptyline*** **(C)(G)** <12 years: not recommended; ≥12 years: 10-20 mg q HS

Tab: 10, 25, 50, 75, 100, 150 mg

▶ ***amoxapine*** **(C)** <12 years: not recommended; ≥12 years: initially 50 mg bid-tid; after 1 week may increase to 100 mg bid-tid; usual effective dose 200-300 mg/day; if total dose exceeds 300 mg/day, give in divided doses (max 400 mg/day); may give as a single bedtime dose (max 300 mg q HS)

Tab: 25, 50, 100, 150 mg

▶ ***clomipramine*** **(C)(G)** <10 years: not recommended; 10-16 years: initially 25 mg daily in divided doses; gradually increase; max 3 mg/kg or 100 mg, whichever is smaller; >16 years: initially 25 mg daily in divided doses; gradually increase to 100 mg during first 2 weeks; max 250 mg/day; total maintenance dose may be given at HS

Anafranil *Cap:* 25, 50, 75 mg

▶ ***desipramine*** **(C)(G)** <12 years: not recommended; ≥12 years: 100-200 mg/day in single or divided doses; max 300 mg/day

Norpramin *Tab:* 10, 25, 50, 75, 100, 150 mg

▶ ***doxepin*** **(C)(G)** <12 years: not recommended; ≥12 years: 75 mg/day; max 150 mg/day

Cap: 10, 25, 50, 75, 100, 150 mg; Oral conc: 10 mg/ml (4 oz w. dropper)

▶ ***imipramine*** **(C)(G)** <12 years: not recommended; ≥12 years:

Tofranil initially 75 mg daily (max 200 mg); adolescents initially 30-40 mg daily (max 100 mg/day); if maintenance dose exceeds 75 mg daily, may switch to **Tofranil PM** for divided or bedtime dose

Tab: 10, 25, 50 mg

Tofranil PM initially 75 mg daily 1 hour before HS; max 200 mg

Cap: 75, 100, 125, 150 mg

▶ ***nortriptyline*** **(D)(G)** <12 years: not recommended; ≥12 years: initially 25 mg tid-qid; max 150 mg/day

Pamelor *Cap:* 10, 25, 50, 75 mg; *Oral soln:* 10 mg/5 ml (16 oz)

▶ ***protriptyline*** **(C)** <12 years: not recommended; ≥12 years: initially 5 mg tid; usual dose 15-40 mg/day in 3-4 divided doses; max 60 mg/day

Vivactil *Tab:* 5, 10 mg

▶ ***trimipramine*** **(C)** <12 years: not recommended; ≥12 years: initially 75 mg/day in divided doses; max 200 mg/day

Surmontil *Cap:* 25, 50, 100 mg

JAPANESE ENCEPHALITIS VIRUS

Comment: Japanese encephalitis is a viral disease spread by the bite of an infected mosquito. It is not spread from person-to-person. Currently there is no cure. A person with encephalitis can experience fever, neck stiffness, seizures, and coma. About 1 person in 4 with encephalitis dies. Up to half of those who don't die have permanent disability. There is one vaccine for Japanese encephalitis, currently licensed in the UK, for use in adults and children >2 months-of-age. The live attenuated vaccine (LAV) is administered in two doses for full protection, with the second dose administered 28 days after the first. The second dose should be given at least a week before travel. Children younger than 3 years-of-age get a smaller dose than patients who are 3 or older. A booster dose might be recommended for anyone 17 or older who was vaccinated more than a year ago and is still at risk of exposure. There is no information yet on the need for a booster dose for children. The vaccine is usually available through the local health department.

JUVENILE IDIOPATHIC ARTHRITIS (JIA) & POLYARTICULAR JUVENILE IDIOPATHIC ARTHRITIS (PJIA) & SYSTEMIC JUVENILE IDIOPATHIC ARTHRITIS (SJIA)

Acetaminophen for IV Infusion *see **Pain** page* 322
NSAIDs *see page* 539
Other Oral Analgesics *see **Pain** page* 324
Topical & Transdermal NSAIDs *see **Pain** page* 323
Parenteral Corticosteroids *see page* 547
Oral Corticosteroids *see page* 546

TOPICAL ANALGESICS

▶ ***capsaicin*** cream **(B)(G)** <2 years: not recommended; 2-12 years: apply sparingly to intact skin bid prn; >12 years: apply tid-qid prn

Axsain *Crm:* 0.075% (1, 2 oz)
Capsin (OTC) *Lotn:* 0.025, 0, 075% (59 ml)
Capzasin-P (OTC) *Crm:* 0.025% (1.5 oz); *Lotn:* 0.025% (2 oz)
Capzasin-HP (OTC) *Crm:* 0.075% (1.5 oz); *Lotn:* 0.075% (2 oz)
Dolorac *Crm:* 0.025% (28 gm)
Double Cap (OTC) *Crm:* 0.05% (2 oz)
R-Gel *Gel:* 0.025% (15, 30 gm)
Zostrix (OTC) *Crm:* 0.025% (0.7, 1.5, 3 oz)
Zostrix HP (OTC) *Emol crm:* 0.075% (1, 2 oz)

Comment: Provides some relief by 1-2 weeks; optimal benefit may take 4-6 weeks. Avoid contact with mucous membranes.

ORAL SALICYLATES

▶ ***indomethacin*** **(C)** <14 years: usually not recommended; >2 years, if risk warranted: 1-2 mg/kg/day in divided doses; max 3-4 mg/kg/day (or 150-200 mg/day, whichever is less); <14 years, ER cap not recommended; ≥14 years: initially 25 mg bid or tid, increase as needed at weekly intervals by 25-50 mg/day; max 200 mg/day

Cap: 25, 50 mg; *Susp;* 25 mg/5 ml (pineapple-coconut, mint) (alcohol 1%); *Supp:* 50 mg; *ER Cap:* 75 mg ext-rel

Comment: ***indomethacin*** is indicated only for acute painful flares. Administer with food and/or antacids. Use lowest effective dose for shortest duration.

▶ ***methotrexate*** (X) <2 years: not recommended; 2-12 years: 10 mg/m^2 once weekly; max 20 mg/m^2; >12 years: 7.5 mg x 1 dose per week or 2.5 mg x 3 at 12 hour intervals once a week; max 20 mg/week; therapeutic response begins in 3-6 weeks; administer ***methotrexate*** injection SC only into the abdomen or thigh

Rasuvo *Autoinjector:* 7.5 mg/0.15 ml, 10 mg/0.20 ml, 12.5 mg/0.25 ml, 15 mg/0.30 ml, 17.5 mg/0.35 ml, 20 mg/0.40 ml, 22.5 mg/0.45 ml, 25 mg/0.50 ml, 27.5 mg/0.55 ml, 30 mg/0.60 ml (solution concentration for SC injection is 50 mg/ml)

Rheumatrex *Tab:* 2.5*mg (5, 7.5, 10, 12.5, 15 mg/week, 4/card unit dose pack)

Trexall *Tab:* 5*, 7.5*, 10*, 15*mg (5, 7.5, 10, 12.5, 15 mg/week, 4/card unit dose pack)

Comment: ***methotrexate*** (MTX) is contraindicated with immunodeficiency, blood dyscrasias, alcoholism, and chronic liver disease.

Interleukin-6 Receptor Antagonist

▶ ***tocilizumab*** (B) <2 years: not recommended; ≥2 years: weight-based dosing according to *SJIA: ≥30 kg:* 8 mg/kg SC every 2 weeks; *<30 kg:* 12 mg/kg SC every 2 weeks; *IV Infusion:* administer over 1 hour; do not administer as bolus or IV push; *PJIA, and SJIA, ≥30 kg:* dilute to 100 mL in 0.9% or 0.45% NaCl. *PJIA and SJIA, <30 kg:* dilute to 50 mL in 0.9% or 0.45% NaCl; ≥18 years: whether used in combination with DMARDs or as monotherapy, the recommended IV infusion starting dose is 4 mg/kg IV every 4 weeks followed by an increase to 8 mg/kg IV every 4 weeks based on clinical response; Max 800 mg per infusion in RA patients; *SC Administration: ≥100 kg:* 162 mg SC once weekly on the same day; *<100 kg:* 162 mg SC every other week on the same day followed by an increase according to clinical response

Actemra *Vial:* 80 mg/4 ml, 200 mg/10 ml, 400 mg/20 ml, single-use, for IV infusion after dilution; *Prefilled syringe:* 162 mg (0.9 ml, single-dose)

Comment: ***tocilizumab*** is an interleukin-6 receptor-α inhibitor indicated for use in moderate-to-severe rheumatoid arthritis (RA) that has not responded to conventional therapy, and also for some subtypes of juvenile idiopathic arthritis (JIA). **Actemra** may be used alone or in combination with ***methotrexate*** and in RA, other DMARDs may be used. Monitor patient for dose related laboratory changes including elevated LFTs, neutropenia, and thrombocytopenia. **Actemra** should not be initiated in patients with an absolute neutrophil count (ANC) below 2000 per mm3, platelet count below 100,000 per mm3, or who have ALT or AST above 1.5 times the upper limit of normal (ULN). Registration in the Pregnancy Exposure Registry (1-877-311-8972) is encouraged for monitoring pregnancy outcomes in women exposed to **Actemra** during pregnancy. The limited available data with **Actemra** in pregnant women are not sufficient to determine whether there is a drug-associated risk for major birth defects and miscarriage. Monoclonal antibodies, such as ***tocilizumab***, are actively transported across the placenta during the third trimester of pregnancy and may affect immune response in the infant exposed *in utero*. It is not known whether ***tocilizumab*** passes into breast milk; therefore, breastfeeding is not recommended while using **Actemra**.

Selective Costimulation Modulator

▶ ***abatacept*** (C) <2 years: not recommended; 2-17 years: administer as an IV infusion over 30 minutes at weeks 0, 2, and 4; then every 4 weeks thereafter; <75 kg, administer 10 mg/kg; same as adult (max 1 gm); administer as an IV infusion over 30 minutes at weeks 0, 2, and 4; then every 4 weeks thereafter; <60 kg, administer 500 mg/dose; 60-100 kg, administer 750 mg/dose; >100 kg, administer 1 gm/dose

Orencia *Vial:* 250 mg pwdr for IV infusion after reconstitution (silicone-free) (preservative-free); *Prefilled syringe:* 125 mg/ml soln for SC injection (preservative-free); *ClickJect Autoinjector:* 125 mg/ml soln for SC injection

Comment: **Orencia** is indicated to reduce signs/symptoms of moderate-to-severe active polyarticular juvenile idiopathic arthritis (PJIA) in patients ≥2 years-of-age as monotherapy or with ***methotrexate***. **Orencia** is also indicated to reduce signs/symptoms, induce major clinical response, inhibit progression of structural damage, and improve physical function in adult patients with moderate-to-severe active RA. **Orencia** may be used as monotherapy or with DMARDs other than TNF antagonists.

JUVENILE RHEUMATOID ARTHRITIS (JRA)

Acetaminophen for IV Infusion *see **Pain** page* 322
NSAIDs *see page* 539
Other Oral Analgesics *see **Pain** page* 324
Topical & Transdermal NSAIDs *see **Pain** page* 323
Parenteral Corticosteroids *see page* 547
Oral Corticosteroids *see page* 546
Juvenile Idiopathic Arthritis (JIA) & Polyarticular Juvenile Idiopathic Arthritis (PJIA) & Systemic Juvenile Idiopathic Arthritis *see page* 264

TOPICAL ANALGESICS

► ***capsaicin*** cream (B)(G) <2 years: not recommended; 2-12 years: apply sparingly to intact skin bid prn; >12 years: apply tid-qid prn

Axsain *Crm:* 0.075% (1, 2 oz)
Capsin (OTC) *Lotn:* 0.025, 0,075% (59 ml)
Capzasin-P (OTC) *Crm:* 0.025% (1.5 oz); *Lotn:* 0.025% (2 oz)
Capzasin-HP (OTC) *Crm:* 0.075% (1.5 oz); *Lotn:* 0.075% (2 oz)
Dolorac *Crm:* 0.025% (28 gm)
Double Cap (OTC) *Crm:* 0.05% (2 oz)
R-Gel *Gel:* 0.025% (15, 30 gm)
Zostrix (OTC) *Crm:* 0.025% (0.7, 1.5, 3 oz)
Zostrix HP (OTC) *Emol crm:* 0.075% (1, 2 oz)

Comment: Provides some relief by 1-2 weeks; optimal benefit may take 4-6 weeks. Avoid contact with mucous membranes.

ORAL SALICYLATE

► ***indomethacin*** (C) <14 years: usually not recommended; ≥2 years, if risk warranted: 1-2 mg/kg/day in divided doses; max 3-4 mg/kg/day (or total 150-200 mg/day, whichever is less); ≤14 years, ER cap not recommended; ≥14 years: initially 25 mg bid-tid, increase as needed at weekly intervals by 25-50 mg/day; max 200 mg/day

Cap: 25, 50 mg; Susp: 25 mg/5 ml (pineapple-coconut, mint; alcohol 1%); Supp: 50 mg; ER Cap: 75 mg ext-rel

Comment: ***indomethacin*** is indicated only for acute painful flares. Administer with food and/or antacids. Use lowest effective dose for shortest duration.

► ***methotrexate*** (X) <2 years: not recommended; 2-12 years: 10 mg/m² once weekly; max 20 mg/m²; >12 years: 7.5 mg x 1 dose per week or 2.5 mg x 3 at 12-hour intervals once a week; max 20 mg/week; therapeutic response begins in 3-6 weeks; administer ***methotrexate*** injection SC only into the abdomen or thigh

Rasuvo *Autoinjector:* 7.5 mg/0.15 ml, 10 mg/0.20 ml, 12.5 mg/0.25 ml, 15 mg/0.30 ml, 17.5 mg/0.35 ml, 20 mg/0.40 ml, 22.5 mg/0.45 ml, 25 mg/0.50 ml, 27.5 mg/0.55 ml, 30 mg/0.60 ml (solution concentration for SC injection is 50 mg/ml)
Rheumatrex *Tab:* 2.5*mg (5, 7.5, 10, 12.5, 15 mg/week, 4/card unit-of-use dose pack)
Trexall *Tab:* 5*, 7.5*, 10*, 15*mg (5, 7.5, 10, 12.5, 15 mg/week, 4/card unit-of-use dose pack)

Comment: ***methotrexate*** **(MTX)** is contraindicated with immunodeficiency, blood dyscrasias, alcoholism, and chronic liver disease.

INTERLEUKIN-6 RECEPTOR ANTAGONIST

▶ ***tocilizumab*** **(B)** <2 years: not recommended; ≥2 years: weight-based dosing according to *SJIA: ≥30 kg:* 8 mg/kg SC every 2 weeks; *<30 kg:* 12 mg/kg SC every 2 weeks; *IV Infusion:* administer over 1 hour; do not administer as bolus or IV push; *PJIA, and SJIA, ≥30 kg:* dilute to 100 mL in 0.9% or 0.45% NaCl. *PJIA and SJIA, <30 kg:* dilute to 50 mL in 0.9% or 0.45% NaCl; ≥18 years: whether used in combination with DMARDs or as monotherapy, the recommended IV infusion starting dose is 4 mg/kg IV every 4 weeks followed by an increase to 8 mg/kg IV every 4 weeks based on clinical response; Max 800 mg per infusion in RA patients; *SC Administration: ≥100 kg:* 162 mg SC once weekly on the same day; *<100 kg:* 162 mg SC every other week on the same day followed by an increase according to clinical response

Actemra *Vial:* 80 mg/4 ml, 200 mg/10 ml, 400 mg/20 ml, single-use, for IV infusion after dilution; *Prefilled syringe:* 162 mg (0.9 ml, single-dose)

Comment: ***tocilizumab*** is an interleukin-6 receptor-α inhibitor indicated for use in moderate-to-severe rheumatoid arthritis (RA) that has not responded to conventional therapy, and also for some subtypes of juvenile idiopathic arthritis (JIA). **Actemra** may be used alone or in combination with ***methotrexate*** and in RA, other DMARDs may be used. Monitor patient for dose related laboratory changes including elevated LFTs, neutropenia, and thrombocytopenia. **Actemra** should not be initiated in patients with an absolute neutrophil count (ANC) below 2000 per mm3, platelet count below 100,000 per mm3, or who have ALT or AST above 1.5 times the upper limit of normal (ULN). Registration in the Pregnancy Exposure Registry (1-877-311-8972) is encouraged for monitoring pregnancy outcomes in women exposed to **Actemra** during pregnancy. The limited available data with **Actemra** in pregnant women are not sufficient to determine whether there is a drug-associated risk for major birth defects and miscarriage. Monoclonal antibodies, such as ***tocilizumab***, are actively transported across the placenta during the third trimester of pregnancy and may affect immune response in the infant exposed *in utero*. It is not known whether ***tocilizumab*** passes into breast milk; therefore, breastfeeding is not recommended while using **Actemra**.

Selective Costimulation Modulator

▶ ***abatacept*** **(C)** <2 years: not recommended; 2-17 years: administer as an IV infusion over 30 minutes at weeks 0, 2, and 4; then every 4 weeks thereafter; <75 kg, administer 10 mg/kg; same as adult (max 1 gm); administer as an IV infusion over 30 minutes at weeks 0, 2, and 4; then every 4 weeks thereafter; <60 kg, administer 500 mg/dose; 60-100 kg, administer 750 mg/dose; >100 kg, administer 1 gm/dose

Orencia *Vial:* 250 mg pwdr for IV infusion after reconstitution (silicone-free) (preservative-free); *Prefilled syringe:* 125 mg/ml soln for SC injection (preservative-free); *ClickJect Autoinjector:* 125 mg/ml soln for SC injection

Comment: **Orencia** is also indicated to reduce signs/symptoms, induce major clinical response, inhibit progression of structural damage, and improve physical function in adult patients with moderate-to-severe active RA. **Orencia** may be used as monotherapy <u>or</u> with DMARDs other than TNF antagonists. **Orencia** is also indicated to reduce signs/symptoms of moderate-to-severe active polyarticular juvenile idiopathic arthritis (PJIA) in patients >2 years-of-age as monotherapy <u>or</u> with ***methotrexate***.

KERATITIS & KERATOCONJUNCTIVITIS: HERPES SIMPLEX

- ***ganciclovir*** **(C)** <2 years: not recommended; ≥2 years: instill 1 drop 5 times per day (every 3 hours) while awake until corneal ulcer heals; then 1 drop tid x 7 days
  Zirgan *Ophth gel:* 0.15% (5 gm) (benzalkonium chloride)
- ***idoxuridine*** **(C)** instill 1 drop q 1 hour during day and every other hour at night <u>or</u> 1 drop every minute for 5 minutes and repeat q 4 hours during day and night
  Herplex *Ophth soln:* 0.1% (15 ml)
- ***trifluridine*** **(C)** <6 years: not recommended; ≥6 years: instill 1 drop q 2 hours while awake (max 9 drops/day until re-epithelialization; then 1 drop q 4 hours x 7 more days (at least 5 drops/day); max 21 days
  Viroptic *Ophth soln:* 1% (7.5 ml) (thimerosal)
- ***vidarabine*** **(C)** <2 years: not recommended; ≥2 years: apply 1/2 inch in lower conjunctival sac 5 x/day q 3 hours until re-epithelialization occurs, then bid x 7 more days
  Vira-A *Ophth oint:* 3% (3.5 gm)

KERATITIS & KERATOCONJUNCTIVITIS: VERNAL

OPHTHALMIC MAST CELL STABILIZERS

Comment: Contact lens wear is contraindicated

- ***cromolyn sodium*** **(B)** <4 years: not recommended; ≥4 years: 1-2 drops 4-6 x/day
  Crolom, Opticrom *Ophth soln:* 4% (10 ml) (benzalkonium chloride)
- ***lodoxamide tromethamine*** **(B)** <2 years: not recommended; ≥2 years: 1-2 drops qid; max 3 months
  Alomide *Ophth susp:* 0.1% (10 ml)

LABYRINTHITIS

- ***meclizine*** **(B)** <12 years: not recommended; ≥12 years: 25 mg tid
  Antivert *Tab:* 12.5, 25, 50*mg
  Bonine (OTC) *Cap:* 15, 25, 30 mg; *Tab:* 12.5, 25, 50 mg; *Chew tab/Film-coat tab:* 25 mg
  Dramamine II (OTC) *Tab:* 25*mg
  Zentrip *Strip:* 25 mg orally disint
- ***promethazine*** **(C)(G)** <2 years: not recommended; 2-12 years 12.5-25 mg q 4-6 hours prn; >12 years: 25-50 mg q 4-6 hours prn
  Phenergan *Tab:* 12.5*, 25*, 50 mg; *Plain syr:* 6.25 mg/5 ml; *Fortis syr:* 25 mg/5 ml; *Rectal supp:* 12.5, 25, 50 mg

  Comment: ***promethazine*** is contraindicated in children with uncomplicated nausea, dehydration, Reye's syndrome, history of sleep apnea, asthma, and lower respiratory disorders in children. ***promethazine*** lowers the seizure threshold in children, may cause cholestatic jaundice, anticholinergic effects, extrapyramidal effects, and potentially fatal respiratory depression.
- ***scopolamine*** **(C)** <12 years: not recommended; ≥12 years: 1 patch behind ear; each patch is effective for 3 days; apply a new patch on behind the opposite ear every 4th day
  Transderm Scop *Transdermal patch:* 1.5 mg (4/carton)

LACTOSE INTOLERANCE

- ***lactase*** enzyme 9,000 FCC units taken with dairy food; adjust based on abatement of symptoms; usual max 18,000 units/dose
  - **Lactaid Drops (OTC)** 5-7 drops to each quart of milk and shake gently; may increase to 10-15 drops if needed; hydrolyzes 70%-99% of lactose at refrigerator temperature in 24 hours
    - *Oral drops:* 1,250 units/5 gtts (7 ml w. dropper)
  - **Lactaid Extra (OTC)** *Cplt:* 4,500 FCC units
  - **Lactaid Fast ACT (OTC)** *Cplt:* 9,000 FCC units; *Chew tab:* 9,000 FCC units (vanilla twist)
  - **Lactaid Original (OTC)** *Cplt:* 3,000 FCC units
  - **Lactaid Ultra (OTC)** *Cplt:* 9,000 FCC units; *Chew tab:* 9,000 FCC units (vanilla twist)

LARVA MIGRANS: CUTANEOUS & VISCERAL

- ***thiabendazole*** **(C)** dosing is bid, is based on weight in pounds, and must be taken with meals; <30 lbs: consult mfr pkg insert; 30 lbs: 250 mg bid; 50 lbs: 500 mg bid; 75 lbs: 750 mg bid; 100 lbs: 1 gm bid; 125 lbs: 1.25 gm bid: ≥150 lbs: 1.5 gm bid; max 3 gm/day; *Cutaneous larva migrans:* treat x 2 days; *Visceral larva migrans:* treat x 7 days
  - **Mintezol** *Chew tab:* 500*mg (orange); *Oral susp:* 500 mg/5 ml (120 ml) (orange)

Comment: ***thiabendazole*** is not for prophylaxis. May impair mental alertness. May not be available in the US.

LEAD POISONING

Comment: Chelation therapy for lead poisoning requires maintenance of adequate hydration, close monitoring of renal and hepatic function, and monitoring for neutropenia; discontinue therapy at first sign of toxicity. Contraindicated with severe renal disease <u>or</u> anuria.

CHELATING AGENTS

- ***deferoxamine mesylate*** **(C)** <3 months: not recommended; ≥3 months: initially 1 gm IM, followed by 500 mg IM every 4 hours x 2 doses; then repeat every 4-12 hours if needed; max 6 gm/day
  - **Desferal** *Vial:* 250 mg/ml after reconstitution (500 mg)
- ***edetate calcium disodium (EDTA)*** **(B)** administer IM <u>or</u> IV; use IM route of administration for children and overt lead encephalopathy; *Serum lead level:* 20-70 mcg/dL: 1 gm/m^2 per day; *IV:* infuse over 8-12 hours; *IM:* divided doses q 8-12 hours; Treat for 5 days; then stop for 2-4 days; may repeat if serum lead level is >70 mcg/dL
  - **Calcium Disodium Versenate** *Amp:* 200 mg/ml (5 ml)
- ***succimer*** **(C)** <12 months: not recommended; ≥12 months: *Serum lead level: >45 mcg/dL:* initially 10 mg/kg (<u>or</u> 350 mg/m^2) every 8 hours for 5 days; then reduce frequency to every 12 hours for 14 more days; allow at least 14 days between courses unless serum lead levels indicate a need for more prompt treatment; for more than 3 consecutive weeks not recommended; may swallow caps whole <u>or</u> put contents onto a small amount of soft food <u>or</u> a spoon and swallow, followed by a fruit drink
  - **Chemet** *Cap:* 100 mg

LEG CRAMPS: NOCTURNAL & RECUMBENCY

▶ ***quinine sulfate*** **(C)(G)** <16 years: not recommended; ≥16 years: 1 tab or cap q HS
Qualaquin *Tab:* 260 mg; *Cap:* 260, 300, 325 mg

Comment: If **hypokalemia** is the cause of leg cramps, treat with potassium supplementation (*see page* 241).

LEISHMANIASIS: CUTANEOUS, MUCOSAL, VISCERAL

Comment: The leishmanial parasite species addressed in this section are: **cutaneous leishmaniasis** (due to ***Leishmania braziliensis, Leishmania guyanensis, Leishmania panamensis***), **mucosal leishmaniasis** (due to ***Leishmania braziliensis***), and **visceral leishmaniasis** (due to ***Leishmania donovani***). The weight-based treatment for adults and adolescents is the same for each of the species, the anti-leishmanial drug ***miltefosine*** **(Impavido)**. Contraindications to this drug include pregnancy, lactation, and Sjogren-Larsson-Syndrome. The contraindication in pregnancy is due to embryo-fetal toxicity, teratogenicity, and fetal death. Obtain a serum or urine pregnancy test for females of reproductive potential and advise females to use effective contraception during therapy and for 5 months following treatment. Breastfeeding is contraindicated while taking this drug and for 5 months following termination of breastfeeding. Potential ASEs include loss of appetite, abdominal pain, nausea, vomiting, diarrhea, headache, dizziness, pruritis, somnolence, elevated liver transaminases, bilirubin, and serum creatinine and thrombocytopenia. ***miltefosine*** is associated with impaired fertility in females and males in animal studies. To report a suspected adverse reaction to this drug, call 1-888-550-6060 or the FDA at 1-800-FDA-1088 or visit www.fda.gov/medwatch.

▶ ***miltefosine*** **(D)(G)** <12 years, <30 kg (60 lbs): not established: ≥12 years: 30-44 kg: one cap bid x 28 consecutive days; >45 kg: one cap tid x 28 consecutive days; take with a full meal
Impavido *Cap:* 50 mg

LISTERIOSIS (*LISTERIA MONOCYTOGENES*)

Comment: *L. monocytogenes* is a potentially lethal foodborne pathogen that is a common contaminant of food and food preparation equipment, and has been isolated in soil, farm environments, produce, raw foods, dairy products, and the feces of asymptomatic people. IV ***ampicillin*** is the mainstay of treatment, but penicillin may be as effective. Some experts recommend combination antibiotic therapy for neuro-invasive *L. monocytogenes*. The most common antimicrobial combination is IV ***ampicillin*** and IV ***gentamycin*** (which is usually discontinued when the patient shows signs of improvement to limit the potential for toxicity). If the patient is penicillin-allergic, IV ***trimethoprim-sulfamethoxazole [TMP-SMX]*** as mono therapy x 14-21 days. Patients with bacteremia but without CNS involvement may be treated with combination (***ampicillin +gentamycin***) therapy for 14 days, but patients with meningitis require a full 21 day combination course of antibiotics. Endocarditis, encephalitis, and brain abscesses may require a longer duration of high dose antimicrobials. Cephalosporins are ineffective. Supportive care and standard isolation precautions are required.

REFERENCES

Kasper, DL, & Fauci, AS. (2017). Listeria monocytogenes infections. In: *Harrison's Infectious Diseases* (3rd ed.). New York: McGraw Hill Education.

McNeill, C, Sisson, W, & Jarrett, A. (2017). Listeriosis: a resurfacing menace. *International Journal of Nursing Practice, 13*(10)647–654.

▶ ***ampicillin*** **(B)(G)** 2 gm IV infusion q 4 hours (in combination with IV gentamycin q 8 hours)
Pediatric: 50 mg/kg IV infusion q 4 hours
Unasyn *Vial:* 1.5, 3 gm

▶ ***gentamicin*** **(C)(G)** 1-2 mg/kg q 8 hours (in combination with IV ampicillin q 4 hours); monitor plasma levels
Pediatric: 2 mg/kg/dose q 8 hours; monitor plasma levels
Geramycin *Vial:* 20, 80 mg/2 ml (2 ml) for dilution and IV infusion

▶ ***trimethoprim-sulfamethoxazole [TMP-SMX]*** **(C)(G)** TMP 5 mg/kg IV infusion q 6 hours; max TMP 160 mg/dose
Pediatric: <2 months: contraindicated: >2 months: 2-5 mg/kg/dose q 8 hours; max TMP 160 mg/dose

Comment: TMP-SMX is contraindicated in the first trimester of pregnancy, the final month of pregnancy, and in infants <8 weeks of age.

▶ ***penicillin g potassium*** **(B)(G)** 4 million units via IV infusion q 4 hours
Pediatric: 65,000 units/kg/dose via IV infusion q 4 hours; max 4 million units/dose; infuse dose over 1-2 hours
Vial: 5, 20 MU pwdr for reconstitution (in D5W or NS) and IV infusion; Pre-mixed bag: 1, 2, 3 MU (50 ml); infuse dose over 1-2 hours

LIVER FLUKES

TREMATODICIDE

Comment: ***praziquantel*** is a trematodicide indicated for the treatment of infections due to all species of Schistosoma (e.g., *Schistosoma mekongi, Schistosoma japonicum, Schistosoma mansoni,* and *Schistosoma hematobium)* and infections due to liver flukes (i.e., *Clonorchis sinensis, Opisthorchis viverrini).* ***praziquantel*** induces a rapid contraction of schistosomes by a specific effect on the permeability of the cell membrane. The drug further causes vacuolization and disintegration of the schistosome tegument.

▶ ***praziquantel*** **(B)** 25 mg/kg tid as a one-day treatment; take the 3 doses at intervals of not less than 4 hours and not more than 6 hours; swallow whole with water during meals; holding the tablets in the mouth leaves a bitter taste which can trigger gagging or vomiting.
Pediatric: <4 years: not established; ≥4 years: same as adult
Biltricide *Tab:* 600mg*** film-coat (3 scores, 4 segments, 150 mg/segment)

Comment: Concomitant administration with strong Cytochrome P450 (P450) inducers, such as ***rifampin***, is contraindicated since therapeutically effective blood levels of ***praziquantel*** may not be achieved. In patients receiving ***rifampin*** who need immediate treatment for schistosomiasis, alternative agents for schistosomiasis should be considered. However, if treatment with ***praziquantel*** is necessary, ***rifampin*** should be discontinued 4 weeks before administration of ***praziquantel***. Treatment with ***rifampin*** can then be restarted one day after completion of ***praziquantel*** treatment. Concomitant administration of other P450 inducers (e.g., antiepileptic drugs such as ***phenytoin***, ***phenobarbital***, ***carbamazepine***) and ***dexamethasone***, may also reduce plasma levels of ***praziquantel***. Concomitant administration of P450 inhibitors (e.g., ***cimetidine***, ***ketoconazole***, ***itraconazole***, ***erythromycin***) may increase plasma levels of ***praziquantel***. Patients should be warned not to drive a car or operate machinery on the day of **Biltricide** treatment and the following day. There are no adequate or well-controlled studies in pregnant women. This drug should be used during pregnancy only if clearly needed. ***praziquantel*** appears in the milk of nursing women at a concentration of about 1/4 that of maternal serum. It is not known whether a pharmacological effect is likely to occur in children. Women should not nurse on the day of **Biltricide** treatment and during the subsequent 72 hours.

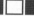

LOW BACK STRAIN

See **Muscle Strain** *page* 287
Acetaminophen for IV Infusion *see* ***Pain*** *page* 322
NSAIDs *see page* 539
Other Oral Analgesics *see* ***Pain*** *page* 324
Topical & Transdermal NSAIDs *see* ***Pain*** *page* 323
Muscle Relaxants *see page* 287
Parenteral Corticosteroids *see page* 547
Oral Corticosteroids *see page* 546

LYME DISEASE (ERYTHEMA CHRONICUM MIGRANS)

Comment: The bite of the deer tick *(Ixodes scapularis)* carries the *Borrelia burgdorferi* organism causing Lyme disease. Proper removal of the tick, and early diagnosis and treatment are essential to effective management of this disease.

STAGE 1

- ***amoxicillin*** (B)(G) <40 kg (88 lb): 20-40 mg/kg/day in 3 divided doses x 10 days or 25-45 mg/kg/day in 2 divided doses x 10 days; *see page* 588 *for dose by weight table;* ≥40 kg: 500-875 mg bid or 250-500 mg tid x 10 days
  - **Amoxil** *Cap:* 250, 500 mg; *Tab:* 875*mg; *Chew tab:* 125, 200, 250, 400 mg (cherry-banana-peppermint) (phenylalanine); *Oral susp:* 125, 250 mg/5 ml (80, 100, 150 ml) (strawberry); 200, 400 mg/5 ml (50, 75, 100 ml) (bubble gum); *Oral drops:* 50 mg/ml (30 ml) (bubble gum)
  - **Moxatag** *Tab:* 775 mg ext-rel
  - **Trimox** *Tab:* 125, 250 mg; *Cap:* 250, 500 mg; *Oral susp:* 125, 250 mg/5 ml (80, 100, 150 ml) (raspberry-strawberry)
- ***clarithromycin*** (C)(G) <6 months: not recommended; ≥6 months-12 years: 7.5 mg/kg bid x 7-14 days; *see page* 602 *for dose by weight table;* >12 years: 500 mg bid or 500 mg ext-rel daily x 7-14 days
  - **Biaxin** *Tab:* 250, 500 mg
  - **Biaxin Oral Suspension** *Oral susp:* 125, 250 mg/5 ml (50, 100 ml)
  - **Biaxin XL** *Tab:* 500 mg ext-rel

Comment: The FDA is advising caution before prescribing ***clarithromycin*** to patients with heart disease because of a potential increased risk of heart problems or death that can occur years later. This recommendation is based on a review of the results of a 10-year follow-up study of patients with coronary heart disease from a large clinical trial that first observed this safety issue. Consider risk benefit and the use of other antibiotics in such patients.

- ***doxycycline*** (D)(G) <8 years: not recommended; ≥8 years, ≤100 lb: 2 mg/lb on first day in 2 divided doses, followed by 1 mg/lb/day in 1-2 divided doses x 14-21 days; ≥8 years, >100 lb: 100 mg bid x 7-14 days; *see page* 605 *for dose by weight table*
  - **Acticlate** *Tab:* 75, 150**mg
  - **Adoxa** *Tab:* 50, 75, 100, 150 mg ent-coat
  - **Doryx** *Tab:* 50, 75, 100, 150, 200 mg del-rel
  - **Doxteric** *Tab:* 50 mg del-rel
  - **Monodox** *Cap:* 50, 75, 100 mg
  - **Oracea** *Cap:* 40 mg del-rel
  - **Vibramycin** *Tab:* 100 mg; *Cap:* 50, 100 mg; *Syr:* 50 mg/5 ml (raspberry-apple) (sulfites); *Oral susp:* 25 mg/5 ml (raspberry)
  - **Vibra-Tab** *Tab:* 100 mg film-coat

Comment: ***doxycycline*** is contraindicated <8 years-of-age, in pregnancy, and lactation (discolors developing tooth enamel). A side effect may be photosensitivity (photophobia). Do not take with antacids, calcium supplements, milk or other dairy, or within 2 hours of taking another drug.

➢ ***minocycline*** **(D)(G)** <8 years: not recommended; ≥8 years, ≤100 lb: 2 mg/lb on first day in 2 divided doses, followed by 1 mg/lb q 12 hours x 9 more days; ≥8 years, >100 lb: 200 mg on first day; then 100 mg q 12 hours x 9 more days

Dynacin *Cap:* 50, 100 mg

Minocin *Cap:* 50, 75, 100 mg; *Oral susp:* 50 mg/5 ml (60 ml) (custard) (sulfites, alcohol 5%)

Comment: ***minocycline*** is contraindicated <8 years-of-age, in pregnancy, and lactation (discolors developing tooth enamel). A side effect may be photosensitivity (photophobia). Do not give with antacids, calcium supplements, milk or other dairy, or within two hours of taking another drug.

➢ ***tetracycline*** **(D)(G)** <8 years: not recommended; ≥8 years, ≤100 lb: 25-50 mg/kg/day in 4 divided doses x 7 days; *see page* 618 *for dose by weight table* , ≥8 years, >100 lb: 250-500 mg qid ac x 21 days

Achromycin V *Cap:* 250, 500 mg

Sumycin *Tab:* 250, 500 mg; *Cap:* 250, 500 mg; *Oral susp:* 125 mg/5 ml (100, 200 ml) (fruit) (sulfites)

Comment: ***tetracycline*** is contraindicated <8 years-of-age, in pregnancy, and lactation (discolors developing tooth enamel). A side effect may be photosensitivity (photophobia). Do not give with antacids, calcium supplements, milk or other dairy, or within two hours of taking another drug.

LYMPHADENITIS

Comment: Therapy should continue for no less than 5 days after resolution of symptoms.

➢ ***amoxicillin+clavulanate*** **(B)(G)**

Augmentin <40 kg: 40-45 mg/kg/day divided tid x 10 days or 90 mg/kg/day divided bid x 10 days; *see page* 590 *for dose by weight table;* ≥40 kg: 500 mg tid or 875 mg bid x 10 days

Tab: 250, 500, 875 mg; *Chew tab:* 125, 250 mg (lemon-lime); 200, 400 mg (cherry-banana) (phenylalanine); *Oral susp:* 125 mg/5 ml (banana), 250 mg/5 ml (75, 100, 150 ml) (orange); 200, 400 mg/5 ml (50, 75, 100 ml) (orange) (phenylalanine)

Augmentin ES-600 <3 months: not recommended; ≥3 months, <40 kg: 90 mg/kg/day divided q 12 hours x 10 days; *see page* 591 *for dose by weight table;* ≥40 kg: not recommended

Oral susp: 600 mg/5 ml (50, 75, 100, 125, 150, 200 ml) (strawberry cream) (phenylalanine)

Augmentin XR <16 years: use other forms; ≥16 years: 2 tabs q 12 hours x 7-10 days

Tab: 1000*mg ext-rel

➢ ***cephalexin*** **(B)(G)** <12 years: 25-50 mg/kg/day in 4 divided doses x 10 days; *see page* 601 *for dose by weight table;* ≥12 years: 500 mg bid x 10 days

Keflex *Cap:* 250, 333, 500, 750 mg; *Oral susp:* 125, 250 mg/5 ml (100, 200 ml) (strawberry)

➢ ***dicloxacillin*** **(B)** <12 years: 12.5-25 mg/kg/day in 4 divided doses x 10 days; *see page* 604 *for dose by weight table;* ≥12 years: 500 mg q 6 hours x 10 days

Dynapen *Cap:* 125, 250, 500 mg; *Oral susp:* 62.5 mg/5 ml (80, 100, 200 ml)

LYMPHOGRANULOMA VENEREUM

Comment: The following treatment regimens are published in the **2015 CDC Sexually Transmitted Diseases Treatment Guidelines.** This section contains treatment regimens for patients ≥18 years only; consult a specialist for treatment of patients < 18 years-of-age. Treatment regimens are presented in alphabetical order by generic drug name, followed by brands and dose forms. Treat all sexual contacts. Persons with both LGV and HIV infection should receive the same treatment regimens as those who are HIV-negative; however, prolonged treatment may be required and delay in resolution of symptoms may occur.

RECOMMENDED REGIMEN

Regimen 1

- ***doxycycline*** 100 mg bid x 21 days

ALTERNATIVE REGIMEN

Regimen 1

- ***erythromycin base*** (B)(G) 500 mg qid x 21 days or ***erythromycin ethylsuccinate*** 400 mg qid x 21 days

RECOMMENDED REGIMENS FOR THE MANAGEMENT OF SEXUAL CONTACTS

Comment: LGV is caused by *C. trachomatis* serovars L1, L2, or L3. Persons who have had sexual contact with a patient who has LGV within 60 days before onset of the patient's symptoms should be examined, tested for urethral or cervical chlamydial infection, and treated with a chlamydia regimen.

Regimen 1

- ***azithromycin*** 1 gm in a single dose

Regimen 2

- ***doxycycline*** 100 mg bid x 7 days

DRUG BRANDS AND DOSE FORMS

- ***azithromycin*** (B)(G)
  - **Zithromax** *Tab:* 250, 500, 600 mg; *Oral susp:* 100 mg/5 ml (15 ml); 200 mg/5 ml (15, 22.5, 30 ml) (cherry); *Pkt:* 1 gm for reconstitution (cherry-banana)
  - **Zithromax Tri-pak** *Tab:* 3 x 500 mg tabs/pck
  - **Zithromax Z-pak** *Tab:* 6 x 250 mg tabs/pck
  - **Zmax** *Oral susp:* 2 gm ext-rel for reconstitution (cherry-banana) (148 mg Na^+)
- ***doxycycline*** (D)(G) <8 years: not recommended; ≥8 years, ≤100 lb: 2 mg/lb on first day in 2 divided doses, followed by 1 mg/lb/day in 1-2 divided doses; ≥8 years, >100 lb: 40-100 mg bid; *see page 605 for dose by weight table*
  - **Acticlate** *Tab:* 75, 150**mg
  - **Adoxa** *Tab:* 50, 75, 100, 150 mg ent-coat
  - **Doryx** *Tab:* 50, 75, 100, 150, 200 mg del-rel
  - **Doxteric** *Tab:* 50 mg del-rel
  - **Monodox** *Cap:* 50, 75, 100 mg
  - **Oracea** *Cap:* 40 mg del-rel

Vibramycin *Tab:* 100 mg; *Cap:* 50, 100 mg; *Syr:* 50 mg/5 ml (raspberry-apple) (sulfites); *Oral susp:* 25 mg/5 ml (raspberry)
Vibra-Tab *Tab:* 100 mg film-coat

Comment: ***doxycycline*** is contraindicated <8 years-of-age, in pregnancy, and lactation (discolors developing tooth enamel). A side effect may be photosensitivity (photophobia). Do not take with antacids, calcium supplements, milk or other dairy, or within 2 hours of taking another drug.

▶ ***erythromycin base*** **(B)(G)**
Ery-Tab *Tab:* 250, 333, 500 mg ent-coat
PCE *Tab:* 333, 500 mg

▶ ***erythromycin ethylsuccinate*** **(B)(G)**
EryPed *Oral susp:* 200 mg/5 ml (100, 200 ml) (fruit); 400 mg/5 ml (60, 100, 200 ml) (banana); *Oral drops:* 200, 400 mg/5 ml (50 ml) (fruit); *Chew tab:* 200 mg wafer (fruit)
E.E.S. *Oral susp:* 200, 400 mg/5 ml (100 ml) (fruit)
E.E.S. Granules *Oral susp:* 200 mg/5 ml (100, 200 ml) (cherry)
E.E.S. 400 Tablets *Tab:* 400 mg

MALARIA (*PLASMODIUM FALCIPARUM, PLASMODIUM VIVAX*)

▶ ***doxycycline*** **(D)(G)** *Treatment:* <8 years: not recommended; ≥8 years, ≤100 lb: 2 mg/lb on first day in 2 divided doses, followed by 1 mg/lb/day in 1-2 divided doses; ≥8 years, >100 lb: 100 mg daily; *Prophylaxis:* initiate 1-2 days prior to travel; take during travel; continue for 4 weeks after leaving the endemic area; *see page* 605 *for dose by weight table*
Acticlate *Tab:* 75, 150**mg
Adoxa *Tab:* 50, 75, 100, 150 mg ent-coat
Doryx *Tab:* 50, 75, 100, 150, 200 mg del-rel
Doxteric *Tab:* 50 mg del-rel
Monodox *Cap:* 50, 75, 100 mg
Oracea *Cap:* 40 mg del-rel
Vibramycin *Tab:* 100 mg; *Cap:* 50, 100 mg; *Syr:* 50 mg/5 ml (raspberry-apple) (sulfites); *Oral susp:* 25 mg/5 ml (raspberry)
Vibra-Tab *Tab:* 100 mg film-coat

Comment: ***doxycycline*** is contraindicated <8 years-of-age, in pregnancy, and lactation (discolors developing tooth enamel). A side effect may be photosensitivity (photophobia). Do not take with antacids, calcium supplements, milk or other dairy, or within 2 hours of taking another drug.

▶ ***minocycline*** **(D)(G)** *Treatment:* <8 years: not recommended; ≥8 years, ≤100 lb: 2 mg/lb on first day in 2 divided doses, followed by 1 mg/lb q 12 hours x 9 more days; ≥8 years, >100 lb: 100 mg daily; *Prophylaxis:* initiate 1-2 days prior to travel; take during travel; continue for 4 weeks after leaving the endemic area
Dynacin *Cap:* 50, 100 mg
Minocin *Cap:* 50, 75, 100 mg; *Oral susp:* 50 mg/5 ml (60 ml) (custard) (sulfites, alcohol 5%)

Comment: ***minocycline*** is contraindicated <8 years-of-age, in pregnancy, and lactation (discolors developing tooth enamel). A side effect may be photosensitivity (photophobia). Do not give with antacids, calcium supplements, milk or other dairy, or within 2 hours of taking another drug.

▶ ***tetracycline*** **(D)(G)** *Treatment:* <8 years: not recommended; ≥8 years, ≤100 lb: 25-50 mg/kg/day in 4 divided doses; *see page* 618 *for dose by weight table*; ≥8 years, >100 lb: 250 mg once daily; *Prophylaxis:* initiate 1-2 days prior to travel; take during travel; continue for 4 weeks after leaving the endemic area

Achromycin V *Cap:* 250, 500 mg

Sumycin *Tab:* 250, 500 mg; *Cap:* 250, 500 mg; *Oral susp:* 125 mg/5 ml (100, 200 ml) (fruit) (sulfites)

Comment: ***tetracycline*** is contraindicated <8 years-of-age, in pregnancy, and lactation (discolors developing tooth enamel). A side effect may be photosensitivity (photophobia). Do not give with antacids, calcium supplements, milk or other dairy, or within 2 hours of taking another drug.

ANTIMALARIALS

▶ ***atovaquone*** (C)(G) <12 years: see mfr pkg insert for weight-based dosing table; ≥12 years: take as a single dose with food or a milky drink at the same time each day; repeat dose if vomited within 1 hour; *Prophylaxis:* 1,500 mg once daily; *Treatment:* 750 mg bid x 21 days

Mepron *Susp:* 750 mg/5 ml (210 ml) (citrus)

▶ ***atovaquone+proguanil*** (C)(G) take as a single dose with food or a milky drink at the same time each day; repeat dose if vomited within 1 hour; *Prophylaxis:* daily dose starting 1-2 days before entering endemic area, during stay, and for 7 days after return; <5 kg: not recommended; 5-20 kg: 1 ped tab; 21-30 kg: 2 ped tabs; 31-40 kg: 3 ped tabs; ≥40 kg: 1 adult tab; *Treatment (acute, uncomplicated):* a single dose once daily x 3 days; <5 kg: not recommended; 5-8 kg: 2 ped tabs; 9-10 kg: 3 ped tabs; 11-20 kg: 1 adult tab; 21-30 kg: 2 adult tabs; 31-40 kg: 3 adult tabs; >40 kg: 4 adult tabs

Malarone *Tab:* atov 250 mg+prog 100 mg

Malarone Pediatric *Tab:* atov 62.5 mg+prog 25 mg

Comment: ***atovaquone*** is antagonized by ***tetracycline*** and ***metoclopramide***. Concomitant ***rifampin*** is not recommended (may elevate LFTs).

▶ ***chloroquine*** (C)(G) *Prophylaxis: <12* years: 8.35 mg/kg (max 500 mg); ≥12 years: 500 mg; a single dose once weekly (on the same day of each week); start 2 weeks prior to exposure, continue while in the endemic area, and continue 4 weeks after departure; *Treatment: <12* years: initially 16.7 mg/kg (max 1 gm); then 8.35 mg/kg (max 500 mg) 6 hours, 24 hours, and 48 hours after initial dose, or initially 6.25 mg/kg IM; may repeat in 6 hours; max 12.5 mg/kg/day; ≥12 years: initially 1 gm; then 500 mg 6 hours, 24 hours, and 48 hours after initial dose or initially 200-250 mg IM; may repeat in 6 hours; max 1 gm in first 24 hours; continue to 1.875 gm in 3 days

Aralen *Tab:* 500 mg; *Amp:* 50 mg/ml (5 ml)

▶ ***hydroxychloroquine*** (C)(G) *Prophylaxis: <12* years: 6.45 mg/kg (max 400 mg); ≥12 years: 400 mg; dose once weekly(on the same day of each week); start weeks prior to arrival, continue while in endemic area, and continue for 4 weeks after departure; *Treatment: <12* years: initially 12.9 mg/kg (max 800 mg); then 6.45 mg/kg (max 400 mg) at 6 hours, 24 hours, and 48 hours after initial dose; ≥12 years: initially 800 mg; then 400 mg at 6 hours, 24 hours, and 48 hours after initial dose

Plaquenil *Tab:* 200 mg

▶ ***mefloquine*** (C) *Prophylaxis:* <6 months: not recommended; ≥6 months-12 years: 3-5 mg/kg (max 250 mg); ≥12 years: 250 mg; dose once weekly (on the same day of each week); start 1 week prior to exposure, continue while in the endemic area, and continue for 4 weeks after departure; *Treatment:* ≥6 months-12 years: 25-50 mg/kg as a single dose (max 250 mg); ≥12 years: 1,250 mg as a single dose

Lariam *Tab:* 250*mg

Comment: ***mefloquine*** is contraindicated with active or recent history of depression, generalized anxiety disorder, psychosis, schizophrenia or any other psychiatric disorder or history of convulsions.

▶ *quinine sulfate* (C)(G) <16 years: not recommended; ≥16 years: 1 tab or cap every 8 hours x 7 days

Tab: 260 mg; *Cap:* 260, 300, 325 mg

Qualaquin *Cap:* 324 mg

Comment: ***Qualaquin*** is indicated in the treatment of uncomplicated *P. falciparum* malaria (including chloroquine-resistant strains).

MASTITIS (BREAST ABSCESS)

ANTI-INFECTIVES

▶ *amoxicillin+clavulanate* (B)(G)

Augmentin <40 kg: 40-45 mg/kg/day divided tid x 10 days or 90 mg/kg/day divided bid x 10 days; *see page* 590 *for dose by weight table;* ≥40 kg: 500 mg tid or 875 mg bid x 10 days

Tab: 250, 500, 875 mg; *Chew tab:* 125, 250 mg (lemon-lime); 200, 400 mg (cherry-banana) (phenylalanine); *Oral susp:* 125 mg/5 ml (banana), 250 mg/5 ml (75, 100, 150 ml) (orange); 200, 400 mg/5 ml (50, 75, 100 ml) (orange) (phenylalanine)

Augmentin ES-600 <3 months: not recommended; ≥3 months, <40 kg: 90 mg/kg/day divided q 12 hours x 10 days; *see page* 591 *for dose by weight table;* ≥40 kg: not recommended

Oral susp: 600 mg/5 ml (50, 75, 100, 125, 150, 200 ml) (strawberry cream) (phenylalanine)

Augmentin XR <16 years: use other forms; ≥16 years: 2 tabs q 12 hours x 7-10 days

Tab: 1000*mg ext-rel

▶ *cefaclor* (B)(G) <1 month: not recommended; 1 month-12 years: 20-40 mg/kg divided bid x 10 days; *see page* 594 *for dose by weight table;* max 1 gm/day; >12 years: 250-500 mg q 8 hours x 10 days; max 2 gm/day

Tab: 500 mg; *Cap:* 250, 500 mg; *Susp:* 125 mg/5 ml (75, 150 ml) (strawberry); 187 mg/5 ml (50, 100 ml) (strawberry); 250 mg/5 ml (75, 150 ml) (strawberry); 375 mg/5 ml (50, 100 ml) (strawberry)

Cefaclor Extended Release <16 years: not recommended; ≥16 years: 500 mg bid x 10 days; (clinically equivalent to 250 mg immed-rel caps tid); swallow whole; take with meals

Tab: 375, 500 mg ext-rel

▶ *ceftriaxone* (B)(G) <12 years: 50 mg/kg IM daily; continue 2 days after signs of infection have disappeared; ≥12 years: 1-2 grams IM daily; continue 2 days after signs of infection have disappeared; max 4 gm/day

Rocephin *Vial:* 250, 500 mg; 1, 2 gm

▶ *cephalexin* (B)(G) <12 years: 25-50 mg/kg/day in 4 divided doses x 10 days; *see page* 601 *for dose by weight table;* ≥12 years: 500 mg bid x 10 days

Keflex *Cap:* 250, 333, 500, 750 mg; *Oral susp:* 125, 250 mg/5 ml (100, 200 ml) (strawberry)

▶ *clindamycin* (B)(G) <12 years: not recommended; ≥12 years: 300 mg tid x 10 days

Cleocin *Cap:* 75 (tartrazine), 150 (tartrazine), 300 mg

Cleocin Pediatric Granules *Oral susp:* 75 mg/5 ml (100 ml) (cherry)

▶ *erythromycin base* (B)(G) <45 kg: 30-40 mg/kg/day in 4 divided doses x 10 days; ≥45 kg: 250-500 mg qid x 10 days

Ery-Tab *Tab:* 250, 333, 500 mg ent-coat

PCE *Tab:* 333, 500 mg

MELASMA/CHLOASMA

SKIN DEPIGMENTING AGENTS

- ***hydroquinone*** **(C)** <12 years: not recommended; ≥12 years: apply a thin film to clean dry affected areas bid; discontinue if lightening does not occur after 2 months
  - **Lustra** *Crm:* hydro 4% (1, 2 oz) (sulfites)
  - **Lustra AF** *Crm:* hydro 4% (1, 2 oz) (sunscreens, sulfites)
- ***hydroquinone+fluocinolone acetonide+tretinoin*** **(C)** <12 years: not recommended; ≥12 years: apply a thin film to clean dry affected areas once daily at least 30 minutes before bedtime
  - **Tri-Luma** *Crm:* hydro 4%+fluo acet 0.01%+tret 0.05% (30 gm) (sulfites, parabens)

MENIERE'S DISEASE

- ***diazepam*** **(D)(IV)(G)** <6 months: not recommended; ≥6 months: initially 1-2.5 mg tid-qid; may increase gradually
  - **Diastat** *Rectal gel delivery system:* 2.5 mg
  - **Diastat AcuDial** *Rectal gel delivery system:* 10, 20 mg
  - **Valium** *Tab:* 2*, 5*, 10*mg
  - **Valium Intensol Oral Solution** *Conc oral soln:* 5 mg/ml (30 ml w. dropper) (alcohol 19%)
  - **Valium Oral Solution** *Oral soln:* 5 mg/5 ml (500 ml) (wintergreen spice)
- ***dimenhydrinate*** **(B)** <2 years: not recommended; 2-6 years: 12.5-25 mg q 6-8 hours; max 75 mg/day; >6-11 years: 25-50 mg q 6-8 hours; max 150 mg/day; >11 years: 50 mg q 4-6 hours
  - **Dramamine (OTC)** *Tab:* 50*mg; *Chew tab:* 50 mg (phenylalanine, tartrazine); *Liq:* 12.5 mg/5 ml (4 oz)
- ***diphenhydramine*** **(B)(OTC)(G)** <2 years: not recommended; 2-6 years: 6.25 mg q 4-6 hours; max 37.5 mg/day; >6-12 years: 12.5-25 mg q 4-6 hours; max 150 mg/day; >12 years: 25-50 mg q 6-8 hours; max 100 mg/day
  - **Benadryl (OTC)** *Chew tab:* 12.5 mg (grape) (phenylalanine); *Liq:* 12.5 mg/5 ml (4, 8 oz); *Cap:* 25 mg; *Tab:* 25 mg; *Dye-free soft gel:* 25 mg; *Dye-free liq:* 12.5 mg/5 ml (4, 8 oz)
- ***diphenhydramine*** injectable **(B)(G)** <12 years: *See mfr pkg insert:* 1.25 mg/kg up to 25 mg IM x 1 dose; then q 6 hours prn; ≥12 years: 25-50 mg IM immediately; then q 6 hours prn
  - **Benadryl Injectable** *Vial:* 50 mg/ml (1 ml single use); 50 mg/ml (10 ml multi-dose); *Amp:* 10 mg/ml (1 ml); *Prefilled syringe:* 50 mg/ml (1 ml)
- ***hydroxyzine*** **(C)(G)** <6 years: 50 mg/day divided qid; 6-12 years: 50-100 mg/day divided qid; >12 years: 50-100 mg qid; max 600 mg/day
  - **Atarax** *Tab:* 10, 25, 50, 100 mg; *Syr:* 10 mg/5 ml (alcohol 0.5%)
  - **Vistaril** *Cap:* 25, 50, 100 mg; *Oral susp:* 25 mg/5 ml (4 oz) (lemon)
- ***meclizine*** **(B)(G)**
  - **Antivert** <12 years: not recommended; ≥12 years: *Tab:* 12.5, 25, 50*mg; *Amp:* 50 mg/ml (1 ml); *Vial:* 50 mg/ml (1 ml single use); 50 mg/ml (10 ml multi-dose)
  - **Bonine (OTC)** <12 years: not recommended; ≥12 years: *Cap:* 15, 25, 30 mg; *Tab:* 12.5, 25, 50 mg; *Chew tab/Film-coat tab:* 25 mg
  - **Dramamine II** <12 years: not recommended; ≥12 years: 25 mg bid; max 50 mg/day
    Tab: 25*mg
  - **Zentrip** <12 years: not recommended; ≥12 years: 25 mg bid; max 50 mg/day *Strip:* 25 mg orally-disint

▶ ***promethazine*** **(C)** <2 years: not recommended; 2-12 years: 0.5 mg/lb or 6.25-25 mg q 4-6 hours PO or rectally; >12 years: 12.5-25 q 4-6 hours PO or rectally

Phenergan *Tab:* 12.5*, 25*, 50 mg; *Plain syr:* 6.25 mg/5 ml; *Fortis syr:* 25 mg/5 ml; *Rectal supp:* 12.5, 25, 50 mg

Comment: ***promethazine*** is contraindicated in children with uncomplicated nausea, dehydration, Reye's syndrome, history of sleep apnea, asthma, and lower respiratory disorders in children. ***Promethazine*** lowers the seizure threshold in children, may cause cholestatic jaundice, anticholinergic effects, extrapyramidal effects, and potentially fatal respiratory depression.

▶ ***scopolamine*** transdermal patch **(C)** <12 years: not recommended; ≥12 years: 1 patch behind ear; each patch is effective for 3 days; change patch every 4th day; alternate sides

Transderm Scop *Patch:* 1.5 mg (4/carton)

MENINGITIS (*NEISSERIA MENINGITIDIS*)

PROPHYLAXIS

Comment: Meningitis vaccine is a 3-dose series (0, 2, 6 month schedule) indicated for persons aged ≥10-25 years. Have epinephrine 1:1,000 readily available and monitor for 15 minutes post-dose of meningitis vaccine.

▶ ***Meningococcal group b vaccine [recombinant, absorbed]*** <10 years: not established; ≥10 years: *First dose:* 0.5 ml IM in the deltoid; *Second dose:* 0.5 ml IM 2 months later; *Third dose:* 0.5 ml IM 6 months after the first dose;

Bexsero *Susp for IM inj:* 0.5 ml single-dose prefilled syringes (1, 10/carton)

Trumenba *Susp for IM inj:* 0.5 ml single-dose prefilled syringes (5, 10/carton)

▶ ***Neisseria meningitides oligosaccharide conjugate*** quadrivalent meningococcal vaccine **(B)** contains *Corynebacterium diphtheria* CRM197 protein; 10 mcg of Group A + 5 mcg each of Group C, Y, and W-135 + 32.7-64.1 mcg of diphtheria CRM197 protein per 0.5 ml pwdr for reconstitution; <2 months: not established; 2 months: administer 4-dose series at 2, 4, 6, and 12 months; 7-23 months: administer 3-dose series with 2nd dose administered in the 2nd year of life and at least 3 months after the 1st dose; ≥2 years: 0.5 ml IM once; 2-5 years, continued high risk: may administer 2nd dose 2 months after the 1st dose

Menveo *Vial multidose:* 5 doses/vial (MenA conjugate component pwdr for reconstitution + 1 vial liquid MenCWY conjugate component for reconstitution) (preservative-free)

▶ ***Neisseria meningitidis polysaccharides*** vaccine **(C)**

Menactra administer in the deltoid only; <9 months: not recommended; *Primary vaccination:* 9-23 months: 0.5 ml administered as a 2-dose series 3 months apart; ≥24 months: 0.5 ml IM once; *Booster vaccination:* ≥15 years: 0.5 ml IM once for those at continued risk if at least 4 years have elapsed since the prior dose

Single-dose prefilled tip-lock syringe: 4 mcg each of group A, C, Y, and W-135 per 0.5 ml soln (preservative-free)

Comment: Latex allergy is a contraindication to **Menactra**.

Menomune-A/C/Y/W-135 <2 years: not recommended (except ≥3 months of age as short-term protection against group A); ≥2 years: same as adult; if at high risk, may revaccinate children first vaccinated ≤4 years-of-age after 2-3 years (older children after 3-5 years)

Vial (single-dose): 50 mcg each of group A, C, Y, and W-135 per 0.5 ml (pwdr for SC inj after reconstitution; preservative-free diluent); *Vial (multi-dose):* 50 mcg each of group A, C, Y, and W-130 per 0.5 ml (pwdr for SC inj after reconstitution [10 doses/vial] [thimerosal-preserved diluent])

Comment: Use precaution with latex allergy.

MENOMETRORRHAGIA (IRREGULAR HEAVY MENSTRUAL BLEEDING) & MENORRHAGIA (HEAVY CYCLICAL MENSTRUAL BLEEDING)

ANTIFIBRINOLYTIC AGENT

➢ ***tranexamic acid*** (B)(G) <18 years: not recommended; ≥18 years: 1,300 mg tid; treat for up to 5 days during menses; *Normal renal function (SCr ≤1.4 mg/dL):* 1,300 mg tid; *SCr ≥1.4-2.8 mg/dL:* 1,300 mg bid; *SCr ≥2.8-5.7 mg/dL:* 1,300 mg once daily; *SCr ≥5.7 mg/dL:* 650 mg once daily
 Lysteda *Tab:* 650 mg

INJECTABLE PROGESTERONE ONLY CONTRACEPTIVES

Combined Oral Contraceptives *see page* 528
Intrauterine Devices *see page* 538

➢ ***medroxyprogesterone*** (X)(G) *Pre-menarche:* not applicable; administer IM in the deltoid or hip; do not massage site; administer first dose within 5 days of onset of normal menses, within 5 days postpartum if not breastfeeding, or at 6 weeks postpartum if breastfeeding exclusively; do not use for >2 years unless other methods are inadequate
 Depo-Provera 150 mg deep IM q 3 months
  Vial: 150 mg/ml (1 ml); *Prefilled syringe:* 150 mg/ml (1 ml)
 Depo-SubQ Provera 104 mg SC q 3 months
  Prefilled syringe: 104 mg/ml (0.65 ml) (parabens)

Comment: Contraindications to injectable ***progesterone*** include: thromboembolic disorders, cerebral vascular disease, breast cancer, significant hepatic disease, undiagnosed vaginal bleeding, pregnancy.

METHAMPHETAMINE-INDUCED PSYCHOSIS

ANTIPSYCHOSIS AGENTS

For more antipsychotics, see **Appendix J: Antipsychotic Drugs** *pages* 557-560
Tardive Dyskinesia *see page* 440

Comment: First-generation antipsychotics (e,g., ***haloperidol*** or ***fluphenazine***) should be used sparingly and cautiously in patients with methamphetamine-induced psychosis because of the risk of developing extrapyramidal symptoms (EPS) and because these patients are prone to develop motor complications as a result of methamphetamine abuse. Second-generation antipsychotics (e.g., ***risperidone*** and ***olanzapine***) may be more appropriate because of the lower risks of EPS. The presence of high norepinephrine levels in some patients with recurrent methamphetamine psychosis suggests that drugs that block norepinephrine receptors (e.g., ***prazosin*** or ***propranolol***) might be of therapeutic benefit although they have not been studied in controlled trials.

REFERENCE

Zarrabi, H, Khalkhali, M, Hamidi, A, *et al.* (2016). Clinical features, course and treatment of methamphetamine-induced psychosis in psychiatric inpatients. *BMC Psychiatry, 16*(44).

➢ ***aripiprazole*** (C)(G) <10 years: not recommended; ≥10-17 years: initially 2 mg/day in a single dose for 2 days; then increase to 5 mg/day in a single dose for 2 days; then increase to target dose of 10 mg/day in a single dose; may increase by 5 mg/day at weekly intervals as needed to max 30 mg/day; >17 years: initially 15 mg once daily; may increase to max 30 mg/day

Abilify *Tab:* 2, 5, 10, 15, 20, 30 mg

Abilify Discmelt *Tab:* 15 mg orally-disint (vanilla) (phenylalanine)

Abilify Maintena *Vial:* 300, 400 mg ext-rel pwdr for IM injection after reconstitution; 300, 400 mg single-dose prefilled dual-chamber syringes w. supplies

▶ ***aripiprazole lauroxil*** **(C)** <18 years: not recommended; ≥18 years: administer by IM injection in the deltoid (441 mg dose only) or gluteal (441 mg, 662 mg, 882 mg or 1064 mg) muscle by a qualified healthcare professional; initiate at a dose of 441 mg, 662 mg or 882 mg administered monthly, or 882 mg every 6 weeks, or 1064 mg every 2 months;

Aristada *Prefilled syringe:* 441, 662, 882, 1064 mg single-use, ext-rel susp

Comment: **Aristada** is an atypical antipsychotic available in 4 doses with 3 dosing duration options for flexible dosing. For patients naïve to ***aripiprazole***, establish tolerability with oral ***aripiprazole*** prior to initiating treatment with **Aristada. Aristada** can be initiated at any of the 4 doses at the appropriate dosing duration option. In conjunction with the first injection, administer treatment with oral ***aripiprazole*** for 21 consecutive days for all 4 dose sizes. The most common adverse event associated with **Aristada** is akathisia. Patients are also at increased risk for developing neuroleptic malignant syndrome, tardive dyskinesia, pathological gambling or other compulsive behaviors, orthostatic hypotension, hyperglycemic, dyslipidemia, and weight gain. Hypersensitive reactions can occur and range from pruritus or urticaria to anaphylaxis. Stroke, transient ischemic attacks, and falls have been reported in elderly patients with dementia-related psychosis who were treated with ***apriprazole***. **Aristada** is not for treatment of people who have lost touch with reality (psychosis) due to confusion and memory loss (dementia). May cause extrapyramidal and/or withdrawal symptoms in neonates exposed in utero in the third trimester of pregnancy. **Aripiprazole** is present in human breast milk; however, there are insufficient data to assess the amount in human milk or the effects on the breastfed infant. The development and health benefits of breastfeeding should be considered along with the mother's clinical need for **Aristada** and any potential adverse effects on the breastfed infant from **Aristada** or from the underlying maternal condition. For more information or to report ASEs, contact the National Pregnancy Registry for Atypical Antipsychotics at 1-866-961-2388 or visit http://womensmentalhealth.org/clinical-and-research-programs/pregnancyregistry/. Limited published data on aripiprazole use in pregnant women are not sufficient to inform any drug-associated risks for birth defects or miscarriage. To report suspected adverse reactions, contact Alkermes at 1-866-274-7823 or FDA at 1-800-FDA-1088 or visit www.fda.gov/medwatch

▶ ***fluphenazine hcl*** [**Prolixin**] **(C)(G)** <18 years: not studied

Tab: 1, 2.5, 5, 10 mg; *Elixer:* 2.5 mg/5 ml; *Conc:* 5 mg/ml; *Vial:* 2.5 mg/ml for injection

▶ ***fluphenazine decanoate*** [**Prolixin Decanoate**] **(C)(G)** <18 years: not studied

Vial: 2.5 mg/ml (5 ml)

Comment: Previously, ***fluphenazine*** was marketed as **Prolixin**, but is currently only available in generic form. Optimal dose and frequency of administration of ***fluphenazine*** must be determined for each patient, since dosage requirements have been found to vary with clinical circumstances as well as with individual response; dosage should not exceed 100 mg; if doses > 50 mg are deemed necessary, the next dose and succeeding doses should be increased cautiously in increments of 12.5 mg. ***fluphenazine decanoate injection*** and ***fluphenazine enanthate injection*** are long-acting parenteral antipsychotic forms intended for use in the management of patients requiring prolonged parenteral neuroleptic therapy. ***fluphenazine*** has activity at all levels of the central nervous system (CNS) as well as on multi ple organ systems. The mechanism whereby its therapeutic action is exerted is unknown. ***fluphenazine*** differs from other phenothiazine derivatives in several respects: it is more potent on a milligram basis, it has less potentiating effect on CNS depressants and anesthetics than do some of the phenothiazines and appears to be less sedating, and it is less likely than some of the older phenothiazines to produce hypotension (nevertheless, appropriate cautions should be observed. Neuroleptic Malignant Syndrome (NMS), a potentially fatal symptom complex, is associated with all antipsychotic drugs. Clinical manifestations of NMS are hyperpyrexia, muscle rigidity, altered mental status and evidence of autonomic instability (irregular pulse or blood pressure, tachycardia, diaphoresis, and cardiac dysrhythmias). Anticholinergic effects may be potentiated with concomitant ***atropine*** and ***fluphenazine.*** Safety and efficacy in children have not been established. Safety during pregnancy has not been established; therefore, the possible hazards should be weighed against the potential benefits when administering this drug to pregnant patients.

➢ ***haloperidol*** (C)(G)

Oral route of administration: Moderate Symptomology: 0.5 to 2 mg orally 2 to 3 times a day; *Severe symptomology:* 3 to 5 mg orally 2 to 3 times a day; initial doses of up to 100 mg/day have been necessary in some severely resistant cases;
Maintenance: after achieving a satisfactory response, the dose should be adjusted as practical to achieve optimum control
Parenteral route of administration: Prompt control of acute agitation: 2 to 5 mg IM every 4 to 8 hours; *Maintenance:* frequency of IM administration should be determined by patient response and may be given as often as every hour; max: 20 mg/day

Haldol *Tab:* 0.5*, 1*, 2*, 5*, 10*, 20*mg
Haldol Lactate *Vial:* 5 mg for IM injection, single-dose

➢ ***mesoridazine*** (C) initially 25 mg tid; max 300 mg/day

Serentil *Tab:* 10, 25, 50, 100 mg; *Conc:* 25 mg/ml (118 ml)

➢ ***olanzapine*** (C) initially 2.5-10 mg daily; increase to 10 mg/day within a few days; then by 5 mg/day at weekly intervals; max 20 mg/day

Zyprexa *Tab:* 2.5, 5, 7.5, 10 mg
Zyprexa Zydis *ODT:* 5, 10, 15, 20 mg (phenylalanine)

➢ ***quetiapine fumarate*** (C)(G)

SeroQUEL initially 25 mg bid, titrate q 2nd or 3rd day in increments of 25-50 mg bid-tid; usual maintenance 400-600 mg/day in 2-3 divided doses
Tab: 25, 50, 100, 200, 300, 400 mg
SeroQUEL XR administer once daily in the PM; *Day 1*: 50 mg; *Day 2*: 100 mg; *Day 3*: 200 mg; *Day 4*: 300 mg; usual range 400-600 mg/day
Tab: 50, 150, 200, 300, 400 mg ext-rel

➢ ***risperidone*** (C) 0.5 mg bid x 1 day; adjust in increments of 0.5 mg bid; usual range 0.5-5 mg/day

Risperdal *Tab:* 1, 2, 3, 4 mg; *Oral soln:* 1 mg/ml (100 ml)
Risperdal M-Tab *Tab:* 0.5, 1, 2 mg

➢ ***thioridazine*** (C)(G) 10-25 mg bid

Mellaril *Tab:* 10, 15, 25, 50, 100, 150, 200 mg; *Oral susp:* 25 mg/5 ml, 100 mg/5 ml; *Oral conc:* 30 mg/ml, 100 mg/ml (4 oz)

MITRAL VALVE PROLAPSE (MVP)

➢ ***propranolol*** (C)(G)

Inderal <12 years: not recommended; ≥12 years: initially 10 mg bid; usual range 160-320 mg/day in divided doses
Tab: 10*, 20*, 40*, 60*, 80*mg
Inderal LA <12 years: not recommended; ≥12 years: initially 80 mg daily in a single dose; increase q 3-7 days; usual range 120-160 mg/day; max 320 mg/day in a single dose
Cap: 60, 80, 120, 160 mg sust-rel

InnoPran XL <12 years: not recommended; ≥12 years: initially 80 mg q HS; max 120 mg/day
Cap: 80, 120 mg ext-rel

MONONUCLEOSIS

Acetaminophen **(B)** *see* ***Fever*** *page* 149
Other Oral Analgesics *see* ***Pain*** *page* 324
Parenteral Corticosteroids *see page* 547
Oral Corticosteroids *see page* 546

▶ ***prednisone*** **(C)** initially 40-80 mg/day, then taper off over 5-7 days
Comment: Corticosteroids are recommended in patients with significant pharyngeal edema.

MOTION SICKNESS

▶ ***dimenhydrinate*** **(B)(OTC)** <2 years: not recommended; 2-6 years: 12.5-25 mg; max 75 mg/day; start 1 hour before travel; may repeat q 6-8 hours; 6-11 years: 25-50 mg; max 150 mg/day; start 1 hour before travel; may repeat q 6-8 hours; ≥12 years 50-100 mg q 4-6 hours; start 1 hour before travel; max 400 mg/day
Dramamine *Tab:* 50*mg; *Chew tab:* 50 mg (phenylalanine, tartrazine); *Liq:* 12.5 mg/5 ml (4 oz)

▶ ***meclizine*** **(B)(G)** 12 years: not recommended; ≥12 years: 25-50 mg 1 hour before travel; may repeat q 24 hours as needed; max 50 mg/day
Antivert *Tab:* 12.5, 25, 50*mg
Bonine (OTC) *Cap:* 15, 25, 50 mg; *Tab:* 12.5, 25, 50 mg; *Chew tab/Film-coat tab:* 25 mg
Dramamine II (OTC) *Tab:* 25 mg
Zentrip *Strip:* 25 mg orally-disint

▶ ***prochlorperazine*** **(C)(G)** 12 years: not recommended; ≥12 years:
Compazine 5-10 mg q 4 hours prn
Tab: 5 mg; *Syr:* 5 mg/5 ml (4 oz; fruit); *Rectal supp:* 2.5, 5, 25 mg
Compazine Spansule 15 mg q AM or 10 mg q 12 hours prn
Spansules: 10, 15 mg sust-rel

▶ ***promethazine*** **(C)(G)** <12 years: not recommended; ≥12 years: 12.5-25 mg 30-60 minutes before travel; may repeat in 8-12 hours
Phenergan *Tab:* 12.5*, 25*, 50 mg; *Plain syr:* 6.25 mg/5 ml; *Fortis syr:* 25 mg/5 ml; *Rectal supp:* 12.5, 25, 50 mg
Comment: ***promethazine*** is contraindicated in children with uncomplicated nausea, dehydration, Reye's syndrome, history of sleep apnea, asthma, and lower respiratory disorders in children. ***Promethazine*** lowers the seizure threshold in children, may cause cholestatic jaundice, anticholinergic effects, extrapyramidal effects, and potentially fatal respiratory depression.

▶ ***scopolamine*** **(C)** <12 years: not recommended; ≥12 years:
Scopace 0.4-0.8 mg 1 hour before travel; may repeat in 8 hours
Tab: 0.4 mg
Transderm Scop 1 patch behind ear at least 4 hours before travel; each patch is effective for 3 days; apply a new patch on the 4th day on the opposite side
Transdermal patch: 1.5 mg (4/carton)

MULTIPLE SCLEROSIS (MS)

NICOTINIC ACID RECEPTOR AGONIST

▶ ***dimethyl fumarate*** **(C)** <18 years: not recommended; ≥18 years: initially 120 mg bid x 7 days; then maintenance 240 mg bid

Tecfidera *Cap:* 120, 240 mg del-rel; *Starter Pack:* 14 x 120 mg, 46 x 240 mg

Comment: The mechanism by which ***dimethyl fumarate*** (DMF) exerts its therapeutic effect in multiple sclerosis is unknown. DMF and the metabolite, ***monomethyl fumarate*** (MMF), have been shown to activate the nuclear factor (erythroid-derived 2)-like 2 (Nrf2) pathway in vitro and in vivo in animals and humans. The Nrf2 pathway is involved in the cellular response to oxidative stress. MMF has been identified as a nicotinic acid receptor agonist in vitro.

POTASSIUM CHANNEL BLOCKER

▶ ***dalfampridine*** **(C)(G)** <18 years: not recommended; ≥18 years: 10 mg q 12 hours

Ampyra *Tab:* 10 mg ext-rel

Comment: ***dalfampridine*** is indicated to improve walking speed.

PYRIMIDINE SYNTHESIS INHIBITOR (DMARD)

▶ ***teriflunomide*** **(X)** <18 years: not recommended; ≥18 years: 7 mg or 14 mg once daily

Aubagio *Tab:* 7, 14 mg

Comment: Contraindicated with severe hepatic impairment and females of childbearing potential not using reliable contraception. Co-administer ***teriflunomide*** with the DMARD ***leflunomide*** (**Arava**).

IMMUNOMODULATORS

Comment: The role of immunomodulators in the treatment of MS is to slow the progression of physical disability and to decrease frequency of clinical exacerbations.

▶ ***alemtuzumab*** **(C)** <18 years: not recommended; ≥18 years: administer two treatment courses: *First treatment course:* 12 mg/day x 5 days (total 60 mg); *Second treatment course:* 12 months later, administer 12 mg/day x 3 days (total 36 mg); complete all immunizations 6 weeks prior to the first treatment; premedicate with 1,000 mg methylprednisolone or equivalent immediately prior to the first 3 treatment days in each treatment course

Lemtrada *Vial:* 12 mg/1.2 ml soln for IV infusion, single-use vial

Comment: **Lemtrada** is indicated for the treatment of patients with relapsing forms of MS. Because of its safety profile, the use of **Lemtrada** should generally be reserved for patients who have had an inadequate response to two or more drugs indicated for the treatment of MS. **Lemtrada REMS** is a restricted distribution program, which allows early detection and management of some of the serious risks associated with its use.

▶ ***fingolimod*** **(C)** <18 years: not recommended; ≥18 years: 0.5 mg once daily

Gilenya *Cap:* 0.5 mg

Comment: First-dose monitoring for bradycardia. In the first 2 weeks, first-dose monitoring is recommended after an interruption of 1 day or more. During weeks 3 and 4, first-dose monitoring is recommended after an interruption of more than 7 days.

▶ ***glatiramer acetate*** **(B)(G)** <18 years: not recommended; ≥18 years: 20-40 mg SC daily

Copaxone *Prefilled syringe:* 20, 40 mg/ml (mannitol, preservative-free)

▶ ***interferon beta-1a*** **(C)** <18 years: not recommended; ≥18 years:

Avonex 30 mcg IM weekly; rotate sites; may titrate to reduce flu-like symptoms; may use concurrent analgesics/antipyretics on treatment days; *Titration Schedule:* 7.5 mcg week 1; 15 mcg week 2; 22.5 mcg week 3; 30 mcg week 4 and ongoing

Vial: 30 mcg pwdr for reconstitution (single-dose w. diluent, 4 vials-kit) (albumin [human], preservative-free); *Prefilled syringe:* 30 mcg single-dose (0.5 ml) (4/dose pck)

Rebif, administer SC 3 x/week (at least 48 hours apart and preferably in the late afternoon <u>or</u> evening); increase over 4 weeks to usual dose 22-44 mcg 3 x/week; *Titration Schedule (22 mcg prescribed dose):* 4.4 mcg weeks 1 & 2; 11 mcg weeks 3 & 4; 22 mcg weeks 5 and ongoing; *Titration Schedule (44 mcg prescribed dose):* 8.8 mcg weeks 1 & 2; 22 mcg weeks 3 & 4; 44 mcg weeks 5 and ongoing

Prefilled syringe: 22, 44 mcg/0.5 ml w. needle (12/carton) (albumin [human], preservative-free); (titration pack, 6 doses of 8.8 mcg [0.2 ml] w. needle per carton) (albumin [human], preservative-free)

Comment: Only prefilled syringes (**Rebif**) can be used to titrate to the 22 mcg prescribed dose. Prefilled syringes <u>or</u> autoinjectors (**Rebif Rebidose**) can be used to titrate to the 44 mcg prescribed dose.

Rebif Rebidose administer SC 3 x/week (at least 48 hours apart and preferably in the late afternoon <u>or</u> evening) after titration to 22 mcg <u>or</u> 44 mcg; *Titration Schedule: see* **Rebif**.

Prefilled autoinjector: 22, 44 mcg/0.5 ml (0.5 ml, 12/carton) (titration pack, 6 doses of 8.8 mcg [0.2 ml] per carton) (albumin [human], preservative-free)

Comment: Only prefilled syringes (**Rebif**) can be used to titrate to the 22 mcg prescribed dose. Prefilled syringes <u>or</u> autoinjectors (**Rebif Rebidose**) can be used to titrate to the 44 mcg prescribed dose.

▶ ***interferon beta-1b*** **(C)** <18 years: not recommended; ≥18 years:

Actimmune *BSA ≤0.5 m^2:* 1.5 mcg/kg SC in a single dose 3 times weekly; *BSA ≥0.5 m^2:* 50 mcg/m^2 SC in a single dose 3 times weekly

Vial: 100 mcg/0.5 ml single-dose for SC injection

Betaseron, Extavia 0.0625 mg (0.25 ml) SC every other day; increase over 6 weeks to 0.25 mg (1 ml) SC every other day

Vial: 0.3 mg pwdr for reconstitution (single-dose w. prefilled diluents syringes) (albumin [human], mannitol, preservative-free)

▶ ***natalizumab*** **(C)** a <18 years: not recommended; ≥18 years: administer 300 mg by IV infusion over 1 hour every 4 weeks; monitor during infusion and for 1 hour post-infusion

Tysabri *Vial:* 300 mg/15 ml (15 ml)

CD20-DIRECTED CYTOLYTIC MONOCLONAL ANTIBODY

▶ ***ocrelizumab*** <18 years: not established; ≥18 years: pre-medicate with corticosteroid and antihistamine, and consider antipyretic, prior to each infusion; initially administer 300 mg by IV infusion followed by another 300 mg infusion 2 weeks later; then administer 600 mg every 6 months; see mfr lit for infusion rates and dose modifications

Ocrevus *Vial: 30 mg/ml (10 ml, single-dose) for dilution (preservative-free)*

Comment: The precise mechanism of action is unknown; however, it is thought to involve binding to CD20, a cell surface antigen present on pre-B and mature B lymphocytes which results in antibody-dependent cellular cytolysis and complement-mediated lysis. ***Ocrevus*** is contraindicated with active HBV infection. Screen for HBV infection (HBsAg and anti-HB) prior to initiation. Concomitant live <u>or</u> attenuated vaccine not recommended during treatment and until B-cell repletion. Administer these at least 6 weeks prior to initiation of treatment. Additive immunosuppressive effects with other immunosupressants. Monitor for infusion reaction (pruritis, rash, urticaria, erythema, throat irritation, bronchospasm). Delay treatment with active infection. Withhold at first sign/symptom of progressive multifocal leukoencephalopathy (PMI) or HBV reactivation. Females of reproductive potential should use effective contraception during treatment and for 6 months after the last dose of **Ocrevus**. It is not known whether ***ocrelizumab*** is excreted in human breast milk or has any effect on the breastfed infant.

PSEUDOBULBAR AFFECT (PBA)

Comment: Pseudobulbar affect (PBA), emotional lability, labile affect, or emotional incontinence refers to a neurologic disorder characterized by involuntary crying or uncontrollable episodes of crying and/or laughing, or other emotional outbursts. PBA occurs secondary to a neurologic disease or brain injury such as traumatic brain injury (TBI), stroke, Parkinson's disease, multiple sclerosis, and amyotrophic lateral sclerosis (ALS, or Lou Gehrig disease).

➢ ***dextromethorphan+quinidine*** (C)(G) <12 years: not recommended; >12 years: 1 cap once daily x 7 days; then starting on day 8, 1 cap bid

Nuedexta *Cap:* dextro 20 mg+quini 10 mg

Comment: ***dextromethorphan hydrobromide*** is an uncompetitive NMDA receptor antagonist and sigma-1 agonist. ***quinidine sulfate*** is a CYP450 2D6 inhibitor. **Nuedexta** is contraindicated with an MAOI or within 14 days of stopping an MAOI, with prolonged QT interval, congenital long QT syndrome, history suggestive of torsades de pointes, or heart failure, complete atrioventricular (AV) block without implanted pacemaker or patients at high risk of complete AV block, and concomitant drugs that both prolong QT interval and are metabolized by CYP2D6 (e.g., ***thioridazine*** or ***pimozide***). Discontinue **Nuedexta** if the following occurs: hepatitis or thrombocytopenia or any other hypersensitivity reaction. Monitor ECG in patients with left ventricular hypertrophy (LVH) or left ventricular dysfunction (LVD). ***desipramine*** exposure increases **Nuedexta** 8-fold; reduce ***desipramine*** dose and adjust based on clinical response. Use of **Nuedexta** with selective serotonin reuptake inhibitors (SSRIs) or tricyclic antidepressants (TCAs) increases the risk of serotonin syndrome. ***paroxetine*** exposure increases **Nuedexta** 2-fold; therefore, reduce ***paroxetine*** dose and adjust based on clinical response (***digoxin*** exposure may increase ***digoxin*** substrate plasma concentration. **Nuedexta** is not recommended in pregnancy or breastfeeding. Safety and effectiveness of **Nuedexta** in children have not been established. To report suspected adverse reactions, contact Avanir Pharmaceuticals at 1-866-388-5041 or FDA at 1-800-FDA-1088 or visit www.fda.gov/medwatch

☐ MUMPS (INFECTIOUS PAROTITIS)

see **Childhood Immunizations** *page* 525
Parenteral Corticosteroids *see page* 547
Oral Corticosteroids *see page* 546
Antipyretics *see Fever page* 149

PROPHYLAXIS VACCINE

➢ ***measles, mumps, rubella, live, attenuated, neomycin vaccine*** (C)

MMR II 25 mcg SC (preservative-free)

Comment: Contraindications: hypersensitivity to ***neomycin*** or eggs, primary or acquired immune deficiency, immunosuppressant therapy, bone marrow or lymphatic malignancy, and pregnancy (within 3 months after vaccination).

MUSCLE STRAIN

Acetaminophen for IV Infusion *see* ***Pain*** *page* 322
Narcotic Analgesics *see* ***Pain*** *page* 335
Parenteral Corticosteroids *see page* 547
Oral Corticosteroids *see page* 546

Comment: Usual length of treatment for acute injury is approximately 5 days.

SKELETAL MUSCLE RELAXANTS

▶ ***baclofen*** (C)(G) <12 years: not recommended; ≥12 years: 5 mg tid; titrate up by 5 mg every 3 days to 20 mg tid; max 80 mg/day
Lioresal *Tab:* 10*, 20*mg
Comment: ***baclofen*** is indicated for muscle spasm pain and chronic spasticity associated with multiple sclerosis and spinal cord injury or disease. Potential for seizures or hallucinations on abrupt withdrawal.

▶ ***carisoprodol*** (C)(G) <12 years: not recommended; ≥12 years: 1 tab tid or qid
Soma *Tab:* 350 mg

▶ ***chlorzoxazone*** (G) <12 years: not recommended; ≥12 years: 1 caplet qid; max 750 mg qid
Parafon Forte DSC *Cplt:* 500*mg

▶ ***cyclobenzaprine*** (B)(G) <15 years: not recommended; ≥15 years: 10 mg tid; usual range 20-40 mg/day in divided doses; max 60 mg/day x 2-3 weeks or 15 mg ext-rel once daily; max 30 mg ext-rel/day x 2-3 weeks
Amrix *Cap:* 15, 30 mg ext-rel
Fexmid *Tab:* 7.5 mg
Flexeril *Tab:* 5, 10 mg

▶ ***dantrolene*** (C) <12 years: 0.5 mg/kg daily x 7 days; then 0.5 mg/kg tid x 7 days; then 1 mg/kg tid x 7 days; then 2 mg/kg tid; max 100 mg qid; ≥12 years: 25 md daily x 7 days; then 25 mg tid x 7 days; then 50 mg tid x 7 days; max 100 mg qid
Dantrium *Tab:* 25, 50, 100 mg
Comment: ***dantrolene*** is indicated for chronic spasticity associated with multiple sclerosis and spinal cord injury or disease.

▶ ***diazepam*** (C)(IV) <6 months: not recommended; >6 months-12 years: initially 1-2.5 mg bid-qid; may increase gradually; ≥12 years: 2-10 mg bid-qid; may increase gradually
Diastat *Rectal gel delivery system:* 2.5 mg
Diastat AcuDial *Rectal gel delivery system:* 10, 20 mg
Valium *Tab:* 2, 5, 10 mg
Valium Intensol Oral Solution *Conc oral soln:* 5 mg/ml (30 ml w. dropper) (alcohol 19%)
Valium Oral Solution *Oral soln:* 5 mg/5 ml (500 ml) (wintergreen spice)

▶ ***metaxalone*** (B) <12 years: not recommended; ≥12 years: 1 tab tid-qid
Skelaxin *Tab:* 800*mg

▶ ***methocarbamol*** (C)(G) <16 years: not recommended; ≥16 years: initially 1.5 gm qid x 2-3 days; maintenance, 750 mg every 4 hours or 1.5 gm 3 x/day; max 8 gm/day
Robaxin *Tab:* 500 mg
Robaxin 750 *Tab:* 750 mg

Robaxin Injection 10 ml IM or IV; max 30 ml/day; max 3 days; max 5 ml/gluteal injection q 8 hours; max IV rate 3 ml/min
Vial: 100 mg/ml (10 ml)

▶ ***nabumetone*** (C) <12 years: not recommended; ≥12 years: initially 1,000 mg as a single dose; titrate as needed; may split dose bid; max 2,000 mg/day
Relafen *Tab:* 500, 750 mg
Relafen 500 *Tab:* 500 mg

▶ ***orphenadrine citrate*** (C)(G) <12 years: not recommended; ≥12 years: 1 tab bid
Norflex *Tab:* 100 mg sust-rel

▶ ***tizanidine*** (C) <12 years: not recommended; ≥12 years: 1-4 mg q 6-8 hours; max 36 mg/day
Zanaflex *Tab:* 2*, 4**mg; *Cap:* 2, 4, 6 mg

SKELETAL MUSCLE RELAXANT+NSAID COMBINATIONS

Comment: ***aspirin***-containing medications are contraindicated with history of allergic type reaction to ***aspirin***, children and adolescents with *Varicella* or other viral illness, and 3rd trimester of pregnancy.

▶ ***carisoprodol+aspirin*** (C)(III)(G) <12 years: not recommended; ≥12 years: 1-2 tabs qid
Soma Compound *Tab:* caris 200 mg+asp 325 mg (sulfites)

▶ ***meprobamate+aspirin*** (D)(IV) <12 years: not recommended; ≥12 years: 1-2 tabs tid or qid
Equagesic *Tab:* mepro 200 mg+asp 325mg*
Comment: ***aspirin***-containing medications are contraindicated with history of allergic-type reaction to ***aspirin***, children and adolescents with *Varicella* or other viral illness, and 3rd trimester of pregnancy.

SKELETAL MUSCLE RELAXANT+NSAID+CAFFEINE COMBINATIONS

▶ ***orphenadrine+aspirin+caffeine*** (D)(G) <12 years: not recommended; ≥12 years:
Norgesic 1-2 tabs tid-qid
Tab: orphen 25 mg+asp 385 mg+caf 30 mg*
Norgesic Forte 1 tab tid or qid; max 4 tabs/day
Tab: orphen 50 mg+asp 770 mg+caf 60 mg*

Comment: ***aspirin***-containing medications are contraindicated with history of allergic-type reaction to ***aspirin***, children and adolescents with *Varicella* or other viral illness, and 3rd trimester of pregnancy.

SKELETAL MUSCLE RELAXANT+NSAID+CODEINE COMBINATIONS

▶ ***carisoprodol+aspirin+codeine*** (D)(III)(G) <12 years: contraindicated; 12-<18: use extreme caution; not recommended for children and adolescents with obesity, asthma, obstructive sleep apnea, or other chronic breathing problem, or for post-tonsillectomy/adenoidectomy pain; ≥18 years: 1-2 tabs qid prn
Soma Compound w. Codeine
Tab: caris 200 mg+asp 325 mg+cod 16 mg (sulfites)
Comment: ***Codeine*** is known to be excreted in breast milk. <12 years: not recommended; 12-<18: use extreme caution; not recommended for children and adolescents with asthma or other chronic breathing problem. The FDA and the European Medicines Agency (EMA) are investigating the safety of using ***codeine*** containing medications to treat pain, cough and colds, in children 12-<18 years because of the potential for serious side effects, including slowed or difficult breathing. ***aspirin***-containing medications are contraindicated with history of allergic-type reaction to ***aspirin***, children and adolescents with *Varicella* or other viral illness, and 3rd trimester of pregnancy.

TOPICAL & TRANSDERMAL NSAIDs

▶ *capsaicin* cream **(B)(G)** <2 years: not recommended; 2-12 years: apply sparingly to intact skin bid prn; >12 years: apply tid-qid prn

Axsain *Crm:* 0.075% (1, 2 oz)
Capsin (OTC) *Lotn:* 0.025, 0,075% (59 ml)
Capzasin-P (OTC) *Crm:* 0.025% (1.5 oz); *Lotn:* 0.025% (2 oz)
Capzasin-HP (OTC) *Crm:* 0.075% (1.5 oz); *Lotn:* 0.075% (2 oz)
Dolorac *Crm:* 0.025% (28 gm)
Double Cap (OTC) *Crm:* 0.05% (2 oz)
R-Gel *Gel:* 0.025% (15, 30 gm)
Zostrix (OTC) *Crm:* 0.025% (0.7, 1.5, 3 oz)
Zostrix HP (OTC) *Emol crm:* 0.075% (1, 2 oz)

Comment: Provides some relief by 1-2 weeks; optimal benefit may take 4-6 weeks. Avoid contact with mucous membranes.

▶ *capsaicin* 8% patch **(B)** <18 years: not recommended; ≥18 years: apply up to 4 patches for one 60-minute application to clean dry skin; may prep area with topical anesthetic; wear non-latex gloves; patches may be cut to size/shape; treatment may be repeated every 3 months; remove with cleansing gel after treatment

Qutenza *Patch:* 8% 1640 mcg/cm (179 mg; 1 or 2 patches, each w. 1-50 gm tube cleansing gel/carton)

▶ *diclofenac epolamine transdermal patch* **(C; D ≥30 wks)** <12 years: not recommended; ≥12 years: apply one patch to affected area bid; remove during bathing; avoid non-intact skin

Flector Patch *Patch:* 180 mg/patch (30/carton)

ORAL NSAIDs

For an expanded list of NSAIDs *see page* 539

▶ *diclofenac* **(C)** <18 years: not recommended; ≥18 years: take on empty stomach; 35 mg tid; *Hepatic impairment:* use lowest dose

Zorvolex *Gelcap: 18, 35 mg*

▶ *diclofenac sodium* **(C)** <18 years: not recommended; ≥18 years:

Voltaren 50 mg bid-qid or 75 mg bid or 25 mg qid with an additional 25 mg at HS if necessary

Tab: 25, 50, 75 mg ent-coat

Voltaren XR 100 mg once daily; rarely, 100 mg bid may be used

Tab: 100 mg ext-rel

ORAL NSAIDs+PPI COMBINATIONS

▶ *esomeprazole/naproxen* **(C; not for use in 3rd)(G)** <18 years: not recommended; ≥18 years: 1 tab bid; use lowest effective dose for the shortest duration; swallow whole; take at least 30 minutes before a meal

Vimovo *Tab:* nap 375 mg+eso 20 mg ext-rel; nap 500 mg+eso 20 mg ext-rel

Comment: **Vimovo** is indicated to improve signs/symptoms, and risk of gastric ulcer in patients at risk of developing NSAID-associated gastric ulcer.

COX-2 INHIBITORS

Comment: Cox-2 inhibitors are contraindicated with history of asthma, urticaria, and allergic-type reactions to ***aspirin***, other NSAIDs, and sulfonamides, 3rd trimester of pregnancy, and coronary artery bypass graft (CABG) surgery.

▶ *celecoxib* **(C)(G)** <18 years: not recommended; ≥18 years: 100-400 mg bid; max 800 mg/day

Celebrex *Cap:* 50, 100, 200, 400 mg

▶ ***meloxicam*** (C)(G)

Mobic <2 years, <60 kg: not recommended; ≥2, >60 kg: 0.125 mg/kg; max 7.5 mg once daily; ≥18 years: initially 7.5 mg once daily; max 15 mg once daily; *Hemodialysis:* max 7.5 mg/day

Tab: 7.5, 15 mg; *Oral susp:* 7.5 mg/5 ml (100 ml) (raspberry)

Vivlodex <18 years: not established; ≥18 years: initially 5 mg qd; may increase to max 10 mg/day; *Hemodialysis:* max 5 mg/day

Cap: 5, 10 mg

TOPICAL & TRANSDERMAL NSAIDs

▶ ***capsaicin*** cream (B)(G) <2 years: not recommended; 2-12 years: apply sparingly to intact skin bid prn; >12 years: apply tid-qid prn

Axsain *Crm:* 0.075% (1, 2 oz)
Capsin (OTC) *Lotn:* 0.025, 0,075% (59 ml)
Capzasin-P (OTC) *Crm:* 0.025% (1.5 oz); *Lotn:* 0.025% (2 oz)
Capzasin-HP (OTC) *Crm:* 0.075% (1.5 oz); *Lotn:* 0.075% (2 oz)
Dolorac *Crm:* 0.025% (28 gm)
Double Cap (OTC) *Crm:* 0.05% (2 oz)
R-Gel *Gel:* 0.025% (15, 30 gm)
Zostrix (OTC) *Crm:* 0.025% (0.7, 1.5, 3 oz)
Zostrix HP (OTC) *Emol crm:* 0.075% (1, 2 oz)

Comment: Provides some relief by 1-2 weeks; optimal benefit may take 4-6 weeks. Avoid contact with mucous membranes.

▶ ***capsaicin*** 8% patch **(B)** <18 years: not recommended; ≥18 years: apply sparingly to intact skin tid-qid prn; apply up to 4 patches for one 60-minute application to clean dry skin; may prep area with topical anesthetic; wear non-latex gloves; patches may be cut to size/shape; treatment may be repeated every 3 months; remove with cleansing gel after treatment

Qutenza *Patch:* 8% 1640 mcg/cm (179 mg; 1 or 2 patches, each w. 1-50 gm tube cleansing gel/carton)

▶ ***diclofenac epolamine transdermal patch*** **(C; D ≥30 wks)** <12 years: not recommended; ≥12 years: apply sparingly tid-qid prn apply one patch to affected area bid; remove during bathing; avoid non-intact skin

Flector Patch *Patch:* 180 mg/patch (30/carton)

▶ ***diclofenac sodium*** **(C; D ≥30 wks)(G)** <18 years: not established; ≥18 years:

Pennsaid 1.5% in 10 drop increments, dispense and rub into front, side, and back of knee: usually; 40 drops (40 mg) qid

Topical soln: 1.5% (150 ml)

Pennsaid 2% apply 2 pump actuations (40 mg) and rub into front, side, and back of knee bid

Topical soln: 2% (20 mg/pump actuation, 112 gm)

Comment: **Pennsaid** <12 years: not recommended; ≥12 years: indicated for the treatment of pain associated with osteoarthritis of the knee

Solaraze Gel *Gel:* 3% (50 gm) (benzyl alcohol)

Comment: Contraindicated with ***aspirin*** allergy. As with other NSAIDs, **Solaraze Gel** should be avoided in late pregnancy (≥30 weeks) because it may cause premature closure of the ductus arteriosus.

Voltaren Gel apply qid; avoid non-intact skin

Gel: 1% (100 gm)

Comment: ***diclofenac*** is contraindicated with ***aspirin*** allergy. As with other NSAIDs, **Voltaren Gel** should be avoided in late pregnancy (≥30 weeks) because it may cause premature closure of the ductus arteriosus.

TOPICAL & TRANSDERMAL LIDOCAINE

▶ ***lidocaine*** transdermal patch **(C)(G)** <12 years: not recommended; ≥12 years: apply one patch to affected area for 12 hours (then off for 12 hours); remove during bathing; avoid non-intact skin

Lidoderm *Patch:* 5% (10 cm x 14 cm; 30/carton)

NARCOLEPSY

STIMULANTS

▶ ***amphetamine sulfate*** **(C)(II)**

Evekeo <6 years: not recommended; 6-12 years: initially 5 mg once or twice daily at the same time(s) each day; may increase by 5 mg/day at weekly intervals; max 40 mg/day; >12-18 years: initially 10 mg once or twice daily at the same time(s) each day; may increase by 10 mg/day at weekly intervals; max 40 mg/day; >18 years: administer first dose on awakening, and additional doses at 4- to 6-hour intervals; usual range 5-60 mg/day

Tab: 5, 10 mg

▶ ***armodafinil*** **(C)(IV)(G)** <17 years: not recommended; ≥17 years: *OSAHS:* 50-250 mg once daily in the AM; *SWSD:* 150 mg 1 hour before starting shift; reduce dose with severe hepatic impairment

Nuvigil *Tab:* 50, 150, 200, 250 mg

▶ ***dextroamphetamine sulfate*** **(C)(II)(G)** <3 years: not recommended; 3-5 years: 2.5 mg daily; may increase by 2.5 mg daily at weekly intervals if needed; 6-12 years: initially 5 mg daily-bid; may increase by 5 mg/day at weekly intervals; usual max 40 mg/day; >12 years: initially 10 mg daily; may increase by mg/day at weekly intervals; max 40 mg/day; initially start with 10 mg daily; increase by 10 mg at weekly intervals if needed; may switch to daily dose with sust-rel spansules when titrated

Dexedrine *Tab:* 5*mg (tartrazine)

Dexedrine Spansule *Cap:* 5, 10, 15 mg sust-rel

Dextrostat *Tab:* 5, 10 mg (tartrazine)

▶ ***dextroamphetamine saccharate+dextroamphetamine sulfate+amphetamine aspartate+amphetamine sulfate*** **(C)(II)(G)**

Adderall <6 years: not indicated; 6-12 years: initially 5 mg daily; may increase weekly by 5 mg/day; usual max 40 mg/day in 2-3 divided doses; >12 years: initially 10 mg daily; may increase weekly by 10 mg/day; usual max 60 mg/day in 2-3 divided doses; first dose on awakening and then q 4-6 hours prn

Tab: 5**, 7.5**, 10**, 12.5**, 15**, 20**, 30**mg

Adderall XR <6 years: not recommended; 6-12 years: initially 10 mg daily in the AM; may increase by 10 mg weekly; max 30 mg/day; >12 years: initially 10 mg daily; may increase to 20 mg/day after 1 week; max 30 mg/day; do not chew; may sprinkle on applesauce

Cap: 5, 10, 15, 20, 25, 30 mg ext-rel

Comment: **Adderall** is also indicated to improve wakefulness in patients with SWSD and OSAHS.

▶ ***dexmethylphenidate*** **(C)(II)(G)** <6 years: not recommended; ≥6 years:

Focalin initially 2.5 mg bid; allow at least 4 hours between doses; may increase at 1 week intervals; max 40 mg/day

Tab: 2.5, 5, 10*mg (dye-free)

Focalin XR 20-40 mg q AM; max 40 mg/day

Tab: 5, 10, 15, 20, 30, 40 mg ext-rel (dye-free)

▶ *methamphetamine* (C)(II)(G)

Desoxyn Gradumet <6 years: not recommended; ≥6 years: initially 5 mg daily bid; may increase by 5 mg/day at weekly intervals; usual effective dose; 20-25 mg/day

Tab: 5, 10, 15 mg sust-rel

▶ ***methylphenidate (regular-acting)*** (C)(II)(G)

Methylin, Methylin Chewable, Methylin Oral Solution <6 years: not recommended; ≥6 years-12 years: initially 5 mg twice daily before breakfast and lunch; may increase 5-10 mg/week; max 60 mg/day; >12 years: usual dose 20-30 mg/day in 2-3 divided doses 30-45 minutes before a meal; may increase to 60 mg/day

Tab: 5, 10*, 20*mg; *Chew tab:* 2.5, 5, 10 mg (grape) (phenylalanine); *Oral soln:* 5, 10 mg/5 ml) (grape)

Ritalin <6 years: not recommended; ≥6-12 years: years: initially 5 mg bid ac (before breakfast and lunch); may gradually increase by 5-10 mg at weekly intervals as needed; max 60 mg/day; >12 years: 10-60 mg/day in 2-3 divided doses 30-45 minutes ac; max 60 mg/day

Tab: 5, 10*, 20*mg

▶ ***methylphenidate (long-acting)*** (C)(II)

Concerta <6 years: not recommended; ≥6 years: initially 18 mg q AM; may increase in 18 mg increments as needed; max 54 mg/day; do not crush or chew

Tab: 18, 27, 36, 54 mg sust-rel

Metadate CD (G) <6 years: not recommended; 6-12 years: initially 20 mg daily; may gradually increase by 20 mg/day at weekly intervals as needed; max 60 mg/day; >12 years: 1 cap daily in the AM; may sprinkle on food; do not crush or chew

Cap: 10, 20, 30, 40, 50, 60 mg immed- and ext-rel beads

Metadate ER <6 years: not recommended; ≥6 years-12 years: use in place of regular-acting ***methylphenidate*** when the 8-hour dose of **Metadate-ER** corresponds to the titrated 8-hour dose of regular-acting ***methylphenidate***: >12 years: 1 tab daily in the AM; do not crush or chew

Tab: 10, 20 mg ext-rel (dye-free)

Ritalin LA <6 years: not recommended; ≥6 years: use in place of regular-acting ***methylphenidate*** when the 8-hour dose of **Ritalin LA** corresponds to the titrated 8-hour dose of regular-acting ***methylphenidate***; 1 cap daily in the AM; max 60 mg/day

Cap: 10, 20, 30, 40 mg ext-rel (immed- and ext-rel beads)

Ritalin SR <6 years: not recommended; ≥6 years: use in place of regular-acting ***methylphenidate*** when the 8-hour dose of **Ritalin SR** corresponds to the titrated 8-hour dose of regular-acting ***methylphenidate***; max 60 mg/day

Tab: 20 mg sust-rel (dye-free)

▶ ***methylphenidate (transdermal patch)*** (C)(II)(G) <6 years: not recommended; ≥6 years: initially 10 mg patch daily in the AM; may increase by 5-10 mg/week; max 60 mg/day

Transdermal patch: 10, 15, 20, 30 mg

▶ ***modafinil*** (C)(IV)(G) <17 years: not recommended; ≥17 years: 100-200 mg q AM; max 400 mg/day

Provigil *Tab:* 100, 200*mg

Comment: **Provigil** also promotes wakefulness in patients with SWSD and excessive sleepiness due to OSAHS.

▶ ***pemoline*** (B)(IV) <6 years: not recommended; ≥6 years: 18.75-112.5 mg/day; usually start with 37.5 mg in AM; increase weekly by 18.75 mg/day if needed; max 112.5 gm/day

Cylert *Tab:* 18.75*, 37.5*, 75*mg

Cylert Chewable *Chew tab:* 37.5*mg

Comment: Monitor baseline serum ALT and repeat every 2 weeks thereafter.

- ➢ ***sodium oxybate*** **(B)(G)** <16 years: not recommended; ≥16 years: take dose at bedtime while in bed and repeat 2.5-4 hours later; titrate to effect; initially 4.5 gm/night in 2 divided doses; may increase by 1.5 gm/night in 2 divided doses; max 9 gm/night

    Xyrem *Oral soln:* 100, 200*mg

    Comment: **Xyrem** is used to reduce the number of cataplexy attacks (sudden loss of muscle strength) and reduce daytime sleepiness in patients with narcolepsy. Contraindicated with ***alcohol*** or CNS depressant (may impair consciousness; may lead to respiratory depression, coma, or death). Prepare both doses prior to bedtime and do not attempt to get out of bed after taking the first dose. Place both doses within reach at the bedside. Set the bedside clock to awaken for the second dose. Dilute each dose in 60 ml (1/4 cup, 4 tbsp) water in child resistant dosing containers. Food significantly reduces the bioavailability of ***sodium oxybate***; take at least 2 hours after ingesting food.

NAUSEA/VOMITING (POST-ANESTHESIA)

RX ANTIEMETICS

- ➢ ***ondansetron*** **(C)(G)** <4 years: not recommended; 4-11 years, moderately emetogenic chemotherapy: 4 mg q 4 hours x 3 doses beginning 30 min prior to start; then 4 mg q 8 hours x 1-2 days following; >11 years: use oral forms: *Highly emetogenic chemotherapy:* 24 mg x 1 dose 30 min prior to start of single-day chemotherapy; *Moderately emetogenic chemotherapy:* 8 mg q 8 hours x 2 doses beginning 30 minutes prior to start of chemotherapy; then 8 mg q 12 hours x 1-2 days following

    Zofran *Tab:* 4, 8, 24 mg

    Zofran ODT *ODT:* 4, 8 mg (strawberry) (phenylalanine)

    Zofran Oral Solution *Oral soln:* 4 mg/5 ml (50 ml) (strawberry) (phenylalanine); *Parenteral form:* see mfr pkg insert

    Zofran Injection *Vial:* 2 mg/ml (2 ml single-dose); 2 mg/ml (20 ml multi-dose); 32 mg/50 ml (50 ml multi-dose); *Prefilled syringe:* 4 mg/2 ml, single-use (24/carton)

    Zuplenz Oral Soluble Film: 4, 8 mg oral-dis (10/carton) (peppermint)

- ➢ ***palonosetron*** **(B)(G)** <1 month: not recommended; 1 month-17 years: 20 mcg/kg; max 1.5 mg single-dose; infuse over 15 minutes beginning 30 minutes prior to administration of chemo; >17 years: *Chemotherapy:* administer 0.25 mg IV over 30 seconds, 30 min prior to administration of chemo; max 1 dose/week or 1 cap 1 hour before chemo; *Post-op:* administer 0.075 mg IV over 10 seconds immediately before induction of anesthesia

    Vial (single-use): 0.075 mg/1.5 ml; 0.25 mg/5 ml (mannitol)

- ➢ ***promethazine*** **(C)** <2 years: not recommended; 2-12 years: 0.5 mg/lb or 6.25-25 mg q 4-6 hours PO or rectally; >12 years: 12.5-25 q 4-6 hours PO or rectally

    Phenergan *Tab:* 12.5*, 25*, 50 mg; *Plain syr:* 6.25 mg/5 ml; *Fortis syr:* 25 mg/5 ml; *Rectal supp:* 12.5, 25, 50 mg

  Comment: ***promethazine*** is contraindicated in children with uncomplicated nausea, dehydration, Reye's syndrome, history of sleep apnea, asthma, and lower respiratory disorders in children. ***Promethazine*** lowers the seizure threshold in children, may cause cholestatic jaundice, anticholinergic effects, extrapyramidal effects, and potentially fatal respiratory depression.

NERVE AGENT POISONING

- ➢ ***atropine sulfate*** **(G)** <15 lb: not recommended; ≥15-40 lb: 0.5 mg IM; ≥40-90 lb: 1 mg IM; >90 lb: 2 mg IM

    AtroPen *Pen (single use):* 0.5, 1, 2 mg (0.5 ml)

NEUTROPENIA: MYELOSUPPRESSION-ASSOCIATED

LEUKOCYTE GROWTH FACTORS

▶ ***pegfilgrastim*** <45 kg: see mfr pkg insert for weight-based dosing Table 1; ≥45 kg: *Patients with Cancer receiving Myelosuppressive Chemotherapy:* 6 mg SC once per chemotherapy cycle; do not administer between 14 days before and 24 hours after administration of cytotoxic chemotherapy; *Patients Acutely Exposed to Myelosuppressive Doses of Radiation.* <45 kg: see mfr pkg insert for weight-based dosing table 1; >45 kg: 6 mg SC x 2 doses one week apart; administer the first dose as soon as possible after suspected or confirmed exposure to myelosuppressive doses of radiation

Neulastin *Prefilled syringe:* 6 mg/0.6 ml, single-dose, for manual use only; 6 mg/0.6 ml, single-dose, co-packaged with the on-body **Neulesta** Auto-injector

Comment: ***pegfilgrastim*** is a leukocyte growth factor, to help reduce the risk/incidence of infection, as manifested by febrile neutropenia, in patients with non-myeloid malignancies receiving myelosuppressive anti-cancer drugs and to increase survival in patients acutely exposed to myelosuppressive doses of radiation (i.e., Hematopoietic Subsyndrome of Acute Radiation Syndrome). Neulasta is not indicated for the mobilization of peripheral blood progenytor cells for hematopoietic stem cell transplantation. Warnings and precautions associated with **Neulasta** include fatal splenic rupture, acute respiratory distress syndrome (ARDS), serious allergic reaction/anaphylaxis, allergic reaction to acrylic adhesive (used to attach the autoinjector), fatal sickle cell crisis; glomerulonephritis, on-body injector failure. There are no adequate or well-controlled studies of **Neulasta** use in pregnancy. Based on animal data, may cause fetal harm. It is not known whether ***pegfilgrastim*** is secreted in human milk. Other recombinant G-CSF products are poorly secreted in breast milk and G-CSF is not orally absorbed by neonates. Caution should be exercised when administered to a nursing female. To report suspected adverse reactions, contact Amgen at 1-800-77-AMGEN (1-800-772-6436) or FDA at 1-800-FDA-1088 or visit www.fda.gov/medwatch

▶ ***pegfilgrastim-jmdb***

Fulphila *Prefilled syringe:* 6 mg/0.6 ml, single-dose, for manual use only

Comment: **Fulphila (*pegfilgrastim-imdb*)** is the first biosimilar to **Neulastin (*pegfilgrastim*). Fulphila** was approved under the FDA category for biosimilars and demonstrated no clinically meaningful differences for use, dosing regimens, strengths, dosage forms, and routes of administration from the FDA-approved biological product **Neulasta**. See ***pegfilgastrim (Neulasta)*** above for full prescribing information. To report suspected adverse reactions, contact Mylan at 1-877-446-3679 (1-877-4-INFO-RX) or FDA at 1-800-FDA-1088 or visit www.fda.gov/medwatch

NON-24 SLEEP-WAKE DISORDER

Comment: For other drug options (stimulants, sedative hypnotics), *see* **Insomnia** *page* 255 or **Sleepiness: Excessive, Shift Work Sleep Disorder** *page* 431

MELATONIN RECEPTOR AGONIST

▶ ***tasimelteon*** (C) <12 years: not established; ≥12 years: 1 gel cap before bedtime at the same time every night; do not take with food

Hetlioz *Gel cap:* 20 mg

OREXIN RECEPTOR ANTAGONIST

▶ ***suvorexant*** (C)(IV) <12 years: not established; ≥12 years: use lowest effective dose; take 30 minutes before bedtime; do not take if unable to sleep for ≥7 hours; max 20 mg

Belsomra *Tab:* 5, 10, 15, 20 mg (30/blister pck)

OBESITY

Comment: Target BMI is 25-30 (≤27 preferred). Approximately 17% of children and adolescents in the US aged 2 to 19 years are obese. Almost 32% of children and adolescents are either overweight or obese, and the proportion of children with severe obesity continues to rise. Obesity in childhood increases the risk of having obesity as an adult and children with obesity are about 5 times more likely to have obesity as adults than children without obesity. The immediate consequences of childhood obesity include increased incidence of psychological issues, asthma, obstructive sleep apnea, orthopedic problems, high blood pressure, elevated lipid levels, and insulin resistance. The US Preventive Services Task Force (USPSTF) recommends that clinicians screen for obesity in children and adolescents 6 years and older and offer or refer them to comprehensive, intensive behavioral interventions (at least 26 hours of contact) to promote improvements in weight status.

REFERENCE

US Preventive Services Task Force. (2017). Screening for obesity in children and adolescents. US preventive services task force recommendation statement. *Journal of the American Medical Association, 317*(23),2417–2426. doi:10.1001/jama.2017.6803

STIMULANTS

▶ ***amphetamine sulfate*** (C)(II) <12 years: not recommended; ≥12 years: initially 5 mg 30-60 minutes before meals; usually up to 30 mg/day

Evekeo *Tab:* 5, 10 mg

LIPASE INHIBITOR

▶ ***orlistat*** (X)(G) <12 years: not recommended; ≥12 years: 1 cap tid 1 hour before or during each main meal containing fat

Alli (OTC) *Cap:* 60 mg

Xenical *Cap:* 120 mg

Comment: For use when BMI >30 kg/m² or BMI >27 kg/m² in the presence of other risk factors (i.e., HTN, DM, dyslipidemia).

ANOREXIGENICS

Sympathomimetics

Comment: ASEs of sympathomimetics include hypertension, tachycardia, restlessness, insomnia, and dry mouth.

▶ ***benzphetamine*** (X)(III) <12 years: not recommended; ≥12 years: initially 25-50 mg daily in the mid-morning or mid-afternoon; may increase to bid-tid as needed

Didrex *Tab:* 50*mg

▶ ***naltrexone+bupropion*** (X)(G) <18 years: not recommended; ≥18 years: swallow whole; avoid high-fat meals; initially 10 mg bid; evaluate weight loss after 12 weeks; discontinue if less than 5% weight loss

Contrave *Tab:* nal 8 mg+bup 900 mg ext-rel

▶ ***methamphetamine*** (C)(II) <12 years: not recommended; ≥12 years: 10-15 mg q AM
Desoxyn *Tab:* 5, 10, 15 mg sust-rel

▶ ***phendimetrazine*** (C)(III)
Bontril PDM <12 years: not recommended; ≥12 years: 35 mg bid-tid 1 hour ac; may reduce to 17.5 mg (1/2 tab/dose); max 210 mg/day in 3 divided doses
Bontril Slow-Release <12 years: not recommended; ≥12 years: 105 mg in the AM 30-60 minutes before breakfast
Cap: 105 mg slow-rel

▶ ***phentermine*** (X)(IV)(G) <16 years: not recommended; ≥16 years:
Adipex-P 1 cap or tab before breakfast or 1/2 tab bid ac
Cap: 37.5 mg; *Tab:* 37.5*mg
Fastin 1 cap before breakfast
Cap: 30 mg
Ionamin cap before breakfast or 10-14 hours prior to HS
Cap: 15, 30 mg
Suprenza ODT dissolve 1 tab on top of tongue once daily in the morning, with or without food; use lowest effective dose
Tab: 15, 30, 37.5 mg orally-disint

Comment: ***phentermine*** is contraindicated with history of cardiovascular disease (e.g., coronary artery disease, stroke, arrhythmias, congestive heart failure, uncontrolled hypertension, during or within 14 days following the administration of an MAOI, hyperthyroidism, glaucoma, agitated states, history of drug abuse, pregnancy, nursing).

Sympathomimetic+Antiepileptic Combination

▶ ***phentermine+topiramate ext-rel*** (X)(IV)(G) <16 years: not established; ≥16 years: initially 3.75 mg/23 mg daily in the AM x 14 days; then, increase to 7.5 mg/46 mg and evaluate weight loss on this dose after 12 weeks; if ≤3% weight loss from baseline, discontinue or increase dose to 11.25 mg/69 mg x 14 days; then, increase to 15 mg/92 mg and evaluate weight loss on this dose after 12 weeks; if ≤5% weight loss from baseline, discontinue by taking a dose every other day for at least one week prior to stopping; max 7.5 mg/46 mg for moderate to severe renal impairment or moderate hepatic impairment.
Qsymia
Cap: **Qsymia 3.75/23** phen 3.75 mg+topir 23 mg ext-rel
Qsymia 7.5/46 phen 7.5 mg+topir 46 mg ext-rel
Qsymia 11.25/69 phen 11.25 mg+topir 69 mg ext-rel
Qsymia 15/92 phen 15 mg+topir 92 mg ext-rel

Comment: Side effects include hypertension, tachycardia, restlessness, insomnia, and dry mouth. Contraindicated with glaucoma, hyperthyroidism, and within 14 days of taking an MAOI. **Qsymia 3.75/23** and **Qsymia 11.25/69** are for titration purposes only.

Serotonin 2C Receptor Agonist

▶ ***lorcaserin*** (X)(G) <18 years: not recommended; ≥18 years: 10 mg bid; discontinue if 5% weight loss is not achieved by week 12
Belviq *Tab:* 10 mg film-coat

Comment: **Belviq** is indicated as an adjunct to a reduced-calorie diet and increased physical activity for chronic weight management in patients ≥18 years with an initial body mass index (BMI) of 30 kg/m^2 or greater (obese) or 27 kg/m^2 or greater (overweight) in the presence of at least one weight-related comorbid condition (e.g., hypertension, dyslipidemia, type 2 diabetes). Serotonin 2C receptor agonists interact with serotonergic drugs (selective serotonin reuptake inhibitors [SSRIs], serotonin-norepinephrine reuptake inhibitors [SNRIs], monoamine oxidase inhibitors [MAOIs], triptans, ***bupropion***, ***dextromethorphan***, ***St. John's wort***); therefore, use with extreme caution due to the risk of *serotonin syndrome*.

GLUCAGON-LIKE PEPTIDE-1 (GLP-1) RECEPTOR AGONIST

▶ ***liraglutide*** (C) <18 years: not recommended; ≥18 years: administer SC in the upper arm, abdomen, or thigh once daily; escalate dose gradually over 5 weeks to 3 mg SC daily; *Week 1:* 0.6 mg SC daily; *Week 2:* 1.2 mg SC daily; *Week 3:* 1.8 mg SC daily; *Week 4:* 2.4 mg SC daily; *Week 5:* 3 mg SC daily

Saxenda Soln for SC inj: 6 mg/ml multi-dose prefilled pen (3 ml; 3, 5 pens/carton)

Comment: **Saxenda** is indicated as an adjunct to a reduced-calorie diet and increased physical activity for chronic weight management in patients ≥18 years with an initial body mass index (BMI) of 30 kg/m^2 or greater (obese) or 27 kg/m^2 or greater overweight) in the presence of at least one weight-related comorbid condition (e.g., hypertension, dyslipidemia, type 2 diabetes). Not indicated for treatment of T2DM. Do not use with **Victoza**, other GLP-1 receptor agonists, or ***insulin***. Contraindicated with personal or family history of medullary thyroid carcinoma (MTC) and multiple endocrine neoplasia syndrome (MENS) type 2. Monitor for signs/symptoms pancreatitis. Discontinue if gastroparesis, renal, or hepatic impairment.

OBSESSIVE-COMPULSIVE DISORDER (OCD)

SELECTIVE SEROTONIN REUPTAKE INHIBITORS (SSRIs)

Comment: Co-administration of SSRIs with TCAs requires extreme caution. Concomitant use of MAOIs and SSRIs is absolutely contraindicated. Avoid other serotonergic drugs. A potentially fatal adverse event is *serotonin syndrome*, caused by serotonin excess. Milder symptoms require HCP intervention to avert severe symptoms that can be rapidly fatal without urgent/emergent medical care. Symptoms include restlessness, agitation, confusion, hallucinations, tachycardia, hypertension, dilated pupils, muscle twitching, muscle rigidity, loss of muscle coordination, diaphoresis, diarrhea, headache, shivering, piloerection, hyperpyrexia, cardiac arrhythmias, seizures, loss of consciousness, coma, death. Abrupt withdrawal or interruption of treatment with an antidepressant medication is sometimes associated with an *antidepressant discontinuation syndrome*, which may be mediated by gradually tapering the drug over a period of two weeks or longer, depending on the dose strength and length of treatment. Common symptoms of the *serotonin discontinuation syndrome* include flu-like symptoms (nausea, vomiting, diarrhea, headaches, sweating), sleep disturbances (insomnia, nightmares, constant sleepiness), mood disturbances (dysphoria, anxiety, agitation), cognitive disturbances (mental confusion, hyperarousal), sensory and movement disturbances (imbalance, tremors, vertigo, dizziness, electric-shock-like sensations in the brain, often described by sufferers as "brain zaps").

▶ ***fluoxetine*** (C)(G)

Prozac <8 years: not recommended; 8-17 years: initially 10 mg/day; may increase after 1 week to 20 mg/day; range 20-60 mg/day; range for lower weight children, 20-30 mg/day; ≥17 years: initially 20 mg daily; may increase after 1 week; doses >20 mg/day should be divided into AM and noon doses; max 80 mg/day

Cap: 10, 20, 40 mg; *Tab:* 30*, 60*mg; *Oral soln:* 20 mg/5 ml (4 oz) (mint)

Prozac Weekly <12 years: not recommended; ≥12 years: following daily ***fluoxetine*** therapy at 20 mg/day for 13 weeks, may initiate **Prozac Weekly** 7 days after the last 20 mg ***fluoxetine*** dose

Cap: 90 mg ent-coat del-rel pellets

▶ ***fluvoxamine*** **(C)(G)**

Luvox <8 years: not recommended; 8-17 years: initially 25 mg q HS; adjust in 25 mg increments q 4-7 days; usual range 50-200 mg/day; over 50 mg/day, divide into 2 doses giving the larger dose at HS; >17 years: initially 50 mg q HS; adjust in 50 mg increments at 4-7 day intervals; range 100-300 mg/day; over 100 mg/day, divide into 2 doses giving the larger dose at HS

Tab: 25, 50*, 100*mg

Luvox CR <18 years: not recommended; ≥18 years: initially 100 mg once daily at HS; may increase by 50 mg increments at 1 week intervals; max 300 mg/day; swallow whole

Cap: 100, 150 mg ext-rel

▶ ***paroxetine maleate*** **(D)(G)**

Paxil <12 years: not recommended; ≥12 years: initially 20 mg daily in AM; may increase by 10 mg/day at weekly intervals as needed; max 60 mg/day

Tab: 10*, 20*, 30, 40 mg

Paxil CR <12 years: not recommended; ≥12 years: initially 25 mg daily in AM; may increase by 12.5 mg at weekly intervals as needed; max 62.5 mg/day

Tab: 12.5, 25, 37.5 mg cont-rel ent-coat

Paxil Suspension <12 years: not recommended; ≥12 years: initially 20 mg daily in AM; may increase by 10 mg/day at weekly intervals as needed; max 60 mg/day

Oral susp: 10 mg/5 ml (250 ml) (orange)

▶ ***paroxetine mesylate*** **(D)(G)** <12 years: not recommended; ≥12 years: initially 7.5 mg daily in AM; may increase by 10 mg/day at weekly intervals as needed; max 60 mg/day

Brisdelle *Cap:* 7.5 mg

▶ ***sertraline*** **(C)** <6 years: not recommended; 6-12 years: initially 25 mg daily; max 200 mg/day; 13-17 years: initially 50 mg daily; max 200 mg/day; >17 years: initially 50 mg daily; increase at 1 week intervals if needed; max 200 mg daily

Zoloft *Tab:* 15*, 50*, 100*mg; *Oral conc:* 20 mg per ml (60 ml [dilute just before administering in 4 oz water, ginger ale, lemon-lime soda, lemonade, <u>or</u> orange juice]) (alcohol 12%)

TRICYCLIC ANTIDEPRESSANTS (TCAs)

Comment: Co-administration of SSRIs and TCAs requires extreme caution.

▶ ***amitriptyline*** **(C)(G)** <12 years: not recommended; ≥12 years: 10-20 mg q HS

Tab: 10, 25, 50, 75, 100, 150 mg

▶ ***amoxapine*** **(C)** <12 years: not recommended; ≥12 years: initially 50 mg bid-tid; after 1 week may increase to 100 mg bid-tid; usual effective dose 200-300 mg/day; if total dose exceeds 300 mg/day, give in divided doses (max 400 mg/day); may give as a single bedtime dose (max 300 mg q HS)

Tab: 25, 50, 100, 150 mg

▶ ***clomipramine*** **(C)(G)** <10 years: not recommended; 10-<16 years: initially 25 mg daily in divided doses; gradually increase; max 3 mg/kg <u>or</u> 100 mg, whichever is smaller; ≥16 years: initially 25 mg daily in divided doses; gradually increase to 100 mg during first 2 weeks; max 250 mg/day; total maintenance dose may be given at HS

Anafranil *Cap:* 25, 50, 75 mg

▶ ***desipramine*** **(C)(G)** <12 years: not recommended; ≥12 years: 100-200 mg/day in single <u>or</u> divided doses; max 300 mg/day

Norpramin *Tab:* 10, 25, 50, 75, 100, 150 mg

▶ ***doxepin*** **(C)(G)** <12 years: not recommended; ≥12 years: 75 mg/day; max 150 mg/day

Cap: 10, 25, 50, 75, 100, 150 mg; Oral conc: 10 mg/ml (4 oz w. dropper)

- *imipramine* (C)(G) <12 years: not recommended; ≥12 years:
  Tofranil initially 75 mg daily (max 200 mg); adolescents initially 30-40 mg daily (max 100 mg/day); if maintenance dose exceeds 75 mg daily, may switch to **Tofranil PM** for divided or bedtime dose
  Tab: 10, 25, 50 mg
  Tofranil PM initially 75 mg daily 1 hour before HS; max 200 mg
  Cap: 75, 100, 125, 150 mg
- *nortriptyline* (D)(G) <12 years: not recommended; ≥12 years: initially 25 mg tid-qid; max 150 mg/day
  Pamelor *Cap:* 10, 25, 50, 75 mg; *Oral soln:* 10 mg/5 ml (16 oz)
- *protriptyline* (C) <12 years: not recommended; ≥12 years: initially 5 mg tid; usual dose 15-40 mg/day in 3-4 divided doses; max 60 mg/day
  Vivactil *Tab:* 5, 10 mg
- *trimipramine* (C) <12 years: not recommended; ≥12 years: initially 75 mg/day in divided doses; max 200 mg/day
  Surmontil *Cap:* 25, 50, 100 mg

ONYCHOMYCOSIS (FUNGAL NAIL)

ORAL AGENTS

- *griseofulvin, microsize* (C)(G) <12 years: <30 lb: 5 mg/lb/day; 30-50 lb: 125-250 mg/day; >50 lb: 250-500 mg/day; 5 mg/lb/day x 4-6 weeks or longer; *see page* 612 *for dose by weight table;* ≥12 years: 500 mg once daily x 4-6 weeks or longer; max 1 gm/day
  Grifulvin V *Tab:* 250, 500 mg; *Oral susp:* 125 mg/5 ml (120 ml; alcohol 0.02%)
- *griseofulvin, ultramicrosize* (C)(G) <2 years: not recommended; 2-12 years: 3.3 mg/lb/day in a single or divided doses x 4-6 weeks or longer; >12 years: 375 mg/day in a single or divided doses x 4-6 weeks or longer
  Gris-PEG *Tab:* 125, 250 mg
- *itraconazole* (C)(G) <12 years: not recommended; ≥12 years: 200 mg daily x 12 consecutive weeks for toenails; 200 mg bid x 1 week, off 3 weeks, then 200 mg bid x 1 additional week for fingernails
  Sporanox *Cap:* 100 mg; *Soln:* 10 mg/ml (150 ml) (cherry-caramel); *Pulse Pack:* 100 mg caps (7/pck)
  Pulse Pack: 100 mg caps (7/pck)
- *terbinafine* (B)(G) <12 years: not recommended; ≥12 years: 250 mg daily x 6 weeks for fingernails; 250 mg daily x 12 weeks for toenails
  Lamisil *Tab:* 250 mg

TOPICAL AGENTS

Comment: File and trim nail while nail is free from drug. Remove unattached infected nail as frequently as monthly. For use with mild to moderate onychomycosis of the fingernails and toenails, without lunula involvement due to *Trichophyton rubrum* immunocompetent patients as part of a comprehensive treatment program. For use on nails and adjacent skin only. Apply evenly to entire onycholytic nail and surrounding 5 mm of skin daily, preferably at HS or 8 hours before washing; apply to nail bed, hyponychium, and under surface of nail plate when it is free of the nail bed; apply over previous coats, then remove with alcohol once per week; treat for up to 48 weeks. <12 years not recommended.

- *ciclopirox* (B)
  Penlac Nail Lacquer *Topical soln (lacquer):* 8% (6.6 ml w. applicator)
- *efinaconazole* (C)
  Jublia *Topical soln:* 5% (10 ml w. brush applicator)

▶ *tavaborole* (C)
Kerydin *Topical soln:* 10% (10 ml w. dropper)

OPHTHALMIA NEONATORUM: CHLAMYDIAL

PROPHYLAXIS

▶ ***erythromycin*** ophthalmic ointment 0.5-1 cm ribbon into lower conjunctival sac of each eye x 1 application
Ilotycin Ophthalmic Ointment *Ophth oint:* 5 mg/gm (1/8 oz)

Comment: The following treatment regimens are published in the **2015 CDC Sexually Transmitted Diseases Treatment Guidelines**. Treatment regimens are presented by generic drug name first, followed by information about brands and dose forms.

RECOMMENDED REGIMENS

Regimen 1

▶ ***erythromycin base*** (B)(G) 50 mg/kg/day in 4 doses x 14 days

Regimen 2

▶ ***erythromycin ethylsuccinate*** (B)(G) 50 mg/kg/day in 4 doses x 14 days

DRUG BRANDS AND DOSE FORMS

▶ ***erythromycin base*** (B)(G)
Ery-Tab *Tab:* 250, 333, 500 mg ent-coat
PCE *Tab:* 333, 500 mg

▶ ***erythromycin ethylsuccinate*** (B)(G) *See page 607 for dose by weight*
EryPed *Oral susp:* 200 mg/5 ml (100, 200 ml) (fruit); 400 mg/5 ml (60, 100, 200 ml (banana); *Oral drops:* 200, 400 mg/5 ml (50 ml) (fruit); *Chew tab:* 200 mg wafer (fruit)
E.E.S. *Oral susp:* 200, 400 mg/5 ml (100 ml) (fruit)
E.E.S. Granules *Oral susp:* 200 mg/5 ml (100, 200 ml) (cherry)

OPHTHALMIA NEONATORUM: GONOCOCCAL

Comment: The following prophylaxis and treatment regimens for gonococcal conjunctivitis are published in the **2015 CDC Sexually Transmitted Diseases Treatment Guidelines.**

REGIMEN 1

▶ ***erythromycin 0.5%*** ophthalmic ointment 0.5-1 cm ribbon into lower conjunctival sac of each eye x 1 application
Ilotycin Ophthalmic Ointment *Ophth oint:* 5 mg/gm (1/8 oz)

REGIMEN 2

▶ ***ceftriaxone*** (B)(G) <12 years: 1 gm IM in a single dose; ≥12 years: 25-50 mg/kg IV or IM in a single dose, not to exceed 125 mg
Rocephin *Vial:* 250, 500 mg; 1, 2 gm

OPIOID DEPENDENCE, OPIOID USE DISORDER, OPIOID WITHDRAWAL SYNDROME

Comment: Healthcare Safety labeling for all immediate-release (IR) opioids has been issued by the FDA. The Black Boxed Warning (BBW) includes serious risks of misuse, abuse, addiction, overdose, and death. The dosing section offers clear steps regarding administration and patient monitoring including initial dose, dose changes, and the abrupt cessation of treatment in physical dependence. Chronic maternal use of opioids during pregnancy can lead to potentially life-threatening neonatal opioid withdrawal. The American Pain Society (APS) has released new evidence-based clinical practice guidelines that include 32 recommendations related to post-op pain management in adults and children. The Transmucosal Immediate Release Fentanyl (TIRF) Risk Evaluation and Mitigation Strategy (REMS) program is an FDA-required program designed to ensure informed risk-benefit decisions before initiating treatment, and while patients are treated to ensure appropriate use of TIRF medicines. The purpose of the TIRF REMS Access program is to mitigate the risk of misuse, abuse, addiction, overdose and serious complications due to medication errors with the use of TIRF medicines. You must enroll in the TIRF REMS Access program to prescribe, dispense, or distribute TIRF medicines. To register, call the TIRF REMS Access program at 1-866-822-1483 or register online at https:/www.tirfremsaccess.com/TirfUI/rems/home.action

SELECTIVE ALPHA 2-ADRENERGIC RECEPTOR AGONIST

Comment: **Lucemyra** ***(lofexidine)*** is the first FDA-approved non-opioid treatment for the management of opioid withdrawal symptoms, for the mitigation of withdrawal symptoms to facilitate abrupt discontinuation of opioids in adults. While **Lucemyra** may lessen the severity of withdrawal symptoms, it may not completely prevent them. This oral selective alpha 2-adrenergic receptor agonist reduces the release of norepinephrine. The actions of norepinephrine in the autonomic nervous system are believed to play a role in many of the symptoms of opioid withdrawal and is only approved for treatment for up to 14 days.

▶ *lofexidine* (C) <17 years: not recommended; ≥17 years: 0.18 mg x 3 tabs taken orally 4 x/day at 5-to 6-hour intervals; max 14 days with dosing guided by symptoms; discontinue with a gradual dose reduction over 2 to 4 days.

Lucemyra *Tab:* 0.18 mg

Comment: **Lucemyra** is not a treatment for Opioid Use Disorder (OUD), per se, but can be used as part of a broader, long-term treatment plan for managing OUD. The most common side effects from treatment with **Lucemyra** include hypotension, bradycardia, somnolence, sedation, and dizziness. **Lucemyra** has also been associated with a few cases of syncope. ***methadone*** and **Lucymra** both prolong the QT interval. Therefore, ECG monitoring is recommended when used concomitantly. Comcomitant use of oral ***naltrexone*** with **Lucemyra** may reduce efficacy of oral naltrexone. Concomitant use of ***paroxetine*** has resulted in increased plasma levels of **Lucemyra**. Monitor for symptoms of orthostasis and bradycardia with concomitant use of CYP2D6 inhibitors. The safety of **Lucymra** in pregnant women has not been established. There is no information regarding the presence of **Lucemyra** or its metabolites in human milk or effects on the breastfed infant.

OPIOID AGONISTS

Methadone Detoxification & Methadone Maintenance

Comment: ***methadone*** is not indicated as an as-needed (prn) analgesic. For use in chronic moderately severe-to-severe pain management (e.g., hospice care), see page 328.

▶ ***methadone*** (C)(II)(G) <12 years: not established; ≥12 years: *Narcotic detoxification:* 15-40 mg daily in decreasing doses not to exceed 21 days; *Narcotic maintenance:* ≥21 days; see mfr pkg insert; clinical stability is most commonly achieved at doses between 80 to 120 mg/day; monitor patients with periodic ECGs (e.g., risk of lethal QT interval prolongation, *torsades de pointes*)

Dolophine *Tab:* 5, 10 mg; *Dispersible tab:* 40 mg (dissolve in 120 ml orange juice or other citrus drink); *Oral soln:* 5, 10 mg/ml; *Oral conc:* 10 mg/ml; *Syr:* 10 mg/30 ml; *Vial:* 10 mg/ml (200 mg/20 ml multi-dose) for injection

Comment: ***methadone*** maintenance is allowed only by approved providers with strict state and federal regulations (as stipulated in 42 CFR 8.12). Black Box Warning (BBW): ***Dolophine*** exposes users to risks of addiction, abuse, and misuse, which can lead to overdose and death. Assess each patient's risk and monitor regularly for development of these behaviors and conditions. Serious, life-threatening, or fatal respiratory depression may occur. The peak respiratory depressant effect of ***methadone*** occurs later, and persists longer than the peak analgesic effect. Accidental ingestion, especially by children, can result in fatal overdose. QT interval prolongation and serious arrhythmia (*torsades de pointes*) have occurred during treatment with ***methadone***. Closely monitor patients with risk factors for development of prolonged QT interval, a history of cardiac conduction abnormalities, and those taking medications affecting cardiac conduction. Neonatal Opioid Withdrawal Syndrome (NOWS) is an expected and treatable outcome of use of methadone use during pregnancy. NOWS may be life-threatening if not recognized and treated in the neonate. The balance between the risks of NOWS and the benefits of maternal ***methadone*** use should be considered and the patient advised of the risk of NOWS so that appropriate planning for management of the neonate can occur. ***methadone*** has been detected in human milk. Concomitant use with CYP3A4, 2B6, 2C19, 2C9 or 2D6 inhibitors or discontinuation of concomitantly used CYP3A4 2B6, 2C19, or 2C9 inducers can result in a fatal overdose of methadone. Concomitant use of opioids with benzodiazepines or other central nervous system (CNS) depressants, including alcohol, may result in profound sedation, respiratory depression, coma, and death.

OPIOID ANTAGONIST

▶ ***naltrexone*** (C)

ReVia <12 years: not established; ≥12 years: 50 mg daily

Tab: 50 mg

Vivitrol <12 years: not established; ≥12 years: 380 mg IM once monthly; alternate buttocks

Vial: 380 mg

OPIOID PARTIAL AGONIST-ANTAGONIST

Comment: **Belbuca, Butrans, Probuphine, Sublocade, and Subutex** maintenance are allowed only by approved providers with strict state and federal regulations. These drugs are potentiated by CYP3A4 inhibitors (e.g, azole antifungals, macrolides, HIV protease inhibitors) and antagonized by CYP3A4 inducers (monitor for opioid withdrawal). Concomitant NNRTIs (e.g., ***efavirenz***, ***nevirapine***, ***etravirine***, ***delavirdine***) or PIs (e.g., ***atazanavir*** with or without ***ritonavir***): monitor. Risk of respiratory or CNS depression with concomitant opioid analgesics, general anesthetics, benzodiazepines, phenothiazines, other tranquilizers, sedative/hypnotics, alcohol, or other CNS depressants. Risk of serotonin syndrome with concomitant SSRIs, SNRIs, TCAs, 5-HT3 receptor antagonists, ***mirtazapine***, ***trazodone***, ***tramadol***, MAO inhibitors.

▶ ***buprenorphine*** (C)(III)

Belbuca <12 years: not established; ≥12 years: apply buccal film to inside of cheek; do not chew or swallow; *Opioid naïve:* initially 75 mcg once daily-q 12 hours x at least 4 days; then, increase to 150 mcg q 12 hours; may increase in increments of 150 mcg q 12 hours no sooner than every 4 days; max 900 mcg q 12 hours; see mfr pkg insert for conversion from other opioids; *Severe hepatic impairment* or *oral mucositis:* reduce initial and titration doses by half

Buccal film: 75, 150, 300, 450, 600, 750, 900 mcg (60/pck) (peppermint)

Butrans Transdermal System <12 years: not established; ≥12 years: apply one patch to clean, dry, hairless, intact skin on the upper outer arm, upper chest, upper back, or side of chest every 7 days; rotate sites and do not reuse a site for at least 21 days; *Opioid naïve* or *oral morphine <30 mg/day* or *equivalent:* one 5 mcg/hour patch; *Converting from oral morphine equivalents 30-80 mg/day:* taper current opioids for up to 7 days to ≤30 mg/day oral morphine equivalents before starting; then initiate with 10 mcg/hour patch; may use a short-acting analgesic until efficacy is attained; increase dose only after exposure to previous dose x at least 72 hours; max one 20 mcg/hour patch/week; *Conversion from higher opioid doses:* not recommended

Transdermal patch: 5, 7.5, 10, 15, 20 mcg/hour (4/pck)

Probuphine <16 years: not established; ≥16 years: initiate when stable on ***buprenorphine*** ≤8 mg/day; insertion site is the inner side of the upper arm; 4 implants are intended to be in place for 6 months; remove the implants by the end of the 6th month and insert four new implants on the same day in the contralateral arm; if a new implant is not inserted on the same day as removal of a previous implant, maintain the patient on the previous dose of transmucosal ***buprenorphine*** (i.e., the dose from which the patient was transferred to **Probuphine** treatment).

Subdermal implant: 74.2 mg of *buprenorphine* (equivalent to 80 mg of ***buprenorphine hcl***)

Comment: Healthcare providers who prescribe, perform insertions, and/or perform removals of **Probuphine** must successfully complete a live training program, and demonstrate procedural competency prior to inserting or removing the implants. Further information: www.ProbuphineREMS.com or 1-844-859-6341.

Subutex (G) <12 years: not established; ≥12 years: 8 mg in a single dose on day 1; then 16 mg in a single dose on day 2; target dose is 16 mg/day in a single dose; dissolve under tongue; do not chew or swallow whole

SL tab (lemon-lime) or *SL film (lime):* 2, 8 mg (30/pck)

Sublocade <12 years: not established; ≥12 years: verify that patient is clinically stable on transmucosal ***buprenorphine*** before initiating **Sublocade**; doses must be prepared by an authorized healthcare provider and administered once monthly only by SC injection in the abdominal region; initially, 300 mg SC once monthly x the first 2 months, followed by 100 mg SC once monthly maintenance dose; increasing the maintenance dose to 300 mg once monthly may be considered for patients in which the benefits outweigh the risks

Prefilled syringe: 100 mg/0.5 ml, 300 mg/1.5 ml sust-rel single-dose w. 19 gauge 5/8-inch needle

Comment: Serious harm or death could result if **Sublocade** is administered intraveniously. Neonatal opioid withdrawal syndrome (NOWS) is an expected and treatable outcome of prolonged use of opioids during pregnancy. (Not recommended with moderate-to-severe hepatic impairment. Monitor liver function tests prior to and during treatment. If diagnosed with adrenal insufficiency, treat with physiologic replacement of corticosteroids, and wean patient off of the opioid. **Sublocade** is only available through the restricted SUBLOCADE REMS Program. Healthcare settings and pharmacies that order and dispense **Sublocade** must be certified in this program. To report suspected adverse reactions, contact Indivior Inc. at 1-877-782-6966 or FDA at 1-800-FDA-1088 or visit www.fda.gov/medwatch

OPIOID PARTIAL AGONIST-ANTAGONIST+OPIOID ANTAGONIST

Comment: **Bunavail, Suboxone, Sucartonone**, *Troxyca ER*, and **Zubsolv** maintenance are allowed only by approved providers with strict state and federal regulations.

➢ ***buprenorphine+naloxone*** (C)(III)

Bunavail <16 years: not recommended; ≥16 years: administer one buccal film once daily at the same time each day; target dose is 8.4/1.4 once daily; place the side of the **Bunavail** film with the text (BN2, BN4, or BN6) against the inside of the cheek; press and hold the film in place for 5 seconds; maintenance is usually 2.1/0.3 to 12.6/2.1 once daily

SL film:

Bunavail 2.1/0.3 bup 2.1 mg+nal 0.3 mg (30/carton) (lime)
Bunavail 4.2/0.7 bup 4.2 mg+nal 0.7 mg (30/carton) (lime)
Bunavail 6.3/1 bup 6.3 mg+nal 1 mg (30/carton) (lime)

Comment: A **Bunavail** 4.2/0.7 buccal film provides equivalent ***buprenorphine*** exposure to a **Sucartonone** 8/2 sublingual tablet.

Suboxone (G) <12 years: not recommended; ≥12 years: adjust dose in increments/decrements of 2/0.5 or 4/1 once daily ***buprenorphine+naloxone***, based on the patient's daily dose of ***buprenorphine***, to a level that suppresses opioid withdrawal signs and symptoms; *Recommended target dosage:* 16/4 as a single daily dose; *Maintenance dose:* generally in the range of 4/1 to 24/6 per day; higher once daily doses have not been demonstrated to provide any clinical advantage

Suboxone

SL tab, SL film:

Suboxone 2/0.5 bup 2 mg+nal 0.5 mg (30/bottle) (lime)
Suboxone 8/2 bup 8 mg+nal 2 mg (30/bottle) (lime)

Sucartonone <12 years: not recommended; ≥12 years: adjust in 2-4 mg of ***buprenorphine***/day in a single dose; usual range is 4-24 mg/day in a single dose; target dose is 6 mg/day in a single dose; dissolve under tongue; do not chew or swallow whole

Sucartonone

SL film:

Sucartonone 2/0.5 bup 2 mg+nal 0.5 mg (30/pck) (lime)
Sucartonone 4/1 bup 4 mg+nal 1 mg (30/pck) (lime)
Sucartonone 8/2 bup 8 mg+nal 2 mg (30/pck) (lime)
Sucartonone 12/3 bup 12 mg+nal 3 mg (30/pck) (lime)

Zubsolv <16 years: not recommended; ≥16 years: initial induction with ***buprenorphine*** sublingual tabs; administer as a single dose once daily; titrate dose in increments of 1.4/0.36 or 2.9/0.72 per day; recommended target dose is 11.4/2.9 per day; usual max 17.2/4.2 per day

Zubsolv

SL tab: **Zubsolv 1.4/0.36** bup 1.4 mg+nal 0.36 mg
Zubsolv 2.9/0.72 bup 2.9 mg+nal 0.71 mg
Zubsolv 5.7/1.4 bup 5.7 mg+nal 1.4 mg
Zubsolv 8.6/2.1 bup 8.6 mg+nal 2.1 mg
Zubsolv 11.4/2.9 bup 11.4 mg+nal 2.9 mg

Comment: One **Subutex 5.7/1.4** SL tab is bioequivalent to one **Sucartonone 8/2** SL film.

➢ ***oxycodone+naloxone*** (C)(II) <18 years: not recommended; ≥18 years: *Opioid-naïve and opioid non-tolerant:* initially 10/1.2 q 12 hours; *Opioid-tolerant:* single doses greater than 40/4.8, or a total daily dose greater than 80/9.6 are only for use in patients for whom tolerance to an opioid of comparable potency has been established; swallow whole, or sprinkle contents on applesauce and swallow immediately without chewing

Troxyca ER

Cap: **Troxyca ER 10/1.2** oxy 10 mg+nalox 1.2 mg ext-rel
Troxyca ER 20/1.2 oxy 20 mg+nalox 2.4 mg ext-rel
Troxyca ER 30/1.2 oxy 30 mg+nalox 3.6 mg ext-rel
Troxyca ER 40/1.2 oxy 40 mg+nalox 4.8 mg ext-rel
Troxyca ER 60/1.2 oxy 60 mg+nalox 7.2 mg ext-rel
Troxyca ER 80/1.2 oxy 80 mg+nalox 9.6 mg ext-rel

Comment: Opioid tolerant patients are those taking, for one week or longer, at least 60 mg oral ***morphine*** per day, 25 mcg transdermal ***fentanyl*** per hour, 30 mg oral ***oxycodone*** per day, 8 mg oral ***hydromorphone*** per day, 25 mg oral ***oxymorphone*** per day, 60 mg oral ***hydrocodone*** per day, or an equianalgesic dose of another opioid.

OPIOID-INDUCED CONSTIPATION (OIC)

▶ ***lubiprostone*** **(C)** <18 years: not established; ≥18 years: swallow whole; take with food and water; initially 24 mcg bid; *Moderate hepatic impairment (Child-Pugh Class B):* 16 mg bid; *Severe hepatic impairment (Child-Pugh Class C):* 8 mg bid

Amitiza *Cap:* 8, 24 mg

▶ ***methylnaltrexone bromide*** **(C)** <18 years: not established; ≥18 years: one oral dose or one weight-based SC dose every other day as needed; max one dose per 24 hours; administer SC inject into the upper arm, abdomen, or thigh; rotate sites

Chronic Non-cancer Pain: 450 mg po once daily in the morning (take with water on an empty stomach at least 30 minutes before the first meal of the day) or 12 mg SC once daily in the morning; *Severe Hepatic Impairment:* <38 kg: 0.075 mg/kg; 38-<62 kg: 4 mg (0.2 ml); 62-114 kg: 6 mg (0.3 ml); >114 kg: 0.075 mg/kg *Advanced Illness, Receiving Palliative Care:* <38 kg: 0.15 mg/kg; 38-<62 kg: 8 mg (0.4 ml); 62-114 kg: 12 mg (0.6 ml); >114 kg: 0.15 mg/kg; *Moderate and Severe Renal Impairment (CrCl<60 mL/min):* <38 kg: 0.075 mg/kg; 38-<62 kg: 4 mg (0.2 ml); 62-114 kg: 6 mg (0.3 ml); >114 kg: 0.075 mg/kg

Relistor *Tab:* 150 mg film-coat; *Vial:* 12 mg single-dose (0.6 ml, 7/carton);
Relistor Injection *Prefilled syringe:* 8 mg (0.4 ml), 12 mg (0.6 ml) (7/carton)

Comment: **Relistor** injection is indicated for patients with advanced illness or pain caused by active cancer who require opioid dosage escalation for palliative care. **Relistor** is an opioid antagonist indicated for the treatment of opioid-induced constipation (OIC) in adult patients with chronic non-cancer pain, including patients with chronic pain related to prior cancer or its treatment who do not require frequent (e.g., weekly) opi-oid dosage escalation. ***methylnaltrexone*** is a selective antagonist of opioid binding at the mu-opioid receptor. As a quaternary amine, the ability of ***methylnaltrexone*** to cross the blood-brain barrier is restricted. This allows ***methylnaltrexone*** to function as a peripherally-acting mu-opioid receptor antagonist in tissues such as the gastrointestinal tract, thereby decreasing the constipating effects of opioids without impacting opioid-mediated analgesic effects on the central nervous system. The pre-filled syringe is only for patients who require a **Relistor** injection dose of 8 mg or 12 mg. Use the vial for patients who require other doses. **Relistor** is contraindicated with known or suspected GI obstruction and patients at increased risk of recurrent obstruction, due to the potential for gastrointestinal perforation. Be within close proximity to toilet facilities once **Relistor** is administered. Discontinue all maintenance laxative therapy prior to initiation. Laxative(s) can be used as needed if there is a suboptimal response after three days. Discontinue if treatment with the opioid pain medication is also discontinued. Safety and effectiveness of **Relistor** have not been established in pediatric patients. Avoid concomitant use with other opioid antagonists because of the potential for additive effects of opioid receptor antagonism and increased risk of opioid withdrawal symptoms (sweating, chills, diarrhea, abdominal pain, anxiety, and yawning). Advise females of reproductive potential, who become pregnant or are planning to become pregnant, that the use of **Relistor** during pregnancy may precipitate opioid withdrawal in a fetus due to the undeveloped blood-brain barrier. Breastfeeding is not recommended during treatment.

➢ ***naldemedine*** **(C)** <12 years: not established; ≥12 years: take one tab once daily; take with or without food; discontinue if opioid pain therapy discontinued

Symproic *Tab:* 0.2 mg

Comment: **Symproic** is contraindicated with known or suspected GI obstruction and patients at increased risk for recurrent obstruction. Avoid with severe hepatic impairment (Child-Pugh Class C). Not recommended in pregnancy and breastfeeding (during and 3 days after final dose). There is risk of perforation in persons with conditions associated with reduction in structural integrity the GI tract wall (e.g., peptic ulcer disease [PUD], Ogilvie's syndrome, diverticulitis disease, infiltrative GI tract malignancies, or peritoneal metastases).

➢ ***naloxegol*** **(C)** <18 years: not established; ≥18 years: swallow whole; take on an empty stomach; initially 25 mg once daily in the AM; discontinue other laxatives; if not tolerated or *CrCl <60 mL/min:* reduce daily dose to 12.5 mg

Movantik *Tab:* 12.5, 25 mg

Comment: **Movantik** is an opioid antagonist indicated for the treatment of opioid-induced constipation (OIC) in adult patients with chronic non-cancer pain, including patients with chronic pain related to prior cancer or its treatment who do not require frequent (e.g., weekly) opioid dosage escalation. Alteration in analgesic dosing regimen prior to starting **Movantik** is not required. Patients receiving opioids for less than 4 weeks may be less responsive to **Movantik.** Take on an empty stomach at least 1 hour prior to the first meal of the day or 2 hours after the meal. For patients who are unable to swallow the **Movantik** tablet whole, the tablet can be crushed and given orally or administered via nasogastric tube (NGT). Avoid consumption of grapefruit or grapefruit juice. Discontinue if treatment with the opioid pain medication is also discontinued.

OPIOID-INDUCED NAUSEA/VOMITING (OINV)

Comment: Opioid analgesics bind to μ (mu), κ (kappa), or δ (delta) opioid receptors in the brain, spinal cord, and digestive tract. However, opioids cause adverse effects that may interfere with their therapeutic use. Opioid-induced nausea/vomiting (OINV) treatment options include serotonin receptor antagonists, dopamine receptor antagonists, and neurokinin-1 receptor antagonists.

SEROTONIN RECEPTOR ANTAGONISTS

➢ ***dolasetron*** **(B)** <2 years: not recommended; 2-16 years: 1.8 mg/kg; >16 years: administer 100 mg IV over 30 seconds; max 100 mg/dose

Anzemet *Tab:* 50, 100 mg; *Amp:* 12.5 mg/0.625 ml; *Prefilled carpuject syringe:* 12.5 mg (0.625 ml); *Vial:* 100 mg/5 ml (single-use); *Vial:* 500 mg/25 ml (multi-dose)

➢ ***granisetron***

Kytril (B) <2 years: not recommended; ≥2 years: 10 mcg/kg; administer IV over 30 seconds; max 1 dose/week

Tab: 1 mg; *Oral soln:* 2 mg/10 ml (30 ml; orange); *Vial:* 1 mg/ml (1 ml single-dose) (preservative-free); 1 mg/ml (4 ml multi-dose) (benzyl alcohol)

Sancuso (B) <12 years: not recommended; ≥12 years: apply 1 patch 24-48 hours before chemo; remove 24 hours (minimum) to 7 days (maximum) after completion of treatment

Transdermal patch: 3.1 mg/day

- ***ondansetron*** **(C)(G)** <4 years: not recommended; 4-11 years: 4 mg q 4 hours x 3 doses; then 4 mg q 8 hours; >11 years: 8 mg q 8 hours x 2 doses; then 8 mg q 12 hours
  - **Zofran** *Tab:* 4, 8, 24 mg
  - **Zofran ODT** *ODT:* 4, 8 mg (strawberry) (phenylalanine)
  - **Zofran Oral Solution** *Oral soln:* 4 mg/5 ml (50 ml) (strawberry) (phenylalanine); *Parenteral form:* see mfr pkg insert
  - **Zofran Injection** *Vial:* 2 mg/ml (2 ml single-dose); 2 mg/ml (20 ml multi-dose); 32 mg/50 ml (50 ml multi-dose); *Prefilled syringe:* 4 mg/2 ml, single-use (24/carton)
  - **Zuplenz Oral Soluble Film**: 4, 8 mg oral-dis (10/carton) (peppermint)
- ***palonosetron*** **(B)(G)** administer 0.25 mg IV over 30 seconds; max 1 dose/week
  Pediatric: <1 month: not recommended; 1 month to 17 years: 20 mcg/kg; max 1.5 mg/single dose; infuse over 15 minutes
  - **Aloxi** *Vial (single-use):* 0.075 mg/1.5 ml; 0.25 mg/5 ml (mannitol)

DOPAMINE RECEPTOR ANTAGONISTS

- ***prochlorperazine*** **(C)(G)**
  - **Compazine** <2 years or <20 lb: not recommended; 20-29 lb: 2.5 mg daily bid prn; max 7.5 mg/day; 30-39 lb: 2.5 mg bid-tid prn; max 10 mg/day; 40-85 lb: 2.5 mg tid or 5 mg bid prn; max 15 mg/day; >85 lb: 5-10 mg tid-qid prn; usual max 40 mg/day
    Tab: 5, 10 mg; *Syr:* 5 mg/5 ml (4 oz) (fruit)
  - **Compazine Suppository** <2 years or <20 lb: not recommended; 20-29 lb: 2.5 mg daily-bid prn; max 7.5; mg/day; 30-39 lb: 2.5 mg bid-tid prn; max 10 mg/day; 40-85 lb: 2.5 mg tid or 5 mg bid prn; max 15 mg/day; >85 lb: 25 mg rectally bid prn; usual max 50 mg/day
    Rectal supp: 2.5, 5, 25 mg
  - **Compazine Injectable** <2 years or <20 lb: not recommended; ≥2 years or ≥20-85 lb: 0.06 mg/kg x 1 dose; >85 lb: 5-10 mg tid or qid prn
    Vial: 5 mg/ml (2, 10 ml)
  - **Compazine Spansule** <12 years: not recommended; ≥12 years: 15 mg q AM prn or 10 mg q 12 hours prn usual max 40 mg/day
    Spansule: 10, 15 mg sust-rel

NEUROKININ-1 RECEPTOR ANTAGONISTS

- ***aprepitant*** **(B)(G)** administer with 5HT-3 receptor antagonist; *Day 1:* 125 mg; *Day 2 & 3:* 80 mg in the morning
  Pediatric: <6 months: years: not recommended; ≥6 months: use oral suspension (see mfr pkg insert for dose by weight)
  - **Emend** *Cap:* 40, 80, 125 mg (2 x 80 mg bi-fold pck; 1 x 25 mg/2 x 80 mg tri-fold pck); *Oral susp:* 125 mg pwdr for oral suspension, single-dose pouch w. dispenser; *Vial:* 150 mg pwdr for reconstitution and IV infusion

OPIOID OVERDOSE

OPIOID ANTAGONISTS

- ***nalmefene*** **(B)** <12 years: not recommended; ≥12 years: initially 0.25 mcg/kg IV, IM, or SC, then incremental doses of 0.25 mcg/kg at 2-5 minute intervals; cumulative max 1 mcg/kg; if opioid dependency suspected use 0.1 mg/70 kg initially and then proceed as usual if no response in 2 minutes
  - **Revex** *Amp:* 100 mcg/ml (1 ml); 1 mg/ml (2 ml)

▶ ***naloxone*** **(B)(G)** <12 years: 0.01 mg/kg initially, repeat in 2-3 minutes at 0.1 mg/kg if response inadequate; ≥12 years: 0.4-2 mg; repeat in 2-3 minutes if no response

Evzio *Prefilled autoinjector:* 0.4 mg/0.4 ml IM/SC only

Comment: **Evzio** 2 mg/0.4 ml comes with 2 autoinjectors and one trainer. This strength is indicated for the emergency treatment of known or suspected opioid overdose manifested by CNS depression.

If the electronic voice instruction system does not operate properly, **Evzio** will still deliver the intended dose of ***naloxone*** when used according to the printed instructions on the flat surface of the autoinjector label. **Evzio** cannot be administered IV. Due to the short duration of action of naloxone, as compared to opioids which are longer acting, monitoring of the patient is critical as the opioid reversal effects of naloxone may wear off before the effects of the opioid.

Narcan *Vial/Amp:* 0.4 mg/ml (1 ml), 1 mg/ml (2 ml); *Prefilled syringe:* 0.4 mg ml (1 ml), 1 mg/ml (2 ml) IV, IM, or SC (parabens-free)

Narcan Nasal Spray position supine with head tilted back; 1 spray in one nostril; if an additional dose is needed, spray into the opposite nostril

Nasal spray: 4 mg/0.1 ml, single-dose, single-use (2 blister pcks, each w a single nasal spray/carton)

ORGAN TRANSPLANT REJECTION PROPHYLAXIS

SELECTIVE IMMUNOMODULATORY AGENTS

Comment: Selective immunosuppressive agents are drugs that suppress the immune system due to a selective point of action. They are used to reduce the risk of rejection in organ transplants, in autoimmune diseases, and can be use as cancer chemotherapy. As immunosuppressive agents lower the immunity, there is increased risk of infection.

MAMMALIAN TARGET OF RAPAMYCIN (mTOR) INHIBITORS (mTORIs)

Comment: The most frequently occurring adverse events associated with mTOR inhibitors (≥30%) include aphthous stomatitis, rash, anemia, fatigue, hyperglycemia, hypertriglyceridemia, hypercholesterolemia, decreased appetite, nausea, diarrhea, abdominal pain, headache, peripheral edema, hypertension, increased serum creatinine, fever, urinary tract infection, arthralgia, pain, thrombocytopenia, and interstitial lung disease. There are no adequate and well-controlled studies in pregnant females. Effective contraception must be initiated before mTORi therapy, continued during therapy, and for 12 weeks after therapy has been stopped. It is not known whether ***serolimus***-based drugs are excreted in human milk. The pharmacokinetic and safety profiles in breastfed infants are not known; therefore, a decision should be made whether to discontinue nursing or to discontinue the drug, taking into account the importance of the drug to the mother.

▶ ***everolimus*** **(C)** <18 years: not established/not recommended; ≥18 years: admininister consistently with or without food at the same time as ***cyclosporine*** or ***tacrolimus***; monitor ***everolimus*** concentrations: adjust maintenance dose to achieve trough concentrations within the 3-8 ng/mL target range (using LC/MS/MS assay method); *Mild hepatic impairment:* reduce initial daily dose by one-third; *Moderate or severe hepatic impairment:* reduce initial daily dose by one-half

Kidney Transplant: indicated for patients at low-moderate immunologic risk; use in combination with ***basiliximab***, ***cyclosporine*** (reduced doses), and ***corticosteroids;*** starting dose is 0.75 mg bid; initiate as soon as possible after transplantation

Liver Transplant: use in combination with ***tacrolimus*** (reduced doses) and ***corticosteroids***; starting dose is 1.0 mg bid; initiate 30 days after transplantation

Zortress *Tab:* 0.25, 0.5, 0.75 mg

Comment: To report suspected adverse reactions, contact Novartis Pharmaceuticals Corporation at 1-888-669-6682 or FDA at 1-800-FDA1088 or visit www.fda.gov/medwatch.

▻ ***serolimus* (C)**

Generic: (for prescribing information, *see* **Rapamune**)

Tab: 1, 2 mg

Rapamune <13 years: not established/not recommended; ≥13 years: administer consistently with or without food at the same time as ***cyclosporine (CsA)***

Low to moderate-immunologic risk: Day 1: 6 mg as a single loading dose; *Day 2:* initiate 2 mg once daily maintenance; use initially with ***cyclosporine*** (CsA) and ***corticosteroids***; initiate CsA withdrawal over 4-8 weeks beginning 2-4 months post-transplantation

High-immunologic risk: Day 1: up to 15 mg as a single loading dose; *Day 2:* initiate 5 mg once daily maintenance; use with CsA for the first 12 months post-transplantation

Tab: 0.5, 1, 2, mg; *Oral soln:* 60 mg/60 ml in amber glass bottle, one oral syringe adapter for fitting into the neck of the bottle, sufficient disposable amber oral syringes and caps for daily dosing, and a carrying case; bottles should be stored protected from light and refrigerated at 2°C to 8°C (36°F to 46°F); once the bottle is opened, the contents should be used within one month; If necessary, bottles may be stored the bottles at room temperatures up to 25°C (77°F) for a short period of time (not more than 15 days)

Comment: To report suspected adverse reactions, contact Pfizer at 1-800-438-1985 or FDA at 1-800-FDA-1088 or visit www.fda.gov/medwatch

OSGOOD–SCHLATTER DISEASE

Acetaminophen for IV Infusion *see **Pain** page* 322
NSAIDs *see page* 539
Other Oral Analgesics *see **Pain** page* 324
Topical & Transdermal NSAIDs *see **Pain** page* 323
Parenteral Corticosteroids *see page* 547
Oral Corticosteroids *see page* 546

OSTEOARTHRITIS, ANKYLOSING SPONDYLITIS

Acetaminophen for IV Infusion *see **Pain** page* 322
NSAIDs *see page* 539
Other Oral Analgesics *see **Pain** page* 324
Topical & Transdermal NSAIDs *see **Pain** page* 323
Parenteral Corticosteroids *see page* 547
Oral Corticosteroids *see page* 546

TOPICAL ANALGESICS

▻ ***capsaicin*** cream **(B)(G)** <2 years: not recommended; 2-12 years: apply sparingly to intact skin bid prn; >12 years: apply tid-qid prn

Axsain *Crm:* 0.075% (1, 2 oz)

Capsin (OTC) *Lotn:* 0.025, 0,075% (59 ml)

Capzasin-P (OTC) *Crm:* 0.025% (1.5 oz); *Lotn:* 0.025% (2 oz)

Capzasin-HP (OTC) *Crm:* 0.075% (1.5 oz); *Lotn:* 0.075% (2 oz)
Dolorac *Crm:* 0.025% (28 gm)
Double Cap (OTC) *Crm:* 0.05% (2 oz)
R-Gel *Gel:* 0.025% (15, 30 gm)
Zostrix (OTC) *Crm:* 0.025% (0.7, 1.5, 3 oz)
Zostrix HP (OTC) *Emol crm:* 0.075% (1, 2 oz)

Comment: Provides some relief by 1-2 weeks; optimal benefit may take 4-6 weeks. Avoid contact with mucous membranes.

ORAL SALICYLATE

▶ ***indomethacin*** (C) <14 years: usually not recommended; ≥2 years, if risk warranted: 1-2 mg/kg/day in divided doses; max 3-4 mg/kg/day (or 150-200 mg/day, whichever is less); <14 years, ER cap not recommended; ≥14 years: initially 25 mg bid to tid, increase as needed at weekly intervals by 25-50 mg/day; max 200 mg/day
Cap: 25, 50 mg; *Susp;* 25 mg/5 ml (pineapple-coconut, mint) (alcohol 1%); *Supp:* 50 mg; *ER Cap:* 75 mg ext-rel

Comment: ***indomethacin*** is indicated only for acute painful flares. Administer with food and/or antacids. Use lowest effective dose for shortest duration.

ORAL NSAIDs

*See more **Oral NSAIDs** page* 539

▶ ***diclofenac*** (C) <18 years: not recommended; ≥18 years: take on empty stomach; 35 mg tid; *Hepatic impairment:* use lowest dose
Zorvolex *Gelcap:* 18, 35 mg

▶ ***diclofenac sodium*** (C) <18 years: not recommended; ≥18 years:
Voltaren 50 mg bid to qid or 75 mg bid or 25 mg qid with an additional 25 mg at HS if necessary
Tab: 25, 50, 75 mg ent-coat
Voltaren XR 100 mg once daily; rarely, 100 mg bid may be used
Tab: 100 mg ext-rel

ORAL NSAIDs+PPI

▶ ***esomeprazole+naproxen*** (C; **not for use in 3rd**)(G) <18 years: not recommended; ≥18 years: 1 tab bid; use lowest effective dose for the shortest duration; swallow whole; take at least 30 minutes before a meal
Vimovo *Tab:* nap 375 mg+eso 20 mg ext-rel; nap 500 mg+eso 20 mg ext-rel
Comment: **Vimovo** is indicated to improve signs/symptoms, and risk of gastric ulcer in patients at risk of developing NSAID-associated gastric ulcer.

COX-2 INHIBITORS

Comment: Cox-2 inhibitors are contraindicated with history of asthma, urticaria, and allergic-type reactions to ***aspirin***, other NSAIDs, and sulfonamides, 3rd trimester of pregnancy, and coronary artery bypass graft (CABG) surgery.

▶ ***celecoxib*** (C)(G) <18 years: not recommended; ≥18 years: 100-400 mg daily bid; max 800 mg/day
Celebrex *Cap:* 50, 100, 200, 400 mg

▶ ***meloxicam*** (C)(G)
Mobic <2 years, <60 kg: not recommended; ≥2, >60 kg: 0.125 mg/kg; max 7.5 mg once daily; ≥18 years: initially 7.5 mg once daily; max 15 mg once daily; *Hemodialysis:* max 7.5 mg/day
Tab: 7.5, 15 mg; *Oral susp:* 7.5 mg/5 ml (100 ml) (raspberry)

Vivlodex <18 years: not established; ≥18 years: initially 5 mg qd; may increase to max 10 mg/day; *Hemodialysis:* max 5 mg/day
Cap: 5, 10 mg

INTRA-ARTICULAR INJECTIONS

▶ ***sodium hyaluronate*** **(B)** <12 years: not recommended; using strict aseptic technique, administer by intra-articular injection (into the synovial space) once weekly for the prescribed number of weeks (see mfr pkg insert); after preparing the injection site and attaining local analgesia, remove joint synovial fluid or effusion prior to injection
Gelsyn-3 *Syringe:* 8.4 mg/ml (2 ml) prefilled
Hyalgan *Vial:* 20 mg (2 ml); *Prefilled syringe:* 20 mg (2 ml)
Hylan *Syringe:* 48 mg/6 ml (6 ml) prefilled
Synvisc One *Syringe:* 46 mg/6 ml (6 ml) prefilled

TUMOR NECROSIS FACTOR (TNF) ALPHA BLOCKERS FOR ANKYLOSING SPONDYLITIS

▶ ***adalimumab-adbm*** **(B)** initially 80 SC; then, 40 mg SC every other week starting one week after initial dose; inject into thigh or abdomen; rotate sites
Pediatric: <18 years: not recommended; ≥18 years: same as adult
Cyltezo *Prefilled syringe:* 40 mg/0.8 ml single-dose (preservative-free)
Comment: **Cyltezo** is biosimilar to **Humira** (***adalimumab***).

▶ ***infliximab*** *(tumor necrosis factor-alpha blocker)* <6 years: not studied; ≥6-17 to years: 5 mg/kg at 0, 2 and 6 weeks, then every 8 weeks; ≥18 years: must be refrigerated at 2°C to 8°C (36°F to 46°F); administer dose intravenously over a period of not less than 2 hours; do not use beyond the expiration date as this product contains no pre-servative; 5 mg/kg at 0, 2 and 6 weeks, then every 8 weeks.
Remicade *Vial:* 100 mg for reconstitution to 10 ml administration volume, single-dose (preservative-free)

Comment: **Remicade** is indicated to reduce signs and symptoms, and induce and maintain clinical remission, in adults and children ≥6 years-of-age with moderately to severely active disease who have had an inadequate response to conventional therapy and reduce the number of draining en-terocutaneous and rectovaginal fistulas, and maintain fistula closure, in adults with fistulizing disease. Common adverse effects associated with **Remicade** included abdominal pain, headache, pharyngitis, sinusitis, and upper respiratory infections. In addition, **Remicade** might increase the risk for serious infections, including tuberculosis, bacterial sepsis, and invasive fungal infections. Available data from published literature on the use of ***infliximab*** products during pregnancy have not reported a clear association with ***infliximab*** products and adverse pregnancy outcomes. ***infliximab*** products cross the placenta and infants exposed in utero should not be administered live vaccines for at least 6 months after birth. Otherwise, the infant may be at increased risk of infection, including disseminated infection which can become fatal. Available information is insufficient to inform the amount of infliximab products present in human milk or effects on the breastfed infant. To report suspected adverse reactions, contact Merck Sharp & Dohme Corp., a subsidiary of Merck & Co. at 1-877-888-4231 or FDA at 1-800-FDA1088 or visit www.fda.gov/medwatch

▶ ***infliximab-abda*** *(tumor necrosis factor-alpha blocker)* **(B)**
Renflexis: see *infliximab* (Remicade) above for full prescribing information

Comment: **Renflexis** is a biosimilar to **Remicade** for the treatment of im-mune-disorders including Crohn's disease, ulcerative colitis, rheumatoid arthritis, ankylosing spondylitis, psoriatic arthritis and plaque psoriasis. **Renflexis** was approved under the FDA category for biosimilars and demonstrated no clinically meaningful differences for use, dosing regimens, strengths, dosage forms, and routes of administration from the FDA-approved biological product **Remicade.**

▶ ***infliximab-dyyb*** *(tumor necrosis factor-alpha blocker)* **(B)**

Inflectra: see ***infliximab*** **(Remicade)** above for full prescribing information

Comment: **Inflectra** is a biosimilar to **Remicade** for the treatment of immune-disorders including Crohn's disease, ulcerative colitis, rheumatoid arthritis, ankylosing spondylitis, psoriatic arthritis and plaque psoriasis. Inflectra was approved under the FDA category for biosimilars and demonstrated no clinically meaningful differences for use, dosing regimens, strengths, dosage forms, and routes of administration from the FDA-approved biological product **Remicade.**

▶ ***infliximab-qbtx*** *(tumor necrosis factor-alpha blocker)* **(B)**

Ifixi: see ***infliximab*** **(Remicade)** above for full prescribing information

Comment: **Ifixi** is a biosimilar to **Remicade** for the treatment of immune disorders including Crohn's disease, ulcerative colitis, rheumatoid arthritis, ankylosing spondylitis, psoriatic arthritis and plaque psoriasis. **Ifixi** was approved under the FDA category for biosimilars and demonstrated no clinically meaningful differences for use, dosing regimens, strengths, dosage forms, and routes of administration from the FDA-approved biological product **Remicade**.

OSTEOPOROSIS

Comment: Prior to initiating, or concomitant prescribing, corticosteroids in patients at risk for, or diagnosed with, osteoporosis, referral to the following ACR guidelines is recommended: Guidelines on Prevention & Treatment of Glucocorticoid-induced Osteoporosis [press release]. Atlanta, GA. American College of Rheumatology; June 7, 2017. https://www.rheumatology.org/About-Us/Newsroom/Press-Releases/ID/812/ACR-Releases-Guideline-on-Prevention-Treatment-of-Glucocorticoid-Induced-Osteoporosis. Indications for bone density screening include: personal history of fragility fracture, presence of high serum markers of bone resorption, smoker, height >67 inches, weight <125 lb, taking a steroid, GnRH agonist, or anti-seizure drug, immobilization, hyperthyroidism, post transplantation, malabsorption syndrome, hyperparathyroidism, prolactinemia. Foods high in calcium include almonds, broccoli, baked beans, salmon, sardines, buttermilk, turnip greens, collard greens, spinach, pumpkin, rhubarb, and bran. *Recommended daily calcium intake:* 1-3 years: 700 mg; 4-8 years: 1,000 mg; 9-18 years: 1,300 mg; >18 years: 1,000 mg; pregnancy or nursing: 1,000-1,300 mg.

CALCIUM SUPPLEMENTS

Comment: Take ***calcium*** supplements with meals to avoid gastric upset. Dosages of calcium over 2000 mg/day have not demonstrated any additional benefit. ***Calcium*** decreases ***tetracycline*** absorption. ***Calcium*** absorption is decreased by corticosteroids.

▶ ***calcitonin-salmon*** **(C)**

Fortical 200 IU intranasally daily; alternate nostrils each day

Nasal spray: 200 IU/actuation (30 doses, 3.7 ml)

Miacalcin Nasal Spray 200 IU spray in one nostril once daily; alternate nostrils each day

Nasal spray: 200 IU/actuation (30 doses, 3.7 ml)

Miacalcin Injection 100 units SC or IM every other day

Vial: 200 units/ml (2 ml)

Comment: Supplement diet with calcium (1 gm/day) and vitamin D (400 IU/day).

▶ ***calcium carbonate*** **(C)(OTC)(G)**

Rolaids chew 2 tabs bid; max 14 tabs/day

Chew tab: 550 mg

Rolaids Extra Strength chew 2 tabs bid; max 8 tabs/day
Chew tab: 1000 mg
Tums chew 2 tabs bid; max 16 tabs/day
Chew tab: 500 mg
Tums Extra Strength chew 2 tabs bid; max 10 tabs/day
Chew tab: 750 mg
Tums Ultra chew 2 tabs bid; max 8 tabs/day
Chew tab: 1000 mg
Os-Cal 500 (OTC) 1-2 tab bid to tid
Chew tab: elemental calcium carbonate 500 mg

▶ ***calcium carbonate+vitamin d*** (C)(G)
Os-Cal 250+D (OTC) 1-2 tab tid
Tab: elemental cal carb 250 mg+vit d 125 IU
Os-Cal 500+D (OTC) 1-2 tab bid-tid
Tab: elemental cal carb 500 mg+vit d 125 IU
Viactiv (OTC) 1 tab tid
Chew tab: elemental calcium 500 mg+vit d 100 IU+vitamin k 40 mcg

▶ ***calcium citrate*** (C)(G)
Citracal (OTC) 1-2 tabs bid
Tab: elemental calcium citrate 200 mg

▶ ***calcium citrate+vitamin d*** (C)(G)
Citracal+D (OTC) 1-2 cplts bid
Cplt: elemental cal cit 315 mg+vit d 200 IU
Citracal 250+D (OTC) 1-2 tabs bid
Tab: elemental cal cit 250 mg+vit d 62.3 IU

VITAMIN D ANALOGS

Comment: Concurrent ***vitamin D*** supplementation is contraindicated for patients taking ***calcitriol*** or ***doxercalciferol*** due to the risk of ***vitamin D*** toxicity.

▶ ***calcitriol*** (C) <12 years: *Predialysis:* <3 years: 10-15 ng/kg/day; ≥3 years: initially 0.25 mcg daily; may increase to 0.5 mcg/day; *Dialysis:* not recommended; *Hypoparathyroidism:* initially 0.25 mcg daily; may increase by 0.25 mcg/day at 2-4 week intervals; usual maintenance (1-5 years) 0.25-0.75 mcg/day, (>6 years) 0.5-2 mcg/day; ≥12 years: *Predialysis:* initially 0.25 mcg daily; may increase to 0.5 mcg daily; *Dialysis:* initially 0.25 mcg daily; may increase by 0.25 mcg/day at 4-8 week intervals; usual maintenance 0.5-1 mcg/day; *Hypoparathyroidism:* initially 0.25 mcg q AM; may increase by 0.25 mcg/day at 4- to 8-week intervals; usual maintenance 0.5-2 mcg/day
Rocaltrol *Cap:* 0.25, 0.5 mcg
Rocaltrol Solution *Soln:* 1 mcg/ml (15 ml, single-use dispensers)

▶ ***doxercalciferol*** (C) <12 years: initially 0.25 mcg daily; may increase by 0.25 mcg; 0.25 mcg/day at 2-4 week intervals; usual maintenance (1-5 years) 0.25-0.75 mcg/day, (≥6 years) 0.5-2 mcg/day; ≥12 weeks: initially 0.25 mcg q AM; may increase by 0.25 mcg/day at 4-8 week intervals; usual maintenance 0.5-2 mcg/day
Hectorol *Cap:* 0.25, 0.5 mcg

BISPHOSPHONATES (CALCIUM MODIFIERS)

Comment: Bisphosphonates should be swallowed whole in the AM with 6-8 oz of plain water 30 minutes before first meal, beverage, or other medications of the day. Monitor serum alkaline phosphatase. Contraindications include abnormalities of the esophagus which delay esophageal emptying such as stricture or achalasia, inability to stand or sit upright for at least 30 minutes post-dose, patients at risk of aspiration, and hypocalcemia. Co-administration of bisphosphonates and ***calcium***, antacids, or oral medications containing multivalent cations will interfere with absorption of the bisphosphonate. Therefore, instruct patients to wait at least half hour after taking the bisphosphonate before taking any other oral medications.

▶ ***alendronate (as sodium)*** (C)(G) <12 years: not recommended; ≥12 years: take once weekly, in the AM, 30 minutes before the first food, beverage, or medication of the day; do not lie down (remain upright) for at least 30 minutes and after the first food of the day; *CrCl <35 mL/min:* not recommended

Binosto dissolve the effervescent tab in 4 oz (120 ml) of plain, room temperature, water (not mineral or flavored); wait 5 minutes after the effervescence has subsided, then stir for 10 seconds, then drink

Tab: 70 mg effervescent for buffered solution (4, 12/carton) (strawberry)

Fosamax (G) swallow tab whole; dosing regimens are the same for males and females; *Prevention:* 5 mg once daily or 35 mg once weekly; *Treatment:* 10 mg once daily or 70 mg once weekly

Tab: 5, 10, 35, 40, 70 mg

▶ ***alendronate+cholecalciferol (vit d3)*** (C)(G) <12 years: not recommended; ≥12 years: take 1 tab once weekly, in the AM, with plain water (not mineral) 30 minutes before the first food, beverage, or medication of the day; do not lie down (remain upright) for at least 30 minutes and after the first food of the day

Fosamax Plus D

Tab: **Fosamax Plus D 70/2800**: alen 70 mg+chole 2,800 IU
Fosamax Plus D 70/5600: alen 70 mg+chole 5,600 IU

▶ ***ibandronate (as monosodium monohydrate)*** (C)(G) <18 years: not recommended; ≥18 years:

Boniva take 2.5 mg once daily or 150 mg once monthly on the same day; take in the AM, with plain water (not mineral) 60 minutes before the first food, beverage, or medication of the day; do not lie down (remain upright) for at least 30 minutes and after the first food of the day

Tab: 2.5, 150 mg

Boniva Injection administer 3 mg every 3 months by IV bolus over 15-30 seconds; if dose is missed, administer as soon as possible; then every 3 months from the date of the last dose

Prefilled syringe: 3 mg/3 ml (5 ml)

Comment: **Boniva Injection** must be administered by a healthcare professional.

▶ ***risedronate (as sodium)*** (C)(G) take in the AM; swallow whole with a full glass of plain water (not mineral); do not lie down (remain upright) for 30 minutes afterward

Actonel <12 years: not recommended; ≥12 years: take at least 30 minutes before any food or drink; *Females:* 5 mg once daily or 35 mg once weekly or 75 mg on two consecutive days monthly or 150 mg once monthly; *Males:* 35 mg once weekly

Tab: 5, 30, 35, 75, 150 mg

Atelvia <12 years: not recommended; ≥12 years: 35 mg once weekly immediately after breakfast

Tab: 35 mg del-rel

▶ ***risedronate+calcium*** (C) <12 years: not recommended; ≥12 years: 1 x 5 mg ***risedronate*** tab weekly plus 1 x 500 mg ***calcium*** tab on days 2-7 weekly

Actonel with Calcium *Tab:* ***risedronate*** 5 mg and *Tab:* ***calcium*** 500 mg (4 ***risedronate*** tabs + 30 ***calcium*** tabs/pck)

▶ ***zoledronic acid*** (D)(G)

Reclast <12 years: not recommended; ≥12 years: administer 5 mg via IV infusion over at least 15 minutes mg once a year (for osteoporosis) or once every 2 years (for osteopenia or prophylaxis)

Bottle: 5 mg/100 ml (single-dose)

Comment: **Reclast** is indicated for the treatment of postmenopausal osteoporosis in females who are at high risk for fracture and to increase bone mass in men with primary or hypogonadal osteoporosis who are at high risk for fracture. Administered by a healthcare professional. Contraindicated in hypocalcemia.

Zometa *Bottle:* 4 mg/5 ml administer 4 mg via IV infusion over at least 15 minutes every 3-4 weeks; optimal duration of treatment not known

Vial: 4 mg/5 ml (single-dose)

Comment: **Zometa** is indicated for the treatment of hypercalcemia of malignancy. The safety and efficacy of **Zometa** in the treatment of hypercalcemia associated with hyperparathyroidism or with other non-tumor-related conditions has not been established.

SELECTIVE ESTROGEN RECEPTOR MODULATOR (SERM)

▶ ***raloxifene*** **(X)(G)** <12 years: not recommended; ≥12 years: 60 mg once daily

Evista *Tab:* 60 mg

Comment: Contraindicated in females who have history of, or current, venous thrombotic event.

HUMAN PARATHYROID HORMONE

▶ ***teriparatide*** (C) <12 years: not recommended; ≥12 years: 20 mcg SC daily in the thigh or abdomen; may treat for up to 2 years

Forteo Multidose Pen *Multidose pen:* 250 mcg/ml (3 ml)

Comment: **Forteo** is indicated for the treatment of postmenopausal osteoporosis in females who are at high risk for fracture and to increase bone mass in men with primary or hypogonadal osteoporosis who are at high risk for fracture.

BIOENGINEERED REPLICA OF HUMAN PARATHYROID HORMONE

▶ ***bioengineered replica of human parathyroid hormone*** (C) <12 years: not recommended; ≥12 years: initially inject mg IM into the thigh once daily; when initiating, decrease dose of active ***vitamin D*** by 50% if serum ***calcium*** is above 7.5 mg/dL; monitor serum ***calcium*** levels every 3 to 7 days after starting or adjusting dose and when adjusting either active ***vitamin D*** or ***calcium*** supplements dose

Natpara *Soln for inj:* 25, 50, 75, 100 mcg (2/pkg) multi-dose, dual-chamber glass cartridge containing a sterile powder and diluent

Comment: **Natpara** is indicated as adjunct to ***calcium*** and ***vitamin D*** in patients with parathyroidism.

OSTEOCLAST INHIBITOR (RANK LIGAND [RANKL] INHIBITOR

▶ ***denosumab*** (X) <18 years: not established; treatment with ***denosumab*** may impair bone growth in children with open growth plates and may inhibit eruption of dentition. ≥18 years: administer 120 mg SC 4 every weeks with additional 120 mg doses on Days 8 and 15 of the first month of therapy and administer ***calcium*** and ***vitamin D*** as necessary to treat or prevent hypocalcemia

Xgeva *Vial:* 120 mg/1.7 ml (70 mg/ml) solution in a single-dose

Comment: ***denosumab*** is indicated for treatment of skeletally mature adolescents with giant cell tumor of bone; CrCl < 30 mL/min or receiving dialysis are at risk for hypocalcemia. Adequately supplement with ***calcium*** and ***vitamin D***. There is no information regarding the presence of ***denosumab*** in human milk or effects on the breastfed infant. To report suspected adverse reactions, contact Amgen Inc. at 1-800-77-AMGEN (1-800-772-6436) or FDA at 1-800-FDA-1088 or visit www.fda.gov/medwatch

OTITIS EXTERNA

OTIC ANALGESIC

▶ ***antipyrine+benzocaine+zinc acetate dihydrate*** (C) fill ear canal with solution; then insert a cotton plug into meatus; may repeat every 1-2 hours prn
  Otozin *Otic soln:* antipyr 5.4%+benz 1%+zinc 1% per ml (10 ml w. dropper)

OTIC ANTI-INFECTIVE

▶ ***chloroxylenol+pramoxine*** (C) <1 year: not recommended; 1-12 years: 5 drops bid x 10 days; >12 years: 4-5 drops tid x 5-10 days
  PramOtic *Otic drops:* chlorox+pramox (5 ml w. dropper)

▶ ***finafloxacin*** (C) <1 year: not recommended; ≥1 year: 4-5 drops tid x 5-10 days
  Xtoro *Otic soln:* 0.3% (5, 8 ml)

▶ ***ofloxacin*** (C)(G) <1 year: not recommended; 1-12 years: 5 drops bid x 10 days; >12 years: 10 drops bid x 10 days
  Floxin Otic *Otic soln:* 0.3% (5, 10 ml w. dropper; 0.25 ml, 5 drop singles, 20/carton)
  Comment: **Floxin Otic** is indicated for patients ≥18 years with perforated tympanic membranes and pediatric patients with PE tubes.

OTIC ANTI-INFECTIVE+CORTICOSTEROID COMBINATIONS

▶ ***chloroxylenol+pramoxine+hydrocortisone*** (C) <12 years: 3 drops tid-qid x 5-10 days; ≥12 years: 4 drops tid-qid x 5-10 days
  Cortane B, Cortane B Aqueous *Otic soln:* chlo 1 mg+pram 10 mg+hydro 10 mg per ml (10 ml w. dropper)
  Comment: **Cortane B Aqueous** may be used to saturate a cotton wick.

▶ ***ciprofloxacin+hydrocortisone*** (C) <1 year: not recommended; ≥1 year: 3 drops bid x 7 days
  Cipro HC Otic *Otic susp:* cipro 0.2%+hydro 1% (10 ml w. dropper)

▶ ***ciprofloxacin+dexamethasone*** (C) <6 months: not recommended; ≥6 months: 4 drops bid x 7 days
  Ciprodex *Otic susp:* cipro 0.3%+dexa 1% (7.5 ml)
  Comment: **Ciprodex** is indicated for the treatment of otitis media in pediatric patients with tympanostomy tubes.

▶ ***colistin+neomycin+hydrocortisone+thonzonium*** (C) <12 years: 4 drops tid-qid x 5-10 days; ≥12 years: 5 drops tid or qid x 5-10 days
  Coly-Mycin S *Otic susp:* 5, 10 ml
  Cortisporin-TC Otic *Otic susp:* colis 3 mg+neo 3.3 mg+hydro 10 mg+thon 0.5 mg per ml (10 ml w. dropper) (thimerosal)

▶ ***polymyxin b+neomycin+hydrocortisone*** (C) <12 years: 3 drops tid-qid; max 10 days; 4 drops tid-qid; ≥12 years: max 10 days
  Cortisporin Otic Suspension *Otic susp:* poly b 10,000 u+neo 3.5 mg+hydro 10 mg per 5 ml (10 ml w. dropper)
  Cortisporin Otic Solution *Otic soln:* poly b 10000 u+neo 3.5 mg+hydro 10 mg per 5 ml (10 ml w. dropper)

OTIC ASTRINGENTS

▶ ***acetic acid 2% in aluminum sulfate*** (C) 4-6 drops q 2-3 hours
  Domeboro Otic *Otic soln:* 60 ml w. dropper

▶ ***acetic acid+propylene glycol+benzethonium chloride+sodium acetate*** (C) 3-5 drops q 4-6 hours
  VoSol *Otic soln:* acet 2% (15, 30 ml)

▶ ***acetic acid+propylene glycol+hydrocortisone+benzethonium chloride+sodium acetate*** (C) 3-5 drops q 4-6 hours
  VoSol HC *Otic soln:* acet 2%+hydro 1% (10 ml)

OTIC ANESTHETIC+ANALGESIC COMBINATIONS

▶ ***antipyrine+benzocaine+glycerine*** (C) fill ear canal and insert cotton plug; may repeat q 1-2 hours
  A/B Otic *Otic soln:* 15 ml w. dropper

▶ ***benzocaine*** (C) <1 year: not recommended; ≥1 year: 4-5 drops q 1-2 hours
  Americaine Otic *Otic soln:* 20% (15 ml w. dropper)
  Benzotic *Otic soln:* 20% (15 ml w. dropper)

SYSTEMIC ANTI-INFECTIVES

Comment: Used for severe disease or with culture.

▶ ***amoxicillin+clavulanate*** (B)(G)
  Augmentin <40 kg: 40-45 mg/kg/day divided tid x 10 days or 90 mg/kg/day divided bid x 10 days; *see page* 590 *for dose by weight table;* ≥40 kg: 500 mg tid or 875 mg bid x 10 days
    Tab: 250, 500, 875 mg; *Chew tab:* 125, 250 mg (lemon-lime); 200, 400 mg (cherry-banana) (phenylalanine); *Oral susp:* 125 mg/5 ml (banana), 250 mg/5 ml (75, 100, 150 ml) (orange); 200, 400 mg/5 ml (50, 75, 100 ml) (orange) (phenylalanine)
  Augmentin ES-600 <3 months: not recommended; ≥3 months, <40 kg: 90 mg/kg/day divided q 12 hours x 10 days; *see page* 591 *for dose by weight table;* ≥40 kg: not recommended
    Oral susp: 600 mg/5 ml (50, 75, 100, 125, 150, 200 ml) (strawberry cream) (phenylalanine)
  Augmentin XR <16 years: use other forms; ≥16 years: 2 tabs q 12 hours x 7-10 days
    Tab: 1000*mg ext-rel

▶ ***cefaclor*** (B)(G) <1 month: not recommended; 1 month-12 years: 20-40 mg/kg in 2 or 3 divided doses x 10 days; *see page* 594 *for dose by weight table;* max 1 gm/day; >12 years: 250-500 mg q 8 hours x 7-10 days; max 2 gm/day
    Tab: 500 mg; *Cap:* 250, 500 mg; *Susp:* 125 mg/5 ml (75, 150 ml) (strawberry); 187 mg/5 ml (50, 100 ml) (strawberry); 250 mg/5 ml (75, 150 ml) (strawberry); 375 mg/5 ml (50, 100 ml) (strawberry)
  Cefaclor Extended Release <16 years: not recommended; ≥16 years: 500 mg bid x 10 days; clinically equivalent to 250 mg immed-rel caps tid; swallow whole; take with meals
    Tab: 375, 500 mg ext-rel

▶ ***dicloxacillin*** (B) <12 years: 12.5-25 mg/kg/day in 4 divided doses x 10 days; *see page* 604 *for dose by weight table;* ≥12 years: 500 mg q 6 hours x 10 days
  Dynapen *Cap:* 125, 250, 500 mg; *Oral susp:* 62.5 mg/5 ml (80, 100, 200 ml)

▶ ***trimethoprim+sulfamethoxazole [TMP-SMX]*** (C)(G)
  Bactrim, Septra <12 years: not recommended; ≥12 years: 2 tabs bid x 10 days
    Tab: trim 80 mg+sulfa 400 mg*
  Bactrim DS, Septra DS <12 years: not recommended; ≥12 years: 1 tab bid x 10 days
    Tab: trim 160 mg+sulfa 800 mg*
  Bactrim Pediatric Suspension, Septra Pediatric Suspension <2 months: not recommended; ≥2 months-12 years: 40 mg/kg/day of ***sulfamethoxazole*** in 2 doses bid; >12 years: use tabs
    Oral susp: trim 40 mg+sulfa 200 mg per 5 ml (100 ml) (cherry) (alcohol 0.3%)

OTITIS MEDIA: ACUTE

OTIC ANALGESIC

▶ ***antipyrine+benzocaine+zinc acetate dihydrate*** otic **(C)** fill ear canal with solution; then insert cotton plug into meatus; may repeat every 1-2 hours prn
Otozin *Otic soln:* antipyr 5.4%+benz 1%+zinc1% per ml (10 ml w. dropper)

SYSTEMIC ANTI-INFECTIVES

▶ ***amoxicillin*** (B)(G) <40 kg (88 lb): 80-100 mg/kg/day divided q 12 hours x 10 days; *see page* 588 *for dose by weight table;* ≥40 kg: 500-875 mg bid or 250-500 mg tid x 10 days
Amoxil *Cap:* 250, 500 mg; *Tab:* 875*mg; *Chew tab:* 125, 200, 250, 400 mg (cherry-banana-peppermint) (phenylalanine); *Oral susp:* 125, 250 mg/5 ml (80, 100, 150 ml) (strawberry); 200, 400 mg/5 ml (50, 75, 100 ml) (bubble gum); *Oral drops:* 50 mg/ml (30 ml) (bubble gum)
Moxatag *Tab:* 775 mg ext-rel
Trimox *Tab:* 125, 250 mg; *Cap:* 250, 500 mg; *Oral susp:* 125, 250 mg/5 ml (80, 100, 150 ml) (raspberry-strawberry)
Comment: Consider 80-90 mg/kg/day in 3 divided doses for resistant for cases

▶ ***amoxicillin+clavulanate*** (B)(G)
Augmentin <40 kg: 40-45 mg/kg/day divided tid x 10 days or 90 mg/kg/day divided bid x 10 days; *see page* 590 *for dose by weight table;* ≥40 kg: 500 mg tid or 875 mg bid x 10 days
Tab: 250, 500, 875 mg; *Chew tab:* 125, 250 mg (lemon-lime); 200, 400 mg (cherry-banana) (phenylalanine); *Oral susp:* 125 mg/5 ml (banana), 250 mg/5 ml (75, 100, 150 ml) (orange); 200, 400 mg/5 ml (50, 75, 100 ml) (orange) (phenylalanine)
Augmentin ES-600 <3 months: not recommended; ≥3 months, <40 kg: 90 mg/kg/day divided q 12 hours x 10 days; *see page* 591 *for dose by weight table;* ≥40 kg: not recommended
Oral susp: 600 mg/5 ml (50, 75, 100, 125, 150, 200 ml) (strawberry cream) (phenylalanine)
Augmentin XR <16 years: use other forms; ≥16 years: 2 tabs q 12 hours x 7-10 days
Tab: 1000*mg ext-rel

▶ ***ampicillin*** (B) <12 years: 50-100 mg/kg/day in 4 divided doses x 10 days; *see page* 592 *for dose by weight table;* ≥12 years: 250-500 mg qid x 10 days
Omnipen, Principen *Cap:* 250, 500 mg; *Oral susp:* 125, 250 mg/5 ml (100, 150, 200 ml) (fruit)

▶ ***azithromycin*** (B)(G) <12 years: 12 mg/kg/day x 5 days; *see page* 593 *for dose by weight table*; max 500 mg/day; ≥12 years: 500 mg x 1 dose on day 1, then 250 mg daily on days 2-5 or 500 mg daily x 3 days or **Zmax** 2 gm in a single dose
Zithromax *Tab:* 250, 500, 600 mg; *Oral susp:* 100 mg/5 ml (15 ml); 200 mg/5 ml (15, 22.5, 30 ml) (cherry); *Pkt:* 1 gm for reconstitution (cherry-banana)
Zithromax Tri-pak *Tab:* 3 x 500 mg tabs/pck
Zithromax Z-pak *Tab:* 6 x 250 mg tabs/pck
Zmax *Oral susp:* 2 gm ext-rel for reconstitution (cherry-banana) (148 mg Na^+)

▶ ***cefaclor*** (B)(G) <1 month: not recommended; 1 month-12 years: 20-40 mg/kg divided bid x 10 days; *see page* 594 *for dose by weight table;* max 1 gm/day; >12 years: 250-500 mg q 8 hours x 10 days; max 2 gm/day
Tab: 500 mg; *Cap:* 250, 500 mg; *Susp:* 125 mg/5 ml (75, 150 ml) (strawberry); 187 mg/5 ml (50, 100 ml) (strawberry); 250 mg/5 ml (75, 150 ml) (strawberry); 375 mg/5 ml (50, 100 ml) (strawberry)

Cefaclor Extended Release <16 years: not recommended; ≥16 years: 500 mg bid x 10 days (clinically equivalent to 250 mg immed-rel caps tid); swallow whole; take with meals

Tab: 375, 500 mg ext-rel

▶ ***cefdinir*** **(B)** <6 months: not recommended; 6 months-12 years: 14 mg/kg/day in 1-2 divided doses x 10 days; *see page* 596 *for dose by weight table;* ≥12 years: 300 mg bid x 10 days or 600 mg daily x 10 days

Omnicef *Cap:* 300 mg; *Oral susp:* 125 mg/5 ml (60, 100 ml) (strawberry)

▶ ***cefixime*** **(B)(G)** <6 months: not recommended; 6 months-12 years, <50 kg: 8 mg/kg/day in 1-2 divided doses x 10 days; *see page* 597 *for dose by weight table;* >12 years, >50 kg: 400 mg once daily x 10 days

Suprax *Tab:* 400 mg; *Cap:* 400 mg; *Oral susp:* 100, 200, 500 mg/5 ml (50, 75, 100 ml) (strawberry)

▶ ***cefpodoxime proxetil*** **(B)** <2 months: not recommended; 2 months-12 years: 10 mg/kg/day (max 400 mg/dose) or 5 mg/kg/day bid (max 200 mg/dose) x 5 days; *see page* 598 *for dose by weight table;* >12 years: 100 mg bid x 5 days

Vantin *Tab:* 100, 200 mg; *Oral susp:* 50, 100 mg/5 ml (50, 75, 100 mg) (lemon creme)

▶ ***cefprozil*** **(B)** ≤6 months: not recommended; 6 months-12 years: 7.5 mg/kg bid x 10 days; *see page* 599 *for dose by weight table;* >12 years: 250-500 mg bid or 500 mg daily x 10 days

Cefzil *Tab:* 250, 500 mg; *Oral susp:* 125, 250 mg/5 ml (50, 75, 100 ml) (bubble gum) (phenylalanine)

▶ ***ceftibuten*** **(B)** <12 years: 9 mg/kg daily x 10 days; max 400 mg/day; *see page* 600 *for dose by weight table;* ≥12 years: 400 mg daily x 10 days

Cedax *Cap:* 400 mg; *Oral susp:* 90 mg/5 ml (30, 60, 90, 120 ml); 180 mg/5 ml (30, 60, 120 ml) (cherry)

▶ ***ceftriaxone*** **(B)(G)** <12 years: 50 mg/kg IM x 1 dose; ≥12 years: 1-2 gm IM x 1 dose; max 4 gm

Rocephin *Vial:* 250, 500 mg; 1, 2 gm

▶ ***cephalexin*** **(B)(G)** <12 years: 25-50 mg/kg/day in 4 divided doses x 10 days; *see page* 601 *for dose by weight table;* ≥12 years: 250 mg qid x 10 days

Keflex *Cap:* 250, 333, 500, 750 mg; *Oral susp:* 125, 250 mg/5 ml (100, 200 ml) (strawberry) roxycodone

▶ ***clarithromycin*** **(C)(G)** <6 months: not recommended; ≥6 months-12 years: 7.5 mg/kg divided bid x 7 days; *see page* 602 *for dose by weight table;* >12 years: 500 mg bid or 500 mg ext-rel daily

Biaxin *Tab:* 250, 500 mg

Biaxin Oral Suspension *Oral susp:* 125, 250 mg/5 ml (50, 100 ml) (fruit punch)

Biaxin XL *Tab:* 500 mg ext-rel

Comment: The FDA is advising caution before prescribing ***clarithromycin*** to patients with heart disease because of a potential increased risk of heart problems or death that can occur years later. This recommendation is based on a review of the results of a 10-year follow-up study of patients with coronary heart disease from a large clinical trial that first observed this safety issue. Consider risk benefit and the use of other antibiotics in such patients.

▶ ***erythromycin+sulfisoxazole*** **(C)(G)** <2 months: not recommended; ≥2 months: 50 mg/kg/day in 3 divided doses x 10 days

Eryzole *Oral susp:* eryth 200 mg+sulf 600 mg per 5 ml (100, 150, 200, 250 ml)

Pediazole *Oral susp:* eryth 200 mg+sulf 600 mg per 5 ml (100, 150, 200 ml) (strawberry-banana)

Comment: ***erythromycin*** may increase INR with concomitant ***warfarin***, as well as increase serum level of ***digoxin***, benzodiazepines, and statins. ***Sulfamethoxazole*** is not recommended in pregnancy or lactation. *CrCl 15-30 mL/min*: reduce dose by 1/2; *CrCl <15 mL/min*: not recommended.

- *loracarbef* (B) <12 years: 30 mg/kg/day in 2 divided doses x 10 days; *see page* 614 *for dose by weight table*; ≥12 years: 400 mg bid x 10 days
  Lorabid *Pulvule:* 200, 400 mg; *Oral susp:* 100 mg/5 ml (50, 100 ml); 200 mg/5 ml (50, 75, 100 ml) (strawberry bubble gum)
- *trimethoprim+sulfamethoxazole [TMP-SMX]* (C)(G)
  Bactrim, Septra <12 years: not recommended; ≥12 years: 2 tabs bid x 10 days
  Tab: trim 80 mg+sulfa 400 mg*
  Bactrim DS, Septra DS <12 years: not recommended; ≥12 years: 1 tab bid x 10 days
  Tab: trim 160 mg+sulfa 800 mg*
  Bactrim Pediatric Suspension, Septra Pediatric Suspension <2 months: not recommended; ≥2 months-12 years: 40 mg/kg/day of in 2 doses bid; >12 years: use tabs
  Oral susp: trim 40 mg+sulfa 200 mg per 5 ml (100 ml) (cherry) (alcohol 0.3%)

OTIC ANTI-INFECTIVE

- *ofloxacin* (C)(G) <6 months: not recommended; 6 months-12 years: 5 drops bid x 14 days; >12 years: 10 drops bid x 14 days
  Floxin Otic *Otic soln:* 0.3% (5, 10 ml w. dropper)

Comment: ***ofloxacin*** may be used with patients with perforated tympanic membrane or tympanostomy tubes.

OTIC ANTI-INFECTIVE+CORTICOSTEROID COMBINATIONS

Comment: ***neomycin*** may cause ototoxicity. Do not use with known or suspected tympanic membrane rupture.

- *chloroxylenol+pramoxine+hydrocortisone* (C) <12 years: 3 drops tid-qid x 5-10 days; ≥12 years: 4 drops tid-qid x 5-10 days
  Cortane Ear Drops, *Otic drops:* 10 ml
- *ciprofloxacin+hydrocortisone* (C) <1 year: not recommended; ≥1 year: 3 drops bid x 7 days
  Cipro HC *Otic susp:* cipro 0.3%+hydroc 0.1% (10 ml)
- *ciprofloxacin+dexamethasone* (C) <6 months: not recommended; ≥6 months: 4 drops bid x 7 days
  Ciprodex *Otic susp:* cipro 0.3%+dexa 1% (7.5 ml)
  Comment: **Ciprodex** is indicated for the treatment of otitis media in pediatric patients with tympanostomy tubes (PE tubes).
- *colistin+neomycin+hydrocortisone+thonzonium* (C) <12 years: 4 drops tid-qid x 5-10 days; ≥12 years: 5 drops tid-qid x 5-10 days
  Coly-Mycin S *Otic susp:* 5, 10 ml
- *polymyxin b+neomycin+hydrocortisone* (C)(G) <12 years: 3 drops tid-qid; max 10 days; ≥12 years: 4 drops tid-qid; max 10 days
  Cortisporin *Otic susp:* 10 ml w. dropper; *Otic soln:* 10 ml w. dropper
  PediOtic *Otic susp:* 7.5 ml w. dropper
- *polymyxin b+neomycin+hydrocortisone+surfactant* (C) <12 years: 3 drops tid-qid; max 10 days; ≥12 years: 4 drops tid-qid
  Cortisporin-TC *Otic susp:* 10 ml w. dropper

OTIC ANESTHETIC+ANALGESIC COMBINATIONS

- *antipyrine+benzocaine+glycerine* (C) fill ear canal and insert cotton plug; may repeat q 1-2 hours as needed
  A/B Otic *Otic soln:* antipy 5.4%+benzo 1.4% 15 ml w. dropper

▶ *benzocaine* (C)(OTC)(G) <1 year: not recommended; ≥1 year: 4-5 drops q 1-2 hours
  Americaine Otic *Otic soln:* 15 ml w. dropper
  Benzotic *Otic soln:* 20% (15 ml w. dropper)

OTITIS MEDIA: SEROUS

Anti-infectives *see* ***Otitis Media: Acute*** *page* 318
Antihistamines and **Decongestants** ***see*** **Drugs for the Management of Allergy, Cough, and Cold Symptoms** *page* 570
Oral Corticosteroids *see page* 546

PAGET'S DISEASE: BONE

Comment: Calcium decreases ***tetracycline*** absorption. **calcium** absorption is decreased by corticosteroids. **calcium** absorption is decreased by foods such as rhubarb, spinach, and bran.

BISPHOSPHONATES (CALCIUM MODIFIERS)

Comment: Bisphosphonates should be swallowed whole in the AM with 6-8 oz of plain water 30 minutes before first meal, beverage, or other medications of the day. Monitor serum alkaline phosphatase. Contraindications include abnormalities of the esophagus, which delay esophageal emptying such as stricture or achalasia, inability to stand or sit upright for at least 30 minutes post-dose, patients at risk of aspiration, and hypocalcemia. Co-administration of bisphosphonates and calcium, antacids, or oral medications containing multivalent cations will interfere with absorption of the bisphosphonate. Therefore, instruct patients to wait at least half hour after taking the bisphosphonate before taking any other oral medications.

▶ ***alendronate (as sodium)*** (C) <12 years: not recommended; ≥12 years: take once weekly, in the AM, 30 minutes before the first food, beverage, or medication of the day; do not lie down (remain upright) for at least 30 minutes and after the first food of the day; not recommended with *CrCl <35 mL/min.*
  Binosto dissolve the effervescent tab in 4 oz (120 ml) of plain, room temperature, water (not mineral or flavored); wait 5 minutes after the effervescence has subsided, then stir for 10 seconds, then drink
    Tab: 70 mg effervescent for buffered solution (4, 12/carton) (strawberry)
  Fosamax (G) swallow tab whole; *Prevention:* 5 mg once daily or 35 mg once weekly; *Treatment:* 10 mg once daily or 70 mg once weekly
    Tab: 5, 10, 35, 40, 70 mg

▶ ***alendronate+cholecalciferol (vit d3)*** (C)(G) 12 years: not recommended; ≥12 years: take 1 tab once weekly, in the AM, with plain water (not mineral) 30 minutes before the first food, beverage, or medication of the day; do not lie down (remain upright) for at least 30 minutes and after the first food of the day
  Fosamax Plus D
    Tab: **Fosamax Plus D 70/2800** alen 70 mg+chole 2800 IU
    Fosamax Plus D 70/5600 alen 70 mg+chole 5600 IU

▶ ***ibandronate (as monosodium monohydrate)*** (C)(G) <12 years: not recommended; ≥12 years:
  Boniva take 2.5 mg once daily or 150 mg once monthly on the same day; take in the AM, with plain water (not mineral) 60 minutes before the first food, beverage, or medication of the day; do not lie down (remain upright) for at least 30 minutes and after the first food of the day
    Tab: 2.5, 150 mg

Boniva Injection administer 3 mg every 3 months by IV bolus over 15-30 seconds; if dose is missed, administer as soon as possible, then every 3 months from the date of the last dose

Prefilled syringe: 3 mg/3 ml (5 ml)

Comment: **Boniva Injection** must be administered by a qualified healthcare professional.

▶ ***risedronate (as sodium)*** **(C)(G)** <12 years: not recommended; ≥12 years: take in the AM; swallow whole with a full glass of plain water (not mineral) do not lie down (remain upright) for 30 minutes afterward

Actonel take at least 30 minutes before any food or drink; *Females:* 5 mg once daily or 35 mg once weekly or 75 mg on two consecutive days monthly or 150 mg once monthly; *Males:* 35 mg once weekly; *Tab:* 5, 30, 35, 75, 150 mg

Atelvia 35 mg once weekly immediately after breakfast

Tab: 35 mg del-rel

▶ ***risedronate+calcium*** **(C)** 1 x 5 mg ***risedronate*** tab weekly and 1 x 500 mg ***calcium*** tab on days 2-7 weekly

Actonel with Calcium *Tab:* ***risedronate*** 5 mg and *Tab:* **calcium** 500 mg (4 ***risedronate*** tabs + 30 ***calcium*** tabs/pck)

▶ ***zoledronic acid*** **(D)(G)** <12 years: not recommended; ≥12 years:

Reclast administer 5 mg via IV infusion over at least 15 minutes mg once a year (for osteoporosis) or once every 2 years (for osteopenia or prophylaxis)

Bottle: 5 mg/100 ml (single-dose)

Comment: **Reclast** is indicated for the treatment of postmenopausal osteoporosis in females who are at high risk for fracture and to increase bone mass in men with primary or hypogonadal osteoporosis who are at high risk for fracture. Must be administered by a qualified healthcare professional. Contraindicated in hypocalcemia.

Zometa administer 4 mg via IV infusion over at least 15 minutes every 3-4 weeks; optimal duration of treatment not known

Bottle: 4 mg/5 ml; *Vial:* 4 mg/5 ml (single-dose)

Comment: **Zometa** is indicated for the treatment of hypercalcemia of malignancy. The safety and efficacy of **Zometa** in the treatment of hypercalcemia associated with hyperparathyroidism or with other nontumor-related conditions has not been established.

PAIN

Antidepressants *see* ***Depression*** *page* 108
Skeletal Muscle Relaxants *see* ***Muscle Strain*** *page* 287

ACETAMINOPHEN FOR IV INFUSION

▶ ***acetaminophen*** injectable **(B)** <2 years: not recommended; 2-<13 years, <50 kg: 15 mg/kg q 6 hours prn or 2.5 mg/kg q 4 hours prn; max single dose 750 mg; max 75 mg/kg per day; ≥13 years: administer by IV infusion over 15 minutes; 1,000 mg q 6 hours prn or 650 mg q 4 hours prn; max 4,000 mg/day

Ofirmev *Vial:* 10 mg/ml (100 ml) (preservative-free)

Comment: The **Ofirmev** vial is intended for single use. If any portion is withdrawn from the vial, use within 6 hours. Discard the unused portion. For pediatric patients, withdraw the intended dose and administer via syringe pump. Do not admix **Ofirmev** with any other drugs. **Ofirmev** is physically incompatible with ***diazepam*** and ***chlorpromazine hydrochloride***.

IBUPROFEN FOR IV INFUSION

▶ ***ibuprofen*** **(B)** <6 months; not recommended; 6 months-<12 years: 10 mg/kg q 4-6 hours prn; max 400 mg/dose; max 40 mg/kg <u>or</u> 2,400 mg/24 hours, whichever is less; 12-<17 years: 400 mg q 4-6 hours prn; max 2,400 mg/24 hours; ≥17 years: dilute dose in 0.9% NS, D5W, <u>or</u> Lactated Ringers (LR) solution; administer by IV infusion over at least 10 minutes; do not administer via IV bolus <u>or</u> IM; 400-800 mg q 6 hours prn; maximum 3,200 mg/day

Caldolor *Vial:* 800 mg/8 ml single-dose

Comment: Prepare **Caldolor** solution for IV administration as follows: 100 mg dose: dilute 1 ml of **Caldolor** in at least 100 ml of diluent (IVF); 200 mg dose: dilute 2 ml of **Caldolor** in at least 100 ml of diluent; 400 mg dose: dilute 4 ml of **Caldolor** in at least 100 ml of diluent; 800 mg dose: dilute 8 ml of **Caldolor** in at least 200 ml of diluent. **Caldolor** is also indicated for management of fever. For patients ≥18 years-of-age with fever, 400 mg via IV infusion, followed by 400 mg q 4-6 hours <u>or</u> 100-200 mg q 4 hours prn.

OCULAR PAIN

▶ ***difluprednate*** **(C)** <12 years: not recommended; ≥12 years: apply 1 drop to affected eye qid; for post-op ocular pain, begin treatment 24 hours post-op and continue x 2 weeks; then bid daily x 1 week; then taper

Durezol *Ophth emul:* 0.05% (5 ml)

Comment: **Durezol** is an ophthalmic steroid.

▶ ***nepafenac*** **(C)** <10 years: not recommended; ≥10 years: apply 1 drop to affected eye tid; for post-op ocular pain, begin treatment 24 hours before surgery and continue day of surgery and for two weeks post-op

Nevanac *Ophth susp:* 0.1% (3 ml) (benzalkonium chloride)

Comment: **Nevanac** is an ophthalmic NSAID.

TOPICAL & TRANSDERMAL NSAIDs

▶ ***capsaicin*** cream **(B)(G)** <2 years: not recommended; 2-12 years: apply sparingly to intact skin bid prn; >12 years: apply tid-qid prn

Axsain *Crm:* 0.075% (1, 2 oz)
Capsin (OTC) *Lotn:* 0.025, 0,075% (59 ml)
Capzasin-P (OTC) *Crm:* 0.025% (1.5 oz); *Lotn:* 0.025% (2 oz)
Capzasin-HP (OTC) *Crm:* 0.075% (1.5 oz); *Lotn:* 0.075% (2 oz)
Dolorac *Crm:* 0.025% (28 gm)
Double Cap (OTC) *Crm:* 0.05% (2 oz)
R-Gel *Gel:* 0.025% (15, 30 gm)
Zostrix (OTC) *Crm:* 0.025% (0.7, 1.5, 3 oz)
Zostrix HP (OTC) *Emol crm:* 0.075% (1, 2 oz)

Comment: Provides some relief by 1-2 weeks; optimal benefit may take 4-6 weeks. Avoid contact with mucous membranes.

▶ ***capsaicin*** 8% patch **(B)** <18 years: not recommended; ≥18 years: apply sparingly tid-qid prn apply up to 4 patches for one 60-minute application to clean dry skin; may prep area with topical anesthetic; wear non-latex gloves; patches may be cut to size/shape; treatment may be repeated every 3 months; remove with cleansing gel after treatment

Qutenza *Patch:* 8% 1640 mcg/cm (179 mg) (1 <u>or</u> 2 patches, each w. 1-50 gm tube cleansing gel/carton)

▶ ***diclofenac epolamine transdermal patch*** **(C; D ≥30 wks)** <12 years: not recommended; ≥12 years: apply one patch to affected area bid; remove during bathing; avoid non-intact skin

Flector Patch *Patch:* 180 mg/patch (30/carton)

▶ ***diclofenac epolamine transdermal patch*** **(C; D ≥30 wks)** <12 years: not recommended; ≥12 years: apply sparingly tid-qid prn apply one patch to affected area bid; remove during bathing; avoid non-intact skin

Flector Patch *Patch:* 180 mg/patch (30/carton)

▶ ***diclofenac sodium*** **(C; D ≥30 wks)(G)**

Comment: ***diclofenac*** is contraindicated with ***aspirin*** allergy and should be avoided in late pregnancy (≥30 weeks) because it may cause premature closure of the ductus arteriosus.

Pennsaid 1.5% <12 years: not recommended; ≥12 years: in 10 drop increments, dispense and rub into front, side, and back of knee: usually; 40 drops (40 mg) qid

Topical soln: 1.5% (150 ml)

Pennsaid 2% <12 years: not recommended; ≥12 years: apply 2 pump actuations (40 mg) and rub into front, side, and back of knee bid

Topical soln: 2% (20 mg/pump actuation, 112 gm)

Comment: **Pennsaid** is indicated for the treatment of pain associated with osteoarthritis of the knee.

Solaraze Gel <12 years: not recommended; ≥12 years:

Gel: 3% (50 gm) (benzyl alcohol)

Voltaren Gel <12 years: not recommended; ≥12 years: apply qid; avoid non-intact skin

Gel: 1% (100 gm)

TOPICAL & TRANSDERMAL LIDOCAINE

▶ ***lidocaine*** transdermal patch **(C)(G)** <12 years: not recommended; ≥12 years: apply one patch to affected area for 12 hours (then off for 12 hours); remove during bathing; avoid non-intact skin; do not reuse

Lidoderm *Patch:* 5% (10 cm x 14 cm, 30/carton)

OPIOID ANALGESICS

▶ ***benzhydrocodone+acetaminophen*** **(II)** <18 years: not recommended; ≥18 years: initiate treatment with at 1-2 tabs every 4 to 6 hours prn; max 12 tabs/24 hours; max 14 days

Apadaz *Tab:* benz 6.12 mg+acet 325 mg

Comment: ***benzhydrocodone*** 6.12 mg is equivalent to 4.54 mg ***hydrocodone*** or 7.5 mg ***hydrocodone bitartrate***. If switching from immediate-release ***hydrocodone bitartrate+acetaminophen***, substitute **Apadaz** 6.12 mg/325 mg for 7.5 mg/325 mg ***hydrocodone bitartrate+acetaminophen***. Dosage of **Apadaz** should be adjusted according to the severity of the pain and the response of the patient. Do not stop **Apadaz** abruptly in the physically-dependent patient.

▶ ***butalbital+acetaminophen*** **(C)(G)** <12 years: not recommended; ≥12 years: 1 tab q 4 hours prn; max 6 tabs/day

Tab: but 50 mg+acet 325 mg

Phrenilin 1-2 tabs q 4 hours prn; max 6 tabs/day

Tab: but 50 mg+acet 325 mg

Phrenilin Forte 1 tab or cap q 4 hours prn; max 6 caps/day

Cap: but 50 mg+acet 325 mg; *Tab:* but 50 mg+acet 325 mg

▶ ***butalbital+acetaminophen+caffeine*** **(C)(G)** <12 years: not recommended; ≥12 years:

Fioricet 1-2 tabs q 4 hours prn; max 6/day

Tab: but 50 mg+acet 325 mg+caf 40 mg

Zebutal 1 cap q 4 hours prn; max 5/day

Cap: but 50 mg+acet 325 mg+caf 40 mg

▶ ***butalbital+aspirin+caffeine*** (C)(III)(G)

Fiorinal <12 years: not recommended; ≥12 years: 1-2 tabs or caps q 4 hours prn; max 6 caps/day

Tab/Cap: but 50 mg+asp 325 mg+caf 40 mg

Comment: ***aspirin***-containing medications are contraindicated with history of allergic-type reaction to ***aspirin***, children and adolescents with *Varicella* or other viral illness, and 3rd trimester of pregnancy.

▶ ***butalbital+aspirin+codeine+caffeine*** (C)(III)(G)

Fiorinal with Codeine <12 years: contraindicated; 12-<18: use extreme caution; not recommended for children and adolescents with obesity, asthma, obstructive sleep apnea, or other chronic breathing problem, or for post-tonsillectomy/adenoidectomy pain; ≥18 years: 1-2 caps q 4 hours prn; max 6 caps/day

Cap: but 50 mg+asp 325 mg+cod 30 mg+caf 40 mg

Comment: ***codeine*** is known to be excreted in breast milk. <12 years: not recommended; 12-<18: use extreme caution; not recommended for children and adolescents with asthma or other chronic breathing problem. The FDA and the European Medicines Agency (EMA) are investigating the safety of using ***codeine*** containing medications to treat pain, cough and colds, in children 12-<18 years because of the potential for serious side effects, including slowed or difficult breathing. ***aspirin***-containing medications are contraindicated with history of allergic-type reaction to ***aspirin***, children and adolescents with *Varicella* or other viral illness, and 3rd trimester of pregnancy.

▶ ***codeine sulfate*** (C)(III)(G) <12 years: contraindicated; 12-<18: use extreme caution; not recommended for children and adolescents with obesity, asthma, obstructive sleep apnea, or other chronic breathing problem, or for post-tonsillectomy/adenoidectomy pain; ≥18 years: 15-60 q 4-6 hours prn; max 60 mg/day

Tab: 15, 30, 60 mg

Comment: ***codeine*** is known to be excreted in breast milk. <12 years: not recommended; 12-<18: use extreme caution; not recommended for children and adolescents with asthma or other chronic breathing problem. The FDA and the European Medicines Agency (EMA) are investigating the safety of using ***codeine*** containing medications to treat pain, cough and colds, in children 12-<18 years because of the potential for serious side effects, including slowed or difficult breathing.

▶ ***codeine+acetaminophen*** (C)(III)(G) <12 years: contraindicated; 12-<18: use extreme caution; not recommended for children and adolescents with obesity, asthma, obstructive sleep apnea, or other chronic breathing problem, or for post-tonsillectomy/adenoidectomy pain; ≥18 years: 15-60 mg of ***codeine*** q 4 hours prn; max 360 mg of ***codeine***/day

Tab: **Tylenol #1** cod 7.5 mg+acet 300 mg (sulfites)
Tylenol #2 cod 15 mg+acet 300 mg (sulfites)
Tylenol #3 cod 30 mg+acet 300 mg (sulfites)
Tylenol #4 cod 60 mg+acet 300 mg (sulfites)

Comment: ***codeine*** is known to be excreted in breast milk. <12 years: not recommended; 12-<18: use extreme caution; not recommended for children and adolescents with asthma or other chronic breathing problem. The FDA and the European Medicines Agency (EMA) are investigating the safety of using ***codeine***-containing medications to treat pain, cough and colds, in children 12-<18 years because of the potential for serious side effects, including slowed or difficult breathing.

Tylenol with Codeine Elixir (C)(III) <12 years: contraindicated; 12-<18: use extreme caution; not recommended for children and adolescents with obesity, asthma, obstructive sleep apnea, or other chronic breathing problem, or for post-tonsillectomy/adenoidectomy pain; ≥18 years: 10 ml tid-qid; ≥12 year: 15-60 mg of ***codeine*** q 4 hours prn; max 360 mg of ***codeine***/day

Elix: cod 12 mg+acet 120 mg per 5 ml (cherry) (alcohol)

Comment: ***codeine*** is known to be excreted in breast milk. <12 years: not recommended; 12-<18: use extreme caution; not recommended for children and adolescents with asthma or other chronic breathing problem. The FDA and the European Medicines Agency (EMA) are investigating the safety of using ***codeine*** containing medications to treat pain, cough and colds, in children 12-<18 years because of the potential for serious side effects, including slowed or difficult breathing.

▶ ***dihydrocodeine+acetaminophen+caffeine*** (C)(III)(G) <18: use extreme caution; not recommended for children and adolescents with obesity, asthma, obstructive sleep apnea, or other chronic breathing problem, or for post-tonsillectomy/adenoidectomy pain; ≥18 years:

Panlor DC 1-2 caps q 4-6 hours prn; max 10 caps/day

Cap: dihydro 16 mg+acet 325 mg+caf 30 mg

Panlor SS 1 tab q 4 hours prn; max 5 tabs/day

Tab: dihydro 32 mg+acet 325 mg+caf 60*mg

Comment: ***codeine*** is known to be excreted in breast milk. <12 years: not recommended; 12-<18: use extreme caution; not recommended for children and adolescents with asthma or other chronic breathing problem. The FDA and the European Medicines Agency (EMA) are investigating the safety of using ***codeine*** containing medications to treat pain, cough and colds, in children 12-<18 years because of the potential for serious side effects, including slowed or difficult breathing.

▶ ***dihydrocodeine+aspirin+caffeine*** (D)(III)(G) <12 years: contraindicated; 12-<18: use extreme caution; not recommended for children and adolescents with obesity, asthma, obstructive sleep apnea, or other chronic breathing problem, or for post-tonsillectomy/adenoidectomy pain; ≥18 years: 1-2 caps q 4 hours prn

Synalgos-DC *Cap:* dihydro 16 mg+asp 356.4 mg+caf 30 mg

Comment: ***codeine*** is known to be excreted in breast milk. <12 years: not recommended; 12-<18: use extreme caution; not recommended for children and adolescents with asthma or other chronic breathing problem. The FDA and the European Medicines Agency (EMA) are investigating the safety of using ***codeine*** containing medications to treat pain, cough and colds, in children 12-<18 years because of the potential for serious side effects, including slowed or difficult breathing. ***aspirin***-containing medications are contraindicated with history of allergic-type reaction to ***aspirin***, children and adolescents with *Varicella* or other viral illness, and 3rd trimester of pregnancy.

▶ ***hydrocodone bitartrate*** (C)(II) <18 years: not recommended; ≥18 year:

Hysingla ER swallow whole; 1 tab once daily at the same time each day

Tab: 20, 30, 40, 60, 80, 100, 120 mg ext-rel

Vantrela ER swallow whole; 1 tab once daily at the same time each day

Tab: 15, 30, 45, 60, 90 mg ext-rel

Zohydro ER swallow whole; *Opioid naïve:* 10 mg q 12 hours; may increase by 10 mg q 12 hours every 3-7 days; when discontinuing, titrate downward every 2-4 days

Cap: 10, 15, 20, 30, 40, 50 mg ext-rel

▶ ***hydrocodone bitartrate+acetaminophen*** (C)(II)(G) <12 years: not recommended; ≥12 years:

Hycet 3 tsp (15 ml) q 4-6 hours prn; max 18 tsp/day

Liq: hydro 7.5 mg+acet 325 mg per 15 ml

Lorcet 1-2 caps q 4-6 hours prn; max 8 caps/day

Cap: hydro 5 mg+acet 325 mg*

Lorcet 10/650 1 tab q 4-6 hours prn; max 6 tabs/day
Tab: hydro 10 mg+acet 325 mg*
Lorcet-HD 1 cap q 4-6 hours prn; max 6 tabs/day
Cap: hydro 5 mg+acet 325 mg*
Lorcet Plus 1 tab q 4-6 hours prn; max 6 tabs/day
Tab: hydro 7.5 mg+acet 325 mg*
Lortab 2.5/500 1-2 tabs q 4-6 hours prn; max 8 tabs/day
Tab: hydro 2.5 mg+acet 325 mg*
Lortab 5/500 1-2 tabs q 4-6 hours prn; max 8 tabs/day
Tab: hydro 5 mg+acet 325 mg*
Lortab 7.5/500 1 tab q 4-6 hours prn; max 6 tabs/day
Tab: hydro 7.5 mg+acet 325 mg*
Lortab 10/500 1 tab q 4-6 hours prn; max 6 tabs/day
Tab: hydro 10 mg+acet 325 mg*
Lortab Elixir 3 tsp q 4-6 hours prn; max 18 tsp/day
Liq: hydro 7.5 mg+acet 300 mg per 15 ml (tropical fruit punch) (alcohol)
Maxidone 1 tab q 4-6 hours prn; max 5 tabs/day
Tab: hydro 10 mg+acet 325 mg*
Norco 5/325 1 tab q 4-6 hours prn; max 8 tabs/day
Tab: hydro 5 mg+acet 325 mg*
Norco 7.5/325 1 tab q 4-6 hours prn; max 6 tabs/day
Tab: hydro 7.5 mg+acet 325 mg*
Norco 10/325 1 tab q 4-6 hours prn; max 6 tabs/day
Tab: hydro 10 mg+acet 325 mg*
Vicodin 1-2 tabs q 4-6 hours prn; max 8 tabs/day
Tab: hydro 5 mg+acet 300 mg*
Vicodin ES 1 tab q 4-6 hours prn; max 6 tabs/day
Tab: hydro 7.5 mg+acet 300 mg*
Vicodin HP 1 tab q 4-6 hours prn; max 6 tabs/day
Tab: hydro 10 mg+acet 300 mg*
Xodol 5/300 1-2 tabs q 4-6 hours prn; max 8 caps/day
Tab: hydro 5 mg+acet 300 mg*
Xodol 7.5/300 1 tab q 4-6 hours prn; max 6 caps/day
Tab: hydro 7.5 mg+acet 300 mg*
Xodol 10/300 1 tab q 4-6 hours prn; max 6 caps/day
Tab: hydro 10 mg+acet 300 mg*
Zamicet 10/325 1-2 tabs q 4-6 hours prn; max 8 caps/day
Liq: hydro 10 mg+acet 325 mg per 15 ml
Zydone 5/400 1-2 tabs q 4-6 hours prn; max 8 caps/day
Tab: hydro 5 mg+acet 400 mg
Zydone 7.5/400 1 tab q 4-6 hours prn; max 6 caps/day
Tab: hydro 7.5 mg+acet 400 mg
Zydone 10/400 1 tab q 4-6 hours prn; max 6 caps/day
Tab: hydro 10 mg+acet 400 mg

► ***hydrocodone+ibuprofen*** **(C; not for use in 3rd)(II)(G)** <12 years: not recommended; ≥12 years:
Ibudone 5/200 1 tab q 4-6 hours prn; max 5 tabs/day
Tab: hydro 5 mg+ibup 200 mg
Ibudone 10/200 1 tab q 4-6 hours prn; max 5 tabs/day
Tab: hydro 10 mg+ibup 200 mg
Reprexain 1 tab q 4-6 hours prn; max 5 tabs/day
Tab: hydro 5 mg+ibup 200 mg
Vicoprofen 1 tab q 4-6 hours prn; max 5 tabs/day
Tab: hydro 7.5 mg+ibup 200 mg

▶ ***hydromorphone*** **(C)(II)(G)** <12 years: not recommended; ≥12 years:
Dilaudid initially 2-4 mg q 4-6 hours prn
Tab: 2, 4, 8 mg (sulfites)
Dilaudid Oral Liquid 2.5-10 mg q 3-6 hours prn
Liq: 5 mg/5 ml (sulfites)
Dilaudid Rectal Suppository 2.5-10 mg q 6-8 hours prn
Rectal supp: 3 mg
Dilaudid Injection initially 1-2 mg SC or IM q 4-6 hours prn
Amp: 1, 2, 4 mg/ml (1 ml)
Dilaudid-HP Injection initially 1-2 mg SC or IM q 4-6 hours prn
Amp: 10 mg/ml (1 ml)
Exalgo initially 8-64 mg once daily
Tab: 8, 12, 16, 32 mg ext-rel (sulfites)

▶ ***meperidine*** **(C; D in 2nd, 3rd)(II)(G)** <12 years: 0.5-0.8 mg/lb q 3-4 hours prn; ≥12 years: 50-150 mg q 3-4 hours prn
Demerol *Tab:* 50, 100 mg; *Syr:* 50 mg/5 ml (banana) (alcohol-free)

▶ ***meperidine+promethazine*** **(C; D in 2nd, 3rd)(II)(G)** <12 years: not recommended; ≥12 years:
Mepergan 1-2 tsp q 3-4 hours prn
Syr: mep 25 mg+prom 25 mg per ml
Mepergan Fortis 1-2 tsp q 4-6 hours prn
Tab: mep 50 mg+prom 25 mg

▶ ***methadone*** **(C)(II)(G)** <18 years: not recommended; ≥18 years: 2.5-10 mg PO, SC, or IM q 3-4 hours; for use only in chronic moderately severe-to-severe pain management (e.g., hospice care). For opioid naïve patients, initiate **Dolophine** tablets with 2.5 mg every 8 to 12 hours; unlike other opioid analgesics, ***methadone*** is not indicated as an as-needed (prn) analgesic, per se; titrate slowly with dose increases no more frequent than every 3 to 5 days; to convert to **Dolophine** tablets from another opioid, use available conversion factors to obtain estimated dose (see mfr pkg insert); do not abruptly discontinue **Dolophine** in a physically dependent patient
Dolophine *Tab:* 5, 10 mg; *Dispersible tab:* 40 mg (dissolve in 120 ml orange juice or other citrus drink); *Oral soln:* 5, 10 mg/ml; *Oral conc:* 10 mg/ml; *Syr:* 10 mg/30 ml; *Vial:* 10 mg/ml (200 mg/20 ml multi-dose) for injection

Comment: ***methadone*** administration is allowed only by approved providers with strict state and federal regulations (as stipulated in 42 CFR 8.12). Black Box Warning (BBW): **Dolophine** exposes users to risks of addiction, abuse, and misuse, which can lead to overdose and death. Assess each patient's risk and monitor regularly for development of these behaviors and conditions. Serious, life-threatening, or fatal respiratory depression may occur. The peak respiratory depressant effect of ***methadone*** occurs later, and persists longer than the peak analgesic effect. Accidental ingestion, especially by children, can result in fatal overdose. QT interval prolongation and serious arrhythmias (*torsades de pointes*) have occurred during treatment with ***methadone***. Closely monitor patients with risk factors for development of prolonged QT interval, a history of cardiac conduction abnormalities, and those taking medications affecting cardiac conduction. Neonatal Opioid Withdrawal Syndrome (NOWS) is an expected and treatable outcome of use of methadone use during pregnancy. NOWS may be life-threatening if not recognized and treated in the neonate. The balance between the risks of NOWS and the benefits of maternal ***methadone*** use should be considered and the patient advised of the risk of NOWS so that appropriate planning for management of the neonate can occur. ***methadone*** has been detected in human milk. Concomitant use with CYP3A4, 2B6, 2C19, 2C9 or 2D6 inhibitors or discontinuation of concomitantly used CYP3A4 2B6,

2C19, or 2C9 inducers can result in a fatal overdose of ***methadone***. Concomitant use of opioids with benzodiazepines or other central nervous system (CNS) depressants, including alcohol, may result in profound sedation, respiratory depression, coma, and death.

➢ ***morphine sulfate*** (C)(II)(G) <18 years: not recommended; ≥18 years: *Tabs:* usually 15-30 mg q 4 hours prn; *Solution:* usually 10-20 mg q 4 hours prn
Tab: 15, 30*mg; Oral soln:* 10 mg/5 ml, 20 mg/5 ml (100, 500 ml), 100 mg/5 ml (30, 120 ml)

➢ ***morphine sulfate (immed- and sust-rel)*** (C)(II) <18 years: not recommended
Comment: Dosage dependent upon previous opioid dosage; see mfr pkg insert for conversion guidelines; not for prn use; swallow whole <u>or</u> sprinkle contents of caps on applesauce (do not crush, chew, <u>or</u> dissolve). Generic ***morphine sulfate*** is available in the following forms: *Tab:* 15*, 30*mg; *Oral soln:* 10, 20 mg/5 ml (100 ml); 100 mg/5 ml (30, 120 ml w. oral syringe)

Arymo ER swallow whole; 1 tab once daily at the same time each day
Tab: 15, 30, 60 mg ext-rel

Duramorph administer per anesthesia
IV/Intrathecal/Epidural: 0.5, 1 mg/ml

Infumorph administer per anesthesia provider
Intrathecal/Epidural: 10, 20 mg/ml

Kadian (G) 1 cap every 12-24 hours
Cap: 10, 20, 30, 50, 60, 80, 100, 200 mg sust-rel

MS Contin (G) 1 tab every 24 hours
Tab: 15, 30, 60, 100, 200 mg sust-rel

MSIR 5-30 mg q 4 hours prn
Tab: 15*, 30*mg; *Cap:* 15, 30 mg

MSIR Oral Solution 5-30 mg q 4 hours prn
Oral soln: 10, 20 mg/5 ml (120 ml)

MSIR Oral Solution Concentrate 5-30 mg q 4 hours prn
Oral conc: 20 mg/ml (30, 120 ml w. dropper)

Oramorph SR 1 cap every 12-24 hours
Tab: 15, 30, 60, 100 mg sust-rel

Roxanol Oral Solution 10-30 mg q 4 hours prn
Oral soln: 20 mg/ml (1, 4, 8 oz)

Roxanol Rescudose
Oral soln: 10 mg/2.5 ml (25 single-dose/carton)

➢ ***morphine sulfate (ext-rel)*** (C)(II) <18 years: not recommended; >18 years:
MorphaBond ER *Tab:* 15, 30, 60, 100 mg ext-*rel*

Comment: **MorphaBond ER** may be prescribed only by a qualified healthcare providers knowledgeable in use of potent opioids for management of chronic pain. Do not abruptly discontinue in a physically dependent patient. Instruct patients to swallow **MorphaBond ER** tablets intact and not to cut, break, crush, chew, <u>or</u> dissolve **MorphaBond ER** to avoid the risk of release and absorption of potentially fatal dose of morphine. **MorphaBond ER** 100 mg tablets, a single dose greater than 60 mg, <u>or</u> a total daily dose >120 mg, are only for use in patients in whom tolerance to an opioid of comparable potency has been established. Patients considered opioid-tolerant are those taking, for one week <u>or</u> longer, at least 60 mg oral ***morphine*** per day, 25 mcg transdermal ***fentanyl*** per hour, 30 mg oral ***oxycodone*** per day, 8 mg oral ***hydromorphone*** per day, 25 mg oral ***oxymorphone*** per day, 60 mg oral ***hydrocodone*** per day, <u>or</u> an equianalgesic dose of another opioid. Use the lowest effective dosage for the shortest duration consistent with individual patient treatment goals. Individualize dosing based on the severity of pain, patient response, prior analgesic experience, and risk factors for addiction, abuse, and misuse.

▶ ***morphine sulfate+naltrexone*** (C)(II) <18 years: not recommended; ≥18 years:
Embeda 1 cap q 12-24 hours
Cap: **Embeda 20/0.8** morph 20 mg+nal 0.8 mg ext-rel
Embeda 30/1.2 morph 30 mg+nal 1.2 mg ext-rel
Embeda 50/2 morph 50 mg+nal 2 mg ext-rel
Embeda 60/2.4 morph 60 mg+nal 2.4 mg ext-rel
Embeda 80/3.2 morph 80 mg+nal 3.2 mg ext-rel
Embeda 100/4 morph 100 mg+nal 4 mg ext-rel

Comment: **Embeda** is not for prn use; for use in opioid-tolerant patients only; swallow whole or sprinkle contents of caps on applesauce (do not crush, chew, or dissolve); do not administer via NG or gastric tube (PEG tube).

▶ ***oxycodone*** (B)(II)(G) <18 years: not recommended; ≥18 year: 5-15 mg q 4-6 hours prn

Comment: Concomitant use of CYP3A4 inhibitors may increase opioid effects and CYP3A4 inducers may decrease effects or possibly cause development of an abstinence syndrome (withdrawal symptoms) in patients who are physically ***oxycodone*** dependent/addicted.

Oxaydo *Tab:* 5, 7.5 mg

Comment: **Oxaydo** is the first and only immediate-release oral ***oxycodone*** that discourages intranasal abuse. **Oxaydo** is formulated with sodium lauryl sulfate, an inactive ingredient that may cause nasal burning and throat irritation when snorted and, thus potentially reducing abuse liability. There is no generic equivalent.

Oxecta *Tab:* 5, 7.5 mg
Oxycodone Oral Solution (G) *Oral soln:* 5 mg/5 ml (15, 30 ml)
OxyIR (G) *Cap:* 5 mg
RoxyBond *Tab:* 5, 15, 30 mg

Comment: **RoxyBond** is the first immediate-release opioid for the management of pain severe enough to require an opioid analgesic and for which alternative treatments are inadequate, with abuse-deterrent labeling (its SentryBond technology makes it difficult to manipulate for misuse and abuse by physical manipulation and chemical extraction).

Roxycodone *Tab:* 5, 15*, 30*mg; *Oral soln:* 5 mg/ml
Roxycodone Intensol *Oral soln:* 20 mg/ml

▶ ***oxycodone cont-rel*** (B)(II)(G) dosage dependent upon previous opioid be taking and tolerating dosages; see mfr pkg insert: <11 years: not recommended; 11-16 years: the child's pain must be severe enough to require around-the-clock, long-term treatment not managed well by other treatments; must already tolerate minimum opium dose equal to ***oxycodone*** 20 mg/day x 5 consecutive days; >16 years: no previous treatment with ***oxycodone*** required

OxyContin dose q 12 hours
Tab: 10, 15, 20, 30, 40, 60, 80 mg cont-rel
OxyFast dose q 6 hours
Oral conc: 20 mg/ml (30 ml w. dropper)
Xtampza ER dose q 12 hours
Cap: 10, 15, 20, 30, 40 mg ext-rel

Comment: May open the **Xtampza ER** capsule and sprinkle in water or on soft food.

▶ ***oxycodone+acetaminophen*** (C)(II)(G) <12 years: not recommended; ≥12 years:

Comment: Maximum 4 grams acetaminophen per day.

Magnacet 2.5/400 1 tab q 6 hours prn; max 10 tabs/day
Tab: oxy 2.5 mg+acet 325 mg
Magnacet 5/400 1 tab q 6 hours prn; max 10 tabs/day
Tab: oxy 5 mg+acet 325 mg

Magnacet 7.5/400 1 tab q 6 hours prn; max 8 tabs/day
Tab: oxy 7.5 mg+acet 325 mg
Magnacet 10/400 1 tab q 6 hours prn; max 6 tabs/day
Tab: oxy 10 mg+acet 325 mg
Percocet 2.5/325 1 tab q 6 hours prn; max 4 gm acet/day
Tab: oxy 2.5 mg+acet 325 mg
Percocet 5/325 1 tab q 6 hours prn; max 4 gm acet/day
Tab: oxy 5 mg+acet 325*mg
Percocet 7.5/325 1 tab q 6 hours prn; max 4 gm acet/day
Tab: oxy 7.5 mg+acet 325 mg
Percocet 7.5/500 1 tabs q 6 hours prn; max 4 gm acet/day
Tab: oxy 7.5 mg+acet 325 mg
Percocet 10/325 1 tabs q 6 hours prn; max 4 gm acet/day
Tab: oxy 10 mg+acet 325 mg
Percocet 10/650 1 tab q 6 hours prn; max 4 gm acet/day
Tab: oxy 10 mg+acet 325 mg
Roxicet 5/325 1 tab/tsp q 6 hours prn
Tab: oxy 5 mg+acet 325 mg; *Oral soln:* oxy 5 mg+acet 325 mg per 5 ml
Roxicet 5/500 1 caplet q 6 hours prn
Cplt: oxy 5 mg+acet 325 mg
Roxicet Oral Solution 1 tsp q 6 hours prn
Oral soln: oxy 5 mg+acet 325 mg per 5 ml (alcohol 0.4%)
Tylox 1 cap q 6 hours prn
Cap: oxy 5 mg+acet 325 mg
Xartemis XR 2 tabs q 12 hours prn
Tab: oxy 7.5 mg+acet 325 mg

➢ ***oxycodone+aspirin*** (D)(II)(G) <12 years: not recommended; ≥12 years:
Percodan 1 tab q 6 hours prn
Tab: oxy 4.8355 mg+asp 325 mg*
Percodan-Demi <6 years: not recommended: 6-12 years: 1/4 tab q 6 hours prn; >12-18 years: 1/2 tab q 6 hours prn; >18 years: 1-2 tabs q 6 hours prn
Tab: oxy 2.25 mg+asp 325 mg

Comment: ***Aspirin***-containing medications are contraindicated with history of allergic-type reaction to ***aspirin***, children and adolescents with *Varicella* or other viral illness, and 3rd trimester of pregnancy.

➢ ***oxycodone+ibuprofen*** (C)(II)(G)
Combunox <12 years: not recommended; ≥12 years: 1 tab q 6 hours prn
Tab: oxy 5 mg+ibu 400 mg*

➢ ***oxycodone+naloxone*** (C)(II) <14 years: not recommended; ≥14 years: 1 tab q 3-4 hours prn
Targiniq
Tab: **Targiniq 10/5** oxy 10 mg+nal 5 mg
Targiniq 20/10 oxy 20 mg+nal 10 mg
Targiniq 40/20 oxy 40 mg+nal 20 mg

➢ ***oxymorphone*** (C)(II)(G) <18 years: not recommended; ≥18 years:
Numorphan 1 supp q 4-6 hours prn
Rectal supp: 5 mg; *Vial:* 1 mg/ml (1 ml), *Amp:* 1.5 mg/ml (10 ml);
Comment: Store in refrigerator in original package. 1 mg of **Numorphan** is approximately equivalent in analgesic activity to 10 mg of ***morphine sulfate***.
Opana 1-1 tab q 4-6 hours prn
Tab: 5, 10 mg
Opana ER 1 tab q 12 hours prn
Tab: 5, 7.5, 10, 15, 20, 30, 40 mg ext-rel crush-resist

Opana Injection initially 0.5 mg IV or IM; 1 x 1 mg IM or IV q 4-6 hours prn
Amp: 1 mg/ml (1 ml) (paraben/sodium dithionite-free)

➢ ***pentazocine+aspirin*** **(D)(IV)** <18 years: not recommended; ≥18 years: 2 cplts tid or qid prn
Talwin Compound *Cplt:* pent 12.5 mg+asp 325 mg

Comment: ***Aspirin***-containing medications are contraindicated with history of allergic-type reaction to ***aspirin***, children and adolescents with *Varicella* or other viral illness, and 3rd trimester of pregnancy.

➢ ***pentazocine+naloxone*** **(C)(IV)** <12 years: not recommended; ≥12 years: 1 tab q 3-4 hours prn
Talwin NX *Tab:* pent 50 mg+nal 0.5 mg*

➢ ***pentazocine lactate*** **(C)(IV)** <1 year: not recommended; >1 year: 0.5 mg/kg IM 30 mg IM, SC, or IV q 3-4 hours; max 360 mg/day
Talwin Injectable *Amp:* 30 mg/ml (1, 1.5, 2 ml)

➢ ***propoxyphene napsylate+acetaminophen*** **(C)(IV)(G)**
Comment: Max 4 gm acetaminophen per day.
Balacet 325 <12 year: not recommended; ≥12 year: 0.5 mg/kg IM 1 tab q 4 hours prn; max 6 tabs/day
Tab: prop 100 mg+acet 325 mg

➢ ***tramadol*** **(C)(IV)(G)**
Comment: ***Tramadol*** is known to be excreted in breast milk. The FDA and the European Medicines Agency (EMA) are investigating the safety of using ***tramadol***-containing medications to treat pain in children 12-18 years because of the potential for serious side effects, including slowed or difficult breathing.
Rybix ODT <12 years: contraindicated; 12-<18: use extreme caution; not recommended for children and adolescents with obesity, asthma, obstructive sleep apnea, or other chronic breathing problem, or for post-tonsillectomy/adenoidectomy pain; ≥18 years: initially 100 mg once daily; may increase by 100 mg every 5 days; max 300 mg/day; *CrCl <30 mL/min or severe hepatic impairment:* not recommended; *Cirrhosis:* max 50 mg q 12 hours
ODT: 50 mg (mint) (phenylalanine)
Ryzolt <12 years: contraindicated; 12-<18: use extreme caution; not recommended for children and adolescents with obesity, asthma, obstructive sleep apnea, or other chronic breathing problem, or for post-tonsillectomy/adenoidectomy pain; ≥18 years: initially 100 mg once daily; may increase by 100 mg every 5 days; max 300 mg/day; *CrCl <30 mL/min or severe hepatic impairment:* not recommended
Tab: 100, 200, 300 mg ext-rel
Ultram <12 years: contraindicated; 12-<18: use extreme caution; not recommended for children and adolescents with obesity, asthma, obstructive sleep apnea, or other chronic breathing problem, or for post-tonsillectomy/adenoidectomy pain; ≥18 years: 50-100 mg q 4-6 hours prn; max 400 mg/day; *CrCl <30 mL/min:* max 100 mg q 12 hours; *Cirrhosis:* max 50 mg q 12 hours
Tab: 50*mg
Ultram ER <12 years: contraindicated; 12-<18: use extreme caution; not recommended for children and adolescents with obesity, asthma, obstructive sleep apnea, or other chronic breathing problem, or for post-tonsillectomy/adenoidectomy pain; ≥18 years: initially 100 mg once daily; may increase by 100 mg every 5 days; max 300 mg/day; *CrCl <30 mL/min or severe hepatic impairment:* not recommended
Tab: 100, 200, 300 mg ext-rel

➢ ***tramadol+acetaminophen*** **(C)(IV)(G)** <12 years: contraindicated; 12-<18: use extreme caution; not recommended for children and adolescents with obesity, asthma, obstructive sleep apnea, or other chronic breathing problem, or for post-tonsillectomy/adenoidectomy pain; ≥18 years: 2 tabs q 4-6 hours; max 8 tabs/day; 5 days; *CrCl <30 mL/min:* max 2 tabs q 12 hours; max 4 tabs/day x 5 days

Ultracet *Tab:* tram 37.5+acet 325 mg

Comment: ***tramadol*** is known to be excreted in breast milk. The FDA and the European Medicines Agency (EMA) are investigating the safety of using ***tramadol***-containing medications to treat pain in children 12-18 years because of the potential for serious side effects, including slowed or difficult breathing.

➢ ***buprenorphine*** (C)(III) <16 years: not recommended; ≥16 years: change patch every 7 days; do not increase the dose until previous dose has been worn for at least 72 hours; after removal, do not reuse the site for at least 3 weeks; do not expose the patch to heat

Butrans Transdermal System *Transdermal patch:* 5, 10, 20 mcg/hour (4/pck)

➢ ***fentanyl*** transdermal system **(C)(II)** <16 years or <110 lb: not recommended; ≥16 years or ≥110 lb: apply to clean, dry, non-irritated, intact, skin; hold in place for 30 seconds; start at lowest dose and titrate upward; *Opioid-naïve:* change patch every 3 days (72 hours)

Duragesic *Transdermal patch:* 12, 25, 37.5, 50, 62.5, 75, 87.5, 100 mcg/hour (5/pck)

TRANSMUCOSAL (SUB-LINGUAL, BUCCAL) OPIOIDS

Comment: For chronic severe pain. For management of breakthrough pain in patients with cancer who are already receiving and who are tolerant to opioid therapy. Opioid-tolerant patients are those taking oral ***morphine*** ≥60 mg/day, transdermal ***fentanyl*** ≥25 mcg/hr, ***oxycodone*** ≥30 mg/day, oral ***hydromorphone*** ≥8 mg/day, or an equianalgesic dose of another opioid, for ≥1 week

ORAL OPIOID PARTIAL AGONIST-ANTAGONIST

➢ ***buprenorphine*** (C)

Subutex <16 years: not recommended; ≥16 years: 8 mg in a single dose on day 1; then 16 mg in a single dose on day 2; target dose is 16 mg/day in a single dose; dissolve under tongue; do not chew or swallow whole

SL tab (lemon-lime) or *SL film (lime):* 2, 8 mg (30/pck)

Comment: The Transmucosal Immediate Release **Fentanyl** (TIRF) Risk Evaluation and Mitigation Strategy (REMS) program is an FDA-required program designed to ensure informed risk-benefit decisions before initiating treatment, and while patients are treated to ensure appropriate use of TIRF medicines. The purpose of the TIRF REMS Access program is to mitigate the risk of misuse, abuse, addiction, overdose and serious complications due to medication errors with the use of TIRF medicines. You must enroll in the TIRF REMS Access program to prescribe, dispense, or distribute TIRF medicines. To register, call the TIRF REMS Access program at 1-866-822-1483 or register online at https://www.tirfremsaccess.com/TirfUI/rems/home.action

➢ ***fentanyl*** buccal soluble film **(C)(II)** <18 years: not recommended; ≥18 years: dissolve 1 film on moistened area inside cheek; initially 200 mcg; no more than 4 doses/day at least 2 hours apart; max 1200 mcg/dose; do not cut film

Onsolis *Buccal film:* 200, 400, 600, 800, 1200 mcg (30 films/pck)

Comment: The Transmucosal Immediate Release **Fentanyl** (TIRF) Risk Evaluation and Mitigation Strategy (REMS) program is an FDA-required program designed to ensure informed risk-benefit decisions before initiating treatment, and while patients are treated to ensure appropriate use of TIRF medicines. The purpose of the TIRF REMS Access program is to mitigate the risk of misuse, abuse, addiction, overdose and serious complications due to medication errors with the use of TIRF medicines. You must enroll in the TIRF REMS Access program to prescribe, dispense, or distribute TIRF medicines. To register, call the TIRF REMS Access program at 1-866-822-1483 or register online at https://www.tirfremsaccess.com/TirfUI/rems/home.action

➢ ***fentanyl citrate*** transmucosal unit **(C)(II)(G)** <18 years: not recommended; ≥18 years: initially one 200 mcg unit placed between cheek and lower gum; move from side to side; suck (not chew); use 6 units before titrating; titrate dose as needed; max 4 units/day

Actiq *Unit:* 200, 400, 600, 800, 1,200, 1,600 mcg (24 units/pck)

Fentora *Unit:* 100, 200, 400, 600, 800 mcg (24 units/pck)

Comment: The Transmucosal Immediate Release **Fentanyl** (TIRF) Risk Evaluation and Mitigation Strategy (REMS) program is an FDA-required program designed to ensure informed risk-benefit decisions before initiating treatment, and while patients are treated to ensure appropriate use of TIRF medicines. The purpose of the TIRF REMS Access program is to mitigate the risk of misuse, abuse, addiction, overdose and serious complications due to medication errors with the use of TIRF medicines. You must enroll in the TIRF REMS Access program to prescribe, dispense, or distribute TIRF medicines. To register, call the TIRF REMS Access program at 1-866-822-1483 or register online at https://www.tirfremsaccess.com/TirfUI/rems/home.action

➢ ***fentanyl*** sublingual tab **(C)(II)** <18 years: not recommended; ≥18 years: initially one 100 mcg dose; if inadequate after 30 minutes, may repeat; titrate in increments of 100 mcg; max 2 doses per episode, up to 4 episodes per day; wait at least 2 hours before treating another episode; *Maintenance:* use only one tablet of appropriate strength; do not chew, suck, or swallow tablets; do not convert from other ***fentanyl*** products on a mcg-per-mcg basis or interchange with other ***fentanyl*** products

Abstral *SL tab:* 100, 200, 300, 400, 600, 800 mcg (32 tabs/pck)

Comment: The Transmucosal Immediate Release **Fentanyl** (TIRF) Risk Evaluation and Mitigation Strategy (REMS) program is an FDA-required program designed to ensure informed risk-benefit decisions before initiating treatment, and while patients are treated to ensure appropriate use of TIRF medicines. The purpose of the TIRF REMS Access program is to mitigate the risk of misuse, abuse, addiction, overdose and serious complications due to medication errors with the use of TIRF medicines. You must enroll in the TIRF REMS Access program to prescribe, dispense, or distribute TIRF medicines. To register, call the TIRF REMS Access program at 1-866-822-1483 or register online at https://www.tirfremsaccess.com/TirfUI/rems/home.action

➢ ***fentanyl sublingual spray*** **(C)(II)** <18 years: not recommended; ≥18 years:

Subsys 100, 200, 400, 600, 800 mcg/SL spray

Comment: **Subsys** is not bioequivalent with other ***fentanyl*** products. Do not convert patients from other ***fentanyl*** products to **Subsys** on a mcg-per-mcg basis. There are no conversion directions available for patients on any other ***fentanyl*** products other than **Actiq**. (Note: This includes oral, transdermal, or parenteral formulations of ***fentanyl***.) The Transmucosal Immediate Release **Fentanyl** (TIRF) Risk Evaluation and Mitigation Strategy (REMS) program is an FDA-required program designed to ensure informed risk-benefit decisions before initiating treatment, and while patients are treated to ensure appropriate use of TIRF medicines. The purpose of the TIRF REMS Access program is to mitigate the risk of misuse, abuse, addiction, overdose and serious complications due to medication errors with the use of TIRF medicines. You must enroll in the TIRF REMS Access program to prescribe, dispense, or distribute TIRF medicines. To register, call the TIRF REMS Access program at 1-866-822-1483 or register online at https://www.tirfremsaccess.com/TirfUI/rems/home.action

PARENTERAL OPIOID AGONIST-ANTAGONIST

➤ ***nalbuphine*** (B)(G) <18 years: not recommended; ≥18 years: 10 mg/70 kg IM, SC, or IV q 3-6 hours prn
Nubain *Amp:* 10, 20 mg/ml (1 ml) (sulfite-free, parabens-free)

➤ ***pentazocine+naloxone*** (C)(IV) <12 years: not recommended; ≥12 years: 1-2 tabs q 3-4 hours prn; max 12 tabs/day
Talwin-NX *Tab:* pent 50 mg/nal 0.5 mg*

TRANSMUCOSAL (INTRA-NASAL) OPIOIDS

➤ ***butorphanol tartrate*** nasal spray **(C)(IV)** <18 years: not recommended; ≥18 years: initially 1 spray (1 mg) in one nostril and may repeat after 60-90 minutes in opposite nostril if needed or 1 spray in each nostril and may repeat q 3-4 hours prn
Butorphanol Nasal Spray *Nasal spray:* 1 mg/actuation (10 mg/ml, 2.5 ml)
Stadol Nasal Spray *Nasal spray:* 1 mg/actuation (10 mg/ml, 2.5 ml)

➤ ***fentanyl*** nasal spray **(C)(II)** <18 years: not recommended; ≥18 years: initially 1 spray (100 mcg) in one nostril and may repeat after 2 hours; when adequate analgesia is achieved, use that dose for subsequent breakthrough episodes; *Titration steps:* 100 mcg using 1 x 100 mcg spray; 200 mcg using 2 x 100 mcg spray (1 spray in each nostril); 400 mcg using 1 x 400 mcg spray; 800 mcg using 2 x 400 mcg (1 spray in each nostril); max 800 mcg; limit to ≤4 doses per day
Lazanda Nasal Spray *Nasal spray:* 100, 400 mcg/100 mcl (8 sprays/bottle)
Comment: **Lazanda Nasal Spray** is available by restricted distribution program. Call 855-841-4234 or visit https://www.fda.gov/downloads/drugs/drugsafety/postmarketdrugsafetyinformationforpatientsandproviders/ucm261983.pdf to enroll. **Lazanda Nasal Spray** is indicated for the management of breakthrough pain in cancer patients who are already receiving and who are tolerant to opioid therapy for their underlying persistent cancer pain. Patients considered opioid tolerant are those who are taking at least 60 mg of oral morphine/day, 25 mcg of transdermal ***fentanyl***/hour, 30 mg oral ***oxycodone***/day, 8 mg oral ***hydromorphone***/day, 25 mg oral ***oxymorphone***/day, or an equianalgesic dose of another opioid for a week or longer. Patients must remain on around-the-clock opioids when using **Lazanda Nasal Spray**. As such, it is contraindicated in the management of acute or post-op pain, including headache/migraine, or dental pain.

Comment: The Transmucosal Immediate Release **Fentanyl** (TIRF) Risk Evaluation and Mitigation Strategy (REMS) program is an FDA-required program designed to ensure informed risk-benefit decisions before initiating treatment, and while patients are treated to ensure appropriate use of TIRF medicines. The purpose of the TIRF REMS Access program is to mitigate the risk of misuse, abuse, addiction, overdose and serious complications due to medication errors with the use of TIRF medicines. You must enroll in the TIRF REMS Access program to prescribe, dispense, or distribute TIRF medicines. To register, call the TIRF REMS Access program at 1-866-822-1483 or register online at https://www.tirfremsaccess.com/TirfUI/rems/home.action

INTRATHECAL OPIOID

➤ ***ziconotide*** intrathecal (IT) infusion **(C)** <12 years: not recommended; ≥12 years: initially no more than 2.4 mcg/day (0.1 mcg/hour) and titrate to upward by up to 2.4 mcg/day (0.1 mcg/day at intervals of no more than 2-3 times per week, up to a recommended maximum of 19.2 mcg/day (0.8 mcg/hr) by Day 21; dose increases in increments of less than 2.4 mcg/day (0.1 mcg/hr) and increases in dose less frequently than 2-3 times per week may be used.
Prialt *Vial:* 25 mcg/ml (20 ml), 100 mcg/ml (1, 2, 5 ml)

Comment: Patients with a pre-existing history of psychosis should not be treated with ***ziconotide***. Contraindications to the use of IT analgesia include conditions such as the presence of infection at the microinfusion injection site, uncontrolled bleeding diathesis, and spinal canal obstruction that impairs circulation of CSF.

PANIC DISORDER

Comment: If possible when considering a benzodiazepine to treat anxiety, a short-acting benzodiazepines should be used only prn to avert intense anxiety and panic for the least time necessary while a different non-addictive antianxiety regimen (e.g., SSRI, SNRI, TCA, ***buspirone***, beta-blocker) is established and effective treatment goals achieved. Co-administration of SSRIs with TCAs requires extreme caution. Concomitant use of MAOIs and SSRIs is absolutely contraindicated. Avoid other serotonergic drugs. A potentially fatal adverse event is *serotonin syndrome*, caused by serotonin excess. Milder symptoms require HCP intervention to avert severe symptoms that can be rapidly fatal without urgent/emergent medical care. Symptoms include restlessness, agitation, confusion, hallucinations, tachycardia, hypertension, dilated pupils, muscle twitching, muscle rigidity, loss of muscle coordination, diaphoresis, diarrhea, headache, shivering, piloerection, hyperpyrexia, cardiac arrhythmias, seizures, loss of consciousness, coma, death. Abrupt withdrawal or interruption of treatment with an antidepressant medication is sometimes associated with an antidepressant discontinuation syndrome (ADS), which may be mediated by gradually tapering the drug over a period of two weeks or longer, depending on the dose strength and length of treatment. Common symptoms of the *serotonin discontinuation syndrome* include flu-like symptoms (nausea, vomiting, diarrhea, headaches, sweating), sleep disturbances (insomnia, nightmares, constant sleepiness), mood disturbances (dysphoria, anxiety, agitation), cognitive disturbances (mental confusion, hyperarousal), sensory and movement disturbances (imbalance, tremors, vertigo, dizziness, electric shock-like sensations in the brain, often described by sufferers as "brain zaps").

SELECTIVE SEROTONIN REUPTAKE INHIBITORS (SSRIs)

▶ ***citalopram*** (C)(G) <12 years: not recommended; ≥12 years: initially 20 mg once daily; may increase after one week to 40 mg once daily; max 40 mg
  Celexa *Tab:* 10, 20, 40 mg; *Oral soln:* 10 mg/5 ml (120 ml) (peppermint) (sugar-free, alcohol-free, parabens)

▶ ***escitalopram*** (C)(G) <12 years: not recommended; 12-17 years: initially 10 mg daily; may increase to 20 mg daily after 3 weeks; >17 years: initially 10 mg daily; may increase to 20 mg daily after 1 week; *Hepatic impairment:* 10 mg once daily
  Lexapro *Tab:* 5, 10*, 20*mg
  Lexapro Oral Solution *Oral soln:* 1 mg/ml (240 ml) (peppermint) (parabens)

▶ ***fluoxetine*** (C)(G)
  Prozac <8 years: not recommended; 8-17 years: initially 10 mg/day; may increase after 1 week to 20 mg/day; range 20-60 mg/day; range for lower weight children, 20-30 mg/day; >17 years: initially 20 mg daily; may increase after 1 week; doses >20 mg/day should be divided into AM and noon doses; max 80 mg/day
    Cap: 10, 20, 40 mg; *Tab:* 30*, 60*mg; *Oral soln:* 20 mg/5 ml (4 oz) (mint)
  Prozac Weekly <12 years: not recommended; ≥12 years: following daily ***fluoxetine*** therapy at 20 mg/day for 13 weeks, may initiate **Prozac Weekly** 7 days after the last 20 mg ***fluoxetine*** dose
    Cap: 90 mg ent-coat del-rel pellets

- ▶ ***levomilnacipran*** (C) <12 years: not recommended; ≥12 years: swallow whole; initially 20 mg once daily for 2 days; then increase to 40 mg once daily; may increase dose in 40 mg increments at intervals of ≥2 days; max 120 mg once daily; *CrCl 30-59 mL/min:* max 80 mg once daily; *CrCl 15-29 mL/min:* max 40 mg once daily
  - **Fetzima** *Cap:* 20, 40, 80, 120 mg ext-rel
- ▶ ***paroxetine maleate*** (D)(G)
  - **Paxil** <12 years: not recommended; ≥12 years: initially 20 mg daily in AM; may increase by 10 mg/day at weekly intervals as needed; max 60 mg/day
    - *Tab:* 10*, 20*, 30, 40 mg
  - **Paxil CR** <12 years: not recommended; ≥12 years: initially 25 mg daily in AM; may increase by 12.5 mg at weekly intervals as needed; max 62.5 mg/day
    - *Tab:* 12.5, 25, 37.5 mg cont-rel ent-coat
  - **Paxil Suspension** <12 years: not recommended; ≥12 years: initially 20 mg daily in AM; may increase by 10 mg/day at weekly intervals as needed; max 60 mg/day
    - *Oral susp:* 10 mg/5 ml (250 ml) (orange)
- ▶ ***paroxetine mesylate*** (D)(G) <12 years: not recommended; ≥12 years: initially 7.5 mg daily in AM; may increase by 10 mg/day at weekly intervals as needed; max 60 mg/day
  - **Brisdelle** *Cap:* 7.5 mg
- ▶ ***sertraline*** (C)(G) <6 years: not recommended; 6-<12 years: initially 25 mg daily; max 200 mg/day; 12-17 years: initially 50 mg daily; max 200 mg/day; >17 years: initially 50 mg daily; increase at 1 week intervals if needed; max 200 mg daily; dilute oral concentrate immediately prior to administration in 4 oz water, ginger ale, lemon-lime soda, lemonade, or orange juice
  - **Zoloft** *Tab:* 25*, 50*, 100*mg; *Oral conc:* 20 mg per ml (60 ml) (alcohol 12%)

SEROTONIN-NOREPINEPHRINE REUPTAKE INHIBITORS (SNRIs)

- ▶ ***desvenlafaxine*** (C)(G) <18 years: not recommended; ≥18 years: swallow whole; initially 50 mg once daily; max 120 mg/day
  - **Pristiq** *Tab:* 50, 100 mg ext-rel
- ▶ ***duloxetine*** (C)(G) <12 years: not recommended; ≥12 years: swallow whole; initially 30 mg once daily x 1 week; then, increase to 60 mg once daily; max 120 mg/day
  - **Cymbalta** *Cap:* 20, 30, 40, 60 mg del-rel
- ▶ ***venlafaxine*** (C)(G)
  - **Effexor** initially <18 years: not recommended; ≥18 years: 75 mg/day in 2-3 divided doses; may increase at 4 day intervals in 75 mg increments to 150 mg/day; max 225 mg/day
    - *Tab:* 37.5, 75, 150, 225 mg
  - **Effexor XR** <18 years: not recommended; ≥18 years: initially 75 mg q AM; may start at 37.5 mg daily x 4-7 days, then increase by increments of up to 75 mg/day at intervals of at least 4 days; usual max 375 mg/day
    - *Tab/Cap:* 37.5, 75, 150 mg ext-rel
- ▶ ***vortioxetine*** (C) <18 years: not established; ≥18 years: initially 10 mg once daily; max 30 mg/day
  - **Brintellix** *Tab:* 5, 10, 15, 20 mg

TRICYCLIC ANTIDEPRESSANTS (TCAs)

Comment: Co-administration of SSRIs and TCAs requires extreme caution.

- ▶ ***amitriptyline*** (C)(G) <12 years: not recommended; ≥12 years: 10-20 mg q HS *Tab:* 10, 25, 50, 75, 100, 150 mg
- ▶ ***amoxapine*** (C) <12 years: not recommended; ≥12 years: initially 50 mg bid-tid; after 1 week may increase to 100 mg bid-tid; usual effective dose 200-300 mg/day; if total

dose exceeds 300 mg/day, give in divided doses (max 400 mg/day); may give as a single bedtime dose (max 300 mg q HS)

Tab: 25, 50, 100, 150 mg

- ***clomipramine*** (C)(G) <10 years: not recommended; 10-<16 years: initially 25 mg daily in divided doses; gradually increase; max 3 mg/kg or 100 mg, whichever is smaller; >16 years: initially 25 mg daily in divided doses; gradually increase to 100 mg during first 2 weeks; max 250 mg/day; total maintenance dose may be given at HS

  Anafranil *Cap:* 25, 50, 75 mg

- ***desipramine*** (C)(G) <12 years: not recommended; ≥12 years: 100-200 mg/day in single or divided doses; max 300 mg/day

  Norpramin *Tab:* 10, 25, 50, 75, 100, 150 mg

- ***doxepin*** (C)(G) <12 years: not recommended; ≥12 years: 75 mg/day; max 150 mg/day

  Cap: 10, 25, 50, 75, 100, 150 mg; Oral conc: 10 mg/ml (4 oz w. dropper)

- ***imipramine*** (C)(G) <12 years: not recommended; ≥12 years:

  Tofranil initially 75 mg daily (max 200 mg); adolescents initially 30-40 mg daily (max 100 mg/day); if maintenance dose exceeds 75 mg daily, may switch to **Tofranil PM** for divided or bedtime dose

  Tab: 10, 25, 50 mg

  Tofranil PM initially 75 mg daily 1 hour before HS; max 200 mg

  Cap: 75, 100, 125, 150 mg

- ***nortriptyline*** (D)(G) <12 years: not recommended; ≥12 years: initially 25 mg tid-qid; max 150 mg/day

  Pamelor *Cap:* 10, 25, 50, 75 mg; *Oral soln:* 10 mg/5 ml (16 oz)

- ***protriptyline*** (C) <12 years: not recommended; ≥12 years: initially 5 mg tid; usual dose 15-40 mg/day in 3-4 divided doses; max 60 mg/day

  Vivactil *Tab:* 5, 10 mg

- ***trimipramine*** (C) <12 years: not recommended; ≥12 years: initially 75 mg/day in divided doses; max 200 mg/day

  Surmontil *Cap:* 25, 50, 100 mg

FIRST GENERATION ANTIHISTAMINE

- ***hydroxyzine*** (C)(G) <6 years: 50 mg/day divided qid; 6-12 years: 50-100 mg/day divided qid; >12 years: 50-100 mg qid; max 600 mg/day

  Atarax *Tab:* 10, 25, 50, 100 mg; *Syr:* 10 mg/5 ml (alcohol 0.5%)

  Vistaril *Cap:* 25, 50, 100 mg; *Oral susp:* 25 mg/5 ml (4 oz) (lemon)

  Comment: ***hydroxyzine*** is contraindicated in early pregnancy and in patients with a prolonged QT interval. It is not known whether this drug is excreted in human milk; therefore, ***hydroxyzine*** should not be given to nursing mothers.

AZAPIRONE

- ***buspirone*** (B) <6 years: not recommended; ≥6 years: initially 7.5 mg bid; may increase by 5 mg/day q 2-3 days; max 60 mg/day

  BuSpar *Tab:* 5, 10, 15*, 30*mg

BENZODIAZEPINES

Short-Acting Benzodiazepines

- ***alprazolam*** (D)(IV)(G)

  Niravam <18 years: not recommended; ≥18 years: initially 0.25-0.5 mg tid; may titrate every 3-4 days; max 4 mg/day

  Tab: 0.25*, 0.5*, 1*, 2*mg orally-disint

Xanax <18 years: not recommended; ≥18 years: initially 0.25-0.5 mg tid; may titrate every 3-4 days; max 4 mg/day

Tab: 0.25*, 0.5*, 1*, 2*mg

Xanax XR <18 years: not recommended; ≥18 years: initially 0.5-1 mg once daily, preferably in the AM; increase at intervals of at least 3-4 days by up to 1 mg/day; taper no faster than 0.5 mg every 3 days; max 10 mg/day; when switching from immed-rel to ext-rel ***alprazolam***, once daily dose of ext-rel equals total daily dose of immed-rel

Tab: 0.5, 1, 2, 3 mg ext-rel

▶ ***oxazepam*** (C)(IV)(G) <12 years: not recommended; ≥12 years: 10-15 mg tid-qid for moderate symptoms; 15-30 mg tid-qid for severe symptoms

Tab: 15 mg; *Cap:* 10, 15, 30 mg

Intermediate-Acting Benzodiazepines

▶ ***lorazepam*** (D)(IV)(G) <18 years: not recommended; ≥18 years: 1-10 mg/day in 2-3 divided doses

Ativan *Tab:* 0.5, 1*, 2*mg

Lorazepam Intensol *Oral conc:* 2 mg/ml (30 ml w. graduated dropper)

Long-Acting Benzodiazepines

▶ ***chlordiazepoxide*** (D)(IV)(G)

Librium <6 years: not recommended; ≥6 years: 5 mg bid-qid; may increase to 10 mg bid-tid; *Moderate symptoms:* 5-10 mg tid-qid; *Severe symptoms:* 20-25 mg tid-qid

Cap: 5, 10, 25 mg

Librium Injectable <18 years: not recommended; ≥18 years: 50-100 mg IM or IV; then 25-50 mg IM tid-qid prn; max 300 mg/day

Inj: 100 mg

▶ ***chlordiazepoxide+clidinium*** (D)(IV) <18 years: not recommended; ≥18 years: 1-2 caps tid-qid: max 8 caps/day

Librax *Cap:* chlor 5 mg+clid 2.5 mg

▶ ***clonazepam*** (D)(IV)(G) <18 years: not recommended; ≥18 years: initially 0.25 mg bid; increase to 1 mg/day after 3 days

Klonopin *Tab:* 0.5*, 1, 2 mg

Klonopin Wafers dissolve in mouth with or without water

Wafer: 0.125, 0.25, 0.5, 1, 2 mg orally-disint

▶ ***clorazepate*** (D)(IV)(G) <9 years: not recommended; ≥9 years: 30 mg/day in divided doses; max 60 mg/day

Tranxene *Tab:* 3.75, 7.5, 15 mg

Tranxene SD do not use for initial therapy

Tab: 22.5 mg ext-rel

Tranxene SD Half Strength do not use for initial therapy

Tab: 11.25 mg ext-rel

Tranxene T-Tab *Tab:* 3.75*, 7.5*, 15*mg

▶ ***diazepam*** (D)(IV)(G) <12 years: not recommended; ≥12 years: 2-10 mg bid to qid

Diastat *Rectal gel delivery system:* 2.5 mg

Diastat AcuDial *Rectal gel delivery system:* 10, 20 mg

Valium *Tab:* 2*, 5*, 10*mg

Valium Injectable *Vial:* 5 mg/ml (10 ml); *Amp:* 5 mg/ml (2 ml); *Prefilled syringe:* 5 mg/ml (5 ml)

Valium Intensol Oral Solution *Conc oral soln:* 5 mg/ml (30 ml w. dropper) (alcohol 19%)

Valium Oral Solution *Oral soln:* 5 mg/5 ml (500 ml) (wintergreen spice)

PHENOTHIAZINES

▶ ***prochlorperazine*** **(C)(G)**
 Compazine 5 mg tid-qid
 Tab: 5 mg; *Syr:* 5 mg/5 ml (4 oz) (fruit); *Rectal supp:* 2.5, 5, 25 mg
 Compazine Spansule 15 mg q AM or 10 mg q 12 hours
 Spansule: 10, 15 mg sust-rel

▶ ***trifluoperazine*** **(C)(G)** <12 years: not recommended; ≥12 years: 1-2 mg bid; max 6 mg/day; max 12 weeks
 Stelazine *Tab:* 1, 2, 5, 10 mg

PARONYCHIA (PERIUNGUAL ABSCESS)

▶ ***cephalexin*** **(B)(G)** <12 years: 25-50 mg/kg/day in 4 divided doses x 10 days; *see page* 601 *for dose by weight table;* ≥12 years: mg bid x 10 days
 Keflex *Cap:* 250, 333, 500, 750 mg; *Oral susp:* 125, 250 mg/5 ml (100, 200 ml) (strawberry)

▶ ***clindamycin*** **(B)(G)** <12 years: 8-16 mg/kg/day in 3-4 divided doses x 10 days; *see page* 603 *for dose by weight table;* ≥12 years: 150-300 mg q 6 hours x 10 days
 Cleocin *Cap:* 75 (tartrazine), 150 (tartrazine), 300 mg
 Cleocin Pediatric Granules *Oral susp:* 75 mg/5 ml (100 ml) (cherry)

▶ ***dicloxacillin*** **(B)(G)** <12 years: 12.5-25 mg/kg/day in 4 divided doses x 10 days; *see page* 604 *for dose by weight table*; ≥12 years: 500 mg q 6 hours x 10 days
 Dynapen *Cap:* 125, 250, 500 mg; *Oral susp:* 62.5 mg/5 ml (80, 100, 200 ml)

▶ ***erythromycin base*** **(B)(G)** <45 kg: 30-50 mg in 2-4 doses x 10 days; ≥45 kg: 500 mg q 6 hours x 10 days
 Ery-Tab *Tab:* 250, 333, 500 mg ent-coat
 PCE *Tab:* 333, 500 mg

▶ ***erythromycin ethylsuccinate*** **(B)(G)** <12 years: 30-50 mg/kg/day in 4 divided doses q 6 hours x 10 days; may double dose with severe infection; max 100 mg/kg/day or 400 mg qid; *see page* 607 *for dose by weight table*
 EryPed *Oral susp:* 200 mg/5 ml (100, 200 ml) (fruit); 400 mg/5 ml (60, 100, 200 ml) (banana); *Oral drops*: 200, 400 mg/5 ml (50 ml) (fruit); *Chew tab*: 200 mg wafer (fruit)
 E.E.S. *Oral susp*: 200, 400 mg/5 ml (100 ml) (fruit)
 E.E.S. Granules *Oral susp:* 200 mg/5 ml (100, 200 ml) (cherry)
 E.E.S. 400 Tablets *Tab:* 400 mg

PEDICULOSIS HUMANUS CAPITIS (HEAD LICE) & PHTHIRUS (PUBIC LICE)

▶ ***ivermectin*** **(C)** <6 months, <33 lbs: not recommended; ≥6 months, ≥33 lbs: same thoroughly wet hair; leave on for 10 minutes; then rinse off with water; do not retreat
 Sklice *Lotn:* 0.5% (4 oz, 117 gm, laminate tube)

▶ ***lindane*** **(C)(G)** <2 years: not recommended; ≥2 years: apply, leave on for 4 minutes, then thoroughly wash off
 Kwell Shampoo *Shampoo:* 1% (60 ml)

▶ ***malathion*** **(B)(G)** <12 years: not recommended; ≥12 years: thoroughly wet hair; allow to dry naturally; shampoo and rinse after 8-12 hours; use a fine tooth comb to remove lice and nits; if lice persist after 7-9 days, may repeat treatment
 Ovide (OTC) *Lotn:* 59% (2 oz)

▶ ***permethrin*** **(B)(G)** <2 months: not recommended; ≥2 months: apply to washed and towel-dried hair; allow to remain on for 10 minutes, then rinse off; repeat after 7 days if needed
 Nix (OTC) *Crm rinse:* 1% (2 oz w. comb)

- *pyrethrins with piperonyl butoxide* (C)(G) <2 months: not recommended; ≥2 months: apply and leave on for 10 minutes, then wash off
  - **A-200** *Shampoo: pyr* 0.33%+*pip but* 3%
  - **Rid Mousse** *Shampoo: pyr* 0.33%+*pip but* 4%
  - **Rid Shampoo** *Shampoo: pyr* 0.33%+*pip but* 3%

Comment: To remove nits, soak hair in equal parts white vinegar and water for 15-20 minutes.

PELVIC INFLAMMATORY DISEASE (PID)

Comment: The following treatment regimens are published in the **2015 CDC Sexually Transmitted Diseases Treatment Guidelines.** Treatment regimens are presented by generic drug name first, followed by information about brands and dose forms. Treat all sexual partners. Because of the high risk for maternal morbidity and preterm delivery, pregnant females who have suspected PID should be hospitalized and treated with parenteral antibiotics. HIV-infected females with PID respond equally well to standard parenteral and antibiotic regimens as HIV-negative females.

OUTPATIENT REGIMENS

Regimen 1

- ***ceftriaxone*** 250 mg IM in a single dose plus ***doxycycline***
- ***doxycycline*** 100 mg bid x 14 days with or without ***metronidazole***
- ***metronidazole*** 500 mg PO bid x 14 days

Regimen 2

- ***cefoxitin*** 2 gm IM in a single dose plus ***probebecid***
- ***probenecid*** 1 gm PO in a single dose administered concurrently plus ***doxycycline*** 100 mg bid x 14 days with or without ***metronidazole***
- ***metronidazole*** 500 mg PO bid x 14 days

Regimen 3

- Other parenteral third-generation cephalosporin (e.g., ***ceftizoxime*** or ***cefotaxime***) in a single dose) plus ***doxycycline***
- ***doxycycline*** 100 mg bid x 14 days with or without ***metronidazole***
- ***metronidazole*** 500 mg PO bid x 14 days

DRUG BRANDS AND DOSE FORMS

- *cefoxitin* (B)(G)
  - **Mefoxin** *Vial:* 1, 2 gm
- *ceftriaxone* (B)(G)
  - **Rocephin** Vials 250, 500 mg: 1, 2 gm
- *doxycycline* (D)(G)
  - **Acticlate** *Tab:* 75, 150**mg
  - **Adoxa** *Tab:* 50, 75, 100, 150 mg ent-coat
  - **Doryx** *Tab:* 50, 75, 100, 150, 200 mg del-rel
  - **Doxteric** *Tab:* 50 mg del-rel
  - **Monodox** *Cap:* 50, 75, 100 mg
  - **Oracea** *Cap:* 40 mg del-rel

Vibramycin *Tab:* 100 mg; *Cap:* 50, 100 mg; *Syr:* 50 mg/5 ml (raspberry-apple) (sulfites); *Oral susp:* 25 mg/5 ml (raspberry)
Vibra-Tab *Tab:* 100 mg film-coat

Comment: ***doxycycline*** is contraindicated <8 years-of-age, in pregnancy, and lactation (discolors developing tooth enamel). A side effect may be photosensitivity (photophobia). Do not take with antacids, calcium supplements, milk or other dairy, or within 2 hours of taking another drug.

▶ ***metronidazole*** **(not for use in 1st; B in 2nd, 3rd)**
Flagyl *Tab:* 250*, 500*mg
Flagyl 375 *Cap:* 375 mg
Flagyl ER *Tab:* 750 mg ext-rel

Comment: Alcohol is contraindicated during treatment with oral ***metronidazole*** and for 72 hours after therapy due to a possible ***disulfiram***-like reaction (nausea, vomiting, flushing, headache).

▶ ***probenecid*** (B)(G)
Benemid *Tab:* 500*mg; *Cap:* 500 mg

PEPTIC ULCER DISEASE (PUD)

Helicobacter pylori **Eradication Regimens** *see page* 188
Antacids *see* **GERD** *page* 158

H2 ANTAGONISTS

▶ ***cimetidine*** (B)(G) <16 years: not recommended; ≥16 years:
Tagamet 800 mg bid or 400 mg qid; max 2.4 gm/day
Tab: 300, 400*, 800*mg
Tagamet HB (OTC) *Prophylaxis:* 1 tab ac; *Treatment:* 1 tab bid
Tab: 200 mg
Tagamet HB Oral Suspension (OTC) *Prophylaxis:* 1 tsp ac; *Treatment:* 1 tsp bid
Oral susp: 200 mg/20 ml (12 oz)
Tagamet Liquid *Liq:* 300 mg/5 ml (mint-peach) (alcohol 2.8%)

▶ ***famotidine*** (B)(G) <12 years: 0.5 mg/kg/day q HS or in 2 divided doses; max 40 mg/day; ≥12 years: 20 mg bid or 40 mg q HS; *max* 6 weeks
Pepcid *Tab:* 20, 40 mg; *Oral susp:* 40 mg/5 ml (50 ml)
Pepcid AC (OTC) *Tab/Rapid dissolv tab:* 10 mg
Pepcid Complete (OTC) *Tab:* fam 10 mg+CaCO2 800 mg+mag hydrox 165 mg
Pepcid RPD *Tab:* 20, 40 mg rapid-dissolv

▶ ***nizatidine*** (B)(G) <12 years: not recommended; ≥12 years: 150 mg bid; max 12 weeks
Axid *Cap:* 150, 300 mg
Axid AR (OTC) 1 tab ac; max 150 mg/day
Tab: 75 mg

▶ ***ranitidine*** (B)(G) <1 month: not recommended; 1 month-16 years: 2-4 mg/kg/day in 2 divided doses; max 300 mg/day; *Duodenal/Gastric Ulcer:* 2-4 mg/kg/day divided bid; max 300 mg/day; *Erosive Esophagitis:* 5-10 mg/kg/day divided bid; max 300 mg/day; >16 years:
Zantac 150 mg bid or 300 mg q HS
Tab: 150, 300 mg
Zantac 75 (OTC) 1 tab ac
Tab: 75 mg
Zantac EFFERdose dissolve 25 mg tab in 5 ml water; dissolve 150 mg tab in 6-8 oz water

Efferdose: 25, 150 mg effervescent (phenylalanine)
Zantac Syrup *Syr:* 15 mg/ml (peppermint) (alcohol 7.5%)

- ***ranitidine bismuth citrate*** **(C)** <12 years: not recommended; ≥12 years: 400 mg bid
  Tritec *Tab:* 400 mg

PROTON PUMP INHIBITORS (PPIs)

Comment: If hepatic impairment, or if patient is Asian, consider reducing the PPI dosage. Research has demonstrated associations between PPI use and fractures of the hip, wrist, and spine, hypomagnesemia, kidney injuries and chronic kidney disease, possible cardiovascular drug interactions, and infections (e.g., *Clostridium difficile* and pneumonia). Reducing the acidity of the stomach allows bacteria to thrive and spread to other organs like the lungs and intestines. This risk is increased with high dose and chronic use and greatest in the elderly. The most recent class-wide FDA warning cites reports of cutaneous and systemic lupus erythematosis (CLS/SLE) associated with PPIs in patients with both new onset and exacerbation of existing autoimmune disease. PPI treatment should be discontinued and the patient should be referred to a specialist.
(http://www.fda.gov/Drugs/DrugSafety/InformationbyDrugClass/ucm213259.htm)

- ***dexlansoprazole*** **(B)(G)** <18 years: not recommended; ≥18 years: 30-60 mg daily for up to 4 weeks
  Dexilant *Cap:* 30, 60 mg ent-coat del-rel granules; may open and sprinkle on applesauce; do not crush or chew granules
  Dexilant SoluTab *Tab:* 30 mg del-rel orally-disint
- ***esomeprazole*** **(B)(OTC)(G)** <1 year: not recommended; 1-11 years: <20 kg: 10 mg; ≥20 kg: 10-20 mg once daily; ≥12 years: 20-40 mg daily; max 8 weeks; take 1 hour before food; swallow whole or mix granules with food or juice and take immediately; do not crush or chew granules
  Nexium *Cap:* 20, 40 mg ent-coat del-rel pellets
  Nexium for Oral Suspension *Oral susp:* 10, 20, 40 mg ent-coat del-rel granules/pkt (30 pkt/carton); mix in 2 tbsp water and drink immediately
- ***lansoprazole*** **(B)(OTC)(G)** year: not recommended; 1-11, <30 kg: 15 mg once daily; ≥12 years: 15-30 mg daily for up to 8 weeks; may repeat course; take before eating
  Prevacid *Cap:* 15, 30 mg ent-coat del-rel granules; swallow whole or mix granules with food or juice and take immediately; do not crush or chew granules; follow with water
  Prevacid for Oral Suspension *Oral susp:* 15, 30 mg ent-coat del-rel granules/pkt; (30 pkt/carton); mix in 2 tbsp water and drink immediately (strawberry)
  Prevacid SoluTab *ODT:* 15, 30 mg (strawberry) (phenylalanine)
  Prevacid 24HR 15 mg ent-coat del-rel granules; swallow whole or mix granules with food or juice and take immediately; do not crush or chew granules; follow with water
- ***omeprazole*** **(C)(OTC)(G)** <1 year: not recommended; 5-<10 kg: 5 mg daily; 10-<20 kg: 10 mg daily; ≥20 kg: 20-40 mg daily; take before eating; swallow whole or mix granules with applesauce and take immediately; do not crush or chew; follow with water
  Prilosec *Cap:* 10, 20, 40 mg del-rel granules
  Prilosec OTC *Tab:* 20 mg del-rel (regular, wild berry)
- ***pantoprazole*** **(B)** <12 years: not recommended; ≥12 years: 40 mg bid
  Protonix (G) *Tab:* 40 mg ent-coat del-rel
  Protonix for Oral Suspension *Oral susp:* 40 mg ent-coat del-rel granules/pkt; mix in 1 tsp apple juice for 5 seconds or sprinkle on 1 tsp applesauce, and swallow immediately; do not mix in water or any other liquid or food; take approximately 30 minutes prior to a meal; 30 pkt/carton

- *rabeprazole* (B)(OTC)(G) 12 years: not recommended; ≥12 years: initially 20 mg daily; then titrate; may take 100 mg daily in divided doses or 60 mg bid; max 8 weeks
    - **AcipHex** *Tab:* 20 mg ent-coat del-rel
    - **AcipHex Sprinkle** *Cap:* 5, 10 mg del-rel

OTHER

- *glycopyrrolate* (B)(G) <12 years: not recommended; ≥12 years: initially 1-2 mg bid-tid; *Maintenance:* 1 mg bid; max 8 mg/day
    - **Robinul** *Tab:* 1 mg (dye-free)
    - **Robinul Forte** *Tab:* 2 mg (dye-free)

  Comment: ***glycopyrrolate*** is an anticholinergic adjunct to PUD treatment.
- *mepenzolate* (B)(G) 25-50 mg divided qid, with meals and at HS
    - **Cantil** *Tab:* 25 mg
- *sucralfate* (B)(G) *Active ulcer:* 1 gm qid; *Maintenance:* 1 gm bid
    - **Carafate** *Tab:* 1 gm; *Oral susp:* 1 gm/10 ml (14 oz)

PROPHYLAXIS

- *misoprostol* (X) <12 years: not recommended; ≥12 years: 200 mg qid with food for prevention of NSAID-induced gastric ulcers
    - **Cytotec** *Tab:* 100, 200 mg

  Comment: ***misoprostol*** is a prostaglandin E1 analog indicated for the prevention of NSAID-induced gastric ulcers. Females of childbearing potential should have a negative serum pregnancy test within 2 weeks before starting and first dose on the 2nd or 3rd day of the next menstrual period. A contraceptive method should be maintained during therapy. Risks to pregnant females include: spontaneous abortion, premature birth, fetal anomalies, and uterine rupture.

PERIPHERAL NEURITIS & DIABETIC NEUROPATHIC PAIN, & PERIPHERAL NEUROPATHIC PAIN

- **Acetaminophen for IV Infusion** *see* ***Pain*** *page* 322
- **Ibuprofen for IV Infusion** *see* ***Pain*** *page* 322
- ***acetaminophen*** (B)(G) *see* ***Fever*** *page* 149
- ***aspirin*** (D)(G) *see* ***Fever*** *page* 150

  Comment: ***aspirin***-containing medications are contraindicated with history of allergic-type reaction to ***aspirin***, children and adolescents with *Varicella* or other viral illness, and 3rd trimester of pregnancy.

ALPHA-2 DELTA LIGAND

- *pregabalin (GABA analog)* (C)(V) <18 years: not recommended; ≥18 years: initially 150 mg daily divided bid-tid; may titrate within one week; max 600 mg divided bid-tid; discontinue over one week
- *pregabalin (GABA analog)* (C)(V) <18 years: not recommended; ≥18 years:
    - **Lyrica** initially 150 mg divided bid-tid; may titrate within one week; max 600 mg divided bid-tid; discontinue over 1 week
        - *Cap:* 25, 50, 75, 100, 150, 200, 225, 300 mg; *Oral soln:* 20 mg/ml
    - **Lyrica CR** *Tab:* usual dose: 165 mg once daily; may increase to 330 mg/day within 1 week; max 660 mg/day; discontinue over 1 week
        - *Tab:* 82.5, 165, 330 mg ext-rel

SEROTONIN-NOREPINEPHRINE REUPTAKE INHIBITOR (SNRI)

▶ ***duloxetine*** **(C)** <12 years: not recommended; ≥12 years: swallow whole; 30-60 mg once daily; may increase by 30 mg at 1 week intervals; usual target 60 mg daily; max 120 mg/day

Cymbalta *Cap:* 20, 30, 60 mg ent-coat pellets

Comment: **Cymbalta** is indicated for chronic pain syndromes (e.g., arthritis, fibromyalgia, low back pain).

TOPICAL & TRANSDERMAL NSAIDs

▶ ***capsaicin*** cream **(B)(G)** <2 years: not recommended; 2-12 years: apply sparingly to intact skin bid prn; >12 years: apply tid-qid prn

Axsain *Crm:* 0.075% (1, 2 oz)
Capsin (OTC) *Lotn:* 0.025, 0, 075% (59 ml)
Capzasin-P (OTC) *Crm:* 0.025% (1.5 oz); *Lotn:* 0.025% (2 oz)
Capzasin-HP (OTC) *Crm:* 0.075% (1.5 oz); *Lotn:* 0.075% (2 oz)
Dolorac *Crm:* 0.025% (28 gm)
Double Cap (OTC) *Crm:* 0.05% (2 oz)
R-Gel *Gel:* 0.025% (15, 30 gm)
Zostrix (OTC) *Crm:* 0.025% (0.7, 1.5, 3 oz)
Zostrix HP (OTC) *Emol crm:* 0.075% (1, 2 oz)

Comment: Provides some relief by 1-2 weeks; optimal benefit may take 4-6 weeks. Avoid contact with mucous membranes.

▶ ***capsaicin 8%*** patch **(B)** <18 years: not recommended; ≥18 years: apply up to 4 patches for one 60-minute application to clean dry skin; may prep area with topical anesthetic; wear non-latex gloves; patches may be cut to size/shape; treatment may be repeated every 3 months; remove with cleansing gel after treatment

Qutenza *Patch:* 8% 1640 mcg/cm (179 mg) (1 or 2 patches, each w. 1-50 gm tube cleansing gel/carton)

▶ ***diclofenac epolamine transdermal patch*** **(C)** <12 years: not recommended; ≥12 years: apply one patch to affected area bid; remove during bathing; avoid non-intact skin

Flector Patch *Patch:* 180 mg/patch (30/carton)

▶ ***capsaicin*** cream **(B)(G)** <2 years: not recommended; 2-12 years: apply sparingly to intact skin bid prn; >12 years: apply tid-qid prn

Axsain *Crm:* 0.075% (1, 2 oz)
Capsin (OTC) *Lotn:* 0.025, 0, 075% (59 ml)
Capzasin-P (OTC) *Crm:* 0.025% (1.5 oz); *Lotn:* 0.025% (2 oz)
Capzasin-HP (OTC) *Crm:* 0.075% (1.5 oz); *Lotn:* 0.075% (2 oz)
Dolorac *Crm:* 0.025% (28 gm)
Double Cap (OTC) *Crm:* 0.05% (2 oz)
R-Gel *Gel:* 0.025% (15, 30 gm)
Zostrix (OTC) *Crm:* 0.025% (0.7, 1.5, 3 oz)
Zostrix HP (OTC) *Emol crm:* 0.075% (1, 2 oz)

Comment: Provides some relief by 1-2 weeks; optimal benefit may take 4-6 weeks. Avoid contact with mucous membranes.

▶ ***capsaicin 8%*** patch **(B)** <18 years: not recommended; ≥18 years: apply up to 4 patches for one 60-minute application to clean dry skin; may prep area with topical anesthetic; wear non-latex gloves; patches may be cut to size/shape; treatment may be repeated every 3 months; remove with cleansing gel after treatment

Qutenza *Patch:* 8% 1640 mcg/cm (179 mg) (1 or 2 patches w. 1-50 gm tube cleansing gel/carton)

▶ ***lidocaine*** 5% patch **(B)(G)** <18 years: not recommended; ≥18 years: apply up to 3 patches at one time for up to 12 hours/24-hour period (12 hours on/12 hours off); patches may be cut into smaller sizes before removal of the release liner; do not reuse

Lidoderm *Patch:* 5% (10 x 14 cm, 30/carton)

ORAL ANALGESICS

▶ ***tramadol*** (C)(IV)(G)

Comment: ***tramadol*** is known to be excreted in breast milk. The FDA and the European Medicines Agency (EMA) are investigating the safety of using ***tramadol***-containing medications to treat pain in children 12-18 years because of the potential for serious side effects, including slowed or difficult breathing.

Rybix ODT <12 years: contraindicated; 12-<18: use extreme caution; not recommended for children and adolescents with obesity, asthma, obstructive sleep apnea, or other chronic breathing problem, or for post-tonsillectomy/adenoidectomy pain; ≥18 years: initially 100 mg once daily; may increase by 100 mg every 5 days; max 300 mg/day; *CrCl <30 mL/min or severe hepatic impairment:* not recommended; *Cirrhosis:* max 50 mg q 12 hours

ODT: 50 mg (mint) (phenylalanine)

Ryzolt <12 years: contraindicated; 12-<18: use extreme caution; not recommended for children and adolescents with obesity, asthma, obstructive sleep apnea, or other chronic breathing problem, or for post-tonsillectomy/adenoid-ectomy pain; ≥18 years: initially 100 mg once daily; may increase by 100 mg every 5 days; max 300 mg/day; *CrCl <30 mL/min or severe hepatic impairment:* not recommended

Tab: 100, 200, 300 mg ext-rel

Ultram <12 years: contraindicated; 12-<18: use extreme caution; not recommended for children and adolescents with obesity, asthma, obstructive sleep apnea, or other chronic breathing problem, or for post-tonsillectomy/adenoidectomy pain; ≥18 years: 50-100 mg q 4-6 hours prn; max 400 mg/day; *CrCl <30 mL/min:* max 100 mg q 12 hours; *Cirrhosis:* max 50 mg q 12 hours

Tab: 50*mg

Ultram ER <12 years: contraindicated; 12-<18: use extreme caution; not recommended for children and adolescents with obesity, asthma, obstructive sleep apnea, or other chronic breathing problem, or for post-tonsillectomy/adenoidectomy pain; ≥18 years: initially 100 mg once daily; may increase by 100 mg every 5 days; max 300 mg/day; *CrCl <30 mL/min: or severe hepatic impairment:* not recommended

Tab: 100, 200, 300 mg ext-rel

▶ ***tramadol+acetaminophen*** (C)(IV)(G) <12 years: contraindicated; 12-<18: use extreme caution; not recommended for children and adolescents with obesity, asthma, obstructive sleep apnea, or other chronic breathing problem, or for post-tonsillectomy/adenoidectomy pain; ≥18 years: 2 tabs q 4-6 hours; max 8 tabs/day; 5 days; *CrCl <30 mL/min:* max 2 tabs q 12 hours; max 4 tabs/day x 5 days

Ultracet *Tab: tram* 37.5+*acet* 325 mg

Comment: ***tramadol*** is known to be excreted in breast milk. The FDA and the European Medicines Agency (EMA) are investigating the safety of using ***tramadol***-containing medications to treat pain in children 12-18 years because of the potential for serious side effects, including slowed or difficult breathing.

MU-OPIOID AGONIST+NOREPINEPHRINE REUPTAKE INHIBITOR COMBINATION

▶ ***tapentadol*** (C) <18 years: not recommended; ≥18 years:

Nucynta 50-100 mg q 4-6 hours prn; max 700 mg/day on the first day; 600 mg/day on subsequent days

Tab: 50, 75, 100 mg

Nucynta ER *Opioid-naïve:* initially 50 mg q 12 hours, then titrate to optimal dose within therapeutic range; usual therapeutic range 100-250 mg q 12 hours; doses >500 mg not recommended; *Converting from Nucynta*: divide total **Nucynta** daily dose into 2 **Nucynta ER** doses and administer q 12 hours; converting from ***oxycodone CR*** and other opioids, see mfr recommendations

Tab: 50, 100, 150, 200, 250 mg ext-rel

PERLECHE/ANGULAR STOMATITIS

Comment: Perleche is a form of intertrigo. This localized tissue inflammation and maceration is characterized by constant exposure to saliva, which normally contains bacteria, yeast, and other organisms, in the natural anatomical furrow at the corners of the mouth. Perleche is often misdiagnosed as yeast infection, but almost never responds to anti-yeast agents. Patients with severe vitamin deficiencies (e.g., chronic alcoholism, malnutrition) are often at increased risk. Sensitivities or allergies to toothpaste (e.g., sodium lauryl sulfate) may be contributing irritants.

Treatment: apply a small amount of a combination of 2.5% ***hydrocortisone*** cream and ***miconazole*** cream (which kills yeast, fungi, and many bacteria) to the affected area twice a day. Once the area is clear, recurrence can be prevented with local application of petroleum jelly.

PERTUSSIS (WHOOPING COUGH)

Prophylaxis *see* ***Childhood Immunizations*** *page* 525

POST-EXPOSURE PROPHYLAXIS AND TREATMENT

Comment: Antibiotics do not alter the course of illness, but they do prevent transmission. Infected persons should be isolated until after the fifth day of antibiotic treatment.

▶ ***azithromycin*** **(B)(G)** <12 years: 12 mg/kg/day x 5 days; *see page* 593 *for dose by weight table*; max 500 mg/day; ≥12 years: 500 mg x 1 dose on day 1, then 250 mg daily on days 2-5 <u>or</u> 500 mg daily x 3 days <u>or</u> **Zmax** 2 gm in a single dose

Zithromax *Tab:* 250, 500, 600 mg; *Oral susp:* 100 mg/5 ml (15 ml); 200 mg/5 ml (15, 22.5, 30 ml) (cherry); *Pkt:* 1 gm for reconstitution (cherry-banana)

Zithromax Tri-pak *Tab:* 3 x 500 mg tabs/pck

Zithromax Z-pak *Tab:* 6 x 250 mg tabs/pck

Zmax *Oral susp:* 2 gm ext-rel for reconstitution (cherry-banana) (148 mg Na^+)

Comment: ***azithromycin*** is the drug of choice for infants <1 month-of-age.

▶ ***clarithromycin*** **(C)(G)** <6 months: not recommended; ≥6 months-12 years: 7.5 mg/kg divided bid x 10 days; *see page* 602 *for dose by weight table;* >12 years: 250 mg bid <u>or</u> 500 mg ext-rel daily x 10 days

Biaxin *Tab:* 250, 500 mg

Biaxin Oral Suspension *Oral susp:* 125, 250 mg/5 ml (50, 100 ml) (fruit punch)

Biaxin XL *Tab:* 500 mg ext-rel

Comment: The FDA is advising caution before prescribing ***clarithromycin*** to patients with heart disease because of a potential increased risk of heart problems or death that can occur years later. This recommendation is based on a review of the results of a 10-year follow-up study of patients with coronary heart disease from a large clinical trial that first observed this safety issue. Consider risk benefit and the use of other antibiotics in such patients.

- ▶ ***erythromycin base*** **(B)(G)** <12 years: 40 mg/kg/day in divided doses x 14 days; ≥12 years: 1 gm/day divided qid x 14 days
  - **Ery-Tab** *Tab:* 250, 333, 500 mg ent-coat
  - **PCE** *Tab:* 333, 500 mg
- ▶ ***erythromycin ethylsuccinate*** **(B)(G)** 40-50 mg/kg/day in 4 divided doses x 14 days; may double dose with severe infection; max 100 mg/kg/day or 400 mg qid; *see page* 607 *for dose by weight table*
  - **EryPed** *Oral susp:* 200 mg/5 ml (100, 200 ml) (fruit); 400 mg/5 ml (60, 100, 200 ml) (banana); Oral drops: 200, 400 mg/5 ml (50 ml) (fruit); *Chew tab:* 200 mg wafer (fruit)
  - **E.E.S.** *Oral susp:* 200, 400 mg/5 ml (100 ml) (fruit)
  - **E.E.S. Granules** *Oral susp:* 200 mg/5 ml (100, 200 ml) (cherry)
  - **E.E.S. 400 Tablets** *Tab:* 400 mg
- ▶ ***trimethoprim+sulfamethoxazole [TMP-SMX]*** **(C)(G)**
  - **Bactrim, Septra** <12 years: not recommended; ≥12 years: 2 tabs bid x 10 days
    - *Tab:* trim 80 mg+sulfa 400 mg*
  - **Bactrim DS, Septra DS** <12 years: not recommended; ≥12 years: 1 tab bid x 10 days
    - *Tab:* trim 160 mg+sulfa 800 mg*
  - **Bactrim Pediatric Suspension, Septra Pediatric Suspension** <2 months: not recommended; 2 months-12 years: 40 mg/kg/day of ***sulfamethoxazole*** in 2 doses bid; >12 years: use tabs
    - *Oral susp:* trim 40 mg+sulfa 200 mg per 5 ml (100 ml) (cherry) (alcohol 0.3%)

PHARYNGITIS: GONOCOCCAL

Comment: Treat all sexual contacts. Empiric therapy requires concomitant treatment for *Chlamydia*. Post-treatment culture recommended with PMHx history rheumatic fever.

PRIMARY THERAPY

- ▶ ***azithromycin*** **(B)(G)** <12 years: 12 mg/kg/day x 5 days; *see page* 593 *for dose by weight table*; max 500 mg/day; ≥12 years: 500 mg x 1 dose on day 1, then 250 mg daily on days 2-5 or 500 mg daily x 3 days or **Zmax** 2 gm in a single dose
  - **Zithromax** *Tab:* 250, 500, 600 mg; *Oral susp:* 100 mg/5 ml (15 ml); 200 mg/5 ml (15, 22.5, 30 ml) (cherry); *Pkt:* 1 gm for reconstitution (cherry-banana)
  - **Zithromax Tri-pak** *Tab:* 3 x 500 mg tabs/pck
  - **Zithromax Z-pak** *Tab:* 6 x 250 mg tabs/pck
  - **Zmax** *Oral susp:* 2 gm ext-rel for reconstitution (cherry-banana) (148 mg Na^+)

  Comment: Per the CDC 2015 STD Treatment Guidelines, ***azithromycin*** should be used with ***ceftriaxone*** 250 mg.
- ▶ ***ceftriaxone*** **(B)(G)** <45 kg: 125 mg IM x 1 dose; ≥45 kg: 250 mg IM x 1 dose
  - **Rocephin** *Vial:* 250, 500 mg; 1, 2 gm

PHARYNGITIS: STREPTOCOCCAL

Comment: Acute rheumatic fever is a rare but serious autoimmune disease that may occur following a group A *streptococcal* throat infection. It causes inflammatory lesions in connective tissue, especially that of the heart, kidneys, joints, blood vessels, and subcutaneous tissue. Prior to the broad availability of penicillin, rheumatic fever was a leading cause of death in children and one of the leading causes of acquired heart disease in adults. Strep throat is highly responsive to the penicillins and cephalosporins.

▶ ***amoxicillin*** **(B)(G)** <40 kg (88 lb): 20-40 mg/kg/day in 3 divided doses x 10 days or 25-45 mg/kg/day in 2 divided doses x 10 days; *see page* 588 *for dose by weight table;* ≥40 kg: 500-875 mg bid or 250-500 mg tid x 10 days

Amoxil *Cap:* 250, 500 mg; *Tab:* 875*mg; *Chew tab:* 125, 200, 250, 400 mg (cherry-banana-peppermint) (phenylalanine); *Oral susp:* 125, 250 mg/5 ml (80, 100, 150 ml) (strawberry); 200, 400 mg/5 ml (50, 75, 100 ml) (bubble gum); *Oral drops:* 50 mg/ml (30 ml) (bubble gum)

Moxatag *Tab:* 775 mg ext-rel

Trimox *Tab:* 125, 250 mg; *Cap:* 250, 500 mg; *Oral susp:* 125, 250 mg/5 ml (80, 100, 150 ml) (raspberry-strawberry)

▶ ***amoxicillin+clavulanate*** **(B)(G)**

Augmentin <40 kg: 40-45 mg/kg/day divided tid x 10 days or 90 mg/kg/day divided bid x 10 days; *see page* 590 *for dose by weight table;* ≥40 kg: 500 mg tid or 875 mg bid x 10 days

Tab: 250, 500, 875 mg; *Chew tab:* 125, 250 mg (lemon-lime); 200, 400 mg (cherry-banana) (phenylalanine); *Oral susp:* 125 mg/5 ml (banana), 250 mg/5 ml (75, 100, 150 ml) (orange); 200, 400 mg/5 ml (50, 75, 100 ml) (orange) (phenylalanine)

Augmentin ES-600 <3 months: not recommended; ≥3 months, <40 kg: 90 mg/kg/day divided q 12 hours x 10 days; *see page* 591 *for dose by weight table;* ≥40 kg: not recommended

Oral susp: 600 mg/5 ml (50, 75, 100, 125, 150, 200 ml) (strawberry cream) (phenylalanine)

Augmentin XR <16 years: use other forms; ≥16 years: 2 tabs q 12 hours x 7-10 days

Tab: 1000*mg ext-rel

▶ ***azithromycin*** **(B)(G)** <12 years: 12 mg/kg/day x 5 days; *see page* 593 *for dose by weight table*; max 500 mg/day; ≥12 years: 500 mg x 1 dose on day 1, then 250 mg daily on days 2-5 or 500 mg daily x 3 days or **Zmax** 2 gm in a single dose

Zithromax *Tab:* 250, 500, 600 mg; *Oral susp:* 100 mg/5 ml (15 ml); 200 mg/5 ml (15, 22.5, 30 ml) (cherry); *Pkt:* 1 gm for reconstitution (cherry-banana)

Zithromax Tri-pak *Tab:* 3 x 500 mg tabs/pck

Zithromax Z-pak *Tab:* 6 x 250 mg tabs/pck

Zmax *Oral susp:* 2 gm ext-rel for reconstitution (cherry-banana) (148 mg Na^+)

▶ ***cefaclor*** **(B)(G)** <1 month: not recommended; 1 month-12 years: 20-40 mg/kg in 2 or 3 divided doses x 10 days; *see page* 594 *for dose by weight table;* max 1 gm/day; >12 years: 375 mg bid x 10 days; max 2 gm/day

Tab: 500 mg; *Cap:* 250, 500 mg; *Susp:* 125 mg/5 ml (75, 150 ml) (strawberry); 187 mg/5 ml (50, 100 ml) (strawberry); 250 mg/5 ml (75, 150 ml) (strawberry); 375 mg/5 ml (50, 100 ml) (strawberry)

Cefaclor Extended Release <16 years: not recommended; ≥16 years: 500 mg bid x 10 days (clinically equivalent to 250 mg immed-rel caps tid); swallow whole; take with meals

Tab: 375, 500 mg ext-rel

▶ ***cefadroxil*** <*12* years: 30 mg/kg/day in 2 divided doses x 10 days; *see page* 595 *for dose by weight table;* ≥12 years: 1-2 gm in a single or 2 divided doses x 10 days

Duricef *Cap:* 500 mg; *Tab:* 1 gm; *Oral susp:* 250 mg/5 ml (100 ml); 500 mg/5 ml (75, 100 ml) (orange-pineapple)

▶ ***cefdinir*** **(B)** <6 months: not recommended; 6 months-12 years: 14 mg/kg/day in 1-2 divided doses x 10 days; *see page* 596 *for dose by weight table;* ≥12 years: 300 mg bid x 10 days or 600 mg daily x 10 days

Omnicef *Cap:* 300 mg; *Oral susp:* 125 mg/5 ml (60, 100 ml) (strawberry)

- ▶ ***cefditoren pivoxil*** **(B)** <12 years: not recommended; ≥12 years: 200 mg bid x 10 days
  Spectracef *Tab:* 200 mg
  Comment: **Spectracef** is contraindicated with milk protein allergy or carnitine deficiency.
- ▶ ***cefixime*** **(B)(G)** <6 months: not recommended; 6 months-12 years, <50 kg: 8 mg/kg/day in 1-2 divided doses x 10 days; >12 years, ≥50 kg: same as adult; *see page* 597 *for dose by weight table;* >12 years: 400 mg daily x 10 days
  Suprax *Tab:* 400 mg; *Cap:* 400 mg; *Oral susp:* 100, 200, 500 mg/5 ml (50, 75, 100 ml) (strawberry)
- ▶ ***cefpodoxime proxetil*** **(B)** <2 months: not recommended; 2 months-12 years: 10 mg/kg/day in 2 divided doses x 5-7 days; *see page* 598 *for dose by weight table;* >12 yours: 100 mg bid x 5-7 days
  Vantin *Tab:* 100, 200 mg; *Oral susp:* 50, 100 mg/5 ml (50, 75, 100 mg) (lemon creme)
- ▶ ***cefprozil*** **(B)** ≤6 months: not recommended; 6 months-12 years: 7.5 mg/kg divided bid x 10 days; *see page* 599 *for dose by weight table;* >12 years: 500 mg daily x 10 days
  Cefzil *Tab:* 250, 500 mg; *Oral susp:* 125, 250 mg/5 ml (50, 75, 100 ml) (bubble gum) (phenylalanine)
- ▶ ***ceftibuten*** **(B)** <12 years: 9 mg/kg daily x 10 days; max 400 mg/day; *see page* 600 *for dose by weight table;* ≥12 years: 400 mg daily x 10 days
  Cedax *Cap:* 400 mg; *Oral susp:* 90 mg/5 ml (30, 60, 90, 120 ml); 180 mg/5 ml (30, 60, 120 ml) (cherry)
- ▶ ***cephalexin*** **(B)(G)** <12 years: 25-50 mg/kg/day in 4 divided doses x 10 days; *see page* 601 *for dose by weight table;* ≥12 years: 500 mg bid x 10 days
  Keflex *Cap:* 250, 333, 500, 750 mg; *Oral susp:* 125, 250 mg/5 ml (100, 200 ml) (strawberry)
- ▶ ***clarithromycin*** **(C)(G)** <6 months: not recommended; ≥6 months-12 years: 7.5 mg/kg divided bid x 10 days; *see page* 602 *for dose by weight table;* >12 years: 250 mg bid or 500 mg ext-rel daily x 10 days
  Biaxin *Tab:* 250, 500 mg
  Biaxin Oral Suspension *Oral susp:* 125, 250 mg/5 ml (50, 100 ml) (fruit punch)
  Biaxin XL *Tab:* 500 mg ext-rel

Comment: The FDA is advising caution before prescribing ***clarithromycin*** to patients with heart disease because of a potential increased risk of heart problems or death that can occur years later. This recommendation is based on a review of the results of a 10-year follow-up study of patients with coronary heart disease from a large clinical trial that first observed this safety issue. Consider risk benefit and the use of other antibiotics in such patients.

- ▶ ***dirithromycin*** **(C)(G)** <12 years: not recommended; ≥12 years: 500 mg daily x 10 days
  Dynabac *Tab:* 250 mg
- ▶ ***erythromycin base*** **(B)(G)** <45 kg: 30-50 mg divided bid-qid x 10 days; ≥45 kg: 500 mg qid x 10 days
  Ery-Tab *Tab:* 250, 333, 500 mg ent-coat
  PCE *Tab:* 333, 500 mg
- ▶ ***erythromycin estolate*** **(B)(G)** <12 years: 20-50 mg/kg divided q 6 hours x 10 days; *see page* 606 *for dose by weight table;* ≥12 years: 250-500 mg qid x 10 days
  Ilosone *Pulvule:* 250 mg; *Tab:* 500 mg; *Liq:* 125, 250 mg/5 ml (100 ml)
- ▶ ***erythromycin ethylsuccinate*** **(B)(G)** 30-50 mg/kg/day in 4 divided doses x 7 days; may double dose with severe infection; max 100 mg/kg/day or 400 mg qid; *see page* 607 *for dose by weight table*
  EryPed *Oral susp:* 200 mg/5 ml (100, 200 ml) (fruit); 400 mg/5 ml (60, 100, 200 ml) (banana); *Oral drops:* 200, 400 mg/5 ml (50 ml) (fruit); *Chew tab:* 200 mg wafer (fruit)

E.E.S. *Oral susp:* 200, 400 mg/5 ml (100 ml) (fruit)
E.E.S. Granules *Oral susp:* 200 mg/5 ml (100, 200 ml) (cherry)
E.E.S. 400 Tablets *Tab:* 400 mg

- ***loracarbef*** **(B)** <12 years: 15 mg/kg/day in 2 divided doses x 5 days; *see page* 614 *for dose by weight table*; ≥12 years: 200 mg bid x 5 days
  Lorabid *Pulvule:* 200, 400 mg; *Oral susp:* 100 mg/5 ml (50, 100 ml); 200 mg/5 ml (50, 75, 100 ml) (strawberry bubble gum)
- ***penicillin g (benzathine)*** **(B)(G)** <60 lb: 300,000-600,000 units IM x 1 dose; ≥60 lb, ≥12-18 years: 900,000 units x 1 dose; ≥18 years: 1.2 million units IM x 1 dose
  Bicillin L-A *Cartridge-needle unit:* 600,000 units (1 ml); 1.2 million units (2 ml)
- ***penicillin g (benzathine and procaine)*** **(B)(G)** <30 lb: 600,000 units IM x 1 dose; 30-<60 lb: 900,000-1.2 million units IM x 1 dose; ≥60 mg, >12 years: 2.4 million units IM x 1 dose
  Bicillin C-R *Cartridge-needle unit:* 600,000 units (1 ml); 1.2 million units (2 ml); 2.4 million units (4 ml)
- ***penicillin v potassium*** **(B)(G)** <12 years: 25-75 mg/kg day divided q 6-8 hours x 10 days; *see page* 616 *for dose by weight table;* ≥12 years: 500 mg bid <u>or</u> 250 mg qid x 10 days
  Pen-Vee K *Tab:* 250, 500 mg; *Oral soln:* 125 mg/5 ml (100, 200 ml); 250 mg/5 ml (100, 150, 200 ml)
  Veetids *Tab:* 250, 500 mg; *Oral soln:* 125, 250 mg/5 ml (100, 200 ml)

PHENYLKETONURIA (PKU)

PHENYLALANINE HYDROXYLASE ACTIVATOR (PHA)

Comment: **Kuvan (sapropterin)** is a phenylalanine hydroxylase activator (PHA) indicated to reduce blood phenylalanine (Phe) levels in patients with hyperphenylalaninemia (HPA) due to tetrahydrobiopterin- (BH4-) responsive Phenylketonuria (PKU). Kuvan is to be used in conjunction with a Phe-restricted diet

- ***sapropterin*** <18 years: not recommended; ≥18 years: recommended starting dose is 10 mg/kg/day taken once daily; doses may be adjusted in the range of 5 to 20 mg/kg taken once daily. Blood Phe must be monitored regularly; take with food to increase absorption; tabs may be swallowed whole <u>or</u> dissolved in 4 to 8 oz (120-240 ml) of water <u>or</u> apple juice; once dissolved, dose should be taken within 15 minutes; pwdr for oral soln should be dissolved in 4 to 8 oz (120-240 m) of water <u>or</u> apple juice and consumed within 30 minutes of preparation
  Kuvan *Tab:* 100 mg; *Pwdr for Oral Soln:* 100 mg/unit dose pkt

PHENYLALANINE-METABOLIZING ENZYME

Comment: **Palynziq** is a phenylalanine-metabolizing enzyme indicated to reduce blood phenylalanine (PHa) concentrations in adult patients with phenylketonuria who have uncontrolled blood phenylalanine concentrations >600 micromol/L on existing management. **Palynziq** is to be used in conjunction with a Phe-restricted diet.

- ***pegvaliase-pqpz*** <18 years: not recommended; ≥18 years: recommended initial dosage is 2.5 mg SC once weekly x 4 weeks; titrate dosage in a step-wise manner over at least 5 weeks based on tolerability to achieve a dosage of 20 mg SC once daily; see mfr pkg insert for titration regimen; consider increasing the dosage to max 40 mg SC once daily in patients who have been on 20 mg once daily continuously for at least 24 weeks and who have not achieved either a 20% reduction in blood phenylalanine concentration from pre-treatment baseline or a blood phenylalanine concentration ≤600 micromol/L; discontinue **Palynziq** in patients who have not achieved at least a 20% reduction in blood phenylalanine concentration from pre-treatment baseline or a blood phenylalanine concentration ≤600 micromol/L after 16 weeks of continuous treatment with the maximum dosage of 40 mg once daily; reduce the dosage and/or modify dietary protein and phenylalanine intake, as needed, to maintain blood phenylalanine concentrations within a clinically acceptable range and >30 micromol/L. ***ALWAYS co-prescribe auto-injectable epinephrine.***

Palynziq *Prefilled syringe:* 2.5, 10 mg/0.5 ml; 20 mg/ml, single-dose (preservative-free)

Comment: Obtain blood phenylalanine concentrations every 4 weeks until a maintenance dosage is established. After a maintenance dosage is established, periodically monitor blood phenylalanine concentrations. Counsel patients to monitor dietary protein and phenylalanine intake, and adjust as directed by their healthcare provider. Anaphylaxis has been reported after administration of **Palynziq** and may occur at any time during treatment. Administer the initial dose under the supervision of a qualified healthcare provider equipped to manage anaphylaxis, and closely observe patients for at least 60 min following injection. Prior to self-injection, confirm patient competency with self-administration, and the patient's and observer's (if applicable) ability to recognize signs and symptoms of anaphylaxis and to administer auto-injectable ***epinephrine***, if needed. Prior to first dose, instruct the patient and observer (if applicable) on its appropriate use. Instruct the patient to seek immediate medical care upon its use. Instruct patients to carry auto-injectable ***epinephrine*** with them at all times during **Palynziq** treatment. **Palynziq** is available only through the restricted Palynziq REMS program. **Palynziq** may cause fetal harm when administered to a pregnant female. Limited available data with ***pegvaliase-pqpz*** use in pregnancy are insufficient to inform a drug-associated risk of adverse developmental outcomes. There are risks to the fetus associated with poorly controlled phenylalanine concentrations in women with PKU during pregnancy including increased risk for miscarriage, major birth defects (including microcephaly, major cardiac malformations), intrauterine fetal growth retardation, and future intellectual disability with low IQ; therefore, phenylalanine concentrations should be closely monitored in women with PKU during pregnancy. There are no data on the presence of ***pegvaliase-pqpz*** in human milk or the effects on the breastfed infant.

PHEOCHROMOCYTOMA

ALPHA-BLOCKER

➤ ***phenoxybenzamine*** (C) initially 10 mg bid; increase every other day as needed; usually 20-40 mg bid-tid

Dibenzyline *Cap:* 10 mg

PINWORM *(ENTEROBIUS VERMICULARIS)*

Comment: Oral bioavailability of anthelmintics is enhanced when administered with a fatty meal (estimated fat content 40 gm). Treatment of all family members is recommended. Some clinicians recommend all household contacts of infected patients receive treatment, especially when multiple or repeated symptomatic infections occur, since such contacts commonly also are infected; retreatment after 14 to 21 days may be needed.

ANTHELMINTICS

Comment: Oral bioavailability of anthelmintics is enhanced when administered with a fatty meal (estimated fat content 40 gm).

- ***albendazole*** **(C)** take with a meal; may crush and mix with food; may repeat in 3 weeks if needed; <2 years: 200 mg bid x 7 days; 2-12 years: 400 mg once daily x 7 days; >12 years: 400 mg bid x 7 days
  Albenza *Tab:* 200 mg
  Comment: ***albendazole*** is a broad-spectrum benzimidazole carbamate anthelmintic.
- ***ivermectin*** **(C)** take with water; chew or crush and mix with food; may repeat in 3 months if needed; <15 kg: not recommended; ≥15 kg: 200 mcg/kg as a single dose
  Stromectol *Tab:* 3, 6*mg
- ***mebendazole*** **(C)(G)** take with a meal; chew or crush and mix with food; may repeat in 3 weeks if needed; <2 years: not recommended; ≥2 years: 100 mg bid x 3 days
  Emverm *Chew tab:* 100 mg
  Vermox *Chew tab:* 100 mg
- ***pyrantel pamoate*** **(C)** take with a meal; may open capsule and sprinkle or mix with food; treat x 3 days; may repeat in 2-3 weeks if needed; treat x 3 days; 11 mg/kg/dose; max 1 gm/dose; <25 lb: not recommended; 25-37 lb: 1/2 tsp/dose; 38-62 lb: 1 tsp/dose; 63-87 lb: 1 tsp/dose; 88-112 lb: 2 tsp/dose; 113-137 lb: 2 tsp/dose; 138-162 lb: 3 tsp/dose; 163-187 lb: 3 tsp/dose; >187 lb: 4 tsp/dose
  Antiminth *Cap:* 180 mg; *Liq:* 50 mg/ml (30 ml); 144 mg/ml (30 ml); *Oral susp:* 50 mg/ml (60 ml)
  Pin-X *Cap:* 180 mg; *Liq:* 50 mg/ml (30 ml); 144 mg/ml (30 ml); *Oral susp:* 50 mg/ml (30 ml)
- ***thiabendazole*** **(C)** take with a meal; may crush and mix with food; treat x 7 days; <30 lb: consult mfr pkg insert; ≥30 lb: 25 mg/kg/dose bid with meals; 30-50 lb: 250 mg bid with meals; >50 lb: 10 mg/lb/dose bid with meals; max 1.5 gm/dose; max 3 gm/day
  Mintezol *Chew tab:* 500*mg (orange); *Oral susp:* 500 mg/5 ml (120 ml) (orange)
  Comment: ***thiabendazole*** is not for prophylaxis. May impair mental alertness. May not be available in the US.

PITYRIASIS ALBA

Topical Corticosteroids *see page* 542

Comment: Pityriasis alba is a chronic skin disorder seen in children with a genetic predisposition to atopic disease. Treatment is directed toward controlling roughness and pruritus. There is no known treatment for the associated skin pigment changes. Pityriasis alba resolves spontaneously and permanently in the 2nd or 3rd decade of life.

COAL TAR PREPARATIONS

- ***coal tar*** **(C)**
  Scytera (OTC) apply qd-qid; use lowest effective dose
  Foam: 2%
  T/Gel Shampoo Extra Strength (OTC) use every other day; max 4 x/week; massage into affected area for 5 minutes; rinse; repeat
  Shampoo: 1%

T/Gel Shampoo Original Formula (OTC) use every other day; max 7 x/week; massage into affected area for 5 minutes; rinse; repeat

Shampoo: 0.5%

T/Gel Shampoo Stubborn Itch Control (OTC) use every other day; max 7 x/week; massage into affected area for 5 minutes; rinse; repeat

Shampoo: 0.5%

EMOLLIENTS AND OTHER MOISTURIZING AGENTS

See **Dermatitis: Atopic** *page* 112

PITYRIASIS ROSEA

Topical Corticosteroids *see page* 542

Antihistamines *see* **Drugs for the Management of Allergy, Cough, and Cold Symptoms** *page* 570

PLAGUE (*YERSINIA PESTIS*)

Comment: *Yersinia pestis* is transmitted via the bite of a flea from an infected rodent or the bite, lick, or scratch of an infected cat. Untreated bubonic plague may progress to secondary pneumonic plague, which may be transmitted via contaminated respiratory droplet spread.

▶ ***streptomycin*** (C)(G) 15 mg/kg IM bid x 10 days

Amp: 1 gm/2.5 ml or 400 mg/ml (2.5 ml)

Comment: For patients with renal impairment, reduce dose of ***streptomycin*** to 20 mg/kg/day if mild and 8 mg/kg/day q 3 days if advanced. For patients who are pregnant or who have hearing impairment, shorten the course of treatment to 3 days after fever has resolved.

▶ ***moxifloxacin*** (C)(G) <18 years: not recommended; ≥18 years: 400 mg daily x 10 days

Avelox *Tab:* 400 mg; IV soln: 400 mg/250 mg (latex-free, preservative-free)

Comment: ***moxifloxacin*** is for prophylaxis as well as treatment for pneumonia and septic plague. ***moxifloxacin*** is contraindicated <18 years-of-age and during pregnancy and lactation. Risk of tendonitis or tendon rupture.

▶ ***tetracycline*** (D)(G) <8 years: not recommended; ≥8 years, ≤100 lb: 25-50 mg/kg/day in 4 divided doses x 10 days; *see page* 618 *for dose by weight table*; ≥8 years, >100 lb: 500 mg qid x 10 days

Achromycin V *Cap:* 250, 500 mg

Sumycin *Tab:* 250, 500 mg; *Cap:* 250, 500 mg; *Oral susp:* 125 mg/5 ml (100, 200 ml) (fruit) (sulfites)

Comment: ***tetracycline*** is contraindicated <8 years-of-age, in pregnancy, and lactation (discolors developing tooth enamel). A side effect may be photosensitivity (photophobia). Do not give with antacids, calcium supplements, milk or other dairy, or within two hours of taking another drug.

PNEUMONIA: BACTERIAL, HOSPITAL-ACQUIRED (HABP)

PARENTERAL CEPHALOSPORIN ANTIBACTERIAL+BETA-LACTIMASE INHIBITOR

▶ ***ceftazidime+avibactam*** (B) <18 years: not recommended; ≥18 years: infuse dose over 2 hours; recommended duration of treatment: 5 to 14 days; *CrCl 31-50 mL/min:* 1.25

gm every 8 hours; *CrCl 16-30 mL/min:* 0.94 gm every 12 hours; *CrCl 6-15 mL/min:* 0.94 gm every 24 hours; *CrCl <5 mL/min:* 0.94 gm every 48 hours; both ***ceftazidime*** and ***avibactam*** are hemodialyzable; thus, administer **Avycaz** after hemodialysis on hemodialysis days

Avycaz *Vial:* 2.5 gm, single-dose, pwdr for reconstitution and IV infusion

Comment: **Avycaz** 2.5 gm contains ***ceftazidime*** (a cephalosporin) 2 grams (equivalent to 2.635 grams of ***ceftazidime pentahydrate/sodium carbonate powder***) and ***avibactam*** (a beta lactam inhibitor) 0.5 grams (equivalent to 0.551 grams of ***avibactam sodium***). As only limited clinical safety and efficacy data for **Avycaz** are currently available, reserve **Avycaz** for use in patients who have limited or no alternative treatment options. To reduce the development of drug-resistant bacteria and maintain the effectiveness of **Avycaz** and other antibacterial drugs. **Avycaz** should be used only to treat infections that are proven or strongly suspected to be caused by susceptible bacteria. Seizures and other neurologic events may occur, especially in patients with renal impairment. Adjust dose in patients with renal impairment. Decreased efficacy in patients with baseline CrCl 30--≤50 mL/min. Monitor CrCl at least daily in patients with changing renal function and adjust the dose of **Avycaz** accordingly. Monitor for hypersensitivity reactions, including anaphylaxis and serious skin reactions. Cross-hypersensitivity may occur in patients with a history of penicillin allergy. If an allergic reaction occurs, discontinue **Avycaz**. *Clostridium difficile*-associated diarrhea (CDAD) has been reported with nearly all systemic antibacterial agents, including **Avycaz**. There are no adequate and well-controlled studies of **Avycaz**, ***ceftazidime***, or ***avibactam*** in pregnant females. ***ceftazidime*** is excreted in human milk in low concentrations. It is not known whether ***avibactam*** is excreted into human milk. There are no studies to inform effects on the breastfed infant.

☐ PNEUMONIA: BACTERIAL, VENTILATOR-ASSOCIATED (VABP)

PARENTERAL CEPHALOSPORIN ANTIBACTERIAL+ BETA-LACTAMASE INHIBITOR

▶ ***ceftazidime+avibactam*** **(B)** <18 years: not recommended; ≥18 years: infuse dose over 2 hours; recommended duration of treatment: 5 to 14 days; *CrCl 31-50 mL/min:* 1.25 gm every 8 hours; *CrCl 16-30 mL/min:* 0.94 gm every 12 hours; *CrCl 6-15 mL/min:* 0.94 gm every 24 hours; *CrCl <5 mL/min:* 0.94 gm every 48 hours; both ***ceftazidime*** and ***avibactam*** are hemodialyzable; thus, administer **Avycaz** after hemodialysis on hemodialysis days

Avycaz *Vial:* 2.5 gm, single-dose, pwdr for reconstitution and IV infusion

Comment: **Avycaz** 2.5 gm contains ***ceftazidime*** (a cephalosporin) 2 grams (equivalent to 2.635 grams of ***ceftazidime pentahydrate/sodium carbonate powder***) and ***avibactam*** (a beta lactam inhibitor) 0.5 grams (equivalent to 0.551 grams of ***avibactam sodium***). As only limited clinical safety and efficacy data for **Avycaz** are currently available, reserve **Avycaz** for use in patients who have limited or no alternative treatment options. To reduce the development of drug-resistant bacteria and maintain the effectiveness of **Avycaz** and other antibacterial drugs. **Avycaz** should be used only to treat infections that are proven or strongly suspected to be caused by susceptible bacteria. Seizures and other neurologic events may occur, especially in patients with renal impairment. Adjust dose in patients with renal impairment. Decreased efficacy in patients with baseline CrCl 30--≤50 mL/min. Monitor CrCl at least daily in patients with changing renal function and adjust the dose of **Avycaz** accordingly. Monitor for hypersensitivity reactions, including anaphylaxis and serious skin reactions. Cross-hypersensitivity may occur in patients with a history of penicillin allergy. If an allergic reaction occurs, discontinue **Avycaz**. *Clostridium difficile*-associated diarrhea

(CDAD) has been reported with nearly all systemic antibacterial agents, including **Avycaz.** There are no adequate and well-controlled studies of **Avycaz**, ***ceftazidime***, or ***avibactam*** in pregnant females. ***ceftazidime*** is excreted in human milk in low concentrations. It is not known whether ***avibactam*** is excreted into human milk. There are no studies to inform effects on the breastfed infant.

PNEUMONIA: CHLAMYDIAL

RECOMMENDED REGIMEN

- ***erythromycin base*** **(B)(G)** <45 kg: 50 mg in 4 divided doses x 10-14 days; ≥45 kg: 500 mg qid hours x 10-14 days
  - **Ery-Tab** *Tab:* 250, 333, 500 mg ent-coat
  - **PCE** *Tab:* 333, 500 mg
- ***erythromycin ethylsuccinate*** **(B)(G)** <45 kg: 50 mg/kg/day in 4 divided doses x 10-14 days; ≥45 kg: same as adult; *see page* 607 *for dose by weight table*
  - **EryPed** *Oral susp:* 200 mg/5 ml (100, 200 ml) (fruit); 400 mg/5 ml (60, 100, 200 ml) (banana); *Oral drops:* 200, 400 mg/5 ml (50 ml) (fruit); *Chew tab:* 200 mg wafer (fruit)
  - **E.E.S.** *Oral susp:* 200, 400 mg/5 ml (100 ml) (fruit)
  - **E.E.S. Granules** *Oral susp:* 200 mg/5 ml (100, 200 ml) (cherry)
  - **E.E.S. 400 Tablets** *Tab:* 400 mg

ALTERNATE REGIMENS

- ***azithromycin*** **(B)(G)** <12 years: 20 mg/kg per dose once daily x 10 days; *see page* 593 *for dose by weight table;* max 500 mg/day; ≥12 years: 500 mg once daily x 10 days
  - **Zithromax** *Tab:* 250, 500, 600 mg; Oral susp: 100 mg/5 ml (15 ml); 200 mg/5 ml (15, 22.5, 30 ml) (cherry); Pkt: 1 gm for reconstitution (cherry-banana)
  - **Zithromax Tri-pak** *Tab:* 3 x 500 mg tabs/pck
  - **Zithromax Z-pak** *Tab:* 6 x 250 mg tabs/pck
  - **Zmax** *Oral susp:* 2 gm ext-rel for reconstitution (cherry-banana) (148 mg Na^+)
- ***levofloxacin*** **(C)** <18 years: not recommended; ≥18 years: *Uncomplicated:* 500 mg daily x 7 days; *Complicated:* 750 mg daily x 7 days
  - **Levaquin** *Tab:* 250, 500, 750 mg; *Oral soln:* 25 mg/ml (480 ml) (benzyl alcohol); *Inj conc:* 25 mg/ml for IV infusion after dilution (20, 30 ml single-use vial) (preservative-free); *Premix soln:* 5 mg/ml for IV infusion (50, 100, 150 ml) (preservative-free)

Comment: ***levofloxacin*** is contraindicated <18 years-of-age, and during pregnancy and lactation. Risk of tendonitis or tendon rupture.

PNEUMONIA: COMMUNITY ACQUIRED (CAP) & COMMUNITY ACQUIRED BACTERIAL (CABP)

Comment: Over 70% of patients with uncomplicated community-acquired pneumonia (CAP) received prescriptions for antibiotics that exceeded national duration recommendations, according to a retrospective study that included 22,128 patients from 18 to 64 years-of-age with private insurance and 130,746 patients aged >65 years with Medicare, who were hospitalized with uncomplicated CAP. Length of antibiotic therapy (LOT) during hospital stay was estimated using the MarketScan Hospital Drug Database and outpatient LOT was determined using prescriptions filled at discharge. The researchers defined excessive duration as a LOT of more than 3 days.

REFERENCE

Yi, S. H., Hatfield, K. M., Baggs, J., Hicks, L. A., Srinivasan, A., Reddy, S., & Jernigan, J. A. (2017). Duration of antibiotic use among adults with uncomplicated community-acquired pneumonia requiring hospitalization in the United States. *Clinical Infectious Diseases*. doi:10.1093/cid/cix986

ANTI-INFECTIVES

▶ ***amoxicillin*** **(B)(G)** <40 kg (88 lb): 80-100 mg/kg/day divided q 12 hours x 3-10 days; *see page* 588 *for dose by weight table;* ≥40 kg: 500-875 mg bid or 250-500 mg tid x 3-10 days

Amoxil *Cap:* 250, 500 mg; *Tab:* 875 mg; *Chew tab:* 125, 200, 250, 400 mg (cherry-banana-peppermint) (phenylalanine); *Oral susp:* 125, 250 mg/5 ml (80, 100, 150 ml) (strawberry); 200, 400 mg/5 ml (50, 75, 100 ml) (bubble gum); *Oral drops:* 50 mg/ml (30 ml) (bubble gum)

Moxatag *Tab:* 775 mg ext-rel

Trimox *Tab:* 125, 250 mg; *Cap:* 250, 500 mg; *Oral susp:* 125, 250 mg/5 ml (80, 100, 150 ml) (raspberry-strawberry)

▶ ***amoxicillin+clavulanate*** **(B)(G)**

Augmentin <40 kg: 45-90 mg/kg/day divided q 12 hours x 3-10 days; *see page* 590 *for dose by weight table;* ≥40 kg: 500 mg tid or 875 mg bid x 10 days

Tab: 250, 500, 875 mg; *Chew tab:* 125, 250 mg (lemon-lime); 200, 400 mg (cherry-banana) (phenylalanine); *Oral susp:* 125 mg/5 ml (banana), 250 mg/5 ml (75, 100, 150 ml) (orange); 200, 400 mg/5 ml (50, 75, 100 ml) (orange) (phenylalanine)

Augmentin ES-600 <3 months: not recommended; ≥3 months, <40 kg: 90 mg/kg/day divided q 12 hours x 3-10 days; *see page* 591 *for dose by weight table;* ≥40 kg: not recommended

Oral susp: 600 mg/5 ml (50, 75, 100, 125, 150, 200 ml) (strawberry cream) (phenylalanine)

Augmentin XR <16 years: use other forms; ≥16 years: 2 tabs q 12 hours x 3-10 days

Tab: 1000*mg ext-rel

▶ ***azithromycin*** **(B)(G)** <6 months: not recommended; ≥6 months: 10 mg/kg x 1 dose on day 1; then 5 mg/kg/day on days 2-5; max 500 mg/day; *see page* 593 *for dose by weight;* >12 years: Day 1, 500 mg as a single dose and *Days 2-5*, 250 mg once daily or 500 mg once daily x 3 days

Zithromax *Tab:* 250, 500, 600 mg; *Oral susp:* 100 mg/5 ml (15 ml); 200 mg/5 ml (15, 22.5, 30 ml) (cherry); *Pkt:* 1 gm for reconstitution (cherry-banana)

Zithromax Tri-pak *Tab:* 3 x 500 mg tabs/pck

Zithromax Z-pak *Tab:* 6 x 250 mg tabs/pck

Zmax *Oral susp:* 2 gm ext-rel for reconstitution (cherry-banana) (148 mg Na^+)

▶ ***cefaclor*** **(B)(G)** <1 month: not recommended; 1 month-12 years: 20-40 mg/kg divided bid x 3-10 days; *see page* 594 *for dose by weight table;* max 1 gm/day; >12 years: 250 mg tid or 375 mg bid x 3-10 days; max 2 gm/day

Tab: 500 mg; *Cap:* 250, 500 mg; *Susp:* 125 mg/5 ml (75, 150 ml) (strawberry); 187 mg/5 ml (50, 100 ml) (strawberry); 250 mg/5 ml (75, 150 ml) (strawberry); 375 mg/5 ml (50, 100 ml) (strawberry)

Cefaclor Extended Release <16 years: not recommended; ≥16 years: 375-500 mg bid x 3-10 days (clinically equivalent to 250 mg immed-rel caps tid); swallow whole; take with meals

Tab: 375, 500 mg ext-rel

▶ ***cefdinir*** **(B)** <6 months: not recommended; 6 months-12 years: 14 mg/kg/day in 1-2 divided doses x 10 days; *see page* 596 *for dose by weight table;* ≥12 years: 300 mg bid x 3-10 days or 600 mg daily x 10 days

Omnicef *Cap:* 300 mg; *Oral susp:* 125 mg/5 ml (60, 100 ml) (strawberry)

▶ ***cefpodoxime proxetil*** **(B)** <2 months: nor recommended; 2 months-12 years: 10 mg/kg/day in 2 doses x 3-10 days; *see page 598 for dose by weight table;* >12 years: 200 mg bid x 14 days

  Vantin *Tab:* 100, 200 mg; *Oral susp:* 50, 100 mg/5 ml (50, 75, 100 mg) (lemon creme)

▶ ***ceftaroline fosamil*** **(B)** <18 years: not recommended; ≥18 years: administer by IV infusion after reconstitution every 12 hours x 3-10 days; *CrCl ≥50 mL/min:* 600 mg; *CrCl >30-<50 mL/min:* 400 mg; *CrCl: >15-<30 mL/min:* 300 mg; ES RD: 200 mg

  Teflaro *Vial:* 400, 600 mg

▶ ***ceftriaxone*** **(B)** 50-75 mg/kg IM in 2 divided doses; max 2 gm/day x 1-3 days

  Rocephin *Vial:* 250, 500 mg; 1, 2 gm

▶ ***clarithromycin*** **(C)** <6 months: not recommended; ≥6 months: 7.5 mg/kg bid x 3-10 days

  Biaxin *Tab:* 250, 500 mg

  Biaxin Oral Suspension *Oral susp:* 125, 250 mg/5 ml (50, 100 ml) (fruit punch)

  Biaxin XL *Tab:* 500 mg ext-rel

Comment: The FDA is advising caution before prescribing ***clarithromycin*** to patients with heart disease because of a potential increased risk of heart problems or death that can occur years later. This recommendation is based on a review of the results of a 10-year follow-up study of patients with coronary heart disease from a large clinical trial that first observed this safety issue. Consider risk benefit and the use of other antibiotics in such patients.

▶ ***dirithromycin*** **(C)(G)** <12 years: not recommended; ≥12 years: 500 mg daily x 3-10 days

  Dynabac *Tab:* 250 mg

▶ ***doxycycline*** **(D)(G)** <8 years: not recommended; ≥8 years, ≤100 lb: 2 mg/lb on first day in 2 divided doses, followed by 1 mg/lb/day in 1-2 divided doses; *see page 605 for dose by weight;* ≥8 years, >100 lb: 100 mg bid x 3-10 days

  Acticlate *Tab:* 75, 150**mg

  Adoxa *Tab:* 50, 75, 100, 150 mg ent-coat

  Doryx *Tab:* 50, 75, 100, 150, 200 mg del-rel

  Doxteric *Tab:* 50 mg del-rel

  Monodox *Cap:* 50, 75, 100 mg

  Oracea *Cap:* 40 mg del-rel

  Vibramycin *Tab:* 100 mg; *Cap:* 50, 100 mg; *Syr:* 50 mg/5 ml (raspberry-apple) (sulfites); *Oral susp:* 25 mg/5 ml (raspberry)

  Vibra-Tab *Tab:* 100 mg film-coat

Comment: ***doxycycline*** is contraindicated <8 years-of-age, in pregnancy, and lactation (discolors developing tooth enamel). A side effect may be photosensitivity (photophobia). Do not take with antacids, calcium supplements, milk or other dairy, or within 2 hours of taking another drug.

▶ ***ertapenem*** **(B)** 1 gm daily; *CrCl <30 mL/min:* 500 mg daily x 3-10 days; may switch to an oral antibiotic after 3 days if warranted; *IV infusion:* administer over 30 minutes; *IM injection:* reconstitute with lidocaine only

  Invanz *Vial:* 1 gm pwdr for reconstitution

▶ ***erythromycin base*** **(B)(G)** <45 kg: 30-50 mg in 2-4 divided doses x 3-10 days; ≥45 kg: 500 mg q 6 hours x 10 days

  Ery-Tab *Tab:* 250, 333, 500 mg ent-coat

  PCE *Tab:* 333, 500 mg

▶ ***erythromycin estolate*** **(B)** <12 years: 30-50 mg/kg/day in divided doses x 3-10 days; *see page 606 for dose by weight table;* ≥12 years: 250 mg q 6 hours or 500 mg bid x 3-10 days

  Ilosone *Pulvule:* 250 mg; *Tab:* 500 mg; *Liq:* 125, 250 mg/5 ml (100 ml)

- ▶ ***gemifloxacin*** **(C)(G)** <18 years: not recommended; ≥18 years: 320 mg daily x 3-10 days
  - **Factive** *Tab:* 320*mg

  Comment: ***gemifloxacin*** is contraindicated <18 years-of-age and during pregnancy and lactation. Risk of tendonitis or tendon rupture.
- ▶ ***levofloxacin*** **(C)** *Uncomplicated:* 500 mg once daily x 3-10 days; *Complicated:* 750 mg once daily x 7-14 days
  - **Levaquin** *Tab:* 250, 500, 750 mg; *Oral soln:* 25 mg/ml (480 ml) (benzyl alcohol); *Inj conc:* 25 mg/ml for IV infusion after dilution (20, 30 ml single-use vial) (preservative-free); *Premix soln:* 5 mg/ml for IV infusion (50, 100, 150 ml) (preservative-free)

  Comment: ***levofloxacin*** is contraindicated <18 years-of-age and during pregnancy and lactation. Risk of tendonitis or tendon rupture.
- ▶ ***linezolid*** **(C)(G)** <5 years: 10 mg/kg q 8 hours x 3-10 days; 5-11 years: 10 mg/kg q 12 hours x 10-14 days; >11 years: 400-600 mg q 12 hours x 3-10 days
  - **Zyvox** *Tab:* 400, 600 mg; *Oral susp:* 100 mg/5 ml (150 ml) (orange) (phenylalanine)

  Comment: ***linezolid*** is indicated to treat susceptible vancomycin-resistant *E. faecium* infections.
- ▶ ***loracarbef*** **(B)** <12 years: 15 mg/kg/day in 2 divided doses x 10 days; *see page* 614 *for dose by weight table*; ≥12 years: 200 mg bid x 3-10 days
  - **Lorabid** *Pulvule:* 200, 400 mg; *Oral susp:* 100 mg/5 ml (50, 100 ml); 200 mg/5 ml (50, 75, 100 ml) (strawberry bubble gum)
- ▶ ***moxifloxacin*** **(C)(G)** <18 years: not recommended; ≥18 years: 400 mg daily x 3-10 days
  - **Avelox** *Tab:* 400 mg; IV soln: 400 mg/250 mg (latex-free, preservative-free)

  Comment: ***moxifloxacin*** is contraindicated during pregnancy and lactation. Risk of tendonitis or tendon rupture.
- ▶ ***ofloxacin*** **(C)(G)** <18 years: not recommended; ≥18 years: 400 mg bid x 3-10 days
  - **Floxin** *Tab:* 200, 300, 400 mg

    Comment: ***ofloxacin*** is contraindicated <18 years-of-age and during pregnancy and lactation. Risk of tendonitis or tendon rupture.
- ▶ ***penicillin v potassium*** **(B)** <12 years: 25-75 mg/kg day divided q 6-8 hours x 3-10 days; *see page 616 for dose by weight table;* ≥12 years: 250-500 mg q 6 hours x 5-7 days
  - **Pen-VK** *Tab:* 250, 500 mg; *Oral soln:* 125 mg/5 ml (100, 200 ml); 250 mg/5 ml (100, 150, 200 ml)
- ▶ ***tedizolid phosphate*** **(B)** administer 200 mg once daily x 6 days, via PO or IV infusion over 1 hour
  - **Sivextro** *Tab:* 200 mg (6/blister pck)

    Comment: **Sivextro** is indicated for the treatment of community acquired bacterial pneumonia (CABP)
- ▶ ***telithromycin*** **(C)** 2 x 400 mg tabs in a single dose daily x 3-10 days
  - **Ketek** *Tab:* 300, 400 mg

  Comment: ***telithromycin*** is contraindicated with PMHx hepatitis or jaundice associated with macrolide use.
- ▶ ***tigecycline*** **(D)(G)** 100 mg once; then 50 mg q 12 hours x 3-10 days; *Severe hepatic impairment (Child Pugh Class C):* 100 mg once; then 25 mg q 12 hours x 3-10 days
  - **Tygacil** *Vial:* 50 mg pwdr for reconstitution and IV infusion (preservative-free)

    Comment: **Tygacil** is indicated only for the treatment of patients ≥18 years-of-age with community acquired bacterial pneumonia (CABP). ***tigecycline*** is contraindicated in pregnancy, and lactation (discolors developing tooth enamel). A side effect may be photosensitivity (photophobia). Do not give with antacids, calcium supplements, milk or other dairy, or within two hours of taking another drug.

▶ ***trimethoprim+sulfamethoxazole [TMP-SMX]*** (C)(G)
Pediatric: <2 months: not recommended; ≥2 months: 40 mg/kg/day of ***sulfamethoxazole*** in 2 doses bid x 3-10 days; *see page 620 for dose by weight*
Bactrim, Septra 2 tabs bid x 10 days
Tab: trim 80 mg+sulfa 400 mg*
Bactrim DS, Septra DS 1 tab bid x 10 days
Tab: trim 160 mg+sulfa 800 mg*
Bactrim Pediatric Suspension, Septra Pediatric Suspension
Oral susp: trim 40 mg+sulfa 200 mg per 5 ml (100 ml) (cherry) (alcohol 0.3%)

PNEUMONIA: LEGIONELLA

▶ ***ciprofloxacin*** (C) <18 years: 20-40 mg/kg/day divided q 12 hours x 14-21 days; ≥18 years: 500 mg bid x 14-21 days; max 1.5 gm/day
Cipro (G) *Tab:* 250, 500, 750 mg; *Oral susp:* 250, 500 mg/5 ml (100 ml) (strawberry)
Cipro XR *Tab:* 500, 1,000 mg ext-rel
ProQuin XR *Tab:* 500 mg ext-rel

▶ ***clarithromycin*** (C)(G) 500 mg bid or 500 mg ext-rel daily x 14-21 days
Biaxin *Tab:* 250, 500 mg
Biaxin Oral Suspension *Oral susp:* 125, 250 mg/5 ml (50, 100 ml) (fruit punch)
Biaxin XL *Tab:* 500 mg ext-rel

Comment: The FDA is advising caution before prescribing ***clarithromycin*** to patients with heart disease because of a potential increased risk of heart problems or death that can occur years later. This recommendation is based on a review of the results of a 10-year follow-up study of patients with coronary heart disease from a large clinical trial that first observed this safety issue. Consider risk benefit and the use of other antibiotics in such patients.

▶ ***dirithromycin*** (C)(G) 500 mg once daily x 14-21 days
Dynabac *Tab:* 250 mg

▶ ***erythromycin base*** (B)(G) <45 kg: 30-50 mg in 2-4 divided doses x 14-21 days; ≥45 kg: 500 mg qid x 14-21 days
Ery-Tab *Tab:* 250, 333, 500 mg ent-coat
PCE *Tab:* 333, 500 mg

▶ ***erythromycin estolate*** (B)(G) <12 years: 30-50 mg/kg/day in divided doses x 14-21 days; *see page 606 for dose by weight table*; ≥12 years: 1-2 gm daily in divided doses x 14-21 days
Ilosone *Pulvule:* 250 mg; *Tab:* 500 mg; *Liq:* 125, 250 mg/5 ml (100 ml)

▶ ***trimethoprim+sulfamethoxazole [TMP-SMX]*** (C)(G)
Bactrim, Septra <12 years: not recommended; ≥12 years: 2 tabs bid x 10 days
Tab: trim 80 mg+sulfa 400 mg*
Bactrim DS, Septra DS <12 years: not recommended; ≥12 years: 1 tab bid x 10 days
Tab: trim 160 mg+sulfa 800 mg*
Bactrim Pediatric Suspension, Septra Pediatric Suspension <2 months: not recommended; ≥2 months-12 years: 40 mg/kg/day of ***sulfamethoxazole*** in 2 doses bid x 10 days; >12 years: use tabs
Oral susp: trim 40 mg+sulfa 200 mg per 5 ml (100 ml) (cherry) (alcohol 0.3%)

PNEUMONIA: MYCOPLASMA

ANTI-INFECTIVES

▶ ***azithromycin*** **(B)(G)** <12 years: 12 mg/kg/day x 5 days; *see page* 593 *for dose by weight table*; max 500 mg/day; ≥12 years: 500 mg x 1 dose on day 1, then 250 mg daily on days 2-5 or 500 mg daily x 3 days or **Zmax** 2 gm in a single dose

Zithromax *Tab:* 250, 500, 600 mg; *Oral susp:* 100 mg/5 ml (15 ml); 200 mg/5 ml (15, 22.5, 30 ml) (cherry); *Pkt:* 1 gm for reconstitution (cherry-banana)

Zithromax Tri-pak *Tab:* 3 x 500 mg tabs/pck

Zithromax Z-pak *Tab:* 6 x 250 mg tabs/pck

Zmax *Oral susp:* 2 gm ext-rel for reconstitution (cherry-banana) (148 mg Na^+)

▶ ***clarithromycin*** **(C)(G)** <6 months: not recommended; ≥6 months-12 years: 7.5 mg/kg bid x 14-21 days; *see page* 602 *for dose by weight table;* >12 years: 500 mg bid or 500 mg ext-rel daily x 14-21 days

Biaxin *Tab:* 250, 500 mg

Biaxin Oral Suspension *Oral susp:* 125, 250 mg/5 ml (50, 100 ml) (fruit punch)

Biaxin XL *Tab:* 500 mg ext-rel

Comment: The FDA is advising caution before prescribing ***clarithromycin*** to patients with heart disease because of a potential increased risk of heart problems or death that can occur years later. This recommendation is based on a review of the results of a 10-year follow-up study of patients with coronary heart disease from a large clinical trial that first observed this safety issue. Consider risk benefit and the use of other antibiotics in such patients.

▶ ***erythromycin base*** **(B)(G)** <45 kg: 30-50 mg in 2-4 doses x 14-21 days; ≥45 kg: 500 mg q 6 hours x 14-21 days

Ery-Tab *Tab:* 250, 333, 500 mg ent-coat

PCE *Tab:* 333, 500 mg

▶ ***erythromycin ethylsuccinate*** **(B)(G)** 30-50 mg/kg/day in 4 divided doses x 14-21 days; may double dose with severe infection; max 100 mg/kg/day or 400 mg qid; *see page* 607 *for dose by weight table*

EryPed *Oral susp:* 200 mg/5 ml (100, 200 ml) (fruit); 400 mg/5 ml (60, 100, 200 ml) (banana); *Oral drops*: 200, 400 mg/5 ml (50 ml) (fruit); *Chew tab*: 200 mg wafer (fruit)

E.E.S. *Oral susp*: 200, 400 mg/5 ml (100 ml) (fruit)

E.E.S. Granules *Oral susp:* 200 mg/5 ml (100, 200 ml) (cherry)

E.E.S. 400 Tablets *Tab:* 400 mg

▶ ***tetracycline*** **(D)(G)** <8 years: not recommended; ≥8 years, ≤100 lb: 25-50 mg/kg/day in 4 divided doses x 14-21 days; *see page* 618 *for dose by weight table*; ≥8 years, >100 lb: 500 mg qid x 14-21 days

Achromycin V *Cap:* 250, 500 mg

Sumycin *Tab:* 250, 500 mg; *Cap:* 250, 500 mg; *Oral susp:* 125 mg/5 ml (100, 200 ml) (fruit) (sulfites)

Comment: ***tetracycline*** is contraindicated <8 years-of-age, in pregnancy, and lactation (discolors developing tooth enamel). A side effect may be photosensitivity (photophobia). Do not give with antacids, calcium supplements, milk or other dairy, or within two hours of taking another drug.

PNEUMONIA: PNEUMOCOCCAL

PROPHYLAXIS

▶ ***pneumococcal*** vaccine **(C)** <2 years: not recommended; ≥2 years: 0.5 ml IM or SC in deltoid x 1 dose

Pneumovax *Vial:* 25 mcg/0.5 ml single-dose (10 carton)
Pnu-Imune 23 *Vial:* 25 mcg/0.5 ml single-dose (5 carton)

Comment: Pneumococcal vaccine contains 23 polysaccharide isolates representing approximately 85-90% of common U.S. isolates. Administer the pneumococcal vaccine in the anterolateral aspect of the thigh for infants and the deltoid for toddlers and children.

TREATMENT

see **CAP/CABP** *page* 356

PNEUMONIA: *PNEUMOCYSTIS JIROVECII*

- ▶ ***atovaquone*** (C) <12 years: see mfr pkg insert for weight-based dosing table; ≥12 years: take as a single dose with food or a milky drink at the same time each day; repeat dose if vomited within 1 hour; *Prophylaxis:* 1,500 mg once daily; *Treatment:* 750 mg bid x 21 days

  Mepron *Susp:* 750 mg/5 ml (citrus)

- ▶ ***trimethoprim+sulfamethoxazole [TMP-SMX]*** (C)(G) <2 months: not recommended; ≥2 months-12 years: 40 mg/kg/day of ***sulfamethoxazole*** in 2 doses bid x 10 days; >12 years: *Prophylaxis:* 1 tab 3 x/week; *Treatment:* 1 tab daily x 3 weeks; ***Septra*** can be given if intolerable to ***Bactrim***

  Bactrim, Septra <12 years: not recommended; ≥12 years: 2 tabs bid x 10 days
  Tab: trim 80 mg+sulfa 400 mg*

  Bactrim DS, Septra DS <12 years: not recommended; ≥12 years: 1 tab bid x 10 days
  Tab: trim 160 mg+sulfa 800 mg*

  Bactrim Pediatric Suspension, Septra Pediatric Suspension <2 months: not recommended; ≥2 months-12 years: 40 mg/kg/day of ***sulfamethoxazole*** in 2 doses bid; >12 years: use tabs
  Oral susp: trim 40 mg+sulfa 200 mg per 5 ml (100 ml) (cherry) (alcohol 0.3%)

POLIOMYELITIS

PROPHYLAXIS

- ▶ ***trivalent poliovirus vaccine, inactivated (type 1, 2, and 3)*** (C) <6 weeks: not recommended; ≥6 weeks: one dose at 2, 4, 6-18 months and 4-6 years-of-age

  Ipol 0.5 ml SC or IM in deltoid area

POLYCYSTIC OVARIAN SYNDROME (PCOS, STEIN-LEVENTHAL DISEASE)

See **Contraceptives** *page* 527
See **Type 2 Diabetes Mellitus** *page* 470

POLYMYALGIA RHEUMATICA

Oral Corticosteroids *see page* 546
Calcium and Vitamin D supplementation, *see* **Hypocalcemia** *page* 238

Comment: Initial treatment is low-dose prednisone at 12-25 mg/day. May attempt a very slow tapering regimen after 2-4 weeks. If relapse occurs, increase the daily dose of corticosteroid to the previous effective dose. Most people with polymyalgia rheumatica need to continue corticosteroid treatment for at least a year. Approximately 30-60% of people will have at least one relapse during corticosteroid tapering. Joint guidelines from the American Academy of Rheumatology (AAR) and the European League Against Rheumatism (ELAR) suggest using concomitant ***methotrexate*** (MTX) along with corticosteroids in some patients. It may be useful early in the course of treatment or later, if the patient relapses or does not respond to corticosteroids. The American Academy of Rheumatology (AAR) recommends the following daily doses for anyone on a chronic oral corticosteroid regimen: ***Calcium*** 1,200-1,500 mg/day and ***vitamin D*** 800-1,000 IU/day.

- ***methotrexate*** (X) <2 years: not recommended; 2-12 years: 10 mg/m^2 once weekly; max 20 mg/m^2; >12 years: 7.5 mg x 1 dose per week or 2.5 mg x 3 at 12 hour intervals once a week; max 20 mg/week; therapeutic response begins in 3-6 weeks; administer ***methotrexate*** injection SC only into the abdomen or thigh

  Rasuvo *Autoinjector:* 7.5 mg/0.15 ml, 10 mg/0.20 ml, 12.5 mg/0.25 ml, 15 mg/0.30 ml, 17.5 mg/0.35 ml, 20 mg/0.40 ml, 22.5 mg/0.45 ml, 25 mg/0.50 ml, 27.5 mg/0.55 ml, 30 mg/0.60 ml (solution concentration for SC injection is 50 mg/ml)

  Rheumatrex *Tab:* 2.5*mg (5, 7.5, 10, 12.5, 15 mg/week, 4/card unit dose pack)

  Trexall R *Tab:* 5*, 7.5*, 10*, 15*mg (5, 7.5, 10, 12.5, 15 mg/week, 4/card unit dose pack)

  Comment: ***methotrexate*** (MTX) is contraindicated with immunodeficiency, blood dyscrasias, alcoholism, and chronic liver disease.

POLYNEUROPATHY, CHRONIC INFLAMMATORY, DEMYELINATING (CIDP)

IMMUNE GLOBULIN, HUMAN

- ***immune globulin subcutaneous [human] 20% liquid*** <18 years: not recommended; ≥18 years: administer once weekly via SC infusion only; *Infusion sites:* abdomen, thigh, upper arm, and/or lateral hip; may use up to 8 injection sites simultaneously, with at least 2 inches between sites; *Infusion volume:* for the first infusion, up to 15 ml per injection site; may increase to 20 ml per site after the fourth infusion; max 25 ml per site as tolerated; *Infusion rate:* first infusion, up to 15 ml/hr per site; may increase, to max 25 ml/hr per site as tolerated; however, maximum flow rate is not to exceed a total of 50 ml/hr for all sites combined; before switching to **Hizentra**, obtain the patient's serum IgG trough level to guide subsequent dose adjustments; adjust the dose: based on clinical response and serum IgG trough levels; initiate therapy 1 week after the last IGIV infusion; recommended subcutaneous dose is 0.2 g/kg (1 ml/kg) per week; in the clinical study after transitioning from IGIV to **Hizentra**, a dose of 0.4 g/kg (2 ml/kg) per week was also safe and effective to prevent CIDP relapse; If CIDP symptoms worsen, consider reinitiating treatment with an IGIV approved for the treatment of CIDP, while discontinuing **Hizentra**; if improvement and stabilization are observed during IGIV treatment, consider reinitiating **Hizentra** at 0.4 g/kg per week, while discontinuing IGIV; if CIDP symptoms worsen on 0.4 g/kg per week, consider reinitiating **Hizentra** therapy with IGIV, while discontinuing **Hizentra**; monitor patient's clinical response and adjust duration of therapy based on patient need

  Hizentra *Vial:* 0.2 mg/ml (20%; 5, 10, 20, 50 ml)

  Comment: IgA-deficient patients with anti-IgA antibodies are at greater risk of severe hypersensitivity and anaphylactic reactions. Thrombosis may occur following treatment with immune globulin products, including **Hizentra**. Aseptic meningitis syndrome has been reported with IGIV and IGSC, including **Hizentra**. Monitor renal function in patients at risk of acute renal failure (ARF). Monitor for clinical signs and symptoms of hemolysis. Monitor for pulmonary adverse reactions (transfusion-related acute lung injury [TRALI]). **Hizentra** is made from human blood and may contain infectious agents (e.g., viruses, the variant Creutzfeldt-Jakob disease (vCJD) agent and, theoretically, the Creutzfeldt-Jakob disease (CJD) agent). Monitor for clinical signs and symptoms of hemolysis. The most common adverse reactions observed in ≥5% of study subjects were local infusion site reactions, headache, diarrhea, fatigue, back pain, nausea, pain in extremity, cough, upper respiratory tract infection, rash, pruritus, vomiting, abdominal pain (upper), migraine, arthralgia, pain, fall and nasopharyngitis. No human or animal reproduction studies have not been conducted with **Hizentra**. It is not known whether **Hizentra** can cause fetal harm when administered during pregnancy. No human data are available to inform maternal use of **Hizentra** on the breastfed infant. Safety and effectiveness of weekly **Hizentra** administration have not been established in children <2 years of age. To report suspected adverse reactions, contact CSL Behring Pharmacovigilance at 1-866-915-6958 or FDA at 1-800-FDA-1088 or www.fda.gov/medwatch

POLYPS, NASAL

LONG-ACTING CORTICOSTEROID SINUS IMPLANT

➢ *mometasone furoate* <18 years: not established: ≥18 years: the **Sinuva Sinus Implant** must be inserted by a physician trained in otolaryngology; the implant is loaded into a sterile delivery system supplied with the implant and placed in the ethmoid sinus under endoscopic visualization; the implant is left in the sinus to gradually release the corticosteroid over 90 days; the implant is removed at Day 90 or earlier at the physician's discretion using standard surgical instruments; repeat administration has not been studied.

Sinuva Sinus Implant *Sinus implant:* 1350 mcg w. sterile delivery system

Comment: **Sinuva** is a corticosteroid-eluting sinus implant indicated for the treatment of recurrent nasal polyp disease in patients who have ethmoid sinus surgery. Monitor nasal mucosa adjacent to the SINUVA Sinus Implant for any signs of bleeding (epistaxis), irritation, infection, or perforation. Avoid use in patients with nasal ulcers or trauma. Monitor patients with a change in vision or with a history of increased intraocular pressure, glaucoma, and/or cataracts closely. Potential worsening of existing tuberculosis; fungal, bacterial, viral, parasitic infection, or ocular herpes simplex. More serious or even fatal course of chickenpox or measles in susceptible patients. If corticosteroid effects such as hypercorticism and adrenal suppression appear in patients, consider sinus implant removal. To report suspected adverse reactions, contact Intersect ENT at 1-866 531-6004 or FDA at 1-800-FDA-1088 or visit www.fda.gov/medwatch

NASAL SPRAY CORTICOSTEROIDS

➢ *beclomethasone dipropionate* (C)

Beconase <6 years: not recommended; 6-12 years: 1 spray in each nostril tid; >12 years: 1 spray in each nostril bid-qid

Nasal spray: 42 mcg/actuation (6.7 gm, 80 sprays; 16.8 gm, 200 sprays)

Beconase AQ <6: not recommended; ≥6 years: 1-2 sprays in each nostril bid

Nasal spray: 42 mcg/actuation (25 gm, 180 sprays)

Beconase Inhalation Aerosol <6: not recommended; 6-12 years: 1 spray in each nostril tid; >12 years: 1-2 sprays in each nostril bid to qid

Nasal spray: 42 mcg/actuation (6.7 gm, 80 sprays; 16.8 gm, 200 sprays)

Vancenase AQ <6 years: not recommended; ≥6 years: 1-2 sprays in each nostril bid

Nasal spray: 84 mcg/actuation (25 gm, 200 sprays)

Vancenase AQ DS <6 years: not recommended; ≥6 years: 1-2 sprays in each nostril once daily

Nasal spray: 84, 168 mcg/actuation (19 gm, 120 sprays)

Vancenase Pockethaler <6: not recommended; 6-12 years: 1 spray in each nostril tid; >12 years: 1 spray in each nostril bid or qid

Pockethaler: 42 mcg/actuation (7 gm, 200 sprays)

QNASL Nasal Aerosol <12 years: 2 sprays, 40 mcg/spray, in each nostril once daily; ≥12 years: 2 sprays, 80 mcg/spray, in each nostril once daily

Nasal spray: 40 mcg/actuation (4.9 gm, 60 sprays); 80 mcg/actuation (8.7 gm, 120 sprays)

▶ ***budesonide*** **(C)**

Rhinocort <6 years: not recommended; ≥6 years: initially 2 sprays in each nostril bid in the AM and PM, or 4 sprays in each nostril in the AM; max 4 sprays each nostril/day; use lowest effective dose

Nasal spray: 32 mcg/actuation (7 gm, 200 sprays)

Rhinocort Aqua Nasal Spray <6 years: not recommended; 6-12 years: initially 1 spray in each nostril once daily; max 2 sprays in each nostril once daily; >12 years: initially 1 spray in each nostril once daily; max 4 sprays in each nostril once daily

Nasal spray: 32 mcg/actuation (10 ml, 60 sprays)

▶ ***ciclesonide*** **(C)**

Omnaris <6 years: not recommended; ≥6 years: 2 sprays in each nostril once daily

Nasal spray: 50 mcg/actuation (12.5 gm, 120 sprays)

Zetonna <6 years: not recommended; ≥6 years: 1-2 sprays in each nostril once daily

Nasal spray: 37 mcg/actuation (6.1 gm, 60 sprays) (HFA)

▶ ***dexamethasone*** **(C)** <6 years: not recommended; ≥6-12 years: 1-2 sprays in each nostril bid; max 8 sprays/day; maintain at lowest effective dose; >12 years: 2 sprays in each nostril bid-tid; max 12 sprays/day; maintain at lowest effective dose

Dexacort Turbinaire *Nasal spray:* 84 mcg/actuation (12.6 gm, 170 sprays)

▶ ***fluticasone furoate*** **(C)** <2 years: not recommended; ≥2-11 years: 1 spray in each nostril once daily; ≥12 years: 2 sprays in each nostril once daily; may reduce to 1 spray each nostril once daily

Veramyst *Nasal spray:* 27.5 mcg/actuation (10 gm, 120 sprays) (alcohol-free)

▶ ***fluticasone propionate*** **(C)**

Flonase (OTC)(G) <4 years: not recommended; 4-12 years: initially 1 spray in each nostril once daily; may increase to 2 sprays in each nostril once daily; maintenance 1 spray in each nostril once daily; max 2 sprays in each nostril/day; >12 years: initially 2 sprays in each nostril once daily or 1 spray bid; maintenance 1 spray once daily

Nasal spray: 50 mcg/actuation (16 gm, 120 sprays)

Xhance <18 years: not established; ≥18 years: 1 spray per nostril bid (total daily dose 372 mcg); 2 sprays per nostril bid may also be effective in some patients (total daily dose 744 mcg)

Nasal spray: 93 mcg/actuation (16 ml, 120 metered sprays)

Comment: Available data from published literature on the use of inhaled or intranasal ***fluticasone propionate*** in pregnant women have not reported a clear association with adverse developmental outcomes. There are no available data on the presence of ***fluticasone propionate*** in human milk or effects on the breastfed child. The safety and efficacy of **Xhance** in <18 years of age patients have not been established.

▶ ***flunisolide*** **(C)** <6 years: not recommended; 6-14 years: initially 1 spray in each nostril tid or 2 sprays in each nostril bid; max 4 sprays/nostril/day; >14 years: 2 sprays in each nostril bid; may increase to 2 sprays in each nostril tid; max 8 sprays/nostril/day

Nasalide *Nasal spray:* 25 mcg/actuation (25 ml, 200 sprays)

Nasarel *Nasal spray:* 25 mcg/actuation (25 ml, 200 sprays)

- ▶ ***mometasone furoate*** (C)(G) <2 years: not recommended; 2-11 years: 1 spray in each nostril once daily; max 2 sprays in each nostril once daily; >11 years: 2 sprays in each nostril once daily
  - **Nasonex** *Nasal spray:* 50 mcg/actuation (17 gm, 120 sprays)
- ▶ ***olopatadine*** (C) <6 years: not recommended; 6-11 years: 1 spray each nostril bid; >11 years: 2 sprays in each nostril bid
  - **Patanase** *Nasal spray:* 0.6%; 665 mcg/actuation (30.5 gm, 240 sprays) (benzalkonium chloride)
- ▶ ***triamcinolone acetonide*** (C)(G) <6 years: not recommended; 6-12 years: 1 spray in each nostril once daily; max 2 sprays in each nostril once daily; >12 years: initially 2 sprays in each nostril once daily; max 4 sprays in each nostril once daily or 2 sprays in each nostril bid or 1 spray in each nostril qid; maintain at lowest effective dose
  - **Nasacort Allergy 24HR (OTC)** *Nasal spray:* 55 mcg/actuation (10 gm, 120 sprays)
  - **Tri-Nasal** *Nasal spray:* 50 mcg/actuation (15 ml, 120 sprays)

POSTHERPETIC NEURALGIA

GAMMA AMINOBUTYRIC ACID ANALOG

- ▶ ***gabapentin*** (C)
  - **Gralise** (C) <18 years: not recommended; ≥18 years: initially 300 mg on Day 1; then 600 mg on Day 2; then 900 mg on Days 3-6; then 1200 mg on Days 7-10; then 1500 mg on Days 11-14; titrate up to 1800 mg on Day 15; take entire dose once daily with the evening meal; do not crush, split, or chew
    - *Tab:* 300, 600 mg
  - **Neurontin** (G) <3 years: not recommended; 3-12 years: initially 10-15 mg/kg/day in 3 divided doses; max 12 hours between doses; titrate over 3 days; 3-4 years: titrate to 40 mg/kg/day; 5-12 years: titrate to 25-35 mg/kg/day; max 50 mg/kg/day; >12 years: 300 mg daily x 1 day, then 300 mg bid x 1 day, then 300 mg tid continuously; max 1,800 mg/day in 3 divided doses; taper over 7 days
    - *Tab:* 600*, 800* mg; *Cap:* 100, 300, 400 mg; *Oral soln:* 250 mg/5 ml (480 ml) (strawberry-anise)
- ▶ ***gabapentin enacarbil*** (C) <18 years: not recommended; ≥18 years: 600 mg once daily at about 5: 00 PM; if dose not taken at recommended time, next dose should be taken the following day; swallow whole; take with food; *CrCl 30-59 mL/min:* 600 mg on Day 1, Day 3, and every day thereafter; *CrCl <30 mL/min:* or on hemodialysis: not recommended
  - **Horizant** *Tab:* 600 ext-rel

TRICYCLIC ANTIDEPRESSANTS (TCAs)

Comment: Co-administration of SSRIs and TCAs requires extreme caution.

- ▶ ***amitriptyline*** (C)(G) <12 years: not recommended; ≥12 years: 10-20 mg q HS *Tab:* 10, 25, 50, 75, 100, 150 mg
- ▶ ***amoxapine*** (C) <12 years: not recommended; ≥12 years: initially 50 mg bid-tid; after 1 week may increase to 100 mg bid-tid; usual effective dose 200-300 mg/day; if total dose exceeds 300 mg/day, give in divided doses (max 400 mg/day); may give as a single bedtime dose (max 300 mg q HS)
  - *Tab:* 25, 50, 100, 150 mg
- ▶ ***clomipramine*** (C)(G) <10 years: not recommended; 10-<16 years: initially 25 mg daily in divided doses; gradually increase; max 3 mg/kg or 100 mg, whichever is smaller; >16 years: initially 25 mg daily in divided doses; gradually increase to 100 mg during first 2 weeks; max 250 mg/day; total maintenance dose may be given at HS
  - **Anafranil** *Cap:* 25, 50, 75 mg

▶ ***desipramine*** **(C)(G)** <12 years: not recommended; ≥12 years: 100-200 mg/day in single or divided doses; max 300 mg/day
  Norpramin *Tab:* 10, 25, 50, 75, 100, 150 mg

▶ ***doxepin*** (C)(G) <12 years: not recommended; ≥12 years: 75 mg/day; max 150 mg/day
  Cap: 10, 25, 50, 75, 100, 150 mg; Oral conc: 10 mg/ml (4 oz w. dropper)

▶ ***imipramine*** (C)(G) <12 years: not recommended; ≥12 years:
  Tofranil initially 75 mg daily (max 200 mg); adolescents initially 30-40 mg daily (max 100 mg/day); if maintenance dose exceeds 75 mg daily, may switch to **Tofranil PM** for divided or bedtime dose
  Tab: 10, 25, 50 mg
  Tofranil PM initially 75 mg daily 1 hour before HS; max 200 mg
  Cap: 75, 100, 125, 150 mg

▶ ***nortriptyline*** (D)(G) <12 years: not recommended; ≥12 years: initially 25 mg tid-qid; max 150 mg/day
  Pamelor *Cap:* 10, 25, 50, 75 mg; *Oral soln:* 10 mg/5 ml (16 oz)

▶ ***protriptyline*** (C) <12 years: not recommended; ≥12 years: initially 5 mg tid; usual dose 15-40 mg/day in 3-4 divided doses; max 60 mg/day
  Vivactil *Tab:* 5, 10 mg

▶ ***trimipramine*** (C) <12 years: not recommended; ≥12 years: initially 75 mg/day in divided doses; max 200 mg/day
  Surmontil *Cap:* 25, 50, 100 mg

ALPHA2-DELTA LIGAND

▶ ***pregabalin (GABA analog)*** (C)(V) <18 years: not recommended; ≥18 years: initially 150 mg daily divided bid-tid and may titrate within one week; max 600 mg divided bid-tid; discontinue over one week
  Lyrica *Cap:* 25, 50, 75, 100, 150, 200, 225, 300 mg; *Oral soln:* 20 mg/ml

▶ ***pregabalin (GABA analog)*** (C)(V) <18 years: not recommended; ≥18 years:
  Lyrica initially 150 mg bid-divided tid; may titrate within one week; max 600 mg divided bid-tid; discontinue over 1 week
  Cap: 25, 50, 75, 100, 150, 200, 225, 300 mg; *Oral soln:* 20 mg/ml
  Lyrica CR *Tab:* usual dose: 165 mg once daily; may increase to 330 mg/day within 1 week; max 660 mg/day; discontinue over 1 week
  Tab: 82.5, 165, 330 mg ext-rel

TOPICAL & TRANSDERMAL ANALGESICS

▶ ***capsaicin*** cream (B)(G) <2 years: not recommended; 2-12 years: apply sparingly to intact skin bid prn; >12 years: apply tid-qid prn
  Axsain *Crm:* 0.075% (1, 2 oz)
  Capsin (OTC) *Lotn:* 0.025, 0, 075% (59 ml)
  Capzasin-P (OTC) *Crm:* 0.025% (1.5 oz); *Lotn:* 0.025% (2 oz)
  Capzasin-HP (OTC) *Crm:* 0.075% (1.5 oz); *Lotn:* 0.075% (2 oz)
  Dolorac *Crm:* 0.025% (28 gm)
  Double Cap (OTC) *Crm:* 0.05% (2 oz)
  R-Gel *Gel:* 0.025% (15, 30 gm)
  Zostrix (OTC) *Crm:* 0.025% (0.7, 1.5, 3 oz)
  Zostrix HP (OTC) *Emol crm:* 0.075% (1, 2 oz)
 Comment: Provides some relief by 1-2 weeks; optimal benefit may take 4-6 weeks. Avoid contact with mucous membranes.

▶ ***diclofenac epolamine*** (C) <12 years: not recommended; ≥12 years: apply one patch to affected area bid; remove during bathing; avoid non-intact skin; do not reuse
  Flector Patch *Patch:* 180 mg/patch (30/carton)

Comment: ***diclofenac*** is contraindicated with ***aspirin*** allergy and late pregnancy.

- ***doxepin*** cream **(B)** <12 years: not recommended; ≥12 years: apply to affected area qid at intervals of at least 3-4 hours; max 8 days
    - **Prudoxin** *Crm:* 5% (45 gm)
    - **Zonalon** *Crm:* 5% (30, 45 gm)
- ***pimecrolimus*** 1% cream (C) <2 years: not recommended; ≥2 years: apply to affected area bid; do not occlude
    - **Elidel** *Crm:* 1% (30, 60, 100 gm)

  Comment: ***pimecrolimus*** is indicated for short-term and intermittent long-term use. Discontinue use when resolution occurs. Contraindicated if the patient is immunosuppressed. Change to the 0.1% preparation or if secondary bacterial infection is present.
- ***tacrolimus*** **(C)** <2 years: not recommended; 2-15 years: use 0.03% strength; apply to affected area bid; continue for 1 week after clearing; >15 years: apply to affected area bid; do not occlude or apply to wet skin; continue for 1 week after clearing
    - **Protopic** *Oint:* 0.03, 0.1% (30, 60, 100 gm)
- ***trolamine salicylate*** <2 years: not recommended; ≥2 years: apply tid-qid prn to intact skin
    - **Mobisyl** *Crm:* 10%

  Comment: Provides some relief by 1-2 weeks; optimal benefit

TOPICAL & TRANSDERMAL ANESTHETICS

- ***lidocaine*** cream **(B)** <12 years: not recommended; ≥12 years:
    - **LidaMantle** *Crm:* 3% (1, 2 oz)
    - **Lidoderm** *Crm:* 3% (85 gm)
- ***lidocaine*** lotion **(B)** <12 years: not recommended; ≥12 years:
    - **LidaMantle** *Lotn:* 3% (177 ml)
- ***lidocaine*** 5% patch **(B)(G)** <12 years: not recommended; ≥12 years: apply up to 3 patches at one time for up to 12 hours/24-hour period (12 hours on/12 hours off); patches may be cut into smaller sizes before removal of the release liner; do not reuse
    - **Lidoderm** *Patch:* 5% (10 x 14 cm, 30/carton)
- ***lidocaine+dexamethasone*** **(B)** <12 years: not recommended; ≥12 years:
    - **Decadron Phosphate with Xylocaine** dexa 4 mg+lido 10 mg per ml (5 ml)
- ***lidocaine+hydrocortisone*** **(B)(G)** <12 years: not recommended; ≥12 years:
    - **LidaMantle HC** *Crm:* lido 3%+hydro 0.5% (1, 3 oz); *Lotn:* (177 ml)

ORAL ANALGESICS

- ***acetaminophen*** (B)(G) *see **Fever** page* 149
- ***aspirin*** (D)(G) *see **Fever** page* 150

  Comment: ***aspirin***-containing medications are contraindicated with history of allergic-type reaction to ***aspirin***, children and adolescents with *Varicella* or other viral illness, and 3rd trimester pregnancy.
- ***tramadol*** (C)(IV)(G)

  Comment: ***tramadol*** is known to be excreted in breast milk. The FDA and the European Medicines Agency (EMA) are investigating the safety of using ***tramadol***-containing medications to treat pain in children 12-18 years because of the potential for serious side effects, including slowed or difficult breathing.

  Rybix ODT <12 years: contraindicated; 12-<18: use extreme caution; not recommended for children and adolescents with obesity, asthma, obstructive sleep apnea, or other chronic breathing problem, or for post-tonsillectomy/adenoidectomy pain; ≥18 years: initially 100 mg once daily; may increase by 100 mg every 5 days; max 300 mg/day; *CrCl <30 mL/min* or *severe hepatic impairment:* not recommended; *Cirrhosis:* max 50 mg q 12 hours

  ODT: 50 mg (mint) (phenylalanine)

Ryzolt <12 years: contraindicated; 12-<18: use extreme caution; not recommended for children and adolescents with obesity, asthma, obstructive sleep apnea, or other chronic breathing problem, or for post-tonsillectomy/adenoidectomy pain; ≥18 years: initially 100 mg once daily; may increase by 100 mg every 5 days; max 300 mg/day; *CrCl <30 mL/min or severe hepatic impairment:* not recommended

Tab: 100, 200, 300 mg ext-rel

Ultram <12 years: contraindicated; 12-<18: use extreme caution; not recommended for children and adolescents with obesity, asthma, obstructive sleep apnea, or other chronic breathing problem, or for post-tonsillectomy/adenoidectomy pain; ≥18 years: 50-100 mg q 4-6 hours prn; max 400 mg/day; *CrCl <30 mL/min:* max 100 mg q 12 hours; *Cirrhosis:* max 50 mg q 12 hours

Tab: 50*mg

Ultram ER <12 years: contraindicated; 12-<18: use extreme caution; not recommended for children and adolescents with obesity, asthma, obstructive sleep apnea, or other chronic breathing problem, or for post-tonsillectomy/adenoidectomy pain; ≥18 years: initially 100 mg once daily; may increase by 100 mg every 5 days; max 300 mg/day; *CrCl <30 mL/min or severe hepatic impairment:* not recommended

Tab: 100, 200, 300 mg ext-rel

▶ ***tramadol+acetaminophen*** (C)(IV)(G) <12 years: contraindicated; 12-<18: use extreme caution; not recommended for children and adolescents with obesity, asthma, obstructive sleep apnea, or other chronic breathing problem, or for post-tonsillectomy/adenoidectomy pain; ≥18 years: 2 tabs q 4-6 hours; max 8 tabs/day; 5 days; *CrCl <30 mL/min:* max 2 tabs q 12 hours; max 4 tabs/day x 5 days

Ultracet *Tab:* tram 37.5+acet 325 mg

Comment: ***tramadol*** is known to be excreted in breast milk. The FDA and the European Medicines Agency (EMA) are investigating the safety of using ***tramadol***-containing medications to treat pain in children 12-18 years because of the potential for serious side effects, including slowed or difficult breathing.

TRICYCLIC ANTIDEPRESSANTS (TCAs)

Comment: Co-administration of SSRIs and TCAs requires extreme caution.

▶ ***amitriptyline*** (C)(G) <12 years: not recommended; ≥12 years: 10-20 mg q HS *Tab:* 10, 25, 50, 75, 100, 150 mg

▶ ***amoxapine*** (C) <12 years: not recommended; ≥12 years: initially 50 mg bid-tid; after 1 week may increase to 100 mg bid-tid; usual effective dose 200-300 mg/day; if total dose exceeds 300 mg/day, give in divided doses (max 400 mg/day); may give as a single bedtime dose (max 300 mg q HS)

Tab: 25, 50, 100, 150 mg

▶ ***clomipramine*** (C)(G) <10 years: not recommended; 10-<16 years: initially 25 mg daily in divided doses; gradually increase; max 3 mg/kg or 100 mg, whichever is smaller; >16 years: initially 25 mg daily in divided doses; gradually increase to 100 mg during first 2 weeks; max 250 mg/day; total maintenance dose may be given at HS

Anafranil *Cap:* 25, 50, 75 mg

▶ ***desipramine*** (C)(G) <12 years: not recommended; ≥12 years: 100-200 mg/day in single or divided doses; max 300 mg/day

Norpramin *Tab:* 10, 25, 50, 75, 100, 150 mg

▶ ***doxepin*** (C)(G) <12 years: not recommended; ≥12 years: 75 mg/day; max 150 mg/day

Cap: 10, 25, 50, 75, 100, 150 mg; Oral conc: 10 mg/ml (4 oz w. dropper)

▶ ***imipramine*** (C)(G) <12 years: not recommended; ≥12 years:

Tofranil initially 75 mg daily (max 200 mg); adolescents initially 30-40 mg daily (max 100 mg/day); if maintenance dose exceeds 75 mg daily, may switch to **Tofranil PM** for divided or bedtime dose

Tab: 10, 25, 50 mg

Tofranil PM initially 75 mg daily 1 hour before HS; max 200 mg
Cap: 75, 100, 125, 150 mg

▶ ***nortriptyline*** (D)(G) <12 years: not recommended; ≥12 years: initially 25 mg tid-qid; max 150 mg/day
Pamelor *Cap:* 10, 25, 50, 75 mg; *Oral soln:* 10 mg/5 ml (16 oz)

▶ ***protriptyline*** (C) <12 years: not recommended; ≥12 years: initially 5 mg tid; usual dose 15-40 mg/day in 3-4 divided doses; max 60 mg/day
Vivactil *Tab:* 5, 10 mg

▶ ***trimipramine*** (C) <12 years: not recommended; ≥12 years: initially 75 mg/day in divided doses; max 200 mg/day
Surmontil *Cap:* 25, 50, 100 mg

POST-TRAUMATIC STRESS DISORDER (PTSD)

Comment: No one pharmacological agent has emerged as the best treatment for PTSD. A combination of pharmacological agents (e.g., antidepressants, non-adrenergic agents, antipsychosis drugs) may comprise an individualized treatment plan to successfully manage core symptoms of PTSD as well as associated anxiety, depression, sleep disturbances, and co-occurring psychiatric disorders.

SELECTIVE SEROTONIN REUPTAKE INHIBITORS (SSRIs)

Comment: The FDA has approved two SSRIs for the treatment of PTSD: (***fluoxetine, citalopram, escitalopram, fluvoxamine***) have been tested in clinical practice. Co-administration of SSRIs with TCAs requires extreme caution. Concomitant use of MAOIs and SSRIs is absolutely contraindicated. Avoid St. John's wort and other serotonergic agents. A potentially fatal adverse event is *serotonin syndrome*, caused by serotonin excess. Milder symptoms require HCP intervention to avert ***paroxetine*** and ***sertraline***. However, the safety and efficacy of other SSRIs severe symptoms that can be rapidly fatal without urgent/emergent medical care. Symptoms include restlessness, agitation, confusion, hallucinations, tachycardia, hypertension, dilated pupils, muscle twitching, muscle rigidity, loss of muscle coordination, diaphoresis, diarrhea, headache, shivering, piloerection, hyperpyrexia, cardiac arrhythmias, seizures, loss of consciousness, coma, and death. Abrupt withdrawal or interruption of treatment with an antidepressant medication is sometimes associated with an antidepressant discontinuation syndrome, which may be mediated by gradually tapering the drug over a period of two weeks or longer, depending on the dose strength and length of treatment. Common symptoms of the *serotonin discontinuation syndrome* include flu-like symptoms (nausea, vomiting, diarrhea, headaches, sweating), sleep disturbances (insomnia, nightmares, constant sleepiness), mood disturbances (dysphoria, anxiety, agitation), cognitive disturbances (mental confusion, hyperarousal), sensory and movement disturbances (imbalance, tremors, vertigo, dizziness, electric-shock-like sensations in the brain, often described by sufferers as "brain zaps").

▶ ***citalopram*** (C)(G) <12 years: not recommended; ≥12 years: initially 20 mg once daily; may increase after one week to 40 mg once daily; max 40 mg
Celexa *Tab:* 10, 20, 40 mg; *Oral soln:* 10 mg/5 ml (120 ml) (pepper mint)(sugar-free, alcohol-free, parabens)

▶ ***escitalopram*** (C)(G) <12 years: not recommended; 12-17 years: initially 10 mg daily; may increase to 20 mg daily after 3 weeks; ≥17 years: initially 10 mg daily; may increase to 20 mg daily after 1 week; *Hepatic impairment:* 10 mg once daily
Lexapro *Tab:* 5, 10*, 20*mg
Lexapro Oral Solution *Oral soln:* 1 mg/ml (240 ml) (peppermint) (parabens)

▶ ***fluoxetine*** (C)(G)

Prozac <8 years: not recommended; 8-17 years: initially 10 mg/day; may increase after 1 week to 20 mg/day; range 20-60 mg/day; range for lower weight children, 20-30 mg/day; ≥17 years: initially 20 mg daily; may increase after 1 week; doses >20 mg/day should be divided into AM and noon doses; max 80 mg/day

Cap: 10, 20, 40 mg; *Tab:* 30*, 60*mg; *Oral soln:* 20 mg/5 ml (4 oz) (mint)

Prozac Weekly <12 years: not recommended; ≥12 years: following daily ***fluoxetine*** therapy at 20 mg/day for 13 weeks, may initiate **Prozac Weekly** 7 days after the last 20 mg ***fluoxetine*** dose

Cap: 90 mg ent-coat del-rel pellets

▶ ***levomilnacipran*** (C) <12 years: not recommended; ≥12 years: swallow whole; initially 20 mg once daily for 2 days; then increase to 40 mg once daily; may increase dose in 40 mg increments at intervals of ≥2 days; max 120 mg once daily; *CrCl 30-59 mL/min:* max 80 mg once daily; *CrCl 15-29 mL/min:* max 40 mg once daily

Fetzima *Cap:* 20, 40, 80, 120 mg ext-rel

▶ ***paroxetine maleate*** (D)(G)

Paxil <12 years: not recommended; ≥12 years: initially 20 mg daily in AM; may increase by 10 mg/day at weekly intervals as needed; max 60 mg/day

Tab: 10*, 20*, 30, 40 mg

Paxil CR <12 years: not recommended; ≥12 years: initially 25 mg daily in AM; may increase by 12.5 mg at weekly intervals as needed; max 62.5 mg/day

Tab: 12.5, 25, 37.5 mg cont-rel ent-coat

Paxil Suspension <12 years: not recommended; ≥12 years: initially 20 mg daily in AM; may increase by 10 mg/day at weekly intervals as needed; max 60 mg/day

Oral susp: 10 mg/5 ml (250 ml) (orange)

▶ ***paroxetine mesylate*** (D)(G) <12 years: not recommended; ≥12 years: initially 7.5 mg daily in AM; may increase by 10 mg/day at weekly intervals as needed; max 60 mg/day

Brisdelle *Cap:* 7.5 mg

▶ ***sertraline*** (C)(G) <6 years: not recommended; 6-<12 years: initially 25 mg daily; max 200 mg/day; 12-17 years: initially 50 mg daily; max 200 mg/day; ≥17 years: initially 50 mg daily; increase at 1 week intervals if needed; max 200 mg daily; dilute oral concentrate immediately prior to administration in 4 oz water, ginger ale, lemon-lime soda, lemonade, <u>or</u> orange juice

Zoloft *Tab:* 25*, 50*, 100*mg; *Oral conc:* 20 mg per ml (60 ml) (alcohol 12%)

ATYPICAL ANTIPSYCHOSIS DRUGS

▶ ***olanzapine*** (C)(G) <13 years: not recommended; 13-17 years: initially 2.5-5 mg once daily at HS; >17 years: initially 5-10 mg once daily at HS; titrate weekly, max 20 mg at HS; usual maintenance 10-20 mg/day

Zyprexa *Tab:* 2.5, 5, 7.5, 10, 15, 20 mg

Zyprexa Zydis *ODT:* 5, 10, 15, 20 mg (phenylalanine)

▶ ***quetiapine*** (C)(G)

SeroQUEL <10 years: not recommended; 10-17 years: initially 25 mg bid, titrate q 2nd <u>or</u> 3rd day in increments of 25-50 mg bid-tid; max 600 mg/day in 2-3 divided doses; >17 years: initially 25 mg bid, titrate q 2nd <u>or</u> 3rd day in increments of 25-50 mg bid-tid; usual maintenance 400-600 mg/day in 2-3 divided doses

Tab: 25, 50, 100, 200, 300, 400 mg

SeroQUEL XR <18 years: not recommended; ≥18 years: swallow whole; administer once daily in the PM; *Day 1:* 50 mg; *Day 2:* 100 mg; *Day 3:* 200 mg; *Day 4:* 300 mg; usual range 400-600 mg/day

Tab: 50, 150, 200, 300, 400 mg ext-rel

▶ *risperidone* (C)

Comment: **Risperdal** tabs, oral solution, and M-tabs are indicated for the short-term monotherapy of acute mania or mixed episodes associated with bipolar I disorder, or in combination with ***lithium*** or ***valproic acid*** in patients >12 years-of-age. **Risperdal Consta** is indicated as monotherapy or adjunctive therapy to ***lithium*** or ***valproic acid*** for the maintenance treatment mania and mixed episodes in bipolar I disorder.

Risperdal <5 years: not established; 5-10 years: initially 0.5 mg once daily at the same time each day adjust at 24 hour intervals by 0.5-1 mg to target dose 2.5 mg/day; usual range 1-6 mg/day; max 6 mg/day; >10 years: *Tab:* initially 2-3 mg once daily; may adjust at 24 hour intervals by 1 mg/day; usual range 1-6 mg/day; max 6 mg/day; *Oral soln:* do not take with cola or tea

Tab: 0.25, 0.5, 1, 2, 3, 4 mg; *Oral soln:* 1 mg/ml (100 ml)

Risperdal Consta <18 years: not established; ≥18 years: administer deep IM in the deltoid or gluteal; give with oral ***risperidone*** or other antipsychotic x 3 weeks; then stop oral form; 25 mg IM every 2 weeks; max 50 mg every 2 weeks

Vial: 12.5, 25, 37.5, 50 mg pwdr for long-acting IM inj after reconstitution, single use w. diluent and supplies

Risperdal M-Tab <10 years: not established; ≥10 years: dissolve on tongue with or without fluid

M-Tab: 0.5, 1, 2, 3, 4 mg orally-disint (phenylalanine)

NON-ADRENERGIC AGENTS

Alpha-1 Antagonists

▶ *prazosin* (C)(G) <12 years: not recommended: ≥12 years: first dose at HS, 1 mg bid-tid; increase dose slowly; usual range 6-15 mg/day in divided doses; max 20-40 mg/day

Minipress *Cap:* 1, 2, 5 mg

Comment: ***prazosin*** is useful in reducing nightmares and other sleep disturbances.

Central Alpha-2A Agonists

▶ *clonidine* (C)

Comment: ***clonidine*** is useful to reduce nightmares, hypervigilance, startle reactions, and outbursts of rage.

Catapres <12 years: not recommended; ≥12 years: initially 0.1 mg bid; usual range 0.2-0.6 mg/day in divided doses; max 2.4 mg/day

Tab: 0.1*, 0.2*, 0.3*mg

Catapres-TTS <12 years: not recommended; ≥12 years: initially 0.1 mg patch weekly; increase after 1-2 weeks if needed; max 0.6 mg/day

Patch: 0.1, 0.2 mg/day (12/carton); 0.3 mg/day (4/carton)

Kapvay (G) <12 years: not recommended; ≥12 years: initially 0.1 mg bid; usual range 0.2-0.6 mg/day in divided doses; max 2.4 mg/day

Tab: 0.1, 0.2 mg

Nexiclon XR <12 years: not recommended; ≥12 years: initially 0.18 mg (2 ml) suspension or 0.17 mg tab once daily; usual max 0.52 mg (6 ml suspension) once daily

Tab: 0.17, 0.26 mg ext-rel; *Oral susp:* 0.09 mg/ml ext-rel (4 oz)

BETA-ADRENERGIC BLOCKER (NON-CARDIOSELECTIVE)

▶ *propranolol* (C)(G)

Comment: ***propranolol*** is useful to mediate hyperarousal. For other non-cardioselective beta-adrenergic blockers, *see* **Hypertension** *page* 221.

Inderal <12 years: not recommended; ≥12 years: initially 10 mg bid; usual range 160-320 mg/day in divided doses

Tab: 10*, 20*, 40*, 60*, 80*mg

Inderal LA <12 years: not recommended; ≥12 years: initially 80 mg daily in a single dose; increase q 3-7 days; usual range 120-160 mg/day; max 320 mg/day in a single dose

Cap: 60, 80, 120, 160 mg sust-rel

InnoPran XL <12 years: not recommended; ≥12 years: initially 80 mg q HS; max 120 mg/day

Cap: 80, 120 mg ext-rel

SEROTONIN-NOREPINEPHRINE REUPTAKE INHIBITORS (SNRIs)

▶ ***desvenlafaxine*** (C)(G) <18 years: not recommended; ≥18 years: swallow whole; initially 50 mg once daily; max 120 mg/day

Pristiq *Tab:* 50, 100 mg ext-rel

▶ ***duloxetine*** (C)(G) <12 years: not recommended; ≥12 years: swallow whole; initially 30 mg once daily x 1 week; then, increase to 60 mg once daily; max 120 mg/day

Cymbalta *Cap:* 20, 30, 40, 60 mg del-rel

▶ ***venlafaxine*** (C)(G)

Effexor <18 years: not recommended; ≥18 years: initially 75 mg/day in 2-3 divided doses; may increase at 4 day intervals in 75 mg increments to 150 mg/day; max 225 mg/day

Tab: 37.5, 75, 150, 225 mg

Effexor XR <18 years: not recommended; ≥18 years: initially 75 mg q AM; may start at 37.5 mg daily x 4-7 days, then increase by increments of up to 75 mg/day at intervals of at least 4 days; usual ax 375 mg/day

Tab/Cap: 37.5, 75, 150 mg ext-rel

▶ ***vortioxetine*** (C) <18 years: not established; ≥18 years: initially 10 mg once daily; max 30 mg/day

Brintellix *Tab:* 5, 10, 15, 20 mg

5HT2/3 RECEPTOR BLOCKERS

▶ ***mirtazapine*** (C) <12 years: not established; ≥12 years: initially 15 mg q HS; increase at intervals of 1-2 weeks; 1-2 weeks; usual range 15-60 mg/day; max 60 mg/day

Remeron *Tab:* 15*, 30*, 45*mg

Remeron SolTab *ODT:* 15, 30, 45 mg (orange) (phenylalanine)

SEROTONIN+ACETYLCHOLINE+NOREPINEPHRINE+DOPAMINE BLOCKER

▶ ***trazodone*** (C)(G) <18 years: not recommended; ≥18 years: initially 150 mg/day in divided doses with food; increase by 50 mg/day q 3-4 days; max 400 mg/day in divided doses <u>or</u> 50-400 mg at HS

Oleptro *Tab:* 50, 100*, 150*, 200, 250, 300 mg

TRICYCLIC ANTIDEPRESSANTS (TCAs)

Comment: Co-administration of SSRIs and TCAs requires extreme caution.

▶ ***amitriptyline*** (C)(G) <12 years: not recommended; ≥12 years: 10-20 mg q HS *Tab:* 10, 25, 50, 75, 100, 150 mg

▶ ***amoxapine*** (C) <12 years: not recommended; ≥12 years: initially 50 mg bid-tid; after 1 week may increase to 100 mg bid-tid; usual effective dose 200-300 mg/day; if total dose exceeds 300 mg/day, give in divided doses (max 400 mg/day); may give as a single bedtime dose (max 300 mg q HS)

Tab: 25, 50, 100, 150 mg

▶ ***clomipramine*** (C)(G) <10 years: not recommended; 10-<16 years: initially 25 mg daily in divided doses; gradually increase; max 3 mg/kg <u>or</u> 100 mg, whichever is smaller; >16 years: initially 25 mg daily in divided doses; gradually increase to 100 mg during first 2 weeks; max 250 mg/day; total maintenance dose may be given at HS

Anafranil *Cap:* 25, 50, 75 mg

- ▶ ***desipramine*** **(C)(G)** <12 years: not recommended; ≥12 years: 100-200 mg/day in single or divided doses; max 300 mg/day

  Norpramin *Tab:* 10, 25, 50, 75, 100, 150 mg

- ▶ ***doxepin*** **(C)(G)** <12 years: not recommended; ≥12 years: 75 mg/day; max 150 mg/day

  Cap: 10, 25, 50, 75, 100, 150 mg; Oral conc: 10 mg/ml (4 oz w. dropper)

- ▶ ***imipramine*** **(C)(G)** <12 years: not recommended; ≥12 years:

  Tofranil initially 75 mg daily (max 200 mg); adolescents initially 30-40 mg daily (max 100 mg/day); if maintenance dose exceeds 75 mg daily, may switch to **Tofranil PM** for divided or bedtime dose

  Tab: 10, 25, 50 mg

  Tofranil PM initially 75 mg daily 1 hour before HS; max 200 mg

  Cap: 75, 100, 125, 150 mg

- ▶ ***nortriptyline*** **(D)(G)** <12 years: not recommended; ≥12 years: initially 25 mg tid-qid; max 150 mg/day

  Pamelor *Cap:* 10, 25, 50, 75 mg; *Oral soln:* 10 mg/5 ml (16 oz)

- ▶ ***protriptyline*** **(C)** <12 years: not recommended; ≥12 years: initially 5 mg tid; usual dose 15-40 mg/day in 3-4 divided doses; max 60 mg/day

  Vivactil *Tab:* 5, 10 mg

- ▶ ***trimipramine*** **(C)** <12 years: not recommended; ≥12 years: initially 75 mg/day in divided doses; max 200 mg/day

  Surmontil *Cap:* 25, 50, 100 mg

MONOAMINE OXIDASE INHIBITORS (MAOIs)

Comment: Many drug and food interactions with this class of drugs; use cautiously. MAOIs should be reserved for refractory depression that has not responded to other classes of antidepressants. Concomitant use of MAOIs and SSRIs is contraindicated. See mfr pkg insert for drug and food interactions. MAOIs have been used to reduce recurrent recollections of the trauma, nightmares, flashbacks, numbing, sleep disturbances, and social withdrawal in PTSD.

- ▶ ***phenelzine*** **(C)(G)** <16 years: not recommended; ≥16 years: initially 15 mg tid; max 90 mg/day

  Nardil *Tab:* 15 mg

- ▶ ***selegiline*** **(C)** <12 years: not recommended; ≥12 years: initially 10 mg tid; max 60 mg/day

  Emsam *Transdermal patch:* 6 mg/24 Hrs, 9 mg/24 Hrs, 12 mg/24 Hrs

  Comment: At the **Emsam** transdermal patch 6 mg/24 Hrs, the dietary restrictions commonly required when using non-selective MAOIs are not necessary.

PRECOCIOUS PUBERTY, CENTRAL (CPP)

Comment: GnRH-dependent CPP is defined by pubertal development occurring before the age of 8 years in girls and 9 years in boys. It is characterized by early pubertal changes such as breast development and start of menses in girls and increased testicular and penile growth in boys, appearance of pubic hair, as well as acceleration of growth velocity and bone maturation and tall stature during childhood, which often results in reduced adult height due to premature fusion of the growth plates.

GONADOTROPIN RELEASING HORMONE (GnRH) AGONIST

- ▶ ***triptorelin*** **(X)** <2 years: not recommended; ≥2 years: administer as a single 22.5 mg IM injection once every 24 weeks; must be administered under the supervision of a physician; monitor response with LH levels after a GnRH or GnRH agonist stimulation test, basal LH, or serum concentration of sex steroid levels beginning 1 to 2 months following initiation of therapy, during therapy as necessary to confirm maintenance of efficacy, and with each subsequent dose; measure height every 3-6 months and monitor bone age periodically; see mfr pkg insert for reconstitution and administration instructions

Triptodur Single-use kit: 1 single-dose vial of **triptorelin** 22.5 mg w. Flip-Off seal containing sterile lyophilized white to slightly yellow powder cake, 1 sterile, glass syringe prefilled with 2 ml of sterile water for injection, 2 sterile 21 gauge, 1½" needles (thin-wall) with safety cover

Comment: **Triptodur** is contraindicated in females who are pregnant since expected hormonal changes that occur with ***triptorelin*** treatment increase the risk for pregnancy loss. Available data with ***triptorelin*** use in pregnant females are insufficient to determine a drug-associated risk of adverse developmental outcomes. Based on mechanism of action in humans and findings of increased pregnancy loss in animal studies, ***triptorelin*** may cause fetal harm when administered to pregnant females. Advise pregnant females of the potential risk to a fetus. The estimated background risk of major birth defects and miscarriage is unknown. There are no data on the presence of ***triptorelin*** in human milk or the effects of the drug on the breastfed infant. The developmental and health benefits of breastfeeding should be considered along with the mother's clinical need for ***triptorelin*** and any potential adverse effects on the breastfed child from ***triptorelin*** or from the underlying maternal condition. During the early phase of therapy, gonadotropins and sex steroids rise above baseline because of the initial stimulatory effect of the drug. Therefore, a transient increase in clinical signs and symptoms of puberty, including vaginal bleeding, may be observed during the first weeks of therapy. Post-marketing reports with this class of drugs include symptoms of emotional lability, such as crying, irritability, impatience, anger, and aggression. Monitor for development or worsening of psychiatric symptoms during treatment with **Triptodur**. Post-marketing reports of convulsions have been observed in patients receiving GnRH agonists, including ***triptorelin***. These included patients with a history of seizures, epilepsy, cerebrovascular disorders, central nervous system anomalies or tumors, and patients on concomitant medications that have been associated with convulsions such as bupropion and SSRIs. Convulsions have also been reported in patients in the absence of any of the conditions mentioned above.

PREGNANCY

Comment: Prenatal vitamins should have at least 400 mcg of folic acid content. Take one dose once daily. It is recommended that prenatal vitamins be started at least 3 months prior to conception to improve preconception nutritional status, and continued throughout pregnancy and the postnatal period, in lactating and non-lactating females, and throughout the childbearing years.

NAUSEA/VOMITING

▶ *doxylamine succinate+pyridoxine* (A)(G)do not crush or chew; take on an empty stomach with water; initially 2 tabs at HS on day 1; may increase to 1 tab AM and 2 tabs at HS day 2; may increase to 1 tab AM, 1 tab mid-afternoon, 2 tabs at HS; max 4 tabs/day

Diclegis *Tab:* doxyl 10 mg+pyri 10 mg del-rel

Comment: **Diclegis** is the only FDA-approved drug for the treatment of morning sickness. It has not been studied in females with hyperemesis gravidarum.

▶ *ondansetron* (C)(G) 4-8 mg bid prn or 8 mg q 8 hours prn

Zofran *Tab:* 4, 8, 24 mg

Zofran Injection *Vial:* 2 mg/ml (2 ml) single-dose; 2 mg/ml (20 ml) multi-dose for IV or IM administration

Zofran ODT *ODT:* 4, 8 mg (strawberry) (phenylalanine)

Zofran Oral Solution *Oral soln:* 4 mg/5 ml (50 ml) (strawberry)

Zuplenz Oral Soluble Film: 4, 8 mg orally-disint (10/carton) (peppermint)

▶ *promethazine* (C) <12 years: 0.5 mg/lb or 6.25-25 mg q 4-6 hours PO or rectally; ≥12 years: 12.5-25 q 4-6 hours PO or rectally

Phenergan *Tab:* 12.5*, 25*, 50 mg; *Plain syr:* 6.25 mg/5 ml; *Fortis syr:* 25 mg/5 ml; *Rectal supp:* 12.5, 25, 50 mg; *Amp:* 25, 50 mg/ml (1 ml)

Comment: ***promethazine*** is contraindicated in children with uncomplicated nausea, dehydration, Reye's syndrome, history of sleep apnea, asthma, and lower respiratory disorders in children. ***Promethazine*** lowers the seizure threshold in children, may cause cholestatic jaundice, anticholinergic effects, extrapyramidal effects, and potentially fatal respiratory depression.

PREMENSTRUAL DYSPHORIC DISORDER (PMDD)

NSAIDs *see page* 539
Other Oral Analgesics *see* ***Pain*** *page* 324
Other Oral Contraceptives *see page* 527

CALCIUM SUPPLEMENT

▶ *calcium* (C) 1200 mg/day

ORAL ESTROGEN+PROGESTERONE COMBINATIONS

Comment: **Rajani** (a generic form of **Beyaz**) and **Yaz,** also available in generic forms (**Gianvi, Ocella, Syeda, Vestura, Yasmin, Zarah**), have an FDA indication for treatment of PMDD in post-menarchal females who choose to use an OCP. Contraindicated with renal and adrenal insufficiency. Monitor K^+ level during the first cycle if the patient is at risk for hyperkalemia for any reason. If the patient is taking a drug that increases serum potassium (e.g., ACEIs, ARBS, NSAIDs, K^+ sparing diuretics), the patient is at risk for hyperkalemia.

▶ ***ethinyl estradiol+drospirenone*** (X)(G) *Pre-menarchal:* not indicated; *Post-menarchal:* 1 tab once daily x 28 days; repeat cycle; start on first Sunday after menses begins or on first day of next menses

Yaz *Tab:* ethin estra 20 mcg+drospir 3 mg

▶ ***ethinyl+estradiol+drospirenone*** **plus** ***levomefolate calcium*** (X)(G) *Pre-menarchal:* not indicated; *Post-menarchal:* 1 tab once daily x 28 days; repeat cycle; start on first Sunday after menses begins or on first day of next menses preceded by a negative pregnancy test

Beyaz *Tab:* ethin estra 20 mcg+drospir 3 mg+levo 0.451 mg

Rajani *Tab:* ethin estra 20 mcg+drospir 3 mg+levo 0.451 mg

DIURETICS

▶ ***spironolactone*** (D) <12 years: not recommended; ≥12 years: initially 50-100 mg once daily or in divided doses; titrate at 2-week intervals

Aldactone (G) *Tab:* 25, 50*, 100*mg

CaroSpir *Oral susp:* 25 mg/5 ml (118, 473 ml) (banana)

SELECTIVE SEROTONIN REUPTAKE INHIBITORS (SSRIs)

▶ ***escitalopram*** (C)(G) <12 years: not recommended; 12-17 years: initially 10 mg daily; may increase to 20 mg daily after 3 weeks; ≥17 years: initially 10 mg daily; may increase to 20 mg daily after 1 week; *Hepatic impairment:* 10 mg once daily

Lexapro *Tab:* 5, 10*, 20*mg

Lexapro Oral Solution *Oral soln:* 1 mg/ml (240 ml) (peppermint) (parabens)

▶ ***fluoxetine*** (C)(G)

Prozac <8 years: not recommended; 8-17 years: initially 10 mg/day; may increase after 1 week to 20 mg/day; range 20-60 mg/day; range for lower weight children, 20-30 mg/day; >17 years: initially 20 mg daily; may increase after 1 week; doses >20 mg/day should be divided into AM and noon doses; max 80 mg/day

Cap: 10, 20, 40 mg; *Tab:* 30*, 60*mg; *Oral soln:* 20 mg/5 ml (4 oz) (mint)

Prozac Weekly <12 years: not recommended; ≥12 years: following daily ***fluoxetine*** therapy at 20 mg/day for 13 weeks, may initiate **Prozac Weekly** 7 days after the last 20 mg ***fluoxetine*** dose

Cap: 90 mg ent-coat del-rel pellets

▶ ***levomilnacipran*** (C) <12 years: not recommended; ≥12 years: swallow whole; initially 20 mg once daily for 2 days; then increase to 40 mg once daily; may increase dose in 40 mg increments at intervals of ≥2 days; max 120 mg once daily; *CrCl 30-59 mL/min:* max 80 mg once daily; *CrCl 15-29 mL/min:* max 40 mg once daily

Fetzima *Cap:* 20, 40, 80, 120 mg ext-rel

▶ ***paroxetine maleate*** (D)(G)

Paxil <12 years: not recommended; ≥12 years: initially 20 mg daily in AM; may increase by 10 mg/day at weekly intervals as needed; max 60 mg/day

Tab: 10*, 20*, 30, 40 mg

Paxil CR <12 years: not recommended; ≥12 years: initially 25 mg daily in AM; may increase by 12.5 mg at weekly intervals as needed; max 62.5 mg/day

Tab: 12.5, 25, 37.5 mg cont-rel ent-coat

Paxil Suspension <12 years: not recommended; ≥12 years: initially 20 mg daily in AM; may increase by 10 mg/day at weekly intervals as needed; max 60 mg/day

Oral susp: 10 mg/5 ml (250 ml) (orange)

▶ ***paroxetine mesylate*** (D)(G) <12 years: not recommended; ≥12 years: initially 7.5 mg daily in AM; may increase by 10 mg/day at weekly intervals as needed; max 60 mg/day

Brisdelle *Cap:* 7.5 mg

▶ ***sertraline*** (C)(G) <6 years: not recommended; 6-<12 years: initially 25 mg daily; max 200 mg/day; 12-17 years: initially 50 mg daily; max 200 mg/day; >17 years: initially 50 mg daily; increase at 1 week intervals if needed; max 200 mg daily; dilute oral concentrate immediately prior to administration in 4 oz water, ginger ale, lemon-lime soda, lemonade, <u>or</u> orange juice

Zoloft *Tab:* 25*, 50*, 100*mg; *Oral conc:* 20 mg per ml (60 ml) (alcohol 12%)

TRICYCLIC ANTIDEPRESSANTS (TCAs)

Comment: Co-administration of SSRIs and TCAs requires extreme caution.

▶ ***amitriptyline*** (C)(G) <12 years: not recommended; ≥12 years: 10-20 mg q HS *Tab:* 10, 25, 50, 75, 100, 150 mg

▶ ***amoxapine*** (C) <12 years: not recommended; ≥12 years: initially 50 mg bid-tid; after 1 week may increase to 100 mg bid-tid; usual effective dose 200-300 mg/day; if total dose exceeds 300 mg/day, give in divided doses (max 400 mg/ day); may give as a single bedtime dose (max 300 mg q HS)

Tab: 25, 50, 100, 150 mg

- ▶ ***clomipramine*** **(C)(G)** <10 years: not recommended; 10-<16 years: initially 25 mg daily in divided doses; gradually increase; max 3 mg/kg or 100 mg, whichever is smaller; >16 years: initially 25 mg daily in divided doses; gradually increase to 100 mg during first 2 weeks; max 250 mg/day; total maintenance dose may be given at HS
  - **Anafranil** *Cap:* 25, 50, 75 mg
- ▶ ***desipramine*** **(C)(G)** <12 years: not recommended; ≥12 years: 100-200 mg/day in single or divided doses; max 300 mg/day
  - **Norpramin** *Tab:* 10, 25, 50, 75, 100, 150 mg
- ▶ ***doxepin*** **(C)(G)** <12 years: not recommended; ≥12 years: 75 mg/day; max 150 mg/day
  - *Cap:* 10, 25, 50, 75, 100, 150 mg; Oral conc: 10 mg/ml (4 oz w. dropper)
- ▶ ***imipramine*** **(C)(G)** <12 years: not recommended; ≥12 years:
  - **Tofranil** initially 75 mg daily (max 200 mg); adolescents initially 30-40 mg daily (max 100 mg/day); if maintenance dose exceeds 75 mg daily, may switch to **Tofranil PM** for divided or bedtime dose
    - *Tab:* 10, 25, 50 mg
  - **Tofranil PM** initially 75 mg daily 1 hour before HS; max 200 mg
    - *Cap:* 75, 100, 125, 150 mg
- ▶ ***nortriptyline*** **(D)(G)** <12 years: not recommended; ≥12 years: initially 25 mg tid-qid; max 150 mg/day
  - **Pamelor** *Cap:* 10, 25, 50, 75 mg; *Oral soln:* 10 mg/5 ml (16 oz)
- ▶ ***protriptyline*** **(C)** <12 years: not recommended; ≥12 years: initially 5 mg tid; usual dose 15-40 mg/day in 3-4 divided doses; max 60 mg/day
  - **Vivactil** *Tab:* 5, 10 mg
- ▶ ***trimipramine*** **(C)** <12 years: not recommended; ≥12 years: initially 75 mg/day in divided doses; max 200 mg/day
  - **Surmontil** *Cap:* 25, 50, 100 mg

CALCIUM SUPPLEMENTS

- ▶ ***calcium*** **(C)** 1200 mg/day

PROCTITIS ACUTE (PROCTOCOLITIS, ENTERITIS)

Comment: The following regimen for the treatment of proctitis, proctocolitis, and enteritis is published in the **2015 CDC Sexually Transmitted Diseases Treatment Guidelines**.

RECOMMENDED REGIMEN

- ▶ ***ceftriaxone*** **(B)(G)** 250 mg IM in a single dose
  - **Rocephin** *Vial:* 250, 500 mg; 1, 2 gm
  - plus
- ▶ ***doxycycline*** **(D)(G)** <8 years: not recommended; ≥8 years, ≤100 lb: 2 mg/lb on first day in 2 divided doses, followed by 1 mg/lb/day in 1-2 divided doses x 7 days; ≥8 years, >100 lb: 100 mg bid x 7 days; *see page 605 for dose by weight table*
  - **Acticlate** *Tab:* 75, 150**-mg
  - **Adoxa** *Tab:* 50, 75, 100, 150 mg ent-coat
  - **Doryx** *Tab:* 50, 75, 100, 150, 200 mg del-rel
  - **Doxteric** *Tab:* 50 mg del-rel
  - **Monodox** *Cap:* 50, 75, 100 mg
  - **Oracea** *Cap:* 40 mg del-rel
  - **Vibramycin** *Tab:* 100 mg; *Cap:* 50, 100 mg; *Syr:* 50 mg/5 ml (raspberry-apple) (sulfites); *Oral susp:* 25 mg/5 ml (raspberry)
  - **Vibra-Tab** *Tab:* 100 mg film-coat

Comment: ***doxycycline*** is contraindicated <8 years-of-age, in pregnancy, and lactation (discolors developing tooth enamel). A side effect may be photosensitivity (photophobia). Do not take with antacids, calcium supplements, milk or other dairy, or within 2 hours of taking another drug.

PROSTATITIS: ACUTE

ANTI-INFECTIVES

▶ ***ciprofloxacin*** (C) <18 years: not recommended; ≥18 years: 500 mg bid x 4-6 weeks; max 1.5 gm/day

Cipro (G) *Tab:* 250, 500, 750 mg; *Oral susp:* 250, 500 mg/5 ml (100 ml) (strawberry)

Cipro XR *Tab:* 500, 1,000 mg ext-rel

ProQuin XR *Tab:* 500 mg ext-rel

Comment: ***ciprofloxacin*** is contraindicated <18 years-of-age, and during pregnancy and lactation. Risk of tendonitis or tendon rupture.

▶ ***norfloxacin*** (C) <18 years: not recommended; ≥18 years: 400 mg bid x 28 days

Noroxin *Tab:* 400 mg

Comment: ***norfloxacin*** is contraindicated <18 years-of-age, and during pregnancy and lactation. Risk of tendonitis or tendon rupture.

▶ ***ofloxacin*** (C)(G) <18 years: not recommended; ≥18 years: 300 mg x bid x 6 weeks

Floxin *Tab:* 200, 300, 400 mg

Comment: ***ofloxacin*** is contraindicated <18 years-of-age, and during pregnancy and lactation. Risk of tendonitis or tendon rupture.

▶ ***trimethoprim+sulfamethoxazole [TMP-SMX]*** (C)(G)

Bactrim, Septra <12 years: not recommended; ≥12 years: 2 tabs bid x 10 days

Tab: trim 80 mg+sulfa 400 mg*

Bactrim DS, Septra DS <12 years: not recommended; ≥12 years: 1 tab bid x 10 days

Tab: trim 160 mg+sulfa 800 mg*

Bactrim Pediatric Suspension, Septra Pediatric Suspension <2 months: not recommended; ≥2 months-12 years: 40 mg/kg/day of ***sulfamethoxazole*** in 2 doses bid x 10 days

Oral susp: trim 40 mg+sulfa 200 mg per 5 ml (100 ml) (cherry) (alcohol 0.3%)

Comment: *CrCl 15-30 mL/min:* reduce dose by 1/2; *CrCl <15 mL/min:* not recommended.

PROSTATITIS: CHRONIC

ANTI-INFECTIVES

▶ ***carbenicillin*** (B) <12 years: not recommended; ≥12 years: 1-2 tabs qid x 7-14 days

Geocillin *Tab:* 382 mg

▶ ***ciprofloxacin*** (C) <18 years: not recommended; ≥18 years: 500 mg bid x 3 or more months; max 1.5 gm/day

Cipro (G) *Tab:* 250, 500, 750 mg; *Oral susp:* 250, 500 mg/5 ml (100 ml) (strawberry)

Cipro XR *Tab:* 500, 1000 mg ext-rel

ProQuin XR *Tab:* 500 mg ext-rel

Comment: ***ciprofloxacin*** is contraindicated <18 years-of-age, and during pregnancy and lactation. Risk of tendonitis or tendon rupture.

▶ ***norfloxacin*** (C) <18 years: not recommended; ≥18 years: 400 mg bid x 4-12 weeks

Noroxin *Tab:* 400 mg

Comment: ***norfloxacin*** contraindicated <18 years-of-age, and during pregnancy and lactation. Risk of tendonitis or tendon rupture.

▶ ***ofloxacin*** **(C)(G)** <18 years: not recommended; ≥18 years: 300 mg bid x 4-12 weeks
  Floxin *Tab:* 200, 300, 400 mg

Comment: ***ofloxacin*** is contraindicated <18 years-of-age, and during pregnancy and lactation. Risk of tendonitis or tendon rupture.

▶ ***trimethoprim+sulfamethoxazole [TMP-SMX]*** **(C)(G)**
  Bactrim, Septra <12 years: not recommended; ≥12 years: 2 tabs bid x 10 days
    Tab: trim 80 mg+sulfa 400 mg*
  Bactrim DS, Septra DS <12 years: not recommended; ≥12 years: 1 tab bid x 10 days
    Tab: trim 160 mg+sulfa 800 mg*
  Bactrim Pediatric Suspension, Septra Pediatric Suspension <2 months: not recommended; ≥2 months-12 years: 40 mg/kg/day of ***sulfamethoxazole*** in 2 doses bid x 10 days
    Oral susp: trim 40 mg+sulfa 200 mg per 5 ml (100 ml) (cherry) (alcohol 0.3%)

SUPPRESSION THERAPY

▶ ***trimethoprim+sulfamethoxazole [TMP-SMX]*** **(C)(G)**
  Bactrim, Septra <12 years: not recommended; ≥12 years: 2 tabs bid x 10 days
    Tab: trim 80 mg+sulfa 400 mg*
  Bactrim DS, Septra DS <12 years: not recommended; ≥12 years: 1 tab bid x 10 days
    Tab: trim 160 mg+sulfa 800 mg*
  Bactrim Pediatric Suspension, Septra Pediatric Suspension <2 months: not recommended; ≥2 months-12 years: 40 mg/kg/day of ***sulfamethoxazole*** in 2 doses bid; >12 years: use tabs
    Oral susp: trim 40 mg+sulfa 200 mg per 5 ml (100 ml) (cherry) (alcohol 0.3%)

PRURITUS

Antihistamines *See* **Drugs for the Management of Allergy, Cough, and Cold Symptoms** *page* 570
Topical Corticosteroids *see page* 542
Parenteral Corticosteroids *see page* 547
Oral Corticosteroids *see page* 546
OTC Antihistamines
OTC Eucerin Products
OTC Lac-Hydrin Products
OTC Lubriderm Products
OTC Aveeno Products

TOPICAL OIL

▶ ***fluocinolone acetamide*** 0.01% topical oil **(C)** <6 years: not recommended; ≥6 years: apply sparingly bid for up to 4 weeks
  Derma-Smoothe/FS Topical Oil apply sparingly tid
    Topical oil: 0.01% (4 oz) (peanut oil)

TOPICAL & TRANSDERMAL ANALGESICS

▶ ***capsaicin*** cream **(B)(G)** <2 years: not recommended; 2-12 years: apply sparingly to intact skin bid prn; >12 years: apply tid-qid prn
  Axsain *Crm:* 0.075% (1, 2 oz)
  Capsin (OTC) *Lotn:* 0.025, 0, 075% (59 ml)

Capzasin-P (OTC) *Crm:* 0.025% (1.5 oz); *Lotn:* 0.025% (2 oz)
Capzasin-HP (OTC) *Crm:* 0.075% (1.5 oz); *Lotn:* 0.075% (2 oz)
Dolorac *Crm:* 0.025% (28 gm)
Double Cap (OTC) *Crm:* 0.05% (2 oz)
Qutenza *Patch:* 8% (1-2, both with 50 gm tube of cleansing gel)
R-Gel *Gel:* 0.025% (15, 30 gm)
Zostrix (OTC) *Crm:* 0.025% (0.7, 1.5, 3 oz)
Zostrix HP (OTC) *Emol crm:* 0.075% (1, 2 oz)

Comment: Provides some relief by 1-2 weeks; optimal benefit may take 4-6 weeks. Avoid contact with mucous membranes.

▶ ***doxepin*** cream **(B)** <12 years: not recommended; ≥12 years: apply to affected area qid at intervals of at least 3-4 hours; max 8 days
Prudoxin *Crm:* 5% (45 gm)
Zonalon *Crm:* 5% (30, 45 gm)

▶ ***pimecrolimus*** 1% cream (C) <2 years: not recommended; ≥2 years: apply to affected area bid; do not apply an occlusive dressing
Elidel *Crm:* 1% (30, 60, 100 gm)

Comment: ***pimecrolimus*** is indicated for short-term and intermittent long-term use. Discontinue use when resolution occurs. Contraindicated if the patient is immunosuppressed. Change to the 0.1% preparation or if secondary bacterial infection is present.

▶ ***tacrolimus*** (C) <2 years: not recommended; 2-15 years: use 0.03% strength; apply to affected area bid; continue for 1 week after clearing; >15 years: apply to affected area bid; do not occlude or apply to wet skin; continue for 1 week after clearing
Protopic *Oint:* 0.03, 0.1% (30, 60, 100 gm)

▶ ***trolamine salicylate*** <2 years: not recommended; ≥2 years: apply tid-qid prn to intact skin
Mobisyl *Crm:* 10%

Comment: Provides some relief by 1-2 weeks; optimal benefit

PSEUDOBULBAR AFFECT (PBA) DISORDER

Comment: Pseudobulbar affect (PBA), emotional lability, labile affect, or emotional incontinence refers by to a neurologic disorder characterized by involuntary crying or uncontrollable episodes of crying and/or laughing, or other emotional outbursts. PBA occurs secondary to a neurologic disease or brain injury such as traumatic brain injury (TBI), stroke, multiple sclerosis.

▶ ***dextromethorphan+quinidine*** **(C)(G)** <12 years: not recommended; ≥12 years: 1 cap once daily x 7 days; then starting on day 8, 1 cap bid
Nuedexta *Cap:* dextro 20 mg+quini 10 mg

Comment: ***dextromethorphan hydrobromide*** is an uncompetitive NMDA receptor antagonist and sigma-1 agonist. ***quinidine sulfate*** is a CYP450 2D6 inhibitor. **Nuedexta** is contraindicated with an MAOI or within 14 days of stopping an MAOI, with prolonged QT interval, congenital long QT syndrome, history suggestive of torsades de pointes, or heart failure, complete atrioventricular (AV) block without implanted pacemaker or patients at high risk of complete AV block, and concomitant drugs that both prolong QT interval and are metabolized by CYP2D6 (e.g., ***thioridazine*** or ***pimozide***). Discontinue **Nuedexta** if the following occurs: hepatitis or thrombocytopenia or any other hypersensitivity reaction. Monitor ECG in patients with left ventricular hypertrophy (LVH) or left ventricular dysfunction (LVD). ***desipramine*** exposure increases **Nuedexta** 8-fold; reduce ***desipramine*** dose and adjust based on clinical response. Use of **Nuedexta** with selective serotonin reuptake inhibitors (SSRIs) or tricyclic antidepressants (TCAs) increases the risk of serotonin syndrome. ***paroxetine*** exposure increases **Nuedexta** 2-fold; therefore, reduce **paroxetine** dose and adjust based on clinical response (***digoxin*** exposure may increase ***digoxin*** substrate plasma concentration. **Nuedexta** is not recommended in pregnancy or breastfeeding. Safety and effectiveness of **Nuedexta** in children have not been established. To report suspected adverse reactions, contact Avanir Pharmaceuticals at 1-866-388-5041 or FDA at 1-800-FDA-1088 or visit www.fda.gov/medwatch

PSEUDOGOUT

Injectable Acetaminophen *see **Pain** page* 322
NSAIDs *see page* 539
Other Oral Analgesics *see **Pain** page* 324
Topical & Transdermal NSAIDs *see **Pain** page* 323
Parenteral Corticosteroids *see page* 547
Oral Corticosteroids *see page* 546

PSEUDOMEMBRANOUS COLITIS

Comment: Staphylococcal enterocolitis and antibiotic-associated pseudomembranous colitis are caused by *C. difficile*.

ANTI-INFECTIVES

- ***metronidazole*** **(not for use in 1st; B in 2nd, 3rd)(G)** 500 mg tid x 14 days
  - **Flagyl** *Tab:* 250*, 500*mg
  - **Flagyl 375** *Cap:* 375 mg
  - **Flagyl ER** *Tab:* 750 mg ext-rel

  Comment: Alcohol is contraindicated during treatment with oral ***metronidazole*** and for 72 hours after therapy due to a possible ***disulfiram***-like reaction (nausea, vomiting, flushing, headache).
- ***vancomycin*** **(B, caps; C, susp)(G)** 40 mg/kg/day in 3-4 doses x 7-10 days; max 2 gm/day; ≥40 kg: 500 mg to 2 gm in 3-4 doses x 7-10 days; max 2 gm/day

GLYCOPEPTIDE ANTIBACTERIAL AGENT

Comment: **Firvanq** ***(vancomycin hcl oral solution)*** is a glycopeptide antibacterial agent FDA approved to treat *C. difficile*-associated diarrhea (CDAD) and entercolitis caused by *Staphylococcus aureus*, including methicillin-resistant strains (MRSA). **Firvanq** should be used only to treat or prevent infections that are proven or strongly suspected to be caused by susceptible bacteria. Orally administered ***vancomycin hcl*** is not effective for treatment of other types of infections. Prescribing **Firvanq** in the absence of a proven or strongly suspected bacterial infection is unlikely to provide benefit to the patient and increases the risk of the development of drug-resistant bacteria.

- ***vancomycin hcl oral solution*** see mfr pkg insert for preparation and important administration information; <18 years: *CDAD and Staphylococcal enterocolitis:* 40 mg/kg orally in 3 or 4 divided doses x 7-10 days; total daily dosage max 2 gm; ≥18 years: *CDAD* 125 mg orally 4 x/day x 10 days; *Staphylococcal enterocolitis:* 500 mg to 2 gm orally in 3 or 4 divided doses x 7-10 days
  - **Firvanq** *Kit w. pwdr for oral soln:* 25, 50 mg/ml (150, 300 ml) equivalent to 3.75, 7.5, 10.5, or 15 gm ***vancomycin hcl***, and grape-flavored diluent

Comment: Nephrotoxicity has occurred following oral ***vancomycin hcl*** therapy and can occur either during or after completion of therapy. The risk is increased in geriatric patients. Monitor renal function. Ototoxicity has occurred in patients receiving ***vancomycin hcl***. Assessment of auditory function may be appropriate in some instances. The most common adverse reactions (≥10%) have been nausea (17%), abdominal pain (15%) and hypokalemia (13%). There are no available data on **Firvanq** use in pregnant women to inform a drug associated risk of major birth defects or miscarriage. Available published data on ***vancomycin hcl*** use in pregnancy during the second and third trimesters have not shown an association with adverse pregnancy related outcomes. There are insufficient data to inform the levels of ***vancomycin hcl*** in human milk. However, systemic absorption of ***vancomycin hcl*** following oral administration is expected to be minimal. There are no data on the effects of **Firvanq** on the breastfed infant.

PSITTACOSIS

ANTI-INFECTIVES

▶ *tetracycline* (D)(G) <8 years: not recommended; ≥8 years, ≤100 lb: 25-50 mg/kg/day in 4 divided doses x 7-14 days; *see page* 618 *for dose by weight table* ; ≥8 years, >100 lb: 250 mg qid or 500 mg tid x 7-14 days

Achromycin V *Cap:* 250, 500 mg

Sumycin *Tab:* 250, 500 mg; *Cap:* 250, 500 mg; *Oral susp:* 125 mg/5 ml (100, 200 ml) (fruit) (sulfites)

Comment: ***tetracycline*** is contraindicated <8 years-of-age, in pregnancy, and lactation (discolors developing tooth enamel). A side effect may be photosensitivity (photophobia). Do not give with antacids or calcium supplements or within two hours of another drug.

PSORIASIS/PLAQUE PSORIASIS

Emollients *see* ***Dermatitis: Atopic*** *page* 112
Topical Corticosteroids *see page* 542

VITAMIN D-3 DERIVATIVES

▶ *calcipotriene* (C) <12 years: not recommended; ≥12 years: apply bid to lesions and gently rub in completely

Dovonex *Crm:* 0.005% (30, 120 gm)

VITAMIN D3 DERIVATIVE+CORTICOSTEROID COMBINATIONS

▶ *calcipotriene+betamethasone dipropionate* (C)(G)

Enstilar <18 years: not recommended; ≥18 years: apply to affected area and gently rub in once daily x up to 4 weeks; limit treatment area to 30% of body surface area; do not occlude; do not use on face, axillae, groin, or atrophic skin; max 100 gm/week

Foam: calci 0.005%+beta 0.064% (60 gm spray can)

Taclonex <18 years: not recommended; ≥18 years: apply to affected area and gently rub in once daily as needed, up to 4 weeks

Taclonex Ointment <18 years: not recommended; ≥18 years: apply bid to lesions and gently rub in completely; limit treatment area to 30% of body surface area; do not occlude; do not use on face, axillae, groin, or atrophic skin; max 100 gm/week

Oint: calci 0.005%+beta 0.064% (60, 100 gm)

Taclonex Scalp Topical Suspension <18 years: not recommended; ≥18 years: apply to affected area and gently rub in once daily x 2 weeks or until cleared; max 8 weeks; limit treatment area to 30% of body surface area; do not occlude; do not use on face, axillae, groin, or atrophic skin; max 100 gm/week

Bottle: 30, 60 gm; 120 gm (2 x 60 gm)

▶ ***Calcitriol*** **(C)** <18 years: not recommended; ≥18 years: apply bid to lesions and gently rub in completely; max weekly dose should not exceed 200 gm

Vectical *Oint:* 3 mcg/gm (100 gm)

IMMUNOSUPPRESSANTS

▶ ***alefacept*** **(B)** <12 years: not recommended; ≥12 years: 7.5 mg IV bolus or 15 mg IM once weekly x 12 weeks; may retreat x 12 weeks

Amevive *IV dose pack:* 7.5 mg single use (w. 10 ml sterile water diluents [use 0.6 ml]; 1, 4/pck); *IM dose pack:* 15 mg single use (w. 10 ml sterile water diluent [use 0.6 ml]; 1, 4/pck)

Comment: $CD4^+$ and T-lymphocyte count should be checked prior to initiating treatment with ***alefacept*** and then monitored. Treatment should be withheld if $CD4^+$ and T-lymphocyte counts are below 250 cells/mcl.

▶ ***cyclosporine*** (C) <18 years: not recommended; ≥18 years: 1.25 mg/kg bid; may increase after 4 weeks by 0.5 mg/kg/day; then adjust at 2-week intervals; max 4 mg/kg/day; administer with meals

Neoral *Cap:* 25, 100 mg (alcohol)

Neoral Oral Solution *Oral soln:* 100 mg/ml (50 ml) may dilute in room temperature apple juice or orange juice (alcohol)

ANTIMITOTICS

▶ ***anthralin*** (C) <12 years: not recommended; ≥12 years: apply once daily

Zithranol-RR *Crm:* 1.2% (15, 45 gm)

RETINOIDS

▶ ***acitretin*** (X)(G) <12 years: not recommended; ≥12 years: 25-50 mg once daily with main meal

Soriatane *Cap:* 10, 25 mg

▶ ***tazarotene*** (X)(G) <12 years: not recommended; ≥12 years: apply once daily at HS

Avage Cream *Crm:* 0.1% (30 gm)

Tazorac Cream *Crm:* 0.05, 0.1% (15, 30, 60 gm)

Tazorac Gel *Gel:* 0.05, 0.1% (30, 100 gm)

COAL TAR PREPARATIONS

▶ ***coal tar*** (C)(G)

Scytera (OTC) apply qd-qid; use lowest effective dose

Foam: 2%

T/Gel Shampoo Extra Strength (OTC) use every other day; max 4 x/week; massage into affected areas for 5 minutes; rinse; repeat

Shampoo: 1%

T/Gel Shampoo Original Formula (OTC) use every other day; max 7 x/week; massage into affected areas for 5 minutes; rinse; repeat

Shampoo: 0.5%

T/Gel Shampoo Stubborn Itch Control (OTC) use every other day; max 7 x/week; massage into affected areas for 5 minutes; rinse; repeat

Shampoo: 0.5%

INTERLEUKIN-17A ANTAGONIST

- ***brodalumab*** **(B)** inject SC into the upper arm, abdomen, or thigh; rotate sites; administer 210 mg SC (as two separate 150 mg SC injections) at weeks 0, 1, and 2; then 210 mg every 2 weeks
  Pediatric: <18 years: not recommended; ≥18 years: same as adult
  Siliq *Prefilled pen:* 210 mg/1.5 ml solution, single-use (2/carton) (preservative-free)

Comment: **Siliq** is currently indicated for plaque psoriasis only. **Siliq** is contraindicated with Crohn's disease. *Black Box Warning (BBW):* Suicidal ideation and behavior, including completed suicides, have occurred in patients treated with **Siliq.** Prior to prescribing, weigh potential risks and benefits in patients with a history of depression and/or suicidal ideation or behavior. Patients with new or worsening suicidal thoughts and behavior should be referred to a mental health professional, as appropriate. Advise patients and caregivers to seek medical attention for manifestations of suicidal ideation or behavior, new onset or worsening depression, anxiety, or other mood changes. Avoid using live vaccines concurrently with **Siliq** therapy. There are no human data on **Siliq** use in pregnant women to inform a drug associated risk. Human IgG antibodies are known to cross the placental barrier; therefore, **Siliq** may be transmitted from the mother to the developing fetus. There are no data on the presence of ***brodalumab*** in human milk or effects on the breastfed infant. **Siliq** is available only through the restricted **Siliq** REMS Program.

- ***secukinumab*** **(B)** <18 years: not recommended; ≥18 years: inject SC into the upper arm, abdomen, or thigh; rotate sites; administer 300 mg SC (as two separate 150 mg SC injections) at weeks 0, 1, 2, 3, and 4; then 300 mg every 4 weeks; for some patients, 150 mg/dose may be sufficient
  Cosentyx *Vial:* 150 mg/ml pwdr for SC inj after reconstitution single use (preservative-free)
  Comment: **Cosentyx** may be used as monotherapy or in combination with ***methotrexate*** (MTX). Avoid using live vaccines concurrently with **Siliq** therapy. For professional preparation and administration only.

HUMANIZED INTERLEUKIN-17A ANTAGONIST

- ***ixekizumab*** <18 years: not recommended; ≥18 years: recommended dose is 160 mg (2 x 80 mg injections) SC at Week 0, followed by 80 mg at weeks 2, 4, 6, 8, 10, and 12, then 80 mg SC every 4 weeks
  Taltz *Prefilled pen/Prefilled autoinjector:* 80 mg/ml (1 ml) single-dose
  Comment: Taltz injection the first and only treatment approved by the FDA for moderate-to-severe plaque psoriasis involving the genital area. This indication is based upon positive results from a randomized, double-blind, placebo-controlled study in moderate-to-severe psoriasis involving the genital area which involved 149 patients with plaque psoriasis who were candidates for phototherapy or systemic therapy but failed to respond to or were intolerant to at least 1 topical therapy. There are no available data on **Taltz** use in pregnancy to inform any drug associated risks. Human IgG is known to cross the placental barrier; therefore, **Taltz** may be transmitted from the mother to the developing fetus. There are no data on the presence of ***ixekizumab*** in human milk or effects on the breastfed infant.

INTERLEUKIN-23 ANTAGONIST

- ***tildrakizumab-asmn*** <18 years: not recommended; ≥18 years: inject SC; rotate sites; recommended dose is 100 mg at Weeks 0, 4, and every 12 weeks thereafter.
  Ilumya *Prefilled syringe:* 100 mg/ml (1 ml) single-use (preservative-free)

Comment: **Ilumya** is an interleukin-23 (IL-23) antagonist indicated for the treatment of adults with moderate-to-severe plaque psoriasis who are candidates for systemic therapy or phototherapy. **Ilumya** acts by selectively binding to the p19 subunit of IL-23 and inhibiting its interaction with the Il-23 receptor, blocking the release of pro-inflammatory cytokines and chemokines. Most common adverse reactions associated with **Ilumya** treatment are upper respiratory infections, injection site reactions, and diarrhea. Avoid use of live vaccines in patients treated with **Ilumya**. If a serious allergic reaction occurs, discontinue **Ilumya** immediately and initiate appropriate therapy. **Ilumya** may increase the risk of infection. Evaluate for TB prior to initiating treatment. Instruct patients to seek medical advice if signs or symptoms of clinically important chronic or acute infection occur. If a serious infection develops, consider discontinuing **Ilumya** until the infection resolves. Limited available data with **Ilumya** use in pregnant women are insufficient to inform a drug associated risk of adverse developmental outcomes. Human IgG is known to cross the placental barrier; therefore, **Ilumya** may be transferred from the mother to the fetus. There are no data on the presence of ***tildrakizumab-asmn*** in human milk or effects on the breastfed infant. To report suspected adverse reactions, contact Merck Sharp & Dohme, a subsidiary of Merck, at 1-877-888-4231 or FDA at 1-800-FDA-1088 or www.fda.gov/medwatch

INTERLEUKIN-12+INTERLEUKIN-23 ANTAGONIST

▶ ***ustekinumab*** **(B)** <18 years: not recommended; ≥18 years: inject SC; rotate sites; <100 kg: 45 mg once; then 4 weeks later; then every 12 weeks; ≥100 kg: 90 mg once; then 4 weeks later; then every 12 weeks

Stelara *Vial:* 45 mg/0.5 ml single use (preservative-free)

Comment: **Stelara** may be used as monotherapy or in combination with *methotrexate* (MTX).

TUMOR NECROSIS FACTOR (TNF) BLOCKERS

▶ ***adalimumab*** **(B)** <18 years: not recommended; ≥18 years: initially 80 mg SC once followed by 40 mg once every other week starting one week after initial dose; inject into thigh or abdomen; rotate sites

Humira *Prefilled syringe:* 20 mg/0.4 ml; 40 mg/0.8 ml single-dose (2/pck; 2, 6/ starter pck) (preservative-free)

▶ ***adalimumab-adbm*** **(B)** initially 80 SC; then, 40 mg SC every other week starting one week after initial dose; inject into thigh or abdomen; rotate sites

Pediatric: <18 years: not recommended; ≥18 years: same as adult

Cyltezo *Prefilled syringe:* 40 mg/0.8 ml single-dose (preservative-free)

Comment: **Cyltezo** is biosimilar to **Humira** (***adalimumab***).

▶ ***etanercept*** **(B)** <18 years: not recommended; ≥18 years: inject SC into thigh, abdomen, or upper arm; rotate sites; initially 50 mg twice weekly (3-4 days apart) for 3 months; then 50 mg/week maintenance or 25 mg or 50 mg per week for 3 months; then 50 mg/week maintenance

Enbrel *Vial:* 25 mg pwdr for SC injection after reconstitution (4/carton w. supplies) (preservative-free, diluent contains benzyl alcohol); *Prefilled syringe:* 50 mg/ml (preservative-free); *SureClick Autoinjector:* 25 mg/ml (preservative-free)

▶ ***golimumab*** **(B)** <18 years: not established; ≥18 years: administer SC or IV infusion (in combination with ***methotrexate*** *[MTX])*

Simponi 50 mg SC once monthly; rotate sites

Prefilled syringe, SmartJect Autoinjector: 50 mg/0.5 ml, single use (preservative-free)

Simponi Aria 2 mg/kg IV infusion week 0 and week 4; then every 8 weeks thereafter

Vial: 50 mg/4 ml, single-use, soln for IV infusion after dilution (latex-free, preservative-free)

▶ ***infliximab*** *(tumor necrosis factor-alpha blocker)* <18 years: not established; ≥18 years: 5 mg/kg at 0, 2 and 6 weeks, then every 8 weeks; must be refrigerated at 2°C to 8°C (36°F to 46°F); administer dose intravenously over a period of not less than 2 hours; do not use beyond the expiration date as this product contains no preservative

Remicade *Vial:* 100 mg for reconstitution to 10 ml administration volume, single-dose (preservative-free)

Comment: **Remicade** is indicated to reduce signs and symptoms, and induce and maintain clinical remission, in adults and children >6 years-of-age with moderately to severely active disease who have had an inadequate response to conventional therapy and reduce the number of draining enterocutaneous and rectovaginal fistulas, and maintain fistula closure, in adults with fistulizing disease. Common adverse effects associated with **Remicade** included abdominal pain, headache, pharyngitis, sinusitis, and upper respiratory infections. In addition, **Remicade** might increase the risk for serious infections, including tuberculosis, bacterial sepsis, and invasive fungal infections. Available data from published literature on the use of ***infliximab*** products during pregnancy have not reported a clear association with ***infliximab*** products and adverse pregnancy outcomes. ***infliximab*** products cross the placenta and infants exposed *in utero* should not be administered live vaccines for at least 6 months after birth. Otherwise, the infant may be at increased risk of infection, including disseminated infection which can become fatal. Available information is insufficient to inform the amount of ***infliximab*** products present in human milk or effects on the breastfed infant. To report suspected adverse reactions, contact Merck Sharp & Dohme Corp., a subsidiary of Merck & Co. at 1-877-888-4231 or FDA at 1-800-FDA-1088 or visit www.fda.gov/medwatch

▶ ***infliximab-abda*** *(tumor necrosis factor-alpha blocker)* **(B)**

Renflexis: see *infliximab* (**Remicade**) above for full prescribing information

Comment: **Renflexis** is a biosimilar to **Remicade** for the treatment of immune-disorders including Crohn's disease, ulcerative colitis, rheumatoid arthritis, ankylosing spondylitis, psoriatic arthritis and plaque psoriasis. **Renflexis** was approved under the FDA category for biosimilars and demonstrated no clinically meaningful differences for use, dosing regimens, strengths, dosage forms, and routes of administration from the FDA-approved biological product **Remicade.**

▶ ***infliximab-qbtx*** *(tumor necrosis factor-alpha blocker)* **(B)**

Ifixi: see ***infliximab*** (**Remicade**) above for full prescribing information

Comment: **Ifixi** is a biosimilar to **Remicade** for the treatment of immune disorders including Crohn's disease, ulcerative colitis, rheumatoid arthritis, ankylosing spondylitis, psoriatic arthritis and plaque psoriasis. **Ifixi** was approved under the FDA category for biosimilars and demonstrated no clinically meaningful differences for use, dosing regimens, strengths, dosage forms, and routes of administration from the FDA-approved biological product **Remicade.**

▶ ***infliximab-dyyb*** *(tumor necrosis factor-alpha blocker)* **(B)**

Inflectra: see ***infliximab*** (**Remicade**) above for full prescribing information

Comment: **Inflectra** is a biosimilar to **Remicade** for the treatment of immune-disorders including Crohn's disease, ulcerative colitis, rheumatoid arthritis, ankylosing spondylitis, psoriatic arthritis and plaque psoriasis. **Inflectra** was approved under the FDA category for biosimilars and demonstrated no clinically meaningful differences for use, dosing regimens, strengths, dosage forms, and routes of administration from the FDA-approved biological product **Remicade.**

Renflexis see ***infliximab*** (**Remicade**) above for full prescribing information

Comment: **Inflectra** is a biosimilar to **Remicade** for the treatment of immune-disorders including Crohn's disease, ulcerative colitis, rheumatoid arthritis, ankylosing spondylitis, psoriatic arthritis and plaque psoriasis. **Inflectra** was approved under the FDA category for biosimilars and demonstrated no clinically meaningful differences for use, dosing regimens, strengths, dosage forms, and routes of administration from the FDA-approved biological product **Remicade.**

MOISTURIZING AGENTS

Aquaphor Healing Ointment (OTC) *Oint:* (1.75, 3.5, 14 oz) (alcohol)
Eucerin Daily Sun Defense (OTC) *Lotn:* 6 oz (fragrance-free)
Comment: **Eucerin Daily Sun Defense** is a moisturizer with SPF 15.
Eucerin Facial Lotion (OTC) *Lotn:* 4 oz
Eucerin Light Lotion (OTC) *Lotn:* 8 oz
Eucerin Lotion (OTC) *Lotn:* 8, 16 oz
Eucerin Original Creme (OTC) *Crm:* 2, 4, 16 oz (alcohol)
Eucerin Plus Creme *Crm:* 4 oz
Eucerin Plus Lotion (OTC) *Lotn:* 6, 12 oz
Eucerin Protective Lotion (OTC) *Lotn:* 4 oz (alcohol)
Comment: **Eucerin Protective Lotion** is a moisturizer with SPF 25.
Lac-Hydrin Cream (OTC) *Crm:* 280, 385 gm
Lac-Hydrin Lotion (OTC) *Lotn:* 225, 400 gm
Lubriderm Dry Skin Scented (OTC) *Lotn:* 6, 10, 16, 32 oz
Lubriderm Dry Skin Unscented (OTC) *Lotn:* 3.3, 6, 10, 16 oz (fragrance-free)
Lubriderm Sensitive Skin Lotion (OTC) *Lotn:* 3.3, 6, 10, 16 oz (lanolin-free)
Lubriderm Dry Skin (OTC) *Lotn (scented):* 2.5, 6, 10, 16 oz; *Lotn (fragrance-free):* 1, 2.5, 6, 10, 16 oz
Lubriderm Bath *Oil:* 1-2 capfuls in bath or rub onto wet skin as needed; then rinse (8 oz)

PSORIATIC ARTHRITIS

Injectable Acetaminophen *see* ***Pain*** *page* 322
NSAIDs *see page* 539
Other Oral Analgesics *see* ***Pain*** *page* 324
Topical & Transdermal NSAIDs *see* ***Pain*** *page* 323
Parenteral Corticosteroids *see page* 547
Oral Corticosteroids *see page* 546

TOPICAL & TRANSDERMAL ANALGESICS

▶ ***capsaicin*** (B)(G) <2 years: not recommended; 2-12 years: apply sparingly to intact skin bid prn; >12 years: apply tid-qid prn

- **Axsain** *Crm:* 0.075% (1, 2 oz)
- **Capsin (OTC)** *Lotn:* 0.025, 0, 075% (59 ml)
- **Capzasin-P (OTC)** *Crm:* 0.025% (1.5 oz); *Lotn:* 0.025% (2 oz)
- **Capzasin-HP (OTC)** *Crm:* 0.075% (1.5 oz); *Lotn:* 0.075% (2 oz)
- **Dolorac** *Crm:* 0.025% (28 gm)
- **Double Cap (OTC)** *Crm:* 0.05% (2 oz)
- **Qutenza (B)** *Patch:* 8% (1-2, both with 50 gm tube of cleansing gel)
- **R-Gel** *Gel:* 0.025% (15, 30 gm)
- **Zostrix (OTC)** *Crm:* 0.025% (0.7, 1.5, 3 oz)
- **Zostrix HP (OTC)** *Emol crm:* 0.075% (1, 2 oz)

Comment: ***capsaicin*** provides some relief by 1-2 weeks; optimal benefit may take 4-6 weeks. Avoid contact with mucous membranes.

▶ ***diclofenac sodium*** **(C; D ≥30 wks)(G)**

Pennsaid 1.5% <12 years: not established; ≥12 years: in 10 drop increments, dispense and rub into front, side, and back of knee: usually; 40 drops (40 mg) qid

Topical soln: 1.5% (150 ml)

Pennsaid 2% <12 years: not established; ≥12 years: apply 2 pump actuations (40 mg) and rub into front, side, and back of knee bid

Topical soln: 2% (20 mg/pump actuation, 112 gm)

Comment: **Pennsaid** is indicated for the treatment of pain associated with osteoarthritis of the knee.

Solaraze Gel *Gel:* 3% (50 gm) (benzyl alcohol)

Comment: Contraindicated with ***aspirin*** allergy. As with other NSAIDs, **Solaraze Gel** should be avoided in late pregnancy (≥30 weeks) because it may cause premature closure of the ductus arteriosus.

Voltaren Gel (G) <12 years: not established; ≥12 years: apply sparingly and rub in

Gel: 1% (100 gm)

Comment: Contraindicated with ***aspirin*** allergy. As with other NSAIDs, **Voltaren Gel** should be avoided in late pregnancy (≥30 weeks) because it may cause premature closure of the ductus arteriosus.

▶ ***trolamine salicylate*** <2 years: not recommended; ≥2 years: apply tid-qid

Mobisyl *Crm:* 10%

Comment: Provides some relief by 1-2 weeks; optimal benefit may take 4-6 weeks.

ORAL SALICYLATE

▶ ***indomethacin*** (C) <14 years: usually not recommended; >2 years, if risk warranted: 1-2 mg/kg/day in divided doses; max 3-4 mg/kg/day <u>or</u> 150-200 mg/day, whichever is less; <14 years, ER cap not recommended; ≥14 years: initially 25 mg bid-tid, increase as needed at weekly intervals by 25-50 mg/day; max 200 mg/day

Cap: 25, 50 mg; *Susp;* 25 mg/5 ml (pineapple-coconut, mint) (alcohol 1%); *Supp:* 50 mg; *ER Cap:* 75 mg ext-rel

Comment: ***indomethacin*** is indicated only for acute painful flares. Administer with food <u>and/or</u> antacids. Use lowest effective dose for shortest duration.

ORAL NSAIDs

See more **Oral NSAIDs** page 539

▶ ***diclofenac sodium*** (C)

Voltaren <12 years: not established; ≥12 years: 50 mg bid-qid <u>or</u> 75 mg bid <u>or</u> 25 mg qid with an additional 25 mg at HS if necessary

Tab: 25, 50, 75 mg ent-coat

Voltaren XR <18 years: not established; ≥18 years: 100 mg once daily; rarely, 100 mg bid may be used

Tab: 100 mg ext-rel

NSAID+PPI

▶ ***esomeprazole+naproxen*** **(C; not for use in 3rd)(G)** <18 years: not recommended; ≥18 years: 1 tab bid; use lowest effective dose for the shortest duration; swallow whole; take at least 30 minutes before a meal

Vimovo *Tab:* nap 375 mg+eso 20 mg ext-rel; nap 500 mg+eso 20 mg ext-rel

Comment: **Vimovo** is indicated to improve signs/symptoms, and risk of gastric ulcer in patients at risk of developing NSAID-associated gastric ulcer.

COX-2 INHIBITORS

Comment: Cox-2 inhibitors are contraindicated with history of asthma, urticaria, and allergic-type reactions to ***aspirin***, other NSAIDs, and sulfonamides, 3rd trimester of pregnancy, and coronary artery bypass graft (CABG) surgery.

- ***celecoxib*** (C)(G) <18 years: not recommended; ≥18 years: 50-400 mg qd-bid; max 800 mg/day
  - **Celebrex** *Cap:* 50, 100, 200, 400 mg
- ***meloxicam*** (C)(G)
  - **Mobic** <2 years, <60 kg: not recommended; ≥2 years, >60 kg: 0.125 mg/kg; max 7.5 mg once daily; ≥18 years: initially 7.5 mg once daily; max 15 mg once daily; *Hemodialysis:* max 7.5 mg/day
    - *Tab:* 7.5, 15 mg; *Oral susp:* 7.5 mg/5 ml (100 ml) (raspberry)
  - **Vivlodex** <18 years: not established; ≥18 years: initially 5 mg qd; may increase to max 10 mg/day; *Hemodialysis:* max 5 mg/day
    - *Cap:* 5, 10 mg

PHOSPHODIESTERASE 4 (PDE4) INHIBITOR

- ***apremilast*** (C) <18 years: not established; ≥18 years: swallow whole; initial titration over 5 days; maintenance 30 mg bid; *Day 1:* 10 mg in AM; *Day 2:* 10 mg AM and 10 mg PM; *Day 3:* 10 mg AM and 20 mg PM; *Day 4:* 20 mg AM and 20 mg PM; *Day 5:* 20 mg AM and 30 mg PM; *Day 6 and ongoing:* 30 mg AM and 30 mg PM
  - **Otezla** *Tab:* 10, 20, 30 mg; *2-Week Starter Pack*

  Comment: Register pregnant patients exposed to by calling 1-877-311-8972.

INTERLEUKIN-12 + INTERLEUKIN-23 ANTAGONIST

- ***ustekinumab*** (B) <18 years: not established; ≥18 years: inject SC; rotate sites; <100 kg: 45 mg once; then 4 weeks later; then every 12 weeks; ≥100 kg: 90 mg once; then 4 weeks later; then every 12 weeks
  - **Stelara** *Vial:* 45 mg/0.5 ml single use (preservative-free)

    Comment: **Stelara** may be used as monotherapy or in combination with ***methotrexate*** (MTX).

TUMOR NECROSIS FACTOR (TNF) BLOCKERS

- ***adalimumab*** (B) <2 years, <10 kg: not recommended; 10-<15 kg: 10 mg every other week; 15-<30 kg: 20 mg every other week; ≥30-40 kg: 40 mg every other week; >40 kg 40 mg SC once every other week; may increase to once weekly without ***methotrexate*** (MTX); administer in abdomen or thigh; rotate sites; 2-17 years, supervise first dose
  - **Humira** *Prefilled syringe:* 20 mg/0.4 ml; 40 mg/0.8 ml single-dose (2/pck; 2, 6/starter pck) (preservative-free)

    Comment: **Humira** may use with ***methotrexate*** **(MTX)**, DMARDs, corticoids, salicylates, NSAIDs, or analgesics.
- ***adalimumab-adbm*** **(B)** initially 80 SC; then, 40 mg SC every other week starting one week after initial dose; inject into thigh or abdomen; rotate sites
  Pediatric: <18 years: not recommended; ≥18 years: same as adult
  - **Cyltezo** *Prefilled syringe:* 40 mg/0.8 ml single-dose (preservative-free)

    Comment: **Cyltezo** is biosimilar to **Humira** (***adalimumab***).
- ***etanercept*** **(B)** <4 years: not recommended; 4-17 years: 0.4 mg/kg SC twice weekly, 72-96 hours apart (max 25 mg/dose) or 0.8 mg/kg SC weekly (max 50 mg/dose); >17 years: 25 mg SC twice weekly, 72-96 hours apart or 50 mg SC weekly; rotate sites

Enbrel *Vial:* 25 mg pwdr for SC injection after reconstitution (4/carton w. supplies) (preservative-free; diluent contains benzyl alcohol); *Prefilled syringe:* 50 mg/ml (preservative-free); *SureClick Autoinjector:* 25 mg/ml (preservative-free)

Comment: ***etanercept*** reduces pain, morning stiffness, and swelling. May be administered in combination with ***methotrexate***. Live vaccines should not be administered concurrently. Do not administer with active infection.

▶ ***golimumab*** **(B)** <18 years: not established; ≥18 years: administer SC or IV infusion (in combination with ***methotrexate*** *[MTX]*)

Simponi 50 mg SC once monthly; rotate sites

Prefilled syringe, SmartJect Autoinjector: 50 mg/0.5 ml, single use (preservative-free)

Simponi Aria 2 mg/kg IV infusion week 0 and week 4; then every 8 weeks thereafter

Vial: 50 mg/4 ml, single-use, soln for IV infusion after dilution (latex-free, preservative-free)

Comment: Corticosteroids, non-biologic DMARDs, and/or NSAIDs may be continued during treatment with ***golimumab***.

▶ ***infliximab*** *(tumor necrosis factor-alpha blocker)* <18 years: not established; ≥18 years: 5 mg/kg at 0, 2 and 6 weeks, then every 8 weeks; must be refrigerated at 2°C to 8°C (36°F to 46°F); administer dose intravenously over a period of not less than 2 hours; do not use beyond the expiration date as this product contains no preservative

Remicade *Vial:* 100 mg for reconstitution to 10 ml administration volume, single-dose (preservative-free)

Comment: **Remicade** is indicated to reduce signs and symptoms, and induce and maintain clinical remission, in adults and children >6 years-of-age with moderately to severely active disease who have had an inadequate response to conventional therapy and reduce the number of draining enterocutaneous and rectovaginal fistulas, and maintain fistula closure, in adults with fistulizing disease. Common adverse effects associated with **Remicade** included abdominal pain, headache, pharyngitis, sinusitis, and upper respiratory infections. In addition, **Remicade** might increase the risk for serious infections, including tuberculosis, bacterial sepsis, and invasive fungal infections. Available data from published literature on the use of ***infliximab*** products during pregnancy have not reported a clear association with ***infliximab*** products and adverse pregnancy outcomes. ***infliximab*** products cross the placenta and infants exposed *in utero* should not be administered live vaccines for at least 6 months after birth. Otherwise, the infant may be at increased risk of infection, including disseminated infection which can become fatal. Available information is insufficient to inform the amount of ***infliximab*** products present in human milk or effects on the breastfed infant. To report suspected adverse reactions, contact Merck Sharp & Dohme Corp., a subsidiary of Merck & Co. at 1-877-888-4231 or FDA at 1-800-FDA1088 or visit www.fda.gov/medwatch

▶ ***infliximab-abda*** *(tumor necrosis factor-alpha blocker)* **(B)**

Renflexis: see *infliximab* (Remicade) above for full prescribing information

Comment: **Renflexis** is a biosimilar to **Remicade** for the treatment of immune-disorders including Crohn's disease, ulcerative colitis, rheumatoid arthritis, ankylosing spondylitis, psoriatic arthritis and plaque psoriasis. **Renflexis** was approved under the FDA category for biosimilars and demonstrated no clinically meaningful differences for use, dosing regimens, strengths, dosage forms, and routes of administration from the FDA-approved biological product **Remicade**.

▶ ***infliximab-dyyb*** *(tumor necrosis factor-alpha blocker)* **(B)**

Inflectra: see ***infliximab*** (**Remicade**) above for full prescribing information

Comment: **Inflectra** is a biosimilar to **Remicade** for the treatment of immune-disorders including Crohn's disease, ulcerative colitis, rheumatoid arthritis, ankylosing spondylitis, psoriatic arthritis and plaque psoriasis. **Inflectra** was approved under the FDA category for biosimilars and demonstrated no clinically meaningful differences for use, dosing regimens, strengths, dosage forms, and routes of administration from the FDA-approved biological product **Remicade**.

▶ ***infliximab-qbtx*** *(tumor necrosis factor-alpha blocker)* **(B)**

Ifixi: see ***infliximab*** **(Remicade)** above for full prescribing information

Comment: **Ifixi** is a biosimilar to **Remicade** for the treatment of immune disorders including Crohn's disease, ulcerative colitis, rheumatoid arthritis, ankylosing spondylitis, psoriatic arthritis and plaque psoriasis. **Ifixi** was approved under the FDA category for biosimilars and demonstrated no clinically meaningful differences for use, dosing regimens, strengths, dosage forms, and routes of administration from the FDA-approved biological product **Remicade.**

SELECTIVE COSTIMULATION MODULATOR

▶ ***abatacept*** (C) <6 years: not recommended; >6 years: administer as an IV infusion over 30 minutes at weeks 0, 2, and 4; then every 4 weeks thereafter; <60 kg, administer 500 mg/dose; 60-100 kg, administer 750 mg/dose; >100 kg, administer 1 gm/dose

Orencia *Vial:* 250 mg pwdr for IV infusion after reconstitution (silicone-free) (preservative-free); *Prefilled syringe:* 125 mg/ml soln for SC injection (preservative-free); *ClickJect Autoinjector:* 125 mg/ml soln for SC injection

CD20 ANTIBODY

▶ ***rituximab*** (C) <6 years: not recommended; ≥6 years: administer corticosteroid 30 minutes prior to each infusion; concomitant ***methotrexate*** therapy, administer a 1,000 mg IV infusion at 0 and 2 weeks; then every 24 weeks or based on response, but not sooner than every 16 weeks.

Rituxan *Vial:* 10 mg/ml (10, 50 ml) (preservative-free)

Comment: ***rituximab*** is a B-cell targeting chimeric monoclonal antibody that acts against CD20 and reduces antibody titers. B-cell depletion by ***rituximab*** may also set the stage for production of interleukin 10–secreting B cells that do not interact with T cells, which further reduces production of antidesmoglein antibodies. ***rituximab*** carries a black box warning regarding fatal infusion reactions, severe mucocutaneous reactions, hepatitis B virus reactivation, and progressive multifocal leukoencephalopathy. However, serious adverse events are rare. There was no evidence of increased mortality with longer exposure to **rituximab** or to multiple courses of therapy.

JANICE KINASE (JAK) INHIBITOR (JAKI)

▶ ***tofacitinib*** (C) <18 years: not established; ≥18 years: 10 mg bid for at least 8 weeks; then 5 or 10 mg bid; discontinue after 16 weeks of 10 mg bid, if adequate therapeutic benefit is not achieved; use the lowest effective dose to maintain response; see mfr pkg insert for dosage adjustments for patients receiving CYP2C19 and/or CYP3A4 inhibitors; in patients with moderate or severe renal impairment or moderate hepatic impairment, and patients with lymphopenia, neutropenia, or anemia; use of **Xeljanz/ Xeljanz XR** in patients with severe hepatic impairment is not recommended in any patient population

Xeljanz *Tab:* 5, 10 mg

Xeljanz XR *Tab:* 11 mg ext-rel

Comment: ***Xeljanz*** is indicated for moderate-to-severe psoriatic arthritis as monotherapy in patients who have inadequate response or intolerance to ***methotrexate*** (MTX). Use of **Xeljanz** in combination with biological DMARDs or potent immunosuppressants, such as ***azathioprine*** and ***cyclosporine***, is not recommended. Avoid use of **Xeljanz/Xeljanz XR** during an active serious infection, including localized infection. Use with caution in patients that may be at increased risk for gastrointestinal perforation. The most common adverse events associated with Xeljanz treatment are diarrhea, elevated cholesterol level, headache, herpes zoster (shingles), increased blood creatine phosphokinase,nasopharyngitis, rash, and upper respiratory tract infection (URI). Patients treated with **Xeljanz** are at increased risk for developing serious infections that may lead to hospitalization or death. **Xeljanz** has a BBW for serious infections (e.g., opportunistic infections), and malignancy (e.g., lymphoma). Avoid live vaccines administration during treatment with **Xeljanz**. Prior to starting **Xeljanz**, perform a test for latent tuberculosis; if it is positive, start treatment for tuberculosis prior to starting **Xeljanz**. Monitor all patients for active tuberculosis during treatment, even if the initial latent tuberculosis test is negative. Recommend lab monitoring due to potential for changes in lymphocytes, neutronphils, hemoglobin, liver enzymes, and lipids. Do not initiate **Xeljanz** if absolute lymphocyte count <500 cells/mm3, an absolute neutrophil count (ANC) <1000 cells/mm3 or Hgb <9 g/dL. The safety and effectiveness of **Xeljanz/Xeljanz XR** in pediatric patients have not been established. Available data with **Xeljanz** use in pregnancy are insufficient to establish a drug associated risk of major birth defects, miscarriage, adverse maternal or fetal outcomes. In animal reproduction studies, fetocidal, and teratogenic effects were noted. There is a pregnancy exposure registry that monitors pregnancy outcomes in females exposed to **Xeljanz/Xeljanz XR** during pregnancy. Consider pregnancy planning and prevention for females of reproductive potential. Patients should be encouraged to enroll in the **Xeljanz/Xeljanz XR** pregnancy registry if they become pregnant. To enroll or obtain information from the registry, patients can call the toll free number 1-877-311-8972. There are no data on the presence of ***tofacitinib*** in human milk or the effects on a breastfed infant; however, patients should be advised not to breastfeed. To report suspected adverse reactions, contact Pfizer at 1-800-438-1985 or FDA at 1-800-FDA-1088 or visit www.fda.gov/medwatch

PULMONARY ARTERIAL HYPERTENSION (PAH) (WHO GROUP I)

ENDOTHELIAL RECEPTOR ANTAGONIST (ERA)

▶ ***bosentan (G)*** <3 years: not established; 3-12: initiate at 62.5 mg orally twice daily; for patients weighing > 40 kg, increase to 125 mg orally twice daily after 4 weeks; >12 years: initiate at 62.5 mg orally twice daily; for patients weighing greater than 40 kg, increase to 125 mg orally twice daily after 4 weeks

Tracleer *Tab:* 62.5, 125 mg film-coat; *Tab for oral suspension:* 32 mg

Comment: ***bosentan*** is an endothelin receptor antagonist (ERA) indicated for the treatment of pulmonary arterial hypertension (PAH) (WHO Group 1). **Tracleer** is the first ERA indicated for the treatment of PAH in patients aged 3 years and older with idiopathic or congenital PAH to improve pulmonary vascular resistance (PVR), which is expected to result in an improvement in exercise ability. The most common adverse events associated with **Tracleer** in clinical trials include respiratory tract infections, headache, edema, chest pain, syncope, flushing, hypotension, sinusitis, arthralgia, abnormal serum aminotransferases, palpitations, and anemia. Monitor hemoglobin levels after 1 and 3 months of treatment, then every 3 months thereafter. If signs of pulmonary edema occur, consider the diagnosis of associated pulmonary veno-occlusive disease (PVOD) and consider discontinuing **Tracleer**. Measure liver aminotransferases prior to initiation of treatment and then monthly. Reduce the dose and closely monitor patients developing aminotransferase elevations >3 x ULN. Co-administration of **Tracleer** with drugs metabolized by CYP2C9 and CYP3A can increase exposure to **Tracleer** and/or the co-administered drug. **Tracleer** use decreases contraceptive exposure and reduces effectiveness. There are no data on the presence of ***bosentan*** in human milk or the effects on the breastfed infant. However, because of the potential for serious adverse reactions, such as fluid retention and hepatotoxicity in breastfed infants, advise women not to breastfeed during treatment with **Tracleer** and pregnancy is contraindicated while taking **Tracleer**. To prevent pregnancy, females of reproductive potential must use two reliable forms of contraception during treatment and for one month after stopping **Tracleer** Due to the risks of hepatotoxicity and birth defects, **Tracleer** includes a boxed warning and is only available through the restricted **Tracleer** Risk Evaluation and Mitigation Strategy REMS Program, a restricted distribution program. Patients, prescribers, and pharmacies must enroll in the program to receive and administer **Tracleer**: http://www.tracleerrems.com/prescribers.aspx. To report adverse side effects, pregnancy, or other complications contact Actelion at 1-866-228-3546 or call 1-800-FDA-1088 or visit www.fda.gov/medwatch

PROSTACYCLIN RECEPTOR AGONIST

▶ ***selexipag*** (X) <12 years: not established; ≥12 years: initially 200 mcg bid; increase by 200 mcg bid to highest tolerated dose up to 1600 mcg bid; *Moderate hepatic impairment (Child-Pugh Class B):* initially 200 mcg once daily; increase by 200 mcg once daily at weekly intervals as tolerated; swallow whole; may take with food to improve tolerability

Uptravi

Tab: 200, 400, 600, 800, 1000, 1200, 1400, 1600 mcg; *Titration pck:* 140 x 200 mcg/60 x 800 mcg)

Comment: Discontinue **Uptravi** if pulmonary veno-occlusive disease is confirmed or severe hepatic impairment (Child-Pugh Class C). May be potentiated by concomitant strong CYP2C8 inhibitors (e.g., gemfibrozil); *Nursing mothers:* not recommended. Discontinue breastfeeding or discontinue the drug.

GUANYLATE CYCLASE STIMULATOR

Endothelin Receptor Antagonist, Selective for the Endothelin Type-A (ETA) Receptor

▶ ***ambrisentan*** (X) <12 years: not established; ≥12 years: 20 mg once daily; at 4-week intervals, either the dose of **Letairis** initially 5 mg once daily, with or without or ***tadalafil*** can be increased, as needed and tolerated, to **Letairis** 10 mg or ***tadalafil*** 40 mg; do not split, crush, or chew.

Letairis *Tab:* 5, 10 mg film-coat

Comment: In patients with PAH, plasma ET-1 concentrations are increased as much as 10-fold and correlate with increased mean right atrial pressure and disease severity. ET-1 and ET-1 mRNA concentrations are increased as much as 9-fold in the lung tissue of patients with PAH, primarily in the endothelium of pulmonary arteries. These findings suggest that ET-1 may play a critical role in the pathogenesis and progression of PAH. When taken with ***tadalafil***, **Letairis** is indicated to reduce the risk of disease progression and hospitalization, to reduce the risk of hospitalization due to worsening PAH, and to improve exercise tolerance. **Letairis** is contraindicated in idiopathic pulmonary fibrosis (IPF). Exclude pregnancy before the initiation of treatment with **Letairis.** Females of reproductive potential must use acceptable methods of contraception during treatment with **Letairis** and for one month after treatment. Obtain monthly pregnancy tests during treatment and 1 month after discontinuation of treatment. Females can only receive **Letairis** through the **Letairis** Risk Evaluation and Mitigation Strategy (REMS) Program, a restricted distribution program, because of the risk of embryo-fetal toxicity: www. Letairisrems.com or 1-866-664-5327.

➢ ***riociguat*** **(X)** <12 years: not recommended; ≥12 years: initially 0.5-1 mg tid; titrate every 2 weeks as tolerated (SBP ≥95 and absence of hypotensive symptoms) to highest tolerated dose; max 2.5 mg tid

Adempas *Tab:* 0.5, 1, 1.5, 2, 2.5 mg

Comment: If **Adempas** is interrupted for ≥3 days, re-titrate. Consider titrating to dosage higher than 2.5 mg tid, if tolerated, in patients who smoke. Consider a starting dose of 0.5 mg tid when initiating **Adempas** in patients receiving strong cytochrome P450 (CYP) and P-glycoprotein/breast cancer resistance protein (P-gp/BCRP) inhibitors such as azole antimycotics (e.g., ***ketoconazole***, ***itraconazole***) or HIV protease inhibitors (e.g., ***ritonavir***). Monitor for signs and symptoms of hypotension with strong CYP and P-gp/BCRP inhibitors. Obtain pregnancy tests prior to initiation and monthly during treatment. **Adempas** has consistently shown to have teratogenic effects when administered to animals. Females can only receive **Adempas** through the Adempas Risk Evaluation and Mitigation Strategy (REMS) Program, a restricted distribution program: **www.AdempasREMS.com** or **855-4 ADEMPAS**. It is not known if **Adempas** is present in human milk; however, ***riociguat*** or its metabolites were present in the milk of rats. Because of the potential for serious adverse reactions in nursing infants from ***riociguat***, discontinue nursing or **Adempas**. In placebo-controlled clinical trials, serious bleeding has occurred (including hemoptysis, hematemesis, vaginal hemorrhage, catheter site hemorrhage, subdural hematoma, and intra-abdominal hemorrhage. Safety and efficacy have not been demonstrated in patients with creatinine clearance <15 mL/min or on dialysis or severe hepatic impairment (Child-Pugh Class C).

Endothelin Receptor Antagonist, Selective for the Endothelin Type-A (ETA) Receptor

PHOSPHODIESTERASE TYPE 5 (PDE5) INHIBITORS, CGMP-SPECIFIC DRUGS

➢ ***sildenafil citrate*** **(B)(G)** <12 years: not established; ≥12 years: *Orally*: initially 5 or 20 mg tid, 4-6 hours apart; max 20 mg tid; *IV bolus:* 2.5 mg or 10 mg bolus injection tid, 4-6 hours apart; max 10 mg tid; the dose does not need to be adjusted for body weight.

Revatio *Tab:* 20 mg film-coat; *Oral susp:* 10 mg/ml pwdr for reconstitution (1.12 gm, 112 ml) (grape) (sorbitol); *Vial:* 10 mg/12.5 ml (0.8 mg/ml)

Comment: A 10 mg IV dose is predicted to provide pharmacological effect equivalent to the 20 mg oral dose. **Revatio** is contraindicated with concomitant nitrate drugs including ***nitroglycerin***, ***isosorbide dinitrate***, isosorbide mononitrate, and some recreational drugs such as "poppers." Taking **Revatio** with a nitrate can cause a sudden and serious decrease in blood pressure. **Revatio** is contraindicated with concomitant guanylate cyclase stimulator drugs such as ***riociguat*** **(Adempas)**. Avoid the use of grapefruit products while taking **Revatio**. Stop **Revatio** and get emergency medical help if sudden vision loss. **Revatio** is contraindicated with other phosphodiesterase type 5 (PDE5) Inhibitors, cGMP-specific drugs such as ***avanafil*** **(Stendra)**, ***tadalafil*** **(Cialis)**, or ***vardenafil*** **(Levitra)**. Caution with history of recent MI, stroke, life-threatening arrhythmia, hypotension, hypertension, cardiac failure, unstable angina, retinitis pigmentosa, CYP3A4 inhibitors (e.g., ***cimetidine***, the azoles, ***erythromycin***, protease inhibitors (e.g., ***ritonavir***), CYP3A4 inducers (e.g., ***rifampin***, ***carbamazepine***, ***phenytoin***, ***phenobarbital***), alcohol, and antihypertensive agents. Side effects include headache, flushing, nasal congestion, rhinitis, dyspepsia, and diarrhea. Use **Revatio** with caution in patients with anatomical deformation of the penis (e.g., angulation, cavernosal fibrosis, or

Peyronie's disease) or in patients who have conditions, which may predispose them to priapism (e.g., sickle cell anemia, multiple myeloma, or leukemia). In the event of an erection that persists longer than 4 hours, the patient should seek immediate medical assistance. If priapism (painful erection greater than 6 hours in duration) is not treated immediately, penile tissue damage and permanent loss of potency could result.

- ***tadalafil*** **(B)(G)** <12 years: not established; ≥12 years: 40 mg once daily; *CrCl 31-80 mL/min:* initially 20 mg once daily; increase to 40 mg once daily if tolerated; *CrCl <30 mL/min:* not recommended; *Mild or moderate hepatic cirrhosis (Child-Pugh Class A or B):* initially 20 mg once daily; *Severe hepatic cirrhosis (Child-Pugh Class C):* not recommended; *use with* ***ritonavir****; Receiving* ***ritonavir*** *for at least 1 week:* initiate ***tadalafil*** at 20 mg once daily; may increase to 40 mg once daily if tolerated; *Already on* ***tadalafil****:* stop ***tadalafil*** at least 24 hours prior to initiating ***ritonavir***; resume ***tadalafil*** at 20 mg once daily after at least 1 week; may increase to 40 mg once daily if tolerated

    Adcirca *Tab:* 20 mg

  Comment: Contraindicated with concomitant organic nitrates and guanylate cyclase stimulators (e.g., ***riociguat***).

- ***treprostinil*** **(B)** <12 years: not established; ≥12 years: swallow whole; take with food

    Orenitram *Tab:* 0.125, 0.25, 1, 2.5 mg ext-rel

    Comment: **Orenitram** is indicated to improve exercise capacity. It is contraindicated with severe hepatic impairment (Child-Pugh Class C). **Orenitram** inhibits platelet aggregation and increases the risk of bleeding. Concomitant administration of **Orenitram** with diuretics, antihypertensive agents, or other vasodilators increases the risk of symptomatic hypotension.

PYELONEPHRITIS: ACUTE

URINARY TRACT ANALGESIA

- ***phenazopyridine*** **(B)(G)** <12 years: not recommended; ≥12 years: 95-200 mg q 6 hours prn; max 2 days

    AZO Standard, Prodium, Uristat (OTC) *Tab:* 95 mg

    AZO Standard Maximum Strength (OTC) *Tab:* 97.5 mg

    Pyridium *Tab:* 100, 200 mg

    Urogesic *Tab:* 100, 200 mg

OUTPATIENT ANTI-INFECTIVE TREATMENT

Comment: Acute pyelonephritis can be treated with a single IM antibiotic administration followed by a PO antibiotic regimen and close follow up. Example: **Rocephin** 1 gm IM followed by **Bactrim DS**, ***cephalexin***, ***ciprofloxacin***, ***levofloxacin***, or ***loracarbef***.

- ***cephalexin*** **(B)(G)** 25-50 mg/kg/day in 4 divided doses x 10-14 days; *see page 601 for dose by weight table;* 1-4 gm/day in 4 divided doses x 10-14 days

    Keflex *Cap:* 250, 333, 500, 750 mg; *Oral susp:* 125, 250 mg/5 ml (100, 200 ml) (strawberry)

- ***ciprofloxacin*** **(C)** <18 years: not recommended; ≥18 years: 500 mg bid or 1000 mg XR once daily x 3-14 days; max 1.5 gm/day

    Cipro (G) *Tab:* 250, 500, 750 mg; *Oral susp:* 250, 500 mg/5 ml (100 ml) (strawberry)

    Cipro XR *Tab:* 500, 1000 mg ext-rel

    ProQuin XR *Tab:* 500 mg ext-rel

  Comment: ***ciprofloxacin*** is contraindicated <18 years-of-age, and during pregnancy and lactation. Risk of tendonitis or tendon rupture.

- ➢ ***levofloxacin*** **(C)** <18 years: not recommended; ≥18 years: *Uncomplicated:* 500 mg once daily x 10 days; *Complicated:* 750 mg once daily x 10 days
  - **Levaquin** *Tab:* 250, 500, 750 mg; *Oral soln:* 25 mg/ml (480 ml) (benzyl alcohol); *Inj conc:* 25 mg/ml for IV infusion after dilution for IV infusion (50, 100, 150 ml) (preservative-free)

  Comment: ***levofloxacin*** is contraindicated <18 years-of-age, and during pregnancy and lactation. Risk of tendonitis or tendon rupture.
- ➢ ***loracarbef*** **(B)** <12 years: 15 mg/kg/day in 2 divided doses x 10 days; *see page 614 for dose by weight table*; ≥12 years: 200 mg bid x 10 days
  - **Lorabid** *Pulvule:* 200, 400 mg; *Oral susp:* 100 mg/5 ml (50, 100 ml); 200 mg/5 ml (50, 75, 100 ml) (strawberry bubble gum)
- ➢ ***trimethoprim+sulfamethoxazole [TMP-SMX]*** **(D)(G)**
  - **Bactrim, Septra** <12 years: not recommended; ≥12 years: 2 tabs bid x 10 days
    - *Tab:* trim 80 mg+sulfa 400 mg*
  - **Bactrim DS, Septra DS** <12 years: not recommended; ≥12 years: 1 tab bid x 10 days
    - *Tab:* trim 160 mg+sulfa 800 mg*
  - **Bactrim Pediatric Suspension, Septra Pediatric Suspension** <2 months: not recommended; ≥2 months-12 years: 40 mg/kg/day of ***sulfamethoxazole*** in 2 doses bid; >12 years: use tabs
    - *Oral susp:* trim 40 mg+sulfa 200 mg per 5 ml (100 ml) (cherry) (alcohol 0.3%)

RABIES (*LYSSAVIRUS*)

PRE-EXPOSURE PROPHYLAXIS (PREP) & POST-EXPOSURE PROPHYLAXIS (PEP)

Comment: Have ***epinephrine*** **1:1000** readily available. Every exposure to possible rabies infection must be individually evaluated. Rabies vaccine and Rabies Immune Globulin (Human) (HRIG) should be given to all persons suspected of exposure to rabies with one exception: persons who have been previously immunized with rabies vaccine and have a confirmed adequate rabies antibody titer should receive only vaccine. Recommendations for use of passive and active immunization after exposure to an animal suspected of having rabies have been detailed by the Health Canada National Advisory Committee on Immunization19 and the U.S. Public Health Service Immunization Practices Advisory Committee (ACIP). HRIG should be used in conjunction with rabies vaccine and can be administered through the seventh day after the first dose of vaccine is administered. Beyond the seventh day, HRIG is not indicated since an antibody response to cell culture vaccine is presumed to have occurred. If the patient has previously received HRIG, and has a confirmed adequate rabies antibody titer, administer only the vaccine. HRIG should be administered as promptly as possible after exposure, but can be administered up to the eighth day after the first dose of vaccine is administered. Repeated doses of rabies immune globulin should not be administered once vaccine treatment has been initiated as this could prevent the full expression of active immunity expected from the rabies vaccine. Administer HRIG via IM injection only. Do not give intravenously. The recommended HRIG dose 20 IU/kg (0.133 mL/kg) of body weight administered at the time of the first vaccine dose. It may also be given through the seventh day after the first dose of vaccine is given. If anatomically feasible, up to one-half the HRIG dose should be thoroughly infiltrated in the area around the wound and the rest should be administered intramuscularly in the gluteal area or lateral thigh muscle using a separate syringe and needle. Because of risk of injury to the sciatic nerve, only the upper, outer quadrant should be used. HRIG should never be administered in the same syringe or needle or in the same anatomical site as vaccine. Because of interference with active antibody production, the recommended dose should not be exceeded. It is not known whether rabies immune globulin can cause fetal harm when administered to a pregnant female or can affect reproduction capacity. It should be administered in pregnancy only if clearly needed. Safety and effectiveness in the pediatric population have not been established.

RABIES IMMUNE GLOBULIN, HUMAN (HRIG)

▶ ***rabies immune globulin, human (HRIG)*** (C) administer 20 IU/kg infiltrated into wound area as much as feasible, then remaining dose administered IM at site remote from vaccine administration

BayRab, KamRAB, Imogam Rabies HT *Vial:* 150 IU/ml (2, 10 ml)

Comment: Administer ***rabies immune globulin, human (HRIG)*** concurrently with a full course of rabies vaccine if the patient have not previously received the rabies vaccine and has confirmed adequate antibodies, administer only the vaccine.

HyperRAB S/D *Vial:* 300 IU/2 ml (2 ml); 1500 IU/10 ml (10 ml), single-dose

Comment: **HyperRAB** is a high-potency rabies immunoglobulin.

RABIES PROPHYLAXIS VACCINE

▶ ***rabies vaccine, human diploid cell [HDVC]*** (C) *Infants and Young Children:* administer IM in the vastus lateralis; *All others:* administer IM in the deltoid; do not inject the vaccine into the gluteal area as administration in this area may result in lower neutralizing antibody titers; *Not previously immunized: Day 0,* administer 1 ml IM as soon as possible after exposure; then repeat on days 7, and 21 or 28; administer 1st dose with rabies immune globulin, human (HRIG); *Previously immunized:* only 2 doses are administered; Day 0, Administer 1 ml IM immediately after exposure and again 3 days later; no HRIG is needed

Imovax, RabAvert *Vial:* 2.5 IU/ml (1 ml) (2.5 IU of freeze-dried vaccine w. diluent) for IM injection after reconstitution (preservative-free)

Comment: Administer vaccine immediately after reconstitution. If not used, discard. It is also not known whether rabies vaccine can cause fetal harm when administered to a pregnant female or can affect reproductive capacity. Rabies vaccine 10 should be given to a pregnant woman only if potential benefits outweigh potential risks. All serious systemic neuroparalytic or anaphylactic reactions to a rabies vaccine should be immediately reported to VAERS at 1-800-822-7967 (http://vaers.hhs.gov) or Sanofi Pasteur at 1-800-VACCINE (1-800-822-2463).

TETANUS PROPHYLAXIS VACCINE

See ***Tetanus*** *page* 445 for patients not within the previous 5 years.

RESPIRATORY SYNCYTIAL VIRUS (RSV)

PROPHYLAXIS

▶ ***palivizumab*** 15 mg/kg IM administered monthly throughout the RSV season

Synagis *Vial:* 100 mg/ml

TREATMENT

See ***Bronchiolitis*** *page* 55

RESTLESS LEGS SYNDROME (RLS)

GAMMA AMINOBUTYRIC ACID ANALOGS

▶ ***gabapentin*** (C)(G) <16 years: not recommended: ≥16 years: 100 mg once daily x 1 day; then 100 mg bid x 1 day; then 100 mg tid thereafter; max 900 mg tid

Gralise (C) initially 300 mg on Day 1; then 600 mg on Day 2; then 900 mg on Days 3-6; then 1200 mg on Days 7-10; then 1500 mg on Days 11-14; titrate up to 1800 mg on Day 15; take entire dose once daily with the evening meal; do not crush, split, or chew

Tab: 300, 600 mg

Neurontin (G) <3 years: not recommended; 3-12 years: initially 10-15 mg/kg/day in 3 divided doses; max 12 hours between doses; titrate over 3 days; 3-4 years: titrate to 40 mg/kg/day; 5-12 years: titrate to 25-35 mg/kg/day; max 50 mg/kg/day; >12 years: 100 mg daily x 1 day, then 100 mg bid x 1 day, then 100 mg tid continuously; max 900 mg tid

▷ ***gabapentin enacarbil*** (C) <16 years: not recommended: ≥16 years: 600 mg once daily at about 5:00 PM; if dose not taken at recommended time, next dose should be taken the following day; swallow whole; take with food; *CrCl 30-59 mL/min:* 600 mg on Day 1, Day 3, and every day thereafter; *CrCl <30 mL/min* or on hemodialysis: not recommended

Horizant *Tab:* 600 ext-rel

Comment: Avoid abrupt cessation of ***gabapentin*** and ***gabapentin enacarbil***. To discontinue, withdraw gradually over 1 week or longer.

DOPAMINE RECEPTOR AGONISTS

▷ ***pramipexole dihydrochloride*** (C)(G) <18 years: not recommended; ≥18 years: initially 0.125 mg once daily 2-3 hours before bedtime; may double dose every 4-7 days; max 0.75 mg/day

Mirapex *Tab:* 0.125, 0.25*, 0.5*, 0.75*, 1*, 1.5*mg

▷ ***ropinirole*** (C) <18 years: not recommended; ≥18 years: take once daily 1-3 hours prior to bedtime; initially 0.25 mg on days 1 and 2; then 0.5 mg on days 3-7; increase by 0.5 mg/day at 1 week intervals to 3 mg; max 4 mg/day

Requip *Tab:* 0.25, 0.5, 1, 2, 3, 4, 5 mg

▷ ***rotigotine*** transdermal patch (C) <12 years: not recommended; ≥12 years: apply to clean, dry, intact skin on abdomen, thigh, hip, flank, shoulder, or upper arm; initially 1mg/24Hrs patch once daily; may increase weekly by 1mg/24Hrs if needed; max 3mg/24Hrs once daily; rotate sites and allow 14 days before reusing site; if hairy, shave site at least 3 days before application to site; avoid abrupt cessation; reduce by 1 mg/24Hrs every other day

Neupro Transdermal Patch *Trans patch:* 1mg/24Hrs, 2mg/24Hrs, 3mg/24Hrs, 4mg/24Hrs, 6mg/24Hrs, 8mg/24Hrs (30/carton) (sulfites)

RETINITIS: CYTOMEGALOVIRUS (CMV)

Comment: ***cidofovir*** *and* ***valganciclovir*** are nucleoside analogs and prodrugs of ***ganciclovir*** indicated for the treatment of AIDS-related *cytomegalovirus* (CMV) retinitis and prevention of CMV disease in patients ≥18 years with kidney, heart, and kidney-pancreas transplant patients at high risk, and for prevention of CMV disease in pediatric kidney and heart transplant patients at high risk.

▷ ***cidofovir*** (C) <12 years: not recommended; ≥12 years: administer via IV infusion over 1 hour; pretreat with oral ***probenecid*** (2 gm, 3 hours prior to starting the ***cidofovir*** infusion and 1 gm, 2 and 8 hours after the infusion is ended) and 1 liter of IV NaCl should be infused immediately before each dose of ***cidofovir*** (a 2nd liter of NaCl should also be infused either during or after each dose of ***cidofovir*** if a fluid load is tolerable); *Induction:* 5 mg/kg once weekly for 2 consecutive weeks; *Maintenance:* 5 mg/kg once every 2 weeks; reduce to 3 mg/kg if serum creatinine (sCr) increases 0.3-0.4 mg/dL above baseline; discontinue if sCr increases to >0.5 mg/dL above baseline or if >3/ proteinuria develops

Vistide *Vial:* 75 mg/ml (5 ml) (preservative-free)

Comment: ***cidofovir*** is a nucleoside analog indicated for treatment of AIDS-related cytomegalovirus (CMV) retinitis.

▶ ***valganciclovir*** **(C)(G)** take with food; <4 months: not recommended; 4 months-16 years: see mfr pkg insert for dosing calculation equation; >16 years: *Induction:* 900 mg bid x 21 days; *Maintenance:* 900 mg daily; *CrCl <60 mL/min:* reduce dose (see mfr pkg insert; hemodialysis or *CrCl <10 mL/min* not recommended (use ***ganciclovir***)

Valcyte *Tab:* 450 mg (preservative-free); *Oral pwdr for reconstitution:* 50 mg/ml (tutti-frutti)

CMV DNA TERMINASE VOMPLRX INHIBITOR

Comment: ***letermovir*** is a CMV DNA terminase complex inhibitor indicated for prophylaxis of CMV infection and disease in adult CMV-seropositive recipients [R+] of an allogeneic hemato-poietic stem cell transplant (HSCT).

▶ ***letermovir*** <18 years: not recommended; ≥18 years: administer dose orally or as an IV infusion over 1 hour; dose is 480 mg once daily through 100 days post-transplant; if co-administered with ***cyclosporine***, decrease the ***letermovir*** dose to 240 mg once daily

Prevymis *Tab:* 240, 450 mg; *Vial:* 240 mg/12 ml (20 mg/ml), 480 mg/24 ml (20 mg/ml), single-dose

Comment: Closely monitor serum creatinine levels in patients with CrCL <50 mL/min using **Prevymis** injection for IV infusion. **Prevymis** is not recommended for patients with severe (Child-Pugh C) hepatic impairment. **Prevymis** is contraindicated with ***pimozide***, ergot alkaloids, and ***pitavastatin*** and ***simvastatin*** when co-administered with ***cyclosporine***. Most common adverse events (10%) have been nausea, diarrhea, vomiting, peripheral edema, cough, head ache, fatigue, and abdominal pain. No adequate human data are available to inform whether **Prevymis** poses a risk to pregnancy outcomes. It is not known whether ***letermovir*** is present in human breast milk or effects the breastfed infant. To report suspected adverse reactions, contact Merck Sharp & Dohme, a subsidiary of Merck, at 1-877-888-4231 or FDA at 1-800-FDA-1088 or visit http://www.fda.gov/www.fda.gov/medwatch

RHEUMATOID ARTHRITIS (RA)

Injectable Acetaminophen *see **Pain** page* 322
NSAIDs *see page* 539
Other Oral Analgesics *see **Pain** page* 324
Topical & Transdermal NSAIDs *see **Pain** page* 323
Parenteral Corticosteroids *see page* 547
Oral Corticosteroids *see page* 546

TOPICAL & TRANSDERMAL ANALGESICS

▶ ***capsaicin*** cream **(B)(G)** <2 years: not recommended; 2-12 years: apply sparingly to intact skin bid prn; >12 years: apply tid-qid prn

Axsain *Crm:* 0.075% (1, 2 oz)
Capsin (OTC) *Lotn:* 0.025, 0, 075% (59 ml)
Capzasin-P (OTC) *Crm:* 0.025% (1.5 oz); *Lotn:* 0.025% (2 oz)
Capzasin-HP (OTC) *Crm:* 0.075% (1.5 oz); *Lotn:* 0.075% (2 oz)
Dolorac *Crm:* 0.025% (28 gm)
Double Cap (OTC) *Crm:* 0.05% (2 oz)

Qutenza *Patch:* 8% (1-2, both with 50 gm tube of cleansing gel)
R-Gel *Gel:* 0.025% (15, 30 gm)s
Zostrix (OTC) *Crm:* 0.025% (0.7, 1.5, 3 oz)
Zostrix HP (OTC) *Emol crm:* 0.075% (1, 2 oz)

Comment: Provides some relief by 1-2 weeks; optimal benefit may take 4-6 weeks. Avoid contact with mucous membranes.

▶ ***trolamine salicylate*** <2 years: not recommended; ≥2 years: apply tid-qid prn to intact skin

Mobisyl *Crm:* 10%

Comment: Provides some relief by 1-2 weeks; optimal benefit may take 4-6 weeks.

ORAL SALICYLATE

▶ ***indomethacin*** **(C)** <14 years: usually not recommended; >2 years, if risk warranted: 1-2 mg/kg/day in divided doses; max 3-4 mg/kg/day (or 150-200 mg/day, whichever is less); <14 years, ER cap not recommended; ≥14 years: initially 25 mg bid-tid, increase as needed at weekly intervals by 25-50 mg/day; max 200 mg/day

Cap: 25, 50 mg; *Susp;* 25 mg/5 ml (pineapple-coconut, mint; alcohol 1%); *Supp:* 50 mg; *ER Cap:* 75 mg ext-rel

Comment: ***indomethacin*** is indicated only for acute painful flares. Administer with food and/or antacids. Use lowest effective dose for shortest duration.

ORAL NSAIDs

See more Oral NSAIDs *page* 539

▶ ***diclofenac sodium*** (C)(G)

Voltaren <12 not recommended; ≥12 years: 50 mg bid-qid or 75 mg bid or 25 mg qid with an additional 25 mg at HS if necessary

Tab: 25, 50, 75 mg ent-coat

Voltaren XR <18: not recommended; ≥18 years: 100 mg once daily; rarely, 100 mg bid may be used

Tab: 100 mg ext-rel

ORAL NSAID+PPI

▶ ***esomeprazole+naproxen*** **(C; not for use in 3rd)(G)** <18 years: not recommended; ≥18 years: 1 tab bid; use lowest effective dose for the shortest duration; swallow whole; take at least 30 minutes before a meal

Vimovo *Tab:* nap 375 mg+eso 20 mg ext-rel; nap 500 mg+eso 20 mg ext-rel

Comment: **Vimovo** is indicated to improve signs/symptoms, and risk of gastric ulcer in patients at risk of developing NSAID-associated gastric ulcer.

COX-2 INHIBITORS

Comment: Cox-2 inhibitors are contraindicated with history of asthma, urticaria, and allergic-type reactions to ***aspirin***, other NSAIDs, and sulfonamides, 3rd trimester of pregnancy, and coronary artery bypass graft (CABG) surgery.

▶ ***celecoxib*** (C)(G) <18 years: not recommended; ≥18 years: 100-400 mg bid; max 800 mg/day

Celebrex *Cap:* 50, 100, 200, 400 mg

▶ ***meloxicam*** (C)(G)

Mobic <2 years, <60 kg: not recommended; ≥2, >60 kg: 0.125 mg/kg; max 7.5 mg once daily; ≥18 years: initially 7.5 mg once daily; max 15 mg once daily; *Hemodialysis:* max 7.5 mg/day

Tab: 7.5, 15 mg; *Oral susp:* 7.5 mg/5 ml (100 ml) (raspberry)

Vivlodex <18 years: not established; ≥18 years: initially 5 mg qd; may increase to max 10 mg/day; *Hemodialysis:* max 5 mg/day
Cap: 5, 10 mg

JANUS KINASE (JAK) INHIBITOR

▶ ***tofacitinib*** (C) <18 years: not established; ≥18 years: 10 mg bid for at least 8 weeks; then 5 or 10 mg bid; discontinue after 16 weeks of 10 mg bid, if adequate therapeutic benefit is not achieved; use the lowest effective dose to maintain response; see mfr pkg insert for dosage adjustments for patients receiving CYP2C19 and/or CYP3A4 inhibitors; in patients with moderate or severe renal impairment or moderate hepatic impairment, and patients with lymphopenia, neutropenia, or anemia; use of **Xeljanz/ Xeljanz XR** in patients with severe hepatic impairment is not recommended in any patient population;

Xeljanz *Tab:* 5, 10 mg
Xeljanz XR *Tab:* 11 mg ext-rel

Comment: **Xeljanz** is indicated for moderate-to-severe RA as monotherapy in patients who have inadequate response or intolerance to ***methotrexate*** (MTX). Use of **Xeljanz** in combination with biologiv DMARDs or potent immunosuppressants, such as ***azathioprine*** and ***cyclosporine***, is not recommended. Avoid use of **Xeljanz/ Xeljanz XR** during an active serious infection, including localized infection. Use with caution in patients that may be at increased risk for gastrointestinal perforation. The most common adverse events associated with ***Xeljanz*** treatment are diarrhea, elevated cholesterol level, headache, herpes zoster (shingles), increased blood creatine phosphokinase, nasopharyngitis, rash, and upper respiratory tract infection (URI). Patients treated with **Xeljanz** are at increased risk for developing serious infections that may lead to hospitalization or death. **Xeljanz** has a BBW for serious infections (e.g., opportunistic infections), and malignancy (e.g., lymphoma). Use of **Xeljanz** in combination with biological therapies for ulcerative colitis or with potent immuno-suppressants, such as ***azathioprine*** and ***cyclosporine***, is not recommended. Avoid live vaccines administration during treatment with **Xeljanz.** Prior to starting **Xeljanz**, perform a test for latent tuberculosis; if it is positive, start treatment for tuberculosis prior to starting **Xeljanz**. Monitor all patients for active tuberculosis during treatment, even if the initial latent tuberculosis test is negative. Recommend lab monitoring due to potential for changes in lymphocytes, neutronphils, hemoglobin, liver enzymes, and lipids. Do not initiate **Xeljanz** if absolute lymphocyte count <500 cells/mm3, an absolute neutrophil count (ANC) <1000 cells/mm3 or Hgb <9 g/dL. The safety and effectiveness of **Xeljanz/Xeljanz XR** in pediatric patients have not been established. Available data with **Xeljanz** use in pregnancy women are insufficient to establish a drug associated risk of major birth defects, miscarriage, adverse maternal or fetal out-comes. In animal reproduction studies, fetocidal, and teratogenic effects were noted. There is a pregnancy exposure registry that monitors pregnancy outcomes in females exposed to **Xeljanz/Xeljanz XR** during pregnancy. Consider pregnancy planning and prevention for females of reproductive potential. Patients should be encouraged to enroll in the **Xeljanz/Xeljanz XR** pregnancy registry if they become pregnant. To enroll or obtain information from the registry, patients can call the toll free number 1-877-311-8972. There are no data on the presence of ***tofacitinib*** in human milk or the effects on a breastfed infant; however, patients should be advised not to breast-feed. To report suspected adverse reactions, contact Pfizer at 1-800-438-1985 or FDA at 1-800-FDA-1088 or visit www.fda.gov/medwatch

DISEASE MODIFYING ANTIRHEUMATIC DRUGS (DMARDs)

Comment: DMARDs are first-line treatment options for RA. DMARDs include penicillamine, gold salts (***auranofin***, ***aurothio-glucose***), immunosuppressants, and

hydroxychloroquine. The DMARDs reduce ESR, reduce RF, and favorably affect the outcome of RA. Immunosuppressants may require 6 weeks to affect benefits and 6 months for full improvement.

- ***auranofin (gold salt)*** **(C)** <12 years: not recommended; ≥12 years: 3 mg bid or 6 mg once daily; if inadequate response after 6 months, increase to 3 mg tid
  Ridaura *Vial:* 100 mg/20 ml
- ***azathioprine*** **(D)** <12 years: not established; ≥12 years: 1 mg/kg/day in a single or divided doses; may increase by 0.5 mg/kg/day q 4 weeks; max 2.5 mg/kg/day; minimum trial to ascertain effectiveness is 12 weeks
  Azasan *Tab* 75*, 100*mg
  Imuran *Tab* 50*mg
- ***cyclosporine (immunosuppressant)*** **(C)** <12 years: not recommended; ≥12 years: 1.25 mg/kg bid; may increase after 4 weeks by 0.5 mg/kg/day; then adjust at 2 week intervals; max 4 mg/kg/day; administer with meals
  Neoral *Cap:* 25, 100 mg (alcohol)
  Neoral Oral Solution *Oral soln:* 100 mg/ml (50 ml) may dilute in room temperature apple juice or orange juice (alcohol)
  Comment: **Neoral** is indicated for RA unresponsive to ***methotrexate*** **(MTX)**.
- ***hydroxychloroquine*** **(C)** <12 years: not recommended; ≥12 years: 400-600 mg/day
  Plaquenil *Tab:* 200 mg

Comment: May require several weeks to achieve beneficial effects. If no improvement in 6 months, discontinue.

- ***leflunomide*** **(X)(G)** <18 years: not recommended; ≥18 years: initially 100 mg once daily x 3 days; maintenance dose 20 mg once daily; max 20 mg daily
  Arava *Tab:* 10, 20, 100 mg
  Comment: **Arava** is contraindicated with breastfeeding.
- ***methotrexate [MTX]*** **(X)** <2 years: not recommended; ≥2 years-12 years: 10 mg/m^2 once weekly; max 20 mg/m^2; >12 years: 7.5 mg x 1 dose per week or 2.5 mg x 3 at 12 hour intervals once a week; max 20 mg/week; therapeutic response begins in 3-6 weeks; administer ***methotrexate*** injection SC only into the abdomen or thigh
  Rasuvo *Autoinjector:* 7.5 mg/0.15 ml, 10 mg/0.20 ml, 12.5 mg/0.25 ml, 15 mg/0.30 ml, 17.5 mg/0.35 ml, 20 mg/0.40 ml, 22.5 mg/0.45 ml, 25 mg/0.50 ml, 27.5 mg/0.55 ml, 30 mg/0.60 ml (solution concentration for SC injection is 50 mg/ml)
  Rheumatrex *Tab:* 2.5*mg (5, 7.5, 10, 12.5, 15 mg/week, 4/card unit-of-use dose pack)
  Trexall *Tab:* 5*, 7.5*, 10*, 15*mg (5, 7.5, 10, 12.5, 15 mg/week, 4/card unit-of-use dose pack)
  Comment: ***methotrexate*** **(MTX)** is contraindicated with immunodeficiency, blood dyscrasias, alcoholism, and chronic liver disease.
- ***penicillamine*** **(D)** <12 years: not recommended; ≥12 years: 125-250 mg once daily initially; may increase by 125-250 mg/day q 1-3 months; max 1.5 gm/day
  Cuprimine *Cap:* 125, 250 mg
  Depen *Tab:* 250 mg
- ***sulfasalazine*** **(C; D in 2nd, 3rd)(G)** <6 years: not recommended; 6-16 years: initially 1/4 to 1/3 of maintenance dose; increase weekly; maintenance 30-50 mg/kg/day in 2 divided doses at regular intervals; max 2 gm/day; >16 years: initially 0.5 gm once daily bid; gradually increase every 4 days; usual maintenance 2-3 gm/day in equally divided doses at regular intervals; max 4 gm/day
  Azulfidine *Tab:* 500 mg
  Azulfidine EN *Tab:* 500 mg ent-coat

TUMOR NECROSIS FACTOR (TNF) BLOCKERS

- ***adalimumab*** **(B)** <2 years, <10 kg: not recommended; ≥2 years: 10-<15 kg: 10 mg every other week; 15-<30 kg: 20 mg every other week; ≥30 kg: 40 mg SC every other week; ≥17 years: may increase to once weekly without ***methotrexate*** **(MTX)**; administer in abdomen or thigh; rotate sites; 2-17 years, supervise first dose

Humira *Prefilled syringe:* 20 mg/0.4 ml; 40 mg/0.8 ml single-dose (2/pck; 2, 6/starter pck) (preservative-free)

Comment: **Humira** may use with ***methotrexate*** **(MTX)**, DMARDs, corticosteroids, salicylates, NSAIDs, or analgesics.

- ***adalimumab-adbm*** **(B)** <18 years: not recommended; ≥18 years: initially 80 SC; then, 40 mg SC every other week starting one week after initial dose; inject into thigh or abdomen; rotate sites

  Cyltezo *Prefilled syringe:* 40 mg/0.8 ml single-dose (preservative-free)

  Comment: **Cyltezo** is biosimilar to **Humira** (***adalimumab***).

- ***certolizumab pegol*** **(B)** <12 years: not recommended; ≥12 years: 400 mg SC on Day 1, at week 2, and at week 4; then 200 give for other week; rotate sites

  Cimzia *Vial:* 200 mg single-dose w. supplies (2/pck, 2, 6/starter pck); *Prefilled syringe:* 200 mg single-dose w. supplies (2/pck, 2, 6/starter pck) (preservative-free)

- ***etanercept*** **(B)** <4 years: not recommended; 4-<17 years: 0.4 mg/kg SC twice weekly, 72-96 hours apart (max 25 mg/dose) or 0.8 mg/kg SC weekly (max 50 mg/dose); ≥17 years: 25 mg SC twice weekly, 72-96 hours apart or 50 mg SC weekly; rotate sites

  Enbrel *Vial:* 25 mg pwdr for SC injection after reconstitution (4/carton w. supplies) (preservative-free; diluent contains benzyl alcohol); *Prefilled syringe:* 50 mg/ml (preservative-free); *SureClick Autoinjector:* 50 mg/ml (preservative-free)

Comment: ***etanercept*** reduces pain, morning stiffness, and swelling. May be administered in combination with ***methotrexate***. Live vaccines should not be administered concurrently. Do not administer with active infection.

- ***golimumab*** **(B)** <18 years: not recommended; ≥18 years: administer SC or IV infusion (in combination with ***methotrexate*** [MTX])

  Simponi 50 mg SC once monthly; rotate sites

  Prefilled syringe, SmartJect Autoinjector: 50 mg/0.5 ml, single use (preservative-free)

  Simponi Aria 2 mg/kg IV infusion week 0 and week 4; then every 8 weeks thereafter

  Vial: 50 mg/4 ml, single-use, soln for IV infusion after dilution (latex-free, preservative-free)

Comment: corticosteroids, non-biologic DMARDs, and/or NSAIDs may be continued during treatment with ***golimumab***.

- ***infliximab*** *(tumor necrosis factor-alpha blocker)* <18 years: not established; ≥18 years: 5 mg/kg at 0, 2 and 6 weeks, then every 8 weeks; must be refrigerated at 2°C to 8°C (36°F to 46°F); administer dose intravenously over a period of not less than 2 hours; do not use beyond the expiration date as this product contains no preservative.

  Remicade *Vial:* 100 mg pwdr for reconstitution and dilution; (preservative-free)

Comment: Use ***infliximab*** concomitantly with ***methotrexate*** when there has been insufficient response to ***methotrexate*** alone. **Remicade** is indicated to reduce signs and symptoms, and induce and maintain clinical remission, in adults and children >6 years-of-age with moderately to severely active disease who have had an inadequate response to conventional therapy and reduce the number of draining enterocutaneous and rectovaginal fistulas, and maintain fistula closure, in adults with fistulizing disease. Common adverse effects associated with **Remicade** included abdominal pain, headache, pharyngitis, sinusitis, and upper respiratory infections. In addition, **Remicade** might increase the risk for serious infections, including tuberculosis, bacterial sepsis, and invasive fungal infections. Available data from published literature on the use of ***infliximab*** products during pregnancy have not reported a clear association with ***infliximab*** products and adverse pregnancy outcomes. ***infliximab*** products cross the placenta and infants exposed *in utero* should not be administered live vaccines for at least 6 months after birth. Otherwise, the infant may be at increased risk of infection, including disseminated infection which can become fatal. Available information is insufficient to inform the amount of ***infliximab*** products present in human milk or effects on the breastfed infant. To report suspected adverse reactions, contact Merck Sharp & Dohme Corp., a subsidiary of Merck & Co. at 1-877-888-4231 or FDA at 1-800-FDA1088 or visit www.fda.gov/medwatch

➢ ***infliximab-abda*** *(tumor necrosis factor-alpha blocker)* **(B)**

Inflectra: *see* ***infliximab*** **(Remicade)** above for full prescribing information

Comment: **Inflectra** is a biosimilar to **Remicade** for the treatment of immune-disorders including Crohn's disease, ulcerative colitis, rheumatoid arthritis, ankylosing spondylitis, psoriatic arthritis and plaque psoriasis. **Inflectra** was approved under the FDA category for biosimilars and demonstrated no clinically meaningful differences for use, dosing regimens, strengths, dosage forms, and routes of administration from the FDA-approved biological product **Remicade.**

Renflexis: *See* ***infliximab*** **(Remicade)** above for full prescribing information

Comment: **Renflexis** is a biosimilar to **Remicade** for the treatment of immune-disorders including Crohn's disease, ulcerative colitis, rheumatoid arthritis, ankylosing spondylitis, psoriatic arthritis and plaque psoriasis. **Renflexis** was approved under the FDA category for biosimilars and demonstrated no clinically meaningful differences for use, dosing regimens, strengths, dosage forms, and routes of administration from the FDA-approved biological product **Remicade.**

INTERLEUKIN-1 RECEPTOR ANTAGONIST

➢ ***anakinra (interleukin-1 receptor antagonist)*** **(B)** <12 years: not recommended; ≥12 years: 100 mg SC once daily; discard any unused portion

Kineret *Prefilled syringe:* 100 mg/single-dose syringe (7, 28/pk) (preservative-free)

INTERLEUKIN-6 RECEPTOR ANTAGONIST

➢ ***sarilumab*** <18 years: not recommended; ≥18 years: 200 mg SC every 2 weeks on the same day; if necessary, the dosage can be reduced 150 mg every 2 weeks to manage potential laboratory abnormalities, such as neutropenia, thrombocytopenia, and liver enzyme elevations; SC injections may be self-administered

Kevzara *Prefilled syringe:* 150, 200 mg (1.4 ml, single-use)

Comment: ***sarilumab*** is a human monoclonal antibody that binds to the interleukin-6 receptor (IL-6R), and has been shown to inhibit IL-6R mediated signaling. IL-6 is a cytokine in the body that, in excess and over time, can contribute to the inflammation associated with RA. **Kevzara** received FDA approval in May, 2017 for use in patients with active moderate-to-severe rheumatoid arthritis (RA) in adults who have had an inadequate response or intolerance to one or more disease modifying antirheumatic drugs (DMARDs). **Kevzara** may be used as monotherapy or in combination with ***methotrexate*** or other conventional DMARDs. Monitor patient for dose related laboratory changes including elevated LFTs, neutropenia, and thrombocytopenia. **Kevzara** should not be initiated in patients with an absolute neutrophil count (ANC) <2000/mm^3, platelet count <150,000/mm^3, or liver transaminases above 1.5 times the upper limit of normal (ULN). Registration in the Pregnancy Exposure Registry (1-877-311-8972) is encouraged for monitoring pregnancy outcomes in women exposed to **Kevzara** during pregnancy. Negative side effects of **Kevzara** should be reported to the FDA at www.fda.gov/medwatch or call 1-800-FDA-1088 or call Sanofi-Aventis at 1-800-633-1610. The limited available data with **Kevzara** in pregnant women are not sufficient to determine whether there is a drug-associated risk for major birth defects and miscarriage. Monoclonal antibodies, such as ***sarilumab***, are actively transported across the placenta during the third trimester of pregnancy and may affect immune response in the infant exposed *in utero*. It is not known whether ***sarilumab*** passes into breast milk; therefore, breastfeeding is not recommended while using **Kevzara**.

▶ ***tocilizumab*** **(B)** <2 years: not recommended; ≥2 years: weight-based dosing according to diagnosis: *PJIA: ≥30 kg*: 8 mg/kg SC every 4 weeks; *<30 kg*: 10 mg/kg SC every 4 weeks; *SJIA: ≥30 kg*: 8 mg/kg SC every 2 weeks; *<30 kg*: 12 mg/kg SC every 2 weeks; *IV Infusion:* administer over 1 hour; do not administer as bolus or IV push; *PJIA, and SJIA, ≥30 kg*: dilute to 100 mL in 0.9% or 0.45% NaCl. *PJIA and SJIA, <30 kg:* dilute to 50 mL in 0.9% or 0.45% NaCl; ≥18 years: whether used in combination with DMARDs or as monotherapy, the recommended IV infusion starting dose is 4 mg/kg IV every 4 weeks followed by an increase to 8 mg/kg IV every 4 weeks based on clinical response; max 800 mg per infusion in RA patients; *SC Administration: ≥100 kg*: 162 mg SC once weekly on the same day; SC injections may be self-administered

Actemra *Vial:* 80 mg/4 ml, 200 mg/10 ml, 400 mg/20 ml, single-use, for IV infusion after dilution; *Prefilled syringe:* 162 mg (0.9 ml, single-dose)

Comment: ***tocilizumab*** is an interleukin-6 receptor-α inhibitor indicated for use in moderate-to-severe rheumatoid arthritis (RA) that has not responded to conventional therapy, and also for some subtypes of juvenile idiopathic arthritis (JIA). **Actemra** may be used alone or in combination with ***methotrexate*** and in RA, other DMARDs may be used. Monitor patient for dose related laboratory changes including elevated LFTs, neutropenia, and thrombocytopenia. **Actemra** should not be initiated in patients with an absolute neutrophil count (ANC) <2000/mm³, platelet count <100,000/mm³, or who have ALT or AST above 1.5 times the upper limit of normal (ULN). Registration in the Pregnancy Exposure Registry (1-877-311-8972) is encouraged for monitoring pregnancy outcomes in women exposed to **Actemra** during pregnancy. The limited available data with **Actemra** in pregnant women are not sufficient to determine whether there is a drug-associated risk for major birth defects and miscarriage. Monoclonal antibodies, such as ***tocilizumab***, are actively transported across the placenta during the third trimester of pregnancy and may affect immune response in the infant exposed *in utero*. It is not known whether ***tocilizumab*** passes into breast milk; therefore, breastfeeding is not recommended while using **Actemra**.

SELECTIVE CO-STIMULATION MODULATOR

▶ ***abatacept*** **(C)** <6 years: not recommended; 6-17 years: administer as an IV infusion over 30 minutes at weeks 0, 2, and 4; then every 4 weeks thereafter; <75 kg, administer 10 mg/kg; max 1 gm; ≥17 years: administer as an IV infusion over 30 minutes at weeks 0, 2, and 4; then every 4 weeks thereafter; <60 kg, administer 500 mg/dose; 60-100 kg, administer 750 mg/dose; >100 kg, administer 1 gm/dose

Orencia *Vial:* 250 mg pwdr for IV infusion after reconstitution (silicone-free) (preservative-free); *Prefilled syringe:* 125 mg/ml soln for SC injection (preservative-free); *ClickJect Autoinjector:* 125 mg/ml soln for SC injection

CD20 ANTIBODY

▶ ***rituximab*** **(C)** <6 years: not recommended; ≥6 years: administer corticosteroid 30 minutes prior to each infusion; concomitant ***methotrexate*** therapy, administer a 1,000 mg IV infusion at 0 and 2 weeks; then every 24 weeks or based on response, but not sooner than every 16 weeks.

Rituxan *Vial:* 10 mg/ml (10, 50 ml) (preservative-free)

Comment: ***rituximab*** is a B-cell targeting chimeric monoclonal antibody that acts against CD20 and reduces antibody titers. B-cell depletion by ***rituximab*** may also set the stage for production of interleukin 10–secreting B cells that do not interact with T cells, which further reduces production of antidesmoglein antibodies. ***rituximab*** carries a black box warning regarding fatal infusion reactions, severe mucocutaneous reactions, hepatitis B virus reactivation, and progressive multifocal leukoencephalopathy. However, serious adverse events are rare. There was no evidence of increased mortality with longer exposure to **rituximab** or to multiple courses of therapy.

INTRA-ARTICULAR INJECTION

➢ ***sodium hyaluronate*** <12 years: not recommended; ≥12 years: 20 mg as intra-articular injection weekly x 5 weeks

Hyalgan *Prefilled syringe:* 20 mg/2 ml

Comment: Remove joint effusion and inject with ***lidocaine*** if possible before injecting **Hyalgan**.

RHINITIS/SINUSITIS: ALLERGIC

Drugs for the Management of Allergy, Cough, and Cold Symptoms *see page* 570
Parenteral Corticosteroids *see page* 547
Oral Corticosteroids *see page* 546

Comment: The Joint Task Force on Practice Parameters, which comprises representatives of the American Academy of Allergy, Asthma and Immunology (AAAAI) and the American College of Allergy, Asthma and Immunology (ACAAI), has provided guidance to healthcare providers on the initial pharmacologic treatment of seasonal allergic rhinitis in patients aged ≥12 years. For initial treatment of seasonal allergic rhinitis in persons aged ≥12 years: routinely prescribe monotherapy with an intranasal corticosteroid rather than an intranasal corticosteroid in combination with an oral antihistamine. For initial treatment of seasonal allergic rhinitis in persons aged ≥15 years: recommend an intranasal corticosteroid over a leukotriene. For initial treatment of seasonal allergic rhinitis in persons aged ≥15 years: recommend an intranasal corticosteroid over a leukotriene receptor antagonist. For initial treatment of moderate to severe seasonal allergic rhinitis in persons aged ≥12 years: recommend a combination of an intranasal corticosteroid and an intranasal antihistamine.

REFERENCE

Wallace, DV, Dykewicz, MS, Oppenheimer, J, *et al.* (2017). Pharmacologic treatment of seasonal allergic rhinitis: synopsis of guidance from the 2017 joint task force on practice parameters. *Annals of Internal Medicine, 167*(12), 876. doi:10.7326/m17-2203

SECOND GENERATION ORAL ANTIHISTAMINES

Comment: Second generation antihistamines are sedating, but much less so than the first generation antihistamines. All antihistamines are excreted into breast milk.

➢ ***cetirizine*** (C)(OTC)(G) <6 years: not recommended; ≥6-<65 years: initially 5-10 mg once daily; ≥65 years: 5 mg once daily

Children's Zyrtec Chewable *Chew tab:* 5, 10 mg (grape)
Children's Zyrtec Allergy Syrup *Syr:* 1 mg/ml (4 oz) (grape, bubble gum) (sugar-free, dye-free)
Zyrtec *Tab:* 10 mg
Zyrtec Hives Relief *Tab:* 10 mg
Zyrtec Liquid Gels *Liq gel:* 10 mg

▶ ***desloratadine*** **(C)**

Clarinex <6 years: not recommended; ≥6 years: 1/2-1 tab once daily

Tab: 5 mg

Clarinex RediTabs <6 years: not recommended; 6-12 years: 2.5 mg once daily; ≥12 years: 5 mg once daily

ODT: 2.5, 5 mg (tutti-frutti) (phenylalanine)

Clarinex Syrup <6 months: not recommended; 6-11 months: 1 mg (2 ml) once daily; 1-5 years: 1.25 mg (2.5 ml) once daily; 6-11 years: 2.5 mg (5 ml) once daily; ≥12 years: 5 mg (10 ml) once daily

Tab: 0.5 mg per ml (4 oz) (tutti-frutti) (phenylalanine)

Desloratadine ODT

▶ ***fexofenadine*** **(C)(OTC)(G)** 6 months-2 years: 15 mg bid; *CrCl ≤90 mL/min:* 15 mg once daily; 2-11 years: 30 mg bid; *CrCl ≤90 mL/min:* 30 mg once daily ≥12 years and older: ≥ 12 years: 60 mg once daily-bid or 180 mg once daily; *CrCl <90 mL/min:* 60 mg once daily **Allegra** *Tab:* 30, 60, 180 mg film-coat

Allegra Allergy *Tab:* 60, 180 mg film-coat

Allegra ODT *ODT:* 30 mg (phenylalanine)

Allegra Oral Suspension *Oral susp:* 30 mg/5 ml (6 mg/ml) (4 oz)

▶ ***levocetirizine*** **(B)(OTC)** administer dose in the PM; *Seasonal Allergic Rhinitis:* <2 years: not recommended; may start at ≥2 years; *Chronic Spontaneous/Idiopathic Urticaria (CSU/CIU), Perennial Allergic Rhinitis:* <6 months: not recommended; may start at ≥ 6 months; *Dosing by Age:* 6 months-5 years: max 1.25 mg once daily; 6-11 years: max 2.5 mg once daily; ≥12 years: 2.5-5 mg once daily; *Renal Dysfunction <12 years:* contraindicated; *Renal Dysfunction ≥12 years: CrCl 50-80 mL/min:* 2.5 mg once daily; *CrCl 30-50 mL/min:* 2.5 mg every other day; *CrCl: 10-30 mL/min:* 2.5 mg twice weekly (every 3-4 days); *CrCl <10 mL/min, ESRD or hemodialysis:* contraindicated

Children's Xyzal Allergy 24HR *Oral soln:* 0.5 mg/ml (150 ml)

Xyzal Allergy 24HR *Tab:* 5*mg

▶ ***loratadine*** **(C)(OTC)(G)** <2 years: not recommended; 2-5 years: 5 mg once daily; ≥6 years: 5 mg bid or 10 mg once daily; *Hepatic or Renal Insufficiency:* (see mfr pkg insert)

Children's Claritin Chewables *Chew tab:* 5 mg (grape) (phenylalanine)

Children's Claritin Syrup 1 mg/ml (4 oz) (fruit) (sugar-free, alcohol-free, dye-free; sodium 6 mg/5 ml)

Claritin *Tab:* 10 mg

Claritin Hives Relief *Tab:* 10 mg

Claritin Liqui-Gels *Lig gel:* 10 mg

Claritin RediTabs 12 Hours *ODT:* 5 mg (mint)

Claritin RediTabs 24 Hours *ODT:* 10 mg (mint)

FIRST GENERATION ANTIHISTAMINES

▶ ***diphenhydramine*** **(B)(G)** <2 years: not recommended; 2-6 years: 6.25 mg q 4-6 hours; max 37.5 mg/day; >6-12 years: 12.5-25 mg q 4-6 hours; max 150 mg/day; >12 years: 25-50 mg q 6-8 hours; max 100 mg/day

Benadryl (OTC) *Chew tab:* 12.5 mg (grape) (phenylalanine); *Liq:* 12.5 mg/5 ml (4, 8 oz); *Cap:* 25 mg; *Tab:* 25 mg; *Dye-free soft gel:* 25 mg; *Dye-free liq:* 12.5 mg/5 ml (4, 8 oz)

▶ ***diphenhydramine*** *injectable* **(B)(G)** <12 years: *See mfr pkg insert:* 1.25 mg/kg up to 25 mg IM x 1 dose; then q 6 hours prn; ≥12 years: 25-50 mg IM immediately; then q 6 hours prn

Benadryl Injectable *Vial:* 50 mg/ml (1 ml single-use); 50 mg/ml (10 ml multi-dose); *Amp:* 10 mg/ml (1 ml); *Prefilled syringe:* 50 mg/ml (1 ml)

▷ ***hydroxyzine*** **(C)(G)** <6 years: 50 mg/day divided qid prn; ≥6 years-12 years: 50 mg/day divided qid prn; >12 years: 50-100 mg/day divided qid prn

Atarax *Tab:* 10, 25, 50, 100 mg; *Syr:* 10 mg/5 ml (alcohol 0.5%)

Vistaril *Cap:* 25, 50, 100 mg; *Oral susp:* 25 mg/5 ml (4 oz) (lemon)

Comment: hydroxyzine is contraindicated in early pregnancy and in patients with a prolonged QT interval. It is not known whether this drug is excreted in human milk; therefore, hydroxyzine should not be given to nursing mothers.

ALLERGEN EXTRACTS

Comment: Allergen extracts (**Grastek, Oralair, Ragwitek**) are not for immediate relief of allergic symptoms. Contraindicated with severe, unstable, and uncontrolled asthma, history of eosinophilic esophagitis, and severe local <u>or</u> systemic reaction. First dose under supervision HCP and observe ≥30 minutes. Subsequent doses may be taken at home.

▷ ***short ragweed pollen allergen extract*** **(C)** <18 years: not recommended; ≥18 years: one SL tab once daily

Ragwitek *SL tab:* ambrosia artemisiifolia 12 amb a 1-unit (30, 90/blister pck)

Comment: Initiate **Ragwitek** at least 12 weeks before onset of ragweed pollen season and continue throughout season.

▷ ***sweet vernal, orchard, perennial rye, timothy, Kentucky blue grass mixed pollen allergen extract*** (C) <10 years: not established; 10-17 years: Day 1: 100 IR; Day 2: 200 IR; Day 3 and thereafter: 300 IR once daily; >17 years: 300 IR once daily

Oralair *SL tab:* 100, 300 IR (index of reactivity) (30/blister pck)

Comment: **Oralair** is indicated for grass pollen-induced allergic rhinitis with <u>or</u> without conjunctivitis confirmed by positive skin test. Initiate **Oralair** at least 4 months before onset of grass pollen season and continue throughout season.

▷ ***Timothy grass pollen allergen extract*** **(C)** <5 years: not established; ≥5 years: one SL tab once daily

Grastek *SL tab:* 2800 bio-equivalent allergy units (BAUS) (30/blister pck)

Comment: **Grastek** is indicated for grass pollen-induced allergic rhinitis with <u>or</u> without conjunctivitis confirmed by positive skin test. Initiate **Grastek** at least 12 weeks before onset of grass pollen season and continue throughout season.

NASAL DECONGESTANTS

▷ ***tetrahydrozoline*** **(C)** <6 years: not recommended; ≥6 years: 2-4 drops <u>or</u> 3-4 sprays in each nostril q 3-8 hours prn

Tyzine Nasal Spray *Nasal spray:* 0.1% (15 ml); *Nasal drops:* 0.1% (30 ml)

Tyzine Pediatric Nasal Drops *Nasal drops:* 0.05% (15 ml)

LEUKOTRIENE RECEPTOR ANTAGONISTS (LRAs)

Comment: The LRAs are indicated for prophylaxis and chronic treatment, only. Not for primary (rescue) treatment of acute asthma attack.

▷ ***montelukast*** **(B)(G)** <12 months: not recommended; 12-23 months: one 4 mg granule pkt daily; 2-5 years: one 4 mg chew tab <u>or</u> granule pkt daily; >5-14 years: one 5 mg chew tab daily; >14 years: 10 mg once daily in the PM; for EIB, take at least 2 hours before exercise; max 1 dose/day

Singulair *Tab:* 10 mg

Singulair Chewable *Chew tab:* 4, 5 mg (cherry) (phenylalanine)

Singulair Oral Granules *Granules:* 4 mg/pkt; take within 15 minutes of opening pkt; may mix with applesauce, carrots, rice, <u>or</u> ice cream

▶ ***zafirlukast*** **(B)** <7 years: not recommended; 7-11 years: 10 mg bid 1 hour ac or 2 hours pc; >11 years: 20 mg bid, 1 hour ac or 2 hours pc

Accolate *Tab:* 10, 20 mg

▶ ***zileuton*** (C)

Zyflo <12 years: not recommended; ≥12 years: 1 tab qid (total 2400 mg/day)

Tab: 600 mg

Zyflo CR <12 years: not recommended; ≥12 years: 2 tabs bid (total 2400 mg/day)

Tab: 600 mg ext-rel

NASAL CORTICOSTEROIDS

▶ ***beclomethasone dipropionate*** (C)

Beconase <6 years: not recommended; 6-12 years: 1 spray in each nostril tid; >12 years: 1 spray in each nostril bid-qid

Nasal spray: 42 mcg/actuation (6.7 gm, 80 sprays; 16.8 gm, 200 sprays)

Beconase AQ <6 years: not recommended; ≥6 years: 1-2 sprays in each nostril bid

Nasal spray: 42 mcg/actuation (25 gm, 180 sprays)

Beconase Inhalation Aerosol <6 years: not recommended; 6-12 years: 1 spray in each nostril tid; >12 years: 1-2 sprays in each nostril bid to qid

Nasal spray: 42 mcg/actuation (6.7 gm, 80 sprays; 16.8 gm, 200 sprays)

Vancenase AQ <6 years: not recommended; ≥6 years: 1-2 sprays in each nostril bid

Nasal spray: 84 mcg/actuation (25 gm, 200 sprays)

Vancenase AQ DS <6 years: not recommended; ≥6 years: 1-2 sprays in each nostril once daily

Nasal spray: 84, 168 mcg/actuation (19 gm, 120 sprays)

Vancenase Pockethaler <6 years: not recommended; ≥6 years: 1 spray in each nostril bid or tid

Pockethaler: 42 mcg/actuation (7 gm, 200 sprays)

QNASL Nasal Aerosol <12 years: 2 sprays, 40 mcg/spray, in each nostril once daily; ≥12 years: 2 sprays, 80 mcg/spray, in each nostril once daily

Nasal spray: 40 mcg/actuation (4.9 gm, 60 sprays); 80 mcg/actuation (8.7 gm, 120 sprays)

▶ ***budesonide*** (C)

Rhinocort <6 years: not recommended; >6 years: initially 2 sprays in each nostril bid in the AM and PM, or 4 sprays in each nostril in the AM; max 4 sprays each nostril/day; use lowest effective dose

Nasal spray: 32 mcg/actuation (7 gm, 200 sprays)

Rhinocort Aqua Nasal Spray <6 years: not recommended; ≥6-12 years: initially 1 spray in each nostril once daily; max 2 sprays in each nostril once daily; >12 years: initially 1 spray in each nostril once daily; max 4 sprays in each nostril once daily

Nasal spray: 32 mcg/actuation (10 ml, 60 sprays)

▶ ***ciclesonide*** (C)

Omnaris <6 years: not recommended; ≥6 years: 2 sprays in each nostril once daily

Nasal spray: 50 mcg/actuation (12.5 gm, 120 sprays)

Zetonna <6 years: not recommended; ≥6 years: 1-2 sprays in each nostril once daily

Nasal spray: 37 mcg/actuation (6.1 gm, 60 sprays) (HFA)

▶ ***dexamethasone*** (C) <6 years: not recommended; ≥6-12 years: 1-2 sprays in each nostril bid; max 8 sprays/day; maintain at lowest effective dose; >12 years: 2 sprays in each nostril bid-tid; max 12 sprays/day; maintain at lowest effective dose

Dexacort Turbinaire *Nasal spray:* 84 mcg/actuation (12.6 gm, 170 sprays)

▶ ***fluticasone furoate*** (C) <2 years: not recommended; ≥2-11 years: 1 spray in each nostril once daily; ≥12 years: 2 sprays in each nostril once daily; may reduce to 1 spray each nostril once daily

Veramyst *Nasal spray:* 27.5 mcg/actuation (10 gm, 120 sprays) (alcohol-free)

▶ ***fluticasone propionate*** (C)(OTC)(G) <4 years: not recommended; >4-12 years: initially 1 spray in each nostril once daily; may increase to 2 sprays in each nostril once daily; maintenance 1 spray in each nostril once daily; max 2 sprays in each nostril/day; >12 years: initially 2 sprays in each nostril once daily or 1 spray bid; maintenance 1 spray once daily
  Flonase *Nasal spray:* 50 mcg/actuation (16 gm, 120 sprays)

▶ ***flunisolide*** (C) <6 years: not recommended; 6-14 years: initially 1 spray in each nostril tid or 2 sprays in each nostril bid; max 4 sprays/nostril/day; >14 years: 2 sprays in each nostril bid; may increase to 2 sprays in each nostril tid; max 8 sprays/nostril/day
  Nasalide *Nasal spray:* 25 mcg/actuation (25 ml, 200 sprays)
  Nasarel *Nasal spray:* 25 mcg/actuation (25 ml, 200 sprays)

▶ ***mometasone furoate*** (C)(G) <2 years: not recommended; 2-11 years: 1 spray in each nostril once daily; max 2 sprays in each nostril once daily; >11 years: 2 sprays in each nostril once daily
  Nasonex *Nasal spray:* 50 mcg/actuation (17 gm, 120 sprays)

▶ ***olopatadine*** (C) <6 years: not recommended; 6-11 years: 1 spray each nostril bid; >11 years: 2 sprays in each nostril bid
  Patanase *Nasal spray:* 0.6%; 665 mcg/actuation (30.5 gm, 240 sprays) (benzalkonium chloride)

▶ ***triamcinolone acetonide*** (C)(G) <6 years: not recommended; ≥6 years-12 years: 1 spray in each nostril once daily; max 2 sprays in each nostril once daily; >12 years: initially 2 sprays in each nostril once daily; max 4 sprays in each nostril once daily or 2 sprays in each nostril bid or 1 spray in each nostril qid; maintain at lowest effective dose
  Nasacort Allergy 24HR (OTC) *Nasal spray:* 55 mcg/actuation (10 gm, 120 sprays)
  Tri-Nasal *Nasal spray:* 50 mcg/actuation (15 ml, 120 sprays)

NASAL MAST CELL STABILIZERS

▶ ***cromolyn sodium*** (B)(OTC) <2 years: not recommended; ≥2 years: 1 spray in each nostril tid-qid; max 6 sprays in each nostril/day
  Children's NasalCrom, NasalCrom *Nasal spray:* 5.2 mg/spray (13 ml, 100 sprays; 26 ml, 200 sprays)

Comment: Begin use 1-2 weeks before exposure to known allergen. May take 2-4 weeks to achieve maximum effect.

NASAL ANTIHISTAMINES

▶ ***azelastine*** (C)
  Astelin Ready Spray <5 years: not recommended; ≥5-12 years: 1 spray in each nostril qd-bid; >12 years: 2 sprays in each nostril bid
    Nasal spray: 137 mcg/actuation (30 ml, 200 sprays) (benzalkonium chloride)
  Astepro 0.15% Nasal Spray <2 years: not recommended; ≥2 years: 1 or 2 sprays each nostril once daily bid
    Nasal spray: 205.5 mcg/actuation (17 ml, 106 sprays; 30 ml, 200 sprays) (benzalkonium chloride)

NASAL ANTIHISTAMINE+CORTICOSTEROID COMBINATION

▶ ***azelastine+fluticasone*** (C) <6 years: not recommended; ≥6 years: 1 spray in each nostril bid
  Dymista *Nasal spray:* azel 137 mcg+flutic 50 mcg per actuation (23 gm, 120 sprays) (benzalkonium chloride)

NASAL ANTICHOLINERGICS

▶ *ipratropium bromide* (B)(G)

Atrovent Nasal Spray 0.03% <6 years: not recommended; ≥6 years: 2 sprays in each nostril bid-tid

Nasal spray: 21 mcg/actuation (30 ml, 345 sprays)

Atrovent Nasal Spray 0.06% 2 <5 years: not recommended; 5-11 years: 2 sprays in each nostril tid; >11 years: sprays in each nostril tid-qid; max 5-7 days

Nasal spray: 42 mcg/actuation (15 ml, 165 sprays)

Comment: Avoid use with narrow-angle glaucoma, prostate hyperplasia, and bladder neck obstruction.

RHINITIS MEDICAMENTOSA

Comment: The nasal/oral regimen selected should be instituted with concurrent weaning from the nasal decongestant.

Nasal Corticosteroids *see* ***Rhinitis, Sinusitis: Allergic*** *page* 392

Oral Corticosteroids *see page* 546

Parenteral Corticosteroids *see page* 547

OTC Oral **Decongestants**

OTC **Oral Antihistamine+Decongestants Combinations**

NASAL ANTICHOLINERGICS

▶ *ipratropium bromide* (B)(G)

Atrovent Nasal Spray 0.03% <6 years: not recommended; ≥6 years: stop nasal decongestant; 2 sprays in each nostril bid-tid with progressive weaning as tolerated

Nasal spray: 21 mcg/actuation (30 ml, 345 sprays)

Atrovent Nasal Spray 0.06% <5 years: not recommended; ≥5-11 years: 2 sprays in each nostril tid; ≥11 years: 2 sprays in each nostril tid-qid with progressive weaning as tolerated

Nasal spray: 42 mcg/actuation (15 ml, 165 sprays)

Comment: Avoid use with narrow-angle glaucoma, prostate hyperplasia, and bladder neck obstruction

NASAL ANTIHISTAMINE

▶ *azelastine* (C) <5 years: not recommended; ≥5-12 years: 1 spray in each nostril bid >12 years: 2 sprays in each nostril bid

Astelin Ready Spray *Nasal spray:* 137 mcg/actuation (30 ml, 200 sprays)

FIRST GENERATION ORAL ANTIHISTAMINES

▶ *diphenhydramine* (B)(G) <2 years: not recommended; 2-6 years: 6.25 mg q 4-6 hours; max 37.5 mg/day; >6-12 years: 12.5-25 mg q 4-6 hours; max 150 mg/day; >12 years: 25-50 mg q 6-8 hours; max 100 mg/day

Benadryl (OTC) *Chew tab:* 12.5 mg (grape) (phenylalanine); *Liq:* 12.5 mg/5 ml (4, 8 oz); *Cap:* 25 mg; *Tab:* 25 mg; *Dye-free soft gel:* 25 mg; *Dye-free liq:* 12.5 mg/5 ml (4, 8 oz)

▶ *hydroxyzine* (C)(G) <6 years: 50 mg/day divided qid prn; ≥6 years: 50-100 mg/day divided qid prn; max 600 mg/day; 25 mg tid prn; max 600 mg/day

Atarax *Tab:* 10, 25, 50, 100 mg; *Syr:* 10 mg/5 ml (alcohol 0.5%)

Vistaril *Cap:* 25, 50, 100 mg; *Oral susp:* 25 mg/5 ml (4 oz) (lemon)

SECOND GENERATION ANTIHISTAMINES

Comment: Second generation antihistamines are sedating, but much less so than the first generation antihistamines. All antihistamines are excreted into breast milk.

- ***cetirizine*** (C)(OTC)(G) <6 years: not recommended; ≥6-<65 years: initially 5-10 mg once daily; ≥65 years: 5 mg once daily
  - **Children's Zyrtec Chewable** *Chew tab:* 5, 10 mg (grape)
  - **Children's Zyrtec Allergy Syrup** *Syr:* 1 mg/ml (4 oz) (grape, bubble gum) (sugar-free, dye-free)
  - **Zyrtec** *Tab:* 10 mg
  - **Zyrtec Hives Relief** *Tab:* 10 mg
  - **Zyrtec Liquid Gels** *Liq gel:* 10 mg
- ***desloratadine*** (C)
  - **Clarinex** <6 years: not recommended; ≥6 years: 1/2-1 tab once daily
    Tab: 5 mg
  - **Clarinex RediTabs** <6 years: not recommended; 6-12 years: 2.5 mg once daily; ≥12 years: 5 mg once daily
    ODT: 2.5, 5 mg (tutti-frutti) (phenylalanine)
  - **Clarinex Syrup** <6 months: not recommended; 6-11 months: 1 mg (2 ml) once daily; 1-5 years: 1.25 mg (2.5 ml) once daily; 6-11 years: 2.5 mg (5 ml) once daily; ≥12 years: 5 mg (10 ml) once daily
    Tab: 0.5 mg per ml (4 oz) (tutti-frutti) (phenylalanine)
  - **Desloratadine ODT**
- ***fexofenadine*** (C)(OTC)(G) 6 months-2 years: 15 mg bid; *CrCl ≤90 mL/min:* 15 mg once daily; 2-11 years: 30 mg bid; *CrCl ≤90 mL/min:* 30 mg once daily ≥12 years and older: ≥12 years: 60 mg once daily-bid <u>or</u> 180 mg once daily; *CrCl <90 mL/min:* 60 mg once daily **Allegra** *Tab:* 30, 60, 180 mg film-coat
  - **Allegra Allergy** *Tab:* 60, 180 mg film-coat
  - **Allegra ODT** *ODT:* 30 mg (phenylalanine)
  - **Allegra Oral Suspension** *Oral susp:* 30 mg/5 ml (6 mg/ml) (4 oz)
- ***levocetirizine*** (B)(OTC) administer dose in the PM; *Seasonal Allergic Rhinitis:* <2 years: not recommended; may start at ≥2 years; *Chronic Spontaneous/Idiopathic Urticaria (CSU/CIU), Perennial Allergic Rhinitis:* <6 months: not recommended; may start at ≥ 6 months; *Dosing by Age:* 6 months-5 years: max 1.25 mg once daily; 6-11 years: max 2.5 mg once daily; ≥12 years: 2.5-5 mg once daily; *Renal Dysfunction <12 years:* contraindicated; *Renal Dysfunction ≥12 years: CrCl 50-80 mL/min:* 2.5 mg once daily; *CrCl 30-50 mL/min:* 2.5 mg every other day; *CrCl: 10-30 mL/min:* 2.5 mg twice weekly (every 3-4 days); *CrCl <10 mL/min, ESRD <u>or</u> hemodialysis:* contraindicated
  - **Children's Xyzal Allergy 24HR** *Oral Soln:* 0.5 mg/ml (150 ml)
  - **Xyzal Allergy 24HR***Tab:* 5*mg
- ***loratadine*** (C)(OTC)(G) <2 years: not recommended; 2-5 years: 5 mg once daily; ≥6 years: 5 mg bid <u>or</u> 10 mg once daily; *Hepatic <u>or</u> Renal Insufficiency:* (see mfr pkg insert)
  - **Children's Claritin Chewables** *Chew tab:* 5 mg (grape) (phenylalanine)
  - **Children's Claritin Syrup** 1 mg/ml (4 oz) (fruit) (sugar-free, alcohol-free, dye-free; sodium 6 mg/5 ml)
  - **Claritin** *Tab:* 10 mg
  - **Claritin Hives Relief** *Tab:* 10 mg
  - **Claritin Liqui-Gels** *Lig gel:* 10 mg
  - **Claritin RediTabs 12 Hours** *ODT:* 5 mg (mint)
  - **Claritin RediTabs 24 Hours** *ODT:* 10 mg (mint)

RHINITIS: VASOMOTOR

NASAL ANTICHOLINERGICS

Comment: Avoid use with narrow-angle glaucoma, prostate hyperplasia, and bladder neck obstruction

▶ *ipratropium bromide* (B)(G)

Atrovent Nasal Spray 0.03% <6 years: not recommended; ≥6 years: stop nasal decongestant; 2 sprays in each nostril bid-tid with progressive weaning as tolerated

Nasal spray: 21 mcg/actuation (30 ml, 345 sprays)

Atrovent Nasal Spray 0.06% <5 years: not recommended; ≥5-11 years: 2 sprays in each nostril tid; >11 years: stop nasal decongestant; 2 sprays in each nostril tid-qid with progressive weaning as tolerated

Nasal spray: 42 mcg/actuation (15 ml, 165 sprays)

ROSEOLA INFANTUM (EXANTHUM SUBITUM)

Antipyretics *see **Fever** page* 149

Comment: Roseola infantum (also known as exanthem subitum, sixth disease, pseudorubella, exanthem criticum, and three-day fever) is a generally mild clinical syndrome, commonly occurring in children ≤3 years-of-age, characterized by sudden onset of high fever (may exceed 40°C [104°F])that lasts 3 days and resolves abruptly, and is followed by development of a rash lasting ≤3 days. Roseola usually is caused by human herpesvirus 6 (HHV-6). Treatment is antipyretics (***aspirin*** is contraindicated) and adequate hydration. Monitor for febrile seizures. As with the common cold, roseola spreads from person to person through contact with an infected person's respiratory secretions <u>or</u> saliva. The disease can occur at any time of year.

ROCKY MOUNTAIN SPOTTED FEVER (*RICKETTSIA RICKETTSII*)

ANTI-INFECTIVES

▶ ***doxycycline*** (D)(G) <8 years: not recommended; ≥8 years, ≤100 lb: 2-2.5 mg/kg q 12 hours x 7-10 days; ≥8 years, >100 lb: 200 mg on first day; then 100 mg bid x 7-10 days

Acticlate *Tab:* 75, 150**mg

Adoxa *Tab:* 50, 75, 100, 150 mg ent-coat

Doryx *Tab:* 50, 75, 100, 150, 200 mg del-rel

Doxteric *Tab:* 50 mg del-rel

Monodox *Cap:* 50, 75, 100 mg

Oracea *Cap:* 40 mg del-rel

Vibramycin *Tab:* 100 mg; *Cap:* 50, 100 mg; *Syr:* 50 mg/5 ml (raspberry-apple) (sulfites); *Oral susp:* 25 mg/5 ml (raspberry)

Vibra-Tab *Tab:* 100 mg film-coat

Comment: ***doxycycline*** contraindicated <8 years-of-age, in pregnancy, and lactation (discolors developing tooth enamel). A side effect may be photosensitivity (photophobia). Do not take with antacids, calcium supplements, milk <u>or</u> other dairy, <u>or</u> within 2 hours of taking another drug.

▶ ***tetracycline*** (D)(G) <8 years: not recommended; ≥8 years, ≤100 lb: 10 mg/kg/day divided q 6 hours x 7-10 days; *see page* 618 *for dose by weight table*; ≥8 years, >100 lb: 500 mg q 6 hours x 7-10 days

Achromycin V *Cap:* 250, 500 mg

Sumycin *Tab:* 250, 500 mg; *Cap:* 250, 500 mg; *Oral susp:* 125 mg/5 ml (100, 200 ml) (fruit) (sulfites)

Comment: ***tetracycline*** is contraindicated <8 years-of-age, in pregnancy, and lactation (discolors developing tooth enamel). A side effect may be photosensitivity (photophobia). Do not give with antacids, calcium supplements, milk or other dairy, or within two hours of taking another drug.

ROTAVIRUS GASTROENTERITIS

PROPHYLAXIS

Comment: **RotaTeq** targets the most common strains of rotavirus (G1, G2, G3, G4), which are responsible for more than 90% of rotavirus disease in the United States.

- ***rotavirus vaccine, live*** <6 weeks or >32 weeks: not recommended; >6 weeks and <32 weeks: administer 1st dose at 6-12 weeks of age; administer 2nd and 3rd doses at 4-10-week intervals for a total of 3 doses; if an incomplete dose is administered, do not administer a replacement dose, but continue with the remaining doses in the recommended series

  RotaTeq *Oral susp:* 2 ml single-use tube (fetal bovine serum [trace], preservative-free, thimerosal-free)

ROUNDWORM (ASCARIASIS)

ANTHELMINTICS

Comment: Oral bioavailability of anthelmintics is enhanced when administered with a fatty meal (estimated fat content 40 gm).

- ***albendazole*** **(C)** take with a meal; may crush and mix with food; may repeat in 3 weeks if needed; <2 years: 200 mg bid x 7 days; 2-12 years: 400 mg once daily x 7 days; >12 years: 400 mg bid x 7 days

  Albenza *Tab:* 200 mg

Comment: ***albendazole*** is a broad-spectrum benzimidazole carbamate anthelmintic.

- ***ivermectin*** **(C)** take with water; chew or crush and mix with food; may repeat in 3 months if needed; <15 kg: not recommended; ≥15 kg: 200 mcg/kg as a single dose

  Stromectol *Tab:* 3, 6*mg

- ***mebendazole*** **(C)(G)** take with a meal; chew or crush and mix with food; may repeat in 3 weeks if needed; <2 years: not recommended; ≥2 years: 100 mg bid x 3 days

  Emverm *Chew tab:* 100 mg

  Vermox *Chew tab:* 100 mg

- ***pyrantel pamoate*** **(C)** take with a meal; may open capsule and sprinkle or mix with food; treat x 3 days; may repeat in 2-3 weeks if needed; treat x 3 days; 11 mg/kg/dose; max 1 gm/dose; <25 lb: not recommended; 25-37 lb: 1/2 tsp/dose; 38-62 lb: 1 tsp/dose; 63-87 lb: 1 tsp/dose; 88-112 lb: 2 tsp/dose; 113-137 lb: 2 tsp/dose; 138-162 lb: 3 tsp/dose; 163-187 lb: 3 tsp/dose; >187 lb: 4 tsp/dose

  Antiminth *Cap:* 180 mg; *Liq:* 50 mg/ml (30 ml); 144 mg/ml (30 ml); *Oral susp:* 50 mg/ml (60 ml)

  Pin-X *Cap:* 180 mg; *Liq:* 50 mg/ml (30 ml); 144 mg/ml (30 ml); *Oral susp:* 50 mg/ml (30 ml)

- ***thiabendazole*** **(C)** take with a meal; may crush and mix with food; treat x 7 days; <30 lb: consult mfr pkg insert; ≥30 lb: 25 mg/kg/dose bid with meals; 30-50 lb: 250 mg bid with meals; >50 lb: 10 mg/lb/dose bid with meals; max 1.5 gm/dose; max 3 gm/day

  Mintezol *Chew tab:* 500*mg (orange); *Oral susp:* 500 mg/5 ml (120 ml) (orange)

Comment: ***thiabendazole*** is not for prophylaxis. May impair mental alertness. May not be available in the US.

RUBELLA (GERMAN MEASLES)

Antipyretics see *Fever* page 149

Comment: Rubella is highly contagious and highly teratogenic. Quarantine is mandatory to prevent a community outbreak. Herd immunity is the best prevention.

PROPHYLAXIS VACCINE

See *Childhood Immunizations* page 525

▶ ***rubella virus, live, attenuated, neomycin*** vaccine (C)
  Meruvax II 25 mcg (0.5 ml)
▶ ***measles, mumps, rubella, live, attenuated, neomycin vaccine*** (C)
  MMR II 25 mcg (preservative-free)

Comment: Contraindications: hypersensitivity to *neomycin* or eggs, primary or acquired immune deficiency, immunosuppressant therapy, bone marrow or lymphatic malignancy, and pregnancy (within 3 months following vaccination).

TREATMENT

▶ ***immune globulin*** (Ig) 0.25 ml/kg IM (0.5 mg/kg in immunocompromised children)

RUBEOLA (RED MEASLES)

Antipyretics see *Fever* page 149

PROPHYLAXIS VACCINE

See *Childhood Immunizations* page 525

▶ ***measles, mumps, rubella, live, attenuated, neomycin vaccine*** (C)
  MMR II 25 mcg (preservative-free)
  Comment: Contraindications: hypersensitivity to ***neomycin*** or eggs (controversial), primary or acquired immune deficiency, immunosuppressant therapy, bone marrow or lymphatic malignancy, and pregnancy (within 3 months following vaccination).

TREATMENT

▶ ***immune globulin*** (Ig) 0.25 ml/kg IM (0.5 mg/kg in immunocompromised children)

SALMONELLOSIS

▶ ***ciprofloxacin*** (C) <18 years: not recommended; ≥18 years: 500 mg bid x 3-5 days; max 1.5 gm/day
  Cipro (G) *Tab:* 250, 500, 750 mg; *Oral susp:* 250, 500 mg/5 ml (100 ml) (strawberry)
  Cipro XR *Tab:* 500, 1000 mg ext-rel
  ProQuin XR *Tab:* 500 mg ext-rel

Comment: ***ciprofloxacin*** is contraindicated <18 years-of-age, and during pregnancy and lactation. Risk of tendonitis or tendon rupture.

▶ ***trimethoprim+sulfamethoxazole [TMP-SMX]*** (D)(G)
  Bactrim, Septra <12 years: not recommended; ≥12 years: 2 tabs bid x 10 days
    Tab: trim 80 mg+sulfa 400 mg*

Bactrim DS, Septra DS <12 years: not recommended; ≥12 years: 1 tab bid x 10 days
Tab: trim 160 mg+sulfa 800 mg*
Bactrim Pediatric Suspension, Septra Pediatric Suspension <2 months: not recommended; ≥2 months-12 years: 40 mg/kg/day of ***sulfamethoxazole*** in 2 doses bid; >12 years: use tabs
Oral susp: trim 40 mg+sulfa 200 mg per 5 ml (100 ml) (cherry) (alcohol 0.3%)

SCABIES (*SARCOPTES SCABIEI*)

Comment: This section presents treatment regimens for scabies infestation published in the **2015 CDC Sexually Transmitted Diseases Treatment Guidelines**, as well as other available treatments.

RECOMMENDED REGIMEN

▶ ***permethrin*** (B)(G) <2 months: not recommended; ≥2 months: massage into skin from head to soles of feet; leave on x 8-14 hours, then rinse off
Acticin, Elimite *Crm:* 5% (60 gm)

ALTERNATIVE REGIMEN

▶ ***lindane*** (B)(G) <2 months: not recommended; ≥2 months: 1 oz of lotion or 30 gm of cream apply to all skin surfaces from neck down to the soles of the feet; leave on x 8 hours, then wash off thoroughly; may repeat if needed in 14 days
Kwell *Lotn:* 1% (60, 473 ml); *Crm:* 1% (60 gm); *Shampoo:* 1% (60, 473 ml)

OTHER TOPICAL TREATMENTS

▶ ***crotamiton*** (C) <12 years: not recommended; ≥12 years: massage into skin from chin down; repeat in 24 hours
Eurax *Lotn:* 10% (60 gm); *Crm:* 10% (60 gm)

SCARLET FEVER (SCARLATINA)

Comment: Microorganism responsible for scarlet fever is Group A beta-hemolytic *Streptococcus* (GABHS). Strep cultures and screens will be positive.

▶ ***azithromycin*** (B)(G) <12 years: 12 mg/kg/day x 5 days; *see page* 593 *for dose by weight table;* max 500 mg/day; ≥12 years: 500 mg x 1 dose on day 1, then 250 mg once daily on days 2-5 or 500 mg once daily x 5 days
Zithromax *Tab:* 250, 500, 600 mg; *Oral susp:* 100 mg/5 ml (15 ml); 200 mg/5 ml (15, 22.5, 30 ml) (cherry); *Pkt:* 1 gm for reconstitution (cherry-banana)
Zithromax Tri-pak *Tab:* 3 x 500 mg tabs/pck
Zithromax Z-pak *Tab:* 6 x 250 mg tabs/pck
Zmax *Oral susp:* 2 gm ext-rel for reconstitution (cherry-banana) (148 mg Na^+)

▶ ***cefadroxil*** <12 years: 30 mg/kg/day in 2 divided doses x 10 days; *see page* 595 *for dose by weight table;* ≥12 years: 1-2 gm in a single or 2 divided doses x 10 days
Duricef *Cap:* 500 mg; *Tab:* 1 gm; *Oral susp:* 250 mg/5 ml (100 ml); 500 mg/5 ml (75, 100 ml) (orange-pineapple)

▶ ***cephalexin*** (B)(G)25-50 mg/kg/day in 2 divided doses x 10 days; *see page* 601 *for dose by weight table*
Keflex *Cap:* 250, 333, 500, 750 mg; *Oral susp:* 125, 250 mg/5 ml (100, 200 ml) (strawberry)

- ***clarithromycin*** **(C)(G)** <6 months: not recommended; ≥6 months-12 years: 7.5 mg/kg bid x 14-21 days; *see page 602 for dose by weight table;* >12 years: 500 mg bid or 500 mg ext-rel daily x 14-21 days

  Biaxin *Tab:* 250, 500 mg
  Biaxin Oral Suspension *Oral susp:* 125, 250 mg/5 ml (50, 100 ml) (fruit punch)
  Biaxin XL *Tab:* 500 mg ext-rel

Comment: The FDA is advising caution before prescribing ***clarithromycin*** to patients with heart disease because of a potential increased risk of heart problems or death that can occur years later. This recommendation is based on a review of the results of a 10-year follow-up study of patients with coronary heart disease from a large clinical trial that first observed this safety issue. Consider risk benefit and the use of other antibiotics in such patients.

- ***clindamycin*** **(B)(G)** <12 years: 8-16 mg/kg/day in 3-4 divided doses x 10 days; *see page 603 for dose by weight table;* ≥12 years: 150-300 mg q 6 hours x 10 days

  Cleocin *Cap:* 75 (tartrazine), 150 (tartrazine), 300 mg
  Cleocin Pediatric Granules *Oral susp:* 75 mg/5 ml (100 ml) (cherry)

- ***erythromycin estolate*** **(B)(G)** <12 years: 20-50 mg/kg q 6 hours x 10 days; *see page 606 for dose by weight table;* ≥12 years: 250 mg q 6 hours x 10 days

  Ilosone *Pulvule:* 250 mg; *Tab:* 500 mg; *Liq:* 125, 250 mg/5 ml (100 ml)

- ***erythromycin ethylsuccinate*** **(B)(G)** 30-50 mg/kg/day in 4 divided doses x 10 days; may double dose with severe infection; max 100 mg/kg/day or 400 mg qid; *see page 607 for dose by weight table*

  EryPed *Oral susp:* 200 mg/5 ml (100, 200 ml) (fruit); 400 mg/5 ml (60, 100, 200 ml) (banana); *Oral drops:* 200, 400 mg/5 ml (50 ml) (fruit); *Chew tab:* 200 mg wafer (fruit)
  E.E.S. *Oral susp:* 200, 400 mg/5 ml (100 ml) (fruit)
  E.E.S. Granules *Oral susp:* 200 mg/5 ml (100, 200 ml) (cherry)
  E.E.S. 400 Tablets *Tab:* 400 mg

- ***penicillin g (benzathine + procaine)*** **(B)(G)** <30 lb: 600,000 units IM x 1 dose; 30-60 lb: 900,000-1.2 million units IM x 1 dose; >60 lbs: 2.4 million units IM x 1 dose

  Bicillin C-R Cartridge-needle unit: 600,000 units (1 ml); 1.2 million units; (2 ml); 2.4 million units (4 ml)

- ***penicillin v potassium*** **(B)** <12 years: 25-75 mg/kg day divided q 6-8 hours x 10 days; *see page 616 for dose by weight table;* ≥12 years: 250 mg tid x 10 days

  Pen-VK *Tab:* 250, 500 mg; *Oral soln:* 125 mg/5 ml (100, 200 ml); 250 mg/5 ml (100, 150, 200 ml)

SCHISTOSOMIASIS

TREMATODICIDE

Comment: ***praziquantel*** is a trematodicide indicated for the treatment of infections due to all species of Schistosoma (e.g., *Schistosoma mekongi, Schistosoma japonicum, Schistosoma mansoni,* and *Schistosoma hematobium)* and infections due to liver flukes (i.e., *Clonorchis sinensis, Opisthorchis viverrini).* ***praziquantel*** induces a rapid contraction of schistosomes by a specific effect on the permeability of the cell membrane. The drug further causes vacuolization and disintegration of the schistosome tegument.

- ***praziquantel*** **(B)** 20 mg/kg tid as a one-day treatment; take the 3 doses at intervals of not less than 4 hours and not more than 6 hours; swallow whole with water during meals; holding the tablets in the mouth leaves a bitter taste which can trigger gagging or vomiting.

  Pediatric: <4 years: not established; ≥4 years: same as adult
  Biltricide *Tab:* 600 mg film-coat

Comment: Concomitant administration with strong Cytochrome P450 (P450) inducers, such as ***rifampin***, is contraindicated since therapeutically effective blood levels of ***praziquantel*** may not be achieved. In patients receiving ***rifampin*** who need immediate treatment for schistosomiasis, alternative agents for schistosomiasis should be considered. However, if treatment with ***praziquantel*** is necessary, ***rifampin*** should be discontinued 4 weeks before administration of ***praziquantel***. Treatment with ***rifampin*** can then be restarted one day after completion of ***praziquantel*** treatment. Concomitant administration of other P450 inducers (e.g., antiepileptic drugs such as ***phenytoin***, ***phenobarbital***, ***carbamazepine***) and ***dexamethasone***, may also reduce plasma levels of ***praziquantel***. Concomitant administration of P450 inhibitors (e.g., ***cimetidine***, ***ketoconazole***, ***itraconazole***, ***erythromycin***) may increase plasma levels of ***praziquantel***. Patients should be warned not to drive a car or operate machinery on the day of **Biltricide** treatment and the following day. There are no adequate <u>or</u> well-controlled studies in pregnant women. This drug should be used during pregnancy only if clearly needed. ***praziquantel*** appears in the milk of nursing women at a concentration of about 1/4 that of maternal serum. It is not known whether a pharmacological effect is likely to occur in children. Women should not nurse on the day of **Biltricide** treatment and during the subsequent 72 hours.

SCHIZOPHRENIA & SCHIZOPHRENIA WITH CO-MORBID PERSONALITY DISORDER

Other Antipsychosis Drugs *see* **Appendix J: Oral and Depot Antipsychotic Drugs** *page* 557
Tardive Dyskinesia *see page* 440

Comment: A team of researchers examined the effects of antipsychotics on mortality risk in schizophrenia patients. They studied data on 29,823 patients with schizophrenia in Sweden, aged 16 to 64 years and found mortality among patients with schizophrenia was 40% lower when they used antipsychotics as compared to when they did not. Long-acting injection (LAI) use was associated with an approximately 33% lower risk of death compared with the oral use of the same medication. The lowest mortality was observed with use of once-monthly paliperidone LAI, oral aripiprazole, and risperidone LAI.

REFERENCE

Taipale, H, Mittendorfer-Rutz, E, Alexanderson, K, *et al.* (2017). Antipsychotics and mortality in a nationwide cohort of 29,823 patients with schizophrenia. *Schizophrenia Research*. doi:10.1016/j.schres.2017.12.010

➢ ***aripiprazole lauroxil*** **(C)** <18 years: not recommended; >18 years: administer by IM injection in the deltoid (441 mg dose only) <u>or</u> gluteal (441 mg, 662 mg, 882 mg <u>or</u> 1064 mg) muscle by a qualified healthcare professional; initiate at a dose of 441 mg, 662 mg <u>or</u> 882 mg administered monthly, <u>or</u> 882 mg every 6 weeks, <u>or</u> 1064 mg every 2 months

Aristada *Prefilled syringe*: 441, 662, 882, 1064 mg single-use, ext-rel susp

Comment: **Aristada** is an atypical antipsychotic available in 4 doses with 3 dosing duration options for flexible dosing. For patients naïve to ***aripiprazole***, establish tolerability with oral ***aripiprazole*** prior to initiating treatment with **Aristada. Aristada** can be initiated at any of the 4 doses at the appropriate dosing duration option. In conjunction with the first injection, administer treatment with oral ***aripiprazole*** for 21 consecutive days for all 4 dose sizes. The most common adverse event associated with **Aristada** is akathisia. Patients are also at increased risk for developing neuroleptic malignant syndrome, tardive dyskinesia, pathological gambling <u>or</u> other compulsive behaviors, orthostatic hypotension, hyperglycemic, dyslipidemia, and weight gain.

Hypersensitive reactions can occur and range from pruritus or urticaria to anaphylaxis. Stroke, transient ischemic attacks, and falls have been reported in elderly patients with dementia-related psychosis who were treated with ***apriprazole***. **Aristada** is not for treatment of people who have lost touch with reality (psychosis) due to confusion and memory loss (dementia). May cause extrapyramidal and/or withdrawal symptoms in neonates exposed in utero in the third trimester of pregnancy. **Aripiprazole** is present in human breast milk; however, there are insufficient data to assess the amount in human milk or the effects on the breastfed infant. The development and health benefits of breastfeeding should be considered along with the mother's clinical need for **Aristada** and any potential adverse effects on the breastfed infant from **Aristada** or from the underlying maternal condition. For more information or to report ASEs, contact the National Pregnancy Registry for Atypical Antipsychotics at 1-866-961-2388 or visit http://womensmentalhealth.org/clinical-and-research-programs/pregnancyregistry Limited published data on aripiprazole use in pregnant women are not sufficient to inform any drug-associated risks for birth defects or miscarriage. To report suspected adverse reactions, contact Alkermes at 1-866-274-7823 or FDA at 1-800-FDA-1088 or visit www.fda.gov/medwatch

☐ SEIZURE DISORDER

Status Epilepticus *see page* 433
Anticonvulsant Drugs *see page* 560

☐ SEXUAL ASSAULT (STD/STI/VD EXPOSURE)

Comment: The following treatment regimens for victims of sexual assault are published in the **2015 CDC Sexually Transmitted Diseases Treatment Guidelines**.

RECOMMENDED PROPHYLAXIS REGIMEN

- ***ceftriaxone*** 250 mg IM in a single dose plus ***metronidazole*** 2 gm in a single dose plus ***azithromycin*** 1 gm in a single dose

ALTERNATE PROPHYLAXIS REGIMENS

Regimen 1

- ***ceftriaxone*** 250 mg IM in a single dose plus ***metronidazole*** 2 gm in a single dose plus ***doxycycline*** 100 mg bid x 7 days

Regimen 2

- ***cefixime*** 400 mg in a single dose plus ***metronidazole*** 2 gm in a single dose plus ***azithromycin*** 1 gm in a single dose

Regimen 3

- ***cefixime*** 400 mg in a single dose plus ***metronidazole*** 2 gm in a single dose plus ***doxycycline*** 100 mg bid x 7 days

Regimen 4

- ***azithromycin*** 1 gm as a single dose plus ***metronidazole*** 2 gm in a single dose

DRUG BRANDS AND DOSE FORMS

▶ *azithromycin* (B)(G)
  Zithromax *Tab:* 250, 500, 600 mg; *Oral susp:* 100 mg/5 ml (15 ml); 200 mg/5 ml (15, 22.5, 30 ml) (cherry); *Pkt:* 1 gm for reconstitution (cherry-banana)
  Zithromax Tri-pak *Tab:* 3 x 500 mg tabs/pck
  Zithromax Z-pak *Tab:* 6 x 250 mg tabs/pck
  Zmax *Oral susp:* 2 gm ext-rel for reconstitution (cherry-banana) (148 mg Na^{+})
▶ *cefixime* (B)(G)
  Suprax *Tab:* 400 mg; *Cap:* 400 mg; *Oral susp:* 100, 200, 500 mg/5 ml (50, 75, 100 ml) (strawberry)
▶ *ceftriaxone* (B)(G)
  Rocephin *Vial:* 250, 500 mg; 1, 2 gm
▶ *doxycycline* (D)(G)
  Acticlate *Tab:* 75, 150**mg
  Adoxa *Tab:* 50, 75, 100, 150 mg ent-coat
  Doryx *Tab:* 50, 75, 100, 150, 200 mg del-rel
  Doxteric *Tab:* 50 mg del-rel
  Monodox *Cap:* 50, 75, 100 mg
  Oracea *Cap:* 40 mg del-rel
  Vibramycin *Tab:* 100 mg; *Cap:* 50, 100 mg; *Syr:* 50 mg/5 ml (raspberry-apple) (sulfites); *Oral susp:* 25 mg/5 ml (raspberry)
  Vibra-Tab *Tab:* 100 mg film-coat

Comment: ***doxycycline*** is contraindicated <8 years-of-age, in pregnancy, and lactation (discolors developing tooth enamel). A side effect may be photosensitivity (photophobia). Do not take with antacids, calcium supplements, milk or other dairy, or within 2 hours of taking another drug.

▶ ***metronidazole*** **(not for use in 1st; B in 2nd, 3rd)**(G)
  Flagyl *Tab:* 250*, 500*mg
  Flagyl 375 *Cap:* 375 mg
  Flagyl ER *Tab:* 750 mg ext-rel

Comment: Alcohol is contraindicated during treatment with oral ***metronidazole*** and for 72 hours after therapy due to a possible ***disulfiram***-like reaction (nausea, vomiting, flushing, headache).

SHIGELLOSIS

ANTI-INFECTIVES

▶ *azithromycin* (B)(G) <6 months: not recommended; ≥6 months-12 years: 10 mg/kg x 1 dose on day 1; then 5 mg/kg/day on days 2-5; *see page 593 for dose by weight table;* max 500 mg/day; >12 years: 500 mg x 1 dose on day 1, then 250 mg once daily on days 2-5 or 500 mg once daily x 3 days or **Zmax** 2 gm in a single dose
  Zithromax *Tab:* 250, 500, 600 mg; *Oral susp:* 100 mg/5 ml (15 ml); 200 mg/5 ml (15, 22.5, 30 ml) (cherry); *Pkt:* 1 gm for reconstitution (cherry-banana)
  Zithromax Tri-pak *Tab:* 3 x 500 mg tabs/pck
  Zithromax Z-pak *Tab:* 6 x 250 mg tabs/pck
  Zmax *Oral susp:* 2 gm ext-rel for reconstitution (cherry-banana) (148 mg Na^{+})
▶ *ciprofloxacin* (C) <18 years: not recommended; ≥18 years: 500 mg bid x 3 days; max 1.5 gm/day
  Cipro (G) *Tab:* 250, 500, 750 mg; *Oral susp:* 250, 500 mg/5 ml (100 ml) (strawberry)

Cipro XR *Tab:* 500, 1000 mg ext-rel
ProQuin XR *Tab:* 500 mg ext-rel

Comment: ***ciprofloxacin*** is contraindicated <18 years-of-age, and during pregnancy and lactation. Risk of tendonitis or tendon rupture.

- ***ofloxacin*** **(C)(G)** <18 years: not recommended; ≥18 years: 400 mg bid x 3 days
  Floxin *Tab:* 200, 300, 400 mg

Comment: ***ofloxacin*** is contraindicated <18 years-of-age, and during pregnancy and lactation. Risk of tendonitis or tendon rupture.

- ***tetracycline*** **(D)(G)** <8 years: not recommended; ≥8 years, ≤100 lb: 25-50 mg/kg/day in 4 divided doses x 5 days; *see page* 618 *for dose by weight table*; ≥8 years, >100 lb: 250-500 mg qid x 5 days
  Achromycin V *Cap:* 250, 500 mg
  Sumycin *Tab:* 250, 500 mg; *Cap:* 250, 500 mg; *Oral susp:* 125 mg/5 ml (100, 200 ml) (fruit) (sulfites)

Comment: ***tetracycline*** is contraindicated <8 years-of-age, in pregnancy, and lactation (discolors developing tooth enamel). A side effect may be photosensitivity (photophobia). Do not give with antacids, calcium supplements, milk or other dairy, or within two hours of taking another drug.

- ***trimethoprim+sulfamethoxazole [TMP-SMX]*** **(D)(G)**
  Bactrim, Septra <12 years: not recommended; ≥12 years: 2 tabs bid x 10 days
  Tab: trim 80 mg+sulfa 400 mg*
  Bactrim DS, Septra DS <12 years: not recommended; ≥12 years: 1 tab bid x 10 days
  Tab: trim 160 mg+sulfa 800 mg*
  Bactrim Pediatric Suspension, Septra Pediatric Suspension <2 months: not recommended; ≥2 months-12 years: 40 mg/kg/day of ***sulfamethoxazole*** in 2 doses bid; >12 years: use tabs
  Oral susp: trim 40 mg+sulfa 200 mg per 5 ml (100 ml) (cherry) (alcohol 0.3%)

SHOCK (SEPTIC AND OTHER DISTRIBUTIVE)

Comment: Septic shock is the most common form of distributive shock and is characterized by considerable mortality (treated, around 30%; untreated, probably >80%). In the United States, septic shock is the leading cause of non-cardiac death in intensive care units. **Giapreza (angiotensin II)** received accelerated review and FDA approval December 2017 to increase blood pressure, when added to conventional interventions used to raise blood pressure, to prevent/treat dangerously low hypotension resulting from septic and other distributive shock states. There is a potential for venous and arterial thrombotic and thromboembolic events in patients who receive **Giapreza**. Therefore, use concurrent venous thromboembolism (VTE) prophylaxis. **Giapreza** is available March 2018.

ANGIOTENSIN II

- ***angiotensin II*** dilute in 0.9% NaCl; must be administered as an IV infusion; initial infusion rate 20 ng/kg/min; titrate as frequently as every 5 minutes by increments of up to 15 ng/kg/min as needed; during the first 3 hours, max 80 ng/kg/min; max maintenance dose 40 ng/kg/min; diluted solution may be stored at room temperature or refrigerated; discard after 24 hours.
  Dilution/Concentration:
  Giapreza 1 ml (2.5 mg/ml) in 500 ml 0.9%NaCl = 5,000 ng/ml
  1 ml (2.5.mg/ml in 250 ml 0.9%NaCl = 10,000 ng/ml
  2 ml (5 mg/ml) in 500 ml 0.9%NaCl = 10,000 ng/ml
  Giapreza Vial: 2.5 mg in ml, 5 mg/2 ml (2.5 mg/ml)

Comment: The safety and efficacy of **Giapreza** in pediatric patients have not been established. It is not known whether ***Giapreza*** is present in human milk and no data are available on the effects of angiotensin II on the breastfed child. The published data on angiotensin II use in pregnant women are not sufficient to determine a drug-associated risk of adverse developmental outcomes. However, Delaying treatment in pregnant women with hypotension associated with septic or other distributive shock is likely to increase the risk of shock-associated maternal and fetal morbidity and mortality.

SICKLE CELL DISEASE (SCD)

▶ *hydroxyurea*

Comment: ***hydroxyurea*** has an FDA-approved "orphan drug" designation for the treatment of sickle cell disease SCD). It is an antimetabolite indicated to reduce the frequency of painful crises and to reduce the need for blood transfusions in patients with sickle cell anemia with recurrent moderate to severe painful crises. ***Black Box Warning (BBW): hydroxyurea*** may cause severe myelosuppression. Do not administer if bone marrow function is markedly depressed. Monitor blood counts at baseline and every 2 weeks throughout treatment. Blood counts within an acceptable range are defined as: *neutrophils* > 2,500 cells/mm3, *platelets* >95,000 cells/mm3, *Hgb* >5.3 gm/dL, *reticulocytes* >95,000 cells/mm3 if the Hgb <9 gm/dL. Discontinue ***hydroxyurea*** until hematologic recovery if blood counts are considered toxic. Treatment may be resumed after reducing the ***hydroxyurea*** dose by 2.5 mg/kg/day from the dose associated with hematological toxicity. *CrCl <60 mL/min:* reduce dose by 50%. ***hydroxyurea*** is carcinogenic. Advise sun protection and monitor patients for malignancies. Avoid live vaccines when using ***hydroyurea***. Discontinue ***hydroxyurea*** if vasculitic toxicity occurs. Risks with concomitant use of antiretroviral drugs: pancreatitis, hepatotoxicity, and neuropathy. Monitor for signs and symptoms in patients with HIV infection using antiretroviral drugs. If patients with HIV infection are treated with ***hydroxyurea***, and in particular, in combination with ***didanosine*** and/or ***stavudine***, close monitoring for signs and symptoms of pancreatitis is recommended. Permanently discontinue ***hydroxyurea*** in patients who develop signs and symptoms of pancreatitis. ***hydroxyurea*** can cause fetal harm (embryotoxic and teratogenic effects in animal studies). Advise patients regarding potential risk to a fetus and use of effecttive contraception during and after treatment with **hydroxyurea** for at least 6 months after therapy is ended. Advise females to immediately report pregnancy. ***Hydroxyurea*** may damage spermatozoa and testicular tissue, resulting in possible genetic abnormalities. Azoospermia or oligospermia, sometimes reversible, has been observed in men. Inform male patients about the possibility of sperm conservation before the initiation of ***hydroxyurea*** therapy. Males with female sexual partners of reproductive potential should use effective contraception during and after treatment for at least 1 year. ***hydroxyurea*** is excreted in human milk. Discontinue breastfeeding during treatment. To report suspected adverse reactions, contact Bristol-Myers Squibb at 1-800-721-5072 or FDA at 1-800-FDA-1088 or visit www.fda.gov/medwatch

Droxia use actual or ideal body weigh (whichever is less) for dosing. ***<18 years: not established: >18 years:*** initially 15 mg/kg once daily; if the blood counts are within an acceptable range, increase the dose by 5 mg/kg/day every 12 weeks to the highest dose that does not produce toxic blood counts over 24 consecutive weeks (dosage should not exceed 35 mg/kg/day).

Cap: 200, 300, 400 mg

Hydrea *(see* **Droxia** *for prescribing information)*

Tab: 500 mg

Siklos use actual or ideal body weight (whichever is less) for dosing <2 years: not recommended; >2 years: initially 20 mg/kg once daily; may be increased by 5 mg/

kg/day every 8 weeks, or sooner if a severe painful crisis occurs, until a maximum tolerated dose or 35 mg/kg/day is reached; reduce the dose of **Siklos** by 50% (10 mg) in patients with CrCl <60 mL/min or with ESRD

*Tab: 100 mg; 1,000***mg*

Comment: Safety and effectiveness of **Siklos** have been established in pediatric patients aged 2-18 years with sickle cell anemia (SSA) with recurrent moderate to severe painful crises and is the only ***hydroxyurea*** approved for use in children. Use of **Siklos** in these age groups is supported by evidence from a non-interventional cohort study, the European Sickle Cell Disease prospective Cohort study, ESCORT-HU, in which 405 pediatric patients ages 2 to <18 were treated with **Siklos**: n=274 children (2-11 years) and n=108 adolescents 12-16 years). Pediatric patients aged 2-16 years had a higher risk of neutropenia than patients >16 years. Continuous follow-up of the growth of treated children is recommended.

AMINO ACID

▶ ***L-glutamine*** **<5 years: not recommended; >5 years:** 5-15 grams (1-3 pkts) twice daily based on body weight; <30 kg (<66 lb): 5 gm bid; 30-65 kg (66-143 lb): 10 gm bid; >65 kg (>143 lb): 15 gm bid; mix each dose in 8 oz. (240 mL) of cold or room temperature beverage or 4-6 oz of food (e.g., applesauce or yogurt) before ingestion; complete dissolution is not required prior to administration

Endari *Oral pwdr: 5 gm/pkt for oral soln (60 pkts/carton)*

Comment: ***L-glutamine*** oral powder is indicated to reduce the acute complications of sickle cell disease (SSD). ***L-glutamine*** is an amino acid that is presumed to work by improving the NAD redox potential in sickle red blood cells through increasing the availability of reduced glutathione. That is, ***L-glutamine*** reduces oxidant damage to red blood cells by improving the redox potential of nicotinamide adenine dinucleotide (NAD), a coenzyme that has been identified as the primary regulator of oxidation. There are no data on the presence of **Endari** in human milk or effect on the breastfed infant. There are no known contraindications. Safety and effectiveness of **Endari** have not been established in patients <5 years. Most common adverse reactions are constipation, nausea, headache, abdominal pain, cough, pain in extremity, back pain, and chest pain. To report suspected adverse reactions, contact Emmaus Medical at 1-877-420-6493 or FDA at 1-800-FDA-1088 or visit www.fda.gov/medwatch

SINUSITIS & RHINOSINUSITIS: ACUTE BACTERIAL (ABRS)

ANTI-INFECTIVES

▶ ***amoxicillin*** (B)(G) <40 kg (88 lb): 20-40 mg/kg/day in 3 divided doses x 10 days or 25-45 mg/kg/day in 2 divided doses x 10 days; *see page* 588 *for dose by weight table;* ≥40 kg: 500-875 mg bid or 250-500 mg tid x 10 days

Amoxil *Cap:* 250, 500 mg; *Tab:* 875*mg; *Chew tab:* 125, 200, 250, 400 mg (cherry-banana-peppermint) (phenylalanine); *Oral susp:* 125, 250 mg/5 ml (80, 100, 150 ml) (strawberry); 200, 400 mg/5 ml (50, 75, 100 ml) (bubble gum); *Oral drops:* 50 mg/ml (30 ml) (bubble gum)

Moxatag *Tab:* 775 mg ext-rel

Trimox *Tab:* 125, 250 mg; *Cap:* 250, 500 mg; *Oral susp:* 125, 250 mg/5 ml (80, 100, 150 ml) (raspberry-strawberry)

▶ ***amoxicillin+clavulanate*** (B)(G)

Augmentin <40 kg: 40-45 mg/kg/day divided tid x 10 days or 90 mg/kg/day divided bid x 10 days; *see page* 590 *for dose by weight table;* ≥40 kg: 500 mg tid or 875 mg bid x 10 days

Tab: 250, 500, 875 mg; *Chew tab:* 125, 250 mg (lemon-lime); 200, 400 mg (cherry-banana) (phenylalanine); *Oral susp:* 125 mg/5 ml (banana), 250 mg/5 ml (75, 100, 150 ml) (orange); 200, 400 mg/5 ml (50, 75, 100 ml) (orange) (phenylalanine)

Augmentin ES-600 <3 months: not recommended; ≥3 months, <40 kg: 90 mg/kg/day divided q 12 hours x 10 days; *see page* 591 *for dose by weight table;* ≥40 kg: use tab

Oral susp: 600 mg/5 ml (50, 75, 100, 125, 150, 200 ml) (strawberry cream) (phenylalanine)

Augmentin XR <16 years: use other forms; ≥16 years: 2 tabs q 12 hours x 7-10 days

Tab: 1000*mg ext-rel

▶ ***cefaclor*** **(B)(G)** <1 month: not recommended; 1 month-12 years: 20-40 mg/kg divided bid x 10 days; *see page* 594 *for dose by weight table;* max 1 gm/day; >12 years: 250-500 mg q 8 hours x 10 days; max 2 gm/day

Tab: 500 mg; *Cap:* 250, 500 mg; *Susp:* 125 mg/5 ml (75, 150 ml) (strawberry); 187 mg/5 ml (50, 100 ml) (strawberry); 250 mg/5 ml (75, 150 ml) (strawberry); 375 mg/5 ml (50, 100 ml) (strawberry)

Cefaclor Extended Release <16 years: not recommended; ≥16 years: 500 mg bid x 10 days (clinically equivalent to 250 mg immed-rel caps tid); swallow whole; take with food

Tab: 375, 500 mg ext-rel

▶ ***cefdinir*** **(B)** <6 months: not recommended; 6 months-12 years: 14 mg/kg/day in a single or 2 divided doses x 10 days; *see page* 596 *for dose by weight table;* >12 years: 300 mg bid or 600 mg once daily x 10 days

Omnicef *Cap:* 300 mg; *Oral susp:* 125 mg/5 ml (60, 100 ml) (strawberry)

▶ ***cefixime*** **(B)(G)** <6 months: not recommended; 6 months-12 years, <50 kg: 8 mg/kg/day in 1-2 divided doses x 10 days; *see page* 597 *for dose by weight table;* >12 years, >50 kg: 400 mg once daily x 10 days

Suprax *Tab:* 400 mg; *Cap:* 400 mg; *Oral susp:* 100, 200, 500 mg/5 ml (50, 75, 100 ml) (strawberry)

▶ ***cefpodoxime proxetil*** <2 months: not recommended; 2 months-12 years: 10 mg/kg/day (max 400 mg/dose) or 5 mg/kg/day bid (max 200 mg/dose) x 10 days; *see page* 598 *for dose by weight table;* >12 years: 200 mg bid x 10 days

Vantin *Tab:* 100, 200 mg; *Oral susp:* 50, 100 mg/5 ml (50, 75, 100 mg) (lemon creme)

▶ ***cefprozil*** **(B)** <6 months: not recommended; 6 months-12 years: *Mild:* 7.5 mg/kg bid x 10 days; *Moderate/Severe:* 15 mg/kg q 12 hours x 10 days; *see page* 599 *for dose by weight table;* >12 years: 250-500 mg bid x 10 days

Cefzil *Tab:* 250, 500 mg; *Oral susp:* 125, 250 mg/5 ml (50, 75, 100 ml) (bubble gum) (phenylalanine)

▶ ***ceftibuten*** **(B)** <12 years: 9 mg/kg once daily x 10 days; max 400 mg/day; *see page* 600 *for dose by weight table;* ≥12 years: 400 mg once daily x 10 days

Cedax *Cap:* 400 mg; *Oral susp:* 90 mg/5 ml (30, 60, 90, 120 ml); 180 mg/5 ml (30, 60, 120 ml) (cherry)

▶ ***ciprofloxacin*** **(C)** <18 years: not recommended; ≥18 years: 500 mg bid x 10 days; max 1.5 gm/day

Cipro (G) *Tab:* 250, 500, 750 mg; *Oral susp:* 250, 500 mg/5 ml (100 ml) (strawberry)

Cipro XR *Tab:* 500, 1000 mg ext-rel

ProQuin XR *Tab:* 500 mg ext-rel

Comment: ***ciprofloxacin*** is contraindicated <18 years-of-age, and during pregnancy and lactation. Risk of tendonitis or tendon rupture.

▶ ***clarithromycin*** **(C)(G)** <6 months: not recommended; ≥6 months-12 years: 7.5 mg/kg bid x 10 days; *see page* 602 *for dose by weight table;* >12 years: 500 mg bid or 500 mg ext-rel daily x 10 days

Biaxin *Tab:* 250, 500 mg

Biaxin Oral Suspension *Oral susp:* 125, 250 mg/5 ml (50, 100 ml) (fruit punch)

Biaxin XL *Tab:* 500 mg ext-rel

Comment: The FDA is advising caution before prescribing ***clarithromycin*** to patients with heart disease because of a potential increased risk of heart problems or death that can occur years later. This recommendation is based on a review of the results of a 10-year follow-up study of patients with coronary heart disease from a large clinical trial that first observed this safety issue. Consider risk benefit and the use of other antibiotics in such patients.

▶ ***levofloxacin*** **(C)** <18 years: not recommended; ≥18 years: *Uncomplicated:* 500 mg once daily x 10-14 days; *Complicated:* 750 mg once daily x 10-14 days

Levaquin *Tab:* 250, 500, 750 mg; *Oral soln:* 25 mg/ml (480 ml) (benzyl alcohol); *Inj conc:* 25 mg/ml for IV infusion after dilution (20, 30 ml single-use vial) (preservative-free); *Premix soln:* 5 mg/ml for IV infusion (50, 100, 150 ml) (preservative-free)

Comment: ***levofloxacin*** is contraindicated <18 years-of-age, and during pregnancy and lactation. Risk of tendonitis or tendon rupture.

▶ ***loracarbef*** **(B)** <12 years: 15 mg/kg/day in 2 divided doses x 10 days; *see page* 614 *for dose by weight table*; ≥12 years: 200 mg bid x 10 days

Lorabid *Pulvule*: 200, 400 mg; *Oral susp:* 100 mg/5 ml (50, 100 ml); 200 mg/5 ml (50, 75, 100 ml) (strawberry bubble gum)

▶ ***moxifloxacin*** **(C)(G)** <18 years: not recommended; ≥18 years: 400 mg daily x 10 days

Avelox *Tab:* 400 mg

Comment: ***moxifloxacin*** is contraindicated <18 years-of-age, and during pregnancy and lactation. Risk of tendonitis or tendon rupture.

▶ ***trimethoprim+sulfamethoxazole [TMP-SMX]*** **(D)(G)**

Bactrim, Septra <12 years: not recommended; ≥12 years: 2 tabs bid x 10 days
Tab: trim 80 mg+sulfa 400 mg*

Bactrim DS, Septra DS <12 years: not recommended; ≥12 years: 1 tab bid x 10 days
Tab: trim 160 mg+sulfa 800 mg*

Bactrim Pediatric Suspension, Septra Pediatric Suspension <2 months: not recommended; ≥2 months-12 years: 40 mg/kg/day of ***sulfamethoxazole*** in 2 doses bid; >12 years: use tabs
Oral susp: trim 40 mg+sulfa 200 mg per 5 ml (100 ml) (cherry) (alcohol 0.3%)

SJÖGREN-LARSSON-SYNDROME (SLS)

Comment: Sjögren-Larsson-Syndrome is a chronic autoimmune disorder that causes the white blood cells to attack the moisture-producing glands. Sjögren's syndrome can occur in association with other autoimmune diseases, including systemic lupus erythematosus, rheumatoid arthritis, scleroderma, systemic sclerosis, cryoglobulinemia, or polyarteritis nodosa. The disease can affect the eyes, mouth, parotid gland, pancreas, gastrointestinal system, blood vessels, lungs, kidneys, skin, and nervous system. Erythrocyte sedimentation rate (ESR) is elevated in 80% of patients. Rheumatoid factor is present in 52% of primary cases and 98% of secondary-type cases. A mild normochromic normocytic anemia is present in 50% of patients, and leukopenia occurs in up to 42% of patients. Creatinine clearance is diminished in up to 50% of patients. Anti-nuclear antibody (ANA) is positive in 70% of patients. SS-A and SS-B are marker antibodies for Sjögren's syndrome—70% of patients are positive for SS-A and 40% are positive for SS-B.

CHOLINERGIC (MUSCARINIC) AGONIST COMBINATION

▶ ***cevimeline*** (C)(G) 30 mg tid
  Evoxac *Cap:* 30 mg
 Comment: ***cevimeline*** is contraindicated in acute iritis, narrow-angle glaucoma, and uncontrolled asthma.

▶ ***pilocarpine*** (C)(G) 5 mg qid or 7.5 mg tid
  Salagen *Tab:* 5, 7.5 mg

ORAL ENZYME RINSE

▶ ***xylitol+solazyme+selectobac*** swish 5 ml for 30 seconds bid-tid
  Orazyme Dry Mouth Rinse *Oral soln:* 1.5, 16 oz

SKIN: CALLOUSED

KERATOLYTICS

▶ ***salicylic acid*** (C)(OTC) <12 years: not recommended; ≥12 years: apply lotion, cream or gel to affected area qd-bid; apply patch to affected area and leave on x 48 hours with max 5 applications/14 days

▶ ***urea*** (C)
  Carmol 40 <12 years: not recommended; ≥12 years: apply to affected area with applicator stick provided once daily-tid; smooth over until cream is absorbed; protect surrounding tissue; may cover with adhesive bandage or gauze secured with adhesive tape
   Crm/Gel: 40% (30 gm)
  Keratol 40 <12 years: not recommended; ≥ 12 years: apply to affected area with applicator stick provided once daily-tid; smooth over until cream is absorbed; protect surrounding tissue; may cover with adhesive bandage or gauze secured with adhesive tape
   Crm: 40% (1, 3, 7 oz); *Gel:* 40% (15 ml); *Lotn:* 40% (8 oz)
 Comment: The moisturizing effect of **Carmol 40** and **Keratol 40** is enhanced by applying while the skin is still moist (after washing or bathing).

SKIN INFECTION: BACTERIAL (CARBUNCLE, FOLLICULITIS, FURUNCLE)

Comment: Abscesses usually require surgical incision and drainage.

ANTIBACTERIAL SKIN CLEANSERS

▶ ***hexachlorophene*** (C) dispense 5 ml into wet hand, work up into lather; then apply to area to be cleansed; rinse thoroughly
  pHisoHex *Liq clnsr:* 5, 16 oz

TOPICAL ANTI-INFECTIVES

▶ ***mupirocin*** (B)(G) apply to lesions bid
  Bactroban *Oint:* 2% (22 gm); *Crm:* 2% (15, 30 gm)
  Centany *Oint:* 2% (15, 30 gm)

▶ ***polymyxin b+neomycin*** (C) *oint:* apply once daily-tid
  Neosporin (OTC) *Oint:* 15 gm

ORAL ANTI-INFECTIVES

- ***amoxicillin*** **(B)(G)** <40 kg (88 lb): 20-40 mg/kg/day in 3 divided doses x 10 days or 25-45 mg/kg/day in 2 divided doses x 10 days; *see page 588 for dose by weight table;* ≥40 kg: 500-875 mg bid or 250-500 mg tid x 10 days
  Amoxil *Cap:* 250, 500 mg; *Tab:* 875*mg; *Chew tab:* 125, 200, 250, 400 mg (cherry-banana-peppermint) (phenylalanine); *Oral susp:* 125, 250 mg/5 ml (80, 100, 150 ml) (strawberry); 200, 400 mg/5 ml (50, 75, 100 ml) (bubble gum); *Oral drops:* 50 mg/ml (30 ml) (bubble gum)
  Moxatag *Tab:* 775 mg ext-rel
  Trimox *Tab:* 125, 250 mg; *Cap:* 250, 500 mg; *Oral susp:* 125, 250 mg/5 ml (80, 100, 150 ml) (raspberry-strawberry)
- ***azithromycin*** **(B)** <6 months: not recommended; ≥6 months-12 years: 10 mg/kg x 1 dose on day 1; then 5 mg/kg/day on days 2-5; *see page 593 for dose by weight table;* max 500 mg/day; >12 years: 500 mg x 1 dose on day 1, then 250 mg once daily on days 2-5 or 500 mg once daily x 3 days or **Zmax** 2 gm in a single dose
  Zithromax *Tab:* 250, 500, 600 mg; *Oral susp:* 100 mg/5 ml (15 ml); 200 mg/5 ml (15, 22.5, 30 ml) (cherry); *Pkt:* 1 gm for reconstitution (cherry-banana)
  Zithromax Tri-pak *Tab:* 3 x 500 mg tabs/pck
  Zithromax Z-pak *Tab:* 6 x 250 mg tabs/pck
  Zmax *Oral susp:* 2 gm ext-rel for reconstitution (cherry-banana) (148 mg Na^+)
- ***cefaclor*** **(B)(G)** <1 month: not recommended; 1 month-12 years: 20-40 mg/kg divided bid or tid x 10 days; *see page 594 for dose by weight table;* max 1 gm/day; >12 years: 375 mg bid x 10 days; max 2 gm/day
  Tab: 500 mg; *Cap:* 250, 500 mg; *Susp:* 125 mg/5 ml (75, 150 ml) (strawberry); 187 mg/5 ml (50, 100 ml) (strawberry); 250 mg/5 ml (75, 150 ml) (strawberry); 375 mg/5 ml (50, 100 ml) (strawberry)
  Cefaclor Extended Release <16 years: not recommended; ≥16 years: 500 mg bid x 10 days (clinically equivalent to 250 mg immed-rel caps tid); swallow whole; take with food
  Tab: 375, 500 mg ext-rel
- ***cefadroxil*** <12 years: 30 mg/kg/day in 2 divided doses x 10 days; *see page 595 for dose by weight table;* ≥12 years: 1-2 gm in a single or 2 divided doses x 10 days
  Duricef *Cap:* 500 mg; *Tab:* 1 gm; *Oral susp:* 250 mg/5 ml (100 ml); 500 mg/5 ml (75, 100 ml) (orange-pineapple)
- ***cefdinir*** **(B)** <6 months: not recommended; 6 months-12 years: 14 mg/kg/day in 1-2 divided doses x 10 days; *see page 596 for dose by weight table;* >12 years: 300 mg bid x 10 days or 600 mg daily x 10 days
  Omnicef *Cap:* 300 mg; *Oral susp:* 125 mg/5 ml (60, 100 ml) (strawberry)
- ***cefditoren pivoxil*** **(B)** <12 years: not recommended; ≥12 years: 200 mg bid x 10 days
  Spectracef *Tab:* 200 mg

Comment: Contraindicated with milk protein allergy or carnitine deficiency.

- ***cefpodoxime proxetil*** **(B)** <2 months: not recommended; 2 months-12 years: 10 mg/kg/day (max 400 mg/dose) or 5 mg/kg/day bid (max 200 mg/dose) x 7-14 days; *see page 598 for dose by weight table;* >12 years: 400 mg bid x 7-14 days
  Vantin *Tab:* 100, 200 mg; *Oral susp:* 50, 100 mg/5 ml (50, 75, 100 mg) (lemon creme)
- ***cefprozil*** **(B)** <2 years: not recommended; 2-12 years: 7.5 mg/kg bid x 10 days; *see page 599 for dose by weight table;* >12 years: 250-500 mg bid or 500 mg once daily x 10 days
  Cefzil *Tab:* 250, 500 mg; *Oral susp:* 125, 250 mg/5 ml (50, 75, 100 ml) (bubble gum) (phenylalanine)
- ***ceftriaxone*** **(B)(G)** <12 years: 50-75 mg/kg IM in 1-2 divided doses; max 2 gm/day; ≥12 years: 1-2 gm IM once daily; max 4 gm/day
  Rocephin *Vial:* 250, 500 mg; 1, 2 gm

▶ ***cephalexin*** **(B)(G)** <12 years*:* 25-50 mg/kg/day in 4 divided doses x 10 days; *see page* 601 *for dose by weight table;* ≥12 years: 500 mg bid x 10 days

  Keflex *Cap:* 250, 333, 500, 750 mg; *Oral susp:* 125, 250 mg/5 ml (100, 200 ml) (strawberry)

▶ ***clarithromycin*** **(C)(G)** <6 months: not recommended; ≥6 months-12 years: 7.5 mg/kg bid x 10 days; *see page* 602 *for dose by weight table;* >12 years: 250-500 mg bid or 500-1000 mg ext-rel once daily x 10 days

  Biaxin *Tab:* 250, 500 mg

  Biaxin Oral Suspension *Oral susp:* 125, 250 mg/5 ml (50, 100 ml) (fruit punch)

  Biaxin XL *Tab:* 500 mg ext-rel

Comment: The FDA is advising caution before prescribing ***clarithromycin*** to patients with heart disease because of a potential increased risk of heart problems or death that can occur years later. This recommendation is based on a review of the results of a 10-year follow-up study of patients with coronary heart disease from a large clinical trial that first observed this safety issue. Consider risk benefit and the use of other antibiotics in such patients.

▶ ***dicloxacillin*** **(B)** <12 years: 12.5-25 mg/kg/day in 4 divided doses x 10 days; *see page* 604 *for dose by weight table;* >12 years: 500 mg qid x 10 days

  Dynapen *Cap:* 125, 250, 500 mg; *Oral susp:* 62.5 mg/5 ml (80, 100, 200 ml)

▶ ***dirithromycin*** **(C)(G)** <12 years: not recommended; ≥12 years: 500 mg once daily x 10 days

  Dynabac *Tab:* 250 mg

▶ ***doxycycline*** **(D)(G)** <8 years: not recommended; ≥8 years, ≤100 lb: 1 mg/lb in a single dose once daily x 9 days; ≥8 years, >100 lb: 100 mg bid x 9 days; *see page* 605 *for dose by weight table*

  Acticlate *Tab:* 75, 150**mg

  Adoxa *Tab:* 50, 75, 100, 150 mg ent-coat

  Doryx *Tab:* 50, 75, 100, 150, 200 mg del-rel

  Doxteric *Tab:* 50 mg del-rel

  Monodox *Cap:* 50, 75, 100 mg

  Oracea *Cap:* 40 mg del-rel

  Vibramycin *Tab:* 100 mg; *Cap:* 50, 100 mg; *Syr:* 50 mg/5 ml (raspberry-apple) (sulfites); *Oral susp:* 25 mg/5 ml (raspberry)

  Vibra-Tab *Tab:* 100 mg film-coat

Comment: ***doxycycline*** is contraindicated <8 years-of-age, in pregnancy, and lactation (discolors developing tooth enamel). A side effect may be photosensitivity (photophobia). Do not take with antacids, calcium supplements, milk or other dairy, or within 2 hours of taking another drug.

▶ ***erythromycin base*** **(B)(G)** <45 kg: 30-50 mg in 2-4 divided doses x 10 days; ≥45 kg: 500 mg q 6 hours x 10 days

  Ery-Tab *Tab:* 250, 333, 500 mg ent-coat

  PCE *Tab:* 333, 500 mg

▶ ***erythromycin estolate*** **(B)(G)** <12 years: 20-50 mg/kg q 6 hours x 10 days; *see page* 606 *for dose by weight table;* ≥12 years: 250-500 mg q 6 hours x 10 days

  Ilosone *Pulvule:* 250 mg; *Tab:* 500 mg; *Liq:* 125, 250 mg/5 ml (100 ml)

▶ ***erythromycin ethylsuccinate*** **(B)(G)** 30-50 mg/kg/day in 4 divided doses x 10 days; may double dose with severe infection; max 100 mg/kg/day or 400 mg qid; *see page* 607 *for dose by weight table*

  EryPed *Oral susp:* 200 mg/5 ml (100, 200 ml) (fruit); 400 mg/5 ml (60, 100, 200 ml) (banana); *Oral drops:* 200, 400 mg/5 ml (50 ml) (fruit); *Chew tab:* 200 mg wafer (fruit)

  E.E.S. *Oral susp:* 200, 400 mg/5 ml (100 ml) (fruit)

  E.E.S. Granules *Oral susp:* 200 mg/5 ml (100, 200 ml) (cherry)

  E.E.S. 400 Tablets *Tab:* 400 mg

▶ ***gemifloxacin*** **(C)(G)** <18 years: not recommended; ≥18 years: 320 mg once daily x 5-7 days

Factive *Tab:* 320*mg

Comment: ***gemifloxacin*** is contraindicated <18 years-of-age, and during pregnancy and lactation. Risk of tendonitis or tendon rupture.

▶ ***levofloxacin*** **(C)** <18 years: not recommended; ≥18 years: *Uncomplicated:* 500 mg once daily x 7-10 days; *Complicated:* 750 mg once daily x 7-10 days

Levaquin *Tab:* 250, 500, 750 mg; *Oral soln:* 25 mg/ml (480 ml) (benzyl alcohol); *Inj conc:* 25 mg/ml for IV infusion after dilution (20, 30 ml single-use vial) (preservative-free); *Premix soln:* 5 mg/ml for IV infusion (50, 100, 150 ml) (preservative-free)

Comment: ***levofloxacin*** is contraindicated <18 years-of-age, and during pregnancy and lactation. Risk of tendonitis or tendon rupture.

▶ ***linezolid*** **(C)(G)** <5 years: 10 mg/kg q 8 hours x 10-14 days; 5-11 years: 10 mg/kg q 12 hours x 10-14 days; >11 years: 400-600 mg q 12 hours x 10-14 days

Zyvox *Tab:* 400, 600 mg; *Oral susp:* 100 mg/5 ml (150 ml) (orange) (phenylalanine)

Comment: ***linezolid*** is indicated to treat susceptible vancomycin-resistant *E. faecium* infections.

▶ ***loracarbef*** **(B)** <12 years: 15 mg/kg/day in 2 divided doses x 7 days; *see page* 614 *for dose by weight table;* ≥12 years: 200 mg bid x 7 days

Lorabid *Pulvule*: 200, 400 mg; *Oral susp:* 100 mg/5 ml (50, 100 ml); 200 mg/5 ml (50, 75, 100 ml) (strawberry bubble gum)

▶ ***minocycline*** **(D)(G)** <8 years: not recommended; ≥8 years, ≤100 lb: 2 mg/lb on first day in 2 divided doses, followed by 1 mg/lb q 12 hours x 9 more days; ≥8 years, >100 lb: 200 mg on first day; then 100 mg q 12 hours x 9 more days

Dynacin *Cap:* 50, 100 mg

Minocin *Cap:* 50, 75, 100 mg; *Oral susp:* 50 mg/5 ml (60 ml) (custard) (sulfites, alcohol 5%)

Comment: ***minocycline*** is contraindicated <8 years-of-age, in pregnancy, and lactation (discolors developing tooth enamel). A side effect may be photosensitivity (photophobia). Do not give with antacids, calcium supplements, milk or other dairy, or within two hours of taking another drug.

▶ ***moxifloxacin*** **(C)(G)** <18 years: not recommended; ≥18 years: 400 mg daily x 10 days

Avelox *Tab:* 400 mg

Comment: ***moxifloxacin*** is contraindicated <18 years-of-age, and during pregnancy and lactation. Risk of tendonitis or tendon rupture.

▶ ***ofloxacin*** **(C)(G)** <18 years: not recommended; ≥18 years: 400 mg bid x 10 days

Floxin *Tab:* 200, 300, 400 mg

Comment: ***ofloxacin*** is contraindicated <18 years-of-age, and during pregnancy and lactation. Risk of tendonitis or tendon rupture.

▶ ***tetracycline*** **(D)(G)** <8 years: not recommended; ≥8 years, ≤100 lb: 25-50 mg/kg/day in 4 divided doses x 10 days; *see page* 618 *for dose by weight table*; ≥8 years, >100 lb: 500 mg qid x 10 days

Achromycin V *Cap:* 250, 500 mg

Sumycin *Tab:* 250, 500 mg; *Cap:* 250, 500 mg; *Oral susp:* 125 mg/5 ml (100, 200 ml) (fruit) (sulfites)

Comment: ***tetracycline*** is contraindicated <8 years-of-age, in pregnancy, and lactation (discolors developing tooth enamel). A side effect may be photosensitivity (photophobia). Do not give with antacids, calcium supplements, milk or other dairy, or within two hours of taking another drug.

SLEEP APNEA: OBSTRUCTIVE (HYPOPNEA SYNDROME)

ANTINARCOLEPTIC AGENTS

- *armodafinil* (C)(IV)(G) <17 years: not recommended; ≥17 years: *OSAHS:* 150-250 mg once daily in the AM; *SWSD:* 150 mg 1 hour before starting shift; reduce dose with severe hepatic impairment
  Nuvigil *Tab:* 50, 150, 200, 250 mg
- *modafinil* (C)(IV) <16 years: not recommended; ≥16 years: 100-200 mg q AM; max 400 mg/day
  Provigil *Tab:* 100, 200*mg

  Comment: ***modafinil*** promotes wakefulness in patients with excessive sleepiness due to obstructive sleep apnea/hypopnea syndrome.

SLEEPINESS: EXCESSIVE & SHIFT WORK SLEEP DISORDER (SWSD)

ANTI-NARCOLEPTIC AGENT

- *armodafinil* (C)(IV)(G) <17 years: not recommended; ≥17 years: *OSAHS:* 150-250 mg once daily in the AM; *SWSD:* 150 mg 1 hour before starting shift; reduce dose with severe hepatic impairment
  Nuvigil *Tab:* 50, 150, 200, 250 mg
- *modafinil* (C)(IV) <16 years: not recommended; ≥16 years: 100-200 mg q AM; max 400 mg/day
  Provigil *Tab:* 100, 200*mg

  Comment: **Provigil** promotes wakefulness in patients with narcolepsy, shift work sleep disorder, and excessive sleepiness due to obstructive sleep apnea/hypopnea syndrome.

SMALLPOX (VARIOLA MAJOR)

PROPHYLAXIS

- *vaccinia virus* **vaccine** ***(dried, calf lymph type)*** (C) <12 months: not recommended; 12 months-18 years, non-emergency: not recommended
  DRYvax
  Kit: vial dried smallpox vaccine (1), 0.25 ml diluent in syringe (1), vented needle (1), 100 individually wrapped bifurcated needles (5 needles/strip, 20 strips) (polymyxin b sulfate+dihydrostreptomycin sulfate+chlortetracycline hcl+neomycin sulfate+glycerin+phenol)

  Comment: **DRYvax** is a dried live vaccine with approximately 100 million *Infectious vaccinia* viruses (pock-forming units [pfu] per ml). Contact with immunosuppressed individuals should be avoided until the scab has separated from the skin (2 to 3 weeks) and/or a protective occlusive dressing covers the inoculation site. Scarification only. Do not inject IV, IM, or SC. Revaccination is recommended every 10 years.

SPINAL MUSCULAR ATROPHY (SMA)

Comment: Spinal muscular atrophy (SMA) is a group of inherited disorders characterized by motor neuron loss in the spinal cord and lower brainstem, muscle weakness, and atrophy. Survival motor neuron (SMN) protein is essential for the maintenance of motor neurons. Because of a defect in, or loss of, the SMN1 gene, patients with SMA do not produce enough SMN protein. It is the most common genetic cause of death in infants, but can affect people at any age. **Spinraza** (***nusinersen***) is the first FDA-approved drug to treat SMA.

SURVIVAL MOTOR NEURON-2 (SMN2)-DIRECTED ANTISENSE OLIGONUCLEOTIDE

▶ ***nusinersen*** 12 mg per intrathecal administration; initially four loading doses: the first 3 loading doses administered at 14-day intervals; the 4th loading dose administered 30 days after the 3rd loading dose; the maintenance dose is administered every 4 months after the 4th loading dose; prior to administration, 5 ml cerebral spinal fluid (CSF) should be removed; the intrathecal bolus injection should be administered over 1-3 minutes using a spinal anesthetic needle.

Comment: At baseline and prior to each dose, obtain a platelet count and coagulation laboratory testing (there is increased risk for thrombocytopenia and coagulation abnormalities) and quantitative spot urine protein testing (to monitor for renal toxicity). Store **Spinraza** in a refrigerator between 2°C to 8°C (36°F to 46°F) in the original carton to protect from light. Do not freeze. Prior to administration, unopened vials of **Spinraza** can be removed from and returned to the refrigerator, if necessary. If removed from the original carton, the total combined time out of refrigeration should not exceed 30 hours at a temperature that does not exceed 25°C (77°F). **Spinraza** has no labeled contraindications. **Spinraza** has not been studied in pregnant or lactating females, or in patients with renal or hepatic impairment.

SPRAIN

Comment: RICE: Rest; Ice; Compression; Elevation.

Injectable Acetaminophen *see* ***Pain*** *page* 322
NSAIDs *see page* 539
Other Oral Analgesics *see* ***Pain*** *page* 324
Topical & Transdermal NSAIDs *see* ***Pain*** *page* 323
Parenteral Corticosteroids *see page* 547
Oral Corticosteroids *see page* 546

STATUS ASTHMATICUS

Inhaled Beta-2 Agonists (Bronchodilators) ***see*** **Asthma** ***page*** 29
Oral Beta-2 Agonists (Bronchodilators) ***see*** **Asthma** ***page*** 36
Inhaled Anticholinergics ***see*** **Asthma** ***page*** 31
Inhaled Anticholinergic+Beta-2 Agonist Combination ***see*** **Asthma** ***page*** 33
Methylxanthines ***see*** **Asthma** ***page*** 36
Parenteral Corticosteroids ***see page*** 547
Oral Corticosteroids ***see page*** 546

EPINEPHRINE

▶ ***epinephrine*** (C)(G) Use 1:1000 solution; may repeat q 20-30 minutes as needed up to 3 doses; <2 years: 0.05-0.1 ml SC; 2-<6 years: 0.1 ml SC; 6-<12 years: 0.2 ml ≥12 years: 0.3-0.5 mg SC

ANAPHYLAXIS EMERGENCY TREATMENT KITS

▶ ***epinephrine*** (C) 0.01 mg/kg SC or IM in thigh; may repeat if needed; <15 kg: not recommended; 15-30 kg: 0.15 mg; ≥30 kg: 0.3 ml IM or SC in thigh; may repeat if needed

AdrenaClick *Autoinjector:* 0.15, 0.3 mg (1 mg/ml, 2/carton) (sulfites)
Auvi-Q *Autoinjector:* 0.15, 0.3 mg (1 mg/ml, 2/carton w. 1 non-active training device) (sulfites)
EpiPen *Autoinjector:* 0.3 mg (epi 1:1000, 0.3 ml (2/carton) (sulfites)
Epi-E-Zpen *Autoinjector:* 0.15 mg (epi 1:2000, 0.3 ml (2/carton) (sulfites)
Twinject *Autoinjector:* 0.15, 0.3 mg (epi 1:1000, 2/carton) (sulfites)

▶ ***epinephrine+chlorpheniramine*** **(C)** infants-2 years: 0.05-0.1 ml SC or IM; 2-<6 years: 0.15 ml SC or IM plus 1 PO tab ***chlorpheniramine;*** 6-<12 years: 0.2 ml SC or IM plus 2 chewable ***chlorpheniramine*** tabs; ≥12 years: ***epinephrine*** 0.3 ml SC or IM plus 4 chewable ***chlorpheniramine*** tabs
Ana-Kit: 0.3 ml syringe of epi 1:1000 (2/carton) for self-injection plus 4 x chlor 2 mg chew tabs

STATUS EPILEPTICUS

Anticonvulsant Drugs *see page* 560

▶ ***diazepam*** injectable **(D)(IV)** <1 months: see mfr pkg insert; 1 month-5 years: 0.2-0.5 mg IV q 2-5 minutes; max 5 mg; >5-<12 years: 1 mg IV q 2-5 minutes; max 10 mg; may repeat in 2-4 hours if needed; ≥12 years: initially 5-10 mg IV in large vein; may repeat q 10-15 minutes; max 30 mg; may repeat in 2-4 hours if needed; do not dilute; may administer IM if IV not accessible
Diastat *Rectal gel delivery system:* 2.5 mg
Diastat AcuDial *Rectal gel delivery system:* 10, 20 mg
Valium Injectable *Vial:* 5 mg/ml (10 ml); *Amp:* 5 mg/ml (2 ml); *Prefilled syringe:* 5 mg/ml (5 ml)
Valium Intensol Oral Solution *Conc oral soln:* 5 mg/ml (30 ml w. dropper) (alcohol 19%)
Valium Oral Solution *Oral soln:* 5 mg/5 ml (500 ml) (wintergreen spice)

▶ ***lorazepam*** injectable **(D)(IV)** <18 years: not recommended; ≥18 years: administer 4 mg IV over 2 minutes (dilute first); may repeat in 10-15 minutes; may give IM if needed (undiluted)
Ativan Injectable *Vial:* 2 mg/ml (1, 10 ml); *Tubex:* 2 mg/ml (0.5 ml); *Cartridge:* 2, 4 mg/ml (1 ml)

▶ ***phenytoin (injectable)*** **(D)(G)** <12 years: 15-20 mg/kg IV, not to exceed 1-2 mg/kg/minute; ≥12 years: 10-15 mg/kg IV, not to exceed 50 mg/minute; follow with 100 mg orally or IV q 6-8 hours; do not dilute in IV fluid
Dilantin *Vial:* 50 mg/ml (2, 5 ml); *Amp:* 50 mg/ml (2 ml)

Comment: Monitor ***phenytoin*** serum levels. Therapeutic serum level: 10-20 gm/ml. Side effects include gingival hyperplasia.

STYE (HORDEOLUM)

OPHTHALMIC ANTI-INFECTIVES

▶ ***erythromycin*** **ophthalmic ointment (B)** 1 cm up to 6 x/day
Ilotycin Ophthalmic Ointment *Ophth oint:* 5 mg/gm (1/8 oz)

▶ ***erythromycin*** ophthalmic solution **(B)** initially 1-2 drops q 1-2 hours; may then increase dose interval
Isopto Cetamide Ophthalmic Solution *Ophth soln:* 15% (15 ml)

▶ ***gentamicin*** ophthalmic ointment **(C)** 1 cm bid-tid
Garamycin Ophthalmic Ointment *Ophth oint:* 3 mg/gm (3.5 gm)
Genoptic Ophthalmic Ointment *Ophth oint:* 3 mg/gm (3.5 gm)
Gentacidin Ophthalmic Ointment *Ophth oint:* 3 mg/gm (3.5 gm)

- ▶ ***polymyxin b+bacitracin*** ophthalmic ointment (C) apply 1/2 inch q 3-4 hours
  Polysporin *Ophth oint:* poly b 10,000 U+bac 500 units per gm (3.75 gm)
- ▶ ***polymyxin B/bacitracin/neomycin*** **ophthalmic ointment** (C)(G) apply 1/2 inch q 3-4 hours
  Neosporin Ophthalmic Ointment *Ophth oint: poly* b 10,000 U+*bac* 400 U+*neo* 3.5 mg/gm (3.75 gm)
- ▶ ***polymyxin b+gramicidin+neomycin*** **ophthalmic solution** (C) 1-2 drops 2-3 times q 1 hour; then 1-2 drops bid-qid x 7-10 days
  Neosporin Ophthalmic Solution
  Ophth soln: poly b 10,000 U+neo 1.75 mg/gm, 0.025 mg/ml (10 ml)
- ▶ ***sodium sulfacetamide*** **ophthalmic solution and ointment** (C)
  Bleph-10 Ophthalmic Solution <2 years: not recommended; ≥2-<12 years: 1-2 drops q 2-3 hours during the day; ≥12 years: 2 drops q 4 hour x 7-14 days
  Ophth soln: 10% (2.5, 5, 15 ml) (benzalkonium chloride)
  Bleph-10 Ophthalmic Ointment <2 years: not recommended; ≥2-<12 years: apply 1/4-1/3 inch qid and HS; ≥12 years: apply 1/2 inch qid and HS
  Ophth oint: 10% (3.5 gm) (phenylmercuric acetate)

SUNBURN

OTC Aloe Vera Gel

- ▶ ***prednisone*** (C)(G) 10 mg qid x 4-6 days if severe and extensive
- ▶ ***silver sulfadiazine*** (B)(G) <12 years: not established; ≥12 years: apply bid
  Silvadene *Crm:* 1% (20 gm tube; 20, 50, 85, 400, 1,000 gm jar)

Comment: ***silver sulfadiazine*** is contradicted in sulfa allergy, late pregnancy, within the first 2 months after birth, premature infants.

SYPHILIS *(TREPONEMA PALLIDUM)*

Comment: The following treatment regimens for *T. pallidum* are published in the **2015 CDC Sexually Transmitted Diseases Treatment Guidelines**. Treat all sexual contacts. Consider testing for other STDs. ***penicillin g***, administered parenterally, is the preferred drug for treating all stages of syphilis. The preparation used (i.e., benzathine, aqueous procaine, or aqueous crystalline), the dosage, and the length of treatment depend on the stage and clinical manifestations of the disease. Combinations of ***benzathine penicillin, procaine penicillin,*** and oral ***penicillin*** preparations are not appropriate (e.g., **Bicillin C-R**). Screen serologically for syphilis early in pregnancy. There are no proven alternatives to penicillin for the treatment of syphilis during pregnancy. Pregnant patients who are allergic to penicillin should be desensitized and treated with ***penicillin***. Sexual transmission of *T. pallidum* is thought to occur only when mucocutaneous syphilis at any stage should be evaluated clinically and serologically and treated with a recommended regimen according to CDC guidelines.

PRIMARY, SECONDARY, AND EARLY LATENT SYPHILIS, <1 YEAR DURATION, ≥12 YEARS-OF-AGE

Regimen 1

- ▶ ***penicillin g (benzathine)*** 2.4 million units IM in a single dose

LATE LATENT, LATENT SYPHILIS OF UNKNOWN DURATION, AND TERTIARY SYPHILIS, ≥12 YEARS-OF-AGE

Regimen 1

- *penicillin g (benzathine)* 2.4 million units IM in a single dose; 7.2 million units total administered in 3 divided doses of 2.4 million units each IM at 1 week intervals

REGIMEN: NEUROSYPHILIS, ≥12 YEARS-OF-AGE

Regimen 1

- *aqueous crystalline penicillin g* 2.4 million units IM in a single dose 18-24 million units per day, administered as 3-4 million units IV every 4 hours or continuous IV infusion, for 10-14 days

ALTERNATIVE REGIMEN: NEUROSYPHILIS, ≥12 YEARS-OF-AGE

Regimen 1

- *penicillin g (procaine)* 2.4 million units IM once daily x 10-14 days plus *probenecid* 500 mg qid x 10-14 days

PRIMARY AND SECONDARY SYPHILIS IN HIV-INFECTED PERSONS

Regimen 1

- *penicillin g (benzathine)* 2.4 million units IM in a single dose

LATENT SYPHILIS AMONG HIV-INFECTED PERSONS ≥12 YEARS-OF-AGE

Comment: Treatment is the same as for HIV-negative persons.

CONGENITAL SYPHILIS, ≥12 YEARS-OF-AGE

Regimen 1

- *aqueous crystalline penicillin g* 100,000-150,000 units/kg/day, administered as 50,000 units IV every 12 hours during the first 7 days of life and every 8 hours thereafter for a total of 10 days

ALTERNATE REGIMENS, ≥12 YEARS-OF-AGE

Regimen 1

- *penicillin g (benzathine)* 50,000 units/kg IM in a single dose

Regimen 2

- *penicillin g (procaine)* 50,000 units/kg/dose IM, administered in a single daily dose x 10 days

INFANTS AND CHILDREN <12 YEARS-OF-AGE

Regimen 1

- *aqueous crystalline penicillin g* 200,000-300,000 units/kg/day, administered as 50,000 units IV every 12 hours during the first 7 days of life and every 4-6 hours thereafter for a total of 10 days

DRUG BRANDS AND DOSE FORMS

▶ *aqueous crystalline penicillin g* (B)(G)

▶ *penicillin g (benzathine)* (B)(G)

Bicillin L-A *Cartridge-needle unit:* 600,000 million units (1 ml); 1.2 million units (2 ml); 2.4 million units (4 ml)

▶ *penicillin g (procaine)* (B)(G)

Bicillin C-R Cartridge-needle unit: 600,000 units (1 ml); 1.2 million units; (2 ml); 2.4 million units (4 ml)

▶ *probenecid* (B)(G)

Benemid *Tab:* 500*mg; *Cap:* 500 mg

SYSTEMIC LUPUS ERYTHEMATOSIS (SLE)

Oral Corticosteroids *see page* 546

Comment: All SLE patients should routinely be given ***hydroxychloroquine*** HCQ and supplemental vitamin D as low levels of vitamin D are associated with higher rates of ESRD; supplemental vitamin D reduces urine protein (the best predictor of future renal failure). Vitamin D insufficiency and deficiency are more common in patients with SLE than in the general population. Vitamin D supplementation may decrease disease activity and improve fatigue. In addition, supplementation may improve endothelial function, which may reduce cardiovascular disease. A disease-modifying anti-rheumatic drug (DMARD) should be added when a patient's prednisone dose cannot be tapered and also when hemolysis is present and hemoglobin is abnormally low in the setting of mild-to-moderate hematological involvement. Other DMARDs, such as **methotrexate** (MTX), ***azathioprine***, ***mycophenolate mofetil*** (MMF), ***cyclosporine*** (CYC), and other calcineurin-inhibitors should be considered in cases of arthritis, cutaneous disease, serositis, vasculitis, or cytopaenias if HCQ is insufficient. For refractory cases, ***belimumab*** **(Benlysta)** or ***rituximab*** **(Rituxan)**, may be considered. The recommended dose of ***rituximab***, if required, is either 750 mg/m2 (to a maximum of 1 gm per day) at day 1 and day 15, or 375 mg/m2 once a week for 4 doses. In patients with SLE without major organ manifestations, glucocorticoids and antimalarial agents may be beneficial. NSAIDs may be used for short periods in patients at low risk for complications from these drugs. Consider immunosuppressive agents (e.g., ***azathioprine***, MMF, MTX) in refractory cases or when steroid doses cannot be reduced to levels for long-term use.

REFERENCES

Gordon, C, Amissah-Arthur, MB, Gayed, M, *et al.* (2017). The British Society for Rheumatology guideline for the management of systemic lupus erythematosus in adults. *Rheumatology*. doi:10.1093/rheumatology/kex286

Groot, N, de Graeff, N, Avcin, T, *et al.* (2017). European evidence-based recommendations for diagnosis and treatment of childhood-onset systemic lupus erythematosus: the SHARE initiative. *Annals of the Rheumatic Diseases, 76*(11), 1788–1796.

Leach, MZ. (2017). First UK guidelines for adults with lupus. Rheumatology Network. http://www.rheumatologynetwork.com/authors/mariah-zebrowski-leach-jd-ms

CD20 ANTIBODY

▶ ***rituximab*** (C) <6 years: not recommended; >6 years: administer corticosteroid 30 minutes prior to each infusion; concomitant ***methotrexate*** therapy, administer a 1000 mg IV infusion at 0 and 2 weeks; then every 24 weeks or based on response, but not sooner than every 16 weeks.

Rituxan *Vial:* 10 mg/ml (10, 50 ml) (preservative-free)

Comment: ***rituximab*** is a B-cell targeting chimeric monoclonal antibody that acts against CD20 and reduces antibody titers. B-cell depletion by ***rituximab*** may also set the stage for production of interleukin 10–secreting B cells that do not interact with T cells, which further reduces production of antidesmoglein antibodies. ***rituximab*** carries a black box warning regarding fatal infusion reactions, severe mucocutaneous reactions, hepatitis B virus reactivation, and progressive multifocal leukoencephalopathy. However, serious adverse events are rare. There was no evidence of increased mortality with longer exposure to **rituximab** or to multiple courses of therapy.

B-LYMPHOCYTE STIMULATOR (BLYS)-S-SPECIFIC INHIBITOR

▶ *belimumab* <18 years: not established; >18 years:

SC administration: 200 mg SC once weekly. May be self-administered by the patient in the home setting.

Comment: ***Benlysta*** was initially approved as an intravenous formulation administered in a hospital or clinic setting as a weight-dosed IV infusion every four weeks. Patients can now self-administer **Benlysta** as a once weekly SC injection after being trained by a healthscare provider.

IV infusion: 10 mg/kg at 2-week intervals for the first 3 doses and at 4-week intervals thereafter; reconstitute, dilute, and administer as an intravenous infusion over a period of 1 hour. Consider administering premedication for prophylaxis against infusion reactions and hypersensitivity reactions. Must be administered in a hospital or clinic setting by a qualified healthcare provider

Benlysta Prefilled syringe: 200 mg/ml (1 ml) single-dose (4/carton); *Autoinjector:* 200 mg (1 ml) single-dose (4/carton); *Vial:* 120 mg/5 ml, 400 mg/20 ml, single-dose, pwdr for reconstitution and IV infusion (4/carton)

Comment: **Benlysta** is indicated for the treatment of patients >18 years-of-age with active, autoantibody-positive, systemic lupus erythematosus who are receiving standard therapy. Common adverse reactions include nausea, diarrhea, pyrexia, nasopharyngitis, bronchitis, insomnia, pain in extremity, depression, migraine, and pharyngitis. The efficacy of **Benlysta** has not been evaluated in patients with severe active lupus nephritis or severe active central nervous system lupus. **Benlysta** has not been studied in combination with other biologics or intravenous ***cyclophosphamide.*** Therefore, use of Benlysta is not recommended in these situations. Limited data on use of **Benlysta** in pregnancy women, from observational studies, published case reports, and post-marketing surveillance, is insufficient to determine whether there is a drug-associated risk for major birth defects or miscarriage. Monoclonal antibodies, such as ***belimumab,*** are actively transported across the placenta during the third trimester of pregnancy and may affect immune response in the in utero-exposed infant. Monoclonal antibodies are increasingly transported across the placenta as pregnancy progresses, with the largest amount transferred during the third trimester. No information is available on the presence of ***belimumab*** in human milk or the effects of the drug on the breastfed infant. As there are risks to the mother and fetus associated with SLE, risks and benefits should be considered prior to administering live or live-attenuated vaccines to infants exposed to **Benlasta** in utero. Monitor the infant of a treated mother for B-cell reduction and other immune dysfunction. There is a pregnancy exposure registry that monitors pregnancy outcomes in females exposed to **Benlysta** during pregnancy. Healthcare professionals are encouraged to register patients by calling 1-877-681-6296. To report suspected adverse reactions, contact GlaxoSmithKline at 1-877-423-6597 or FDA at 1-800-FDA-1088 or visit www.fda.gov/medwatch

DISEASE MODIFYING ANTI-RHEUMATIC DRUGS (DMARDs)

Comment: DMARDs include ***penicillamine***, gold salts (***auranofin, aurothio- glucose***), immunosuppressants, and ***hydroxychloroquine***. The DMARDs reduce ESR, reduce RF, and favorably affect SLE symptoms. Immunosuppressants may require 6 weeks to affect benefits and 6 months for full improvement.

- ***auranofin (gold salt)*** **(C)** <12 years: not recommended; ≥12 years: 3 mg bid or 6 mg once daily; if inadequate response after 6 months, increase to 3 mg tid
  - **Ridaura** *Vial:* 100 mg/20 ml
- ***azathioprine*** **(D)** <12 years: not recommended; ≥12 years: 1 mg/kg/day in a single or divided doses; may increase by 0.5 mg/kg/day q 4 weeks; max 2.5 mg/kg/day; minimum trial to ascertain effectiveness is 12 weeks
  - **Azasan** *Tab* 75*, 100*mg
  - **Imuran** *Tab* 50*mg
- ***cyclosporine (immunosuppressant)*** **(C)** <12 years: not recommended; ≥12 years: 1.25 mg/kg bid; may increase after 4 weeks by 0.5 mg/kg/day; then adjust at 2 week intervals; max 4 mg/kg/day; administer with meals
  - **Neoral** *Cap:* 25, 100 mg (alcohol)
  - **Neoral Oral Solution** *Oral soln:* 100 mg/ml (50 ml) may dilute in room temperature apple juice or orange juice (alcohol)
  - Comment: **Neoral** is indicated for RA unresponsive to ***methotrexate*** **(MTX)**.
- ***leflunomide*** **(X)(G)** <18 years: not recommended; ≥18 years: initially 100 mg once daily x 3 days; maintenance dose 20 mg once daily; max 20 mg daily
  - **Arava** *Tab:* 10, 20, 100 mg
  - Comment: **Arava** is contraindicated with breastfeeding.
- ***methotrexate*** **(X)** <2 years: not recommended; ≥2-12 years: 10 mg/m2 once weekly; max 20 mg/m2; ≥12 years: 7.5 mg x 1 dose per week or 2.5 mg x 3 at 12 hour intervals once a week; max 20 mg/week; therapeutic response begins in 3-6 weeks; administer ***methotrexate*** injection SC only into the abdomen or thigh
  - **Rasuvo** *Autoinjector:* 7.5 mg/0.15 ml, 10 mg/0.20 ml, 12.5 mg/0.25 ml, 15 mg/0.30 ml, 17.5 mg/0.35 ml, 20 mg/0.40 ml, 22.5 mg/0.45 ml, 25 mg/0.50 ml, 27.5 mg/0.55 ml, 30 mg/0.60 ml (solution concentration for SC injection is 50 mg/ml)
  - **Rheumatrex** *Tab:* 2.5*mg (5, 7.5, 10, 12.5, 15 mg/week, 4/card unit-of-use dose pack)
  - **Trexall** *Tab:* 5*, 7.5*, 10*, 15*mg (5, 7.5, 10, 12.5, 15 mg/week, 4/card unit-of-use dose pack)

  Comment: ***methotrexate*** **(MTX)** is contraindicated with immunodeficiency, blood dyscrasias, alcoholism, and chronic liver disease.
- ***penicillamine*** **(D)** <12 years: not recommended; ≥12 years: 125-250 mg once daily initially; may increase by 125-250 mg/day q 1-3 months; max 1.5 gm/day
  - **Cuprimine** *Cap:* 125, 250 mg
  - **Depen** *Tab:* 250 mg
- ***sulfasalazine*** **(C; D in 2nd, 3rd)(G)** initially 0.5 gm once daily bid; gradually increase every 4 days; usual maintenance 2-3 gm/day in equally divided doses at regular intervals; max 4 gm/day

  Pediatric: <6 years: not recommended; 6-16 years: initially 1/4 to 1/3 of maintenance dose; increase weekly; maintenance 30-50 mg/kg/day in 2 divided doses at regular intervals; max 2 gm/day
  - **Azulfidine** *Tab:* 500 mg
  - **Azulfidine EN** *Tab:* 500 mg ent-coat

ANTIMALARIALS

▶ ***atovaquone*** (C)(G) <13 years: not established; ≥13 years: take as a single dose with food or a milky drink at the same time each day; repeat dose if vomited within 1 hour; *Prophylaxis:* 1,500 mg once daily; *Treatment:* 750 mg bid x 21 days
  Mepron *Susp:* 750 mg/5 ml

▶ ***atovaquone+proguanil*** (C)(G) <5 kg: not recommended; 5-40 kg: *Prophylaxis:* daily dose starting 1-2 days before entering endemic area, during stay, and for 7 days after return; 5-20 kg: 1 ped tab; 21-30 kg: 2 ped tabs; 31-40 kg: 3 ped tabs; ≥40 kg: same as adult; *Treatment (acute, uncomplicated):* daily dose x 3 days; 5-8 kg: 2 ped tabs; 9-10 kg: 3 ped tabs; 11-20 kg: 1 adult tab; 21-30 kg: 2 adult tabs; 31-40 kg: 3 adult tabs; >40 kg: take as a single dose with food or a milky drink at the same time each day; repeat dose if vomited within 1 hour; *Prophylaxis:* 1 tab daily starting 1-2 days before entering endemic area, during stay, and for 7 days after return; *Treatment (acute, uncomplicated):* 4 tabs daily x 3 days
  Malarone *Tab:* atov 250 mg+prog 100 mg
  Malarone Pediatric *Tab:* atov 62.5 mg+prog 25 mg
 Comment: ***atovaquone*** is antagonized by ***tetracycline*** and ***metoclopramide***. Concomitant ***rifampin*** is not recommended (may elevate LFTs).

▶ ***chloroquine*** (C)(G) *Prophylaxis:* 500 mg once weekly (on the same day of each week); start 2 weeks prior to exposure, continue while in the endemic area, and continue 4 weeks after departure; *Treatment:* initially 1 gm; then 500 mg 6 hours, 24 hours, and 48 hours after initial dose or initially 200-250 mg IM; may repeat in 6 hours; max 1 gm in first 24 hours; continue to 1.875 gm in 3 days
 Suppression: 8.35 mg/kg (max 500 mg) weekly (on the same day of each week); *Treatment:* initially 16.7 mg/kg (max 1 gm); then 8.35 mg/kg (max 500 mg) 6 hours, 24 hours, and 48 hours after initial dose, or initially 6.25 mg/kg IM; may repeat in 6 hours; max 12.5 mg/kg/day
  Aralen *Tab:* 500 mg; *Amp:* 50 mg/ml (5 ml)

▶ ***hydroxychloroquine*** (C)(G) <12 years: not recommended; ≥12 years: 400-600 mg/day
  Plaquenil *Tab:* 200 mg

Comment: May require several weeks to achieve beneficial effects. If no improvement in 6 months, discontinue.

▶ ***mefloquine*** (C) <6 months: not recommended; *Prophylaxis:* ≥6 months: 3-5 mg/kg (max 250 mg) weekly (on the same day of each week); start 1 week prior to exposure, continue while in the endemic area, and continue for 4 weeks after departure; *Treatment:* ≥6 months: 25-50 mg/kg as a single dose; max 250 mg as a single dose
  Lariam *Tab:* 250*mg
 Comment: ***mefloquine*** is contraindicated with active or recent history of depression, generalized anxiety disorder, psychosis, schizophrenia or any other psychiatric disorder or history of convulsions.

▶ ***quinine sulfate*** (C)(G) <16 years: not recommended; ≥16 years: 1 tab or cap every 8 hours x 7 days
  Tab: 260 mg; *Cap:* 260, 300, 325 mg
  Qualaquin *Cap:* 324 mg
  Comment: ***Qualaquin*** is indicated in the treatment of uncomplicated *P. falciparum* malaria (including chloroquine-resistant strains).

TAPEWORM (CESTODE)

ANTHELMINTICS

Comment: Oral bioavailability of anthelmintics is enhanced when administered with a fatty meal (estimated fat content 40 gm).

▶ ***albendazole*** (C) take with a meal; may crush and mix with food; may repeat in 3 weeks if needed; <2 years: 200 mg bid x 7 days; 2-12 years: 400 mg once daily x 7 days; >12 years: 400 mg bid x 7 days

Albenza *Tab:* 200 mg

Comment: ***albendazole*** is a broad-spectrum benzimidazole carbamate anthelmintic.

TARDIVE DYSKINESIA

Comment: Tardive dyskinesia is a treatable, albeit irreversible, neurological disorder characterized by repetitive involuntary movements, usually of the jaw, lips and tongue, such as grimacing, sticking out the tongue and smacking the lips. Some affected people also experience involuntary movement of the extremities or difficulty breathing. This condition is most often an adverse side effect associated with the older "typical" antipsychotic drugs. Risk is decreased with the newer "atypical" antipsychotic drugs. The first and only FDA-approved treatment for this disorder is ***valbenazine*** **(Ingrezza),** a vesicular monoamine transporter 2 (VMAT2) inhibitor.

REFERENCE

Davis, MC, Miller, BJ, Kalsi, JK, *et al.* (2017). Efficient trial design—FDA approval of valbenazine for tardive dyskinesia. *The New England Journal of Medicine, 376*(26), 2503–2506.

▶ ***amantadine*** <18 years: not recommended; ≥18 years: <18 years: not recommended; ≥18 years: initial dose 129 mg orally once daily in the morning; may be increase dose in weekly intervals; max daily dose 322 mg in the morning; dose frequency reduction and monitoring required for renal impairment; swallow whole; do not chew, crush, or divide

Osmolex ER *Tab:* 129, 193, 258 mg ext-rel

Comment: **Osmolex ER** is not interchangeable with other ***amantadine*** immediate- or extended-release products. Most common adverse reactions (incidence ≥ 5%) are nausea, dizziness/ lightheadedness, and insomnia. **Osmolex ER** is contraindicated in patients with end-stage renal disease (ESRD). Advise patients prior to treatment about potential for falling asleep during activities of daily living (ADLs) and somnolence and discontinue **Osmolex ER** if occurs. Monitor patients for depressed mood, depression, and suicidal ideation or behavior. Patients with major psychotic disorder should ordinarily not be treated with **Osmolex ER**; observe patients throughout treatment for the occurrence of hallucinations, especially at initiation and after dose increases. Monitor patients for dizziness and orthostatic hypotension, especially after starting **Osmolex ER** or increasing the dose. Avoid sudden withdrawal/discontinuation due to risk of Withdrawal-Emergent Hyperpyrexia and confusion: Monitor patient for development of impulse control/compulsive behaviors. Ask patients about increased gambling urges, sexual urges, uncontrolled spending or other urges and consider dose reduction or discontinuation if any occur. Increased risk of anticholinergic effects may require reduction of **Osmolex ER** or dose of the anticholinergic drug(s). Excretion of ***amantadine*** increases with acidic urine resulting in possible accumulation with urine change towards alkaline. Live Attenuated Influenza Vaccines (LAVs) are not recommended during treatment with **Osmolex ER**. Concomitant use of alcohol is not recommended due to increased potential for CNS effects. There are no adequate data on the developmental risk associated with use of ***amantadine*** in pregnant women. Animal studies suggest a potential risk for fetal harm with ***amantadine***. ***Amantadine*** is excreted in human milk, but amounts have not been quantified. There is no information on the risk to the breastfed infant. To report suspected reactions, contact Vertical Pharmaceuticals, LLC at 1-877-482-3788 or FDA at 1-800-FDA-1088 or www.fda.gov/medwatch

VESICULAR MONOAMINE TRANSPORTER 2 (VMAT2) INHIBITOR

▶ *valbenazine* <18 years: not established; ≥18 years: initially 40 mg once daily; after one week, increase to the recommended 80 mg once daily; take with or without food; recommended dose for patients with moderate or severe hepatic impairment is 40 mg once daily; consider dose reduction based on tolerability in known CYP2D6 poor metabolizers; concomitant use of strong CYP3A4 inducers is not recommended; avoid concomitant use of MAOIs

Ingrezza *Cap:* 40 mg

Comment: The limited available data on **Ingrezza** use in pregnant females are insufficient to inform a drug-associated risk. There is no information regarding the presence of **Ingrezza** or its metabolites in human milk or the effects on the breastfed infant. However, females are advised not to breastfeed during treatment and for 5 days after the final dose. To report suspected adverse reactions, contact Neurocrine Biosciences, Inc at 1-877-641-3461 or FDA at 1-800-FDA-1088 or visit www.fda.gov/medwatch.

TEMPOROMANDIBULAR JOINT (TMJ) DISORDER

Injectable Acetaminophen *see* **Pain** *page* 322
NSAIDs *see page* 539
Other Oral Analgesics see ***Pain*** *page* 324
Topical & Transdermal NSAIDs *see* ***Pain*** *page* 323
Parenteral Corticosteroids *see page* 547
Oral Corticosteroids *see page* 546

SKELETAL MUSCLE RELAXANTS

▶ ***baclofen*** (C)(G) <12 years: not recommended; ≥12 years: 5 mg tid; titrate up by 5 mg every 3 days to 20 mg tid; max 80 mg/day

Lioresal *Tab:* 10*, 20*mg

Comment: ***baclofen*** is indicated for muscle spasm pain and chronic spasticity associated with multiple sclerosis and spinal cord injury or disease. Potential for seizures or hallucinations on abrupt withdrawal.

▶ ***carisoprodol*** (C)(G) <12 years: not recommended; ≥12 years: 1 tab tid or qid

Soma *Tab:* 350 mg

▶ ***chlorzoxazone*** (G) <12 years: not recommended; ≥12 years: 1 caplet qid; max 750 mg qid

Parafon Forte DSC *Cplt:* 500*mg

▶ ***cyclobenzaprine*** (B)(G) <15 years: not recommended; ≥15 years: 10 mg tid; usual range 20-40 mg/day in divided doses; max 60 mg/day x 2-3 weeks or 15 mg ext-rel once daily; max 30 mg ext-rel/day x 2-3 weeks

Amrix *Cap:* 15, 30 mg ext-rel
Fexmid *Tab:* 7.5 mg
Flexeril *Tab:* 5, 10 mg

▶ ***dantrolene*** (C) <12 years: 0.5 mg/kg daily x 7 days; then 0.5 mg/kg tid x 7 days; then 1 mg/kg tid x 7 days; then 2 mg/kg tid; max 100 mg qid; ≥12 years: 25 md daily x 7 days; then 25 mg tid x 7 days; then 50 mg tid x 7 days; max 100 mg qid

Dantrium *Tab:* 25, 50, 100 mg

Comment: ***dantrolene*** is indicated for chronic spasticity associated with multiple sclerosis and spinal cord injury or disease.

- ▶ ***diazepam*** (C)(IV) <6 months: not recommended; >6 months-12 years: initially 1-2.5 mg bid-qid; may increase gradually; ≥12 years: 2-10 mg bid-qid; may increase gradually
  - **Diastat** *Rectal gel delivery system:* 2.5 mg
  - **Diastat AcuDial** *Rectal gel delivery system:* 10, 20 mg
  - **Valium** *Tab:* 2, 5, 10 mg
  - **Valium Intensol Oral Solution** *Conc oral soln:* 5 mg/ml (30 ml w. dropper) (alcohol 19%)
  - **Valium Oral Solution** *Oral soln:* 5 mg/5 ml (500 ml) (wintergreen spice)
- ▶ ***metaxalone*** (B) <12 years: not recommended; ≥12 years: 1 tab tid-qid
  - **Skelaxin** *Tab:* 800*mg
- ▶ ***methocarbamol*** (C)(G) <16 years: not recommended; ≥16 years: initially 1.5 gm qid x 2-3 days; maintenance, 750 mg every 4 hours or 1.5 gm 3 x/day; max 8 gm/day
  - **Robaxin** *Tab:* 500 mg
  - **Robaxin 750** *Tab:* 750 mg
  - **Robaxin Injection** 10 ml IM or IV; max 30 ml/day; max 3 days; max 5 ml/gluteal injection q 8 hours; max IV rate 3 ml/min
    - *Vial:* 100 mg/ml (10 ml)
- ▶ ***nabumetone*** (C) <12 years: not recommended; ≥12 years: initially 1,000 mg as a single dose; titrate as needed; may split dose bid; max 2,000 mg/day
  - **Relafen** *Tab:* 500, 750 mg
  - **Relafen 500** *Tab:* 500 mg
- ▶ ***orphenadrine citrate*** (C)(G) <12 years: not recommended; ≥12 years: 1 tab bid
  - **Norflex** *Tab:* 100 mg sust-rel
- ▶ ***tizanidine*** (C) <12 years: not recommended; ≥12 years: 1-4 mg q 6-8 hours; max 36 mg/day
  - **Zanaflex** *Tab:* 2*, 4**mg; *Cap:* 2, 4, 6 mg

SKELETAL MUSCLE RELAXANT+NSAID COMBINATIONS

Comment: ***aspirin***-containing medications are contraindicated with history of allergic type reaction to ***aspirin***, children and adolescents with *Varicella* or other viral illness, and 3rd trimester pregnancy.

- ▶ ***carisoprodol+aspirin*** (C)(III)(G) <12 years: not recommended; ≥12 years: 1-2 tabs qid
  - **Soma Compound** *Tab: caris* 200 mg+*asp* 325 mg (sulfites)
- ▶ ***meprobamate+aspirin*** (D)(IV) <12 years: not recommended; ≥12 years: 1-2 tabs tid or qid
  - **Equagesic** *Tab: mepro* 200 mg+*asp* 325 mg*

SKELETAL MUSCLE RELAXANT+NSAID+CAFFEINE COMBINATIONS

- ▶ ***orphenadrine+aspirin+caffeine*** (D)(IV)(G) <12 years: not recommended; ≥12 years:
  - **Norgesic** 1-2 tabs tid-qid
    - *Tab: orphen* 25 mg+*asp* 385 mg+*caf* 30 mg*
  - **Norgesic Forte** 1 tab tid or qid; max 4 tabs/day
    - *Tab: orphen* 50 mg+*asp* 770 mg+*caf* 60 mg*

Comment: ***aspirin***-containing medications are contraindicated with history of allergic-type reaction to ***aspirin***, children and adolescents with *Varicella* or other viral illness, and 3rd trimester of pregnancy.

SKELETAL MUSCLE RELAXANT+NSAID+CODEINE COMBINATIONS

▶ ***carisoprodol+aspirin+codeine*** (D)(III)(G) <12 years: contraindicated; 12-<18: use extreme caution; not recommended for children and adolescents with obesity, asthma, obstructive sleep apnea, or other chronic breathing problem, or for post-tonsillectomy/adenoidectomy pain; ≥18 years:

Soma Compound w. Codeine 1-2 tabs qid

Tab: caris 200 mg+*asp* 325 mg+*cod* 16 mg (sulfites)

Comment: ***Codeine*** is known to be excreted in breast milk. <12 years: not recommended; 12-<18: use extreme caution; not recommended for children and adolescents with asthma or other chronic breathing problem. The FDA and the European Medicines Agency (EMA) are investigating the safety of using ***codeine*** containing medications to treat pain, cough and colds, in children 12-<18 years because of the potential for serious side effects, including slowed or difficult breathing. ***aspirin***-containing medications are contraindicated with history of allergic-type reaction to ***aspirin***, children and adolescents with *Varicella* or other viral illness, and 3rd trimester of pregnancy.

☐ TESTOSTERONE DEFICIENCY, HYPOTESTOSTERONEMIA, HYPOGONADISM

Comment: ***testosterone*** is contraindicated in male breast cancer and prostate cancer. ***Testosterone*** replacement therapy is indicated in males with primary hypogonadism (congenital or acquired due to cryptorchidism, bilateral torsion, orchitis, vanishing testis syndrome, or orchidectomy), or hypogonadotropic hypogonadism (congenital or acquired), and delayed puberty not secondary to a pathological disorder (x-ray of the hand and wrist to determine bone age should be obtained every 6 months to assess the effect of treatment on the epiphyseal centers).

ORAL ANDROGENS

▶ ***fluoxymesterone*** (X)(III) *Hypogonadism:* <12 years: use by specialist only; *Puberty:* 5-20 mg once daily; *Delayed puberty:* use low dose and limit duration to 4-6 months

Halotestin *Tab:* 2*, 5*, 10*mg (tartrazine)

▶ ***methyltestosterone*** (X)(III) *Hypogonadism:* <12 years: use by specialist only; *Puberty:* usually 10-50 mg once daily; *Delayed puberty:* use low dose and limit duration to 4-6 months

Android *Cap:* 10 mg

Methitest *Tab:* 10*mg

Testred *Cap:* 10 mg

▶ ***testosterone*** (X)(III) <18 years: not recommended; ≥18 years: 30 mg q 12 hours to gum region, just above the incisor tooth on either side of the mouth; hold system in place for 30 seconds; rotate sites with each application

Striant *Buccal tab:* 30 mg (6 blister pcks; 10 buccal systems/blister pck)

Comment: Serum total ***testosterone*** concentrations may be checked 4 to 12 weeks after initiating treatment with **Striant**. To capture the maximum serum concentration, an early morning sample (just prior to applying the AM dose) is recommended.

TOPICAL ANDROGENS

Comment: Topical androgens are not recommended under 18 years-of-age. Wash hands after application. Allow solution to dry before it touches clothing. Do not wash site for at least 2 hours after application. Pregnant and nursing females, and children, must avoid skin contact with application sites. If there is contact, wash the area as soon as possible with soap and water.

▶ ***testosterone*** (X)(III)

AndroGel 1% (G) <18 years: not recommended; ≥18 years: initially apply 25 mg once daily in the AM to clean, dry, intact skin of the shoulders, upper arms, and/or abdomen; do not apply to scrotum; may increase to 75 mg/day and then to 100 mg/day if needed

Gel: 25 mg/2.5 gm pkt (30 pkts/carton); 50 mg/5 gm pkt (30 pkts/carton)

AndroGel 1.62% (G) <18 years: not recommended; ≥18 years: initially apply 25 mg once daily in the AM to clean, dry, skin of the shoulders and upper arms intact skin of the upper arms; do not apply to abdomen or genitals; may adjust dose between 1 and 4 pump actuations based on the pre-dose morning serum testosterone concentration at approximately 14 and 28 days after starting treatment or adjusting dose

Gel: 20.25 mg/1.25 gm pkt; 40.5 mg/2.5 gm pkt; 20.25 mg/1.25 gm pump actuation (60 metered dose actuations)

Axiron <18 years: not recommended; ≥18 years: apply to clean dry intact skin of the axillae; do not apply to the scrotum, penis, abdomen, shoulders, or upper arms; initially apply 60 mg (30 mg/axilla) once daily in the AM; adjust dose based on serum testosterone concentration 2 to 8 hours after applying and at least 14 days after starting therapy or following dose adjustment; may increase dose in 30 mg increments if serum testosterone <300 ng/dL up to 120 mg; reduce dose to 30 mg if levels >1050 ng/dL; discontinue if serum testosterone remains at >1050 ng/dL; to apply a 120 mg dose, apply 30 mg to each axilla and allow to dry, then repeat

Soln: 30 mg/1.5 ml pump actuation (60 metered dose actuations) (alcohol, latex-free)

Fortesta (G) <18 years: not recommended; ≥18 years: initially 40 mg of testosterone (4 pump actuations) applied to the thighs once daily in the AM; may adjust between 10 mg minimum and 70 mg maximum

Gel: 10 mg/0.5 gm pump actuation (120 metered dose actuations) (ethanol)

Comment: The **Fortesta** dose should be based on the serum ***testosterone*** concentration 2 hours after applying **Fortesta** and at approximately 14 days and 35 days after starting treatment or following dose adjustment. Dose adjustment criteria: ≤500 ng/dL, increase daily dose by 10 mg; 500-≤1250 ng/dL, no change; 1250-≤2500 ng/dL, decrease daily dose by 10 mg; ≥2500 ng/dL, decrease daily dose by 20 mg.

Testim (G) <18 years: not recommended; ≥18 years: initially apply 5 gm once daily in the AM to clean, dry, intact skin of the shoulders and/or upper arms; do not apply to the genitals or abdomen; may increase to 10 gm after 2 weeks

Gel: 1%, clear, hydroalcoholic (50 mg/5 gm pkt, 30 pkts/carton)

Vogelxo Gel (G) <18 years: not recommended; ≥18 years: 1% initially apply 5 gm once daily in the AM to clean, dry, intact skin of the shoulders, upper arms, and/or abdomen; do not apply to scrotum; may increase to 7.5 gm/day and then to 10 gm/day if needed

Gel: 50 mg/5 gm pkt (30 pkts/carton); 50 mg/5 gm tube (30 tubes/ carton); *Pump:* 12.5 mg/1.25 gm pump actuation, 60 metered dose actuations)

INTRANASAL ANDROGENS

▶ ***testosterone (nasal gel)*** **(X)(III)** <18 years: not established; ≥18 years: initially one pump actuation each nostril (33 mg) 3 x/day, at least 6-8 hours apart, at the same times each day max: 6 pump actuations/day

Natesto *Gel:* 5.5 mg/0.122 gm pump actuation (60 metered dose actuations)

TRANSDERMAL ANDROGEN PATCH

▶ *testosterone* (X)(III)
Androderm <15 years: not recommended; ≥15 years: initially apply 4 mg nightly at approximately 10 PM to clean, dry area of the arm, back, or upper buttocks; leave on x 24 hours; may increase to 7.5 mg or decrease to 2.5 mg based on confirmed AM serum testosterone concentrations
Transdermal patch: 2, 4 mg/24 Hr

TETANUS (*CLOSTRIDIUM TETANI*)

PROPHYLAXIS

See **Childhood Immunizations** *page* 525

POSTEXPOSURE PROPHYLAXIS IN PREVIOUSLY NON-IMMUNIZED PERSONS

▶ ***tetanus immune globulin, human*** (C) <7 years: not recommended; ≥7 years: 250 mg deep IM in a single dose
BayTET, HyperTET *Vial:* 250 unit single-dose; *Prefilled syringe:* 250 units
▶ ***tetanus toxoid* vaccine** (C) 0.5 ml IM x 3 dose series
Vial: 5 Lf units/0.5 ml (0.5, 5 ml); *Prefilled syringe:* 5 Lf units/0.5 ml (0.5 ml)

Comment: Dose of **BayTET/HyperTET** S/D is calculated as 4 units/kg. However, it may be advisable to administer the entire contents of the syringe of **BayTET/HyperTET** S/D (250 units) regardless of the child's size, since theoretically the same amount of toxin will be produced in the child's body by the infecting tetanus organism as it will in an adult's body. At the same time but in a different extremity and with a different syringe, administer Diphtheria and Tetanus Toxoids and Pertussis Vaccine Adsorbed (DTP) or Diphtheria and Tetanus Toxoids Adsorbed (For Pediatric Use) (DT), if pertussis vaccine is contraindicated, should be administered per mfr pkg insert. Tetanus immune globulin may interact with live viral vaccines such as measles, mumps, rubella, and polio. It is also unknown if **BayTET/HyperTET** can cause fetal harm when administered to a pregnant female or can affect reproduction capacity. The single injection of tetanus toxoid only initiates the series for producing active immunity in the recipient. The patient will need further toxoid injections in 1 month and 1 year; otherwise the active immunization series is incomplete. If a contraindication to using tetanus toxoid-containing preparations exists for a person who has not completed a primary series of tetanus toxoid immunization, and that person has a wound that is neither clean nor minor, only passive immunization should be administered using tetanus immune globulin.

THREADWORM (*STRONGYLOIDES STERCORALIS*)

ANTHELMINTICS

Comment: Oral bioavailability of anthelmintics is enhanced when administered with a fatty meal (estimated fat content 40 gm).

▶ ***albendazole*** (C) take with a meal; may crush and mix with food; may repeat in 3 weeks if needed; <2 years: 200 mg bid x 7 days; 2-12 years: 400 mg once daily x 7 days; >12 years: 400 mg bid x 7 days
Albenza *Tab:* 200 mg
Comment: ***albendazole*** is a broad-spectrum benzimidazole carbamate anthelmintic.
▶ ***ivermectin*** (C) take with water; chew or crush and mix with food; may repeat in 3 months if needed; <15 kg: not recommended; ≥15 kg: 200 mcg/kg as a single dose
Stromectol *Tab:* 3, 6*mg

- ***mebendazole*** (C)(G) take with a meal; chew or crush and mix with food; may repeat in 3 weeks if needed; <2 years: not recommended; ≥2 years: 100 mg bid x 3 days
  Emverm *Chew tab:* 100 mg
  Vermox *Chew tab:* 100 mg
- ***pyrantel pamoate*** (C) take with a meal; may open capsule and sprinkle or mix with food; treat x 3 days; may repeat in 2-3 weeks if needed; treat x 3 days; 11 mg/kg/dose; max 1 gm/dose; <25 lb: not recommended; 25-37 lb: 1/2 tsp/dose; 38-62 lb: 1 tsp/dose; 63-87 lb: 1 tsp/dose; 88-112 lb: 2 tsp/dose; 113-137 lb: 2 tsp/dose; 138-162 lb: 3 tsp/dose; 163-187 lb: 3 tsp/dose; >187 lb: 4 tsp/dose
  Antiminth *Cap:* 180 mg; *Liq:* 50 mg/ml (30 ml); 144 mg/ml (30 ml); *Oral susp:* 50 mg/ml (60 ml)
  Pin-X *Cap:* 180 mg; *Liq:* 50 mg/ml (30 ml); 144 mg/ml (30 ml); *Oral susp:* 50 mg/ml (30 ml)
- ***thiabendazole*** (C) take with a meal; may crush and mix with food; treat x 7 days; <30 lb: consult mfr pkg insert; ≥30 lb: 25 mg/kg/dose bid with meals; 30-50 lb: 250 mg bid with meals; >50 lb: 10 mg/lb/dose bid with meals; max 1.5 gm/dose; max 3 gm/day
  Mintezol *Chew tab:* 500*mg (orange); *Oral susp:* 500 mg/5 ml (120 ml) (orange)
  Comment: ***thiabendazole*** is not for prophylaxis. May impair mental alertness. May not be available in the US.

THROMBOCYTOPENIA

THROMBOPOIETIN (TPO) RECEPTOR AGONIST

Comment: **Doptelet *(avatrombopage)*** is the first oral thrombopoietin (TPO) receptor agonist approved by the FDA for the treatment of adults with chronic liver disease who are scheduled to undergo a procedure. **Doptelet** is a second generation, once-daily, orally administered TPO receptor agonist that works by increasing platelet counts to the target level of greater or equal to 50,000 per microliter.

- ***avatrombopag*** <18 years: not recommended; ≥18 years: begin dosing 10 to 13 days prior to a scheduled procedure; the patient should undergo the procedure within 5 to 8 days after the last dose; take with food, as a single dose x 5 consecutive days; PLT count <40 x 10^9/L: 60 mg (3 tabs) once daily x 5 days; PLT count 40-50 x 10^9/L: 40 mg (2 tabs) once daily x 5 days
  Doptelet *Tab:* 20 mg film-coat
  Comment: TPO receptor agonists have been associated with thrombotic and thromboembolic complications in patients with chronic liver disease. Monitor platelet counts and for thromboembolic events and institute treatment promptly. Potential adverse reactions include pyrexia, abdominal pain, nausea, headache, fatigue, and peripheral edema. Based on animal studies, ***avatrombopag*** may cause fetal harm when administered to a pregnant female. There are no information regarding the presence of ***avatrombopag*** in human milk or effects on the breastfed infant. However, breastfeeding is not recommended during treatment with **Doptelet** and for at least 2 weeks after the last dose. Safety and effectiveness in patients (<18 years-of-age) have not been established. To report suspected adverse reactions, contact Dova Pharmaceuticals at 1-844-506-3682 or FDA at 1-800-FDA-1088 or visit www.fda.gov/medwatch

TINEA CAPITIS

Comment: Tinea capitis must be treated with an oral antifungal.

FOR SEVERE KERION PRURITUS

▶ *prednisone* (C) 1 mg/kg/day for 7-14 days
See ***Oral Corticosteroids*** *page* 546

SYSTEMIC ANTIFUNGALS

▶ ***griseofulvin, microsize*** (C)(G) <12 years: <30 lb: 5 mg/lb/day; 30-50 lb: 125-250 mg/day; >50 lb: 250-500 mg/day; 5 mg/lb/day x 4-6 weeks or longer; *see page* 612 *for dose by weight table;* >12 years: 500 mg once daily x 4-6 weeks or longer; max 1 gm/day
Grifulvin V *Tab:* 250, 500 mg; *Oral susp:* 125 mg/5 ml (120 ml) (alcohol 0.02%)

▶ ***griseofulvin, ultramicrosize*** (C)(G) <2 years: not recommended; 2-12 years: 3.3 mg/lb/day in a single or divided doses x 4-6 weeks or longer; >12 years: 375 mg/day in a single or divided doses x 4-6 weeks or longer
Gris-PEG *Tab:* 125, 250 mg

Comment: ***griseofulvin*** should be taken with fatty foods (e.g., milk, ice cream). Liver enzymes should be monitored.

▶ ***ketoconazole*** (C)(G) <2 years: not recommended; ≥2 years-12 years: 3.3-6.6 mg/kg once daily x 4 weeks; >12 years: initially 200 mg once daily; max 400 mg/day x 4 weeks
Nizoral ***Tab:*** 200 mg

Comment: Caution with ***ketoconazole*** due to potential for hepatotoxicity.

TINEA CORPORIS (RINGWORM)

TOPICAL ANTI-FUNGALS

▶ ***butenafine*** (C)(G) <12 years: not recommended; ≥12 years: apply bid x 1 week or once daily x 4 weeks
Lotrimin Ultra (OTC) *Crm:* 1% (12, 24 gm)
Mentax *Crm:* 1% (15, 30 gm)

Comment: ***butenafine*** is a benzylamine, not an azole. Fungicidal activity continues for at least 5 weeks after last application.

▶ ***ciclopirox*** (B)
Loprox Cream <10 years: not recommended; ≥10 years: apply bid; max 4 weeks
Crm: 0.77% (15, 30, 90 gm)
Loprox Lotion <10 years: not recommended; ≥10 years: apply bid; max 4 weeks
Lotn: 0.77% (30, 60 ml)
Loprox Gel <16 years: not recommended; ≥16 years: apply bid; max 4 weeks
Gel: 0.77% (30, 45 gm)

▶ ***clotrimazole*** (B)(G) apply to affected area bid x 14 days
Lotrimin *Crm:* 1% (15, 30, 45 gm)
Lotrimin AF (OTC) *Crm:* 1% (12 gm); *Lotn:* 1% (10 ml); *Soln:* 1% (10 ml)

▶ ***econazole*** (C) apply once daily x 14 days
Spectazole *Crm:* 1% (15, 30, 85 gm)

▶ ***ketoconazole*** (C) apply to affected area bid x 14 days
Nizoral Cream *Crm:* 2% (15, 30, 60 gm)

▶ ***luliconazole*** (C) <18 years: not recommended; ≥18 years: apply to affected area and 1 inch into the immediate surrounding area(s) once daily
Luzu Cream 1% *Crm:* 1% (30, 60 gm)

▶ ***miconazole*** **2%** (C) <12 years: not recommended; ≥12 years: apply qd-bid x 2 weeks
Lotrimin AF Spray Liquid (OTC) *Spray liq:* 2% (113 gm) (alcohol 17%)
Lotrimin AF Spray Powder (OTC) *Spray pwdr:* 2% (90 gm) (alcohol 10%)
Monistat-Derm *Crm:* 2% (1, 3 oz); *Spray liq:* 2% (3.5 oz); *Spray pwdr:* 2% (3 oz)

▶ ***naftifine*** (B)(G)

Naftin Cream <12 years: not recommended; ≥12 years: apply once daily x 14 days

Crm: 1% (15, 30, 60 gm)

Naftin Gel apply <12 years: not recommended; ≥12 years: bid x 14 days

Gel: 1% (20, 40, 60 gm)

▶ ***oxiconazole nitrate*** (B)(G) <12 years: not recommended; ≥12 years: apply qd-bid x 2 weeks

Oxistat *Crm:* 1% (15, 30, 60 gm); *Lotn:* 1% (30 ml)

▶ ***sulconazole*** (C) <12 years: not recommended; ≥12 years: apply qd-bid x 3 weeks

Exelderm *Crm:* 1% (15, 30, 60 gm); *Lotn:* 1% (30 mg)

▶ ***terbinafine*** (B)(G)

Lamisil Cream (OTC) <12 years: not recommended; ≥12 years: apply to affected and surrounding area qd-bid x 1-4 weeks until significantly improved

Crm: 1% (15, 30 gm)

Lamisil AT Cream (OTC) apply to affected and surrounding area qd-bid x 1-4 weeks until significantly improved

Crm: **1% (15, 30 gm)**

Lamisil Solution (OTC) <12 years: not recommended; ≥12 years: apply to affected and surrounding area once daily x 1 week

Soln: 1% (30 ml spray bottle)

TOPICAL ANTIFUNGAL+STEROID COMBINATION

▶ ***clotrimazole+betamethasone*** (C)(G) <12 years: not recommended; ≥12 years: apply bid x 2 weeks; max 4 weeks

Lotrisone ***Crm:*** clotrim 10 mg+beta 0.5 mg (15, 45 gm); *Lotn:* clotrim 10 mg+ beta 0.5 mg (30 ml)

SYSTEMIC ANTIFUNGALS

▶ ***griseofulvin, microsize*** (C)(G) <12 years: <30 lb: 5 mg/lb/day; 30-50 lb: 125-250 mg/day; >50 lb: 250-500 mg/day; 5 mg/lb/day x 4-6 weeks <u>or</u> longer; *see page* 612 *for dose by weight table;* ≥12 years: 500 mg once daily x 4-6 weeks <u>or</u> longer; max 1 gm/day

Grifulvin V *Tab:* 250, 500 mg; *Oral susp:* 125 mg/5 ml (120 ml) (alcohol 0.02%)

▶ ***griseofulvin, ultramicrosize*** (C)(G) <2 years: not recommended; 2-12 years: 3.3 mg/lb/day in a single <u>or</u> divided doses x 4-6 weeks <u>or</u> longer; >12 years: 375 mg/day in a single <u>or</u> divided doses x 4-6 weeks <u>or</u> longer

Gris-PEG *Tab:* 125, 250 mg

Comment: ***griseofulvin*** should be taken with fatty foods (e.g., milk, ice cream). Liver enzymes should be monitored.

▶ ***ketoconazole*** (C)(G) <2 years: not recommended; ≥2 years-12 years: 3.3-6.6 mg/kg once daily x 4 weeks; >12 years: initially 200 mg once daily; max 400 mg/day x 4 weeks

Nizoral *Tab:* 200 mg

Comment: Caution with ***ketoconazole*** due to potential for hepatotoxicity.

TINEA CRURIS (JOCK ITCH)

TOPICAL ANTIFUNGALS

▶ ***butenafine*** (B)(G) <12 years: not recommended; ≥12 years: apply bid x 1 week <u>or</u> once daily x 4 weeks

Lotrimin Ultra (C)(OTC) *Crm:* 1% (12, 24 gm)

Mentax *Crm:* 1% (15, 30 gm)

Comment: ***butenafine*** is a benzylamine, not an azole. Fungicidal activity continues for at least 5 weeks after last application.

- ***ciclopirox*** (B)
  - **Loprox Cream** <10 years: not recommended; ≥10 years: apply bid; max 4 weeks
    - *Crm:* 0.77% (15, 30, 90 gm)
  - **Loprox Lotion** <10 years: not recommended; ≥10 years: apply bid; max 4 weeks
    - *Lotn:* 0.77% (30, 60 ml)
  - **Loprox Gel** <16 years: not recommended; ≥16 years: apply bid; max 4 weeks
    - *Gel:* 0.77% (30, 45 gm)
- ***clotrimazole*** **(B)(G)** apply to affected area bid x 7 days
  - **Lotrimin** *Crm:* 1% (15, 30, 45 gm)
  - **Lotrimin AF (OTC)** *Crm:* 1% (12 gm); *Lotn:* 1% (10 ml); *Soln:* 1% (10 ml)
- ***econazole*** **(C)** apply once daily x 2 weeks
  - **Spectazole** *Crm:* 1% (15, 30, 85 gm)
- ***ketoconazole*** **(C)** apply to affected area bid x 2 weeks
  - **Nizoral Cream** *Crm:* 2% (15, 30, 60 gm)
- ***luliconazole*** (C) <18 years: not recommended; ≥18 years: apply to affected area and 1 inch into the immediate surrounding area(s) once daily
  - **Luzu Cream 1%** *Crm:* 1% (30, 60 gm)
- ***miconazole*** **2%** (C)(G) apply qd-bid x 2 weeks
  - **Lotrimin AF Spray Liquid (OTC)** *Spray liq:* 2% (113 gm) (alcohol 17%)
  - **Lotrimin AF Spray Powder (OTC)** *Spray pwdr:* 2% (90 gm) (alcohol 10%)
  - **Monistat-Derm** *Crm:* 2% (1, 3 oz); *Spray liq:* 2% (3.5 oz); *Spray pwdr:* 2% (3 oz)
- ***naftifine*** (B)(G)
  - **Naftin Cream** <12 years: not recommended; ≥12 years: apply once daily x 2 weeks
    - *Crm:* 1% (15, 30, 60 gm)
  - **Naftin Gel** <12 years: not recommended; ≥12 years: apply bid x 2 weeks
    - *Gel:* 1% (20, 40, 60 gm)
- ***oxiconazole nitrate*** **(B)(G)** apply qd-bid x 2 weeks
  - **Oxistat** *Crm:* 1% (15, 30, 60 gm); *Lotn:* 1% (30 ml)
- ***sulconazole*** **(C)** <12 years: not recommended; ≥12 years: apply qd-bid x 3 weeks
  - **Exelderm** *Crm:* 1% (15, 30, 60 gm); *Lotn:* 1% (30 mg)
- ***terbinafine*** (B)(G)
  - **Lamisil Cream (OTC)** <12 years: not recommended; ≥12 years: apply bid x 1-4 weeks
    - *Crm:* 1% (15, 30 gm)
  - **Lamisil AT Cream (OTC)** <12 years: not recommended; ≥12 years: apply to affected and surrounding area qd-bid x 1-4 weeks until significantly improved
    - *Crm:* 1% (15, 30 gm)
  - **Lamisil Solution (OTC)** <12 years: not recommended; ≥12 years: apply to affected and surrounding area once daily x 1 week
    - *Soln:* 1% (30 ml spray bottle)
- ***tolnaftate*** (C)(OTC)(G) <2 years: not recommended; ≥2 years: apply sparingly bid x 2-4 weeks
  - **Tinactin** *Crm:* 1% (15, 30 gm); *Pwdr:* 1% (45, 90 gm); *Soln:* 1% (10 ml); *Aerosol liq:* 1% (4 oz); *Aerosol pwdr:* 1% (3.5, 5 oz)
- ***undecylenate acid*** apply bid x 4 weeks
  - **Desenex (OTC)** *Pwdr:* 25% (1.5, 3 oz); *Spray pwdr:* 25% (2.7 oz); *Oint:* 25% (0.5, 1 oz)

TOPICAL ANTIFUNGAL+STEROID COMBINATION

- ***clotrimazole+betamethasone*** (C)(G) <12 years: not recommended; ≥12 years: apply bid x 4 weeks; max 4 weeks

Lotrisone *Crm: clotrim* 10 mg+*beta* 0.5 mg (15, 45 gm); *Lotn: clotrim* 10 mg+ *beta* 0.5 mg (30 ml)

SYSTEMIC ANTIFUNGALS

▶ ***griseofulvin, microsize*** **(C)(G)** <12 years: <30 lb: 5 mg/lb/day; 30-50 lb: 125-250 mg/day; >50 lb: 250-500 mg/day; 5 mg/lb/day x 4-6 weeks or longer; *see page 612 for dose by weight table;* ≥12 years: 500 mg once daily x 4-6 weeks or longer; max 1 gm/day

Grifulvin V *Tab:* 250, 500 mg; *Oral susp:* 125 mg/5 ml (120 ml) (alcohol 0.02%)

▶ ***griseofulvin, ultramicrosize*** **(C)(G)** <2 years: not recommended; 2-12 years: 3.3 mg/lb/day in a single or divided doses x 4-6 weeks or longer; >12 years: 375 mg/day in a single or divided doses x 4-6 weeks or longer

Gris-PEG *Tab:* 125, 250 mg

Comment: ***griseofulvin*** should be taken with fatty foods (e.g., milk, ice cream). Liver enzymes should be monitored.

▶ ***ketoconazole*** **(C)(G)** <2 years: not recommended; ≥2 years-12 years: 3.3-6.6 mg/kg once daily x 4 weeks; >12 years: initially 200 mg once daily; max 400 mg/day x 4 weeks

Nizoral *Tab:* 200 mg

Comment: Caution with ***ketoconazole*** due to potential for hepatotoxicity.

TINEA PEDIS (ATHLETE'S FOOT)

TOPICAL ANTIFUNGALS

▶ ***butenafine*** **(B)(G)** <12 years: not recommended; ≥12 years: apply bid x 1 week or once daily x 4 weeks

Lotrimin Ultra (C)(OTC) *Crm:* 1% (12, 24 gm)

Mentax *Crm:* 1% (15, 30 gm)

Comment: ***butenafine*** is a benzylamine, not an azole. Fungicidal activity continues for at least 5 weeks after last application.

▶ ***ciclopirox*** **(B)**

Loprox Cream <10 years: not recommended; ≥10 years: apply bid; max 4 weeks
Crm: 0.77% (15, 30, 90 gm)

Loprox Lotion <10 years: not recommended; ≥10 years: apply bid; max 4 weeks
Lotn: 0.77% (30, 60 ml)

Loprox Gel <16 years: not recommended; ≥16 years: apply bid; max 4 weeks
Gel: 0.77% (30, 45 gm)

▶ ***clotrimazole*** **(C)(G)** <12 years: not recommended; ≥12 years: apply bid to affected area x 4 weeks

Desenex *Crm:* 1% (0.5 oz)

Lotrimin *Crm:* 1% (15, 30, 45, 90 gm); *Lotn:* 1% (30 ml); *Soln:* 1% (10, 30 ml)

Lotrimin AF (OTC) *Crm:* 1% (15, 30, 45, 90 gm); *Lotn:* 1% (20 ml); *Soln:* 1% (20 ml)

▶ ***econazole*** **(C)** apply once daily x 4 weeks

Spectazole *Crm:* 1% (15, 30, 85 gm)

▶ ***ketoconazole*** **(C)** apply to affected area bid x 4 weeks

Nizoral Cream *Crm:* 2% (15, 30, 60 gm)

▶ ***luliconazole*** **(C)** <18 years: not recommended; ≥18 years: apply to affected area and 1 inch into the immediate surrounding area(s) once daily

Luzu Cream 1% *Crm:* 1% (30, 60 gm)

▶ ***miconazole*** **2% (C)(G)** apply bid x 4 weeks

Lotrimin AF Spray Liquid (OTC) *Spray liq:* 2% (113 gm) (alcohol 17%)

Lotrimin AF Spray Powder (OTC) *Spray pwdr:* 2% (90 gm) (alcohol 10%)
Monistat-Derm *Crm:* 2% (1, 3 oz); *Spray liq:* 2% (3.5 oz); *Spray pwdr:* 2% (3 oz)

▶ ***naftifine*** **(B)(G)**
Naftin Cream <12 years: not recommended; ≥12 years: apply once daily x 4 weeks
Crm: 1% (15, 30, 60 gm)
Naftin Gel <12 years: not recommended; ≥12 years: apply bid x 4 weeks
Gel: 1% (20, 40, 60 gm)

▶ ***oxiconazole nitrate*** **(B)(G)** apply qd-bid x 4 weeks
Oxistat *Crm:* 1% (15, 30, 60 gm); *Lotn:* 1% (30 ml)

▶ ***sertaconazole*** **(C)** <12 years: not recommended; ≥12 years: apply qd-bid x 4 weeks
Ertaczo *Crm:* 2% (15, 30 gm)

▶ ***sulconazole*** **(C)** <12 years: not recommended; ≥12 years: apply qd-bid x 4 weeks
Exelderm *Crm:* 1% (15, 30, 60 gm); *Lotn:* 1% (30 mg)

▶ ***terbinafine*** **(B)(G)**
Lamisil Cream (OTC) <12 years: not recommended; ≥12 years: apply bid x 1-4 weeks
Crm: 1% (15, 30 gm)
Lamisil AT Cream (OTC) <12 years: not recommended; ≥12 years: apply to affected and surrounding area qd-bid x 1-4 weeks until significantly improved
Crm: 1% (15, 30 gm)
Lamisil Solution (OTC) <12 years: not recommended; ≥12 years: apply to affected and surrounding area bid x 1 week
Soln: 1% (30 ml spray bottle)

▶ ***tolnaftate*** **(C)(OTC)(G)** <2 years: not recommended; ≥2 years: apply sparingly bid x 2-4 weeks
Tinactin *Crm:* 1% (15, 30 gm); *Pwdr:* 1% (45, 90 gm); *Soln:* 1% (10 ml); *Aerosol liq:* 1% (4 oz); *Aerosol pwdr:* 1% (3.5, 5 oz)

TOPICAL ANTIFUNGAL+STEROID COMBINATION

▶ ***clotrimazole/betamethasone*** **(C)(G)** 12 years: not recommended; ≥12 years: apply bid x 4 weeks; max 4 weeks
Lotrisone *Crm:* clotrim 10 mg+beta 0.5 mg (15, 45 gm); *Lotn:* clotrim 10 mg+ beta 0.5 mg (30 ml)

SYSTEMIC ANTIFUNGALS

▶ ***griseofulvin, microsize*** **(C)(G)** <12 years: <30 lb: 5 mg/lb/day; 30-50 lb: 125-250 mg/day; >50 lb: 250-500 mg/day; 5 mg/lb/day x 4-6 weeks or longer; *see page 612 for dose by weight table;* ≥12 years: 500 mg once daily x 4-6 weeks or longer; max 1 gm/day
Grifulvin V *Tab:* 250, 500 mg; *Oral susp:* 125 mg/5 ml (120 ml) (alcohol 0.02%)

▶ ***griseofulvin, ultramicrosize*** **(C)(G)** <2 years: not recommended; 2-12 years: 3.3 mg/lb/day in a single or divided doses x 4-6 weeks or longer; >12 years: 375 mg/day in a single or divided doses x 4-6 weeks or longer
Gris-PEG *Tab:* 125, 250 mg

Comment: ***griseofulvin*** should be taken with fatty foods (e.g., milk, ice cream). Liver enzymes should be monitored.

▶ ***ketoconazole*** **(C)(G)** <2 years: not recommended; ≥2 years-12 years: 3.3-6.6 mg/kg once daily x 4 weeks; >12 years: initially 200 mg once daily; max 400 mg/day x 4 weeks
Nizoral *Tab:* 200 mg

Comment: Caution with ***ketoconazole*** due to potential for hepatotoxicity.

TINEA VERSICOLOR

Comment: Resolution may take 3-6 months.

TOPICAL ANTIFUNGALS

- ***butenafine*** (G) <12 years: not recommended; ≥12 years: apply once daily x 2 weeks
  - **Lotrimin Ultra (C)(OTC)** *Crm:* 1% (12, 24 gm)
  - **Mentax (B)** *Crm:* 1% (15, 30 gm)

  Comment: ***butenafine*** is a benzylamine, not an azole. Fungicidal activity continues for at least 5 weeks after last application.
- ***ciclopirox*** (B)
  - **Loprox Cream** <10 years: not recommended; ≥10 years: apply bid; max 4 weeks
    Crm: 0.77% (15, 30, 90 gm)
  - **Loprox Lotion** <10 years: not recommended; ≥10 years: apply bid; max 4 weeks
    Lotn: 0.77% (30, 60 ml)
  - **Loprox Gel** <16 years: not recommended; ≥16 years: apply bid; max 4 weeks
    Gel: 0.77% (30, 45 gm)
- ***clotrimazole*** (B)(G) apply bid x 7 days
  - **Lotrimin** ***Crm:*** 1% (15, 30, 45 gm)
  - **Lotrimin AF (OTC)** *Crm:* 1% (12 gm); *Lotn:* 1% (10 ml); *Soln:* 1% (10 ml)
- ***econazole*** (C) apply once daily x 2 weeks
  - **Spectazole** *Crm:* 1% (15, 30, 85 gm)
- ***miconazole*** **2%** (C)(G) apply once daily x 2 weeks
  - **Lotrimin AF Spray Liquid (OTC)** *Spray liq:* 2% (113 gm) (alcohol 17%)
  - **Lotrimin AF Spray Powder (OTC)** *Spray pwdr:* 2% (90 gm) (alcohol 10%)
  - **Monistat-Derm** *Crm:* 2% (1, 3 oz); Spray liq: 2% (3.5 oz); Spray *pwdr: 2%* (3 oz)
- ***ketoconazole*** (C) apply to affected area once daily x 2 weeks
  - **Nizoral Cream** *Crm:* 2% (15, 30, 60 gm)
  - **Nizoral Shampoo** lather into area and leave on 5 minutes x 1 application
    Shampoo: 2% (4 oz)
- ***oxiconazole nitrate*** (B)(G) apply once daily x 2 weeks
  - **Oxistat** *Crm:* 1% (15, 30, 60 gm); *Lotn:* 1% (30 ml)
- ***selenium sulfide*** shampoo (C)(G) apply after shower, allow to dry, leave on overnight; then scrub off vigorously in AM; repeat in 1 week and again q 3 months until resolution occurs
  - **Selsun Blue** *Shampoo:* 1% (120, 210, 240, 330 ml); 2.5% (120 ml)
- ***sulconazole*** (C) <12 years: not recommended; ≥12 years: apply qd-bid x 3 weeks
  - **Exelderm** *Crm:* 1% (15, 30, 60 gm); *Lotn:* 1% (30 mg)
- ***terbinafine*** (B) <12 years: not recommended; ≥12 years: apply bid to affected and surrounding area x 1 week
  - **Lamisil Solution (OTC)** *Soln:* 1% (30 ml spray bottle)

ORAL ANTIFUNGALS

- ***ketoconazole*** (C)(G) <2 years: not recommended; ≥2 years-12 years: 3.3-6.6 mg/kg once daily x 4 weeks; >12 years: initially 200 mg once daily; max 400 mg/day x 4 weeks
  - **Nizoral** *Tab:* 200 mg

Comment: Caution with ***ketoconazole*** due to potential for hepatotoxicity.

TOBACCO DEPENDENCE, TOBACCO CESSATION, & NICOTINE WITHDRAWAL SYNDROME

Comment: According to findings from the Population Assessment of Tobacco and Health (PATH) Study (respondents=10, 384, mean age=14.3, any use of e-cigarettes, hookah, non-cigarette combustible tobacco, or smokeless tobacco was independently associated with traditional cigarette smoking 1 year later and use of more than 1 of these products increases the odds of progressing to traditional cigarette use.

REFERENCE

Watkins, SL, Glantz, SA, & Chaffee, BW. (2018). Association of noncigarette tobacco product use with future cigarette smoking among youth in the population assessment of tobacco and health (PATH) study, 2013-2015. *JAMA Pediatrics, 172*(2), 181. doi:10.1001/jamapediatrics.2017.4173

NON-NICOTINE PRODUCTS

Alpha 4-Beta 4 Nicotinic Acetylcholine Receptor Partial Agonist

▶ ***varenicline*** (C) <18 years: not recommended; ≥18 years: set target quit date; begin therapy 1 week prior to target quit date; take after eating with a full glass of water; initially 0.5 mg once daily for 3 days; then 0.5 mg bid x 4 days; then 1 mg bid; treat x 12 weeks; may continue treatment for 12 more weeks

Chantix *Tab:* 0.5, 1 mg; *Starting Month Pak:* 0.5 mg x 11 tabs + 1 mg x 42 tabs; *Continuing Month Pak:* 1 mg x 56 tabs

Comment: Caution with **Chantix** due to potential risk for anxiety or suicidal ideation.

AMINOKETONES

▶ ***bupropion HBr*** (C)(G) <18 years: not recommended; ≥18 years: initially 100 mg bid for at least 3 days; may increase to 375 or 400 mg/day after several weeks; then after at least 3 more days, 450 mg in 4 divided doses; max 450 mg/day, 174 mg/single-dose

Aplenzin *Tab:* 174, 348, 522 mg

▶ ***bupropion HCl*** (B)(G)

Forfivo XL do not use for initial treatment; use immediate-release bupropion forms for initial titration; switch to **Forfivo XL** 450 mg once daily when total dose/day reaches 450 mg; may switch to **Forfivo XL** when total dose/day reaches 300 mg for 2 weeks and patient needs 450 mg/day to reach therapeutic target; swallow whole, do not crush or chew

Tab: 450 mg ext-rel

Wellbutrin <18 years: not recommended; ≥18 years: initially 100 mg bid for at least 3 days; may increase to 375 or 400 mg/day after several weeks; then after at least 3 more days, 450 mg in 4 divided doses; max 450 mg/day, 150 mg/single-dose

Tab: 75, 100 mg

Wellbutrin SR <18 years: not recommended; ≥18 years: initially 150 mg in AM for at least 3 days; may increase to 150 mg bid if well tolerated; usual dose 300 mg/day; max 400 mg/day

Tab: 100, 150 mg sust-rel

Wellbutrin XL <18 years: not recommended; ≥18 years: initially 150 mg in AM for at least 3 days; increase to 150 mg bid if well tolerated; usual dose 300 mg/day; max 400 mg/day

Tab: 150, 300 mg sust-rel

Zyban <18 years: not recommended; ≥18 years: 150 mg once daily x 3 days; then 150 mg bid x 7-12 weeks; max 300 mg/day

Tab: 150 mg sust-rel

Comment: Contraindications to ***bupropion*** include seizure disorder, disorder, concurrent MAOI and alcohol use. Smoking should be discontinued after the 7th day of therapy with ***bupropion***. Avoid bedtime dose.

TRANSDERMAL NICOTINE SYSTEMS (D)

Habitrol (OTC) <12 years: not recommended; ≥12 years: initially one 21 mg/24 Hr patch/day x 4-6 weeks; then one 14 mg/24 Hr patch/day x 2-4 weeks; then one 7 mg/24 Hr patch/day x 2-4 weeks; then discontinue

Transdermal patch: 7, 14, 21 mg/24 Hr

Nicoderm CQ (OTC) <12 years: not recommended; ≥12 years: initially one 21 mg/24 Hr patch/day x 6 weeks, then one 14 mg/24 Hr patch/day x 2 weeks; then one 7 mg/24 Hr patch/day x 2 weeks

Transdermal patch: 7, 14, 21 mg/24 hour

Comment: **Nicoderm CQ** is available as a clear patch.

Nicotrol Step-down Patch (OTC) <12 years: not recommended; ≥12 years: 1 patch/day x 6 weeks

Transdermal patch: 5, 10, 15 mg/16 Hr (7/pck)

Nicotrol Transdermal (OTC) <12 years: not recommended; ≥12 years: 1 patch/day x 6 weeks

Transdermal patch: 15 mg/16 hour (7/pck)

Prostep <12 years: not recommended; ≥12 years: initially one 22 mg/24 Hr patch/day x 4-8 weeks; then discontinue or one 11 mg/24 Hr patch/day x 2-4 additional weeks

Transdermal patch: 11, 22 mg/24 Hr (7/pck)

NICOTINE GUM

▶ ***nicotine polacrilex*** (D) <12 years: not recommended; ≥12 years: chew one piece of gum slowly and intermittently over 30 minutes q 1-2 hours x 6 weeks; then q 2-4 hours x 3 weeks; then q 4-8 hours x 3 weeks; max 24 pieces/day; 2 mg if smoked <25 cigarettes/day; 4 mg if smoked >24 cigarettes/day

Nicorette (OTC) *Gum squares:* 2, 4 mg (108 piece starter kit and 48 piece refill) (orange, mint, or original) (sugar-free)

NICOTINE LOZENGE

▶ ***nicotine polacrilex*** (X)(OTC)(G) <18 years: not recommended; ≥18 years: dissolve over 20-30 minutes; minimize swallowing; do not eat or drink for 15 min before and during use; use 2 mg lozenge if first cigarette smoked >30 minutes after waking; use 4 mg lozenge if first cigarette smoked within 30 min of waking; 1 lozenge q 1-2 hours (at least 9/day) x 6 weeks; then q 2-4 hours x 3 weeks; then q 4-8 hours x 3 weeks; then stop; max 5 lozenges/6 hours and 20 lozenges/day

Commit Lozenge *Loz:* 2, 4 mg (72/pck) (phenylalanine)

Nicorette Mini Lozenge (G) *Loz:* 2, 4 mg (72/pck) (mint) (phenylalanine)

NICOTINE INHALATION PRODUCTS

▶ ***nicotine*** 0.5 mg aqueous nasal spray (D)

Nicotrol NS 12 years: not recommended; ≥12 years: 1-2 doses/hour nasally; max 5 doses/hour or 40 doses/day; usual max 3 months

Nasal spray: 0.5 mg/spray; 10 mg/ml (10 ml, 200 doses)

▶ ***nicotine*** (D) <12 years: not recommended; ≥12 years: 10 mg inhalation system

Nicotrol Inhaler individualize therapy; at least 6 cartridges/day x 3-6 weeks; max 16 cartridges/day x first 12 weeks; then reduce gradually over 12 more weeks

Inhaler: 10 mg/cartridge, 4 mg delivered (42 cartridges/pck) (menthol)

Comment: **Nicotrol Inhaler** is a smoking replacement; to be used with decreasing frequency. Smoking should be discontinued before starting therapy. Side effects include cough, nausea, mouth, or throat irritation. This system delivers nicotine, but no tars or carcinogens. Each cartridge lasts about 20 minutes with frequent continuous puffing and provides nicotine equivalent to 2 cigarettes.

TONSILLITIS: ACUTE

▶ ***amoxicillin*** **(B)(G)** <40 kg (88 lb): 20-40 mg/kg/day in 3 divided doses x 10 days or 25-45 mg/kg/day in 2 divided doses x 10 days; *see page* 588 *for dose by weight table;* ≥40 kg: 500-875 mg bid or 250-500 mg tid x 10 days

Amoxil *Cap:* 250, 500 mg; *Tab:* 875*mg; *Chew tab:* 125, 200, 250, 400 mg (cherry-banana-peppermint) (phenylalanine); *Oral susp:* 125, 250 mg/5 ml (80, 100, 150 ml) (strawberry); 200, 400 mg/5 ml (50, 75, 100 ml) (bubble gum); *Oral drops:* 50 mg/ml (30 ml) (bubble gum)

Moxatag *Tab:* 775 mg ext-rel

Trimox *Tab:* 125, 250 mg; *Cap:* 250, 500 mg; *Oral susp:* 125, 250 mg/5 ml (80, 100, 150 ml) (raspberry-strawberry)

▶ ***azithromycin*** **(B)(G)** <12 years: 12 mg/kg/day x 5 days; *see page* 593 *for dose by weight table;* max 500 mg/day; ≥12 years: 500 mg x 1 dose on day 1, then 250 mg once daily on days 2-5 or 500 mg once daily x 3 days or **Zmax** 2 gm in a single dose

Zithromax *Tab:* 250, 500, 600 mg; *Oral susp:* 100 mg/5 ml (15 ml); 200 mg/5 ml (15, 22.5, 30 ml) (cherry); *Pkt:* 1 gm for reconstitution (cherry-banana)

Zithromax Tri-pak *Tab:* 3 x 500 mg tabs/pck

Zithromax Z-pak *Tab:* 6 x 250 mg tabs/pck

Zmax *Oral susp:* 2 gm ext-rel for reconstitution (cherry-banana) (148 mg Na^+)

▶ ***cefaclor*** **(B)(G)** <1 month: not recommended; 1 month-12 years: 20-40 mg/kg divided bid x 10 days; *see page* 594 *for dose by weight table;* max 1 gm/day; >12 years: 250-500 mg q 8 hours x 10 days; max 2 gm/day

Tab: 500 mg; *Cap:* 250, 500 mg; *Susp:* 125 mg/5 ml (75, 150 ml) (strawberry); 187 mg/5 ml (50, 100 ml) (strawberry); 250 mg/5 ml (75, 150 ml) (strawberry); 375 mg/5 ml (50, 100 ml) (strawberry)

Cefaclor Extended Release <16 years: not recommended; ≥16 years: 500 mg bid x 10 days (clinically equivalent to 250 mg immed-rel caps tid); swallow whole; take with meals

Tab: 375, 500 mg ext-rel

▶ ***cefadroxil*** <12 years: 30 mg/kg/day in 2 divided doses x 10 days; *see page* 595 *for dose by weight table;* ≥12 years: 1-2 gm in a single or 2 divided doses x 10 days

Duricef *Cap:* 500 mg; *Tab:* 1 gm; *Oral susp:* 250 mg/5 ml (100 ml); 500 mg/5 ml (75, 100 ml) (orange-pineapple)

▶ ***cefdinir*** **(B)** <6 months: not recommended; 6 months-12 years: 14 mg/kg/day in 1-2 divided doses x 10 days; *see page* 596 *for dose by weight table;* ≥12 years: 300 mg bid x 10 days or 600 mg daily x 10 days

Omnicef *Cap:* 300 mg; *Oral susp:* 125 mg/5 ml (60, 100 ml) (strawberry)

▶ ***cefditoren pivoxil*** **(B)** <12 years: not recommended; ≥12 years: 200 mg bid x 10 days

Spectracef *Tab:* 200 mg

Comment: Contraindicated with milk protein allergy or carnitine deficiency.

▶ ***ceftibuten*** **(B)** <12 years: 9 mg/kg daily x 10 days; max 400 mg/day; *see page* 600 *for dose by weight table;* ≥12 years: 400 mg daily x 10 days

Cedax *Cap:* 400 mg; *Oral susp:* 90 mg/5 ml (30, 60, 90, 120 ml); 180 mg/5 ml (30, 60, 120 ml) (cherry)

- ▶ ***cefixime*** **(B)(G)** <6 months: not recommended; 6 months-12 years, <50 kg: 8 mg/kg/day in 1-2 divided doses x 10 days; *see page 597 for dose by weight table;* >12 years, >50 kg: 400 mg once daily x 10 days
  Suprax *Tab:* 400 mg; *Cap:* 400 mg; *Oral susp:* 100, 200, 500 mg/5 ml (50, 75, 100 ml) (strawberry)
- ▶ ***cefpodoxime proxetil*** **(B)** <2 months: not recommended; 2 months-12 years: 10 mg/kg/day (max 400 mg/dose) or 5 mg/kg/day bid (max 200 mg/dose) x 5-7 days; *see page 598 for dose by weight table;* >12 years: 200 mg bid x 5-7 days
  Vantin *Tab:* 100, 200 mg; *Oral susp:* 50, 100 mg/5 ml (50, 75, 100 mg) (lemon creme)
- ▶ ***cefprozil*** **(B)** <2 years: not recommended; 2-12 years: 7.5 mg/kg bid x 10 days; *see page 599 for dose by weight table;* >12 years: 500 mg once daily x 10 days
  Cefzil *Tab:* 250, 500 mg; *Oral susp:* 125, 250 mg/5 ml (50, 75, 100 ml) (bubble gum) (phenylalanine)
- ▶ ***cephalexin*** **(B)(G)** <12 years: 25-50 mg/kg/day in 4 divided doses x 10 days; *see page 601 for dose by weight table;* ≥12 years: 250 mg tid x 10 days
  Keflex *Cap:* 250, 333, 500, 750 mg; *Oral susp:* 125, 250 mg/5 ml (100, 200 ml) (strawberry)
- ▶ ***clarithromycin*** **(C)(G)** <6 months: not recommended; ≥6 months-12 years: 7.5 mg/kg bid x 10 days; *see page 602 for dose by weight table;* >12 years: 250 mg bid or 500 mg ext-rel once daily 10 days
  Biaxin *Tab:* 250, 500 mg
  Biaxin Oral Suspension *Oral susp:* 125, 250 mg/5 ml (50, 100 ml) (fruit punch)
  Biaxin XL *Tab:* 500 mg ext-rel

Comment: The FDA is advising caution before prescribing ***clarithromycin*** to patients with heart disease because of a potential increased risk of heart problems or death that can occur years later. This recommendation is based on a review of the results of a 10-year follow-up study of patients with coronary heart disease from a large clinical trial that first observed this safety issue. Consider risk benefit and the use of other antibiotics in such patients.

- ▶ ***dirithromycin*** **(C)(G)** <12 years: not recommended; ≥12 years: 500 mg once daily x 10 days
  Dynabac *Tab:* 250 mg
- ▶ ***erythromycin base*** **(B)(G)** <45 kg: 30-50 mg in 2-4 divided doses x 10 days; ≥45 kg: 500 mg q 6 hours x 10 days
  Ery-Tab *Tab:* 250, 333, 500 mg ent-coat
  PCE *Tab:* 333, 500 mg
- ▶ ***erythromycin ethylsuccinate*** **(B)(G)** 30-50 mg/kg/day in 4 divided doses x 7 days; may double dose with severe infection; max 100 mg/kg/day or 400 mg qid; *see page 607 for dose by weight table*
  EryPed *Oral susp:* 200 mg/5 ml (100, 200 ml) (fruit); 400 mg/5 ml (60, 100, 200 ml) (banana); *Oral drops:* 200, 400 mg/5 ml (50 ml) (fruit); *Chew tab:* 200 mg wafer (fruit)
  E.E.S. *Oral susp:* 200, 400 mg/5 ml (100 ml) (fruit)
  E.E.S. Granules *Oral susp:* 200 mg/5 ml (100, 200 ml) (cherry)
  E.E.S. 400 Tablets *Tab:* 400 mg
- ▶ ***loracarbef*** **(B)** <12 years: 15 mg/kg/day in 2 divided doses x 10 days; *see page 614 for dose by weight table*; ≥12 years: 200 mg bid x 10 days
  Lorabid *Pulvule:* 200, 400 mg; *Oral susp:* 100 mg/5 ml (50, 100 ml); 200 mg/5 ml (50, 75, 100 ml) (strawberry bubble gum)
- ▶ ***penicillin v potassium*** **(B)(G)** <12 years: 25-75 mg/kg day divided q 6-8 hours x 10 days; *see page 616 for dose by weight table;* ≥12 years: 250 mg tid x 10 days

Pen-VK *Tab:* 250, 500 mg; *Oral soln:* 125 mg/5 ml (100, 200 ml); 250 mg/5 ml (100, 150, 200 ml)

TRICHINOSIS (*TRICHINELLA SPIRALIS*)

Comment: Trichinosis is caused by eating raw or undercooked pork or wild game infected with the larvae of a parasitic worm, *Trichinella spiralis*. The initial symptoms are abdominal discomfort, nausea, vomiting, diarrhea, fatigue, and fever beginning one to two days following ingestion. These parasites then invade other organs (e.g., muscles) causing muscle aches, itching, fever, chills, and joint pains that begins about two to eight weeks after ingestion. The treatment is oral anthelmintics, which may cause abdominal pain, diarrhea, and (rarely) hypersensitivity reactions, convulsions, neutropenia, agranulocytosis, and hepatitis.

ANTHELMINTICS

Comment: Oral bioavailability of anthelmintics is enhanced when administered with a fatty meal (estimated fat content 40 gm).

▶ ***albendazole*** **(C)** take with a meal; may crush and mix with food; may repeat in 3 weeks if needed; <2 years: 200 mg bid x 7 days; 2-12 years: 400 mg once daily x 7 days; >12 years: 400 mg bid x 7 days
  Albenza *Tab:* 200 mg
  Comment: ***albendazole*** is a broad-spectrum benzimidazole carbamate anthelmintic.

▶ ***ivermectin*** **(C)** take with water; chew or crush and mix with food; may repeat in 3 months if needed; <15 kg: not recommended; ≥15 kg: 200 mcg/kg as a single dose
  Stromectol *Tab:* 3, 6*mg

▶ ***mebendazole*** **(C)(G)** take with a meal; chew or crush and mix with food; may repeat in 3 weeks if needed; <2 years: not recommended; ≥2 years: 100 mg bid x 3 days
  Emverm *Chew tab:* 100 mg
  Vermox *Chew tab:* 100 mg

▶ ***pyrantel pamoate*** **(C)** take with a meal; may open capsule and sprinkle or mix with food; treat x 3 days; may repeat in 2-3 weeks if needed; treat x 3 days; 11 mg/kg/dose; max 1 gm/dose; <25 lb: not recommended; 25-37 lb: 1/2 tsp/dose; 38-62 lb: 1 tsp/dose; 63-87 lb: 1 tsp/dose; 88-112 lb: 2 tsp/dose; 113-137 lb: 2 tsp/dose; 138-162 lb: 3 tsp/dose; 163-187 lb: 3 tsp/dose; >187 lb: 4 tsp/dose
  Antiminth *Cap:* 180 mg; *Liq:* 50 mg/ml (30 ml); 144 mg/ml (30 ml); *Oral susp:* 50 mg/ml (60 ml)
  Pin-X *Cap:* 180 mg; *Liq:* 50 mg/ml (30 ml); 144 mg/ml (30 ml); *Oral susp:* 50 mg/ml (30 ml)

▶ ***thiabendazole*** **(C)** take with a meal; may crush and mix with food; treat x 7 days; <30 lb: consult mfr pkg insert; ≥30 lb: 25 mg/kg/dose bid with meals; 30-50 lb: 250 mg bid with meals; >50 lb: 10 mg/lb/dose bid with meals; max 1.5 gm/dose; max 3 gm/day
  Mintezol *Chew tab:* 500*mg (orange); *Oral susp:* 500 mg/5 ml (120 ml) (orange)
  Comment: ***thiabendazole*** is not for prophylaxis. May impair mental alertness. May not be available in the US.

TRICHOMONIASIS (*TRICHOMONAS VAGINALIS*)

Comment: The following treatment regimens for *Trichomoniasis* are published in the **2015 CDC Sexually Transmitted Diseases Treatment Guidelines**. Treat all sexual contacts. A multi-dose treatment regimen should be considered in HIV-positive females.

RECOMMENDED REGIMENS (NON-PREGNANT)

Regimen 1

- ***metronidazole*** 2 gm once in a single dose

Regimen 2

- ***tinidazole*** 2 gm once in a single dose

RECOMMENDED ALTERNATE REGIMEN

Regimen 1

- ***metronidazole*** 500 mg bid x 7 days

DRUG BRANDS AND DOSE FORMS

- ***metronidazole*** **(not for use in 1st; B in 2nd, 3rd)(G)**
  Flagyl *Tab:* 250*, 500*mg
  Flagyl 375 *Cap:* 375 mg
  Flagyl ER *Tab:* 750 mg ext-rel
  Comment: Alcohol is contraindicated during treatment with oral ***metronidazole*** and for 72 hours after therapy due to a possible ***disulfiram***-like reaction (nausea, vomiting, flushing, headache).
- ***tinidazole*** **(not for use in 1st; B in 2nd, 3rd)**
  Tindamax *Tab:* 250*, 500*mg

RECOMMENDED REGIMENS: PREGNANCY/LACTATION

Comment: All pregnant females should be considered for treatment. They can be treated with 2 gm ***metronidazole*** in a single dose at any stage of pregnancy. Lactating females who are administered ***metronidazole*** should be instructed to interrupt breastfeeding for 12-24 hours after receiving the 2 gm dose of ***metronidazole***.

TRICHOTILLOMANIA

Comment: Trichotillomania is on the obsessive-compulsive spectrum within the larger DS-5 category, Anxiety Disorders, and depression is frequently a co-morbid disorder. Hence, medications used to treat OCD can be helpful in treating trichotillomania. Recommended psychotropic agents include ***clomipramine*** (**Anafranil**) and ***fluvoxamine*** (**Luvox**). Other medications that research suggests may have some benefit include the SSRIs ***fluoxetine*** (**Prozac**), ***sertraline*** (**Zoloft**), ***paroxetine*** (**Paxil**), the mood stabilizer ***lithium carbonate*** (**Lithobid, Eskalith**), the OTC supplement **N-acetylcysteine**, an amino acid that influences neurotransmitters related to mood, ***olanzapine*** (**Zyprexa**), an atypical anti-psychotic, and ***valproate*** (**Depakote**), an anticonvulsant.

TRICYCLIC ANTIDEPRESSANT (TCA)

- ***clomipramine*** (C)(G) <10 years: not recommended; 10-<16 years: initially 25 mg daily in divided doses; gradually increase; max 3 mg/kg <u>or</u> 100 mg, whichever is smaller; >16 years: initially 25 mg daily in divided doses; gradually increase to 100 mg during first 2 weeks; max 250 mg/day; total maintenance dose may be given at HS
  Anafranil *Cap:* 25, 50, 75 mg

SELECTIVE SEROTONIN REUPTAKE INHIBITORS (SSRIs)

▶ *fluoxetine* (C)(G)

Prozac <8 years: not recommended; 8-17 years: initially 10 or 20 mg/day; start lower weight children at 10 mg/day; if starting at 10 mg/day, may increase after 1 week to 20 mg/day; >17 years: initially 20 mg daily; may increase after 1 week; doses >20 mg/day should be divided into AM and noon doses; max 80 mg/day

Tab: 10*mg; *Cap:* 10, 20, 40 mg; *Oral soln:* 20 mg/5 ml (4 oz) (mint)

Prozac Weekly <8 years: not recommended; ≥8 years: following daily ***fluoxetine*** therapy at 20 mg/day for 13 weeks, may initiate **Prozac Weekly** 7 days after the last 20 mg ***fluoxetine*** dose

Cap: 90 mg ent-coat del-rel pellets

Sarafem <8 years: not recommended; ≥8 years: administer daily or 14 days before expected menses and through first full day of menses; initially 20 mg/day; max 80 mg/day

Tab: 10, 15, 20 mg; *Cap:* 20 mg

▶ *fluvoxamine* (C)(G)

Luvox <8 years: not recommended; 8-17 years: initially 25 mg q HS; adjust in 25 mg increments q 4-7 days; usual range 50-200 mg/day; over 50 mg/day, divide into 2 doses giving the larger dose at HS; >17 years: initially 50 mg q HS; adjust in 50 mg increments at 4-7 day intervals; range 100-300 mg/day; over 100 mg/day, divide into 2 doses giving the larger dose at HS

Tab: 25, 50*, 100*mg

Luvox CR <18 years: not recommended; ≥18 years: initially 100 mg once daily at HS; may increase by 50 mg increments at 1 week intervals; max 300 mg/day; swallow whole

Cap: 100, 150 mg ext-rel

▶ ***paroxetine maleate*** **(D)(G)** <12 years: not recommended; ≥12 years:

Paxil initially 20 mg daily in AM; may increase by 10 mg/day at weekly intervals as needed; max 60 mg/day

Tab: 10*, 20*, 30, 40 mg

Paxil CR initially 25 mg daily in AM; may increase by 12.5 mg at weekly intervals as needed; max 62.5 mg/day

Tab: 12.5, 25, 37.5 mg cont-rel ent-coat

Paxil Suspension initially 20 mg daily in AM; may increase by 10 mg/day at weekly intervals as needed; max 60 mg/day

Oral susp: 10 mg/5 ml (250 ml) (orange)

▶ ***paroxetine mesylate*** **(D)(G)** <12 years: not recommended; ≥12 years: initially 7.5 mg daily in AM; may increase by 10 mg/day at weekly intervals as needed; max 60 mg/day

Brisdelle *Cap:* 7.5 mg

▶ ***sertraline*** **(C)(G)** <6 years: not recommended; 6-12 years: initially 25 mg daily; max 200 mg/day; 13-17 years: initially 50 mg daily; max 200 mg/day; >17 years: initially 50 mg daily; increase at 1 week intervals if needed; max 200 mg daily; dilute oral concentrate immediately prior to administration in 4 oz water, ginger ale, lemon-lime soda, lemonade, or orange juice

Zoloft *Tab:* 25*, 50*, 100*mg; *Oral conc:* 20 mg per ml (60 ml) (alcohol 12%)

Lithium Salts Mood Stabilizer

▶ ***lithium carbonate*** **(D)(G)** <12 years: not recommended; ≥12 years: swallow whole; *Usual maintenance:* 900-1200 mg/day in 2-3 divided doses

Lithobid *Tab:* 300 mg slow-rel

Comment: Signs and symptoms of ***lithium*** toxicity can occur below 2 mEq/L and include blurred vision, tinnitus, weakness, dizziness, nausea, abdominal pains, vomiting, diarrhea to (severe) hand tremors, ataxia, muscle twitches, nystagmus, seizures, slurred speech, decreased level of consciousness, coma, death.

Valproate Mood Stabilizer

➢ ***divalproex sodium*** (D)(G) <12 years: not recommended; ≥12 years: take once daily; swallow ext-rel form whole; initially 25 mg/kg/day in divided doses; max 60 mg/kg/day;

Depakene *Cap:* 250 mg; *Syr:* 250 mg/5 ml (16 oz)
Depakote *Tab:* 125, 250 mg
Depakote ER *Tab:* 250, 500 mg ext-rel
Depakote Sprinkle *Cap:* 125 mg

ANTIPSYCHOTIC

➢ ***olanzapine*** (C) <13 years: not recommended; 13-17 years: initially 2.5-5 mg once daily at HS; >17 years: initially 5-10 mg once daily at HS; titrate weekly, max 20 mg at HS; usual maintenance 10-20 mg/day

Zyprexa *Tab:* 2.5, 5, 7.5, 10 mg
Zyprexa Zydis *ODT:* 5, 10, 15, 20 mg (phenylalanine)

TRIGEMINAL NEURALGIA (TIC DOULOUREUX)

➢ ***baclofen*** (C)(G) <12 years: not recommended; ≥12 years: initially 5-10 mg tid with food; usual dose 10-80 mg/day

Lioresal *Tab:* 10*, 20*mg

Comment: Potential for seizures or hallucinations on abrupt withdrawal of ***baclofen***.

➢ ***carbamazepine*** (C)

Carbatrol <12 years: max <35 mg/kg/day; use ext-rel form above 400 mg/day; 12-15 years: max 1 gm/day in 2 divided doses; >15-18 years: usual maintenance 1.2 gm/day in 2 divided doses; >18 years: initially 200 mg bid; may increase weekly as needed by 200 mg/day; usual maintenance 800 mg-1.2 gm/day

Cap: 200, 300 mg ext-rel

Tegretol(G) <6 years: initially 10-20 mg/kg/day in 2 divided doses; increase weekly as needed in 3-4 divided doses; max 35 mg/kg/day in 3-4 divided doses; ≥6 years-12 years: initially 100 mg bid; increase weekly as needed by 100 mg/day in 3-4 divided doses; max 1 gm/day in 3-4 divided doses; >12 years: initially 100 mg bid or 1/2 tsp susp qid; may increase dose by 100 mg q 12 hours or by 1/2 tsp susp q 6 hours; usual maintenance 400-800 mg/day; max 200 mg/day

Tab: 200*mg; *Chew tab:* 100*mg; *Oral susp:* 100 mg/5 ml (450 ml) (citrus-vanilla)

Tegretol XR (G) <6 years: use other forms; 6-12 years: initially 100 mg bid; may increase weekly by 100 mg/day in 2 divided doses; max 1 gm/day; >12 years: initially 200 mg bid; may increase weekly by 200 mg/day in 2 divided doses

Tab: 100, 200, 400 mg ext-rel

➢ ***clonazepam*** (D)(IV)(G) <10 years, <30 kg: initially 0.1-0.3 mg/kg/day; may increase up to 0.05 mg/kg/day bid-tid; usual maintenance 0.1-0.2 mg/kg/day tid; ≥10 years: initially 0.25 mg bid; increase to 1 mg/day after 3 days

Klonopin *Tab:* 0.5*, 1, 2 mg

Klonopin Wafers dissolve in mouth with or without water
Wafer: 0.125, 0.25, 0.5, 1, 2 mg orally-disint

- ***divalproex sodium*** **(D)** <10 years: not recommended; ≥10 years: initially 250 mg bid; gradually increase to max 1000 mg/day if needed
  Depakene *Cap:* 250 mg; *Syr:* 250 mg/5 ml
  Depakote *Tab:* 125, 250 mg
  Depakote ER *Tab:* 250, 500 mg ext-rel
  Depakote Sprinkle *Cap:* 125 mg
- ***phenytoin*** **(D)** 400 mg/day in divided doses
  Dilantin *Cap:* 30, 100 mg; *Oral susp:* 125 mg/5 ml (8 oz); *Infatab:* 50 mg
  Comment: Monitor ***phenytoin*** serum levels. Therapeutic serum level: 10-20 gm/ml. An ASE is gingival hyperplasia.
- ***valproic acid*** **(D)** initially 15 mg/kg/day; may increase weekly by 5-10 mg/kg/day; max 60 mg/kg/day or 250 mg/day
  Depakene *Cap:* 250 mg; *Syr:* 250 mg/5 ml

TRICYCLIC ANTIDEPRESSANTS (TCAs)

Comment: Co-administration of SSRIs and TCAs requires extreme caution.

- ***amitriptyline*** **(C)(G)** <12 years: not recommended; ≥12 years: 10-20 mg q HS
  Tab: 10, 25, 50, 75, 100, 150 mg
- ***amoxapine*** **(C)** <12 years: not recommended; ≥12 years: initially 50 mg bid-tid; after 1 week may increase to 100 mg bid-tid; usual effective dose 200-300 mg/day; if total dose exceeds 300 mg/day, give in divided doses (max 400 mg/day); may give as a single bedtime dose (max 300 mg q HS)
  Tab: 25, 50, 100, 150 mg
- ***clomipramine*** **(C)(G)** <10 years: not recommended; 10-<16 years: initially 25 mg daily in divided doses; gradually increase; max 3 mg/kg or 100 mg, whichever is less; >16 years: initially 25 mg daily in divided doses; gradually increase to 100 mg during first 2 weeks; max 250 mg/day; total maintenance dose may be given at HS
  Anafranil *Cap:* 25, 50, 75 mg
- ***desipramine*** **(C)(G)** <12 years: not recommended; ≥12 years: 100-200 mg/day in single or divided doses; max 300 mg/day
  Norpramin *Tab:* 10, 25, 50, 75, 100, 150 mg
- ***doxepin*** **(C)(G)** <12 years: not recommended; ≥12 years: 75 mg/day; max 150 mg/day
  Cap: 10, 25, 50, 75, 100, 150 mg; *Oral conc:* 10 mg/ml (4 oz w. dropper)
- ***imipramine*** **(C)(G)** <12 years: not recommended; ≥12 years:
  Tofranil initially 75 mg daily (max 200 mg); adolescents initially 30-40 mg daily (max 100 mg/day); if maintenance dose exceeds 75 mg daily, may switch to **Tofranil PM** for divided or bedtime dose
  Tab: 10, 25, 50 mg
  Tofranil PM initially 75 mg daily 1 hour before HS; max 200 mg
  Cap: 75, 100, 125, 150 mg
- ***nortriptyline*** **(D)(G)** <12 years: not recommended; ≥12 years: initially 25 mg tid-qid; max 150 mg/day
  Pamelor *Cap:* 10, 25, 50, 75 mg; *Oral soln:* 10 mg/5 ml (16 oz)
- ***protriptyline*** **(C)** <12 years: not recommended; ≥12 years: initially 5 mg tid; usual dose 15-40 mg/day in 3-4 divided doses; max 60 mg/day
  Vivactil *Tab:* 5, 10 mg
- ***trimipramine*** **(C)** <12 years: not recommended; ≥12 years: initially 75 mg/day in divided doses; max 200 mg/day
  Surmontil *Cap:* 25, 50, 100 mg

TUBERCULOSIS (TB): PULMONARY *(MYCOBACTERIUM TUBERCULOSIS)*

SCREENING

- ***purified protein derivative (PPD)*** (C) 0.1 ml intradermally; examine inoculation site for induration at 48 to 72 hours.
  Aplisol, Tubersol *Soln:* 5 US units/0.1 ml (1, 5 ml)

PROPHYLAXIS VACCINE

The only tuberculosis vaccine uses attenuation of the related organism *Mycobacterium bovis* by culture in bile-containing media to create the *Bacillus Calmette-Guerin* (BCG) vaccination strain. It was first used experimentally in 1921 by Albert Calmette and Camille Guerin and is currently in widespread use outside of the United States. It is not available in the US. The BCG vaccine protects newborns against tuberculosis-related meningitis and other systemic tuberculosis infections, but it has limited protection against active pulmonary disease. Once vaccinated, the patient will be PPD positive.

ANTI-TUBERCULAR AGENTS

Comment: Avoid ***streptomycin*** in pregnancy. ***pyridoxine*** (***vitamin*** B_6) 25 mg once daily x 6 months should be administered concomitantly with *INH* for prevention of side effects. ***Rifapentine*** produces red-orange discoloration of body tissues and body fluids and may stain contact lenses.

- ***bedaquiline*** (B)(G)
  Sirturo *Tab:* 100 mg
  Comment: ***bedaquiline*** is a diarylquinoline antimycobacterial ATP synthase for the treatment of pulmonary multidrug resistant TB (MDR-TB).
- ***ethambutol (EMB)*** (B)(G)
  Myambutol *Tab:* 100, 400*mg
- ***isoniazid (INH)*** (C) *Tab:* 300*mg
- ***pyrazinamide (PZA)*** (C) *Tab:* 500*mg
- ***rifampin (RIF)*** (C)(G)
  Rifadin, Rimactane *Cap:* 150, 300 mg
- ***rifapentine*** (C)
  Priftin *Tab:* 150 mg (24, 32/pck)
  Comment: The 32-count packs of **Priftin** are intended for patients with active tuberculosis infection (TB). The 24-count packs are intended for patients with latent tuberculosis infection (LTBI) who are at high risk for progression to tuberculosis disease. **Priftin** for active TB is indicated for patients ≥12 years-of-age. **Priftin** for LTBI is indicated for patients ≥2 years-of-age.
- ***rilpivirine*** (C) *Tab:* 25 mg
  Rifabutin *Cap:* 150 mg
- ***streptomycin (SM)*** (C)(G) *Amp:* 1 gm/2.5 ml or 400 mg/ml (2.5 ml)

COMBINATION AGENTS

- ***rifampin+isoniazid*** (C)
  Rifamate *Cap:* rif 300 mg+iso 150 mg
- ***rifampin/isoniazid/pyrazinamide*** (C)
  Rifater *Tab:* rif 120 mg+iso 50 mg/pyr 300 mg

PROPHYLAXIS AFTER EXPOSURE TO TUBERCULOSIS, WITH NEGATIVE PPD

- ***isoniazid*** (C) <12 years: 10-20 mg/kg/day x 9 months; ≥12 years: 300 mg once daily in a single dose x at least 6 months

PROPHYLAXIS AFTER EXPOSURE, WITH NEW PPD CONVERSION

- ***isoniazid*** (C) <12 years: 10-20 mg/kg/day x 9 months; ≥12 years: 300 mg once daily in a single dose x 12 months
  Tab: 100, 300*mg; *Syr:* 50 mg/5 ml; *Inj:* 100 mg/ml
- ***rifampin*** (C) <12 years: ***rifampin*** 10-20 mg/kg + ***isoniazid*** 10-20 mg/kg once daily x 4 months; ≥12 years: 600 mg once daily + ***isoniazid*** 300 mg once daily x 4 months
- ***rifapentine*** (C) <12 years: ≤12 years: Treat x 12 weeks; 10-14 kg: ***rifapentine*** 300 mg once weekly + ***isoniazid*** 25 mg/kg (max 900 mg) once weekly; 14.1-25 kg: ***rifapentine*** 450 mg once weekly + ***isoniazid*** 25 mg/kg (max 900 mg) once weekly; 25.1-32 kg: ***rifapentine*** 600 mg once weekly + ***isoniazid*** 25 mg/kg (max 900 mg) once weekly; 32.1-50 kg: ***rifapentine*** 750 mg once weekly + ***isoniazid*** 25 mg/kg (max 900 mg) once weekly; >50 kg: ***rifapentine*** 900 mg once weekly + ***isoniazid*** 25 mg/kg (max 900 mg) once weekly; ≥12 years: 600 mg once weekly + ***isoniazid*** 300 mg once weekly x 12 weeks

TREATMENT REGIMENS (<12 YEARS-OF-AGE)

Regimen 1

- ***rifampin*** 10-20 mg/kg + ***isoniazid*** 10-20 mg/kg + ***pyrazinamide*** 15-20 mg/kg + ***ethambutol*** 15-25 mg/kg <u>or</u> ***streptomycin*** 20-40 mg/kg once daily x 8 weeks; then ***isoniazid*** 10-20 mg/kg + ***rifampin*** 10-20 mg/kg once daily x 16 weeks <u>or</u> ***isoniazid*** 20-40 mg/kg + ***rifampin*** 10-20 mg/kg 2-3 x/week x 16 weeks

Regimen 2

- ***rifampin*** 10-20 mg/kg + ***isoniazid*** 10-20 mg/kg + ***pyrazinamide*** 15-30 mg/kg + ***ethambutol*** 15-25 mg/kg <u>or</u> ***streptomycin*** 20-40 mg/kg once daily x 2 weeks; then ***rifampin*** 10-20 mg/kg + ***isoniazid*** 20-40 mg/kg + ***pyrazinamide*** 50-70 mg/kg + ***ethambutol*** 50 mg/kg <u>or</u> ***streptomycin*** 25-30 mg/kg 2 x/week x 6 weeks; then ***isoniazid*** 10-20 mg/kg + ***rifampin*** 10-20 mg/kg once daily x 16 weeks <u>or</u> ***rifampin*** 10-20 mg/kg + ***isoniazid*** 20-40 mg/kg 2 x/week x 16 weeks

Regimen 3

- ***rifampin*** 10-20 mg/kg + ***isoniazid*** 20-40 mg/kg + ***pyrazinamide*** 50-70 mg/kg + ***ethambutol*** 25-30 mg/kg <u>or</u> ***streptomycin*** 25-30 mg/kg 3 x/week x 6 months

Regimen 4 (When Pyrazinamide Is Contraindicated)

- ***rifampin*** 10-20 mg/kg + ***isoniazid*** 10-20 mg/kg + ***ethambutol*** 15-25 mg/kg + ***streptomycin*** 20-40 mg/kg once daily x 4-8 weeks; then ***isoniazid*** 10-20 mg/kg + ***rifampin*** 10-20 mg/kg once daily x 24 weeks <u>or</u> ***rifampin*** 10-20 mg/kg + ***isoniazid*** 20-40 mg/kg 2 x/week x 24 weeks

TREATMENT REGIMENS (≥12 YEARS-OF-AGE)

Regimen 1

- ***rifampin*** 600 mg + ***isoniazid*** 300 mg + ***pyrazinamide*** 2 gm + ***ethambutol*** 15-25 mg/kg <u>or</u> ***streptomycin*** 1 gm once daily x 8 weeks; then ***isoniazid*** 300 mg + ***rifampin*** 600 mg once daily x 16 weeks <u>or</u> ***isoniazid*** 900 mg + ***rifampin*** 600 mg 2-3 x/week x 16 weeks

Regimen 2

- ***rifampin*** 600 mg + ***isoniazid*** 300 mg + ***pyrazinamide*** 2 gm + ***ethambutol*** 15-25 mg/kg or ***streptomycin*** 1 gm once daily x 2 weeks; then ***rifampin*** 600 mg + ***isoniazid*** 900 mg + ***pyrazinamide*** 4 gm + ***ethambutol*** 50 mg/kg or ***streptomycin*** 1.5 gm 2 x/week x 6 weeks; then ***isoniazid*** 300 mg + ***rifampin*** 600 mg once daily x 16 weeks or 2 x/week x 16 weeks ***rifampin*** 600 mg once daily x 16 weeks or 2 x/week x 16 weeks

Regimen 3

- ***rifampin*** 600 mg + ***isoniazid*** 900 mg + ***pyrazinamide*** 3 gm + ***ethambutol*** 25-30 mg/kg or ***streptomycin*** 1.5 gm 3 x/week x 6 months

Regimen 4 (Smear and Culture Negative for Pulmonary TB ≥12 Years-of-Age)

- **Options 1, 2,** or **3** x 8 weeks; then ***isoniazid*** 300 mg + ***rifampin*** 600 mg once daily x 16 weeks; then ***rifampin*** 600 mg + ***isoniazid*** 300 mg + ***pyrazinamide*** 2 gm + ***ethambutol*** 15-25 mg/kg or ***streptomycin*** 1 gm once daily x 8 weeks or 2-3 x/week x 8 weeks

Regimen 5 (Smear and Culture Negative for Pulmonary TB ≥12 Years-of-Age)

- ***rifapentine*** 600 mg twice weekly x 2 months (at least 72 hours between doses) + once daily ***isoniazid*** 300 mg, ***ethambutol*** 15-25 mg/kg + ***pyrazinamide*** 2 g; then ***rifapentine*** 600 mg once weekly x 4 months + once daily ***isoniazid*** 300 mg + another appropriate antituberculosis agent for susceptible organisms

Regimen 6 (When Pyrazinamide Is Contraindicated)

- ***rifampin*** 600 mg + ***isoniazid*** 300 mg + ***ethambutol*** 15-25 mg/kg + ***streptomycin* 1 gm** once daily x 4-8 weeks; then ***isoniazid*** 300 mg + ***rifampin*** 600 mg once daily x 24 weeks or 2 x/week x 24 weeks

POLYPEPTIDE ANTIBIOTIC ISOLATED FROM STREPTOMYCES CAPREOLUS

Comment: ***capreomycin sulfate*** is a complex of 4 microbiologically active components which have been characterized in part; however, complete structural determination of all the components has not been established. **Capastat Sulfate**, which is to be used concomitantly with other appropriate anti-tuberculosis agents, is indicated in pulmonary infections caused by ***capreomycin***-susceptible strains of *M. tuberculosis* when the primary agents (i.e., ***isoniazid***, ***rifampin***, ***ethambutol***, ***aminosalicylic acid***, and ***streptomycin***) have been ineffective or cannot be used because of toxicity or the presence of resistant tubercle bacilli.

- ***capreomycin sulfate*** (C)(G) <18 years: not recommended; ≥18 years: may be administered deep IM in a large muscle mass after reconstitution with 2 ml 0.9%NS or sterile water or via IV infusion over 60 minutes after reconstitution and dilution in 100 ml 0.9%NS; usual dose is 1 gm daily (not to exceed 20 mg/kg/day) via IM or IV infusion for 60 to 120 days; see mfr pkg insert for dosage table based on kg body weight and toute of administration

    Capastat *Vial:* 1 gm pwdr for reconstitution with 2 ml 0.9%NS or sterile water

Comment: Black Box Warning (BBW): The use of ***capreomycin sulfate*** in patients with renal insufficiency or preexisting auditory impairment must be undertaken with great caution, and the risk of additional cranial nerve VIII impairment or renal injury should be weighed against the benefits to be derived from therapy. Since other parenteral antituberculosis agents (e.g., ***streptomycin***, ***viomycin***) also have similar and sometimes irreversible toxic effects, particularly on cranial nerve VIII and renal function, simultaneous administration of these agents with **Capastat Sulfate** is not recommended. Use with non-antituberculosis drugs (e.g., ***polymyxin A sulfate***, ***colistin sulfate***, ***amikacin***, ***gentamicin***, ***tobramycin***, ***vancomycin***, ***kanamycin***, and ***neomycin***) having ototoxic or nephrotoxic potential should be undertaken only with great caution. Audiometric measurements and assessment of vestibular function should be performed prior to initiation of therapy with **Capastat Sulfate** and at regular intervals during treatment. Renal injury, with tubular necrosis, elevation of the blood urea nitrogen (BUN) or serum creatinine, and abnormal urinary sediment, has been noted. Slight elevation of the BUN and serum creatinine (sCr) has been observed in a significant number of patients receiving prolonged therapy. The appearance of casts, red cells, and white cells in the urine has been noted in a high percentage of these cases. The safety of the use of **Capastat Sulfate** in pregnancy has not been determined. Safety and effective ness in pediatric patients have not been established. It is not known whether this drug is excreted in human milk.

TYPE 1 DIABETES MELLITUS (T1DM)

Comment: Target glycosylated hemoglobin (HbA1c) is <7%. Addition of daily ACE-I and/or ARB therapy is strongly recommended for renal protection. Insulin may be indicated in the management of Type 2 diabetes with or without concomitant oral antidiabetic agents.

TREATMENT FOR ACUTE HYPOGLYCEMIA

- ***glucagon (recombinant)*** **(B)** administer SC, IM, or IV; if patient does not respond in 15 minutes, may administer a single dose or 2 divided doses; <20 kg: 0.5 mg or 20-30 mg/kg; ≥20 kg: 1 mg

INHALED INSULIN

Rapid-Acting Inhalation Powder Insulin

- ***insulin human (inhaled)*** (C) <18 years: not established; ≥18 years: one inhaler may be used for up to 15 days, then discard; dose at meal times as follows: *insulin-naïve:* initially 4 units at each meal; adjust according to blood glucose monitoring

  Conversion from SC to inhaled mealtime insulin:

  SC 1-4 units: inhal 4 units
  SC 5-8 units: inhal 8 units
  SC 9-12 units: inhal 12 units
  SC 13-16 units: inhal 16 units
  SC 17-20 units: inhal 20 units
  SC 21-24 units: inhal 24 units

  Afrezza Inhalation Powder administer at the beginning of the meal; *Mealtime **insulin**-naïve:* initially 4 units at each meal; *Using SC prandial **insulin**:* convert dose to **Afrezza** using a conversion table (see mfr pkg insert); *Using SC pre-mixed:* divide 1/2 of total daily injected premixed ***insulin*** equally among 3 meals of the day; administer 1/2 total injected premixed dose as once daily injected basal ***insulin*** dose

  Inhal: 4, 8, 12 unit single-inhalation color-coded cartridges (30, 60, 90/pkg w. 2 disposable inhalers)

  Comment: **Afrezza** is not a substitute for long-acting ***insulin***. **Afrezza** must be used in combination with long-acting ***insulin*** in patients with T1DM. **Afrezza** is not recommended for the treatment of diabetic ketoacidosis. **Afrezza** is contraindicated with chronic lung disease because of the risk of acute bronchospasm. The use of **Afrezza** is not recommended in patients who smoke or who have recently stopped smoking. Each card contains 5 blister strips with 3 cartridges each (total 15 cartridges). The doses are color-coded. **Afrezza** is contraindicated with chronic respiratory disease (e.g., asthma, COPD) and patients prone to episodes of hypoglycemia.

INJECTABLE INSULINS

Rapid-Acting Insulins

▶ ***insulin aspart (recombinant)***

Fiasp <18 years: not recommended; ≥18 years: administer at the beginning of a meal or within 20 minutes after starting a meal

Vial: 100 U/ml (10 ml); *FlexTouvh pen:* 100 U/ml (3 ml, 5/pck) (zinc, niacinamide)

Comment: **Fiasp** is a new formulation of **NovoLog**, in which the addition of niacinamide (vitamin B3) helps to increase the speed of the initial ***insulin*** absorption, resulting in an onset of appearance in the blood in approximately 2.5 minutes.

NovoLog <2 years: not recommended; 2-4 years: use SC only; >4 years: may use SC or ***insulin*** pump (CSII); onset ≤15 minutes; peak 1-3 hours; duration 3-5 hours; administer 5-10 minutes prior to a meal; SC or infusion pump or IV infusion

Vial: 100 U/ml (10 ml); *PenFill cartridge:* 100 U/ml (3 ml, 5/pck) (zinc, m-cresol)

▶ ***insulin glulisine (rDNA origin)*** **(C)** <4 years: not recommended; ≥4 years: SC only; may administer via ***insulin*** pump; do not dilute or mix with other ***insulin*** in pump; onset <15 minutes; peak 1 hour; duration 2-4 hours; administer up to 15 minutes before, or within 20 minutes after starting a meal; use with an intermediate or long-acting ***insulin***

Apidra *Vial:* 100 U/ml (10 ml); *Cartridge:* 100 U/ml (3 ml, 5/pck) (m-cresol)

▶ ***insulin lispro (recombinant)*** **(B)** <3 years: not recommended; ≥3 years: administer up to 15 minutes before, or immediately after, a meal; SC or IV infusion pump only onset ≤15 minutes; peak 1 hour; duration 3.5-4.5 hours

Admelog *Vial:* 100 U/ml (10 ml) *(zinc, m-cresol); Prefilled disposable So-loStar pen (disposable)*: 100 U/ml (3 ml) (5/carton) *(zinc, m-cresol)*

Humalog *Vial:* 100 U/ml (10 ml); *Prefilled disposable KwikPen:* 100 U/ml (3 ml, 5/pck) (zinc, m-cresol); *HumaPen Memoir* and *HumaPen Luxura* HD inj device for *Humalog cartridges* (100 U/ml, 3 ml 5/pck) (zinc, m-cresol)

▶ ***insulin regular*** **(B)**

Humulin R U-100 *(human, recombinant)* (OTC) onset 30 minutes; peak 2-4 hours; duration up to 6-8 hours; SC or IV or IM

Vial: 100 U/ml (10 ml)

Humulin R U-500 *(human, recombinant)* onset 30 minutes; peak 1.75-4 hours; duration up to 24 hours; SC only; for in-hospital use only

Vial: 500 U/ml (20 ml) (m-cresol); *KwikPen:* 3 ml (2, 5/carton)

Comment: **Humulin R U-500** formulation is 5 times more concentrated than standard U-100 concentration, indicated for patient's ≥18 years-of-age and children who require ≥200 units of ***insulin***/day, allowing patients to inject 80% less liquid to receive the desired dose.

Iletin II Regular *(pork)* (OTC) onset 30 minutes; peak 2-4 hours; duration 6-8 hours; SC or IV or IM

Vial: 100 U/ml (10 ml)

Novolin R *(human)* (OTC) onset 30 minutes; peak 2.5-5 hours; duration 8 hours; SC or IV or IM

Vial: 100 U/ml (10 ml); *PenFill cartridge:* 100 U/ml (1.5 ml, 5/pck); *Prefilled syringe:* 100 U/ml (1.5 ml, 5/pck)

▶ ***pramlintide*** *(amylin analog/amylinomimetic)* **(C)** <12 years: not recommended; ≥12 years: administer immediately before major meals (≥250 kcal or ≥30 gm carbohydrates); initially 15 mcg; titrate in 15 mcg increments for 3 days if no significant nausea occurs; if nausea occurs at 45 or 60 mcg, reduce to 30 mcg; if not tolerated, consider discontinuing therapy; *Maintenance:* 60 mcg (30 mcg *only* if 60 mcg not tolerated)

Symlin *Vial:* 0.6 mg/ml (5 ml) (m-cresol, mannitol)

Comment: **Symlin** is indicated as adjunct to mealtime ***insulin*** with or without a sulfonylurea and blood glucose control is suboptimal despite optimal ***insulin*** therapy. Do not mix with ***insulin***. When initiating **Symlin**, reduce preprandial short/rapid-acting ***insulin*** dose by 50% and monitor pre- and postprandial and bedtime blood glucose. Do not use in patients with poor compliance, HgbA1c is >9%, recurrent hypoglycemia requiring assistance in the previous 6 months, or if taking a prokinetic drug. With Type 2 DM, initial therapy is 60 mcg/dose and max is 120 mcg/dose.

RAPID-ACTING & INTERMEDIATE-ACTING INSULIN

Insulin Aspart Protamine Suspension+Insulin Aspart Combinations

▶ ***insulin aspart protamine suspension 70%+insulin aspart 30%*** *(recombinant)* **(B)(G)** <12 years: not recommended; do not mix with other ***insulin***; SC only; onset 15 min; peak 2.4 hours; duration up to 24 hours

NovoLog Mix 70/30 (OTC) *Vial:* 100 U/ml (10 ml)

NovoLog Mix 70/30 FlexPen (OTC) *Prefilled disposable pen:* 100 U/ml (3 ml, 5/pck); *PenFill cartridge:* 100 U/ml (3 ml, 5/pck)

LONG-ACTING INSULINS

▶ ***insulin detemir (human)*** **(B)** <2 years: not recommended; ≥2 years: administer SC once daily with evening meal or at HS as a basal ***insulin***; may administer twice daily (AM/PM); administer in the deltoid, abdomen, or thigh; onset 1-2 hours; peak 6-8 hours; duration 24 hours; switching from another basal ***insulin***, dose should be the same on a unit-to-unit basis; may need more ***insulin detemir*** when switching from **NPH**; *Type 1:* starting dose 1/3 of total daily ***insulin*** requirements; rapid-acting or short-acting, pre-meal ***insulin*** should be used to satisfy the remainder of daily ***insulin*** requirements; *Type 2 (inadequately controlled on oral antidiabetic agents):* initially 10 units or 0.1-0.2 units/kg, once daily in the evening or divided twice daily (AM/PM); do not add-mix or dilute ***insulin detemir*** with other ***insulins***.

Levemir *Vial:* 100 U/ml (10 ml); *FlexPen:* 100 U/ml (3 ml, 5/pck) (zinc, m-cresol)

▶ ***insulin glargine (recombinant)*** **(C)** <6 years: not established; ≥6 years: do not mix or dilute with other ***insulins***

Basaglar administer SC once daily, at the same time each day, as a basal ***insulin*** in the deltoid, abdomen, or thigh; onset 1-1.5 hours, no pronounced peak, duration 20-24 hours; *T1DM (adults, adolescents, and children >6 years-of-age):* initially 1/3 of total daily ***insulin*** dose; administer the remainder of the total dose as short- or rapid-acting preprandial ***insulin***; *T2DM (≥18 years only):* initially 2 units/kg or up to 10 units once daily; *Switching from once daily insulin glargine 300 units/ml (i.e., **Toujeo**) to 100 units/ml:* initially 80% of the ***insulin glargine*** 300 units/ml; *Switching from twice daily NPH:* initially 80% of the total daily NPH dose; do not add-mix or dilute ***insulin glargine*** with other ***insulins***.

Prefilled KwikPen (disposable), 100 U/ml (3 ml) (5/carton)

Lantus <6 years: not recommended; ≥6 years: administer SC once daily at the same time each day as a basal ***insulin***; onset 1-1.5 hours, no pronounced peak, duration 20-24 hours; initial average starting dose 10 units for ***insulin***-naïve patients; *Switching from once daily **NPH** or **Ultralente insulin***: initial dose of ***insulin glargine*** should be on a unit-for-unit basis; *Switching from twice daily **NPH insulin***: start at 20% lower than the total daily ***NPH*** dose

Vial: 100 U/ml (10 ml); *Cartridge:* 100 U/ml (3 ml, for use in the *OptiPen One **Insulin** Delivery Device*) (5/carton) (m-cresol); *SoloStar pen (disposable):* 100 U/ml (3 ml) (5/carton)

Toujeo <18 years: not established; ≥18 years: administer SC once daily at the same time each day as a basal ***insulin***; in the upper arm, abdomen, or thigh; onset of action 6 hours; duration 20-24 hours; *T2DM, **insulin** naïve:* initially 0.2 units/kg; titrate every 3-4 days; *T1DM, insulin-naïve:* initially 1/3-1/2 total daily ***insulin*** dose; remainder as short-acting ***insulin*** divided between each meal; *Switch from once daily long- or intermediate-acting **insulin**:* on a unit-for-unit basis; *Switching from **Lantus**:* a higher daily dose is expected; *Switching from twice daily **NPH**:* reduce initial dose by 20% of total daily NPH dose

Soln for SC injection: 300 units/ml prefilled disposable SoloStar Pen (1.5 ml, 3-5/carton)

▶ ***insulin isophane suspension (NPH)*** **(B)** <18 years: not recommended; ≥18 years:

Humulin N *(human, recombinant)* (OTC) onset 1-2 hours; peak 6-12 hours; duration 18-24 hours; SC only

Vial: 100 U/ml (10 ml); *Prefilled disposable pen:* 100 U/ml (3 ml, 5/pck)

Novolin N *(recombinant)* (OTC) onset 1.5 hours; peak 4-12 hours; duration 24 hours; SC only

Vial: 100 U/ml (10 ml); *PenFill cartridge:* 1.5 ml (5/pck); *KwikPens:* 1.5 ml (5/pck)

Iletin II NPH *(pork)* (OTC) onset 1-2 hours; peak 6-12 hours; duration 18-26 hours; SC only

Vial: 100 U/ml (10 ml)

▶ ***insulin zinc suspension*** *(lente)* **(B)** <18 years: not recommended; ≥18 years:

Humulin L *(human)* (OTC) onset 1-3 hours; peak 6-12 hours; duration 18-24 hours; SC only

Vial: 100 U/ml (10 ml)

Iletin II Lente *(pork)* (OTC) onset 1-3 hours; peak 6-12 hours; duration 18-26 hours; SC only

Vial: 100 U/ml (10 ml)

Novolin L *(human)* (OTC) onset 2.5 hours; peak 7-15 hours; duration 22 hours; SC only

Vial: 100 U/ml (10 ml)

ULTRA LONG-ACTING INSULINS

▶ ***insulin degludec (insulin analog)*** **(C)** <1 year: not established; ≥1 year: administer by SC injection once daily at any time of day, with or without food, into the upper arm, abdomen, or thigh; titrate every 3-4 days; ***Insulin**-naïve with type 1 diabetes:* initially 1/3-1/2 of total daily ***insulin*** dose, usually 0.2-0.4 units/kg; administer the remainder of the total dose as short-acting ***insulin*** divided between each daily meal; ***Insulin**-naive with type 2 diabetes:* initially 10 units once daily; adjust dose of concomitant oral antidiabetic agent; *Already on insulin (type 1 or type 2):* initiate at same unit dose as total daily long- or intermediate-acting ***insulin*** unit dose

Tresiba FlexTouch *Pen:* 100 U/ml (3 ml, 5 pens/carton); 200 U/ml (3 ml, 5 pens/carton) (zinc, m-cresol)

Comment: **Tresiba U-200 FlexTouch** is the only long-acting ***insulin*** in a 160-unit pen allowing up to 160 units in a single injection. The U-200 dose counter always shows the desired dose (i.e., no conversion from U/100 to U-200 is required)

- ***insulin extended zinc suspension (Ultralente, human)*** (B) <18 years: not recommended; ≥18 years: SC only; onset 4-6 hours; peak 8-20 hours; duration 24-48 hours
  Humulin U (OTC) *Vial:* 100 U/ml (10 ml)

Insulin Lispro Protamine+Insulin Lispro Combinations

- ***insulin lispro protamine*** **75%+*insulin lispro*** **25%** (B) <18 years: not recommended; ≥18 years:
  Humalog Mix 75/25 *(human)* onset 15 minutes; peak 30 minutes to 1 hour; duration 24 hours; SC only
  Vial: 100 U/ml (10 ml); *Prefilled disposable KwikPen:* 100 U/ml (3 ml, 5/carton) (zinc, m-cresol); *HumaPen Memoir* and *HumaPen Luxura* HD inj device for *Humalog cartridges* (100 U/ml, 3 ml, 5/carton) (zinc, m-cresol)
- ***insulin lispro protamine*** **50%+*insulin lispro*** **50%** (B) <18 years: not recommended; ≥18 years:
  Humalog Mix 50/50 ***(recombinant)*** (B) onset 15 minutes; peak 2.3 hours; range 1-5 hours; SC only
  Vial: 100 U/ml (10 ml); *Prefilled disposable KwikPen:* 100 U/ml (3 ml, 5/carton) (zinc, m-cresol); *HumaPen Memoir* and *HumaPen Luxura* HD inj device for *Humalog cartridges* (100 U/ml, 3 ml, 5/carton) (zinc, m-cresol)

Insulin Isophane Suspension (NPH)+Insulin Regular Combinations

- ***NPH*** **70%+*regular*** **30%** (B) <18 years: not recommended; ≥18 years:
  Humulin 70/30 *(human, recombinant)* **(OTC)** onset 30 minutes; peak 2-12 hours; duration up to 24 hours; SC only
  Vial: 100 U/ml (10 ml)
  Novolin 70/30 *(recombinant)* **(OTC)** onset 30 minutes; peak 2-12 hours; duration up to 24 hours; SC only
  Vial: 100 U/ml (10 ml)
- ***NPH*** **50%+*regular*** **50%** (B) <18 years: not recommended; ≥18 years:
  Humulin 50/50 *(human)* **(OTC)** onset 30 minutes; peak 3-5 hours; duration up to 24 hours; SC only
  Vial: 100 U/ml (10 ml)

Insulin Lispro Protamine+Insulin Lispro Combinations

- ***insulin lispro protamine*** **75%+*insulin lispro*** **25%** (B) <18 years: not recommended; ≥18 years:
  Humalog Mix 75/25 *(recombinant)* onset 15 minutes; peak 30-90 minutes; duration 24 hours; SC only
  Vial: 100 U/ml (10 ml); *Prefilled disposable KwikPen:* 100 U/ml (3 ml, 5/carton) (zinc, m-cresol); *HumaPen Memoir* and *HumaPen Luxura* HD inj device for *Humalog cartridges* (100 U/ml, 3 ml, 5/carton) (zinc, m-cresol)
- ***insulin lispro protamine*** **50%+*insulin lispro*** **50%** (B) <18 years: not recommended; ≥18 years:
  Humalog Mix 50/50 *(recombinant)* onset 15 minutes; peak 1 hour; duration up to 16 hours; SC only
  Vial: 100 U/ml (10 ml); *Prefilled disposable KwikPen:* 100 U/ml (3 ml, 5/carton) (zinc, m-cresol); *HumaPen Memoir* and *HumaPen LUXURA* HD inj device for *Humalog cartridges* (100 U/ml, 3 ml, 5/carton) (zinc, m-cresol); U/ml (3 ml,

5/pck) (zinc, m-cresol); *HumaPen Memoir* and *HumaPen LUXURA* HD inj device for *Humalog cartridges* (100 U/ml, 3 ml, 5/carton) (zinc, m-cresol); (100 U/ml, 3 ml 5/carton (zinc, m-cresol)

Basal Insulin+GLP-1 RA Combinations

▶ ***insulin degludec (insulin analog)+liraglutide*** **(C)** for treatment of type 2 diabetes only in adults inadequately controlled on <50 units of basal insulin daily or ≤1.8 mg of ***liraglutide*** daily; administer by SC injection once daily, with or without food, into the upper arm, abdomen, or thigh; titrate every 3-4 days
Pediatric: <18 years: not recommended; ≥18 years: same as adult
Xultophy Prefilled pen: 100/3.6 U/ml (3 ml, 5 pens/carton)

▶ ***insulin glargine (insulin analog)+lixisenatide*** **(C)** for treatment of type 2 diabetes only in adults inadequately controlled on <60 units of basal insulin daily or ***lixisenatide***; administer by SC injection once daily, with or without food, into the upper arm, abdomen, or thigh; titrate every 3-4 days
Pediatric: <18 years: not recommended; ≥18 years: same as adult
Soliqua Prefilled pen: 100/33 U/ml (3 ml, 5 pens/carton) covering 15-60 mg ***insulin glargine*** 100 units/ml and 15-20 mcg of ***lixisenatide (m-cresol)***

TYPE 2 DIABETES MELLITUS (T2DM)

For insulins see ***Type 1 Diabetes Mellitus*** *page* 465

Comment: Normal fasting glucose is <100 mg/dL. Impaired glucose tolerance is a risk factor for type 2 diabetes and a marker for cardiovascular disease risk; it occurs early in the natural history of these two diseases. Impaired fasting glucose is ≥100 mg/dL and <125 mg/dL. Impaired glucose tolerance is OGTT, 2 hour post-load 75 gm glucose >140 mg/dL and <200 mg/dL. Target pre-prandial glucose is 80 mg/dL to 120 mg/dL. Target bedtime glucose is 100 mg/dL to 140 mg/dL. Target glycosylated HbA1c is <7.0%. Additional medications to be considered for initiation at onset of T2DM, particularly in the presence of hypertension, include an angiotensin-converting enzyme inhibitor (ACEI), angiotensin II receptor blocker (ARB), thiazide-like diuretic, or a calcium channel blocker (CCB). Consider diabetes screening at age 25 years for persons in high-risk groups (non-Caucasian, positive family history for DM, obesity). Hypertension and hyperlipidemia are common comorbid conditions. Macrovascular complications include cerebral vascular disease, coronary artery disease, and peripheral vascular disease. Microvascular complications include retinopathy, nephropathy, neuropathy, and cardiomyopathy. Oral hypoglycemics are contraindicated in pregnancy.

REFERENCE

American Diabetes Association. (2017). Standards of Medical Care in Diabetes—2017. *Diabetes Care, 40*(Suppl 1), S1–S135.

TREATMENT FOR ACUTE HYPOGLYCEMIA

▶ ***glucagon (recombinant)*** **(B)** <20 kg: 0.5 mg or 20-30 mg/kg; ≥20 kg: 1 mg; administer SC or IM or IV; if patient does not respond in 15 minutes, may administer a single or 2 divided doses

SULFONYLUREAS

Comment: Sulfonylureas are secretagogues (i.e., stimulate pancreatic insulin secretion); therefore, the patient taking a sulfonylurea should be alerted to the risk for hypoglycemia. Action is dependent on functioning beta cells in the pancreatic islets.

First Generation Sulfonylureas

▶ ***chlorpropamide*** (C)(G) <12 years: not recommended; ≥12 years: initially 250 mg/day with breakfast; max 750 mg
Diabinese *Tab:* 100*, 250*mg

▶ ***tolazamide*** (C)(G) <12 years: not recommended; ≥12 years: initially 100-250 mg/day with breakfast; increase by 100-250 mg/day at weekly intervals; maintenance 100 mg 1 gm/day; max 1 gm/day
Tolinase *Tab:* 100, 250, 500 mg

▶ ***tolbutamide*** (C) <12 years: not recommended; ≥12 years: initially 1-2 gm in divided doses; max 2 gm/day
Tab: 500 mg

Second Generation Sulfonylureas

▶ ***glimepiride*** (C) <12 years: not recommended; ≥12 years: initially 1-2 mg once daily with breakfast; after reaching dose of 2 mg, increase by 2 mg at 1-2 week intervals as needed; usual maintenance 1-4 mg once daily; max 8 mg/day
Amaryl *Tab:* 1*, 2*, 4*mg

▶ ***glipizide*** (C)(G) <12 years: not recommended; ≥12 years:
Glucotrol initially 5 mg before breakfast; increase by 2.5-5 mg every few days if needed; max 15 mg/day; max 40 mg/day in divided doses
Tab: 5*, 10*mg
Glucotrol XL initially 5 mg with breakfast; usual range 5-10 mg/day; max 20 mg/day
Tab: 2.5, 5, 10 mg ext-rel

▶ ***glyburide*** (C)(G) <12 years: not recommended; ≥12 years: initially 2.5-5 mg/day with breakfast; increase by 2.5 mg at weekly intervals; maintenance 1.25-20 mg/day in a single or 2 divided doses; max 20 mg/day
DiaBeta, Micronase *Tab:* 1.25*, 2.5*, 5*mg

▶ ***glyburide, micronized*** (B) <12 years: not recommended; ≥12 years:
Glynase PresTab initially 1.5-3 mg/day with breakfast; increase by 1.5 mg at weekly intervals if needed; usual maintenance 0.75-12 mg/day in single or divided doses; max 12 mg/day
Tab: 1.5*, 3*, 6*mg

ALPHA-GLUCOSIDASE INHIBITORS

Comment: Alpha-glucosidase inhibitors block the enzyme that breaks down carbohydrates in the small intestine, delaying digestion and absorption of complex carbohydrates, and lowering peak postprandial glycemic concentrations. Use as monotherapy or in combination with a sulfonylurea. Contraindicated in inflammatory bowel disease, colon ulceration, and intestinal obstruction. Side effects include flatulence, diarrhea, and abdominal pain.

▶ ***acarbose*** (B) <12 years: not recommended; ≥12 years: initially 25 mg tid ac, increase at 4-8 week intervals; or initially 25 mg once daily, increase gradually to 25 mg tid; usual range 50-100 mg tid; max 100 mg tid
Precose *Tab:* 25, 50, 100 mg

▶ ***miglitol*** (B)(G) <12 years: not recommended; ≥12 years: initially 25 mg tid at the start of each main meal, titrated to 50 mg tid at the start of each main meal; max 100 mg tid
Glyset *Tab:* 25, 50, 100 mg

BIGUANIDES

Comment: Biguanides decrease gluconeogenesis by the liver in the presence of insulin. Action is dependent on the presence of circulating insulin. Lower hepatic glucose production leads to lower overnight, fasting, and pre-prandial plasma glucose levels. Common side effects include GI distress, nausea, vomiting, bloating, and flatulence, which usually eventually resolve. May be used as monotherapy (≥12 years only) or with a sulfonylurea or ***insulin***.

▶ ***metformin*** (B)(G) take with meals

Comment: ***metformin*** is contraindicated with renal impairment, metabolic acidosis, and ketoacidosis. Suspend ***metformin***, prior to, and for 48 hours after, surgery or receiving IV iodinated contrast agents.

Fortamet <17 years: not recommended; ≥17 years: initially 1000 mg once daily; may increase by 500 mg/day at 1 week intervals; max 2.5 gm/day

Tab: 500, 1000 mg ext-rel

Glucophage <10 years: not recommended; 10-16 years: use only as monotherapy; >16 years: initially 500 mg bid; may increase by 500 mg/day at 1 week intervals; max 1 gm bid or 2.5 gm in 3 divided doses; or initially 850 mg once daily in AM; may increase by 850 mg/day in divided doses at 2 week intervals; max 2000 mg/day; take with meals

Tab: 500, 850, 1000*mg

Glucophage XR <10 years: not recommended; 10-16 years: use immediate release form; >16 years: initially 500 mg by mouth every evening; may increase by 500 mg/day at 1 week intervals; max 2 gm/day

Tab: 500, 750 mg ext-rel

Glumetza ER (G) <18 years: not recommended; ≥18 years: initially 1000 mg once daily; may increase by 500 mg/day at weekly intervals; max 2 gm/day

Tab: 500, 1000 mg ext-rel

Riomet XR <10 years: not recommended; ≥10 years: monotherapy only; initially 500 mg once daily; may increase by 500 mg/day at 1 week intervals; max 2 gm/day in divided doses; take with meals

Oral soln: 500 mg/ml (4 oz) (cherry)

MEGLITINIDES

Comment: Meglitinides are secretagogues (i.e., stimulate pancreatic insulin secretion) in response to a meal. Action is dependent on functioning beta cells in the pancreatic islets. Use as monotherapy or in combination with ***metformin***.

▶ ***nateglinide*** (C) <12 years: not recommended; ≥12 years: 60-120 mg tid ac 1-30 minutes prior to start of the meal

Starlix *Tab:* 60, 120 mg

▶ ***repaglinide*** (C)(G) <12 years: not recommended; ≥12 years: initially 0.5 mg with 2-4 meals/day; take 30 minutes ac; titrate by doubling dose at intervals of at least 1 week; range 0.5-4 mg with 2-4 meals/day; max 16 mg/day

Prandin *Tab:* 0.5, 1, 2 mg

THIAZOLIDINEDIONES (TZDs)

Comment: The TZDs decrease hepatic gluconeogenesis and reduce insulin resistance (i.e., increase glucose uptake and utilization by the muscles). Liver function tests are indicated before initiating these drugs. Do not start if ALT more than 3 times greater than normal. Recheck ALT monthly for the first six months of therapy; then, every two months for the remainder of the first year and periodically thereafter. Liver function tests should be obtained at the first symptoms suggestive of hepatic dysfunction (nausea, vomiting, fatigue, dark urine, anorexia, abdominal pain).

▶ ***pioglitazone*** (C)(G) <18 years: not recommended; ≥18 years: initially 15-30 mg once daily; max 45 mg/day as a monotherapy; usual max 30 mg/day in combination with ***metformin***, ***insulin***, or a sulfonylurea

Actos *Tab:* 15, 30, 45 mg

▶ ***rosiglitazone*** (C)(G) <18 years: not recommended; ≥18 years: initially 4 mg/day in a single <u>or</u> 2 divided doses; may increase after 8-12 weeks; max 8 mg/day as a monotherapy <u>or</u> combination therapy with ***metformin*** <u>or</u> a sulfonylurea; not for use with ***insulin***

Avandia *Tab:* 2, 4, 8 mg

DIPEPTIDYL PEPTIDASE-4 (DPP-4) INHIBITOR+THIAZOLIDINEDIONE COMBINATION

Comment: The FDA has reported that ***alogliptin***-containing drugs may increase the risk of heart failure, especially in patients who already have cardiovascular <u>or</u> renal disease. The drug **Oseni** (***alogliptin+pioglitazone***) is in this risk group.

▶ ***alogliptin+pioglitazone*** (C) <18 years: not recommended; ≥18 years: take 1 dose once daily with first meal of the day; max: ***rosiglitazone*** 8 mg and max ***glimepiride*** per day; same precautions as ***alogliptin*** and ***pioglitazone***

Oseni

Tab: **Oseni 12.5/15** alo 12.5 mg+pio 15 mg
Oseni 12.5/30 alo 12.5 mg+pio 30 mg
Oseni 12.5/45 alo 12.5 mg+pio 45 mg
Oseni 25/15 alo 25 mg+pio 15 mg
Oseni 25/30 alo 25+pio 30 mg
Oseni 25/45 alo 25 mg+pio 45 mg

SECOND GENERATION SULFONYLUREA+BIGUANIDE COMBINATIONS

Comment: **Metaglip** and **Glucovance** are combination secretagogues (sulfonylureas) and insulin sensitizers (biguanides). *Sulfonylurea:* Action is dependent on functioning beta cells in the pancreatic islets; patient should be alerted to the risk for hypoglycemia. Common side effects of the biguanide include GI distress, nausea, vomiting, bloating, and flatulence, which usually eventually resolve. Take with food. ***metformin*** is contraindicated with renal impairment, metabolic acidosis, and ketoacidosis. Suspend ***metformin***, prior to, and for 48 hours after, surgery <u>or</u> receiving IV iodinated contrast agents.

▶ ***glipizide/metformin*** (C) <12 years: not recommended; ≥12 years: take with meals; *Primary therapy:* 2.5/250 once daily <u>or</u> if FBS is 280-320 mg/dL, may start at 2.5/250 bid; may increase by 1 tab/day every 2 weeks; max 10/2,000 per day in 2 divided doses; *Second-Line Therapy:* 2.5/500 <u>or</u> 5/500 bid; may increase by up to 5/500 every 2 weeks; max: 20/2000 per day; same precautions as ***glipizide*** and ***metformin***

Metaglip

Tab: **Metaglip 2.5/250** glip 2.5 mg+met 250 mg
Metaglip 2.5/500 glip 2.5 mg+met 500 mg
Metaglip 5/500 glip 5 mg+met 500 mg

▶ ***glyburide+metformin*** (B) <12 years: not recommended; ≥12 years: take with meals; *Primary therapy (initial therapy if HgbA1c <9.0%):* initially 1.25/250 once daily; max ***glyburide*** 20 mg and ***metformin*** 2,000 mg per day; *Primary therapy (initial therapy if HbA1c >9.0% <u>or</u> FBS >200):* initially 1.25/250 bid; max ***glyburide*** 20 mg and ***metformin*** 2000 mg per day; *Second-line therapy (initial therapy if HbA1c >7.0%):* initially 2.5/500 <u>or</u> 5/500 bid; max ***glyburide*** 20 mg and ***metformin*** 2,000 mg per day; *Previously treated with a sulfonylurea and **metformin**:* dose to approximate total daily doses of ***glyburide*** and ***metformin*** already being taken; max: ***glyburide*** 20 mg and ***metformin*** 2000 mg per day; same precautions as ***glyburide*** and ***metformin***

Glucovance

Tab: **Glucovance 1.25/250** glyb 1.25 mg+met 250 mg
Glucovance 2.5/500 glyb 2.5 mg+met 500 mg
Glucovance 5/500 glyb 5 mg+met 500 mg

Comment: ***metformin*** is contraindicated with renal impairment, metabolic acidosis, and ketoacidosis. Suspend ***metformin***, prior to, and for 48 hours after, surgery or receiving IV iodinated contrast agents.

THIAZOLIDINEDIONE+BIGUANIDE COMBINATIONS

➢ ***pioglitazone/metformin*** (C) <12 years: not recommended; ≥12 years: take in divided doses with meals; *Previously on metformin alone:* initially 15/500 or 15/850 once or twice daily; *Previously on **pioglitazone** alone:* initially 15/500 bid; *Previously on **pioglitazone** and metformin:* switch on a mg/mg basis; may increase after 8-12 weeks; max: ***pioglitazone*** 45 mg and ***metformin*** 2000 mg per day; same precautions as ***pioglitazone*** and ***metformin***

Actoplus Met, Actoplus Met R (G)

Tab: **Actoplus Met 15/500** pio 15 mg+met 500 mg
Actoplus Met 15/850 pio 15 mg+met 850 mg
Actoplus Met XR 15/1000 pio 15 mg+met 1000 mg
Actoplus Met XR 30/1000 pio 30 mg+met 1000 mg

Comment: ***metformin*** is contraindicated with renal impairment, metabolic acidosis, ketoacidosis. Suspend ***metformin***, prior to, and for 48 hours after, surgery or receiving IV iodinated contrast agents.

➢ ***rosiglitazone/metformin*** (C)(G) <12 years: not recommended; ≥12 years: take in divided doses with meals; *Previously on **metformin** alone:* add ***rosiglitazone*** 4 mg/day; may increase after 8-12 weeks; *Previously on **rosiglitazone** alone:* add ***metformin*** 1000 mg/day; may increase after 1-2 weeks; *Previously on **rosiglitazone** and **metformin**:* switch on a mg/mg basis; may increase ***rosiglitazone*** by 4 mg and/or ***metformin*** by 500 mg per day; max: ***rosiglitazone*** 8 mg and ***metformin*** 2,000 mg per day; same precautions as ***rosiglitazone*** and ***metformin***

Avandamet

Tab: **Avandamet 2/500** rosi 2 mg+met 500 mg
Avandamet 2/1,000 rosi 2 mg+met 1000 mg
Avandamet 4/500 rosi 4 mg+met 500 mg
Avandamet 4/1,000 rosi 4 mg+met 1000 mg

Comment: ***rosiglitazone*** has been withdrawn from retail pharmacies. In order to enroll and receive ***rosiglitazone***, healthcare providers and patients must enroll in the *Avandia-Rosiglitazone Medicines Access Program.* The program limits the use of ***rosiglitazone*** to patients already being treated successfully, and those whose blood sugar cannot be controlled with other antidiabetic medicines. ***Metformin*** is contraindicated with renal impairment, metabolic acidosis, and ketoacidosis. Suspend ***metformin***, prior to, and for 48 hours after, surgery or receiving IV iodinated contrast agents.

THIAZOLIDINEDIONE+SULFONYLUREA COMBINATIONS

➢ ***pioglitazone/glimepiride*** (C) <18 years: not recommended; ≥18 years: take 1 dose daily with first meal of the day; *Previously on sulfonylurea alone:* initially 30 mg/2 mg; *Previously on **pioglitazone** and **glimepiride**:* switch on a mg/mg basis; max: ***pioglitazone*** 30 mg and ***glimepiride*** 4 mg per day; Same precautions as ***pioglitazone*** and ***glimepiride***

Duetact

Tab: **Duetact 30/2** pio 30 mg+glim 2 mg
Duetact 304 pio 30 mg+glim 4 mg

➢ ***rosiglitazone+glimepiride*** (C) <18 years: not recommended; ≥18 years: take 1 dose daily with first meal of the day; max: ***rosiglitazone*** 8 mg and ***glimepiride*** 4 mg per day; same precautions as ***rosiglitazone*** and ***glimepiride***

Avandaryl

Tab: **Avandaryl 4/1** rosi 4 mg+glim 1 mg
Avandaryl 4/2 rosi 4 mg+glim 2 mg
Avandaryl 4/4 rosi 4 mg+glim 4 mg
Avandaryl 8/2 rosi 8 mg+glim 2 mg
Avandaryl 8/4 rosi 8 mg+glim 4 mg

GLUCAGON-LIKE PEPTIDE-1 (GLP-1) RECEPTOR AGONISTS

Comment: GLP-1 receptor agonists act as an agonist at the GLP-1 receptors. They have a longer half-life than the native protein allowing them to be dosed once daily. They increase intracellular cAMP resulting in ***insulin*** release in the presence of increased serum concentration, decrease ***glucagon*** secretion, and delay gastric emptying, thus, reducing fasting, pre-meal, and postprandial glucose throughout the day. GLP-1 receptor agonists are not a substitute for ***insulin***, not for treatment of DKA, and not for postprandial administration.

▶ ***dulaglutide*** **(C)** <18 years: not recommended; ≥18 years: administer by SC injection into the upper arm, abdomen, or thigh once weekly on the same day and the same time of day, with or without food; initially 0.75 mg SC once weekly; may increase to 1.5 mg SC once weekly

Trulicity *Prefilled pen/syringe:* 0.75, 1.5 mg/0.5 ml single-dose (4/carton)

▶ ***exenatide*** **(C)** <18 years: not recommended; ≥18 years: administer by SC injection into the upper arm, abdomen, or thigh

Bydureon administer 2 mg SC once weekly inject immediately after mixing; at any time of day; with or without meals; if switching from **Byetta,** discontinue **Byetta** and instead administer **Bydureon** and continue the same once weekly administration schedule

Vial: 2 mg w. 0.65 ml diluent, single-dose; *Prefilled pen:* 2 mg w. 0.65 ml diluent, single-dose

Bydureon BCise administer 2 mg by subcutaneous injection once weekly; at any time of day; with or without meals; if switching from **Byetta,** discontinue **Byetta** and start **Bydureon BCise** and continue the same once weekly administration schedule

Autoinjector: 2 mg (0.85 ml) single-dose

Byetta inject within 60 minutes before AM and PM meals, or before the 2 main meals of the day, approx ≥6 hours apart; initially 5 mcg/dose; may increase to 10 mcg/dose after one month

Prefilled pen: 250 mcg/ml (5, 10 mcg/dose; 60 doses) (needles not included) (m-cresol, mannitol)

▶ ***liraglutide*** **(C)** <18 years: not recommended; ≥18 years: administer by SC injection into the upper arm, abdomen, or thigh once daily; initially 0.6 mg/day for 1 week; then 1.2 mg/day; may increase to 1.8 mg/day

Victoza *Prefilled pen:* 6 mg/ml (3 ml) (needles not included)

▶ ***lixisenatide*** **(C)** <18 years: not established; ≥18 years: administer SC in the upper arm, abdomen, or thigh once daily; initially 10 mcg SC x 14 days; maintenance: 20 mcg beginning on day 15; administer within one hour of the first meal of the day and the same meal of the day

Adlyxin Soln for SC inj; *Starter Pen:* 50 mcg/ml (14 doses of 10 mcg; 3 ml); *Maintenance Pen:* 100 mcg/ml (14 doses of 20 mcg); *Starter Pack:* 1 prefilled starter pen + 1 prefilled maintenance pen; *Maintenance Pack:* 2 prefilled maintenance pens

Comment: **Adlyxin** is indicated as an adjunct to diet and exercise for T2DM. Not indicated for treatment of T1DM. Do not use with **Victoza, Saxenda,** other GLP-1 receptor agonists, or ***insulin***. Contraindicated with gastroparesis and GFR <15 mL/min. Poorly controlled diabetes in pregnancy increases the maternal risk for diabetic ketoacidosis, pre-eclampsia, spontaneous abortions, preterm delivery, stillbirth and delivery complications. Poorly controlled diabetes increases the fetal risk for major birth defects, stillbirth, and macrosomia related morbidity. **Adlyxin** should be used during pregnancy only if the potential benefit justifies the potential risk to the fetus. Estimated background risk of major birth defects and miscarriage in clinically recognized pregnancies is 2-4% and 15-20% respectively.

- ***semaglutide*** <18 years: not recommended: ≥18 years: administer SC in the upper arm, abdomen, or thigh once weekly at any time of day, with or without meals; initially 0.25 mg once weekly; after 4 weeks, increase the dose to 0.5 mg once weekly; if after at least 4 weeks additional glycemic control is needed, increase to 1 mg once weekly (usual main-maintenance dose); if a dose is missed, administer within 5 days of the missed dose

  Ozempic *Prefilled pen:* 2 mg/1.5 ml (1.34 mg/ml) single-patient-use; 0.25, 0.5, 1 mg/injection

  Comment: ***semaglutide*** is contraindicated with personal or family history of medullary thyroid carcinoma or with multiple endocrine neoplasia syndrome type 2. **Ozempic** has not been studied in patients with a history of pancreatitis. Consider another antidiabetic therapy. **Ozempic** is not recommended in females or males with reproductive potential. Discontinue in women at least 2 months before a planned pregnancy due to the long washout period for ***semaglutide***. Not recommended as first-line therapy for patients inadequately controlled on diet and exercise. There are no data on the presence of ***semaglutide*** in human milk or the effects on the breastfed infant.

BASAL INSULIN+GLP-1 RA COMBINATIONS

- ***insulin degludec (insulin analog)+liraglutide*** (C) <18 years: not recommended; ≥18 years: for treatment of type 2 diabetes only when inadequately controlled on <50 units of basal ***insulin*** daily or ≤1.8 mg of ***liraglutide*** daily; administer by SC injection once daily, with or without food, into the upper arm, abdomen, or thigh; titrate every 3-4 days

  Xultophy *Prefilled pen:* 100/3.6 U/ml (3 ml, 5 pens/carton)

- ***insulin glargine (insulin analog)+lixisenatide*** (C) <18 years: not recommended; ≥18 years: for treatment of type 2 diabetes only when inadequately controlled on <60 units of basal ***insulin*** daily or *lixisenatide*; administer by SC injection once daily, with or without food, into the upper arm, abdomen, or thigh; titrate every 3-4 days

  Soliqua *Prefilled pen:* 100/33 U/ml (3 ml, 5 pens/carton) covering 15-60 mg ***insulin glargine*** 100 units/ml and 15-20 mcg of ***lixisenatide (m-cresol)***

SODIUM-GLUCOSE CO-TRANSPORTER 2 (SGLT2) INHIBITORS

Comment: SGLT2 inhibitors block the SGLT2 protein involved in 90% of glucose reabsorption in the proximal renal tubule, resulting in increased renal glucose excretion (typically >2000 mg/dL), and lower blood glucose levels (low risk of hypoglycemia), modest weight loss, and mild reduction in blood pressure (probably due to sodium loss). These agents probably also increase ***insulin*** sensitivity, decrease gluconeogenesis, and improve ***insulin*** release from pancreatic beta cells. SGLT2 inhibitors are contraindicated in T1DM, and dose is decreased or contraindicated with decreased GFR, increased SCr, renal failure, ESRD, renal dialysis, metabolic acidosis, and diabetic ketoacidosis. The most common ASEs are increased urination, UTI, and female genital mycotic infection (due to the glycosuria). These effects may be managed with adequate oral hydration and post-voiding genital hygiene. OTC **Vagisil** wet wipes are recommended to completely remove any post-voiding glucose film, and, thus, reduce potential risk of UTI and vaginal candidiasis, and reverse initial signs/symptoms of candida vaginalis. The SGLT2 inhibitors are not recommended in nursing females. There is potential for a hypersensitivity reaction to include angioedema and anaphylaxis. Caution with SGLT2 use due to reports of increased risk of treatment-emergent bone fractures.

- ***canagliflozin*** **(C)** <18 years: not recommended; ≥18 years: take one tab before the first meal of the day; initially 100 mg; may titrate up to max 300 mg once daily; *GFR <45 mL/min:* do not initiate

    Invokana *Tab:* 100, 300 mg

    Comment: **Invokana** is contraindicated with GFR <45 mL/min. If GFR 45 ≤ 60 mL/min: max 100 mg once daily or consider other antihyperglycemic agents.

- ***dapagliflozin*** **(C)** <18 years: not recommended; ≥18 years: take one tab before the first meal of the day; initially 5 mg; may increase to max 10 mg once daily

    Farxiga *Tab:* 5, 10 mg

    Comment: **Farxiga** is contraindicated with GFR <60 mL/min.

- ***empagliflozin*** **(C)** <18 years: not recommended; ≥18 years: take one tab before the first meal of the day; initially 10 mg; may increase to max 25 mg once daily

    Jardiance *Tab:* 10, 25 mg

    Comment: **Jardiance** is contraindicated with GFR <45 mL/min.

- ***ertugliflozen*** **(C)** <18 years: not established; ≥18 years: take one tab before the initially 5 mg; may increase to max 15 mg once daily

    Steglatro *Tab:* 5, 15 mg

SODIUM-GLUCOSE CO-TRANSPORTER 2 (SGLT2) INHIBITOR+BIGUANIDE COMBINATIONS

Comment: Caution with **SGLT2** use due to reports of increased risk of treatment-emergent bone fractures. ***metformin*** is contraindicated with renal impairment, metabolic acidosis, and ketoacidosis. Suspend ***metformin***, prior to, and for 48 hours after, surgery or receiving IV iodinated contrast agents.

- ***canagliflozin/metformin*** **(C)** <18 years: not recommended; ≥18 years: take 1 dose twice daily with meals; max daily dose 300/2000; *GFR 45-≤60 mL/min:* ***canagliflozin*** max 100 mg once daily or consider other antihyperglycemic agents; *GFR <45 mL/min:* do not initiate

    Invokamet

    Tab: **Invokamet 50/500** cana 50 mg+met 500 mg
    Invokamet 50/1000 cana 50 mg+met 1000 mg
    Invokamet 150/500 cana 150 mg+met 500 mg
    Invokamet 150/1000 cana 150 mg+met 1000 mg

- ***dapagliflozin/metformin*** **(C)** <18 years: not recommended; ≥18 years: swallow whole; do not crush or chew; take once daily first meal of the day; max daily dose 10/2000

    Xigduo XR

    Tab: **Xigduo XR 5/500** dapa 5 mg+met 500 mg ext-rel
    Xigduo XR 5/1000 dapa 5 mg+met 1000 mg ext-rel
    Xigduo XR 10/500 dapa 10 mg+met 500 mg ext-rel
    Xigduo XR 10/1000 dapa 10 mg+met 1000 mg ext-rel

    Comment: **Xigduo** is contraindicated with GFR <60 *mL/min*, SCr >1.5 (males) or SCr >1.4 (females)

- ***empagliflozin+metformin*** **(C)** <18 years: not recommended; ≥18 years: take 1 dose twice daily with meals; max daily dose 25/2000

    Synjardy

    Tab: **Synjardy 5/500** empa 5 mg+met 500 mg
    Synjardy 5/1000 empa 5 mg+met 1000 mg

Synjardy 12.5/500 empa 12.5 mg+met 500 mg
Synjardy 12.5/1000 empa 12.5 mg+met 1000 mg

Synjardy XR
Tab: **Synjardy XR 5/1000** empa 5 mg+met 1000 mg
Synjardy XR 12.5/1000 empa 12.5 mg+met 1000 mg
Synjardy XR 10/1000 empa 10 mg+met 1000 mg
Synjardy XR 25/1000 empa 25 mg+met 1000 mg

Comment: **Synjardy** is contraindicated with *GFR <45 mL/min*, *SCr* >1.5 (males), or *SCr* >1.4 (females).

▶ ***ertugliflozin+metformin*** (C) <18 years: not established; ≥18 years: take 1 dose twice daily with meals; max daily dose 15/2000

Segluormet
Tab: **Segluormet 2.5/500** ertu 2.5 mg+met 500 mg
Segluormet 2.5/1000 ertu 2.5 mg+met 1000 mg
Segluormet 7.5/500 ertu 7.5 mg+met 500 mg
Segluormet 7.5/1000 ertu 7.5 mg+met 1000 mg

SODIUM-GLUCOSE CO-TRANSPORTER 2 (SGLT2) INHIBITOR+DIPEPTIDYL PEPTIDASE-4 (DPP-4) INHIBITOR COMBINATIONS

Comment: Caution with **SGLT2** use due to reports of increased risk of treatment-emergent bone fractures. DPP-4 inhibitors have been associated with a risk of developing and exacerbating acute pancreatitis.

▶ ***dapagliflozin+saxagliptin*** (C) <18 years: not established; ≥18 years: initially 5/10 once daily, at any time of day, with or without food; if a dose is missed and it is ≥12 hours until the next dose, the dose should be taken; if a dose is missed and it is <12 hours until the next dose, the missed dose should be skipped and the next dose taken at the usual time.

Qtern *Tab: dapa* 10 mg+*saxa* 5 mg film-coat

Comment: **Qtern** should not be used during pregnancy. If pregnancy is detected, treatment with **Qtern** should be discontinued. It is unknown whether **Qtern** and/or its metabolites are excreted in human milk. Do not use with CrCl <60 mL/min or eGFR <60 mL/min/1.73 m² or ESRD or severe hepatic impairment or history of pancreatitis.

▶ ***empagliflozin+linagliptin*** (C) <18 years: not recommended; ≥18 years: initially 10/5 once daily with the first meal of the day; max daily dose 25/5; GFR *<45 mL/min:* contraindicated

Glyxambi
Tab: **Glyxambi 10/5** empa 10 mg+lina 5 mg
Glyxambi 25/5 empa 25 mg+lina 5 mg

▶ ***ertugliflozin+sitagliptin*** (C) <18 years: not established; ≥18 years: initially 5/100 once daily with the first meal of the day; max daily dose 15/100

Steglujan
Tab: **Steglujan 5/100** ertu 5 mg+sita 100 mg
Steglujan 15/100 ertu 15 mg+sita 100 mg

Comment: **Steglujan** is contraindicated with GFR <45 mL/min.

DIPEPTIDYL PEPTIDASE-4 (DPP-4) INHIBITORS

Comment: DPP-4 is an enzyme that degrades incretin hormones glucagon-like peptide-1 (GLP-1) and glucose-dependent insulinotropic polypeptide (GIP). Thus, DPP-4 inhibitors increase the concentration of active incretin hormones, stimulating the release of ***insulin*** in a glucose-dependent manner and decreasing the levels of circulating ***glucagon***. The FDA has reported that ***saxagliptin***- and ***alogliptin***-containing drugs may increase the risk of heart failure, especially in patients who already have cardiovascular or renal disease. Drugs in this risk group include **Nesina** (***alogliptin***) and **Onglyza** (***saxagliptin***)

▻ ***alogliptin*** **(B)** <18 years: not recommended; ≥18 years: take twice daily with meals; max 25 mg/day
  Nesina *Tab:* 6.25, 12.5, 25 mg

▻ ***linagliptin*** **(B)** <18 years: not recommended; ≥18 years: 5 mg once daily
  Tradjenta *Tab:* 5 mg

▻ ***saxagliptin*** **(B)** <18 years: not recommended; ≥18 years: 2.5-5 mg once daily
  Onglyza *Tab:* 2.5, 5 mg

▻ ***sitagliptin*** **(B)** <18 years: not recommended; ≥18 years: as monotherapy or as combination therapy with ***metformin*** or a TZD
  Januvia 25-100 mg once daily
    Tab: 25, 50, 100 mg

DIPEPTIDYL PEPTIDASE-4 (DPP-4) INHIBITOR+BIGUANIDE COMBINATIONS

Comment: DPP-4 inhibitor+***metformin*** combinations are contraindicated with renal impairment (males: SCr ≥1.5 mg/dL; females: SCr ≥1.4 mg/dL) or abnormal CrCl, metabolic acidosis, ketoacidosis, or history of angioedema. Suspend ***metformin***, prior to, and for 48 hours after, surgery or receiving IV iodinated contrast agents. Avoid in the malnourished, dehydrated, or with clinical or lab evidence of hepatic disease. For other DPP-4 and/or ***metformin*** precautions, see mfr pkg insert. The FDA has reported that ***saxagliptin***- and ***alogliptin***-containing drugs may increase the risk of heart failure, especially in patients who already have cardiovascular or renal disease. These drugs include: **Onglyza** (***saxagliptin***), **Kombiglyze XR** (***saxagliptin/metformin***), **Nesina** (***alogliptin***), **Kazano** (***alogliptin+metformin***), and **Oseni** (***alogliptin+pioglitazone***).

▻ ***alogliptin+metformin*** **(B)** <18 years: not recommended; ≥18 years: take twice daily with meals; max ***alogliptin*** 25 mg/day, max ***metformin*** 2000 mg/day
  Kazano
    Tab: **Kazano 12.5/500** algo 12.5 mg+met 500 mg
      Kazano 2.5/1000: algo 12.5 mg+met 1000 mg

▻ ***linagliptin+metformin*** **(B)** <18 years: not recommended; ≥18 years:
  Jentadueto take twice daily with meals; max ***linagliptin*** 5 mg/day, max ***metformin*** 2000 mg/day
    Tab: **Jentadueto 2.5/500** lina 2.5 mg+met 500 mg film-coat
      Jentadueto 2.5/850 lina 2.5 mg+met 850 mg film-coat
      Jentadueto 2.5/1000 lina 2.5 mg+met 1,000 mg film-coat
  Jentadueto XR *Currently not treated with* ***metformin:*** initiate **Jentadueto XR 5/1000** once daily; *Already treated with* ***metformin:*** initiate **Jentadueto XR** 5 mg ***linagliptin*** total daily dose and a similar total daily dose of ***metformin*** once daily; *Already treated with* ***linagliptin*** *and* ***metformin*** or ***Jentadueto:*** switch to **Jentadueto XR** containing 5 mg of ***linagliptin*** total daily dose and a similar total daily dose of ***metformin*** once daily; max ***linagliptin*** *5 mg* and ***metformin*** 2,000 mg*;* take as a single dose once daily; take with food; do not crush or chew; *eGFR <30 mL/min:* contraindicated; *eGFR 30-45 mL/min:* not recommended
    Tab: **Jentadueto 2.5/1000** lina 2.5 mg+met 1000 mg film-coat ext-rel
      Jentadueto 5/1000 lina 5 mg+met 1000 mg film-coat ext-rel

▻ ***saxagliptin+metformin*** **(B)** <18 years: not recommended; ≥18 years: take once daily with meals; max ***saxagliptin*** 5 mg/day, max ***metformin*** 2000 mg/day; do not crush or chew
  Kombiglyze XR
    Tab: **Kombiglyze XR 5/500** saxa 5 mg+met 500 mg
      Kombiglyze XR 2.5/1000 saxa 2.5 mg+met 1000 mg
      Kombiglyze XR 5/1000 saxa 5 mg+met 1000 mg

Comment: The FDA has reported that ***saxagliptin***-containing drugs may increase the risk of heart failure, especially in patients who already have cardiovascular or renal disease. The drug **Kombiglyze XR** (***saxagliptin/metformin***) is in this risk group. ***metformin*** is contraindicated with renal impairment, metabolic acidosis, and ketoacidosis. Suspend ***metformin***, prior to, and for 48 hours after, surgery or receiving IV iodinated contrast agents.

- ***sitagliptin+metformin*** **(B)** <18 years: not recommended; ≥18 years: take twice daily with meals; max ***sitagliptin*** 100 mg/day, max *metformin* 2000 mg/day

  Janumet

  Tab: **Janumet 50/500** sita 50 mg+met 500 mg
  Janumet 50/1000 sita 50 mg+met 1000 mg

  Janumet XR

  Tab: **Janumet XR 50/500** sita 50 mg+met 500 mg ext-rel
  Janumet XR 50/1000 sita 50 mg+met 1000 mg ext-rel
  Janumet XR 100/1000 sita 100 mg+met 1000 mg ext-rel

  Comment: ***metformin*** is contraindicated with renal impairment, metabolic acidosis, and ketoacidosis. Suspend ***metformin***, prior to, and for 48 hours after, surgery or receiving IV iodinated contrast agents.

MEGLITINIDE+BIGUANIDE COMBINATIONS

- ***repaglinide+metformin*** **(C)(G)** <12 years: not recommended; ≥12 years: take in 2-3 divided doses within 30 minutes before food; max 4/1000 per meal and 10/2000 per day

  Prandimet

  Tab: **Prandimet 1/500** repa 1 mg+met 500 mg
  Prandimet 2/500 repa 2 mg+met 500 mg

  Comment: ***metformin*** is contraindicated with renal impairment, metabolic acidosis, and ketoacidosis. Suspend ***metformin***, prior to, and for 48 hours after, surgery or receiving IV iodinated contrast agents.

DIPEPTIDYL PEPTIDASE-4 (DPP-4) INHIBITOR+HMG-COA REDUCTASE INHIBITOR COMBINATIONS

- ***sitagliptin/simvastatin*** **(B)** <18 years: not recommended; ≥18 years: take once daily in the PM; swallow whole; adjust dose if needed after 4 weeks; *Concomitant* ***verapamil*** or ***diltiazem***: max 100/10 once daily; *Concomitant* ***amiodarone***, ***amlodipine***, or ***ranolazine***: max 100/20 once daily; *HoFH:* max 100/40 once daily; *Chinese patients taking lipid-modifying doses (>1 gm/day niacin) of niacin-containing products:* caution with 100/40 dose; increase risk of myopathy

  Juvisync

  Tab: **Juvisync 100/10** sita 100 mg+simva 10 mg
  Juvisync 100/20 sita 100 mg+simva 20 mg
  Juvisync 100/40 sita 100 mg+simva 40 mg

DOPAMINE RECEPTOR AGONIST

- ***bromocriptine mesylate*** **(B)** <12 years: not recommended; ≥12 years: take with food in the morning within 2 hours of waking; initially 0.8 mg once daily; may increase by 0.8 mg/week; max 4.8 mg/week; *Severe psychotic disorders:* not recommended

  Cycloset *Tab:* 0.8 mg

  Comment: **Cycloset** is an adjunct to diet and exercise to improve glycemic control. Contraindicated with syncopal migraines, nursing mothers, and other ergot-related drugs.

ADJUNCTIVE TREATMENT: BILE ACID SEQUESTRANT

▶ ***colesevelam*** **(B)** <12 years: not recommended; ≥12 years: *Monotherapy:* 3 tabs bid or 6 tabs once daily or one 1.875 gm pkt bid or one 3.75 gm pkt once daily
  WelChol *Tab:* 625 mg; *Pwdr for oral susp:* 1.875 gm pwdr pkts (60/carton); 3.75 gm pwdr pkts (30/carton) (citrus) (phenylalanine)

Comment: ***colesevelam*** **(WelChol)** is indicated as an adjunctive therapy to improve glycemic control in older adolescents ≥18 years with T2DM. It can be added to ***metformin***, sulfonylureas, or ***insulin*** alone or in combination with other antidiabetic agents.

TYPHOID FEVER (*SALMONELLA TYPHI*)

PRE-EXPOSURE PROPHYLAXIS

▶ ***typhoid*** **vaccine, oral, live, attenuated strain**
  Vivotif Berna <6 years: not recommended; ≥6 years: 1 cap every other day, 1 hour before a meal, with a lukewarm (not > body temperature) or cold drink for a total of 4 doses; do not crush or chew; complete therapy at least 1 week prior to expected exposure; re-immunization recommended every 5 years if repeated exposure
    Cap: ent-coat

▶ ***typhoid vi polysaccharide*** **vaccine (C)** <2 years: not recommended; ≥2 years:
  Typhim Vi 0.5 ml IM in deltoid; re-immunization recommended every 2 years if repeated exposure
    Vial: 20, 50 dose; *Prefilled syringe:* 0.5 ml

Comment: Febrile illness may require delaying administration of the vaccine; have *epinephrine* 1:1000 readily available.

TREATMENT

▶ ***azithromycin*** **(B)(G)** 8-10 mg/kg/day; max 500 mg/day; *Mild Illness:* treat x 7 days; *Severe Illness:* treat x 14 days; *see page 593 for dose by weight table*
  Zithromax *Tab:* 250, 500, 600 mg; *Oral susp:* 100 mg/5 ml (15 ml); 200 mg/5 ml (15, 22.5, 30 ml) (cherry); *Pkt:* 1 gm for reconstitution (cherry-banana)
  Zithromax Tri-pak *Tab:* 3 x 500 mg tabs/pck
  Zithromax Z-pak *Tab:* 6 x 250 mg tabs/pck
  Zmax *Oral susp:* 2 gm ext-rel for reconstitution (cherry-banana) (148 mg Na^+)

▶ ***cefixime*** **(B)(G)** <6 months: not recommended; 6 months-12 years, <50 kg: 8 mg/kg/day in 1-2 divided doses x 10 days; *see page 597 for dose by weight table;* >12 years, >50 kg: *Mild illness:* 15-20 mg/kg/day x 7-14 days; *Severe illness:* 20 mg/kg/day x 10-14 days
  Suprax *Tab:* 400 mg; *Cap:* 400 mg; *Oral susp:* 100, 200, 500 mg/5 ml (50, 75, 100 ml) (strawberry)

▶ ***ciprofloxacin*** **(C)** <18 years: not recommended; ≥18 years: 15 mg/kg/day; *Mild illness:* treat x 5-7 days; *Severe illness:* treat x 10-14 days; max 1.5 gm/day
  Cipro (G) *Tab:* 250, 500, 750 mg; *Oral susp:* 250, 500 mg/5 ml (100 ml) (strawberry)
  Cipro XR *Tab:* 500, 1000 mg ext-rel
  ProQuin XR *Tab:* 500 mg ext-rel

Comment: ***ciprofloxacin*** is contraindicated <18 years-of-age, and during pregnancy and lactation. Risk of tendonitis or tendon rupture.

- ***ofloxacin*** (C) <18 years: not recommended; ≥18 years: 15 mg/kg/day; *Mild Illness:* treat x 5-7 days; *Severe Illness:* treat x 10-14 days
    Floxin *Tab:* 200, 300, 400 mg
  Comment: ***ofloxacin*** is contraindicated <18 years-of-age, and during pregnancy and lactation. Risk of tendonitis or tendon rupture.
- ***cefotaxime*** 80 mg/kg/day IM/IV x 10-14 days; max 2 gm/day
    Claforan *Vial:* 500 mg; 1, 2 gm
- ***ceftriaxone*** (B)(G) 75 mg/kg/day IM/IV x 10-14 days; max 2 gm/day
    Rocephin *Vial:* 250, 500 mg; 1, 2 gm
- ***trimethoprim+sulfamethoxazole [TMP-SMX]*** (D)(G)
    Bactrim, Septra <12 years: not recommended; ≥12 years: 2 tabs bid x 10 days
      Tab: trim 80 mg+sulfa 400 mg*
    Bactrim DS, Septra DS <12 years: not recommended; ≥12 years: 1 tab bid x 10 days
      Tab: trim 160 mg+sulfa 800 mg*
    Bactrim Pediatric Suspension, Septra Pediatric Suspension <2 months: not recommended; ≥2 months-12 years: 40 mg/kg/day of ***sulfamethoxazole*** in 2 doses bid; >12 years: use tabs
      Oral susp: trim 40 mg+sulfa 200 mg per 5 ml (100 ml) (cherry) (alcohol 0.3%)

ULCER: DIABETIC, NEUROPATHIC, VENOUS INSUFFICIENCY (LOWER EXTREMITY)

NUTRITIONAL SUPPLEMENT

- ***L-methylfolate calcium (as metafolin)+pyridoxyl 5-phosphate+methylcobalamin*** <12 years: not recommended; ≥12 years: take 1 cap daily
    Metanx *Cap:* metafo 3 mg+pyrid 35 mg+methyl 2 mg (gluten-free, yeast-free, lactose-free)
    Comment: **Metanx** is indicated as adjunct treatment of endothelial dysfunction and/or hyperhomocysteinemia in patients who have lower extremity ulceration.

DEBRIDING+CAPILLARY STIMULANT AGENT

- ***trypsin+balsam peru/castor oil*** apply at least twice daily; may cover with a wet dressing
    Granulex *Aerosol liq:* tryp 0.12 mg+bal peru 87 mg+cast 788 mg per 0.82 ml

GROWTH FACTOR

- ***becaplermin*** (C) apply once daily with a cotton swab or tongue depressor; then, cover with saline moistened gauze dressing; rinse after 12 hours; then, re-cover with a clean saline dressing
    Regranex *Gel:* 0.01% (2, 7.5, 15 gm) (parabens)
  Comment: Store in refrigerator; do not freeze. Not for use with wounds that close by primary intention.

ULCER: PRESSURE, DECUBITUS

DEBRIDING+CAPILLARY STIMULANT AGENT

Granulex (***trypsin* 0.1 mg+*balsam peru* 72.5 mg+castor oil 650 mg per 0.82 ml**) apply at least twice daily; may cover with a wet dressing
  Aerosol liq: (2, 4 oz)

GROWTH FACTOR

▶ ***becaplermin*** **(C)** apply once daily with a cotton swab or tongue depressor; then cover with saline moistened gauze dressing; rinse after 12 hours; then recover with a clean saline dressing

Regranex *Gel:* 0.01% (2, 7.5, 15 gm) (parabens)

Comment: Store in refrigerator; do not freeze. Not for use in wounds that close by primary intention.

ULCERATIVE COLITIS (UC)

Comment: Standard treatment regimen is anti-infective, antispasmodic, and bowel rest; progressing to clear liquids; then to high fiber.

Parenteral Corticosteroids *see page* 547

Oral Corticosteroids *see page* 546

▶ ***budesonide micronized*** (C)(G) <12 years: not recommended; ≥12 years: 9 mg once daily in the AM for up to 8 weeks; may repeat an 8-week course; *Maintenance of remission:* 6 mg once daily for up to 3 months; taper other systemic steroids when transferring to ***budesonide***

Entocort EC *Cap:* 3 mg ent-coat granules

Uceris *Tab:* 9 mg ext-rel

RECTAL CORTICOSTEROIDS

▶ ***hydrocortisone*** **rectal** (C) <12 years: not recommended; ≥12 years:

Anusol-HC Suppositories 1 supp rectally 3 x/day or 2 supp rectally 2 x/day x 2 weeks; max 8 weeks

Rectal supp: 25 mg (12, 24/pck)

Cortenema 1 enema q HS x 21 days or until symptoms controlled

Enema: 100 mg/60 ml (1, 7/pck)

Cortifoam 1 applicator full qd-bid x 2-3 weeks and every 2nd day thereafter until symptoms are controlled

Aerosol: 80 mg/applicator (14 applications/container)

Proctocort 1 supp rectally in AM and PM x 2 weeks; for more severe cases, may increase to 1 supp rectally 3 times daily or 2 supp rectally twice daily; max 4-8 weeks

Rectal supp: 30 mg (12, 24/pck)

Comment: Use ***hydrocortisone*** foam as adjunctive therapy in the distal portion of the rectum when ***hydrocortisone*** enemas cannot be retained.

RECTAL CORTICOSTEROID+ANESTHETIC

Hydrocortisone+Pramoxine

Proctofoam HC apply to anal/rectal area 3-4 times daily; max 4-8 weeks

Rectal foam: hydrocort 1%+pram 1% (10 gm w. applicator)

SALICYLATES

▶ ***balsalazide disodium*** **(B)**

Comment: ***balsalazide*** 6.75 gm provides 2.4 gm of ***mesalazine*** to the colon.

Colazal <5 years: not recommended; ≥5 years: 1 x 750 mg cap 3 x/day (2.25 gm/day), with or without food for up to 8 weeks or 3 x 750 mg caps/day (6.75 gm/day), with or without food, x 8 weeks; swallow whole or may be opened and sprinkled on applesauce, then chewed or swallowed immediately

Cap: 750 mg

Comment: **Colazal** is a locally-acting aminosalicylate indicated for the treatment of mildly to moderately active ulcerative colitis in patients ≥5 years. Safety and effectiveness of **Colazal** >8 weeks in children (5-17 years) and >12 weeks in patients ≥18 years has not been established.

Giazo <18 years: not recommended; ≥18 years; males only: take 3 x 1.1 gm tabs bid (6.6 gm/day) for up to 8 weeks

Tab: 1.1 gm (sodium 126 mg/tab) film-coat

Comment: **Giazo** is a locally-acting aminosalicylate indicated for the treatment of mildly to moderately active ulcerative colitis only in male patients ≥18 years; Effectiveness of **Giazo** in female patients has not been demonstrated in clinical trials. Safety and effectiveness of **Giazo** > 8 weeks has not been established.

▻ ***mesalamine* (B)**

Apriso <18 years: not recommended; ≥18 years: *Maintenance: of Remission* 4 x 0.375 gm caps (1.5 gm/day) once daily in the morning, for maintenance of remission with or without food; do not co-administer with antacids

Cap: 0.375 gm ext-rel (phenylalanine 0.56 mg/cap)

Comment: **Apriso** is a locally-acting aminosalicylate indicated for the maintenance of remission of ulcerative colitis in adults.

Asacol HD (G) <18 years: not recommended; ≥18 years: *Induction of Remission:* 2 x 800 mg tab (1600 mg) tid x 6 weeks; *Maintenance of Remission:* 1.6 gm/day in divided doses; take on an empty stomach, at least 1 hour before or 2 hours after a meal; swallow whole; do not crush, break, or chew

Tab: 800 mg del-rel

Comment: **Asacol HD** is an aminosalicylate indicated for the treatment of moderately active ulcerative colitis in adults. Do not substitute one **Asacol HD 800** tablet for two **mesalamine** delayed-release 400 mg oral products

Canasa <18 years: not recommended; ≥18 years: 1 x 1,000 mg suppository administered rectally once daily at bedtime for 3 to 6 weeks.

Rectal supp: 1 gm del-rel (30, 42/pck)

Comment: **Canasa** is an aminosalicylate indicated in adults for the treatment of mildly to moderately active ulcerative proctitis. Safety and effectiveness of **Canasa** beyond 6 weeks have not been established.

Delzicol <5 years: not recommended; ≥5-17 years: twice daily dosing for 6 weeks; see mfr pkg insert for weight-based dosing table; ≥18 years: *Treatment:* 2 x 400 mg caps (800 mg/day) 3 x/day x 6 weeks; *Maintenance:* 4 x 400 mg caps (1.6 gm/day) in 2-4 divided doses once daily; swallow whole; take with or without food; do not crush or chew

Cap: 400 mg del-rel

Comment: 2 x 400 mg **Dezlicol** caps have not been shown to be interchangeable or substitutable with one ***mesalamine*** delayed-release 800 mg tablet. Evaluate renal function prior to initiation of **Dezlicol**.

Lialda (G) <18 years: not recommended; ≥18 years: *Induction of Remission:* 2-4 x 1.2 gm tabs (2.4-4.8 gm) once daily for up to 8 weeks; *Maintenance: of Remission:* 2 x 1.2 gm tabs (2.4 gm) once daily; swallow whole; do not crush or chew

Tab: 1.2 gm del-rel

Comment: **Lialda** is a locally-acting 5-aminosalicylic acid (5-ASA) indicated for the induction of remission in adults with active, mild to moderate ulcerative colitis and for the maintenance of remission of ulcerative colitis. Safety and effectiveness of **Lialda** in pediatric patients have not been established.

Pentasa <18 years: not recommended; ≥18 years: Induction of Remission: 1 gm qid for up to 8 weeks

Cap: 250, 500 mg ext-rel

Comment: **Pentasa** is an aminosalicylate indicated for the induction of remission and for the treatment of patients with mildly to moderately active ulcerative colitis.

Rowasa Rectal Suspension Enema <18 years: not recommended; ≥18 years: 4 gm (60 ml) rectally by enema q HS; retain for 8 hours x 3-6 weeks (sulfite-free)

Enema: 4 gm/60 ml (7, 14, 28/pck; kit, 7, 14, 28/pck w. wipes)

Comment: **Rowasa Rectal Suspension Enema** is indicated for the treatment of active mild to moderate distal ulcerative colitis, proctosigmoiditis, and proctitis.

Rowasa Suppository <18 years: not recommended; ≥18 years: 1 supp rectally bid x 3-6 weeks; retain for 1-3 hours or longer

Rectal supp: 500 mg (12, 24/pck)

- ***olsalazine*** **(C)** <18 years: not recommended; ≥18 years: *Maintenance of Remission:* 1 gm/day in 2 divided doses; take with food

  Dipentum *Cap:* 250 mg

  Comment: ***osalazine*** is the sodium salt of a salicylate, disodium 3,3'-azobis (6-hydroxybenzoate) a compound that is effectively bioconverted to 5-amino-salicylic acid (5-ASA), which has anti-inflammatory activity in ulcerative colitis. The conversion of ***olsalazine*** to ***mesalamine*** (5-ASA) in the colon is similar to that of ***sulfasalazine***, which is converted into ***sulfapyridine*** and ***mesalamine***. ***olsalazine*** is indicated for the maintenance of remission of ulcerative colitis in patients who are intolerant of ***sulfasalazine***.

- ***sulfasalazine*** **(B; D in 2nd, 3rd)(G)** <2 years: not recommended; 2-16 years: initially 40-60 mg/kg/day in 3 to 6 divided doses; max 30 mg/kg/day in 4 divided doses; max 2 gm/day in divided doses; >16 years: *Induction of Remission:* 3-4 gm/day in evenly divided doses with dosage intervals not exceeding eight hours; in some cases, it is advisable to initiate therapy with a smaller dosage, e.g., 1-2 gm/day, to reduce possible gastrointestinal intolerance. If daily doses exceeding 4 gm are required to achieve desired effects, the increased risk of toxicity should be kept in mind; *Maintenance of Remission:* 4 gm/day in divided doses

  Azulfidine *Tab:* 500*mg

  Azulfidine EN-Tabs *Tab:* 500 mg ent-coat

TUMOR NECROSIS FACTOR (TNF) BLOCKER

- ***adalimumab*** **(B)** <18 years: not recommended; ≥18 years: initially 180 mg SC (as 4 injections in 1 day or divided over 2 days) on week 0; then 80 mg at week 2; start 40 mg every other week maintenance at week 4; only continue if evidence of clinical remission by 8 weeks; administer in abdomen or thigh; rotate sites

  Humira *Prefilled syringe:* 20 mg/0.4 ml; 40 mg/0.8 ml single-dose (2/pck; 2, 6/ starter pck) (preservative-free)

- ***adalimumab-adbm*** **(B)** ***First dose*** <18 years: not recommended; >18 years: *(Day 1):* 160 mg SC (4 x 40 mg injections in one day or 2 x 40 mg injections per day for two consecutive days); *Second dose two weeks later (Day 15):* 80 mg SC; *Two weeks later (Day 29):* begin a maintenance dose of 40 mg SC every other week (only continue in patients who have shown evidence of clinical remission by eight weeks (Day 57) of therapy.

  Cyltezo *Prefilled syringe:* 40 mg/0.8 ml single-dose (preservative-free)

  Comment: **Cyltezo** is biosimilar to **Humira** (***adalimumab***).

- ***infliximab*** *(tumor necrosis factor-alpha blocker)* <6 years: not recommended; ≥6 years: administer 5 mg/kg at 0, 2 and 6 weeks, then every 8 weeks; administer dose via IV infusion over a period of not less than 2 hours; must be refrigerated at 2°C to 8°C (36°F to 46°F); do not use beyond the expiration date as this product contains no preservative

Remicade *Vial:* 100 mg for reconstitution to 10 ml administration volume, single-dose (preservative-free)

Comment: **Remicade** is indicated to reduce signs and symptoms, and induce and maintain clinical remission, in adults and children ≥6 years-of-age with moderately to severely active disease who have had an inadequate response to conventional therapy and reduce the number of draining enterocutaneous and rectovaginal fistulas, and maintain fistula closure, in adults with fistulizing disease. Common adverse effects associated with **Remicade** included abdominal pain, headache, pharyngitis, sinusitis, and upper respiratory infections. In addition, **Remicade** might increase the risk for serious infections, including tuberculosis, bacterial sepsis, and invasive fungal infections. Available data from published literature on the use of ***infliximab*** products during pregnancy have not reported a clear association with ***infliximab*** products and adverse pregnancy outcomes. ***infliximab*** products cross the placenta and infants exposed *in utero* should not be administered live vaccines for at least 6 months after birth. Otherwise, the infant may be at increased risk of infection, including disseminated infection which can become fatal. Available information is insufficient to inform the amount of ***infliximab*** products present in human milk or effects on the breastfed infant. To report suspected adverse reactions, contact Merck Sharp & Dohme Corp., a subsidiary of Merck & Co. at 1-877-888-4231 or FDA at 1-800-FDA-1088 or visit www.fda.gov/medwatch

▶ ***infliximab-abda*** *(tumor necrosis factor-alpha blocker)* **(B)**

Renflexis: see *infliximab* (Remicade) above for full prescribing information

Comment: **Renflexis** is a biosimilar to **Remicade** for the treatment of immune-disorders including Crohn's disease, ulcerative colitis, rheumatoid arthritis, ankylosing spondylitis, psoriatic arthritis and plaque psoriasis. **Renflexis** was approved under the FDA category for biosimilars and demonstrated no clinically meaningful differences for use, dosing regimens, strengths, dosage forms, and routes of administration from the FDA-approved biological product **Remicade.**

▶ ***infliximab-dyyb*** *(tumor necrosis factor-alpha blocker)* **(B)**

Inflectra: see ***infliximab*** **(Remicade)** above for full prescribing information

Comment: **Inflectra** is a biosimilar to **Remicade** for the treatment of immune-disorders including Crohn's disease, ulcerative colitis, rheumatoid arthritis, ankylosing spondylitis, psoriatic arthritis and plaque psoriasis. **Inflectra** was approved under the FDA category for biosimilars and demonstrated no clinically meaningful differences for use, dosing regimens, strengths, dosage forms, and routes of administration from the FDA-approved biological product **Remicade.**

▶ ***infliximab-qbtx*** *(tumor necrosis factor-alpha blocker)* **(B)**

Ifixi: see ***infliximab*** **(Remicade)** above for full prescribing information

Comment: **Ifixi** is a biosimilar to **Remicade** for the treatment of immune disorders including Crohn's disease, ulcerative colitis, rheumatoid arthritis, ankylosing spondylitis, psoriatic arthritis and plaque psoriasis. **Ifixi** was approved under the FDA category for biosimilars and demonstrated no clinically meaningful differences for use, dosing regimens, strengths, dosage forms, and routes of administration from the FDA-approved biological product **Remicade.**

INTEGRIN RECEPTOR ANTAGONIST (IMMUNOMODULATOR)

▶ ***vedolizumab*** **(B)** <18 years: not recommended; ≥18 years: administer by IV infusion over 30 minutes; 300 mg at weeks 0, 2, 6; then once every 8 weeks

Entyvio *Vial:* 300 mg (20 ml) single-dose, pwdr for IV infusion after reconstitution (preservative-free)

Comment: To report suspected adverse reactions, contact Takeda Pharmaceuticals at 1-877-TAKEDA-7 (1-877-825-3327) or FDA at 1-1800-FDA-1088 or visit www.fda.gov/medwatch

CD20 ANTIBODY

➢ ***rituximab*** (C) <6 years: not recommended; ≥6 years: administer corticosteroid 30 minutes prior to each infusion; concomitant ***methotrexate*** therapy, administer a 1,000 mg IV infusion at 0 and 2 weeks; then every 24 weeks or based on response, but not sooner than every 16 weeks.

Rituxan *Vial:* 10 mg/ml (10, 50 ml) (preservative-free)

Comment: ***rituximab*** is a B-cell targeting chimeric monoclonal antibody that acts against CD20 and reduces antibody titers. B-cell depletion by ***rituximab*** may also set the stage for production of interleukin 10–secreting B cells that do not interact with T cells, which further reduces production of antidesmoglein antibodies. ***rituximab*** carries a black box warning regarding fatal infusion reactions, severe mucocutaneous reactions, hepatitis B virus reactivation, and progressive multifocal leukoencephalopathy. However, serious adverse events are rare. There was no evidence of increased mortality with longer exposure to **rituximab** or to multiple courses of therapy.

JANUS KINASE (JAK) INHIBITOR (JAKI)

➢ ***tofacitinib*** (C) <18 years: not established; ≥18 years: 10 mg bid for at least 8 weeks; then 5 or 10 mg bid; discontinue after 16 weeks of 10 mg bid, if adequate therapeutic benefit is not achieved; use the lowest effective dose to maintain response; see mfr pkg insert for dosage adjustments for patients receiving CYP2C19 and/or CYP3A4 inhibitors; in patients with moderate or severe renal impairment or moderate hepatic impairment, and patients with lymphopenia, neutropenia, or anemia; use of **Xeljanz/ Xeljanz XR** in patients with severe hepatic impairment is not recommended in any patient population;

Xeljanz *Tab:* 5, 10 mg
Xeljanz XR *Tab:* 11 mg ext-rel

Comment: **Xeljanz** is the first oral JAKI approved for chronic treatment of moderately-to-severely active UC. Other FDA-approved treatments for the treatment of moderately-to-severely active UC must be administered through an IV infusion or SC injection. Use with caution in patients that may be at increased risk for gastrointestinal perforation. The most common adverse events associated with Xeljanz treatment for UC are diarrhea, elevated cholesterol level, headache, herpes zoster (shingles), increased blood creatine phosphokinase, nasopharyngitis, rash, and upper respiratory tract infection (URI). Avoid use of **Xeljanz/Xeljanz XR** during an active serious infection, including localized infection. Patients treated with **Xeljanz** are at increased risk for developing serious infections that may lead to hospitalization or death. **Xeljanz** has a BBW for serious infections (e.g., opportunistic infections), and malignancy (e.g., lymphoma). Use of **Xeljanz** in combination with biological therapies for ulcerative colitis or with potent immunosuppressants, such as ***azathioprine*** and ***cyclosporine***, is not recommended. Avoid live vaccines administration during treatment with **Xeljanz.** Prior to starting **Xeljanz**, perform a test for latent tuberculosis; if it is positive, start treatment for tuberculosis prior to starting **Xeljanz**. Monitor all patients for active tuberculosis during treatment, even if the initial latent tuberculosis test is negative. Recommend lab monitoring due to potential for changes in lymphocytes, neutronphils, hemoglobin, liver enzymes, and lipids. Do not initiate **Xeljanz** if absolute lymphocyte count <500 cells/mm^3, an absolute neutrophil count (ANC) <1000 cells/mm3 or Hgb <9 g/dL. The safety and effectiveness of **Xeljanz/Xeljanz XR** in pediatric patients have not been established. Available data with **Xeljanz** use in pregnancy are insufficient to establish a drug associated risk of major birth defects, miscarriage, or adverse maternal or fetal outcomes. In animal reproduction studies, fetocidal, and teratogenic effects were noted. There is a pregnancy exposure registry that monitors pregnancy outcomes in women exposed to **Xeljanz/Xeljanz XR** during pregnancy. Consider pregnancy planning and prevention for females of reproductive potential. Patients should be encouraged to enroll in the **Xeljanz/Xeljanz XR** pregnancy registry if they become pregnant. To enroll or obtain information from the registry, patients can call the toll free number 1-877-311-8972. There are no data on the presence of ***tofacitinib*** in human milk or the effects on a breastfed infant; however, patients should be advised not to breastfeed. To report suspected adverse reactions, contact Pfizer at 1-800-438-1985 or FDA at 1-800-FDA-1088 or visit www.fda.gov/medwatch

ANTIDIARRHEAL AGENTS

- ***difenoxin+atropine*** (C) 2 tabs; then 1 tab after each loose stool or 1 tab q 3-4 hours; max 8 tabs/day x 2 days
  - **Motofen** *Tab:* dif 1 mg+atro 0.025 mg
- ***diphenoxylate+atropine*** (C)(G) 2 tabs or 10 ml qid
  - **Lomotil** *Tab:* diphen 2.5 mg+atro 0.025 mg; *Liq:* diphen 2.5 mg+atro 0.025 mg/5 ml (2 oz w. dropper)
- ***loperamide*** (B)(G)
  - **Imodium (OTC)** 4 mg initially; then 2 mg after each loose stool; max 16 mg/day
    - *Cap:* 2 mg
  - **Imodium A-D (OTC)** 4 mg initially; then 2 mg after each loose stool; usual max 8 mg/day x 2 days
    - *Cplt:* 2 mg; *Liq:* 1 mg/5 ml (2, 4 oz)
- ***loperamide+simethicone*** (B)(G)
  - **Imodium Advanced (OTC)** 2 tabs chewed after first loose stool; then 1 after the next loose stool; max 4 tabs/day
    - *Chew tab:* loper 2 mg+simeth 125 mg

URETHRITIS: NON-GONOCOCCAL (NGU)

Comment: The following treatment regimens for NGU are published in the **2015 CDC Sexually Transmitted Diseases Treatment Guidelines.** Treatment regimens are for patients ≥18 years-of-age; consult a specialist for treatment of patients <18 years-of-age. Treatment regimens are presented by generic drug name first, followed by information about brands and dose forms. All persons who have confirmed or suspected urethritis should be tested for gonorrhea and chlamydia. Males treated for NGU should be instructed to abstain from sexual intercourse for 7 days after a single-dose regimen or until completion of a 7-day regimen.

RECOMMENDED REGIMEN: UNCOMPLICATED NGU

- ***azithromycin*** 1 gm in a single dose or 100 mg orally bid x 7 days
  - plus
- ***doxycycline*** 100 mg bid x 7 days

PERSISTENT-RECURRENT NGU

Males Initially Treated With Azithromycin+Doxycycline

- ***azithromycin*** 1 gm PO in a single dose

Males Who Fail a Regimen of Azithromycin

- ***moxifloxacin*** 400 mg PO once daily x 7 days

Heterosexual Males Who Live in Areas Where T. Vaginalis is Highly Prevalent

- *metronidazole* 2 gm PO in a single dose
  or
- *tinidazole* 2 gm PO in a single dose

ALTERNATIVE REGIMENS

- *erythromycin base* 500 mg PO qid x 7 days
  or
- *erythromycin ethylsuccinate* 800 mg PO qid x 7 days
  or
- *levofloxacin* 500 mg once daily x 7 days
  or
- *ofloxacin* 300 mg PO bid x 7 days

DRUG BRANDS AND DOSE FORMS

- *azithromycin* (B)(G)
  Zithromax *Tab:* 250, 500, 600 mg; *Oral susp:* 100 mg/5 ml (15 ml); 200 mg/5 ml (15, 22.5, 30 ml) (cherry); *Pkt:* 1 gm for reconstitution (cherry-banana)
  Zithromax Tri-pak *Tab:* 3 x 500 mg tabs/pck
  Zithromax Z-pak *Tab:* 6 x 250 mg tabs/pck
  Zmax *Oral susp:* 2 gm ext-rel for reconstitution (cherry-banana) (148 mg Na^+)
- *doxycycline* (D)(G)
  Acticlate *Tab:* 75, 150**mg
  Adoxa *Tab:* 50, 75, 100, 150 mg ent-coat
  Doryx *Tab:* 50, 75, 100, 150, 200 mg del-rel
  Doxteric *Tab:* 50 mg del-rel
  Monodox *Cap:* 50, 75, 100 mg
  Oracea *Cap:* 40 mg del-rel
  Vibramycin *Tab:* 100 mg; *Cap:* 50, 100 mg; *Syr:* 50 mg/5 ml (raspberry-apple) (sulfites); *Oral susp:* 25 mg/5 ml (raspberry)
  Vibra-Tab *Tab:* 100 mg film-coat

  Comment: ***doxycycline*** is contraindicated <8 years-of-age, in pregnancy, and lactation (discolors developing tooth enamel). A side effect may be photosensitivity (photophobia). Do not take with antacids, calcium supplements, milk or other dairy, or within 2 hours of taking another drug.
- *erythromycin base* (B)
  Ery-Tab *Tab:* 250, 333, 500 mg ent-coat
  PCE *Tab:* 333, 500 mg
- *erythromycin ethylsuccinate* (B)(G)
  EryPed *Oral susp:* 200 mg/5 ml (100, 200 ml) (fruit); 400 mg/5 ml (60, 100, 200 ml) (banana); *Oral drops:* 200, 400 mg/5 ml (50 ml) (fruit); *Chew tab:* 200 mg wafer (fruit)
  E.E.S. *Oral susp:* 200, 400 mg/5 ml (100 ml) (fruit)
  E.E.S. Granules *Oral susp:* 200 mg/5 ml (100, 200 ml) (cherry)
  E.E.S. 400 Tablets *Tab:* 400 mg
- *levofloxacin* (C)
  Levaquin *Tab:* 250, 500, 750 mg; *Oral soln:* 25 mg/ml (480 ml) (benzyl alcohol); *Inj conc:* 25 mg/ml for IV infusion after dilution (20, 30 ml single-use vial) (preservative-free); *Premix soln:* 5 mg/ml for IV infusion (50, 100, 150 ml) (preservative-free)

  Comment: ***levofloxacin*** is contraindicated <18 years-of-age, and during pregnancy and lactation. Risk of tendonitis or tendon rupture.

▶ ***metronidazole* (not for use in 1st; B in 2nd, 3rd)(G)**
  Flagyl *Tab*: 250*, 500*mg
  Flagyl 375 *Cap*: 375 mg
  Flagyl ER *Tab*: 750 mg ext-rel

Comment: Alcohol is contraindicated during treatment with oral ***metronidazole*** and for 72 hours after therapy due to a possible ***disulfiram***-like reaction (nausea, vomiting, flushing, headache).

▶ ***moxifloxacin*** (C)(G)
  Avelox *Tab*: 400 mg

Comment: ***moxifloxacin*** is contraindicated <18 years-of-age, and during pregnancy and lactation. Risk of tendonitis or tendon rupture.

▶ ***ofloxacin*** (C)(G)
  Floxin *Tab*: 200, 300, 400 mg

Comment: ***ofloxacin*** is contraindicated <18 years-of-age, and during pregnancy and lactation. Risk of tendonitis or tendon rupture.

▶ ***tinidazole* (not for use in 1st; B in 2nd, 3rd)**
  Tindamax *Tab*: 250*, 500*mg

URINARY RETENTION: UNOBSTRUCTIVE

▶ ***bethanechol*** (C) 10-30 mg tid
  Urecholine *Tab*: 5, 10, 25, 50 mg

Comment: Contraindicated in presence of urinary obstruction. ***Atropine*** 0.4 mg administered SC reverses the effects of ***bethanechol***.

URINARY TRACT INFECTION (UTI, ACUTE CYCTITIS)
URINARY TRACT INFECTION, COMPLICATED (cUTI)

URINARY TRACT ANALGESIA

Comment: Except when contraindicated, ***ibuprofen*** or other inflammatory agent of choice is a recommended adjunct or monotherapy in the treatment of UTI dysuria, frequency, and urgency which is due to inflammation and associated smooth muscle spasms/colic.

OTC AZO Standard
OTC AZO Standard Maximum Strength
OTC Prodium
OTC Uristat

▶ ***phenazopyridine*** (B)(G) <12 years: not recommended; ≥12 years: 100-200 mg q 6 hours prn; max 2 days
  Pyridium *Tab*: 100, 200 mg
  Urogesic *Tab*: 100, 200 mg

ANTISPASMODIC AGENT

▶ ***flavoxate*** (B)(G) <12 years: not recommended; >12 years: 100-200 mg tid-qid
  Urispas *Tab*: 100 mg

Comment: ***flavoxate*** hydrochloride tablets are indicated for symptomatic relief of dysuria, urgency, nocturia, suprapubic pain, frequency and incontinence as may occur in cystitis, prostatitis, urethritis, urethrocystitis/urethrotrigonitis. ***flavoxate*** is not indicated for definitive treatment, but is compatible with drugs used for the treatment of UTI. ***flavoxate*** is contraindicated in patients who have any of the following obstructive conditions: pyloric or duodenal obstruction, obstructive intestinal lesions, ileus, achalasia, GI hemorrhage, and obstructive uropathies of the lower urinary tract. Used with caution with glaucoma. It is not known whether ***flavoxate*** is excreted in human milk.

URINARY TRACT ANALGESIC-ANTISPASMODIC AGENTS

▶ *hyoscyamine* (C)(G)

Anaspaz <2 years: not recommended; ≥2-12 years: 0.0625-0.125 mg q 4 hours prn; max 0.75 mg/day; >12 years: 1-2 tabs q 4 hours prn; max 12 tabs/day

Tab: 0.125*mg

Levbid <12 years: not recommended; ≥12 years: 1-2 tabs q 12 hours prn; max 4 tabs/day

Tab: 0.375*mg ext-rel

Levsin <6 years: not recommended; 6-12 years: 1 tab q 4 hours prn; ≥12 years: 1-2 tabs q 4 hours prn; max 12 tabs/day

Tab: 0.125*mg

Levsin Drops 3.4 kg: 4 drops q 4 hours prn; max 24 drops/day; 5 kg: 5 drops q 4 hours prn; max 30 drops/day; 7 kg: 6 drops q 4 hours prn; max 36 drops/day; 10 kg: 8 drops q 4 hours prn; max 40 drops/day

Oral drops: 0.125 mg/ml (15 ml) (orange) (alcohol 5%)

Levsin Elixir <10 kg: use drops; 10-19 kg: 1.25 ml q 4 hours prn; 20-39 kg: 2.5 ml q 4 hours prn; 40-49 kg: 3.75 ml q 4 hours prn; >50 kg: 5 ml q 4 hours prn

Elix: 0.125 mg/5 ml (16 oz) (orange) (alcohol 20%)

Levsinex SL <2 years: not recommended; 2-12 years: 1 tab q 4 hours; max 6 tabs/day; >12 years: 1-2 tabs q 4 hours SL or PO; max 12 tabs/day

Tab: 0.125 mg sublingual

Levsinex Timecaps <2 years: not recommended; 2-12 years: 1 cap q 12 hours; max 2 caps/day; >12 years: 1-2 caps q 12 hours; may adjust to 1 cap q 8 hours

Cap: 0.375 mg time-rel

NuLev <2 years: not recommended; 2-12 years: dissolve 1 tab on tongue, with or without water, q 4 hours prn; max 6 tabs/day; >12 years: dissolve 1-2 tabs on tongue, with or without water, q 4 hours prn; max 12 tabs/day

ODT: 0.125 mg (mint) (phenylalanine)

▶ ***methenamine+phenyl salicylate+methylene blue+benzoic acid+atropine sulfate+hyoscyamine*** (C)(G) <6 years: not recommended; ≥6 years: 2 tabs qid prn

Urised *Tab:* meth 40.8 mg+phenyl salic 18.1 mg+meth blue 5.4 mg+benz acid 4.5 mg+atro sulf 0.03 mg+hyoscy 0.03 mg

Comment: **Urised** imparts a blue-green color to urine which may stain fabrics.

▶ ***methenamine+phenyl salicylate+methylene blue+sod phosphate monobasic+hyoscyamine*** (C) <6 years: not recommended; ≥6 years: 1 cap qid prn

Uribel *Cap:* meth 118 mg+phenyl salic 36 mg+meth blue 10 mg+sod phos mono 40.8 mg+hyoscy 0.12 mg

▶ ***methenamine+phenyl salicylate+methylene blue+sod biphosphate+hyoscyamine*** (C) <6 years: not recommended; ≥6 years: 1 tab qid prn

Urelle *Cap:* meth 81 mg+phenyl salic 32.4 mg+meth blue 10.8 mg+sod biphos 40.8 mg+hyoscy 0.12 mg

▶ ***phenazopyridine*** (B)(G) <12 years: not recommended; ≥12 years: 95-200 mg q 6 hours prn; max 2 days

AZO Standard, Prodium, Uristat (OTC) *Tab:* 95 mg

AZO Standard Maximum Strength (OTC) *Tab:* 97.5 mg

Pyridium, Urogesic *Tab:* 100, 200 mg

Comment: ***phenazopyridine*** imparts an orange-red color to urine which may stain fabrics.

ANTI-INFECTIVES

▶ ***acetyl sulfisoxazole*** (C)(G)

Gantrisin <12 years: not recommended; ≥12 years: initially 2-4 gm in a single or divided doses; then, 4-8 gm/day in 4-6 divided doses x 3-10 days

Tab: 500 mg

Gantrisin<2 months: not recommended; ≥2 months: initial dose 75 mg/kg/ day; then 150 mg/kg/day in 4-6 divided doses x 3-10 days; max 6 gm/day

Oral susp: 500 mg/5 ml (4, 16 oz); *Syr:* 500 mg/5 ml (16 oz)

▶ ***amoxicillin*** (B)(G) <40 kg (88 lb): 20-40 mg/kg/day in 3 divided doses x 3-10 days or 25-45 mg/kg/day in 2 divided doses x 3-10 days; *see page* 588 *for dose by weight table;* ≥40 kg: 500-875 mg bid or 250-500 mg tid x 3-10 days

Amoxil *Cap:* 250, 500 mg; *Tab:* 875*mg; *Chew tab:* 125, 200, 250, 400 mg (cherry-banana-peppermint) (phenylalanine); *Oral susp:* 125, 250 mg/5 ml (80, 100, 150 ml) (strawberry); 200, 400 mg/5 ml (50, 75, 100 ml) (bubble gum); *Oral drops:* 50 mg/ml (30 ml) (bubble gum)

Moxatag *Tab:* 775 mg ext-rel

Trimox *Tab:* 125, 250 mg; *Cap:* 250, 500 mg; *Oral susp:* 125, 250 mg/5 ml (80, 100, 150 ml) (raspberry-strawberry)

▶ ***amoxicillin+clavulanate*** (B)(G)

Augmentin <40 kg: 40-45 mg/kg/day divided tid x 3-10 days or 90 mg/kg/day divided bid x 3-10 days; *see page* 590 *for dose by weight table;* ≥40 kg: 500 mg tid or 875 mg bid x 3-10 days

Tab: 250, 500, 875 mg; *Chew tab:* 125, 250 mg (lemon-lime); 200, 400 mg (cherry-banana) (phenylalanine); *Oral susp:* 125 mg/5 ml (banana), 250 mg/5 ml (75, 100, 150 ml) (orange); 200, 400 mg/5 ml (50, 75, 100 ml) (orange) (phenylalanine)

Augmentin ES-600 <3 months: not recommended; ≥3 months, <40 kg: 90 mg/kg/day divided q 12 hours x 3-10 days; *see page* 591 *for dose by weight table;* ≥40 kg: not recommended

Oral susp: 600 mg/5 ml (50, 75, 100, 125, 150, 200 ml) (strawberry cream) (phenylalanine)

Augmentin XR <16 years: use other forms; ≥16 years: 2 tabs q 12 hours x 3-10 days

Tab: 1000*mg ext-rel

▶ ***ampicillin*** (B) <12 years: 50-100 mg/kg/day in 4 divided doses x 3-10 days; *see page* 592 *for dose by weight table;* ≥12 years: 500 mg qid x 3-10 days

Omnipen, Principen *Cap:* 250, 500 mg; *Oral susp:* 125, 250 mg/5 ml (100, 150, 200 ml) (fruit)

▶ ***carbenicillin*** (B) <12 years: not recommended; ≥12 years: 1-2 tabs qid x 3-10 days

Geocillin *Tab:* 382 mg

▶ ***cefaclor*** (B)(G) <1 month: not recommended; 1 month-12 years: 20-40 mg/kg divided bid x 10 days; *see page* 594 *for dose by weight table;* max 1 gm/day; ≥12 years: 250-500 mg q 8 hours x 3-10 days; max 2 gm/day

Tab: 500 mg; *Cap:* 250, 500 mg; *Susp:* 125 mg/5 ml (75, 150 ml) (straw-berry); 187 mg/5 ml (50, 100 ml) (strawberry); 250 mg/5 ml (75, 150 ml) (strawberry); 375 mg/5 ml (50, 100 ml) (strawberry)

Cefaclor Extended Release <16 years: not recommended; ≥16 years: 500 mg bid x 10 days (clinically equivalent to 250 mg immed-rel caps tid); swallow whole; take with meals

Tab: 375, 500 mg ext-rel

▶ ***cefadroxil*** (B) <12 years: 30 mg/kg/day in 2 divided doses x 3-10 days; *see page* 595 *for dose by weight table;* ≥12 years: 1-2 gm in a single or 2 divided doses x 3-10 days

Duricef *Cap:* 500 mg; *Tab:* 1 gm; *Oral susp:* 250 mg/5 ml (100 ml); 500 mg/ 5 ml (75, 100 ml) (orange-pineapple)

▶ ***cefixime*** **(B)(G)** <6 months: not recommended; 6 months-12 years, <50 kg: 8 mg/kg/day in 1-2 divided doses x 3-10 days; *see page* 597 *for dose by weight table;* >12 years, >50 kg: 400 mg once daily x 5 days

Suprax *Tab:* 400 mg; *Cap:* 400 mg; *Oral susp:* 100, 200, 500 mg/5 ml (50, 75, 100 ml) (strawberry)

▶ ***cefpodoxime proxetil*** **(B)** <2 months: not recommended; 2 months-12 years: 10 mg/kg/day (max 400 mg/dose) or 5 mg/kg/day bid (max 200 mg/dose) x 3-10 days: *see page* 598 *for dose by weight table;* ≥12 years: 100 mg bid x 3-10 days

Vantin *Tab:* 100, 200 mg; *Oral susp:* 50, 100 mg/5 ml (50, 75, 100 mg) (lemon creme)

▶ ***cephalexin*** **(B)(G)** <12 years: 25-50 mg/kg/day in 4 divided doses x 3-10 days; *see page* 601 *for dose by weight table;* ≥12 years: 500 mg bid x 3-10 days

Keflex *Cap:* 250, 333, 500, 750 mg; *Oral susp:* 125, 250 mg/5 ml (100, 200 ml) (strawberry)

▶ ***ciprofloxacin*** **(C)** <18 years: not recommended; ≥18 years: 500 mg bid or 1000 mg XR once daily x 3-7 days

Cipro (G) *Tab:* 250, 500, 750 mg; *Oral susp:* 250, 500 mg/5 ml (100 ml) (strawberry)

Cipro XR *Tab:* 500, 1000 mg ext-rel

ProQuin XR *Tab:* 500 mg ext-rel

Comment: ***ciprofloxacin*** is contraindicated <18 years-of-age, and during pregnancy and lactation. Risk of tendonitis or tendon rupture.

▶ ***doxycycline*** **(D)(G)** <8 years: not recommended; ≥8 years, <100 lb: 2 mg/lb on first day in 2 divided doses, followed by 1 mg/lb/day in a single or 2 divided doses x 3-10 days; ≥8 years, ≥100 lb: 100 mg bid x 3-10 days

Acticlate *Tab:* 75, 150**mg

Adoxa *Tab:* 50, 75, 100, 150 mg ent-coat

Doryx *Tab:* 50, 75, 100, 150, 200 mg del-rel

Doxteric *Tab:* 50 mg del-rel

Monodox *Cap:* 50, 75, 100 mg

Oracea *Cap:* 40 mg del-rel

Vibramycin *Tab:* 100 mg; *Cap:* 50, 100 mg; *Syr:* 50 mg/5 ml (raspberry-apple) (sulfites); *Oral susp:* 25 mg/5 ml (raspberry)

Vibra-Tab *Tab:* 100 mg film-coat

Comment: ***doxycycline*** is contraindicated <8 years-of-age, in pregnancy, and lactation (discolors developing tooth enamel). A side effect may be photosensitivity (photophobia). Do not take with antacids, calcium supplements, milk or other dairy, or within 2 hours of taking another drug.

▶ ***enoxacin*** **(C)** <18 years: not recommended; ≥18 years: 200 mg q 12 hours x 3-10 days

Penetrex *Tab:* 200, 400 mg

Comment: ***enoxacin*** is contraindicated <18 years-of-age, and during pregnancy and lactation. Risk of tendonitis or tendon rupture.

▶ ***fosfomycin tromethamine*** **(B) take as a single dose on an empty stomach;** <12 years: not established; ≥12 years: **dissolve** 1 sachet pkt in 3-4 oz cold water and drink immediately

Monurol *Single-dose sachet pkts:* 3 gm (mandarin orange) (saccharin, sucrose)

Comment: ***fosfomycin tromethamine*** is a single-dose synthetic, broad spectrum, bactericidal antibiotic for treatment of uncomplicated UTI. Repeat dosing does not improve clinical efficacy. Safety and effectiveness in children age 12 years and under have not been established in adequate and well-controlled studies.

▶ ***levofloxacin*** **(C)** <18 years: not recommended; ≥18 years: 250 mg once daily x 3-7 days

Levaquin *Tab:* 250, 500, 750 mg; *Oral soln:* 25 mg/ml (480 ml) (benzyl alcohol); *Inj conc:* 25 mg/ml for IV infusion after dilution (20, 30 ml single-use vial) (preservative-free); *Premix soln:* 5 mg/ml for IV infusion (50, 100, 150 ml) (preservative-free)

Comment: ***levofloxacin*** is contraindicated <18 years-of-age, and during pregnancy and lactation. Risk of tendonitis or tendon rupture.

▶ ***lomefloxacin*** **(C)** <18 years: not recommended; ≥18 years: 400 mg once daily 3-7 days

Maxaquin *Tab:* 400 mg

Comment: ***lomefloxacin*** is contraindicated <18 years-of-age, and during pregnancy and lactation. Risk of tendonitis or tendon rupture.

▶ ***minocycline*** **(D)(G)** <8 years: not recommended; ≥8 years, <100 lb: 2 mg/lb on first day in 2 divided doses, followed by 1 mg/lb q 12 hours 3-10 days; ≥8 years, ≥100 lb: 100 mg q 12 hours x 3-10 days

Dynacin *Cap:* 50, 100 mg

Minocin *Cap:* 50, 75, 100 mg; *Oral susp:* 50 mg/5 ml (60 ml) (custard) (sulfites, alcohol 5%)

Comment: ***minocycline*** is contraindicated <8 years-of-age, in pregnancy, and lactation (discolors developing tooth enamel). A side effect may be photossensitivity (photophobia). Do not give with antacids, calcium supplements, milk or other dairy, or within two hours of taking another drug.

▶ ***nalidixic acid*** **(B)** <3 months: not recommended; ≥3 months-<12 years: 25 mg/lb/day in 4 divided doses x 7-14 days; ≥12 years: 1 gm qid x 3-10 days

NegGram *Tab:* 250, 500 mg; 1 gm; *Cap:* 250, 500 mg; *Oral susp:* 250 mg/5 ml

▶ ***nitrofurantoin*** **(B)(G)**

Furadantin <1 month: not recommended; ≥1 month-12 years: 3-10 mg/kg/ day in 4 divided doses x 3-10 days; *see page 615 for dose by weight table;* >12 years: 50-100 mg qid x 3-10 days

Oral susp: 25 mg/5 ml (60 ml)

Macrobid <12 years: not recommended; ≥12 years: 100 mg q 12 hours x 3-10 days

Cap: 100 mg

Macrodantin <12 years: not recommended; ≥12 years: 50-100 mg qid x 3-10 days; long-term use 50-100 mg q HS

Cap: 25, 50, 100 mg

▶ ***norfloxacin*** **(C)** <18 years: not recommended; ≥18 years: 400 mg once daily x 3-7 days

Noroxin *Tab:* 400 mg

Comment: ***norfloxacin*** is contraindicated <18 years-of-age, and during pregnancy and lactation. Risk of tendonitis or tendon rupture.

▶ ***ofloxacin*** **(C)(G)** <18 years: not recommended; ≥18 years: 200 mg q 12 hours x 3-7 days

Floxin *Tab:* 200, 300, 400 mg

Floxin UroPak *Tab:* 200 mg (6/pck)

Comment: ***ofloxacin*** is contraindicated <18 years-of-age, and during pregnancy and lactation. Risk of tendonitis or tendon rupture.

▶ ***trimethoprim*** **(C)(G)**

Primsol <6 months: not recommended; ≥6 months-12 years: 10 mg/kg/day in 2 divided doses x 10 days; >12 years: 100 mg q 12 hours or 200 mg once daily x 10 days

Oral soln: 50 mg/5 ml (bubble gum) (dye-free, alcohol-free)

Proloprim <12 years: not recommended; ≥12 years: 100 mg q 12 hours or 200 mg once daily x 10 days

Tab: 100, 200 mg

Trimpex <12 years: not recommended; ≥12 years: 100 mg q 12 hours or 200 mg once daily x 10 days
Tab: 100 mg

▶ ***trimethoprim+sulfamethoxazole [TMP-SMX]*** (D)(G)
Bactrim, Septra <12 years: not recommended; ≥12 years: 2 tabs bid x 10 days
Tab: trim 80 mg+*sulfa* 400 mg*
Bactrim DS, Septra DS <12 years: not recommended; ≥12 years: 1 tab bid x 10 days
Tab: trim 160 mg+*sulfa* 800 mg*
Bactrim Pediatric Suspension, Septra Pediatric Suspension <2 months: not recommended; ≥2 months-12 years: 40 mg/kg/day of ***sulfamethoxazole*** in 2 doses bid; >12 years: use tabs
Oral susp: trim 40 mg+*sulfa* 200 mg per 5 ml (100 ml) (cherry) (alcohol 0.3%)

PARENTERAL THERAPY FOR COMPLICATED UTI (cUTI)

Penem Antibacterial

▶ ***ertapenem*** (B) <18 years: not recommended; ≥18 years: 1 gm once daily; *CrCl <30 mL/min:* 500 mg once daily; treat x 10-14 days; may switch to an oral antibiotic after 3 days if warranted; *IV infusion:* administer over 30 minutes; *IM injection:* reconstitute
Invanz *Vial:* 1 gm pwdr for reconstitution and IV infusion

Penem Antibacterial+Beta-Lactamase Inhibitor

▶ ***meropenem+vaborbactam*** <18 years: not recommended; ≥18 years: administer 4 gm (***meropenem*** 2 gm and ***vaborbactam*** 2 gm) every 8 hours by IV infusion; administer over 3 hours; treat for up to 14 days; monitor urine cultures and eGFR; *eGFR 30-49 mL/min:* 2 gm (***meropenem*** 1 gm and ***vaborbactam*** 1 gm) every 8 hours; *eGFR 15-29 mL/min:* 2 gm (***meropenem*** 1 gm and ***vaborbactam*** 1 gm) every 12 hours; *eGFR <15 mL/min:* 1 gm (***meropenem*** 0.5 gm and ***vaborbactam*** 0.5 gm) every 12 hours; *ESRD:* administer 1 gm (***meropenem*** 0.5 gm and ***vaborbactam*** 0.5 gm) every 12 hours *after* dialysis
Vabomere *Vial:* mero 1 gm+vabor 1 gm pwdr for reconstitution and dilution
Comment: **Vabomere** (formerly **Carbavance**) is a carbapenem *(**meropenpenem**)* and beta-lactamase inhibitor *(**vaborbactam**)* combination indicated for the treatment of complicated urinary tract infections (cTIs). Administer **Vabomere** with caution with history of hyper-sensitivity to penicillin, cephalosporin, other betalactams or other allergens. Discontinue immedately if allergic reaction occurs. Vabomere is not recommended with con-comitant ***valproic acid*** or ***divalproex sodium***. Discontinue **Vabomere** if *C. difficile*-associated diarrhea is suspected or confirmed. Monitor, and re-evaluate risk/ benefit if signs of neuromotor impairment (e.g., seizures, focal tremors, myoclonus, delirium, paresthesias), renal impairment, thrombocytopenia, and/or superinfection.

LONG-TERM PROPHYLACTIC-SUPPRESSION THERAPY

▶ ***methenamine hippurate*** (C) <6 years: 0.25 gm/30 lb once daily; 6-12 years: 25-50 mg/kg/day once daily or 0.5-1 gm once daily; >12 years: 1 gm once daily
Hiprex *Tab:* 1 gm; *Oral susp:* 500 mg/5 ml (480 ml)
Urex *Tab:* 1 gm; *Oral susp:* 500 mg/5 ml (480 ml)

▶ ***nitrofurantoin*** (B)(G)
Furadantin <12 years: not recommended; ≥12 years: 50-100 mg once daily
Oral susp: 25 mg/5 ml (60 ml)
Macrobid <12 years: not recommended; ≥12 years: 100 mg once daily
Cap: 100 mg

Macrodantin <12 years: not recommended; ≥12 years: 2-100 mg once daily
Cap: 25, 50, 100 mg

UROLITHIASIS (RENAL CALCULI, KIDNEY STONES)

Parenteral Opioid Analgesics *see* ***Pain*** *page* 335
Opioids and Other Oral Analgesics *see* ***Pain*** *page* 324

PREVENTION OF CALCIUM STONES

- ***chlorothiazide*** **(B)(G)** <6 months: up to 15 mg/lb/day in 2 divided doses; ≥6 months-12 years: 10 mg/lb/day in 2 divided doses; max 375 mg/day; >12 years: 50 mg bid
  Diuril *Tab:* 250*, 500*mg; *Oral susp:* 250 mg/5 ml (237 ml)
- ***hydrochlorothiazide*** **(B)(G)** <12 years: not recommended; ≥12 years: 50 mg bid
  Esidrix *Tab:* 25, 50 mg
  Microzide *Cap:* 12.5 mg

PREVENTION OF CYSTINE STONES

- ***penicillamine*** **(D)** <12 years: not recommended; ≥12 years: 1-4 gm/day
  Cuprimine *Cap:* 125, 250 mg
  Depen *Titratable tab:* 250 mg
- ***potassium citrate*** **(C)(G)** 30 mEq qid
  Urocit-K *Tab:* 5, 10, 15 mEq ext-rel

Comment: ***potassium citrate*** is contraindicated in hyperkalemia. Encourage patients to limit salt intake and maintain liberal hydration (urine volume should be at least 2 liters/day). Target urine pH is 6.0-7.0 and urine citrate at least 320 mg/day and close to the normal mean of 640 mg/day. Take with food.

PREVENTION OF URIC ACID STONES

- ***allopurinol*** **(C)(G)** <6 years: max 150 mg/day; 6-10 years: max 400 mg/day; >10 years: 200-300 mg in 1-3 doses; max 800 mg/day; max single dose 300 mg
  Zyloprim *Tab:* 100*, 300*mg
- ***potassium citrate*** **(C)(G)** <12 years: not recommended; ≥12 years: 30 mEq qid
  Urocit-K *Tab:* 5, 10, 15 mEq ext-rel

Comment: ***potassium citrate*** is contraindicated in hyperkalemia. Encourage patients to limit salt intake and maintain liberal hydration (urine volume should be at least 2 liters/day). Target urine pH is 6.0-7.0 and urine citrate at least 320 mg/day and close to the normal mean of 640 mg/day. Take with food.

ALPHA-1A BLOCKERS

Comment: Alpha-1A blockers facilitate stone passage.

- ***alfuzosin*** **(B)(G)** <18 years: not recommended; ≥18 years: 10 mg once daily taken immediately after the same meal each day
  UroXatral *Tab:* 10 mg ext-rel
- ***tamsulosin*** **(B)(G)** ≤18 years: with radiopaque lower ureteral stones of 10-12 mm or smaller have received the following doses: ***tamsulosin*** 0.2 mg PO at bedtime (≤4 years) and 0.4 mg PO at bedtime (>4 years); administer x 28 days or until definite stone passage (i.e., evidence of stone on urine straining); ≥18 years: initially 0.4 mg once daily; may increase to 0.8 mg once daily after 2-4 weeks if needed
  Flomax *Cap:* 0.4 mg

Comment: ***tamsulosin*** 0.4 mg may be taken with **Avodart** 0.5 mg once daily as combination therapy. ***tamsulosin*** is taken with standard analgesia (e.g., ibuprofen); mild somnolence is common. If pain is controlled with oral analgesia, clear liquids are tolerated, and there is no evidence of infection, monitor closely for spontaneous passage for 3 to 4 weeks prior to definitive therapy, since most data demonstrate safe lower ureteral stone expulsion in the first 10 days of conservative medical management. **Flomax** 0.4 mg should not be used with strong inhibitors of CYP3A4 (e.g., ***ketoconazole***). **Flomax** should be used with caution in combination with moderate inhibitors of CYP3A4 (e.g., ***erythromycin***), in combination with strong (e.g., ***paroxetine***) or moderate (e.g., ***terbinafine***) inhibitors of CYP2D6, or in patients known to be CYP2D6 poor metabolizers, particularly at a dose higher than 0.4 mg (i.e., 0.8 mg. Concomitant use of PDE5 inhibitors with ***tamsulosin*** can potentially cause symptomatic hypotension.

ANTISPASMODIC AGENT

▶ ***flavoxate*** **(B)(G)** <12 years: not recommended; >12 years: 100-200 mg tid-qid

Urispas Tab: 100 mg

Comment: ***flavoxate*** hydrochloride tablets are indicated for symptomatic relief of dysuria, urgency, nocturia, suprapubic pain, frequency and incotinence as may occur in cystitis, prostatitis, urethritis, urethrocystitis/urethrotrigonitis. ***flavoxate*** is not indicated for definitive treatment, but is compatible with drugs used for the treatment of UTI. ***flavoxate*** is contraindicated in patients who have any of the following obstructive condtions: pyloric or duodenal obstruction, obstructive intestinal lesions, ileus, achalasia, GI hemorrhage, and obstructive uropathies of the lower urinary tract. Used with caution with glaucoma. It is not known whether ***flavoxate*** is excreted in human milk.

ACETAMINOPHEN FOR IV INFUSION

▶ ***acetaminophen*** injectable **(B)** <2 years: not recommended; 2-<13 years, <50 kg: 15 mg/kg q 6 hours prn or 2.5 mg/kg q 4 hours prn; max single dose 750 mg; max 75 mg/kg per day; ≥13 years: administer by IV infusion over 15 minutes; 1,000 mg q 6 hours prn or 650 mg q 4 hours prn; max 4,000 mg/day

Ofirmev *Vial:* 10 mg/ml (100 ml) (preservative-free)

Comment: The **Ofirmev** vial is intended for single use. If any portion is withdrawn from the vial, use within 6 hours. Discard the unused portion. For pediatric patients, withdraw the intended dose and administer via syringe pump. Do not admix **Ofirmev** with any other drugs. **Ofirmev** is physically incompatible with ***diazepam*** and ***chlorpromazine hydrochloride***.

IBUPROFEN FOR IV INFUSION

▶ ***ibuprofen*** **(B)** <6 months; not recommended; 6 months-<12 years: 10 mg/kg q 4-6 hours prn; max 400 mg/dose; max 40 mg/kg or 2,400 mg/24 hours, whichever is less; 12-17 years: 400 mg q 4-6 hours prn; max 2,400 mg/24 hours; dilute dose in 0.9% NS, D5W, or Lactated Ringers (LR) solution; administer by IV infusion over at least 10 minutes; do not administer via IV bolus or IM; 400-800 mg q 6 hours prn; maximum 3,200 mg/day

Caldolor *Vial:* 800 mg/8 ml single-dose

Comment: Prepare **Caldolor** solution for IV administration as follows: 100 mg dose: dilute 1 ml of **Caldolor** in at least 100 ml of diluent (IVF); 200 mg dose: dilute 2 ml of **Caldolor** in at least 100 ml of diluent; 400 mg dose: dilute 4 ml of **Caldolor** in at least 100 ml of diluent; 800 mg dose: dilute 8 ml of **Caldolor** in at least 200 ml of diluent. **Caldolor** is also indicated for management of fever. For adults with fever, 400 mg via IV infusion, followed by 400 mg q 4-6 hours <u>or</u> 100-200 mg q 4 hours prn.

MU OPIOID ANALGESICS

▶ ***tramadol*** (C)(IV)(G)

Comment: ***tramadol*** is known to be excreted in breast milk. The FDA and the European Medicines Agency (EMA) are investigating the safety of using ***tramadol***-containing medications to treat pain in children 12-18 years because of the potential for serious side effects, including slowed <u>or</u> difficult breathing.

Rybix ODT <12 years: contraindicated; 12-<18: use extreme caution; not recommended for children and adolescents with obesity, asthma, obstructive sleep apnea, <u>or</u> other chronic breathing problem, <u>or</u> for post-tonsillectomy/adenoidectomy pain; ≥18 years: initially 100 mg once daily; may increase by 100 mg every 5 days; max 300 mg/day; *CrCl <30 mL/min* <u>or</u> *severe hepatic impairment:* not recommended; *Cirrhosis:* max 50 mg q 12 hours

ODT: 50 mg (mint) (phenylalanine)

Ryzolt <12 years: contraindicated; 12-<18: use extreme caution; not recommended for children and adolescents with obesity, asthma, obstructive sleep apnea, <u>or</u> other chronic breathing problem, <u>or</u> for post-tonsillectomy/adenoidectomy pain; ≥18 years: initially 100 mg once daily; may increase by 100 mg every 5 days; max 300 mg/day; *CrCl <30 mL/min* <u>*or*</u> *severe hepatic impairment:* not recommended

Tab: 100, 200, 300 mg ext-rel

Ultram <12 years: contraindicated; 12-<18: use extreme caution; not recommended for children and adolescents with obesity, asthma, obstructive sleep apnea, <u>or</u> other chronic breathing problem, <u>or</u> for post-tonsillectomy/adenoidectomy pain; ≥18 years: 50-100 mg q 4-6 hours prn; max 400 mg/day; *CrCl <30 mL/min:* max 100 mg q 12 hours; *Cirrhosis:* max 50 mg q 12 hours

Tab: 50*mg

Ultram ER <12 years: contraindicated; 12-<18: use extreme caution; not recommended for children and adolescents with obesity, asthma, obstructive sleep apnea, <u>or</u> other chronic breathing problem, <u>or</u> for post-tonsillectomy/adenoidectomy pain; ≥18 years: initially 100 mg once daily; may increase by 100 mg every 5 days; max 300 mg/day; *CrCl <30 mL/min:* <u>or</u> *severe hepatic impairment:* not recommended

Tab: 100, 200, 300 mg ext-rel

▶ ***tramadol+acetaminophen*** (C)(IV)(G) <12 years: contraindicated; 12-<18: use extreme caution; not recommended for children and adolescents with obesity, asthma, obstructive sleep apnea, <u>or</u> other chronic breathing problem, <u>or</u> for post-tonsillectomy/adenoidectomy pain; ≥18 years: 2 tabs q 4-6 hours; max 8 tabs/day; 5 days; *CrCl <30 mL/min:* max 2 tabs q 12 hours; max 4 tabs/day x 5 days

Ultracet *Tab: tram* 37.5+*acet* 325 mg

Other Oral Analgesics *see* ***Pain*** *page* 324

INTRANASAL (TRANSMUCOSAL) OPIOID ANALGESICS

▶ ***butorphanol tartrate*** nasal spray (C)(IV) <18 years: not recommended; ≥18 years: initially 1 spray (1 mg) in one nostril and may repeat after 60-90 minutes in opposite nostril if needed <u>or</u> 1 spray in each nostril and may repeat q 3-4 hours prn

Butorphanol Nasal Spray *Nasal spray:* 1 mg/actuation (10 mg/ml, 2.5 ml)

Stadol Nasal Spray *Nasal spray:* 1 mg/actuation (10 mg/ml, 2.5 ml)

▶ ***fentanyl*** nasal spray (C)(II) <18 years: not recommended; ≥18 years: initially 1 spray (100 mcg) in one nostril and may repeat after 2 hours; when adequate analgesia is achieved, use that dose for subsequent breakthrough episodes; *Titration steps:* 100 mcg using 1 x 100 mcg spray; 200 mcg using 2 x 100 mcg spray (1 spray in each nostril); 400 mcg using 1 x 400 mcg spray; 800 mcg using 2 x 400 mcg (1 spray in each nostril); max 800 mcg; limit to ≤4 doses per day

Lazanda Nasal Spray *Nasal spray:* 100, 400 mcg/100 mcl (8 sprays/bottle)

Comment: **Lazanda Nasal Spray** is available by restricted distribution program. Call 855-841-4234 or visit https:/www.fda.gov/downloads/drugs/drugsafety/postmarketdrugsafetyinformationforpatientsandproviders/ucm261983.pdf to enroll. **Lazanda Nasal Spray** is indicated for the management of breakthrough pain in cancer patients who are already receiving and who are tolerant to opioid therapy for their underlying persistent cancer pain. Patients considered opioid tolerant are those who are taking at least 60 mg of oral morphine/day, 25 mcg of transdermal ***fentanyl***/hour, 30 mg oral ***oxycodone***/day, 8 mg oral ***hydromorphone***/day, 25 mg oral ***oxymorphone***/day, or an equianalgesic dose of another opioid for a week or longer. Patients must remain on around-the-clock opioids when using **Lazanda Nasal Spray**. As such, it is contraindicated in the management of acute or post-op pain, including headache/migraine, or dental pain.

Comment: The Transmucosal Immediate Release **Fentanyl** (TIRF) Risk Evaluation and Mitigation Strategy (REMS) program is an FDA-required program designed to ensure informed risk-benefit decisions before initiating treatment, and while patients are treated to ensure appropriate use of TIRF medicines. The purpose of the TIRF REMS Access program is to mitigate the risk of misuse, abuse, addiction, overdose and serious complications due to medication errors with the use of TIRF medicines. You must enroll in the TIRF REMS Access program to prescribe, dispense, or distribute TIRF medicines. To register, call the TIRF REMS Access program at 1-866-822-1483 or register online at https:/www.tirfremsaccess.com/TirfUI/rems/home.action

URTICARIA: MILD-TO-ACUTE HIVES & CHRONIC SPONTANEOUS/IDIOPATHIC URTICARIA (CSU/CIU)

Topical Corticosteroids *see page* 542
Oral Corticosteroids *see page* 546
Parenteral Corticosteroids *see page* 547

MILD-TO-MODERATE URTICARIA (HIVES, ANGIOEDEMA)

Second Generation Oral Antihistamines

Comment: The following drugs are second generation antihistamines. As such they minimally sedating, much less so than the first generation antihistamines. All antihistamines are excreted into breast milk.

▶ ***cetirizine*** (C)(OTC)(G) <6 years: not recommended; ≥6-<65 years: initially 5-10 mg once daily; ≥65 years: 5 mg once daily

Children's Zyrtec Chewable *Chew tab:* 5, 10 mg (grape)
Children's Zyrtec Allergy Syrup *Syr:* 1 mg/ml (4 oz) (grape, bubble gum) (sugar-free, dye-free)
Zyrtec *Tab:* 10 mg
Zyrtec Hives Relief *Tab:* 10 mg
Zyrtec Liquid Gels *Liq gel:* 10 mg

▶ ***desloratadine*** (C)

Clarinex <6 years: not recommended; ≥6 years: 1/2-1 tab once daily
Tab: 5 mg

Clarinex RediTabs <6 years: not recommended; 6-12 years: 2.5 mg once daily; ≥12 years: 5 mg once daily
ODT: 2.5, 5 mg (tutti-frutti) (phenylalanine)
Clarinex Syrup <6 months: not recommended; 6-11 months: 1 mg (2 ml) once daily; 1-5 years: 1.25 mg (2.5 ml) once daily; 6-11 years: 2.5 mg (5 ml) once daily; ≥12 years: 5 mg (10 ml) once daily
Tab: 0.5 mg per ml (4 oz) (tutti-frutti) (phenylalanine)
Desloratadine ODT

- ▶ ***fexofenadine*** **(C)(OTC)(G)** 6 months-2 years: 15 mg bid; *CrCl ≤90 mL/min:* 15 mg once daily; 2-11 years: 30 mg bid; *CrCl ≤90 mL/min:* 30 mg once daily ≥12 years and older: ≥ 12 years: 60 mg once daily-bid or 180 mg once daily; *CrCl <90 mL/min:* 60 mg once daily **Allegra** *Tab:* 30, 60, 180 mg film-coat
  Allegra Allergy *Tab:* 60, 180 mg film-coat
  Allegra ODT *ODT:* 30 mg (phenylalanine)
  Allegra Oral Suspension *Oral susp:* 30 mg/5 ml (6 mg/ml) (4 oz)
- ▶ ***levocetirizine*** **(B)(OTC)** administer dose in the PM; *Seasonal Allergic Rhinitis:* <2 years: not recommended; may start at ≥2 years; *Chronic Spontaneous/Idiopathic Urticaria (CSU/CIU), Perennial Allergic Rhinitis:* <6 months: not recommended; may start at ≥ 6 months; *Dosing by Age:* 6 months-5 years: max 1.25 mg once daily; 6-11 years: max 2.5 mg once daily; ≥12 years: 2.5-5 mg once daily; *Renal Dysfunction <12 years:* contraindicated; *Renal Dysfunction ≥12 years: CrCl 50-80 mL/min:* 2.5 mg once daily; *CrCl 30-50 mL/min:* 2.5 mg every other day; *CrCl: 10-30 mL/min:* 2.5 mg twice weekly (every 3-4 days); *CrCl <10 mL/min, ESRD or hemodialysis:* contraindicated;
  Children's Xyzal Allergy 24HR *Oral soln:* 0.5 mg/ml (150 ml)
  Xyzal Allergy 24HR *Tab:* 5*mg
- ▶ ***loratadine*** **(C)(OTC)(G)** <2 years: not recommended; 2-5 years: 5 mg once daily; ≥6 years: 5 mg bid or 10 mg once daily; *Hepatic or Renal Insufficiency:* (see mfr pkg insert)
  Children's Claritin Chewables *Chew tab:* 5 mg (grape) (phenylalanine)
  Children's Claritin Syrup 1 mg/ml (4 oz) (fruit) (sugar-free, alcohol-free, dye-free, sodium 6 mg/5 ml)
  Claritin *Tab:* 10 mg
  Claritin Hives Relief *Tab:* 10 mg
  Claritin Liqui-Gels *Liq gel:* 10 mg
  Claritin RediTabs 12 Hours *ODT:* 5 mg (mint)
  Claritin RediTabs 24 Hours *ODT:* 10 mg (mint)

FIRST GENERATION ORAL ANTIHISTAMINES

- ▶ ***diphenhydramine*** **(B)(G)** <2 years: not recommended; 2-6 years: 6.25 mg q 4-6 hours; max 37.5 mg/day; >6-12 years: 12.5-25 mg q 4-6 hours; max 150 mg/day; >12 years: 25-50 mg q 6-8 hours; max 100 mg/day
  Benadryl (OTC) *Chew tab:* 12.5 mg (grape) (phenylalanine); *Liq:* 12.5 mg/5 ml (4, 8 oz); *Cap:* 25 mg; *Tab:* 25 mg; *Dye-free soft gel:* 25 mg; *Dye-free liq:* 12.5 mg/5 ml (4, 8 oz)
- ▶ ***hydroxyzine*** **(C)(G)** <6 years: 50 mg/day divided qid prn; ≥6 years: 50-100 mg/day divided qid prn; max 600 mg/day; 25 mg tid prn; max 600 mg/day
  AtaraxR *Tab:* 10, 25, 50, 100 mg; *Syr:* 10 mg/5 ml (alcohol 0.5%)
  VistarilR *Cap:* 25, 50, 100 mg; *Oral susp:* 25 mg/5 ml (4 oz) (lemon)

SEVERE URTICARIA

Parenteral Antihistamine

- ▶ ***diphenhydramine*** **injectable (B)(G)** <12 years: *See mfr pkg insert:* 1.25 mg/kg up to 25 mg IM x 1 dose; then q 6 hours prn; ≥12 years: 25-50 mg IM immediately; then q 6 hours prn

Benadryl Injectable *Vial:* 50 mg/ml (1 ml single-use); 50 mg/ml (10 ml multi-dose); *Amp:* 10 mg/ml (1 ml); *Prefilled syringe:* 50 mg/ml (1 ml)

Parenteral Epinephrine

▶ ***epinephrine*** **(C)** 1:1000 0.01 ml/kg SC; max 0.3 ml

CHRONIC SPONTANEOUS/IDIOPATHIC URTICARIA

IgE Blocker (IgG1K Monoclonal Antibody)

Comment: **Xolair *(omalizumab)*** is a humanized monoclonal antibody that specifically binds to free immunoglobulin E in the blood and on the surface of selected B lymphocytes, but not on the surface of mast cells, antigen-presenting dendritic cells, or basophils. In the US ***omalizumab*** is approved for adults at 150 mg or 300 mg subcutaneously administered every 4 weeks for the treatment of CSU not responsive to high-dose antihistamines. In three published, pivotal, phase 3 randomized trials, the clinical response rate to ***omalizumab*** at 300 mg every 4 weeks, as defined by a weekly 7-day Urticaria Activity Score (UAS7) ≤6 at 12 weeks, was 52% in ASTERIA I, 66% in ASTERIA II, and 52% in GLACIAL. Good control of disease activity was defined as a UAS7 score of ≤6 on the 0- to 42-point UAS7, which correlates well with minimal or no patient symptoms

REFERENCE

Finlay, AY, Kaplan, AP, Beck, LA, *et al.* (2017). Omalizumab substantially improves dermatology-related quality of life in patients with chronic spontaneous urticaria. *Journal of the European Academy of Dermatology and Venereology, 31*(10), 1715–1721.

Comment: A multicenter open-label study of 286 adult patients with CSU, conducted by the Catalan and Balearic Chronic Urticaria Network (XUrCB) at 15 hospitals, found about two-thirds of patients with CSU treated with the approved dose of ***omalizumab*** achieved good disease control. Three-quarters of the non-responders achieved good disease control upon up-dosing to 450 or 600 mg (twice the approved dose) every 4 weeks, without increase in adverse events.

REFERENCE

https:/www.mdedge.com/familypracticenews/article/155732/urticaria/updosing-omalizumab-chronic-urticaria-pays

▶ ***omalizumab*** **(B)** <12 years: not recommended; ≥12 years: 30-90 kg + IgE >30-100 IU/ml 150 mg q 4 weeks; 90-150 kg + IgE >30-100 IU/ml or 30-90 kg + IgE >100-200 IU/ml or 30-60 kg + IgE >200-300 IU/ml 300 mg q 4 hours; >90-150 kg + IgE >100-200 IU/ml or >60-90 kg + IgE >200-300 IU/ml or 30-70 kg + IgE >300-400 IU/ml 225 mg q 2 weeks; >90-150 kg + IgE >200-300 IU/ml or >70-90 kg + IgE >300-400 IU/ml or 30-70 kg + IgE >400-500 IU/ml or 30-60 kg + IgE >500-600 IU/ml or 30-60 kg + IgE >600-700 IU/ml 375 mg q 2 weeks

Xolair *Vial:* 150 mg pwdr for SC injection after reconstitution (preservative-free)

VAGINAL IRRITATION: EXTERNAL

▶ **OTC Replens Vaginal Moisturizer**

▶ **OTC Vagisil Intimate Moisturizer**

Comment: **Vagisil** has no effect on condom integrity.

VERTIGO

- ***meclizine*** **(B)(G)** <12 years: not recommended; ≥12 years: 25-100 mg/day in divided doses
  - **Antivert** *Tab:* 12.5, 25, 50*mg
  - **Bonine (OTC)** *Cap:* 15, 25, 30 mg; *Tab:* 12.5, 25, 50 mg; *Chew tab/Film-coat tab:* 25 mg
  - **Dramamine II (OTC)** *Tab:* 25*mg
  - **Zentrip** *Strip:* 25 mg orally-disint
- ***methscopolamine bromide*** **(B)** <12 years: not recommended; ≥12 years: 1 tab q 6 hours prn
  - **Pamine** *Tab:* 2.5 mg
  - **Pamine Forte** *Tab:* 5 mg
- ***scopolamine*** **(C)** <12 years: not recommended; ≥12 years: 0.4-0.8 mg tab (may repeat in 8 hours) or 1 x 1.5 mg transdermal patch behind ear (effective x 3 days; may replace every 4th day)
  - **Scopace** *Tab:* 0.4 mg
  - **Transderm Scop** *Transdermal patch:* 1.5 mg (4/carton)

VITILIGO

RE-PIGMENTATION AGENTS

- ***methoxsalen*** **(C)** <12 years: not recommended; ≥12 years: apply to well-defined area of vitiligo; then expose area to source of UVA (ultraviolet A) or sunlight; initial exposure no more than 1/2 predicted minimal erythemal dose; repeat weekly
  - **Oxsoralen** *Lotn:* 1% (30 ml)

  Comment: ***methoxsalen*** may only be applied by a healthcare provider. Do not dispense to patient.
- ***trioxsalen*** **(C)** <12 years: not recommended; ≥12 years: 10 mg daily, taken 2-4 hours before ultraviolet light exposure; max 14 days and 28 tabs
  - **Trisoralen** *Tab:* 5 mg
  - **Depigmenting Agents** *see* ***Hyperpigmentation*** *page* 220

DEPIGMENTING AGENTS

- ***hydroquinone*** **(C)(G)** apply sparingly to affected area and rub in bid
  - **Lustra** *Crm:* 4% (1, 2 oz) (sulfites)
  - **Lustra AF** *Crm:* 4% (1, 2 oz) (sunscreen, sulfites)
- ***monobenzone*** **(C)** apply sparingly to affected area and rub in bid-tid; depigmentation occurs in 1-4 months
  - **Benoquin** *Crm:* 20% (1.25 oz)
- ***tazarotene*** **(X)(G)** <12 years: not recommended; ≥12 years: apply daily at HS
  - **Avage Cream** *Crm:* 0.1% (30 gm)
  - **Tazorac Cream** *Crm:* 0.05, 0.1% (15, 30, 60 gm)
  - **Tazorac Gel** *Gel:* 0.05, 0.1% (30, 100 gm)
- ***tretinoin*** **(C)(G)** <12 years: not recommended; ≥12 years: apply daily at HS
  - **Atralin Gel** *Gel:* 0.05% (45 gm)
  - **Avita** *Crm:* 0.025% (20, 45 gm); *Gel:* 0.025% (20, 45 gm)
  - **Renova** *Crm:* 0.02% (40 gm); 0.05% (40, 60 gm)
  - **Renova** *Crm:* 0.02% (40 gm); 0.05% (40, 60 gm)
  - **Retin-A Cream** *Crm:* 0.025, 0.05, 0.1% (20, 45 gm)
  - **Retin-A Gel** *Gel:* 0.01, 0.025% (15, 45 gm) (alcohol 90%)

Retin-A Liquid *Soln:* 0.05% (alcohol 55%)
Retin-A Micro Gel *Gel:* 0.04, 0.08, 0.1% (20, 45 gm)
Tretin-X Cream *Crm:* 0.075% (35 gm) (parabens-free, alcohol-free, propylene glycol-free)
Retin-A Micro *Microspheres:* 0.04, 0.1% (20, 45 gm)

COMBINATION AGENTS

- ***hydroquinone+fluocinolone+tretinoin*** (C) <12 years: not recommended; ≥12 years: apply sparingly to affected area and rub in daily at HS
  Tri-Luma *Crm: hydro* 4%+*fluo* 0.01%+*tretin* 0.05% (30 gm) (parabens, sulfites)
- ***hydroquinone+padimate o+oxybenzone+octyl methoxycinnamate*** (C) <12 years: not recommended; ≥12 years: apply sparingly to affected area and rub in bid
  Glyquin *Crm:* 4% (1 oz jar)
- ***hydroquinone+ethyl dihydroxypropyl PABA+dioxybenzone+oxybenzone*** (C) <12 years: not recommended; ≥12 years: apply sparingly to affected area and rub in bid; max 2 months
  Solaquin *Crm: hydro* 2%+*PABA* 5%+*dioxy* 3%+*oxy* 2% (1 oz) (sulfites)
- ***hydroquinone+padimate+dioxybenzone+oxybenzone*** (C) <12 years: not recommended; ≥12 years: apply sparingly to affected area and rub in bid; max 2 months
  Solaquin Forte *Crm: hydro* 4%+*pad* 0.5%+*dioxy* 3%+*oxy* 2% (1 oz) (sunscreen, sulfites)
- ***hydroquinone+padimate+dioxybenzone*** (C) <12 years: not recommended; ≥12 years: apply sparingly to affected area and rub in bid; max 2 months
  Solaquin Forte Gel: *hydro* 4%+*pad* 0.5%+*dioxy* 3% (1 oz) (alcohol, sulfites)

WART: COMMON (*VERRUCA VULGARIS*)

- ***salicylic acid*** (G)
  Duo Film (OTC) apply daily-bid; max 12 weeks; *Liq:* 17% (1/2 oz w. applicator)
  Duo Film Patch for Kids (OTC) apply 1 patch q 48 hours; max 12 weeks
    Patch: 40% (18/pck)
  Occlusal HP (OTC) apply daily-bid; max 12 weeks
    Liq: 17% (10 ml w. applicator)
  Wart-Off (OTC) apply one drop at a time to sufficiently cover wart, let dry; repeat 1-2 times daily; max 12 weeks
    Liq: 17% (0.45 oz)
- ***trichloroacetic acid*** apply after wart is pared and repeat weekly
- Cryotherapy with liquid nitrogen or cryoprobe or cryospray; repeat applications every 1-2 weeks as needed to destroy lesion
  Histofreeze (see pkg insert for application freeze times

ORAL RETINOID

- ***acitretin*** (X)(G) <18 years: not recommended; ≥18 years: 25-50 mg once daily with main meal
  Soriatane *Cap:* 10, 25 mg

REFERENCE

Can Oral Retinoids Have An Impact For Recalcitrant Warts? https:/www.podiatrytoday.com/blogged/can-oral-retinoids-have-impact-recalcitrant-warts

WART: PLANTAR (*VERRUCA PLANTARIS*)

- *salicylic acid* (G)
  Duo Plant Gel (OTC) apply daily bid; max 12 weeks
  Gel: 17% (1/2 oz)
  Mediplast cut to size of wart and apply; remove q 1-2 days, peel keratin, and reapply; repeat as often as needed
  Occlusal-HP (OTC) apply qd-bid; max 12 weeks
  Liq: 17% (10 ml w. applicator)
  Wart-Off (OTC) apply one drop at a time to sufficiently cover wart, let dry; repeat 1-2 times daily; max 12 weeks
  Liq: 17% (0.45 oz)
- ***trichloroacetic acid*** apply after wart is pared/cored and repeat weekly
- Cryotherapy with liquid nitrogen or cryoprobe or cryospray; repeat applications every 1-2 weeks as needed to destroy lesion
  Histofreeze (see pkg insert for application freeze time)

REFERENCE

Joshipura, D, Goldminz, A, Greb, J, *et al*. Acitretin for the treatment of recalcitrant plantar warts. *Dermatol Online J*. 2017:23(3).

WART: VENEREAL, HUMAN PAPILLOMAVIRUS (HPV, *CONDYLOMA ACUMINATA*)

Comment: This section contains treatment regimens for genital warts published in the **2015 CDC Sexually Transmitted Diseases Treatment Guidelines** as well as other treatment options. Due to the increased risk of cervical cancer with HPV, Pap smears should be done q 3 months during active disease and then q 3-6 months for the next 2 years.

PATIENT-APPLIED AGENTS

Regimen 1

- *imiquimod* (C) <12 years: not recommended; ≥12 years:
  Aldara (G) rub into lesions before bedtime and remove with soap and water 6-10 hours later; treat 3 times per week; max 16 weeks
  Crm: 5% (12 single-use pkts/carton)
  Zyclara rub into lesions before bedtime and remove with soap and water 8 hours later; treat 3 times per week; max 1 packet per treatment; max 8 weeks
  Crm: 3.75% (28 single-use pkts/carton) (parabens)

Regimen 2

- ***podofilox 0.5% cream*** (C) apply bid (q 12 hours) x 3 days; then discontinue for 4 days; may repeat if needed; max 4 treatment cycles
  Condylox *Soln:* 0.5% (3.5 ml); *Gel:* 0.5% (3.5 gm)

Regimen 3

- ***sinecatechins 15% ointment*** (C) apply to each lesion tid for up to 16 weeks
  Veregen *Oint:* 15% (15, 30 gm)

PROVIDER-ADMINISTERED AGENTS

Regimen 1

Cryotherapy with liquid nitrogen or cryoprobe; repeat applications every 1-2 weeks as needed

Regimen 2

➢ ***trichloroacetic acid 80-90%*** (C) apply to warts; repeat weekly if needed
Comment: TCA is the preferred treatment during pregnancy. Immediate application of sodium bicarbonate paste following treatment decreases pain.

Regimen 3

➢ ***podofilox 0.5% cream*** (C) apply bid (q 12 hours) x 3 days; then discontinue for 4 days; may repeat if needed; max 4 treatment cycles
Condylox *Soln:* 0.5% (3.5 ml); *Gel:* 0.5% (3.5 gm)

Regimen 4

➢ ***interferon alfa-n3*** (C) 0.05 ml injected into base of wart twice weekly for up to 8 weeks; max 0.5 ml/session (20 warts/session)
Alferon N *Vial:* 5 million units/ml (1 ml)

Regimen 5

➢ ***interferon alfa-2b*** (C) 0.1 ml injected into base of wart three times weekly for up to 3 weeks; max 0.5 ml/session (5 warts/session)
Intron A *Vial:* 1 million units/0.1 ml (0.5, 1 ml)

Regimen 6

Surgical removal either by tangential scissor excision, tangential shave excision, curettage, or electrosurgery

WEST NILE VIRUS

Comment: The principal route of human infection with West Nile virus is through the bite of an infected mosquito. Additional routes of infection have become apparent during the 2002 West Nile epidemic. It is important to note that these other methods of transmission represent a very small proportion of cases. Other methods of transmission include blood transfusion, organ transplantation, mother-to-child (ingestion of breast milk and transplacental) and occupational. Symptoms of mild disease will generally last a few days. Symptoms of severe disease may last several weeks, although neurological effects may be permanent. There is no specific treatment for West Nile virus infection; treatment is symptomatic and supportive. About 8 in 10 infected with West Nile virus do not develop any symptoms. About 1 in 5 develop a fever with other symptoms such as headache, body aches, joint pains, vomiting, diarrhea, or rash. Most people with this level of disease recover completely, but fatigue and weakness can last for weeks to months. About 1 in 150 people who are infected develop a severe illness affecting the central nervous system (encephalitis meningitis). Symptoms of severe illness include high fever, headache, neck stiffness, stupor, disorientation, coma, tremors, convulsions, muscle weakness, vision loss, numbness and paralysis. About 1 in 10 who develop severe illness affecting the central nervous system die. There is currently no preventive vaccine available. However, the National Institutes of Health have announced that an experimental vaccine to protect against West Nile Virus has entered human trial. The developers say because the vaccine uses inactivated virus it should be suitable for a wide range of people. The trial tests safety of the vaccine, called **HydroVax-001**, and its ability to produce an immune response in human subjects. The randomized, placebo-controlled, double-blind clinical trial was conducted by researchers at Duke University School of Medicine, Durham, NC, and enrolled 50 healthy volunteers, men and women 18-50 years-of-age. Participants were randomly assigned to one of the three groups. One group of volunteers (n=20) received a low dose of the vaccine (1 mcg), another group (n=20) received a higher dose (4 mcg), and a third group (n=10) received a placebo. All participants received their doses via IM injection on day 1 and day 29 of the trial and are followed for 14 months. Results of the completed trial are pending.

REFERENCE

https:/www.cdc.gov/westnile/symptoms/index.html

WHIPWORM (TRICHURIASIS)

ANTHELMINTICS

Comment: Oral bioavailability of anthelmintics is enhanced when administered with a fatty meal (estimated fat content 40 gm).

- ▶ ***albendazole*** (C) take with a meal; may crush and mix with food; may repeat in 3 weeks if needed; <2 years: 200 mg bid x 7 days; 2-12 years: 400 mg once daily x 7 days; >12 years: 400 mg bid x 7 days
  - **Albenza** *Tab:* 200 mg

  Comment: ***albendazole*** is a broad-spectrum benzimidazole carbamate anthelmintic.
- ▶ ***ivermectin*** (C) take with water; chew <u>or</u> crush and mix with food; may repeat in 3 months if needed; <15 kg: not recommended; ≥15 kg: 200 mcg/kg as a single dose
  - **Stromectol** *Tab:* 3, 6*mg
- ▶ ***mebendazole*** (C)(G) take with a meal; chew <u>or</u> crush and mix with food; may repeat in 3 weeks if needed; <2 years: not recommended; ≥2 years: 100 mg bid x 3 days
  - **Emverm** *Chew tab:* 100 mg
  - **Vermox** *Chew tab:* 100 mg
- ▶ ***pyrantel pamoate*** (C) take with a meal; may open capsule and sprinkle <u>or</u> mix with food; treat x 3 days; may repeat in 2-3 weeks if needed; treat x 3 days; 11 mg/kg/dose; max 1 gm/dose; <25 lb: not recommended; 25-37 lb: 1/2 tsp/dose; 38-62 lb: 1 tsp/dose; 63-87 lb: 1 tsp/dose; 88-112 lb: 2 tsp/dose; 113-137 lb: 2 tsp/dose; 138-162 lb: 3 tsp/dose; 163-187 lb: 3 tsp/dose; >187 lb: 4 tsp/dose
  - **Antiminth** *Cap:* 180 mg; *Liq:* 50 mg/ml (30 ml); 144 mg/ml (30 ml); *Oral susp:* 50 mg/ml (60 ml)
  - **Pin-X** *Cap:* 180 mg; *Liq:* 50 mg/ml (30 ml); 144 mg/ml (30 ml); *Oral susp:* 50 mg/ml (30 ml)
- ▶ ***thiabendazole*** (C) take with a meal; may crush and mix with food; treat x 7 days; <30 lb: consult mfr pkg insert; ≥30 lb: 25 mg/kg/dose bid with meals; 30-50 lb: 250 mg bid with meals; >50 lb: 10 mg/lb/dose bid with meals; max 1.5 gm/dose; max 3 gm/day
  - **Mintezol** *Chew tab:* 500*mg (orange); *Oral susp:* 500 mg/5 ml (120 ml) (orange)

  Comment: ***thiabendazole*** is not for prophylaxis. May impair mental alertness. May not be available in the US.

WOUND: INFECTED, NON-SURGICAL, MINOR

TETANUS PROPHYLAXIS

Previously Immunized (Within Previous 5 Years)

▶ ***tetanus toxoid*** vaccine (C) 0.5 ml IM x 1 dose
Vial: 5 Lf units/0.5 ml (0.5, 5 ml); *Prefilled syringe:* 5 Lf units/0.5 ml (0.5 ml)

Not Previously Immunized

see Tetanus *page* 445

TOPICAL ANTI-INFECTIVES

▶ ***mupirocin*** (B)(G) <12 years: not recommended; ≥12 years: apply to lesions bid
Bactroban *Oint:* 2% (22 gm); *Crm:* 2% (15, 30 gm)
Centany *Oint:* 2% (15, 30 gm)

ORAL ANTI-INFECTIVES

▶ ***azithromycin*** (B)(G) <12 years: 10 mg/kg x 1 dose on day 1, then 5 mg/kg/day on days 2-5; *see page* 593 *for dose by weight table;* max 500 mg/day; ≥12 years: 500 mg x 1 dose on day 1, then 250 mg daily on days 2-5 or 500 mg daily x 3 days or **Zmax** 2 gm in a single dose
Zithromax *Tab:* 250, 500, 600 mg; *Oral susp:* 100 mg/5 ml (15 ml); 200 mg/5 ml (15, 22.5, 30 ml) (cherry); *Pkt:* 1 gm for reconstitution (cherry-banana)
Zithromax Tri-pak *Tab:* 3 x 500 mg tabs/pck
Zithromax Z-pak *Tab:* 6 x 250 mg tabs/pck
Zmax *Oral susp:* 2 gm ext-rel for reconstitution (cherry-banana) (148 mg Na^+)

▶ ***amoxicillin+clavulanate*** (B)(G)
Augmentin <40 kg: 40-45 mg/kg/day divided tid x 10 days or 90 mg/kg/day divided bid x 10 days; *see page* 590 *for dose by weight table;* ≥40 kg: 500 mg tid or 875 mg bid x 10 days
Tab: 250, 500, 875 mg; *Chew tab:* 125, 250 mg (lemon-lime); 200, 400 mg (cherry-banana) (phenylalanine); *Oral susp:* 125 mg/5 ml (banana), 250 mg/5 ml (75, 100, 150 ml) (orange); 200, 400 mg/5 ml (50, 75, 100 ml) (orange) (phenylalanine)
Augmentin ES-600 <3 months: not recommended; ≥3 months, <40 kg: 90 mg/kg/day divided q 12 hours x 10 days; *see page* 591 *for dose by weight table;* ≥40 kg: not recommended
Oral susp: 600 mg/5 ml (50, 75, 100, 125, 150, 200 ml) (strawberry cream) (phenylalanine)
Augmentin XR <16 years: use other forms; ≥16 years: 2 tabs q 12 hours x 7-10 days
Tab: 1000*mg ext-rel

▶ ***cefaclor*** (B)(G) <1 month: not recommended; 1 month-12 years: 20-40 mg/kg divided bid x 10 days; *see page* 594 *for dose by weight table;* max 1 gm/day; ≥12 years: 250-500 mg q 8 hours x 10 days; max 2 gm/day
Tab: 500 mg; *Cap:* 250, 500 mg; *Susp:* 125 mg/5 ml (75, 150 ml) (strawberry); 187 mg/5 ml (50, 100 ml) (strawberry); 250 mg/5 ml (75, 150 ml) (strawberry); 375 mg/5 ml (50, 100 ml) (strawberry)
Cefaclor Extended Release <16 years: not recommended; ≥16 years: 500 mg bid x 10 days (clinically equivalent to 250 mg immed-rel caps tid); swallow whole; take with meals
Tab: 375, 500 mg ext-rel

- ▶ ***cefadroxil*** <12 years: 30 mg/kg/day in 2 divided doses x 10 days; *see page* 595 *for dose by weight table;* ≥12 years: 1-2 gm in a single or 2 divided doses x 10 days
  Duricef *Cap:* 500 mg; *Tab:* 1 gm; *Oral susp:* 250 mg/5 ml (100 ml); 500 mg/5 ml (75, 100 ml) (orange-pineapple)
- ▶ ***cefdinir*** **(B)** <6 months: not recommended; 6 months-12 years: 14 mg/kg/day in 1-2 divided doses x 10 days; *see page* 596 *for dose by weight table;* ≥12 years: 300 mg bid x 10 days or 600 mg daily x 10 days
  Omnicef *Cap:* 300 mg; *Oral susp:* 125 mg/5 ml (60, 100 ml) (strawberry)
- ▶ ***cefpodoxime proxetil*** **(B)** <2 months: not recommended; 2 months-12 years: 10 mg/kg/day (max 400 mg/dose) or 5 mg/kg/day bid (max 200 mg/dose) x 7-14 days; *see page* 598 *for dose by weight table;* >12 years: 400 mg bid x 7-14 days
  Vantin *Tab:* 100, 200 mg; *Oral susp:* 50, 100 mg/5 ml (50, 75, 100 mg) (lemon creme)
- ▶ ***cefprozil*** **(B)** <2 years: not recommended; 2-12 years: 7.5 mg/kg-15 mg/kg q 12 hours x 10 days; *see page* 599 *for dose by weight table;* >12 years: 250-500 mg q 12 hours or 500 mg daily x 10 days
  Cefzil *Tab:* 250, 500 mg; *Oral susp:* 125, 250 mg/5 ml (50, 75, 100 ml) (bubble gum) (phenylalanine)
- ▶ ***cephalexin*** **(B)(G)** <12 years: 50 mg/kg/day in 4 divided doses x 10 days; *see page* 601 *for dose by weight table;* ≥12 years: 2 gm 1 hour before procedure
  Keflex *Cap:* 250, 333, 500, 750 mg; *Oral susp:* 125, 250 mg/5 ml (100, 200 ml) (strawberry)
- ▶ ***clarithromycin*** **(C)(G)** <6 months: not recommended; ≥6 months-12 years: 7.5 mg/kg bid x 7-10 days; *see page* 602 *for dose by weight table;* >12 years: 500 mg bid or 500 mg ext-rel daily x 7-10 days
  Biaxin *Tab:* 250, 500 mg
  Biaxin Oral Suspension *Oral susp:* 125, 250 mg/5 ml (50, 100 ml) (fruit punch)
  Biaxin XL *Tab:* 500 mg ext-rel

Comment: The FDA is advising caution before prescribing ***clarithromycin*** to patients with heart disease because of a potential increased risk of heart problems or death that can occur years later. This recommendation is based on a review of the results of a 10-year follow-up study of patients with coronary heart disease from a large clinical trial that first observed this safety issue. Consider risk benefit and the use of other antibiotics in such patients.

- ▶ ***dirithromycin*** (C)(G) <12 years: not recommended; ≥12 years: 500 mg daily x 7 days
  Dynabac *Tab:* 250 mg
- ▶ ***erythromycin base*** **(B)(G)** <45 kg: 30-50 mg in 2-4 divided doses x 7 days; ≥45 kg: 500 mg q 6 hours x 7 days
  Ery-Tab *Tab:* 250, 333, 500 mg ent-coat
  PCE *Tab:* 333, 500 mg
- ▶ ***erythromycin ethylsuccinate*** (B)(G) 30-50 mg/kg/day in 4 divided doses x 7 days; may double dose with severe infection; max 100 mg/kg/day or 400 mg qid; *see page* 607 *for dose by weight table*
  EryPed *Oral susp:* 200 mg/5 ml (100, 200 ml) (fruit); 400 mg/5 ml (60, 100, 200 ml) (banana); *Oral drops:* 200, 400 mg/5 ml (50 ml) (fruit); *Chew tab:* 200 mg wafer (fruit)
  E.E.S. *Oral susp:* 200, 400 mg/5 ml (100 ml) (fruit)
  E.E.S. Granules *Oral susp:* 200 mg/5 ml (100, 200 ml) (cherry)
  E.E.S. 400 Tablets *Tab:* 400 mg
- ▶ ***gemifloxacin*** (C)(G) <18 years: not recommended; ≥18 years: 320 mg once daily x 5-7 days
  Factive *Tab:* 320*mg

  Comment: ***gemifloxacin*** is contraindicated <18 years-of-age, and during pregnancy and lactation. Risk of tendonitis or tendon rupture.

- ▶ ***levofloxacin*** **(C)** <18 years: not recommended; ≥18 years: *Uncomplicated:* 500 mg daily x 7 days; *Complicated:* 750 mg daily x 7 days
  - **Levaquin** *Tab:* 250, 500, 750 mg

  Comment: ***levofloxacin*** is contraindicated <18 years-of-age, and during pregnancy and lactation. Risk of tendonitis or tendon rupture.
- ▶ ***loracarbef*** **(B)** <12 years: 15 mg/kg/day in 2 divided doses x 7 days; *see page 614 for dose by weight table*; ≥12 years: 200 mg bid x 7 days
  - **Lorabid** *Pulvule:* 200, 400 mg; *Oral susp:* 100 mg/5 ml (50, 100 ml); 200 mg/5 ml (50, 75, 100 ml) (strawberry bubble gum)
- ▶ ***ofloxacin*** **(C)(G)** <18 years: not recommended; ≥18 years: 400 mg bid x 10 days
  - **Floxin** *Tab:* 200, 300, 400 mg

  Comment: ***ofloxacin*** is contraindicated <18 years-of-age, and during pregnancy and lactation. Risk of tendonitis or tendon rupture.

XEROSIS

MOISTURIZING AGENTS

Aquaphor Healing Ointment (OTC) *Oint:* 1.75, 3.5, 14 oz (alcohol)
Eucerin Daily Sun Defense (OTC) *Lotn:* 6 oz (fragrance-free)
Comment: **Eucerin Daily Sun Defense** is a moisturizer with SPF-15 sunscreen.
Eucerin Facial Lotion (OTC) *Lotn:* 4 oz
Eucerin Light Lotion (OTC) *Lotn:* 8 oz
Eucerin Lotion (OTC) *Lotn:* 8, 16 oz
Eucerin Original Creme (OTC) *Crm:* 2, 4, 16 oz (alcohol)
Eucerin Plus Creme (OTC) *Crm:* 4 oz
Eucerin Plus Lotion (OTC) *Lotn:* 6, 12 oz
Eucerin Protective Lotion (OTC) *Lotn:* 4 oz (alcohol)
Comment: **Eucerin Protective** is a moisturizer with SPF-25 sunscreen.
Lac-Hydrin Cream (OTC) *Crm:* 280, 385 gm
Lac-Hydrin Lotion (OTC) *Lotn:* 225, 400 gm
Lubriderm Dry Skin Scented (OTC) *Lotn:* 6, 10, 16, 32 oz
Lubriderm Dry Skin Unscented (OTC) *Lotn:* 3.3, 6, 10, 16 oz (fragrance-free)
Lubriderm Sensitive Skin Lotion (OTC) *Lotn:* 3.3, 6, 10, 16 oz (lanolin-free)
Lubriderm Dry Skin (OTC) *Lotn:* 2.5, 6, 10, 16 oz (scented); 1, 2.5, 6, 10, 16 oz (fragrance-free)
Lubriderm Bath & Shower Oil (OTC) 1-2 capfuls in bath or rub onto wet skin as needed, then rinse
Oil: 8 oz
Moisturel apply as needed
Crm: 4, 16 oz; *Lotn:* 8, 12 oz; *Clnsr:* 8.75 oz

Topical Oil

- ▶ ***fluocinolone acetamide*** 0.01% topical oil **(C)** <6 years: not recommended; ≥6 years: apply sparingly bid for up to 4 weeks
  - **Derma-Smoothe/FS Topical Oil** apply sparingly tid
    - *Topical oil:* 0.01% (4 oz; peanut oil)

ZIKA VIRUS (CONGENITAL ZIKA SYNDROME, CZS)

Comment: The Zika virus is transmitted via the bite of an infected mosquito and is associated with severe teratogenicity: a unique and distinct pattern of birth defects, called Congenital Zika Syndrome (CZS), characterized by the following five features: (1) Severe microcephaly in which the skull has partially collapsed; (2) Decreased brain tissue with a specific pattern of brain damage, including subcortical calcifications; (3) Damage to the back of the eye, including macular scarring and focal pigmentary retinal mottling; (4) Congenital contractures, such as clubfoot and arthrogryposis; (5) Hypertonia restricting body movement. Congenital Zika virus infection has also been associated with other abnormalities, including but not limited to brain atrophy and asymmetry, abnormally formed or absent brain structures, hydrocephalus, and neuronal migration disorders. Other anomalies include excessive and redundant scalp skin. Reported neurologic findings include, hyperreflexia, irritability, tremors, seizures, brainstem dysfunction, and dysphagia. Reported eye abnormalities include, but are not limited to, focal pigmentary mottling and chorioretinal atrophy in the macula, optic nerve hypoplasia, cupping, and atrophy, other retinal lesions, iris colobomas, congenital glaucoma, microphthalmia, lens subluxation, cataracts, and intraocular calcifications. **A synthetic DNA-based preventive vaccine showed promising immune responses with no severe adverse reactions in humans,** an interim analysis of a phase I trial found. Following three doses of vaccine, 100% of patients produced binding antibodies, and 95% of patients produced binding antibodies following two doses of the vaccine, Examining immunogenicity, 41% of participants had detectable binding antibody responses 4 weeks after the first dose, the authors said, with a 74% antibody response at week 6 (2 weeks after the second dose). **The vaccine is not yet available to the public.** The FDA formally approved Roche's cobas Zika molecular test for use on whole donor blood and blood products and living organ donors; it's the first such approval granted.

REFERENCES

Paz-Bailey, GM, *et al.* Zika virus persistence in body fluids, final report in body fluids-Final report. ASTMH 2017. Paper presented at the 66th Annual Meeting of the American Society of Tropical Medicine and Hygiene, November 5-9, Baltimore, MD

Rosenberg, E, *et al.* Prevalence and incidence of Zika virus infection among household contacts of Zika patients, Puerto Rico, 2016-2017. ASTMH 2017

Tebas, P, Roberts, CC, Muthumani, K, *et al.* (2017). Safety and immunogenicity of an anti–zika virus dna vaccine—preliminary report. New *England Journal of Medicine.* doi:10.1056/nejmoa1708120

ZOLLINGER–ELLISON SYNDROME

PROTON PUMP INHIBITORS

Comment: If hepatic impairment, or if patient is Asian, consider reducing the PPI dose.

- ***dexlansoprazole*** (B)(G) <18 years: not recommended; ≥18 years: 30-60 mg daily for up to 4 weeks

  Dexilant *Cap:* 30, 60 mg ent-coat del-rel granules; may open and sprinkle on applesauce; do not crush or chew granules

  Dexilant SoluTab *Tab:* 30 mg del-rel orally-disint

- ***esomeprazole*** (B)(OTC)(G) <1 year: not recommended; 1-11 years, <20 kg: 10 mg once daily; >20 kg: 10-20 mg once daily; 12-17 years: 20-40 mg once daily; >17 years: 20-40 mg daily; max 8 weeks; take 1 hour before food; swallow whole or mix granules with food or juice and take immediately; do not crush or chew granules; max 8 weeks

  Nexium *Cap:* 20, 40 mg ent-coat del-rel pellets

  Nexium for Oral Suspension *Oral susp:* 10, 20, 40 mg ent-coat del-rel granules/pkt; mix in 2 tbsp water and drink immediately; 30 pkt/carton

▶ ***esomeprazole+aspirin*** **(D)** <18 years: not recommended; ≥18 years: take one dose daily; max 8 weeks; take 1 hour before food

Yosprala

Tab: **Yosprala 40/81** esom 40 mg+asp 81 mg del-rel

Yosprala 40/325 esom 40 mg+asp 325 mg del-rel

Comment: ***aspirin***-containing medications are contraindicated with history of allergic-type reaction to ***aspirin***, children and adolescents with *Varicella* or other viral illness, and 3rd trimester of pregnancy.

▶ ***lansoprazole*** (B)(OTC)(G) <1 year: not recommended; 1-11 years, <30 kg: 15 mg once daily; >11 years: 15-30 mg daily for up to 8 weeks; may repeat course; take before eating

Prevacid *Cap:* 15, 30 mg ent-coat del-rel granules; swallow whole or mix granules with food or juice and take immediately; do not crush or chew granules; follow with water

Prevacid for Oral Suspension *Oral susp:* 15, 30 mg ent-coat del-rel granules/pkt; mix in 2 tbsp water and drink immediately; 30 pkt/carton (strawberry)

Prevacid SoluTab *ODT:* 15, 30 mg (strawberry) (phenylalanine)

Prevacid 24HR *Oral granules*: 15 mg ent-coat del-rel granules; swallow whole or mix granules with food or juice and take immediately; do not crush or chew granules; follow with water

▶ ***omeprazole*** (C)(OTC)(G) <1 year: not recommended; 5-<10 kg: 5 mg daily; 10-<20 kg: 10 mg daily; ≥20 kg: 20-40 mg daily; take before eating; swallow whole or mix granules with applesauce and take immediately; do not crush or chew; follow with water

Prilosec *Cap:* 10, 20, 40 mg ent-coat del-rel granules

Prilosec *Tab:* 20 mg del-rel (regular, wild berry)

▶ ***pantoprazole*** (B) <12 years: not recommended; ≥12 years: initially 40 mg bid

Protonix (G) *Tab:* 40 mg ent-coat del-rel

Protonix for Oral Suspension *Oral susp:* 40 mg ent-coat del-rel granules/pkt; mix in 1 tsp apple juice for 5 seconds or sprinkle on 1 tsp applesauce, and swallow immediately; do not mix in water or any other liquid or food; take approximately 30 minutes prior to a meal; 30 pkt/carton any other liquid or food; take approximately 30 minutes prior to a meal; 30 pkt/carton

▶ ***rabeprazole*** (B)(OTC)(G) <12 years: not recommended; ≥12-18 years: 20 mg once daily; max 8 week; >18 years: initially 20 mg daily; then titrate; may take 10 mg daily in divided doses or 60 mg bid

AcipHex *Tab:* 20 mg ent-coat del-rel

AcipHex Sprinkle *Cap:* 5, 10 mg del-rel

SECTION II

APPENDICES

APPENDIX A. BLOOD PRESSURE GUIDELINES (JNC-8)

APPENDIX A.1. BLOOD PRESSURE CLASSIFICATIONS (≥18 YEARS)¶

Classification	SBP mmHg		DBP mmHg
Normal	<120	and	<80
Elevated BP	120-129	and	<80
Stage I Hypertension	130-139	or	80-89
Stage 2 Hypertension	>140	or	>90
Hypertensive Crisis	>180	and/or	>120

¶Adapted from: Vogt, C. New AHA/ACC guidelines lower high BP threshold. *Consultant360.* November 14, 2017. https://www.consultant360.com/exclusives/new-ahaacc-guidelines-lower-high-bp-threshold
2017 ACC/AHA/AAPA/ABC/ACPM/AGS/APhA/ASH/ASPC/NMA/PCNA Guideline for the Prevention, Detection, Evaluation, and Management of High Blood Pressure in Adults: A report of the American College of Cardiology/American Heart Association Task Force on Clinical Practice Guidelines
http://hyper.ahajournals.org/content/hypertensionaha/early/2017/11/10/HYP.0000000000000065.full.pdf

APPENDIX A.2. BLOOD PRESSURE CLASSIFICATIONS (<18 YEARS)¶

Age Group	Significant		Severe	
	SBP	DBP	SBP	DBP
Newborn <7 days	>96		>106	
Newborn 8-30 days	>104		>110	
Infant 30 days-2 years	>112	>74	>118	>82
Children 3-5 years	>116	>76	>124	>84
Children 6-9 years	>122	>78	>130	>86
Children 10-12 years	>126	>82	>134	>90
Adolescents 13-15 years	>136	>86	>144	>92
Adolescents 16-18 years	>142	>92	>150	>98

¶Adapted from American Pharmacists Association. (2015). *Pediatric and neonatal dosage handbook: A universal resource for clinicians treating pediatric and neonatal patients* (22nd ed.). Hudson, Ohio: Lexicomp.

APPENDIX A.3. PATIENT-SPECIFIC FACTORS TO CONSIDER WHEN SELECTING DRUG TREATMENT FOR HYPERTENSION (JNC-8* AND ASH**)

JNC-8:

- Non-Black, including those with diabetes: thiazide, CCB, ACEI, or ARB
- African American, including those with diabetes: thiazide or CCB
- CKD; regimen should include an ACEI or ARB (including African Americans)
- Can initiate with two agents, especially if systolic >20 mmHg above goal or diastolic >10 mmHg above goal
- If goal not reached: stress adherence to medication and lifestyle, increase dose or add a second or third agent from one of the recommended classes
- Choose a drug outside of the classes recommended above only if these options have been exhausted. Consider specialist referral.

ASH:

- **Non-Black <60 years-of-age:** *First-line:* ACEI or ARB; *Second-line (add-on):* CCB or thiazide; *Third-line:* CCB plus ACEI or ARB plus thiazide
- **Non-Black 60 years-of-age and older:** *First-line:* CCB or thiazide preferred, ACEI, or ARB; *Second-line (add-on):* CCB, thiazide, ACEI, or ARB (do not use ACEI plus ARB); *Third-line:* CCB plus ACEI or ARB plus thiazide
- **African American:** *First-line:* CCB or thiazide; *Second-line (add-on):* ACEI or ARB. *Third-line:* CCB plus ACEI or ARB plus thiazide

Comorbidities (ASH):

- **Diabetes:** *First-line:* ACEI or ARB (can start with CCB or thiazide in African Americans); *Second-line:* add CCB or thiazide (can add ACEI or ARB in African Americans); *Third-line:* CCB plus ACEI or ARB plus thiazide
- **CKD:** *First-line:* ARB or ACEI (ACEI for African Americans); *Second-line (add-on):* CCB or thiazide; *Third-line:* CCB plus ACEI or ARB plus thiazide
- **CAD:** *First-line:* BB plus ARB or ACEI; *Second-line (add-on):* CCB or thiazide; *Third-line:* BB plus ARB or ACEI plus CCB plus thiazide
- **Stroke history:** *First-line:* ACEI or ARB; *Second-line:* add CCB or thiazide; *Third-line:* CCB plus ACEI or ARB plus thiazide
- **Heart failure:** ACEI or ARB plus BB plus diuretic plus aldosteronism antagonist. **Amlodipine** can be added for additional BP control (Start with ACEI, BB, diuretic. Can add BB even before ACE-I optimized. Use diuretic to manage fluid.)
- In patients 60 years of age or older who do not have diabetes or chronic kidney disease, the goal blood pressure level is now <150/90 mmHg
- In patients 18 to 59 years-of-age without major comorbidities, and in patients 60 years-of-age or older who have diabetes, chronic kidney disease, or both conditions, the new goal blood pressure level is <140/90 mmHg

APPENDIX A.4. BLOOD PRESSURE TREATMENT RECOMMENDATIONS (JNC-8)¶

- First-line and later-line treatments should now be limited to 4 classes of medications: thiazide-type diuretics, calcium channel blockers (CCBs), ACEIs, and ARBs
- Second- and third-line alternatives included higher doses <u>or</u> combinations of ACEIs, ARBs, thiazide-type diuretics, and CCBs
- Several medications are now designated as later-line alternatives, including the following:
- Beta-blockers
- Alpha-blockers
- Alpha1/beta-blockers (e.g., ***carvedilol***)
- Vasodilating beta-blockers (e.g., ***nebivolol***)
- Central alpha2-adrenergic agonists (e.g., ***clonidine***)
- Direct vasodilators (e.g., ***hydralazine***)
- Loop diuretics (e.g., ***furosemide***)
- Aldosterone antagonists (e.g., ***spironolactone***)
- Peripherally acting adrenergic antagonists (e.g., ***reserpine***)
- When initiating therapy, patients of African descent without chronic kidney disease should use CCBs and thiazides instead of ACEIs
- Use of ACEIs and ARBs is recommended in all patients with chronic kidney disease regardless of ethnic background, either as first-line therapy <u>or</u> in addition to first-line therapy
- ACEIs and ARBs should not be used in the same patient simultaneously
- CCBs and thiazide-type diuretics should be used instead of ACEIs and ARBs in patients over the age of 75 with impaired kidney function due to the risk of hyperkalemia, increased creatinine, and further renal impairment

¶Adapted from PL Detail-Document. (2014, February). Treatment of hypertension: JNC 8 and more. *Pharmacist's Letter/Prescriber's Letter*. Retrieved from https://www.scribd.com/doc/290772273/JNC-8-guideline-summary

APPENDIX B. TARGET LIPID RECOMMENDATIONS (ATP-IV)¶

APPENDIX B.1. TARGET TC, TRG, HDL-C, NON-HDL-C

Total cholesterol (TC)	<200 mg/dL
Triglyceride (TRG)	<150 mg/dL
High-density lipoprotein (HDL-C)	>40 mg/dL (male) >50 mg/dL (female)
Non-high-density lipoprotein (Non-HDL-C)	<130 mg/dL; 30 mg/dL above the LDL-treatment target

¶Adapted from the National Cholesterol Education Program Expert Panel on Detection, Evaluation, and Treatment of High Blood Cholesterol in Adults (Adult Treatment Panel IV, 2012)

APPENDIX B.2. TARGET LDL-C (ATP IV)[†]

Risk Assessment[††]	LDL Target	Initiate TLC[†††]	Initiate Drug Therapy
0-1	<160 mg/dL	≥160 mg/dL	≥190 mg/dL (optional at 160-189 mg/dL)
2 or more plus 10-year risk <10%	<130 mg/dL	≥130 mg/dL	≥160 mg/dL
2 or more plus 10-year risk <20%	<130 mg/dL <100 mg/dL (optional)	≥130 mg/dL	≥130 mg/dL
CHD or CHD risk equivalents 10-year risk >20%	<100 mg/dL <70 mg/dL (optional)	≥100 mg/dL	≥100 mg/dL

[†]Treatment decisions based on LDL-C
[††]Risk factors include age (men ≥45 years and women ≥55 years)
[†††]Therapeutic lifestyle changes (e.g., exercise, weight loss, low fat diet)

APPENDIX B.3. NON-HDL-C CLASSIFICATIONS (ATP-IV)[¶]

Desirable	<130 mg/dL	Non-HDL-C is calculated as total cholesterol minus HDL-C. The addition of non-HDL-C to the Lipid Panel reflects the recognition of this calculated value as a predictive factor in cardiovascular disease based on the National Cholesterol Education III studies. The reference ranges for non-HDL-C are based on National Cholesterol Education III guidelines: Non-HDL-C is thought to be a better predictor of CVD than LDL-C; treatment goal for non-HDL-C is usually 30 mg/dL above the LDL-C treatment target. For example, if the LDL-C treatment goal is <70 mg/dL, then Non-HDL-C treatment target would be <100 mg/dL.
Borderline high	139-159 mg/dL	
High	160-189 mg/dL	
Very high	≥190 mg/dL	

[¶]Adapted from the National Cholesterol Education Program Expert Panel on Detection, Evaluation, and Treatment of High Blood Cholesterol in Adults (Adult Treatment Panel IV, 2012).

APPENDIX C. GLYCOSYLATED HEMOGLOBIN (HgbA1c) & AVERAGE BLOOD GLUCOSE EQUIVALENT

HbA1c and Average Blood Glucose Equivalent			
HbA1c (%)	GLU	HbA1c (%)	GLU
4	60 mg/dL	14	360 mg/dL
5	90 mg/dL	15	390 mg/dL
6	120 mg/dL	16	420 mg/dL
7	150 mg/dL	17	450 mg/dL
8	180 mg/dL	18	480 mg/dL
9	210 mg/dL	19	510 mg/dL
10	240 mg/dL	20	540 mg/dL
11	270 mg/dL	21	570 mg/dL
12	300 mg/dL	22	600 mg/dL
13	330 mg/dL	23	630 mg/dL

APPENDIX D. ROUTINE IMMUNIZATION RECOMMENDATIONS

APPENDIX D.1. ADMINISTRATION OF VACCINES¶

- Prior to 1 year-of-age, administer IM vaccinations in the vastus lateralis muscle
- After 1 year-of-age, administer vaccinations in the posterolateral upper arm
- Influenza vaccine should be administered annually for all ages ≥6 months
- Inactivated vaccines (e.g., pneumococcal, meningococcal, and inactivated influenza vaccines) are generally acceptable and live vaccines are generally avoided, in persons with immune deficiencies <u>or</u> immunocompromising conditions
- Additional information about routine vaccinations, unknown vaccination status, travel vaccinations, vaccinations in pregnancy, and other vaccines, is available at:
    - **www.cdc.gov/vaccines/hcp/acip-recs/index.html**
    - **wwwnc.cdc.gov/travel/destinations/list**
- **DTaP** (diphtheria-tetanus-toxoid, acellular pertussis); minimum age 6 wks
- **DTaP** should <u>not</u> be administered at <u>or</u> after the 7th birthday
- The 4th dose of **DTaP** vaccine can be administered as early as age 12 months, provided that the interval between doses 3 and 4 is at least 6 months
- **DTaP** and **IPV** should be administered at <u>or</u> before school entry
- **HAV** (*hepatitis A vaccine*) is recommended for all children at 1 year (12-23 months) of age
- **HAV** 2-dose series should be administered at least 6 months apart
- **HBV** (*hepatitis B vaccine*) is a 3-dose series initiated at birth; administer 2nd dose at 1-2 months; administer the 3rd dose at age 6 months (<u>not</u> before ≥24 weeks)

(*continued*)

(*continued*)

- **HBV** should be offered to all children who have not received the full series
- Infants born to HBsAg-positive mothers should be tested for HBsAG and antibody to HBsAg after completion of the **HBV** series (at age 9-18 months)
- **Hib** (*Haemophilus influenza* type b conjugate vaccine) minimum age 6 months
- **Hib** is not recommended if age >5 years
- **HPV** (*human papillomavirus vaccine*) vaccine should be administered anytime between 11 and 12 years-of-age
- **HPV** is a 3-series vaccine administered at months 0, 1, 6; females may receive HPV/4 or HPV/2; males should receive HPV/2
- **HPV** if not previously received at 11 or 12 years-of-age, may be initiated at any time between 13 and 26 years-of-age
- **IIV** (*inactivated influenza vaccine*) can be administered >6 months (use age-appropriate formulation), pregnant women, and persons with hives-only allergy to eggs
- **IHD** (*influenza high dose*) (**Fluzone High Dose**) may be recommended to persons ≥65 years of age
- **IPV** (inactivated poliovirus vaccine) minimum age 4 weeks
- An all-**IPV** schedule is recommended to eliminate the risk of vaccine-associated paralytic polio (VAPP) associated with **OPV** (*oral poliovirus vaccine*)
- **LAIV** (*live attenuated influenza vaccine*) may be administered intranasally (**FluMist**)
- **Men** (*meningococcal vaccine*) should be administered to all children at the 11-12 year old visit as well as to unvaccinated adolescents 15 years-of-age (usually at high school entry)
- **Men** should be administered to all college freshmen living in dormitories
- Use MPSV4 for children aged 2-10 years and MCV4 for older children, although MPSV4 is an acceptable alternative for prophylaxis in men
- **MMR** (*mumps-measles-rubella*) should be administered at age 12 months in high-risk areas; if indicated, tuberculin testing can be done at the same visit
- **MMR** should be administered at age 11-12 years unless 2 doses were given after the first birthday; the interval between doses should be at least 4 weeks
- **MMR** adults born <1957 are generally considered immune to measles and mumps; all adults born ≥1957 should have documentation of at least 1 dose of MMR vaccine unless there is a medical contraindication or laboratory evidence of immunity to each of the 3 disease components; documentation of provider-diagnosed diseases not acceptable evidence of immunity to any of the 3 disease components
- **PCV-13** (*pneumococcal vaccine*) does not replace 23-valent pneumococcal polysaccharide in children age ≥24 months
- **PCV-13** when PCV-13 and PCV-23 are indicated, administer PCV-13 first; do not administer PCV-13 and PCV-23 in the same visit
- **PCV-13** adults ≥65 years-of-age, who have not received PCV-13 or PCV-23, should receive PCV-13 followed by PCV-23 6-12 months later
- **PCV-23** (pneumococcal vaccine 23 trivalent) minimum age 6 weeks
- **PCV-23** adults ≥65 years of age, who have received **PCV-23**, but not received PCV-13, should receive. **PCV-13** at least I year later; adults ≥65 years of age, who have not received **PCV-23**, should receive

(*continued*)

(*continued*)

- **PCV-13** followed by **PCV-23** 6-12 months later
- **RIV** (*recombinant influenza vaccine*; **FluBlok**) may be administered to any adult >18 years-of-age, including pregnant women
- **RIV** does not contain any egg protein; can be administered to anyone with egg allergy at any severity
- Older infants and children previously vaccinated with **PCV** should receive 3 doses (if age 7-11 months), 2 doses (if age 12-23 months), or 1 dose (if age >24 months)
- **Rot** (*rotavirus vaccine*) is a live attenuated oral vaccine for infants aged >6 weeks or <32 weeks *only*; administer the 1st dose at 6-12 weeks-of-age; administer 2nd and 3rd doses at 4-10-week intervals for a total of 3 doses
- **Rot** If an incomplete dose is administered, *do not* administer a replacement dose, but continue with the remaining doses in the recommended series
- **Td** (*tetanus-diphtheria vaccine*) should be repeated every 10 years throughout life (or if at-risk injury ≥5 years after previous dose)
- **Td** should *not be* administered until minimum age ≥7 years
- **TdaP** (*tetanus-diphtheria-acellular pertussis*) administer 1 dose to pregnant women during each pregnancy, preferably during 27-36 weeks gestation, regardless of interval since prior Td or TdaP
- **TdaP** persons ≥11 years-of-age who have not received **TdaP** vaccine or for whom vaccine status is unknown, should receive 1 dose of **TdaP** followed by a **Td** booster every 10 years
- **Var** should be administered to children at age 11-12 years who have not had chickenpox or who report having had chickenpox but do not have laboratory documentation of immunity
- **Var** If not received between age 11 and 12 years, administer 2 doses at least 4 weeks apart any time after 12 years-of-age or a 2nd dose if previously only received 1 dose
- **VarZ** (*herpes zoster vaccine*) should be administered in a single dose once at ≥60 years-of-age, whether or not the person reports a prior episode of active herpes zoster infection
- **VarZ** is contraindicated in pregnancy and immune deficiency
- **DTaP** and **IPV** can be initiated as early as 4 weeks in areas of high endemicity or outbreak.

¶Adapted from DHHS CDC 2018.

APPENDIX D.2. CONTRAINDICATIONS TO VACCINES¶

All vaccines	Previous anaphylactic reaction to the vaccine Moderate or severe illness with or without fever
TdaP/DTaP, Td	Encephalopathy within 7 days of administration of previous dose
Hib	Previous anaphylactic reaction to the vaccine Moderate or severe illness with or without fever
HBV	Anaphylactic reaction to baker's yeast
HAV	Previous anaphylactic reaction to the vaccine Moderate or severe illness with or without fever

(*continued*)

Influenza	Allergy to eggs (*except* **FluBlok,** which does not contain any egg protein)
IPV	Anaphylactic reaction to neomycin or streptomycin
Pneumococcal	Hypersensitivity to diphtheria toxoid
MMR	Pregnancy, immunodeficiency, anaphylactic reaction to eggs or neomycin
Meningococcal	Encephalopathy within 7 days of administration of previous dose
Rotavirus	<6 months or >32 months
HPV	Pregnancy; pregnancy testing is not required; however, if administered, defer the remaining dose(s) until completion or termination of pregnancy
Varicella	Pregnancy
Herpes zoster	Pregnancy

¶Adapted from DHHS CDC 2018.

APPENDIX D.3. ROUTE OF ADMINISTRATION AND DOSE OF VACCINES¶

Vaccine	Route	Dose
Single Vaccines		
Diphtheria-Tetanus-Pertussis (DTaP, Dtap, DT)	IM	0.5 ml
Haemophilus influenza type b (Hib)	IM	0.5 ml
Hepatitis A vaccine (HAV)	IM	0.5 ml: age <18 yrs 1.0 ml: age ≥19 yrs
Hepatitis B vaccine (HBV)	IM	0.5 ml: age <18 yrs 1.0 ml: age ≥19 yrs
Human Papillomavirus (HPV)	IM	0.5 ml
Influenza **(Fluzone Intradermal)**	ID	0.5 ml
Influenza, inactivated (IIV), recombinant (RIV)	IM	0.25 ml: age 6-35 months 0.5 ml: age ≥3 yrs
Influenza, live attenuated (LAIV)	NS	0.2 ml; 0.1 ml in each nostril
Meningococcal conjugate	IM	0.5 ml
Meningococcal polysaccharide (MPSV)	SC	0.5 ml
Meningococcal serogroup B (Men B)	IM	0.5 ml

(*continued*)

(*continued*)

Vaccine	Route	Dose
Mumps-Measles-Rubella (MMR)	SC	0.5 ml
Pneumococcal conjugate (PCV)	IM	0.5 ml
Pneumococcal polysaccharide (PPSV)	IM/SC	0.5 ml
Polio, Inactivated (IPV)	IM/SC	0.5 ml
Rotavirus (**Rotarix**)	PO	1 ml
Rotavirus (**Rotateq**)	PO	2 ml
Tetanus (Td)	IM	0.5 ml
Varicella	SC	0.5 ml
Herpes Zoster	SC	0.65 ml: age ≥60 yrs
Combination Vaccines		
MMR-Var (**ProQuad**)	SC	0.5 ml: age ≤12 yrs
HBV-HAV (**Twinrix**)	IM	1 ml: >18 yrs
DTaP-HBV-IPV (**Pediarix**)	IM	0.5 ml
DTaP-IPV-Hib (**Pentacel**)	IM	0.5 ml
DTaP-IPV (**Kinrix, Quadracel**)	IM	0.5 ml
Hib-HBV (**Comvax**)	IM	0.5 ml
Hib-MenCY (**MenHibrix**)	IM	0.5 ml

¶Adapted from DHHS CDC 2018.

APPENDIX D.4. MINIMUM INTERVAL BETWEEN VACCINE DOSES¶

Type	#1 to #2	#2 to #3	#3 to #4	#4 to #5
HBV	4 weeks	5 months		
HAV	6 months			
DTaP	4 weeks	4 weeks	6 months	6 months
IPV	4 weeks	4 weeks	4 weeks	
MMR	4 weeks			
Var	4 weeks			
Rotavirus	4 weeks	4 weeks; do not administer >32 weeks of age		

(*continued*)

Type	#1 to #2	#2 to #3	#3 to #4	#4 to #5
PCV-13	4 weeks (if #1 at age <12 months and current age <24 months); 8 weeks (as last dose if #1 at age>12 months <u>or</u> current age 24-59 months); No more doses needed if healthy and #1 at age ≥24 months	4 weeks if age <12 months; 8 weeks (as last dose if age ≥12 months); No more doses needed if healthy and previous dose at age ≥24 months	8 weeks (as last dose; only necessary for age 12 months to 5 years who received 3 doses before age 12 months)	
Hib	4 weeks (if #1 at age <12 months); 8 weeks (as last dose if #1 at age 12-14 months); No more doses needed if healthy and #1 at age ≥15 months	4 weeks if age 12 months; 8 weeks (as last dose if age ≥12 months); No more doses needed if previous dose at age ≥15 months	8 weeks (as last dose; only necessary for age 12 months to 2 years who received 3 doses before age 12 months)	
HPV	4 weeks	20 weeks (24 weeks after #1		

¶Adapted from DHHS CDC 2015.

APPENDIX D.5. RECOMMENDED CHILDHOOD (BIRTH-12 YEARS) IMMUNIZATION SCHEDULE¶

Type	Birth	1 month	2 months	4 months	6 months	6-18 months	12-15 months	15-18 months	4-6 years	11-12 years
HBV	✓	✓			✓					
DTaP			✓	✓	✓		✓		✓	
IPV			✓	✓		✓			✓	
Hib			✓	✓	✓		✓			
Rotavirus			✓	✓	✓					
MMR							✓		✓	
TdaP										✓
Varicella							✓		✓	
PVC-13			✓	✓	✓		✓			
HAV							✓	✓		
Meningitis										✓
HPV•										✓✓✓

¶Adapted from DHHS CDC 2018.

✓Shaded box = immunization due.

✓✓✓HPV 3-dose series, months 0, 1, 6.

APPENDIX D.6. RECOMMENDED CHILDHOOD (BIRTH-12 YEARS) IMMUNIZATION CATCH-UP SCHEDULE¶

Vaccine	Minimum Interval Between Doses			
	#1 to #2	#2 to #3	#3 to #4	#4 to #5
HBV	4 weeks	8 weeks (16 weeks after #1)		
DTaP	4 weeks	4 weeks	6 months	6 months
IPV	4 weeks	4 weeks	4 weeks	
MMR	4 weeks			
Var	4 weeks			
Rotavirus	4 weeks	4 weeks; do not administer >32 weeks of age		
PCV	2 months	2 months	2 months	6-15 months
HPV	4 weeks	20 weeks (24 weeks after #1		

¶Adapted from DHHS CDC 2018.

APPENDIX D.7. RECOMMENDED SCHEDULE FOR MISSED CHILDHOOD IMMUNIZATIONS (13-21 YEARS)¶

Influenza	1 dose annually
HBV	3 dose series: months 0, 1, 6
Td/TdaP	Substitute Tdap for Td one time; then continue Td once every 10 years
MMR*	2 doses, 4 weeks apart
Varicella*	Without evidence of immunity: 2 doses, 4 weeks apart
HAV	Single antigen, 2 doses: months 0, 6-12 (**Havrix**); 0, 6-18 (**Vaqta**)
Meningitis	1 or more doses
HPV (female)*β	3 doses; months 0, 1, 6
HPV (male)β	3 doses; months 0, 1, 6

¶Adapted from DHHS CDC 2018

* Contraindicated in pregnancy

β Only if not previously vaccinated between 11-12 years-of-age

APPENDIX E. CONTRACEPTIVES

APPENDIX E.1. CONTRACEPTIVE CONTRAINDICATIONS AND RECOMMENDATIONS

- All contraceptives are pregnancy category X
- No non-barrier contraceptives protect against STDs
- **Absolute Contraindications:**
  - HTN >35 years-of-age
  - DM >35 years-of-age
  - LDL-C >160 or TG >250
  - Known or suspected pregnancy
  - Known or suspected carcinoma of the breast
  - Known or suspected carcinoma of the endometrium
  - Known or suspected estrogen-dependent neoplasia
  - Undiagnosed abnormal genital bleeding
  - Cerebral vascular or coronary artery disease
  - Cholestatic jaundice of pregnancy or jaundice with prior use
  - Hepatic adenoma or carcinoma or benign liver tumor
  - Active or past history of thrombophlebitis or thromboembolic disorder
- **Relative Contraindications:**
  - Lactation
  - Asthma
  - Ulcerative colitis
  - Migraine or vascular headache
  - Cardiac or renal dysfunction
  - Gestational diabetes, prediabetes, diabetes mellitus
  - Diastolic BP 90 mmHg or greater or hypertension by any other criteria
  - Psychic depression
  - Varicose veins
  - Smoker >35 years-of-age
  - Sickle-cell or sickle-hemoglobin C disease
  - Cholestatic jaundice during pregnancy, active gallbladder disease
  - Hepatitis or mononucleosis during the preceding year
  - First-order family history of fatal or non-fatal rheumatic CVD or diabetes prior to age 50 years
  - Drug(s) with known interaction(s)
  - Elective surgery or immobilization within 4 weeks
  - Age >50 years
- **Recommendations:**
  - Start the first pill on the first Sunday after menses begins. Thereafter, each new pill pack will be started on a Sunday.
  - Take each daily pill in the same 3-hour window (e.g., 9A-12N, 12N-3P; a 4-hour window prior to bedtime is not recommended).
  - If 1 pill is missed, take it as soon as possible and the next pill at the regular time.
  - If 2 pills are missed, take both pills as soon as possible and then two pills the following day. A barrier method should be used for the remainder of the pill pack.

(*continued*)

(*continued*)

- If 3 pills are missed before 10th cycle day, resume taking OCs on a regular schedule and take precautions.
- If 3 pills are missed after the 10th cycle day, discard the current pill pack and begin a new one 7 days after the last pill was taken.
- If very low-dose OCs are used or if combination OCs are begun after the 5th day of the menstrual cycle, an additional method of birth control should be used for the first 7 days of OC use.
- If nausea occurs as a side effect, select an OC with *lower* ***estrogen*** content.
- If breakthrough bleeding occurs during the first half of the cycle, select an OC with *higher* ***progesterone*** content.
- Symptoms of a serious nature include loss of vision, diplopia, unilateral numbness, weakness, or tingling, severe chest pain, severe pain in left arm or neck, severe leg pain, slurring of speech, and abdominal tenderness or mass.

APPENDIX E.2. 28-DAY ORAL CONTRACEPTIVES WITH ESTROGEN AND PROGESTERONE CONTENT

Comment: **Beyaz, Loryna, Syeda, Safyral, Yasmin**, and **Yaz** are contraindicated with renal and adrenal insufficiency. Monitor k^+ level during the first cycle if the patient is at risk for hyperkalemia for any reason. If the patient is taking drugs that increase potassium (e.g., ACEIs, ARBS, NSAIDs, K^+ sparing diuretics), the patient is at risk for hyperkalemia.

Combined Oral Contraceptive	Estrogen (mcg)	Progesterone (mg)
Alesse-21, Alesse-28 (X)(G) *ethinyl estradiol/levonorgestrel*	20	0.1
Altavera (X) *ethinyl estradiol/levonorgestrel*	30	0.15
Apri (X)(G) *ethinyl estradiol+desogestrel*	30	0.15
Aranelle (X)(G) *ethinyl estradiol+norethindrone*	35	0.5 1 0.5
Aviane (X)(G) *ethinyl estradiol/levonorgestrel*	20	0.1
Balziva (X)(G) *ethinyl estradiol+norethindrone*	35	0.4
Beyaz (X)(G) *ethinyl estradiol+drospirenone* plus levomefolate calcium 0.451 mcg (28 tabs)	20	3

(*continued*)

(*continued*)

Combined Oral Contraceptive	Estrogen (mcg)	Progesterone (mg)
Blisovi 24 Fe (X)(G) *ethinyl estradiol/norethindrone* <u>plus</u> *ferrous fumarate* 75 mg (4 tabs)	20	1
Brevicon-21, Brevicon-28 (X)(G) *ethinyl estradiol+norethindrone*	35	0.5
Camrese (X) *ethinyl estradiol/levonorgestrel*	30 10	0.15
Camrese Lo (X) *ethinyl estradiol/levonorgestrel*	20 10	0.1
Cesia (X)(G) *ethinyl estradiol+desogestrel*	25 25 25	0.1 0.125 0.15
Cryselle (X)(G) *ethinyl estradiol/norgestrel*	30	0.3
Cyclessa (X)(G) *ethinyl estradiol+desogestrel*	25 25 25	0.1 0.125 0.15
Demulen 1/35-21, Demulen 1/35-28 (X)(G) *ethinyl estradiol+ethynodiol diacetate*	35	1
Demulen 1/50-21, Demulen 1/50-28 (X)(G) *ethinyl estradiol+ethynodiol diacetate*	50	1
Desogen (X)(G) *ethinyl estradiol+desogestrel diacetate*	30	0.15
Enpresse (X)(G) *ethinyl estradiol/levonorgestrel*	30 40 30	0.05 0.075 0.125
Estrostep Fe (X) *ethinyl estradiol+norethindrone* <u>plus</u> *ferrous fumarate* 75 mg	20 30 35	1 1 1
Femcon Fe (X)(G) *ethinyl estradiol+norethindrone* <u>plus</u> *ferrous fumarate* 75 mg	35	0.4
Generess Fe Chew tab (X)(G) *ethinyl estradiol+norethindrone* <u>plus</u> *ferrous fumarate* 75 mg	25	0.8

(*continued*)

(*continued*)

Combined Oral Contraceptive	Estrogen (mcg)	Progesterone (mg)
Genora (X)(G) *ethinyl estradiol+norethindrone*	35 35 35	0.5 1 0.5
Gianvi (X)(G) *ethinyl estradiol+drospirenone*	20	3
Gildess 1.5/30 (X)(G) *ethinyl estradiol+norethindrone*	30	1.5
Introvale (X) *ethinyl estradiol/levonorgestrel*	30	0.15
Jenest-28 (X) *ethinyl estradiol+norethindrone*	35 35	0.5 1
Jolessa (X)(G) *ethinyl estradiol+levonorgestrel*	30	0.15
Junel 1/20 (X)(G) *ethinyl estradiol+norethindrone*	20	1
Junel 1.5/30 (X)(G) *ethinyl estradiol+norethindrone*	30	1.5
Junel Fe 1/20 (X)(G) *ethinyl estradiol+norethindrone* plus *ferrous fumarate* 75 mg	20	1
Junel Fe 1.5/30 (X)(G) *ethinyl estradiol+norethindrone* plus *ferrous fumarate* 75 mg	30	1.5
Kaitlib Fe Chew Tab (X)(G) *ethinyl estradiol+norethindrone* plus *ferrous fumarate* 75 mg	25	0.8
Kariva (X)(G) *ethinyl estradiol+desogestrel*	20 10	0.15 0.15
Kelnor 1/35 (X)(G) *ethinyl estradiol+ethynodiol diacetate*	35	1
Leena (X) *ethinyl estradiol+norethindrone*	35 35 35	0.5 1 0.5
Lessina 28 (X)(G) *ethinyl estradiol+levonorgestrel*	20	0.1

(*continued*)

(*continued*)

Combined Oral Contraceptive	Estrogen (mcg)	Progesterone (mg)
Levlen 21, Levlen 28 (X)(G) *ethinyl estradiol+levonorgestrel*	30	0.15
Levlite 28 (X)(G) *ethinyl estradiol+levonorgestrel*	20	0.1
Levora-21, Levora-28 (X)(G) *ethinyl estradiol+levonorgestrel*	30	0.15
Loestrin 21 1/20 (X)(G) *ethinyl estradiol+norethindrone*	20	1
Loestrin 21 1.5/30 (X)(G) *ethinyl estradiol+norethindrone*	30	1.5
Loestrin Fe 1/20 (X)(G) *ethinyl estradiol+norethindrone* plus *ferrous fumarate* 75 mg	20	1
Loestrin Fe 1.5/30 (X)(G) *ethinyl estradiol/norethindrone* plus *ferrous fumarate* 75 mg (4 tabs)	30	1.5
Loestrin 24 Fe (X)(G) *ethinyl estradiol/norethindrone* plus *ferrous fumarate* 75 mg (4 tabs)	20	1
Lo Loestrin Fe (X) *ethinyl estradiol/norethindrone* plus *ferrous fumarate* 75 mg (2 tabs)	10	1
Lomedia 24 Fe (X)(G) *ethinyl estradiol+norethindrone* plus *ferrous fumarate* 75 mg	20	1
Lo/Ovral-21, Lo/Ovral-28 (X)(G) *ethinyl estradiol/norgestrel*	30	0.3
Loryna (X) *ethinyl estradiol+drospirenone*	20	3
Low-Ogestrel-21, Low-Ogestrel-28 (X)(G) *ethinyl estradiol+norgestrel*	30	0.3
Lutera (X)(G) *ethinyl estradiol+levonorgestrel*	20	0.1
Lybrel (X) *ethinyl estradiol+levonorgestrel*	20	0.09

(*continued*)

(continued)

Combined Oral Contraceptive	Estrogen (mcg)	Progesterone (mg)
Mibelas 24 FE (X)(G) *ethinyl estradiol+norethindrone* plus *ferrous fumarate* 75 mg	20	1
Microgestin 1/20 (X)(G) *ethinyl estradiol+norethindrone*	20	1
Microgestin Fe 1/20 (X)(G) *ethinyl estradiol+norethindrone* plus *ferrous fumarate* 75 mg	20	1
Microgestin 1.5/30 (X)(G) *ethinyl estradiol+norethindrone*	30	1.5
Microgestin Fe 1.5/30 (X)(G) *ethinyl estradiol+norethindrone* plus *ferrous fumarate* 75 mg	30	1.5
Minastrin 24 FE (X)(G) *ethinyl estradiol+norethindrone* plus *ferrous fumarate* 75 mg	20	1
Mircette (X)(G) *ethinyl estradiol+desogestrel diacetate*	20 10	0.15
Modicon 0.5/35-28 (X)(G) *ethinyl estradiol+norethindrone*	35	0.5
MonoNessa (X)(G) *ethinyl estradiol+norgestimate*	35	0.25
Natazia (X)(G) *estradiol valerate+dienogest*	30 20 20 10	— 2 3 —
Necon 0.5/35-21, Necon 0.5/35-28 (X)(G) *ethinyl estradiol+norethindrone*	35	0.5
Necon 1/35-21, Necon 1/35-28 (X)(G) *ethinyl estradiol+norethindrone*	35	0.5
Necon 10/11-21, Necon 10/11-28 (X)(G) *ethinyl estradiol+norethindrone*	35 35	0.5 1
Necon 1/50-21, Necon 1/50-28 (X)(G) *mestranol+norethindrone*	50	1
Nelova 0.5/35-21, Nelova 0.5/35-28 (X)(G) *ethinyl estradiol+norethindrone*	35	0.5

(continued)

(*continued*)

Combined Oral Contraceptive	Estrogen (mcg)	Progesterone (mg)
Nelova 1/35-21, Nelova 1/35-28 (X)(G) *ethinyl estradiol+norethindrone*	35	1
Nelova 10/11-21, Nelova 10/11-28 (X)(G) *ethinyl estradiol+norethindrone*	35 35	0.5 1
Nelova 1/50-21, Nelova 1/50-28 (X)(G) *mestranol+norethindrone*	50	1
Neocon 7/7/7 (X)(G) *ethinyl estradiol+norethindrone*	35 35 35	0.5 0.75 1
Nordette-21, Nordette-28 (X)(G) *ethinyl estradiol+levonorgestrel*	30	0.15
Norinyl 1+35-21, Norinyl 1+35-28 (X)(G) *ethinyl estradiol+norethindrone*	35	1
Norinyl 1+50-21, Norinyl 1+50-28 (X)(G) *mestranol+norethindrone*	50	1
Nortrel 0.5/35 (X)(G) *ethinyl estradiol+norethindrone*	35	0.5
Nortrel 1/35-21, Nortrel 1/35-28 (X)(G) *ethinyl estradiol+norethindrone*	35	1
Nortrel 7/7/7-28 (X)(G) *ethinyl estradiol+norethindrone*	35 35 35	0.5 0.75 1
Ocella (X)(G) *ethinyl estradiol+drospirenone*	30	3
Ortho-Cept 28 (X)(G) *ethinyl estradiol+desogestrel*	30	0.15
Ortho-Cyclen 28 (X)(G) *ethinyl estradiol+norgestimate*	35	0.25
Ortho-Novum 1/35-21, Ortho-Novum 1/35-28 (X)(G) *ethinyl estradiol+norethindrone*	35	1
Ortho-Novum 1/50-21, Ortho-Novum 1/50-28 (X)(G) *mestranol+norethindrone*	50	1
Ortho-Novum 7/7/7-28 (X)(G) *ethinyl estradiol+norethindrone*	35 35 35	0.5 0.75 1

(*continued*)

(*continued*)

Combined Oral Contraceptive	Estrogen (mcg)	Progesterone (mg)
Ortho-Novum 10/11-28 (X) *ethinyl estradiol+norethindrone*	35 35	0.5 1
Ortho Tri-Cyclen 21, Ortho Tri-Cyclen 28 (X)(G) *ethinyl estradiol+norgestimate*	35 35 35	0.18 0.215 0.25
Ortho Tri-Cyclen Lo (X)(G) *ethinyl estradiol+norgestimate*	25 25 25	0.18 0.215 0.25
Ovcon 35 (X)(G) *ethinyl estradiol+norethindrone*	35	1
Ovcon 35 Fe (X)(G) *ethinyl estradiol/norethindrone* plus *ferrous fumarate* (7 inert tabs)	35	0.4
Ovral-21, Ovral-28 (X)(G) *ethinyl estradiol+norgestrel*	50	0.5
Portia (X)(G) *ethinyl estradiol+levonorgestrel*	30	0.15
Previfem (X) *ethinyl estradiol+norgestimate*	35	0.25
Quasense (X) *ethinyl estradiol+levonorgestrel*	30	0.15
Reclipsen (X)(G) *ethinyl estradiol/desogestrel* plus *ferrous fumarate* 75 mg (4 tabs)	30	0.15
Safyral (X)(G) *ethinyl estradiol+drospirenone* plus *levomefolate calcium* 0.451 mg	30	3
Sprintec 28 (X)(G) *ethinyl estradiol+norgestimate*	35	0.25
Syeda (X) *ethinyl estradiol+drospirenone*	30	3
Tarina Fe 1/20 (X)(G) *ethinyl estradiol/norethindrone* plus *ferrous fumarate* 75 mg (7 tabs)	20	1
Taytulla Fe 1/20 (X)(G) (Softgel caps) *ethinyl estradiol+norethindrone* plus *ferrous fumarate* 75 mg (4 Softgel caps)	20	1

(*continued*)

(*continued*)

Combined Oral Contraceptive	Estrogen (mcg)	Progesterone (mg)
Tilia Fe (X)(G) *ethinyl estradiol/norethindrone* plus *ferrous fumarate* 75 mg (7 tabs)	20 30 35	1 1 1
Tri-Legest 21 (X)(G) *ethinyl estradiol+norethindrone*	20 30 35	1 1 1
Tri-Legest Fe (X)(G) *ethinyl estradiol/norethindrone* plus *ferrous fumarate* 75 mg (7 tabs)	20 30 35	1 1 1
Tri-Levlen 21, Tri-Levlen 28 (X)(G) *ethinyl estradiol+levonorgestrel*	30 40 30	0.05 0.075 0.125
Tri-Lo-Estarylla (X)(G) *ethinyl estradiol+norgestimate*	25 25 25	0.18 0.215 0.25
Tri-Lo-Sprintec (X)(G) *ethinyl estradiol+norgestimate*	25 25 25	0.18 0.215 0.25
TriNessa (X)(G) *ethinyl estradiol+norgestimate*	35 35 35	0.18 0.215 0.25
Tri-Norinyl 21, Tri-Norinyl 28 (X)(G) *ethinyl estradiol+norethindrone*	35 35 35	0.5 1 0.5
Triphasil-21, Triphasil-28 (X)(G) *ethinyl estradiol+levonorgestrel*	30 40 30	0.050 0.075 0.125
Tri-Previfem (X)(G) *ethinyl estradiol+norgestimate*	35 35 35	0.18 0.215 0.25
Tri-Sprintec (X)(G) *ethinyl estradiol+norgestimate*	35 35 35	0.18 0.215 0.25
Trivora (X)(G) *ethinyl estradiol+levonorgestrel*	30 40 30	0.05 0.075 0.125

(*continued*)

(*continued*)

Combined Oral Contraceptive	Estrogen (mcg)	Progesterone (mg)
Velivet (X)(G) *ethinyl estradiol+desogestrel*	25 25 25	0.1 0.125 0.15
Yasmin (X)(G) *ethinyl estradiol+drospirenone*	30	3
Yaz (X)(G) *ethinyl estradiol+drospirenone*	20	3
Zovia 1/35E-28 (X)(G) *ethinyl estradiol+ethynodiol diacetate*	35	1
Zovia 1/50E-28 (X)(G) *ethinyl estradiol+ethynodiol diacetate*	50	1

APPENDIX E.3. EXTENDED-CYCLE ORAL CONTRACEPTIVES

91 Day

▶ ***ethinyl estradiol+levonorgestrel*** (X) 1 tab daily x 91 days; repeat (no tablet-free days)

Ashlyna (G) *Tab: levonorgest* 15 mcg/*eth est* 30 mcg (84) + *eth est* 10 mcg (7) (91 tabs/pck)

Jolessa (G) *Tab: levonorgest* 15 mcg/*eth est* 30 mcg (84) + inert tabs (7) (91 tabs/pck)

LoSeasonique *Tab: levnorgest* 0.1 mcg/*eth est* 20 mcg (84) + *eth est* 10 mcg (7) (91 tabs/pck)

Quartette (G) *Tab: levonorgest* 15 mcg/*eth est* 30 mcg (84) + *eth est* 10 mcg (7) (91 tabs/pck)

Quasense (G) *Tab: levonorgest* 15 mcg/*eth est* 30 mcg (84) + inert tabs (7) (91 tabs/pck)

Seasonale (G) *Tab: levonorgest* 15 mcg/*eth est* 30 mcg (84) + inert tabs (7) (91 tabs/pck)

Seasonique (G) *Tab: levnorgest* 15 mcg/*eth est* 30 mcg (84) + *eth est* 10 mcg (7) (91 tabs/pck)

365 Day

▶ ***ethinyl estradiol+levonorgestrel*** (X) 1 tab daily x 28 days; repeat (no tablet-free days)

Lybrel *Tab: levnorgest* 0.09 mcg/*eth est* 20 mcg (28 tabs/pck)

APPENDIX E.4. PROGESTERONE-ONLY ORAL CONTRACEPTIVES ("MINI-PILL")

Brand	Progesterone	mcg
Comment: Take progestin-only pills at the same time each day (within a 3-hour time window). If a pill is missed, another method of contraception should be used for the remainder of the pill pack.		
Camila (X)(G)	*norethindrone*	35
Errin (X)(G)	*norethindrone*	35
Jolivette (X)(G)	*norethindrone*	35
Micronor (X)(G)	*norethindrone*	35
Nora-BE (X)(G)	*norethindrone*	35
Nor-QD (X)(G)	*norethindrone*	35
Ortho Micronor	*norethindrone*	35
Ovrette (X)	*norgestrel*	7.5

APPENDIX E.5. INJECTABLE PROGESTERONE

90 Day

Comment: Administer first dose within 5 days of onset of normal menses, within 5 days postpartum if not breastfeeding, or at 6 weeks postpartum if breastfeeding exclusively. Do not use for >2 years unless other methods are inadequate.

▶ *medroxyprogesterone* (X)(G)

Depo-Provera 150 mg deep IM q 3 months

Vial: 150 mg/ml (1 ml); *Prefilled syringe:* 150 mg/ml

Depo-SubQ 104 mg SC q 3 months

Prefilled syringe: 104 mg/ml (0.65 ml) (parabens)

APPENDIX E.6. TRANSDERMAL CONTRACEPTIVE

Ethinyl Estradiol/Norelgestromin

Comment: Apply the transdermal patch to the abdomen, buttock, upper-outer arm, or upper torso. *Do* not apply the transdermal patch to the breast. Rotate the site (however, may use the same anatomical area).

▶ *ethinyl estradiol+levonorgestrel* (X)(G) apply one patch once weekly x 3 weeks; then 1 patch-free week; then repeat sequence

Climara Pro ***Transdermal patch:*** *eth est* 0.045 mg+levonorgest 0.15 mg per day (3/pck)

▶ *ethinyl estradiol+norethindrone* (X)(G) apply one patch twice weekly x 3 weeks; then 1 patch-free week; then repeat sequence

Combipatch Transdermal patch: eth est 0.05 mg/noreth 0.14 mg per day (6/pck)

APPENDIX E.7. CONTRACEPTIVE VAGINAL RINGS

Ethinyl Estradiol+Etonogestrel

Comment: The vaginal ring should be inserted prior to, or on 5th day, of the menstrual cycle. Use of a backup method is recommended during the first week. When switching from oral contraceptives, the vaginal ring should be inserted anytime within 7 days after the last active tablet and no later than the day a new pill pack would have been started (no backup method is needed). If the ring is accidently expelled for less than 3 hours, it should be rinsed with cool to lukewarm water and reinserted promptly. If ring removal lasts for more than 3 hours, an additional contraceptive method should be used. If the ring is lost, a new ring should be inserted and the regimen continued without alteration.

▶ ***etonogestrel+ethinyl estradiol*** (X) insert 1 ring vaginally and leave in place for 3 weeks; then remove for 1 ring-free week; then repeat

NuvaRing *Vag ring: eth est* 15 mcg/*eton* 120 mcg per day (1, 3/pck)

APPENDIX E.8. SUBDERMAL CONTRACEPTIVES

Comment: Implants must be inserted within 7 days of the onset of menses. A complete physical examination is required annually. Remove if pregnancy, thromboembolic disorder including thrombophlebitis, jaundice, visual disturbances. Not for use by patients with hypertension, diabetes, hyperlipidemia, impaired liver function, epilepsy, asthma, migraine, depression, cardiac or renal insufficiency, thromboembolic disorder including thrombophlebitis, prolonged immobilization, or who are smokers.

▶ ***etonogestrel*** (X) implant rod subdermally in the upper inner non-dominant arm; remove and replace at the end of 3 years

Implanon, Nexplanon

Implantable rod: 68 mg implant for subdermal insertion (w. insertion device; latex-free)

▶ ***levonorgestrel*** (X) implant rods subdermally in the upper inner non-dominant arm; remove and replace at the end of 5 years

Norplant

Implantable rods: 6-36 mg implants (total 216 mg) for subdermal insertion (1 kit w. sterile supplies)

APPENDIX E.9. INTRAUTERINE CONTRACEPTIVES

Comment: Indicated in females who have had at least one child and who are in a stable, mutually monogamous relationship. Re-examine after menses within 3 months (recommend 4-6 weeks) to check placement.

▶ ***levonorgestrel*** (X)

Kyleena *IUD:* 19.5 mg (replace at least every 5 years)
Liletta *IUD:* 52 mg (replace at least every 3 years)
Mirena *IUD:* 52 mg (replace at least every 5 years)
Skyla *IUD:* 13.5 mg (replace at least every 3 years)

(*continued*)

APPENDIX E.10. EMERGENCY CONTRACEPTION

Comment: Emergency contraception must be started within 72 hours after unprotected intercourse following a negative urine hCG pregnancy test. If vomiting occurs within 1 hour of taking a dose, repeat the dose.

▷ ***ethinyl estradiol+levonorgestrel*** **(X)** 2 tabs as soon as possible after unprotected intercourse or contraceptive failure, then 2 more 12 hours after first dose
Premenarchal: not applicable
Preven *Tab: eth est* 50 mcg+*lev* 250 mcg (4/pck)+*Pregnancy test:* 1 hCG home pregnancy test
Yuzpe Regimen *Tab: eth est* 50 mcg+*lev* 250 mcg (4/pck)

▷ ***levonorgestrel*** **(X)(OTC)(G)** take 1 tab as soon as possible, within 72 hours, after unprotected sex or suspected contraceptive failure
Premenarchal: not applicable; <17 years-of-age (prescription required); ≥17 years-of-age (OTC)
My Way *Tab:* 1.5 mg (1/pck)
Plan B One Step
Tab: 1.5 mg (1/pck)
EContra EZ take 1 tab within 72 hours after unprotected sex or suspected contraceptive failure
Tab: 1.5 mg (1/pck)

▷ ***ulipristal*** **(X)(G)** take 1 tab as soon as possible within 120 hours (5 days) after unprotected sex or contraceptive failure; may repeat dose if vomiting occurs within 3 hours
Premenarchal: not applicable
Ella
Tab: 30 mg (1/pck)
Logilia *Tab:* 30 mg (1/pck)

APPENDIX F. NSAIDs

Comment: NSAIDs should be taken with food to decrease gastric upset. Dosing of NSAIDs should be scheduled rather than PRN for maximal benefit. NSAIDs are contraindicated with sulfonamide or ***aspirin*** allergy, 3rd trimester pregnancy (causes premature closure of the ductus arteriosus), and coronary artery bypass graft (CABG) surgery. Concomitant use of ***misoprostol*** **(Cytotec)** with NSAIDs reduces gastric upset and potential for ulceration; however, ***misoprostol*** is pregnancy category X. Administration of ***misoprostol*** in pregnancy can cause spontaneous abortion, premature birth, birth defects, and uterine rupture (beyond the 8th week of pregnancy). NSAIDs and ***warfarin*** **(Coumadin)** are synergistic. With all patients, use the lowest effective dose for the shortest time necessary. NSAIDs should be taken with food to reduce the risk of gastrointestinal adverse side effects (GIASE).

Legend: GI Adverse Side Effects:
(+) mild; (++) frequent; (+++) more frequent/severe

(*continued*)

(*continued*)

▶ ***celecoxib*** **(C/D)(G)(+)** <2 years: not recommended; 2-12 years, >10-<25 kg: 50 mg bid;≥25 kg: 100 mg once daily; >12 years: 100 mg bid or 200 mg once daily or 200 mg bid or 400 mg once daily; <50 kg, start at lowest dose
Celebrex *Cap:* 50, 100, 200, 400 mg

▶ ***diclofenac potassium*** **(C/D)(G)(+++)** <12 years: not recommended; ≥12 years: 50 mg tid or qid or 25 mg tid or qid and may add 25 mg at HS
Cataflam *Tab:* 50 mg
Zipsor *Gel cap:* 25 mg

▶ ***diclofenac sodium*** **(D)(+++)** <12 years: not recommended; ≥12 years:
Dyloject administer 37.5 mg IV bolus over 15 seconds q 6 hours; max 150 mg/day
Vial: 37.5 mg/ml (25/box)
Pennsaid 1% in 10 drop increments, dispense and rub into front, side, and back of knee: usually 40 drops (40 mg) qid
Topical soln: 1.5% (150 ml)
Pennsaid 2% apply 2 pump actuations (40 mg) and rub into front, side, and back of knee bid
Topical soln: 2% (20 mg/pump actuation; 112 gm)
Solaraze Gel apply to affected areas bid
Gel: 3% (30 mg (100 gm)
Voltaren 50 mg bid or qid or 75 mg bid or 25 mg qid with an additional 25 mg at HS if necessary
Tab: 25, 50, 75 mg ent-coat
Voltaren XR 100 mg once daily; rarely, 100 mg bid may be used
Tab: 100 mg ext-rel
Zorvolex 35 mg tid
Gelcap: 18, 35 mg ext-rel

▶ ***diclofenac sodium*** plus ***misoprostol*** **(X)(++)** <18 years: not recommended; ≥18 years: 50-75 mg bid
Arthrotec *Tab:* 50, 75 mg

▶ ***diflunisal*** **(C/D)(G)(+++)** <12 years: not recommended; >12 years: initially 1 gm as a single dose followed by 500 mg q 8-12 hours or 500 mg as a single dose followed by 250 mg q 8-12 hours
Dolobid *Tab:* 500*mg

▶ ***etodolac*** **(C/D)(G)(+)** <12 years: not recommended; ≥12 years:
Lodine initially 600 mg to 1 gm/day in 2-3 divided doses; usual max 1 gm/day in divided doses; may increase to 1.2 gm/day when needed
Tab: 400, 500 mg; *Cap:* 200, 300 mg
Lodine XL 400 mg to 1 gm once daily; max 1.2 gm/day
Tab: 400, 500, 600 mg ext-rel

▶ ***fenoprofen*** **(B/D)(++)** <12 years: not recommended; ≥12 years: 300-600 mg tid-qid; max 3.2 gm/day
Nalfon *Tab:* 200 mg

(*continued*)

(*continued*)

▶ ***flurbiprofen*** (B/D)(G)(++) <12 years: not recommended; ≥12 years: 200-300 mg/day in 2-4 divided doses; max single dose 100 mg; reduce dosage for renal impairment
Ansaid *Tab:* 50, 100 mg

▶ ***ibuprofen+famotidine*** (B/D)(++) <12 years: not recommended; ≥12 years: 1 tab tid; swallow whole; use lowest effective dose for the shortest duration
Duexis *Tab: ibu* 800 mg/*fam* 26.6 mg

▶ ***indomethacin*** (B/D)(G)(+++) <14 years: not recommended; ≥14 years: 75-100 mg daily in 3-4 divided doses; max 200 mg/day
Indocin *Cap:* 25, 50 mg; *Rectal supp:* 50 mg; *Oral susp:* 25 mg/5 ml; *Vial:* 1 mg pwdr for reconstitution
Indocin SR *Cap:* 75 mg ext-rel
Tivorbex *Cap:* 20, 40 mg

▶ ***ketoprofen*** (C/D)(G)(++) <18 years: not recommended; ≥18 years: 75 mg tid <u>or</u> 50 mg qid; max 300 mg/day
Orudis *Cap:* 50, 75 mg
Oruvail *Cap:* 100, 150, 200 mg ext-rel

▶ ***ketorolac tromethamine*** (C/D)(G)(+++)
Sprix <17 years: not recommended; ≥17 years: 1 spray each nostril (total dose 31.5 mg) every 6-8 hours prn; max 4 doses/24 hours (total daily dose 126 mg); *renal impairment* <u>or</u> *<50 kg:* 1 spray in one nostril (total dose 15.75 mg) every 6-8 hours; max 4 doses/24 hours (63 mg); discard used bottle after 24 hours
Nasal spray: 15.75 mg/100 mcl nasal spray (8 sprays, 1.7 gm)
Toradol <17 years: not recommended; ≥17 years: 60 mg as a single IM dose; max 30 mg as a single IV dose; may administer 30 mg IV and 30 mg IM as a single dose; oral dosing is indicated <u>*only*</u> as continuation therapy to IM <u>or</u> IV dosing; oral formulation should <u>*never*</u> be administered as an initial dose; initiate oral dosing at 20 mg followed by 10 mg q 4-6 hours prn; max oral dosing 40 mg/day; the combined duration of IV/IM/PO dosing is not to exceed 5 days
Tab: 10 mg; *Inj* 15, 30, 60 mg/ml

▶ ***magnesium chol salicylate*** (C/D)(G)(+) <12 kg: not recommended; 12-37 kg: 50 mg/kg/day in 2 divided doses; >37 kg: 2.25 gm/day in 2 divided doses; ≥18 years: 3 gm daily at bedtime <u>or</u> in 2 divided doses
Trilisate *Tab:* 500*, 750*mg; 1*gm; *Oral susp:* 5 mg/5 ml (cherry cordial)

▶ ***meclofenamate sodium*** (B/D)(G)(++) <14 years: not recommended; ≥14 years: 50-100 mg q 4-6 hours <u>or</u> 300-400 mg/day in 3-4 equal doses; max 400 mg/day
Meclofen *Cap:* 50, 100 mg

▶ ***mefenamic acid*** (C)(G)(++) <14 years: not recommended; ≥14 years: 500 mg once; then, 250 mg q 6 hours
Ponstel *Cap:* 250 mg

▶ ***meloxicam*** (C/D)(G)(+) <2 years: not recommended; ≥2-14 years: years: 0.125 mg/kg; max 7.5 mg once daily; >14 years: 7.5-15 mg once daily; max 15 mg/day; hemodialysis max 7.5 mg/day
Mobic *Tab:* 7.5, 15 mg; *Oral susp:* 7.5 mg/5 ml (100 ml) (raspberry)

(*continued*)

(*continued*)

➢ ***nabumetone*** (C/D)(G)(+) <12 years: not recommended; ≥12 years: 1-2 gm/day in a single dose or 2 divided doses; max 2 gm/day; <50 kg: max 1 gm/day
Tab: 500, 750 mg

➢ ***naproxen*** (B)(G)(++) <2 years: not recommended; ≥2-12 years: 5 mg/kg bid; max 15 mg/kg/day has been used; use suspension; 275-550 mg bid or 275 mg every 6-8 hours; max 1.375 gm first day; then, max 1.1 gm/day; *Acute gout:* 825 mg once, then 275 mg every 8 hours
Naprosyn *Tab:* 250, 375, 500 mg
Naprosyn Suspension *Oral susp:* 125 mg/5 ml

➢ ***naproxen+esomeprazole (as magnesium trihydrate)*** (C/D)(++)(G) <18 years: not recommended; ≥18 years: one 375/20 or one 500/20 tab bid; take at least 30 minutes before meals; take lowest effective dose
Vimovo 375/20 *Tab: nap* 375 mg/*eso* 20 mg
Vimovo 500/20 *Tab: nap* 500 mg/*eso* 20 mg

➢ ***oxaprozin*** (C/D)(++) <6 years: not recommended; 6-16 years, 21-31 kg: 600 mg once daily; 32-54 kg: 900 mg once daily; ≥55 kg: 1.2 gm once daily; >16 years: 1.2 gm once daily; max 1.8 gm or 26 mg/kg, whichever is less, in divided doses; low body weight, milder disease, or on dialysis: initially 600 mg once daily; max 1.2 gm/day
Daypro *Tab:* 600*

➢ ***piroxicam*** (C/D)(G)(+++) <12 years: not recommended; ≥12 years: 20 mg once daily
Feldene *Cap:* 10, 20 mg
Comment: Because of the long half-life, steady state blood levels of ***piroxicam*** are not reached for 7-12 days. Therefore, expect a progressive response over several weeks.

➢ ***salsalate*** (C/D)(G)(+) <12 years: not recommended; ≥12 years: 1.5 gm bid or 1 gm tid
Tab: 500*, 750*mg; *Cap:* 500 mg

➢ ***sulindac*** (B/D)(G)(+++) <18 years: not recommended; ≥18 years: 150-200 mg bid; max 400 mg/day; usually x 7-14 days
Tab: 150*, 200*mg

➢ ***tolmetin*** (C/D)(G)(+++) <2 years: not recommended; ≥2 years: 20 mg/kg divided tid to qid; usual range 15-30 mg/kg/day divided tid to qid: max 30 mg/kg/day initially 400 mg tid; usual range 600 mg to 1.8 gm/day in divided doses; max 1,800 mg/day
Tab: 200*mg

APPENDIX G. GLUCOCORTICOSTEROIDS

APPENDIX G.1. TOPICAL STEROIDS BY POTENCY

Comment: All topical, oral, and parenteral corticosteroids are pregnancy category C. Use with caution in infants and children. Steroids should be applied sparingly and for the shortest time necessary. Do not use in the diaper area. Do not use an occlusive dressing.

(*continued*)

(*continued*)

Systemic absorption of topical corticosteroids can induce reversible hypothalamic-pituitary-adrenal (HPA) axis suppression with the potential for clinical glucocorticoid insufficiency.

Potency guide: Face: Low potency
- Ears/scalp margin: Intermediate potency
- Eyelids: Hydrocortisone in ophthalmic ointment base 1%
- Chest/back: Intermediate potency
- Skin folds: Low potency

Generic	Brand/Formulation/ Frequency	Strength/Volume
Low Potency		
alclometasone dipropionate (C)	**Aclovate** Crm bid-tid **Aclovate** Oint bid-tid	0.05% (15, 45, 60 gm) 0.05% (15, 45, 60 gm)
fluocinolone acetonide (C)	**Synalar** Crm bid-qid	0.025% (15, 60 gm)
hydrocortisone base or *acetate* (C)(G)	**Anusol-HC** Crm bid-qid **Hytone** Crm bid-qid **Hytone** Oint bid-qid **Hytone** Lotn bid-qid **Hytone** Crm bid-qid **Hytone** Oint bid-qid **Hytone** Lotn bid-qid **U-cort** Crm bid-qid	2.5% (30 gm) 1% (1, 2 oz) 1% (1 oz) 1% (2 oz) 2.5% (1, 2 oz) 2.5% (1 oz) 2.5% (1 oz) 1% (7, 28, 35 gm)
triamcinolone acetonide (C)(G)	**Kenalog** Crm bid-qid **Kenalog** Lotn bid-qid **Kenalog** Oint bid-qid	0.025% (15, 80 gm) 0.025% (60 ml) 0.025% (15, 60, 80 gm)
Intermediate Potency		
betamethasone valerate (C)(G)	**Luxiq** Foam bid	0.12% (100 gm)
clocortolone pivalate (C)	**Cloderm** Crm tid	0.1% (30, 45, 75, 90 gm)
desonide (C)(G)	**Desonate** Gel/Formulation bid-tid **DesOwen** Crm bid-tid **DesOwen** Lotn bid-tid **DesOwen** Oint bid-tid **Tridesilon** Crm bid-qid **Tridesilon** Oint bid-qid **Verdeso** Foam	0.05% (15, 60 gm) 0.05% (15, 60 gm) 0.05% (2, 4 fl oz) 0.05% (15, 60 gm) 0.05% (15, 60 gm) 0.05% (15, 60 gm)
desoximetasone (C)(G)	**Topicort-LP** Emol Crm bid	0.05% (15, 60 gm, 4 oz)

(*continued*)

(*continued*)

Generic	Brand/Formulation/ Frequency	Strength/Volume
fluocinolone acetonide **(C)(G)**	**Capex** Shampoo **Derma-Smoothe/FS** Oil tid **Derma-Smoothe/FS** Shampoo **Synalar** Crm bid-qid **Synalar** Oint bid-qid	0.01% (4 oz) 0.01% (4 oz) 0.01% (4 oz) 0.025% (15, 30, 60 gm) 0.025% (15, 60 gm)
flurandrenolide **(C)(G)**	**Cordran-SP** Crm bid to tid **Cordran** Oint bid-tid **Cordran-SP** Crm bid-tid **Cordran** Lotn bid-tid **Cordran** Oint bid-tid	0.025% (30, 60 gm) 0.025% (30, 60 gm) 0.05% (15, 30, 60 gm) 0.05% (15, 60 ml) 0.05% (15, 30, 60 gm)
fluticasone propionate **(C)(G)**	**Cutivate** Oint bid **Cutivate** Crm qd-bid **Cutivate** Lotn qd-bid	0.005% (15, 30, 60 gm) 0.05% (15, 30, 60 gm) 0.05%
hydrocortisone probutate **(C)**	**Pandel** Crm qd-bid	0.1% (15, 45 gm)
hydrocortisone butyrate **(C)(G)**	**Locoid** Crm bid-tid **Locoid** Oint bid-tid **Locoid** Soln bid-tid	0.1% (15, 45 g) 0.1% (15, 45 gm) 0.1% (30, 60 ml)
hydrocortisone valerate **(C)(G)**	**Westcort** Crm bid-tid **Westcort** Oint bid-tid	0.2% (15, 45, 60, 120 gm) 0.2% (15, 45, 60 gm)
mometasone furoate **(C)**	**Elocon** Crm qd **Elocon** Lotn qd **Elocon** Oint qd	0.1% (15, 45 gm) 0.1% (30, 60 ml) 0.1% (15, 45 gm)
prednicarbate **(C)**	**Dermatop** Emol Crm bid **Dermatop** Oint bid	0.1% (15, 60 gm)
triamcinolone acetonide **(C)(G)**	**Kenalog** Crm bid-tid **Kenalog** Lotn bid-tid **Kenalog** Emul Spray bid-tid	0.1% (15, 60, 80 gm) 0.1% (60 ml) 0.2% (63, 100 gm)
High Potency		
amcinonide **(C)(G)**	Crm bid-tid Lotn bid Oint bid	0.1% (15, 30, 60 gm) 0.1% (20, 60 ml) 0.1% (15, 30, 60 gm)
betamethasone dipropionate **(C)**	**Sernivo Spray** Emul Spray bid	0.05% (60, 120 ml)

(*continued*)

(*continued*)

Generic	Brand/Formulation/ Frequency	Strength/Volume
betamethasone dipropionate, augmented **(C)**	**Diprolene AF** Emol Crm qd-bid **Diprolene** Lotn qd-bid	0.05% (15, 50 gm) 0.05% (30, 60 ml)
desoximetasone **(C)(G)**	**Topicort** Spray bid **Topicort** Gel bid **Topicort** Emol Crm bid **Topicort** Oint bid	0.25% (30, 50, 100 ml) 0.05% (15, 60 gm) 0.25% (15, 60 gm) 0.25% (15, 60 gm)
diflorasone diacetate **(C)**	**Psorcon e** Emol Crm bid **Psorcon e** Emol Oint qd-tid	0.05% (15, 30, 60 gm) 0.05% (15, 30, 60 gm)
fluocinonide **(C)**	**Lidex** Crm bid-qid **Lidex** Gel bid-qid **Lidex** Oint bid-qid **Lidex** Soln bid-qid **Lidex-E** Emol Crm bid-qid	0.05% (15, 30, 60, 120 gm) 0.05% (15, 30, 60 gm) 0.05% (15, 30, 60, 120 gm) 0.05% (20, 60 ml) 0.05% (15, 30, 60 gm)
flurandrenolide **(C)**	**Cordran** Oint bid-tid **Cordran** Crm bid-tid	0.05% (15, 30, 60 gm) 0.025% (30, 60, 120 gm) 0.05% (15, 30, 60, 120 gm)
halcinonide **(C)**	**Halog** Crm bid-tid **Halog** Oint bid-tid **Halog** Soln bid-tid **Halog-E** Emol Crm qd-tid	0.1% (15, 30, 60, 240 gm) 0.1% (15, 30, 60, 120 gm) 0.1% (20, 60 ml) 0.1% (15, 30, 60 gm)
triamcinolone acetonide **(C)(G)**	**Kenalog** Crm bid-tid	0.5% (20 gm)
Super High Potency		
betamethasone dipropionate, augmented **(C)**	**Diprolene** Oint qd-bid **Diprolene** Gel qd-bid	0.05% (15, 50 gm) 0.05% (15, 50 gm)
clobetasol propionate **(C)(G)**	**Clobex** Shampoo daily **Clobex** Spray bid **Cormax** Oint bid **Cormax** Scalp App **Olux** Foam **Olux E** Foam **Temovate** Crm bid	0.05% (4 oz) 0.05% (2, 4.5 oz) 0.05% (15, 45 gm) 0.05% (15, 45 gm) 0.05% (50, 100 gm) 0.05% (50, 100 gm) 0.05% (15, 30, 45, 60 gm)

(*continued*)

(*continued*)

Generic	Brand/Formulation/ Frequency	Strength/Volume
	Temovate Gel bid **Temovate** Oint bid **Temovate Scalp** App bid **Temovate-E** Emol Crm bid	0.05% (15, 30, 60 gm) 0.05% (15, 30, 45, 60 gm) 0.05% (25, 50 ml) 0.05% (15, 30, 60 gm)
fluocinonide **(C)(G)**	**Vanos** Oint qd-tid	0.1% (30, 60, 120 gm)
flurandrenolide **(C)**	**Cordran** Tape q 12 hours	4 mcg/sq cm (roll of 3″ x 80″)
halobetasol propionate **(C)**	**Ultravate** Crm qd-bid **Ultravate** Oint qd to bid	0.05% (15, 45 gm) 0.05% (15, 45 gm)

APPENDIX G.2. ORAL STEROIDS

Comment: Systemic corticosteroids increase glucose intolerance, reduce the action of insulin and oral hypoglycemic agents, reduce adrenal cortex activity, decrease immunity, mask signs of infection, impair wound healing, suppress growth in children, and promote osteoporosis, fluid retention, and weight gain. Use systemic steroids with caution, using the lowest possible dose to affect clinical response, and withdraw (wean) gradually in tapering doses to avoid adrenal insufficiency. The American Academy of Rheumatology (AAR) recommends the following daily doses of ***calcium*** and ***vitamin D*** for anyone on a chronic systemic corticosteroid regimen: ***calcium*** 1,200-1,500 mg/day and ***vitamin D*** 800-1,000 IU/day.

▶ ***betamethasone*** (C)(G) initially 0.6-7.2 mg daily
  Celestone *Tab:* 0.6 mg; *Syr:* 0.6 mg/5 ml (120 ml)

▶ ***cortisone*** (D)(G) <12 years: not recommended; ≥12 years: initially 25-300 mg daily or every other day
  Cortone Acetate *Tab:* 25 mg

▶ ***dexamethasone*** (C)(G)<12 years: not recommended; ≥12 years: initially 0.75-9 mg/day
  Decadron *Tab:* 0.5*, 0.75*, 4*mg; *Syr:* 0.5 mg/5 ml (100 ml)
  Decadron 5-12 Pak *Tabs:* 0.75*mg (12/pck)

▶ ***hydrocortisone*** (C)(G) <12 years: 2-8 mg/day; ≥12 years: 20-240 mg/daily
  Cortef *Tab:* 5, 10, 20 mg; *Oral susp:* 10 mg/5 ml
  Hydrocortone *Tab:* 10 mg

▶ ***methylprednisolone*** (C)(G) 4-48 mg/day
  Medrol *Tab:* 2*, 4*, 8*, 16*, 24*, 32*mg
  Medrol Dosepak *Dosepak:* 4*mg tabs (21/pck, 42 pck)

▶ ***prednisolone*** (C)(G) <12 years: 0.14-2 mg/kg/day in 3-4 doses x 3-5 days; ≥12 years: initially 5-60 mg/day in 1-2 doses x 3-5 days
  Flo-Pred *Susp:* 5, 15 mg/5 ml

(*continued*)

(*continued*)

Orapred *Soln:* 15 mg/5 ml (grape) (dye-free, alcohol 2%)
Orapred ODT *Tab:* 10, 15, 30 mg orally disint (grape)
Pediapred *Soln:* 5 mg/5 ml (raspberry) (sugar-, alcohol-, dye-free)
Prelone *Syr:* 15 mg/5 ml

Comment: **Flo-Pred** does not require refrigeration or shaking prior to use.

➢ ***prednisone*** **(C)(G)** <12 years: 0.14-2 mg/kg/day in 3-4 doses x 3-5 days; >12 years: initially 5-60 mg/day in 1-2 doses x 3-5 days
Deltasone *Tab:* 2.5*, 5*, 10*, 20*, 50*mg

➢ ***prednisone (delayed release)*** **(C)(G)** <12 years: 0.14-**2 mg**/kg/day in 3-4 divided doses x 3-5 days; ≥12 years: initially 5-60 mg/day in 1-2 doses x 3-5 days
RAYOS *Tab:* 1, 2, 5 mg del-rel

➢ ***triamcinolone*** **(C)(G)** <12 years: 0.14-2 mg/kg/day in 3-4 divided doses x 3-5 days; ≥12 years: initially 4-48 mg/day in 1-2 divided doses x 3-5 days
Aristocort *Tab:* 4*mg
Aristocort Forte *Susp:* 40 mg/ml (benzoyl alcohol)
Aristocort Aristopak *Tab:* 4*mg (16/pck)

APPENDIX G.3. PARENTERAL STEROIDS

➢ ***betamethasone*** **(C)(G)**
Celestone 0.5-9 mg IM/IV x 1 dose
Vial: 3 mg/ml (10 ml)
Celestone Sol span 0.5-9 mg IM/IV x 1 dose; usual IM dose 6 mg
Vial: 6 mg/ml (10 ml)

➢ ***cortisone*** **(D)(G)** <12 years: not recommended;≥12 years: 20-300 mg IM
Cortone Acetate *Vial:* 50 mg/ml (10 ml)

➢ ***dexamethasone*** **(C)(G)** initially 0.5-9 mg IM/IV daily
Decadron *Vial:* 4, 24 mg/ml for IM use (5 ml) (sulfites)
Dalalone D.P. *Vial:* 16 mg/ml (1, 5 ml)
Decadron-LA *Vial:* 8 mg/ml (1, 5 ml)

➢ ***hydrocortisone*** **(C)(G)** <12 years: 2-8 mg/kg loading dose (max 250 mg); then 8 mg/kg/day: >12 years: initially 100-500 mg IM/IV daily
Hydrocortone *Vial:* 50 mg/ml (5 ml)
Solu-Cortef *Vial:* 100 mg (2 ml); 250 mg (2 ml); 500 mg (4 ml); 1 gm (8 ml)

➢ ***hydrocortisone phosphate*** **(C)(G)** for IM, IV, and SC injection
Hydrocortone *Vial:* 50 mg/ml (2 ml)

➢ ***methylprednisolone*** **(C)(G)** 40-120 mg IM/week for 1-4 weeks
Depo-Medrol *Vial:* 20 mg/ml (5 ml); 40 mg/ml (5, 10 ml); 80 mg/ml (5 ml)

➢ ***methylprednisolone sodium succinate*** **(C)(G)** <12 years: 1-2 mg/kg loading dose; then 1.6 mg/kg/day in divided doses at least 6 hours apart; ≥12 years: 10-40 mg IV initially; then, IM or IV
Solu-Medrol *Vial:* 40 mg (1 ml), 125 mg (2 ml), 500 mg (4 ml); 1 gm (8 ml); 2 gm (8 ml)

(*continued*)

(*continued*)

▶ *triamcinolone* (C)(G) 40 mg IM/week
Aristocort *Vial:* 25 mg/ml (5 ml)
Aristocort Forte *Vial:* 40 mg/ml (1, 5 ml)*(do* not *administer IV)*
Aristospan *Vial:* 5 mg/ml (5 ml); 20 mg/ml (1, 5 ml)
TAC-3 *Vial:* 3 mg/ml (5 ml) for intralesional and intradermal use

PARENTERAL STEROID+ANESTHETIC

▶ *dexamethasone+lidocaine* (C) 0.1-0.75 ml into painful area
Decadron Phosphate with Xylocaine *Vial:* dexa 4 mg+lido 10 mg per ml (5 ml)

APPENDIX G.4. INHALATIONAL STEROIDS

Comment: Inhaled corticosteroids are indicated for the long-term control of asthma. Inhaled corticosteroids are not indicated for exercise induced asthma or for relief of acute symptoms (i.e., "rescue"). Low doses are indicated for mild persistent asthma, medium doses are indicated for moderate persistent asthma, and high doses are reserved for severe cases. Titrate to lowest effective dose. To reduce the potential for adverse effects with inhalers, the patient should use a spacer or holding chamber and rinse the mouth and spit after every inhalation treatment. Linear growth should be monitored in children. When inhaled doses exceed 1,000 mcg/day, consider supplements of calcium (1-1.5 g/day), vitamin D (400 IU/day).

▶ *beclomethasone* (C)
Beclovent <6 years: not recommended; 6-12 years: 1-2 inhalations tid-qid or 4 inhalations bid; max 10 inhalations/day; >12 years: 2 inhalations tid-qid or 4 inhalations bid; max 20 inhalations/day
Inhaler: 42 mcg/actuation (6.7 gm, 80 inh); 16.8 gm (200 inh)
Qvar <12 years: not recommended; ≥12 years: *Previously using only bronchodilators:* initiate 40-80 mcg bid; max 320 mcg/day; *Previously using an inhaled corticosteroid:* initiate 40-160 mcg bid; max 320 mcg/day; *Previously taking a systemic corticosteroid:* attempt to wean off the systemic drug after approximately 1 week after initiating **Qvar**
Inhaler: 40, 80 mcg/actuation metered-dose aerosol w. dose counter (8.7 gm, 120 inh) (CFC-free)
Vanceril <6 years: not recommended; 6-12 years: 1-2 inhalations tid-qid; >12 years: 2 inhalations tid to qid or 4 inhalations bid
Inhaler: 42 mcg/actuation (16.8 gm, 200 inh)
Vanceril Double Strength <6 years: not recommended; 6-12 years: 1-2 inhalations bid; >12 years: 2 inhalations bid
Inhaler: 84 mcg/actuation (12.2 gm, 120 inh)

▶ *budesonide* (B)(G)
Pulmicort Respules use turbuhaler; <12 months: not recommended; ≥12 months-8 years: *Previously using only bronchodilators:* initiate 0.5 mg/day once daily or in 2 divided doses; may start at 0.25 mg/day; *Previously using inhaled corticosteroids:* initiate 0.5 mg/day daily or in 2 divided doses; max 1 mg/day; *Previously using oral corticosteroids:* initiate 1 mg/day daily or in 2 divided doses
Inhal susp: 0.25 mg/2 ml (30/box)

(*continued*)

(*continued*)

Pulmicort Turbuhaler <6 years: not recommended; ≥6-12 years: 1-2 inhalations bid; >12 years: 1-2 inhalations bid; *Previously on oral corticosteroids:* 2-4 inhalations bid

Turbuhaler: 200 mcg/actuation (200 inh)

▷ ***flunisolide*** (C)(G)

AeroBid, AeroBid M <6 years: not recommended; 6-15 years: 2 inhalations bid; ≥16 years: initially 2 inhalations bid; max 8 inhalations/day

Inhaler: 250 mcg/actuation (7 gm, 100 inh)

▷ ***fluticasone*** (C)(G)

Flovent HFA use **Rotadisk**: initially 50-88 mcg inh bid; <4 years: not recommended; 4-11 years: initially 50-88 mcg bid; >11 years: initially 100 mcg bid; *If previously using an inhaled corticosteroid:* initially 100-200 mcg bid; *Previously taking an oral corticosteroid:* initially 1000 mcg bid

Inhaler: 44 mcg/actuation (7.9 gm, 60 inh; 13 gm, 120 inh); 110 mcg/actuation (13 gm, 120 inh); 220 mcg/actuation (13 gm, 120 inh)

Rotadisk ≥11 years: initially 88 mcg bid; *If previously using an inhaled corticosteroid:* initially 88-220 mcg bid; *If previously taking an oral corticosteroid;* initially 880 mcg/day

Rotadisk: 50 mcg/actuation (60 blisters/disk); 100 mcg/actuation (60 blisters/disk); 250 mcg/actuation (60 blisters/disk)

▷ ***mometasone furoate*** (C) <12 years: not recommended; ≥12 years: *Previously using a bronchodilator or inhaled corticosteroid:* 220 mcg q PM or bid; max 440 mcg q PM or 220 mcg bid; *Previously using an oral corticosteroid:* 440 mcg bid; max 880 mcg/day

Asmanex Twisthaler

Inhaler: 220 mcg/actuation (6.7 gm, 80 inh); 16.8 gm (200 inh)

APPENDIX H. ANTIARRHYTHMIC DRUGS

Antiarrhythmics by Classification/Indications and Dose Forms		
Brand/*generic* Pregnancy Category	**Class/Indication(s)**	**Dose Form(s)**
Betapace *sotalol* **(B)**	*Class:* Class II and III Antiarrhythmic *Indications:* Documented life-threatening ventricular arrhythmias	*Tab:* 80*, 120*, 160*, 240*mg
Betapace AF *sotalol* **(B)**	*Class:* Class II and III Antiarrhythmic *Indications:* Maintenance of normal sinus rhythm in patients with highly symptomatic atrial fibrillation or atrial flutter who are currently in sinus rhythm	*Tab:* 80*, 120*, 160*mg

(*continued*)

(*continued*)

Antiarrhythmics by Classification/Indications and Dose Forms		
Brand/*generic* **Pregnancy Category**	**Class/Indication(s)**	**Dose Form(s)**
Calan *verapamil* **(C)(G)**	*Class:* Calcium Channel Blocker *Indications:* Control (with *digitalis*) of ventricular rate in patients with chronic atrial fibrillation or atrial flutter; prophylaxis of repetitive paroxysmal supraventricular tachycardia	*Tab:* 40, 80*, 120*mg
Codarone *amiodarone* **(D)(G)**	*Class:* Class III Antiarrhythmic *Indications:* Documented life-threatening recurrent refractory ventricular fibrillation or hemodynamically unstable ventricular tachycardia	*Tab:* 200*mg
Inderal *propranolol* **(C)(G)** **Inderal XL** *propranolol ext-rel* **(C)(G)** **InnoPran XL** *propranolol ext-rel* **(C)**	*Class:* Beta-Blocker *Indications:* Atrial and ventricular arrhythmias; tachyarrhythmias due to *digitalis* intoxication; reduce mortality and risk of reinfarction in stabilized patients after myocardial infarction	*Tab:* 10*, 20*, 40*, 60*, 80*mg *Cap:* 60, 80, 120, 160 mg sust-rel *Cap:* 80, 120 mg ext-rel
Mexitil *mexiletine* **(C)**	*Class:* Class IB Antiarrhythmic *Indications:* Documented life-threatening ventricular arrhythmias	*Cap:* 150, 200, 250 mg
Multaq *dronedarone* **(C)**	*Class:* IB Antiarrhythmic *Indications:* Paroxysmal or persistent atrial fibrillation or atrial flutter	*Tab:* 400 mg
Nexterone *amiodarone* **(D)(G)**	*Class:* Class III Antiarrhythmic *Indications:* Documented life-threatening recurrent refractory ventricular fibrillation or hemodynamically unstable ventricular tachycardia	*Premixed:* 360 mg/200 ml; *Vial:* 150 mg/3 ml, 450 mg/9 ml, 900/19 ml; *Prefilled syringe:* 150 mg/3 ml;
Norpace *disopyramide* **(C)**	*Class:* Class I Antiarrhythmic *Indications:* Documented life-threatening ventricular arrhythmias	*Cap:* 100, 150 mg

(*continued*)

Antiarrhythmics by Classification/Indications and Dose Forms		
Brand/*generic* Pregnancy Category	**Class/Indication(s)**	**Dose Form(s)**
Pacerone *amiodarone* **(D)(G)**	*Class:* Class III Antiarrhythmic *Indications:* Documented life-threatening recurrent refractory ventricular fibrillation or hemodynamically unstable ventricular tachycardia	*Tab:* 100, 200 mg
Procanbid *procainamide* **(C)(G)**	*Class:* Class IA Antiarrhythmic *Indications:* Life-threatening ventricular arrhythmias	*Tab:* 500, 1000 mg ext-rel
Quinaglute *quinidine gluconate* **(C)(G)**	*Class:* Class I Antiarrhythmic *Indications:* Atrial and ventricular arrhythmias	*Tab:* 324 mg ext-rel
Quinidex *quinidine sulfate* **(C)(G)**	*Class:* Class I Antiarrhythmic *Indications:* Atrial and ventricular arrhythmias	*Tab:* 300 mg ext-rel
Rythmol *propafenone* **(C)(G)**	*Class:* Class IC Antiarrhythmic *Indications:* Documented life-threatening ventricular arrhythmias; prolonged recurrence of paroxysmal atrial fibrillation <u>and/or</u> atrial flutter <u>or</u> paroxysmal supraventricular tachycardia associated with disabling symptoms in patients without structural heart disease	*Tab:* 150*, 225*, 300*mg *Cap:* 225, 325, 425 mg ext-rel
Sectral *acebutolol* **(B)(G)**	*Class:* Beta-Blocker *Indications:* Ventricular arrhythmias	*Cap:* 200, 400 mg
Sotylize *sotalol* **(B)**	*Class:* Class II and III Antiarrhythmic *Indications:* Documented life-threatening ventricular arrhythmias, and highly symptomatic AFlutter/AFib	*Oral soln:* 5 mg/ml
Tambocor *flecainide acetate* **(C)(G)**	*Class:* Class IC Antiarrhythmic *Indications:* Documented life-threatening ventricular arrhythmias; paroxysmal atrial fibrillation <u>and/or</u> atrial flutter <u>or</u> paroxysmal supraventricular tachycardia in patients without structural heart disease	*Tab:* 50, 100*, 150*mg

(*continued*)

(*continued*)

Antiarrhythmics by Classification/Indications and Dose Forms		
Brand/*generic* Pregnancy Category	**Class/Indication(s)**	**Dose Form(s)**
Tenormin *atenolol* **(C)(G)**	*Class:* Beta-Blocker *Indications:* Reduce mortality and in stabilized patients after myocardial infarction	*Tab:* 25, 50, 100 mg *Inj:* 5 mg/10 ml for IV administration
timolol maleate **(C)(G)**	*Class:* Beta-Blocker *Indications:* Reduce mortality and in stabilized patients after myocardial infarction	*Tab:* 5, 10*, 20*mg
dofetilide **(C)(G)**	*Class:* Class III Antiarrhythmic *Indications:* Maintenance of normal sinus rhythm in patients with atrial fibrillation or atrial flutter of >1 week duration who were converted to normal sinus rhythm (only for highly symptomatic patients); conversion to normal sinus rhythm	*Cap:* 125, 250, 500 mcg
Tonocard *tocainide* **(C)(G)**	*Class:* Class I Antiarrhythmic *Indications:* Documented life-threatening ventricular arrhythmias	*Tab:* 400*, 600*mg
Toprol XL *metoprolol* **(C)(G)**	*Class:* Beta-Blocker *Indications:* Ischemic, hypertensive, or cardiomyopathic heart failure	*Tab:* 25*, 50*, 100*, 200*mg

APPENDIX I. ANTINEOPLASIA DRUGS

Antineoplasia Drugs with Classification and Dose Forms		
Brand/*generic* Pregnancy Category	**Class/Indications**	**Dose Forms**
Alecensa *alectinib*	Kinase Inhibitor	*Cap: 150 mg*
Aliqopa *copanlisib*	Kinase Inhibitor	*Vial: 60 mg pwdr for injection, single dose*
Alkeran (D)(G) *melphalan*	Alkylating Agent	*Tab:* 2*mg
Alunbrig *brigatinib*	Kinase Inhibitor	*Tab:* 30, 90 mg

(*continued*)

(*continued*)

Antineoplasia Drugs with Classification and Dose Forms		
Brand/*generic* Pregnancy Category	**Class/Indications**	**Dose Forms**
Arimidex (D) *anastrozole*	Aromatase Inhibitor	*Tab:* 1 mg
Aromasin (D) *exemestane*	Aromatase Inactivator	*Tab:* 25 mg
Arranon (D) *nelarabine*	Nucleoside Analog	*Vial:* 250 mg for IV infusion
Bavencio *avelumab*	Programmed Death Ligand-1 (PD-L1) Blocking Antibody	*Vial:* 200 mg/10 ml (20 mg/ml), single-dose)
Bevyxxa *betrixiban*	Factor Xa (FXa) Inhibitor	*Cap:* 40, 80 mg
Blincyto *blinatumomab*	**Bispecific CD19-directed CD3 T-cell Engager**	*Vial:* 35 mcg pwdr for reconstitution, single-dose.
Cabometyx *cabozantinib*	Kinase Inhibitor	*Cap: 20, 40, 60 mg*
Calquence *acalabrutinib*	Kinase Inhibitor	*Cap: 100 mg*
Casodex (X) *bicalutamide*	Antiandrogen	*Tab:* 50 mg
Clolar (G) *clofarabine*	Purine Nucleoside Metabolic Inhibitor	*Vial: 20 mg/20 ml single-dose*
Cytoxan *cyclophosphamide* **(D)**	Alkylating Agent	*Tab:* 25, 50 mg
Daralex *daratumumab*	Human CD38-directed Monoclonal Antibody	*Vial:* 100 mg/5 ml, 400 mg/20 ml, single-dose
Taxotere *Docetaxel*		*Vial:* 20 mg/2 ml (10 mg/ml) single-dose; 80 mg/8 ml (10 mg/ml), 160 mg/10 ml (10 mg/ml) multi-dose
Eligard *leuprolide acetate* **(X)**	GnRH Analog	*Inj:* 7.5 mg ext-rel per monthly SC injection
Endari *L-glutamine*	Amino Acid	*Oral Pwdr*: 5 grams of L-glutamine pwdr per paper-foil-plastic laminate pkt

(*continued*)

(*continued*)

Antineoplasia Drugs with Classification and Dose Forms		
Brand/*generic* Pregnancy Category	**Class/Indications**	**Dose Forms**
Eulexin (D) *flutamide*	Antiandrogen	*Cap:* 125 mg
Faslodex (D)(G) *fulvestrant*	Estrogen Receptor Antagonist	*Prefilled syringe for IM inj:* 50 mg/ml (2.5, 5 ml/syringe)
Femara (D) *letrozole*	Aromatase Inhibitor	*Tab:* 2.5 mg
Gleevec (D) *imatinib mesylate*	Signal Transduction Inhibitor	*Cap:* 100 mg
Hydrea (D)(G) *hydroxyurea*	Substituted Urea	*Cap:* 500 mg
Ibrance *palbociclib*	Kinase Inhibitor	*Cap:* 75, 100, 150 mg
Imbruvica *imbrutinib*	Kinase Inhibitor	*Tab:* 140 mg
Imfinzi *durvalumab*	Programmed Death Ligand-1 (PD-L1) Blocking Antibody	*Vial:* 120 mg/2.4 ml (50 mg/ml, single-dose; 500 mg/10 ml (50 mg/ml, single-dose)
Idhifa *enasidenib*	Isocitrate Dehydrogenase-2 Inhibitor	*Tab:* 50, 100 mg
Iressa (D) *gefitinib*	Epidermal Growth Factor receptor tyrosine kinase inhibitor	*Tab:* 250 mg
Keytruda *pembrolizumab*	Programmed Death Receptor-1 (PD-1)-Blocking Antibody	*Vial:* 50 mg, single-dose for reconstitution; 100 mg/4 ml (25 mg/ml, single dose
Kisquali Femara Co-Pack *ribocyclib+letrozole*	Cyclin-dependent Kinase Inhibitor/Aromatase Inhibitor	*Tab:* 600/2.5, 400/2.5, 200/2.5 mg
Kymriah *tisagenlecleucel*	CD19-directed Genetically Modified Autologous T cell Immunotherapy	*IV bag:* frozen suspension for IV infusion after thawing
Kyprolis *carfilzomib*	Protease Inhibitor	*Vial: 30, 60 mg, single-dose, pwdr for reconstitution*

(*continued*)

(*continued*)

Antineoplasia Drugs with Classification and Dose Forms		
Brand/*generic* Pregnancy Category	**Class/Indications**	**Dose Forms**
Lartruvo *olaratumab*	Platelet-derived Growth Factor Receptor Alpha (PDGFR-α) Blocking Antibody	*Vial:* 500 mg/50 ml (10 mg/ ml, single-dose)
Lemvina *lenvatinib*	Kinase Inhibitor	*Cap:* 4, 10 mg
Leukeran (D)(G) *chlorambucil*	Alkylating Agent	*Tab:* 2 mg
Lupron (X) *leuprolide*	GnRH Analog	*Susp for IM inj:* 1 mg (daily); 7.5 mg depot (monthly); 22.5 mg depot (every 3 months); 30 mg depot (every 4 months)
Lynparza *olaparib*	Poly (ADP-ribose) Polymerase (PARP)-Inhibitor	*Tab:* 100, 150 mg
Megace, Megace Oral Suspension, Megace ES (D)(G) *megestrol acetate*	Progestin	*Tab:* 20*, 40*mg; *Susp:* 40 mg/ ml; ES concentrate: 125 mg/ml, 625 mg/5 ml
Mekinist *trametinib*	Kinase Inhibitor	*Tab:* 0.5, 2 mg
Nerlynx *neratinib*	Kinase Inhibitor	*Tab:* 40 mg
Nexavar (D) *sorafenib*	Multikinase Inhibitor	*Tab:* 200 mg
Nolvadex (D)(G) *tamoxifen citrate*	Anti-estrogen	*Tab:* 10, 20 mg
Opdivo *nivolumab*	Programmed Death Receptor-1 (PD-1)-Blocking Antibody	*Vial:* 40 mg/4 ml, 100 mg/10 ml (10 mg/ml, single dose)
Revlimid *lenalidomide*	Thalidomide Analogue	*Cap:* 2.5, 5, 10, 15, 20, 25 mg
Responsa *inotuzumab ozogamicin*	CD22-directed Antibody-Drug Conjugade (ADC)	*Vial: 0.9 mg, single-dose, for reconstitution*

(*continued*)

(*continued*)

Antineoplasia Drugs with Classification and Dose Forms		
Brand/*generic* Pregnancy Category	**Class/Indications**	**Dose Forms**
Rituxan Hyclea *rituximab+ hyaluronidase*	Combination of *rituximab*, a CD20-Directed Cytolytic Antibody and *hyaluronidase human*, an endoglycosidase	*Vial:* 1,400 mg *rituximab* and 23,400 Units *hyaluronidase human* per 11.7 ml (120 mg/2,000 Units per ml) single-dose; 1,600 mg *rituximab* and 26,800 Units *hyaluronidase human* per 13.4 ml (120 mg/2,000 Units per ml) single-dose
Rubraca *rucaparib*	Poly ADP-ribose Polymerase (PARP)-Inhibitor	*Tab:* 200, 300 mg
Rydapt *midostaurin*	Kinase Inhibitor	*Tab:* 40 mg
Stivarga *regorafenib*	Kinase Inhibitor	*Tab:* 40 mg
Sutent *sunitinib malate*	Kinase Inhibitor	*Cap: 12.5, 25, 37.5, 50 mg*
Tagrisso *osimertinib*	Kinase Inhibitor	*Tab:* 40, 80 mg
Tarceva (D) *erlotinib*	Kinase Inhibitor	*Tab:* 25, 100, 150 mg
Tecentriq *atezolizumab*	Programmed Death Ligand-1 (PD-L1) Blocking Antibody	*Vial:* 1,200 mg/20 ml (60 mg/ml, single-dose)
Treanda *bendamustine*	Alkylating Agent	*Vial:* 45 mg/0.5 ml, 180 mg/2 ml solution, single dose; 25, 100 mg pwdr for reconstitution, single dose
Vectibix *panitumumab*	Epidermal growth factor receptor (EGFR) antagonist	*Vial:* 100 mg/5 ml, 200 mg/10 ml, 400 mg/20 ml (20 mg/ml, single-use
Velcade (D) *bortezomib*	Proteasome Inhibitor	*Vial:* 3.5 mg (pwdr for IV injection after reconstitution)

(*continued*)

(*continued*)

Antineoplasia Drugs with Classification and Dose Forms		
Brand/*generic* **Pregnancy Category**	**Class/Indications**	**Dose Forms**
Viadur (X) *leuprolide acetate*	GnRH Analog	*SC implant:* 65 mg depot (replace every 12 months)
Vyxeos, *daunorubicin+ cytarabine*	*daunorubicin:* anthracycline topoisomerase inhibitor; *cytarabine:* nucleoside metabolic inhibitor	*Vial: daun 44 mg+cytar 100 mg (pwdr for IV injection after reconstitution)*
Xeloda (D) *capecitabine*	Fluoropyrimidine (prodrug of *5-fluorouracil*)	*Tab:* 150, 500 mg
Yescarta *axicabtagene ciloleucel*	Chimeric Antigen Receptor T Cell (CAR T) Therapy	*Infusion bag: (68 ml)*
Zejula *niraparib*	Poly ADP-ribose Polymerase (PARP)-Inhibitor	*Cap:* 100 mg
Zoladex (D) *goserelin acetate*	GnRH Analog	*SC implant:* 3.6 mg depot (28 days), 10.8 mg depot (3-month)
Zometa (D) *zoledronic acid*	Bisphosphonate	*Vial:* 4 mg pwdr for reconstitution for IV infusion, single dose
Zykadia *ceritinib*	Kinase Inhibitor	*Cap:* 150 mg

APPENDIX J. ANTIPSYCHOSIS DRUGS

Comment: Patients receiving an antipsychotic agent should be monitored closely for the following adverse side effects: neuroleptic malignant syndrome, extrapyramidal reactions, tardive dyskinesia, blood dyscrasias, anticholinergic effects, drowsiness, hypotension, photo-sensitivity, retinopathy, and lowered seizure threshold. Use lower doses for elderly or debilitated patients. Prescriptions should be written for the smallest practical amount. Foods and beverages containing alcohol are contraindicated for patients receiving any psychotropic drug. *Neuroleptic Malignant Syndrome* (NMS) and *Tardive Dyskinesia* (TD) are adverse side effects (ASEs) most often associated with the older antipsychotic drugs. Risk is decreased with the newer "atypical" antipsychotic drugs. However, these syndromes can develop, although

(*continued*)

(*continued*)

much less commonly, after relatively brief treatment periods at low doses. Given these considerations, antipsychotic drugs should be prescribed in a manner that is most likely to minimize the occurrence. NMS, a potentially fatal symptom complex, is characterized by hyperpyrexia, muscle rigidity, altered mental status and evidence of autonomic instability (irregular pulse or blood pressure, tachycardia, diaphoresis, and cardiac dysrhythmia). Additional signs may include elevated creatine phosphokinase (CPK), myoglobinuria (rhabdomyolysis), and acute renal failure (ARF). TD is a syndrome consisting of potentially irreversible, involuntary, dyskinetic movements that can develop in patients with antipsychotic drugs. Characteristics include repetitive involuntary movements, usually of the jaw, lips and tongue, such as grimacing, sticking out the tongue and smacking the lips. Some affected people also experience involuntary movement of the extremities or difficulty breathing. The syndrome may remit, partially or completely, if antipsychotic treatment is withdrawn. If signs and symptoms of NMS and/or TD appear in a patient, management should include immediate discontinuation of antipsychotic drugs and other drugs not essential to concurrent therapy, intensive symptomatic treatment, medical monitoring, and treatment of any concomitant serious medical problems. The risk of developing NMS and/or TD, and the likelihood that either syndrome will become irreversible, is believed to increase as the duration of treatment and the total cumulative dose of antipsychotic drugs administered to the patient increase. The first and only FDA-approved treatment for TD is ***valbenazine*** (**Ingrezza**) (*see page* 440).

ANTIPSYCHOSIS DRUGS WITH DOSE FORMS

▶ ***aripiprazole*** (C)(G)

Abilify *Tab:* 2, 5, 10, 15, 20, 30 mg; *Oral soln:* 1 mg/ml (150 ml) (orange cream) (parabens)

Abilify Discmelt *Tab:* 15 mg orally disintegrating (vanilla) (phenylalanine)

Abilify Maintena *Vial:* 300, 400 mg ext-rel pwdr for IM injection after reconstitution; 300, 400 mg single-dose prefilled dual chamber syringes w. supplies

Aristada *Prefilled syringe:* 441, 662, 882, 1064 mg, ext-rel susp for IM injection, single-dose w. safety needle

▶ ***asenapine*** (C)

Saphris *SL tab:* 2.5, 5, 10 mg

▶ ***brexpiprazole*** (C)

Rexulti *Tab:* 0.25, 0.5, 1, 2, 3, 4 mg

▶ ***bupropion*** (C)

Forfivo XL *Tab:* 450 mg ext-rel

▶ ***cariprazine***

Vraylar *Cap:* 1.5, 3, 4.5, 6 mg

▶ ***chlorpromazine*** (C)(G)

Thorazine *Tab:* 10, 25, 50, 100, 200 mg; *Cap:* 30, 75, 150 mg sust-rel; *Syr:* 10 mg/5 ml (4 oz, orange-custard); *Vial/Amp:* 25 mg/ml (1, 2 ml) (sulfites)

▶ ***clozapine*** (B)(G)

Clozapine ODT (G) *ODT:* 150, 200 mg

Clozaril (G) *Tab:* 25*, 100*mg; *ODT:* 150, 200 mg

FazaClo ODT (G) *ODT:* 12.5, 25, 100, 150, 200 mg (phenylalanine)

Versacloz *Oral susp:* 50 mg/ml (100 ml)

(*continued*)

(*continued*)

▶ ***fluphenazine*** (C)(G)
Prolixin *Tab:* 1, 2.5, 5*, 10 mg (tartrazine); *Conc:* 5 mg/ml (4 oz w. calib dropper) (alcohol 14%); *Elix:* 5 mg/ml (2 oz w. calib dropper) (alcohol 14%); *Vial:* 25 mg/ml (10 ml)

▶ ***fluphenazine decanoate*** (C)(G)
Prolixin Decanoate *Vial:* 25 mg/ml (5 ml) (benzyl alcohol)

▶ ***fluphenazine*** (C)(G)
Prolixin Ethanate *Vial:* 25 mg (5 ml) (benzyl alcohol)

▶ ***fluphenazine decanoate*** (C)(G)
Prolixin Decanoate *Vial:* 25 mg/ml (5 ml) (benzyl alcohol)

▶ ***haloperidol*** (B)(G)
Haldol *Tab:* 0.5*, 1*, 2*, 5*, 10*, 20*mg
Haldol Lactate *Vial:* 5 mg for IM injection, single-dose
Haldol Decanoate *Vial:* 50, 100 mg for IM injection, single-dose

▶ ***iloperidone*** (C)(G)
Fanapt *Tab:* 1, 2, 4, 6, 8, 10, 12 mg

▶ ***loxapine*** (C)
Adasuve *Oral inhal pwdr:* 10 mg single-use disposable inhaler (5/box)

▶ ***lurasidone*** (B)
Latuda *Tab:* 20, 40, 80 mg

▶ ***olanzapine fumarate*** (C)(G)
Zyprexa *Tab:* 2.5, 5, 7.5, 10, 15, 20 mg
Zyprexa Zydis *ODT:* 5, 10, 15, 20 mg (phenylalanine)

▶ ***paliperidone palmitate*** (C)(G)
Invega *Tab:* 3, 6, 9 mg ext-rel
Invega Sustenna *Prefilled syringe:* 39, 78, 117, 156, 234 mg ext-rel suspension w. needle
Invega Trinza *Prefilled syringe:* 273, 410, 546, 819 mg ext-rel suspension

▶ ***pimozide*** (C)(G)
Orap *Tab:* 1, 2 mg

▶ ***prochlorperazine*** (C)(G)
Compazine *Tab:* 5, 10 mg; *Cap:* 10, 15 mg sus-rel; *Syr:* 5 mg/5 ml (4 oz) (fruit); *Supp:* 2.5, 5, 25 mg

▶ ***quetiapine*** (C)(G)
Seroquel *Tab:* 25, 100, 200, 300 mg
Seroquel XR *Tab:* 50, 150, 200, 300, 400 mg ext-rel

▶ ***risperidone*** (C)(G)
Risperdal *Tab:* 0.25, 0.5, 1, 2, 3, 4 mg; *Soln:* 1 mg/ml (30 ml w. pipette);*Consta (Inj)*: 25, 37.5, 50 mg
Risperdal M-Tabs *M-tab:* 0.5, 1, 2, 3, 4 mg orally-disint (phenylalanine)

▶ ***thioridazine*** (C)(G) *Tab:* 10, 25, 50, 100 mg

(*continued*)

(*continued*)

▶ ***trifluoperazine*** (C)(G)
Stelazine *Tab:* 1, 2, 5, 10 mg; *Conc:* 10 mg/ml; (2 oz w. calib dropper (banana-vanilla) (sulfites); *Vial:* 2 mg/ml (10 ml)

▶ ***ziprasidone*** (C)(G)
Geodon *Cap:* 20, 40, 60, 80 mg

APPENDIX K. ANTICONVULSANT DRUGS

ANTICONVULSANT DRUGS WITH DOSE FORMS

▶ ***brivaracetam*** (C)
Briviact *Tab:* 10, 25, 50, 75, 100 mg; *Oral soln:* 10 mg/ml (300 ml); *Vial:* 50 mg/5 ml single dose for IV inj

▶ ***carbamazepine*** (D)(G)
Carbatrol *Cap:* 200, 300 mg ext-rel
Carnexiv *Vial:* 200 mg/20 ml (10 mg/ml) single-dose for IV infusion
Equetro *Cap:* 100, 200, 300 mg ext-rel
Tegretol *Tab:* 100*, 200*mg; *Chew tab:* 100*mg
Tegretol Suspension *Oral susp:* 100 mg/5 ml (450 ml) (citrus vanilla) (sorbitol)
Tegretol-XR *Tab:* 100, 200, 400 mg ext-rel

▶ ***clobazam*** (C)(IV)
Onfi *Tab:* 10*, 20*mg
Onfi Oral Suspension *Oral susp:* 2.5 mg/ml (120 ml w. 2 dosing syringes)(berry)

▶ ***clonazepam*** (D)(IV)(G)
Clonazepam ODT *ODT:* 0.125, 0.25, 0.5, 1, 2, oral-dis
Klonopin *Tab:* 0.5*, 1, 2 mg

▶ ***diazepam*** (D)(IV)(G)
Diastat *Rectal gel delivery system:* 2.5 mg
Diastat AcuDial *Rectal gel delivery system:* 10, 20 mg
Valium *Tab:* 2*, 5*, 10*mg
Valium Injectable *Vial:* 5 mg/ml (10 ml); *Amp:* 5 mg/ml (2 ml); *Prefilled syringe:* 5 mg/ml (5 ml)
Valium Intensol *Conc oral soln:* 5 mg/ml (30 ml w. dropper) (alcohol 19%)
Valium Oral Solution *Oral soln:* 5 mg/5 ml (500 ml) (winter green-spice)

▶ ***divalproex sodium*** (D)(G)
Depakene *Cap:* 250 mg; *Syr:* 250 mg/5 ml (16 oz)
Depakote *Tab:* 125, 250, 500 mg
Depakote ER *Tab:* 250, 500 mg ext-rel
Depakote Sprinkle *Cap:* 125 mg

▶ ***eslicarbazepine*** (C)
Aptiom *Tab:* 200*, 400, 600*, 800*mg

▶ ***ethosuccimide*** (C)(G)
Zarontin *Cap:* 250 mg; *Oral soln:* 250 mg/5 ml (raspberry)

(*continued*)

(*continued*)

▶ *ezogabine* (C)
Potiga *Tab:* 50, 200, 300, 400 mg

▶ *felbamate* (C)(G)
Felbatol *Tab:* 400*, 600*mg
Felbatol Oral Suspension *Oral susp:* 600 mg/5 ml (4, 8, 32 oz)
Peganone *Tab:* 250, 500 mg

▶ *gabapentin* (C)
Horizant *Tab:* 300, 600 ext-rel
Neurontin (G) *Cap:* 100, 300, 400 mg; *Tab:* 600*, 800*mg
Neurontin Oral Solution *Oral soln:* 250 mg/5 ml (480 ml) (strawberry-anise)

▶ *lacosamide* (C)(V)(G)
Vimpat *Tab:* 50, 100, 150, 200 mg; *Oral soln:* 10 mg/ml (200, 465 ml); *Vial:* 10 mg/ml soln for IV infusion, single use (20 ml)

▶ *lamotrigine* (C)(G)
Lamictal *Tab:* 25*, 100*, 150*, 200*mg
Lamictal Chewable Dispersible Tab *Chew tab:* 2, 5, 25, 50 mg (black current)
Lamictal ODT *ODT:* 25, 50, 100, 200 mg oral-disint
Lamictal XR *Tab:* 25, 50, 100, 200, 250, 300 mg ext-rel

▶ *levetiracetam* (C)(G)
Elepsia *Tab:* 1000, 1500 mg ext-rel
Keppra *Tab:* 250*, 500*, 750*, 1000*mg
Keppra Oral Solution *Oral soln:* 100 mg/ml (16 oz) (grape) (dye-free)
Keppra XR *Tab:* 500, 750 mg ext-rel
Levetiracetam IV *Pre-mixed:* 500, 1,000, 1,500 mg/100 ml for IV infusion
Roweepra *Tab:* 250, 500, 750 mg; 1 gm

▶ *mephobarbital* (D)(II)
Mebaral *Tab:* 32, 50, 100 mg

▶ *methsuximide* (C)
Celontin Kapseals *Cap:* 150, 300 mg

▶ *oxcarbazepine* (C)(G)
Trileptal *Tab:* 150, 300, 600 mg; *Oral susp:* 300 mg/5 ml (lemon) (alcohol)
Oxtellar XR *Tab:* 150, 300, 600 mg ext-rel

▶ *perampanel* (C)(III)
Fycompa *Tab:* 2, 4, 6, 8, 10, 12 mg
Fycompa Oral Suspension *Oral susp:* 0.5 mg/ml (340 ml w. dosing syringe)

▶ *phenytoin* (D)(G)
Dilantin *Cap:* 30, 100 mg ext-rel
Dilantin Infatabs *Chew tab:* 50 mg
Dilantin Oral Suspension *Oral susp:* 125 mg/5 ml (237 ml) (alcohol 6%)
Phenytek *Cap:* 200, 300 mg ext-rel

▶ *pregabalin* (C)(V)
Lyrica *Cap:* 25, 50, 75, 100, 200, 225, 300 mg
Lyrica CR *Tab:* 82.5, 165, 330 mg ext-rel
Lyrica Oral Solution *Oral soln:* 20 mg/ml

(*continued*)

(*continued*)

▶ *primidone* (C)
Mysoline *Tab:* 50*, 250*mg
Mysoline Oral Solution *Oral susp:* 250 mg/5 ml (8 oz)

▶ *rufinamide* (C)(G)
Banzel *Tab:* 200*, 400*mg
Banzel Oral Solution *Susp:* 40 mg/ml (orange) (lactose-free, gluten-free, dye-free)

▶ *tiagabine* (C)(G)
Gabitril *Tab:* 2, 4, 12, 16 mg

▶ *topiramate* (D)(G)
Topamax *Tab:* 25, 50, 100, 200 mg
Topamax Sprinkle Caps *Cap:* 15, 25, 50 mg
Trokendi XR *Cap:* 100, 200 mg ext-rel
Qudexy *Tab:* 25, 50, 100, 150, 200 mg ext-rel
Qudexy XR *Cap:* 25, 50, 100, 150, 200 mg ext-rel

▶ *vigabatrin* (C)(G)
Sabril *Tab:* 500 mg
Sabril for Oral Solution 500 mg/pkt pwdr for reconstitution

▶ *zonisamide* (C)
Zonegran *Cap:* 25, 50, 100 mg

APPENDIX L. ANTI-HIV DRUGS

ANTI-HIV DRUGS WITH DOSE FORMS

▶ **Aptivus** (C) ***tipranavir***
Gel cap: 250 mg (alcohol); *Oral soln:* 100 mg/ml (95 ml w. dosing syringe) (Vit E 116 IU/ml) (buttermint-butter, toffee)
Comment: ***valganciclovir*** is indicated for the treatment of AIDS-related cytomegalovirus (CMV) retinitis.

▶ **Atripla** (D) ***efavirenz+emtricitabine+tenofovir disoproxil***
Tab: efa 600 mg+emtri 200 mg+teno diso 300 mg

▶ **Biktarvy** (G) ***bictegravir+emtricitabine+tenofovir alafenamide***
Tab: bict 50 mg+emtr 200 mg+teno ala 25 mg

▶ **Cimduo** ***lamivudine+tenofovir disoproxil fumarate***
Tab: lam 300 mg+teno teno diso 300 mg

▶ **Combivir** (C)(G) ***lamivudine+zidovudine***
Tab: lami 150+zido 300 mg

▶ **Complera** (B) ***emtricitabine+tenofovir disoproxil fumarate+rilpivirine***
Tab: emtri 200 mg+teno diso 300 mg+rilpiv 25 mg

▶ **Crixivan** (C) ***indinavir sulfate***
Cap: 100, 200, 333, 400 mg

(*continued*)

(*continued*)

➢ **Cytovene (C)(G)** ***ganciclovir***
Cap: 250, 500 mg; *Vial:* 50 mg/ml single-dose (500 mg, 10 ml)

➢ **Descovy (D)** ***emtricitabine+tenofovir alafenamide+rilpivirine***
Tab: emtri 200 mg+teno ala 25 mg

➢ **Edurant (B)** ***rilpivirine***
Tab: 25 mg

➢ **Emtriva (B)** ***emtricitabine***
Cap: 200 mg; *Oral soln:* 10 mg/ml (170 ml) (cotton candy)

➢ **Epivir (C)(G)** ***lamivudine***
Tab: 150*, 300 mg; *Oral soln:* 10 mg/ml (240 ml) (strawberry-banana) (sucrose 3 gm/15 ml)

➢ **Epzicom (B)** ***abacavir sulfate+lamivudine***
Tab: aba 600 mg+lami 300 mg

➢ **Evotaz (B)** ***atazanavir+cobicistat***
Tab: ataz 300+cobi 150 mg

➢ **Fortovase (B)** ***saquinavir***
Soft gel cap: 200 mg

➢ **Fuzeon (B)** ***enfuvirtide***
Vial: 90 mg/ml pwdr for SC inj after reconstitution (1 ml, 60 vials/kit) (preservative-free)

➢ **Genvoya (B)** ***elvitegravir+cobicistat+emtricitabine+tenofovir alafenamide (TAF)***
Tab: elv 150 mg+cob 150 mg+emtri 200 mg+teno alafen 10 mg

➢ **Intelence (C)** ***etravirine***
Tab: 25*, 100, 200 mg

➢ **Invirase (B)** ***saquinavir mesylate***
Hard gel cap: 200 mg

➢ **Isentress (C)** ***raltegravir (potassium)***
Tab: 400 mg film-coat; *Chew tab:* 25, 100*mg (orange-banana) (phenylalanine); *Oral susp:* 100 mg/pkt pwdr for oral susp (banana)

➢ **Juluca** ***dolutegravir+trilpivirine***
Tab: dolu 50 mg+tril 25 mg

➢ **Kaletra (C)(G)** ***lopinavir+ritonavir***
Cap: lopin 100 mg+riton 25 mg, lopin 200 mg+riton 50 mg; Oral soln: lopin 80 mg+riton 20 mg per ml (160 ml w. dose cup) (cotton candy) (alcohol 42%)
Hard gel cap: 200 mg

➢ **Lexiva (C)(G)** ***fosamprenavir***
Tab: 700 mg; *Oral soln:* 50 mg/ml (grape, bubble gum) (peppermint)

➢ **Norvir (B)** ***ritonavir***
Soft gel cap: 100 mg (alcohol); *Oral soln:* 80 mg/ml (8 oz) (peppermint-caramel) (alcohol)

(*continued*)

(*continued*)

▶ **Odefsey (D)** ***emtricitabine+rilpivirine+tenofovir alafenamide***
Tab: emtri 200 mg+rilpiv 25 mg+tenof alafen 25 mg

▶ **Prezcobix (B)** ***darunavir+cobicistat***
Tab: daru 800 mg+cobi 150 mg

▶ **Prezista (C)(G)** ***darunavir***
Tab: 75, 150, 600, 800 mg; *Oral susp:* 100 mg/ml (200 ml) (strawberry cream)

▶ **Rescriptor (C)** ***delavirdine mesylate***
Tab: 100, 200 mg

▶ **Retrovir (C)(G)** ***zidovudine***
Tab: 300 mg; *Cap:* 100 mg; *Syr:* 50 mg/5 ml (240 ml) (strawberry); *Vial:* 10 mg/ml (20 ml for IV infusion) (preservative-free)

▶ **Reyataz (B)** ***atazanavir***
Cap: 100, 150, 200, 300 mg

▶ **Selzentry (B)** ***maraviroc***
Tab: 150, 300 mg

▶ **Stribild (B)** ***elvitegravir+cobicistat+emtricitabine+tenofovir disoproxil fumarate***
Tab: elv 150 mg+cob 150 mg+emtri 200 mg+teno diso fumar 300 mg

▶ **Sustiva (C)** ***efavirenz***
Tab: 75, 150, 600, 800 mg; *Cap:* 50, 200 mg

▶ **Symfi** ***efavirenz+lamivudine+tenofovir disoproxil fumarate***
Tab: efav 600 mg+lami 300 mg+teno diso fum 300 mg

▶ **Symfi Lo** ***efavirenz+lamivudine+tenofovir disoproxil fumarate***
Tab: efav 400 mg+lami 300 mg+teno diso fum 300 mg

▶ **Tivicay (B)** ***dolutegravir***
Tab: 10, 25, 50 mg

▶ **Triumeq (C)** ***abacavir sulfate+dolutegravir+lamivudine***
Tab: aba 600 mg+dilu 50 mg+lami 300 mg

▶ **Trizivir (C)(G)** ***abacavir sulfate+lamivudine+zidovudine***
Tab: aba 300 mg+lami 150 mg+zido 300 mg

▶ **Trogarzo** ***ibalizumab-uiyk***
Vial: 200 mg/1.33 ml (1.33 ml), single-dose

▶ **Truvada (B)(G)** ***emtricitabine+tenofovir disoproxil fumarate***
Tab: emt 100 mg+teno diso fum 150 mg; 133 mg+teno diso fum 200 mg; emt 167 mg+teno diso fum 250 mg; emt 200 mg+teno diso fum 300 mg

▶ **Valcyte (C)(G)** ***valganciclovir***
Tab: 450 mg

▶ **Videx EC (C)(G)** ***didanosine***
Cap: 125, 200, 250, 400 mg ent-coat del-rel; *Chew tab:* 25, 50, 100, 150, 200 mg (mandarin orange) (buffered with calcium carbonate and magnesium hydroxide, phenylalanine); *Pwdr for oral soln:* 2 gm (120 ml); 4 gm (240 ml)

(*continued*)

(*continued*)

▶ **Videx Pediatric Pwdr for Oral Solution (C) *didanosine***
Pwdr for oral soln: 2 gm (120 ml); 4 gm (240 ml)

▶ **Viracept (B) *nelfinavir mesylate***
Tab: 250, 625 mg; *Pwdr for oral soln:* 50 mg/gm (144 gm) (phenylalanine)

▶ **Viramune (C)(G) *nevirapine***
Tab: 200*mg; *Oral susp:* 50 mg/5 ml (240 ml)

▶ **Viramune XR (C) *nevirapine***
Tab: 100, 400 mg ext-rel

▶ **Viread (C) *tenofovir disoproxil fumarate***
Tab: 150, 200, 250, 300 mg; *Oral pwdr:* 40 mg/1 gm pwdr (60 gm w. dosing scoop)

▶ **Vistide (C) *cidofovir***
Inj: 75 mg/ml (5 ml vials for IV infusion) (preservative-free)
Comment: ***cidofovir*** is indicated for the treatment of AIDS-related cytomegalovirus (CMV) retinitis.

▶ **Vitekta (C) *elvitegravir***
Inj: 75 mg/ml (5 ml vials for IV infusion) (preservative-free)
Comment: ***cidofovir*** is indicated for the treatment of AIDS-related cytomegalovirus (CMV) retinitis.

▶ **Zerit (C)(G) *stavudine***
Cap: 15, 20, 30, 40 mg; *Oral soln:* 1 mg/ml pwdr for reconstitution (200 ml) (fruit) (dye-free)

▶ **Ziagen (C)(G) *abacavir sulfate***
Tab: 300*mg; *Oral soln:* 20 mg/ml (240 ml) (strawberry-banana) (parabens, propylene glycol)

APPENDIX M. ANTICOAGULANT AND ANTIPLATELET DRUGS

APPENDIX M.1. COUMADIN (WARFARIN)

▶ ***warfarin*** (X)(G) <18 years: not recommended; ≥18 years: dosage initially 2-5 mg/day; usual maintenance 2-10 mg/day; adjust dosage to maintain INR in therapeutic range:
Venous thrombosis: 2.0-3.0
Atrial fibrillation: 2.0-3.0
Post MI: 2.5-3.5
Mechanical and bioprosthetic heart valves: 2.0-3.0 for 12 weeks after valve insertion, then 2.5-3.5 long-term
Coumadin *Tab:* 1*, 2*, 2.5*, 3*, 4*, 5*, 6*, 7.5*, 10*mg
Coumadin for Injection *Vial:* 2 mg/ml (2.5 ml)
Comment: **Coumadin for Injection** is for peripheral IV administration only.

APPENDIX M.2. COUMADIN OVER-ANTICOAGULATION REVERSAL

▶ ***phytonadione (vitamin K)*** (G) 2.5-10 mg PO or IM; max 25 mg
AquaMEPHYTON *Vial:* 1 mg/0.5 ml (0.5 ml), 10 mg/ml (1, 2.5, 5 ml)
Mephyton *Tab:* 5 mg

APPENDIX M.3. AGENTS THAT INHIBIT COUMADIN'S ANTICOAGULATION EFFECTS

Increase Metabolism	Decrease Absorption	Other Mechanism(s)
azathioprine	***azathioprine***	**coenzyme Q10**
carbamazepine	***cholestyramine***	**estrogen**
dicloxacillin	***colestipol***	***griseofulvin***
ethanol	***sucralfate***	**oral contraceptives**
griseofulvin		***ritonavir***
nafcillin		***spironolactone***
pentobarbital		***trazodone***
phenobarbital		**vitamin C (high dose)**
phenytoin		**vitamin K**
primidone		
rifabutin		
rifampin		

APPENDIX M.4. LOW MOLECULAR WEIGHT HEPARINS (LMWHs)

Comment: Administer by subcutaneous injection *only*, in the abdomen, and rotate sites. Avoid concomitant drugs that affect hemostasis (e.g., oral anticoagulants and platelet aggregation inhibitors, including ***aspirin***, NSAIDs, ***dipyridamole***, ***sulfinpyrazone, ticlopidine***). Not recommended <18 years-of-age.

▶ ***dalteparin*** (B)
Fragmin *Prefilled syringe:* 2500 IU/0.2 ml, 5000 IU/0.2 ml (10/box) (preservative-free); *Multi-dose vial:* 1,000 IU/ml (95,000 IU, 9.5 ml) (benzyl alcohol)

▶ ***danaparoid*** (B)
Orgaran *Amp:* 750 anti-Xa units/0.6 ml (0.6 ml, 10/box); *Prefilled syringe:* 750 anti-Xa units/0.6 ml (0.6 ml, 10/box) (sulfites)

▶ ***enoxaparin*** (B)(G)
Lovenox *Prefilled syringe:* 30 mg/0.3 ml, 40 mg/0.4 ml, 60 mg/0.6 ml, 80 mg/0.8 ml (100 mg/ml) (preservative-free); *Vial:* 100 mg/ml (3 ml)

▶ ***tinzaparin*** (B)
Innohep *Vial:* 20,000 *anti-Factor Xa* IU/ml (2 ml) (sulfites, benzyl alcohol)

APPENDIX M.5. FACTOR XA INHIBITORS & REVERSAL AGENT

▶ ***apixaban*** **(C)** <12 years: not recommended; >12 years: 5 mg bid; reduce to 2.5 mg bid if any two of the following: ≥80 years, ≤60 kg, serum Cr ≥1.5
Eliquis *Tab:* 2.5, 5 mg
Comment: **Eliquis** is indicated to reduce the risk of stroke and systemic embolism in patients with non-valvular atrial fibrillation (NVAF).

(*continued*)

(*continued*)

▶ ***edoxaban*** **(C)** <12 years: not recommended; ≥12 years: transition to and from **Savaysa**; assess CrCl prior to initiation: *NVAF CrCl >50 mL/min:* 60 mg once daily; *CrCl 15-50 mL/min:* 30 mg once daily; *DVT/PE CrCl >50 mL/min:* 60 mg once daily following initial parental anticoagulant; *CrCl 15-50 mL/min, <60 kg, or concomitant Pgp inhibitors:* 30 mg once daily

Savaysa *Tab:* 15, 30, 60 mg

Comment: **Savaysa** is indicated to reduce the risk of stroke and systemic embolism in patients with non-valvular atrial fibrillation (NVAF), treatment of DVT and pulmonary embolism (PE) following 5-10 days of initial therapy with parenteral anticoagulant. Not for use in persons with NVAF with *CrCl >95 mL/min.*

▶ ***fondaparinux*** **(B)** <12 years: not established; ≥12 years: administer SC; administer first dose no earlier than 6-8 hours after hemostasis is achieved, start warfarin usually within 72 hours of last dose of ***fondaparinux***

Post-op: 2.5 mg once daily x 5-9 days; *Hip/Knee Replacement:* once daily x 11 days *Hip Fracture:* once daily x 32 days; *Abdominal Surgery:* once daily x 10 days *Prophylaxis:* do not use <50 kg; *Treatment:* once daily for at least 5 days until INR = 2-3 (usually 5-9 days); max 26 days; <50 kg: 5 mg; 50-100 kg: 7.5 mg; >100 kg: 10 mg

Arixtra *Soln for SC inj:* 2.5 mg/0.5 ml, 5 mg/0.4 ml, 7.5 mg/0.6 ml, 10 mg/0.8 ml *prefilled syringe* (10/box) (preservative-free)

▶ ***prasugrel*** **(B)(G)** <12 years: not recommended; ≥12 years: *Loading dose:* 60 mg once in a single dose; *Maintenance:* 10 mg once daily; <60 kg: consider 5 mg once daily; take with ***aspirin*** 75-325 mg once daily

Effient *Tab:* 5, 10 mg

Comment: **Effient** is indicated to reduce the risk of thrombotic cardiovascular events in persons with acute coronary syndrome (ACS) who are to be managed with percutaneous coronary intervention (PCI) including unstable angina, non-ST elevation myocardial infarction (NSTEMI) and STEMI. Do not start if active pathological bleeding (e.g., peptic ulcer, intracranial hemorrhage), prior TIA or stroke, or if patient likely to undergo urgent CABG. Discontinue 7 days before surgery and if TIA or stroke occurs.

▶ ***rivaroxaban*** **(C)** take with food; <12 years: not recommended; ≥12 years:

Treatment of DVT or PE: 15 mg twice daily for the first 21 days; then 20 mg once daily

Reduction in risk of DVT or PE recurrence: 20 mg once daily with the evening meal; *CrCl <30 mL/min*: avoid

Prophylaxis of DVT: take 6-10 hours after surgery when hemostasis established, then 10-20 mg once daily with the evening meal; *CrCl 30-50 mL/min:* 10 mg; *CrCl <30 mL/min:* avoid; discontinue if acute renal failure develops; monitor closely for blood loss

Hip: treat for 35 days; *Knee:* treat for 12 days

Non-valvular AF: take once daily with the evening meal; *CrCl >50 mL/min:* 20 mg; *CrCl 15-50 mL/min:* 15 mg; *CrCl >15 mL/min:* avoid

Xarelto *Cap:* 10, 15, 20 mg

Comment: **Xarelto** is indicated to reduce the risk of stroke and systemic embolism in non-valvular atrial fibrillation (AF), to treat deep vein thrombosis (DVT) and pulmonary embolism (PE), to reduce the risk of recurrence of DVT and/or PE following 6 months treatment for DVT and/or PE, and prophylaxis

(*continued*)

(*continued*)

of DVT which may lead to PE in patients undergoing knee or hip replacement surgery. **Xarelto** eliminates the need for bridging with heparin or LMWH; no need for routine monitoring of INR or other coagulation parameters; no need for dose adjustments for age, weight, or gender; no known dietary restrictions. Switching from ***warfarin*** or other anticoagulant, see mfr pkg insert.

FACTOR XA INHIBITOR REVERSAL AGENT

Comment: **Andexxa *(coagulation factor Xa [recombinant] inactivated-zhzo)*** is indicated to reverse the anticoagulation effects of factor Xa inhibitors (i.e., reversal agent specific to ***rivaroxaban*** **[Xarelto]**, ***apixaban*** **[Eliquis]**) when needed due to life-threatening or uncontrolled bleeding or emergency surgery. **Andexxa** was approved under the FDA's accelerated approval pathway based on effects in healthy volunteers, and continued approval may be contingent on post-marketing studies to demonstrate an improvement in hemostasis in patients. A clinical trial comparing this agent or usual care is scheduled to start in 2019 and to be reported in 2023.

▶ ***coagulation factor Xa [recombinant] inactivated-zhzo*** <18 years: not studied; ≥18 years: administer as an IV bolus, with a target rate of 30 mg/min, followed by continuous infusion for up to 120 minutes; select a high dose or low dose regimen based on the specific FXa inhibitor, dose of FXa inhibitor, and time since the patient's last dose of FXa inhibitor (see mfr pkg insert); resume anticoagulant therapy as soon as medically appropriate following treatment with **Andexxa**

High Dose Regimen: Initial IV Bolus: 800 mg at a target rate of 30 mg/min; *Follow-on IV infusion:* 8 mg/min for up to 120 min

Low Dose Regimen: Initial IV Bolus: 400 mg at a target rate of 30 mg/min; *Follow-on IV infusion:* 4 mg/min for up to 120 min

Andexxa *Vial:* 100 mg, single dose, pwdr for reconstitution and IV infusion

Comment: There are no adequate and well-controlled studies of **Andexxa** in pregnant women to inform patients of associated risks. The safety and effectiveness of **Andexxa** during labor and delivery have not been evaluated. There is no information regarding the presence of **Andexxa** in human milk or effects on the breastfed infant. Safety and efficacy of **Andexxa** in the pediatric population have not been studied. BBW: Treatment with **Andexxa** has been associated with serious and life-threatening adverse events, including arterial and venous thromboembolic events, ischemic events, including myocardial infarction and ischemic stroke, cardiac arrest, and sudden deaths.

APPENDIX M.6. DIRECT THROMBIN INHIBITORS & REVERSAL AGENT

▶ ***aspirin*** **(D)** <12 years: not recommended; ≥12 years: one single dose once daily

Durlaza *Cap:* 162.5 mg 24-hr ext-rel (30, 90/bottle)

▶ ***dabigatran etexilate mesylate*** **(C)** <12 years: not recommended; ≥12 years: swallow whole; *CrCl >30 mL/min:* 150 mg bid; *CrCl 15-30 mL/min:* 75 mg bid; *CrCl <15 mL/min:* not recommended

Pradaxa *Cap:* 75, 150 mg

Comment: **Pradaxa** is indicated to reduce the risk of stroke and systemic embolism in non-valvular AF, DVT prophylaxis, PE prophylaxis in patients who have undergone hip replacement surgery, treatment of DVT and PE in

(*continued*)

(*continued*)

patients who have been treated with a parenteral anticoagulant for 5-10 days, and to reduce the risk of recurrent DVT and PE in patients who have been previously treated. **Pradaxa** is contraindicated in patients with a mechanical prosthetic heart valve.

▶ ***desirudin (recombinant hirudin)*** **(C)** <12 years: not recommended; ≥12 years: 15 mg SC every 12 hours, preferably in the abdomen or thigh, starting up to 5-15 minutes before surgery (after induction of regional block anesthesia, if used); may continue for 9-12 days post-op; *CrCl <60 mL/min:* reduce dose (see mfr pkg insert)

Iprivask *Pwdr for SC inj after reconstitution:* 15 mg/single-use vial (10/box) (preservative-free, diluent contains mannitol)

Comment: **Iprivask** is indicated for DVT prophylaxis in patients undergoing hip replacement surgery. It is not interchangeable with other hirudins.

DIRECT THROMBIN INHIBIOR REVERSAL AGENT

▶ ***idarucizumab*** **(NE)** <12 years: not established; ≥12 years: administer 5 gm (2 vials) IV drip or push; administer within 1 hour of removal from vial

Praxbind *Vial:* 2.5 gm/50 ml, single use (preservative-free)

Comment: ***idarucizumab*** **(Praxbind)** is a specific reversal agent for ***dabigatran*** **(Pradaxa)**. It is a humanized monoclonal antibody fragment (Fab) that binds to ***dabigatran*** and its acylglucuronide metabolites with higher affinity than the binding affinity of ***dabigatran*** to thrombin, neutralizing its anticoagulant effects. Presently, there is inadequate human and animal data to assess risk of ***idarucizumab*** use in pregnancy. Risk/benefit should be considered prior to use.

APPENDIX M.7. PLATELET AGGREGATION INHIBITORS

▶ ***cilostazol*** **(B)** <12 years: not recommended; ≥12 years: 100 mg bid

Pletal *Tab:* 50, 100 mg

Comment: **Pletal** is an (antiplatelet/vasodilator [PDE III inhibitor]).

▶ ***clopidogrel*** **(B)** <12 years: not recommended; ≥12 years: 75 mg once daily

Plavix *Tab:* 75, 300 mg

Comment: **Plavix** is indicated for the reduction of atherosclerotic events in recent MI or stroke, established PAD, non-ST-segment elevation acute coronary syndrome (unstable angina/non-STEMI), or STEMI.

▶ ***dipyridamole*** **(B)(G)** <12 years: not recommended; ≥12 years: 75-100 mg qid

Persantine *Tab:* 25, 50, 75 mg

Comment: ***dipyridamole*** is indicated as an adjunct to oral anticoagulants after cardiac valve replacement surgery to prevent thromboembolism.

▶ ***dipyridamole+aspirin*** **(B)(G)** <12 years: not recommended; ≥12 years: swallow whole; one cap bid

Aggrenox *Cap:* dipyr 200 mg+asa 25 mg

(*continued*)

(continued)

➢ ***pentoxifylline*** **(C)** (hemorrhologic [xanthine]) <12 years: not recommended; ≥12 years: 400 mg once daily
Trental *Tab:* 400 mg sust-rel

➢ ***prasugrel*** **(C)(G)** <12 years: not recommended; ≥12 years: 5-10 mg once daily
Effient *Tab:* 5, 10 mg
Comment: **Effient** is indicated to reduce the risk of cardiovascular events in patients with acute coronary syndrome (ACS) who are to be managed with percutaneous coronary intervention (unstable angina or non-STEMI), and STEMI when managed with either primary or delayed PCI.

➢ ***ticagrelor*** **(C)** <12 years: not recommended; ≥12 years: initiate 180 mg loading dose once in a single dose with aspirin 325 mg loading dose in a single dose; maintenance 90 mg twice daily with aspirin 75-100 mg once daily; ACS patients may start ***ticagrelor*** after a loading dose of ***clopidogrel***
Brilinta *Tab:* 90 mg
Comment: **Effient** is indicated to reduce the risk of cardiovascular events in patients with acute coronary syndrome (ACS) (unstable angina, non-ST elevation (NSTEMI), myocardial infarction, or STEMI).

➢ ***ticlopidine*** **(B)** <12 years: not recommended; ≥12 years: 250 mg bid
Ticlid *Tab:* 250 mg
Comment: **Ticlid** is indicated to reduce the risk of thrombotic stroke in selected patients intolerant of aspirin.

APPENDIX M.8. PROTEASE-ACTIVATED RECEPTOR-1 (PAR-1) INHIBITOR

➢ ***vorapaxar*** **(B)** <12 years: not established; ≥12 years: administer 2.08 mg once daily; use with ***aspirin*** or ***clopidogrel***
Zontivity *Tab:* 2.08 mg (equivalent to 2.5 mg ***vorapaxar sulfate***)
Comment: **Zontivity** is indicated to reduce thrombotic cardiovascular events in patients with a history of myocardial infarction or with peripheral arterial disease (PAD). Contraindicated with active pathological bleeding (e.g., peptic ulcer, intracranial hemorrhage), prior TIA or stroke. Not recommended with severe hepatic impairment.

APPENDIX N. DRUGS FOR THE MANAGEMENT OF ALLERGY, COUGH, AND COLD SYMPTOMS

Comment: Oral prescription drugs for the management of allergy symptoms, cough, and symptoms of the common cold are listed in alphabetical order by brand/trade name.

Legend:	acriv	*acrivastine*
	benzo	*benzonatate*
	brom	*bromopheniramine*
	barb	*carbinoxamine*
	carbeta	*carbetapentane*
	cetir	*cetirazine*

(continued)

(*continued*)

chlor	*chlorpheniramine*
cod	*codeine*
cypro	*cyproheptadine*
deslorat	*desloratadine*
dexchlo	*dexchlorpheniramine*
dextro	*dextromethorphan*
diphen	*diphenhydramine*
fedxo	*fexophenadine*
guaiac	*potassium guaiacolsulfonate*
guaif	*guaifenesin*
homat	*homatropine*
hydro	*hydrocodone*
hydrox	*hydroxyzine*
levocetir	*levocetirizine*
meth	*methscopolamine*
phenyle	*phenylephrine*
prometh	*promethazine*
pseud	*pseudoephedrine*
pyril	*pyrilamine tannate*

- **Allegra (C)(G)(OTC)** <12 years: 60 mg once daily; ≥12 years: 60 mg twice daily or 180 mg once daily
  Tab: fexo 60, 180 mg
- **Allegra-D 12 Hours (C)(G)(OTC)** <18 years: not recommended; ≥18 years: 1 tab once daily
  Tab: fexo 60 mg+pseudo 120 mg ext-rel
- **Allegra-D 24 Hours (C)(G)(OTC)** <18 years: not recommended; ≥18 years: 1 tab once daily
  Tab: fexo 60 mg+pseudo 240 mg ext-rel
- **Atarax (B)(G)** <2 years: not recommended; 2-6 years: 6.25 mg q 4-6 hours prn; 6-12 years: 12.5-25 mg q 4-6 hours prn; >12 years: 25 mg tid or qid prn
  Tab: hydrox 10, 25, 50, 100 mg; *Syr:* 10 mg/5 ml (alcohol 0.5%)
- **Bromfed DM** (C)(G) <2 years: not recommended; 2-6 years: 1/2 tsp q 4 hours prn; 6-12 years: 1 tsp q 4 hours prn; >12 years: 2 tsp q 4 hours prn: max 6 doses/day
  Susp: brom 2 mg+pseudo 30 mg+dextro 10 mg per 5 ml (butterscotch; alcohol 0.95%)
- **Clarinex (C)** <6 years: not recommended; ≥6-12 years: 1/2-1 tab once daily; >12 years: 1 tab daily prn
  Tab: deslorat 5 mg
- **Claritin (C)(G)(OTC)** <6 years: not recommended; ≥6-12 years: 1/2-1 tab once daily; >12 years: 1 tab or 1 liq gel daily prn
  Tab/Liq gel: lorat 10 mg
- **Claritin-D 12 Hours (C)(G)(OTC)** <18 years: not recommended; ≥18 years: 1 tab twice daily
  Tab: lorat 5 mg+pseudo 120 mg ext-rel

(*continued*)

(*continued*)

- **Claritin-D 24 Hours (C)(G)(OTC)** <18 years: not recommended; ≥18 years: 1 tab daily
  Tab: lorat 5 mg+pseudo 240 mg ext-rel
- **Claritin RediTabs 12 Hour (C)(G)(OTC)** <2 years: not recommended; 2-5 years: 1/2 tab twice daily; ≥6 years: 1 tab twice daily
  ODT: lorat 5 mg orally-desint (mint)
- **Claritin RediTabs 24 Hour (C)(G)(OTC)** <5 years: not recommended; 6-11 years: 1/2 tab once daily; ≥12 years: 1 tab once daily
  ODT: lorat 10 mg orally-desint (mint)
- **Claritin Syrup (C)(OTC)** <2 years: not recommended; 2-5 years: 2.5 mg (2.5 ml) once daily; 6-11 years: 5 mg (5 ml) once daily prn; ≥12 years: 10 mg (10 ml) once daily
  Tab: lorat 1 mg per ml (4 oz) (grape, fruit) (alcohol-free, dye-free)
  Comment: **Claritin Syrup** is also available in a (grape, fruit) (sugar-free, alcohol-free, dye-free, sodium 6 mg/5 ml) formulation.
- **Flowtuss Oral Solution (C)(II)(G)** <18 years: not recommended; >18 years: 1-2 tsp q 4-6 hours prn; max 6 tsp/24 hours
  Oral soln: hydro 2.5 mg+guaif 200 mg per 5 ml (black raspberry)
  Comment: ***hydrocodone*** is known to be excreted in human milk. Current FDA recommendations are to limit the minimum age for hydrocone use to 18 years.
- **Hycodan (C)(III)** <6 years: not recommended; 6-12 years: 1/2 tab q 4-6 hours prn; max 3 tabs/day; >12 years: 1 tab q 4-6 hours prn; max 6 tabs/day
  Tab: hydro 5 mg+homat 1.5 mg
  Comment: ***hydrocodone*** is known to be excreted in human milk. Current FDA recommendations are to limit the minimum age for hydrocone use to 18 years.
- **Hycodan Syrup (C)(II)(G)** <6 years: not recommended; 6-12 years: 1/2 tsp q 4-6 hours prn; max 15 ml/day; >12 years: 1 tsp q 4-6 hours prn
  Syr: hydro 5 mg+homat 1.5 mg per 5 ml
  Comment: ***hydrocodone*** is known to be excreted in human milk. Current FDA recommendations are to limit the minimum age for hydrocone use to 18 years.
- **Hycofenix (C)(II)** <18 years: not recommended; >18 years: 10 ml q 6 hours prn
  Oral soln: hydro 2.5 mg+pseudo 30 mg+quaf 200 mg per 5 ml (black raspberry)
  Comment: ***hydrocodone*** is known to be excreted in human milk. Current FDA recommendations are to limit the minimum age for hydrocone use to 18 years.
- **Obredon (C)(II)** <18 years: not recommended; ≥18 years: 10 ml q 4-6 hours prn cough; max 60 ml/day
  Oral soln: hydro 2.5 mg+guaif 200 mg per 5 ml
  Comment: **Obredon** is indicated only for short term treatment of cough due to the common cold. Obredon is not indicated for persistent or chronic cough such as occurs with smoking, asthma, chronic bronchitis, or emphysema, or where cough is accompanied by excessive phlegm. Use with caution in patients with diabetes, thyroid disease, Addison's disease, BPH or urethral stricture, and asthma. Obredon is contraindicated with paralytic ileus, anticholinergics, TCAs, and within 14 days of an MAOI. ***hydrocodone*** is known to be excreted in human milk. There is no FDA-approved generic form of ***hydrocodone+guaifenesin***. Current FDA recommendations are to limit the minimum age for hydrocone use to 18 years.
- **Periactin (B)(G)** <2 years: not recommended; 2-6 years: 2 mg 2-3 x/day: max 12 mg daily; 7-14 years: 4 mg 2-3 x/day: max 16 mg daily; >14 years: initially 4 mg tid prn, then adjust as needed; usual range 12-16 mg/day; max 32 mg/day
  Tab: cypro 4*mg; *Syr:* cypro 2 mg per 5 ml
- **Phenergan (C)(G)** <2 years: not recommended; 2-12 years: 0.5 mg/lb or 6.25-25 mg po or rectally tid; >12 years: 25 mg po or rectally tid ac and HS prn

(*continued*)

(*continued*)

Tab: 12.5*, 25*, 50 mg; *Syr:* prom 6.25 mg per 5 ml; *Syr fortis:* prom 25 mg per 5 ml; *Rectal supp:* prom 12.5, 25, 50 mg

- **Promethazine DM (C)(V)(G)** <6 years: not recommended; 6-12 years: 1/2-1 tsp q 4-6 hours prn; >12 years: 1 tsp q 4-6 hours prn
  Syr: prometh 6.25 mg+dex 15 mg per 5 ml (alcohol 7%)
  Comment: Not recommended for adolescents with asthma or other chronic breathing problem.
- **Promethazine w. Codeine (C)(V)(G)** <6 years: not recommended; 6-12 years: 1/2-1 tsp q 4-6 hours prn; >12 years: 1 tsp q 4-6 hours prn
  Liq: prometh 6.25 mg/cod 10 mg per 5 ml (alcohol 7%)
  Comment: ***codeine*** is known to be excreted in breast milk. <12 years: not recommended; 12-<18: use extreme caution; not recommended for children and adolescents with asthma or other chronic breathing problem. The FDA and the European Medicines Agency (EMA) are investigating the safety of using ***codeine***-containing medications to treat pain, cough and colds, in children 12-<18 years because of the potential for serious side effects, including slowed or difficult breathing. Current FDA recommendations are to limit the minimum age for ***codeine*** use to 18 years.
- **Promethazine VC (C)(V)(G)** <18 years: not recommended; ≥18 years: 1 tsp q 4-6 hours prn; max 30 ml/day
  Syr: prometh 6.25 mg+phenyle 5 mg per 5 ml (alcohol 7%)
  Comment: Not recommended for adolescents with asthma or other chronic breathing problem.
- **Promethazine VC w. Codeine (C)(V)(G)** <18 years: not recommended; ≥18 years: 1 tsp q 4-6 hours prn; max 30 ml/day
  Syr: prometh 6.25 mg+phenyle 5 mg+cod 10 mg per 5 ml (alcohol 7%)
  Comment: ***codeine*** is known to be excreted in breast milk. Not recommended for adolescents with asthma or other chronic breathing problem. The FDA and the European Medicines Agency (EMA) are investigating the safety of using ***codeine***-containing medications to treat pain, cough and colds, in children 12-<18 years because of the potential for serious side effects, including slowed or difficult breathing. Current FDA recommendations are to limit the minimum age for ***codeine*** use to 18 years.
- **Robitussin AC (C)(III)(G)** <2 years: not recommended; 2-6 years: 1/4-1/2 tsp q 4 hours prn; 6-12 years: 1 tsp q 4 hours prn; >12 years: 2 tsp q 4 hours prn; max 60 ml/day
  Liq: cod 10 mg+guaif 100 mg per 5 ml
  Comment: ***codeine*** is known to be excreted in breast milk. <12 years: not recommended; 12-<18: use extreme caution; not recommended for children and adolescents with asthma or other chronic breathing problem. The FDA and the European Medicines Agency (EMA) are investigating the safety of using ***codeine***-containing medications to treat pain, cough and colds, in children 12-<18 years because of the potential for serious side effects, including slowed or difficult breathing. Current FDA recommendations are to limit the minimum age for ***codeine*** use to 18 years.
- **Rondec Syrup (C)(G)** <2 years: not recommended; 2-5 years: 1/4 tsp q 4-6 hours prn; max 7.5 ml/day; 6-11 years: 1/2 tsp q 4-6 hours prn; max 15 ml/day; >11 years: 1 tsp qid prn; max 30 ml/day
  Syr: phenyle 12.5 mg+chlor 4 mg per 5 ml (bubblegum) (sugar-free, alcohol-free)
- **Semprex-D (B)** <12 years: not recommended; ≥12 years: 1 cap q 4-6 hours prn; max 4 doses/day
  Cap: acriv 8 mg+pseud 60 mg

(*continued*)

(*continued*)

- ▶ **Tessalon Caps (C)** <10 years: not recommended; ≥10 years: 100-200 mg tid prn; max 600 mg/day
  Cap: benzo 200 mg
  Comment: Swallow whole. Do not suck or chew.
- ▶ **Tessalon Perles (C)** <10 years: not recommended; ≥10 years: 100-200 mg tid prn; max 600 mg/day
  Perles: benzo 100 mg
  Comment: Swallow whole. Do not suck, crush, or chew.
- ▶ **TussiCaps 5 mg/4 mg (C)(III)** <6 years: not recommended; 6-11 years: 1 cap q 12 hours prn; max 2 caps/day; >11 years: 2 caps q 12 hours prn; max 4 caps/day
  Cap: hydro 5 mg+chlor 4 mg ext-rel (alcohol)
  Comment: ***hydrocodone*** is known to be excreted in human milk. Current FDA recommendations are to limit the minimum age for ***hydrocone*** use to 18 years.
- ▶ **TussiCaps 10 mg/8 mg (C)(III)** <12 years: not recommended; ≥12 years: 1 cap q 12 hours prn; max 2 caps/day
  Cap: hydro 10 mg+chlor 8 mg ext-rel (alcohol)
  Comment: ***hydrocodone*** is known to be excreted in human milk. Current FDA recommendations are to limit the minimum age for ***hydrocone*** use to 18 years.
- ▶ **Tussionex (C)(III)** <6 years: not recommended; 6-12 years: 1/2 tsp q 12 hours prn; >12 years: 1 tsp q 12 hours prn
  Susp: hydro 10 mg+chlor 8 mg per 5 ml ext-rel
  Comment: ***hydrocodone*** is known to be excreted in human milk. Current FDA recommendations are to limit the minimum age for ***hydrocone*** use to 18 years.
- ▶ **Tuzistra XR (C)(III)** <18 years: not recommended: >18 years: 1-2 tsp q 12 hours prn; max 20 ml/day
  Liq: cod 14.7 mg+chlor 2.8 mg per 5 ml (cherry)
- ▶ **Vistaril (C)(G)** <6 years: 50 mg/day prn; 6-12 years: 50-100 mg daily prn; >12 years: 25 mg tid or qid prn
  Cap: hydrox 25, 50, 100 mg; *Susp:* hydrox 25 mg/5 ml (lemon)
- ▶ **Xyzal, Xyzal Oral Solution (B)** <2 years: not recommended; 2-5 years: 1.25 mg (2.5 ml) once daily in the PM prn; 6-11 years: max 2.5 mg (5 ml) once daily in the PM prn; ≥12 years: 5 mg once daily in the PM; *CrCl 30-50 mL/min:* 2.5 mg every other day; *CrCl 10-30 mL/min:* 2.5 mg twice weekly; *CrCl <10 mL/min or hemodialysis:* contraindicated
  Tab: levocetir 5*mg film-coat; *Oral soln:* levocetir 2.5 mg/5 ml (tutti-frutti) (sodium 3 mg/5 ml) (150 ml)
- ▶ **Zyrtec (C)(G)(OTC)** <2 years: not recommended; ≥2-6 years: 5 mg once daily; daily; >12 years: 10 mg once daily
  Tab/Liq gel: cetir 10 mg; *Chewtab:* 5, 10 mg (grape)
- ▶ **Zyrtec-D 12 Hours (C)(G)(OTC)** <18 years: not recommended; ≥18 years: 1 tab twice daily
  Tab: cetir 5 mg+pseudo 120 mg ext-rel
- ▶ **Zyrtec Syrup (C)(OTC)** <2 years: not recommended; 2-5 years: 2.5 mg (2.5 ml) once daily; 6-11 years: 5 mg (5 ml) once daily prn; ≥12 years: 10 mg (10 ml) once daily
  Tab: cetir 1 mg per ml (4 oz) (grape, bubble gum) (alcohol-free, dye-free)
  Comment: Zyrtec Syrup is available in a (grape, bubble gum) (dye-free, alcohol-free, sugar-free, sodium 6 mg/5 ml) formulation.

APPENDIX O. SYSTEMIC ANTI-INFECTIVE DRUGS

Comments:

- Adverse effects of aminoglycosides include nephrotoxicity and ototoxicity.
- Use cephalosporins with caution in persons with penicillin allergy due to potential cross allergy.
- Sulfonamides are contraindicated with sulfa allergy and G6PD deficiency. A high fluid intake is indicated during sulfonamide therapy.
- Tetracyclines should be taken on an empty stomach to facilitate absorption. Tetracyclines should not be taken with milk.
- Tetracyclines are contraindicated during pregnancy and breastfeeding, and in children <8 years of age, due to the risk of developing tooth enamel discoloration.
- Systemic quinolones and fluoroquinolones are contraindicated in pregnancy and children <18 years of age due to the risk of joint dysplasia

Systemic Anti-infectives by Drug Class		
Generic Name	**Brand Name**	**Dose Form/Volume**
Amebicides		
chloroquine phosphate **(C)**	**Aralen**	*Tab:* 500 mg; *Inj:* 50 mg/ml (5 ml)
iodoquinol **(C)**	**Yodoxin**	*Tab:* 210, 650 mg
metronidazole **(not for use in 1st; B in 2nd, 3rd)(G)**	**Flagyl**	*Tab:* 250*, 500*mg
	Flagyl 375	*Cap:* 375 mg
	Flagyl ER	*Tab:* 750 mg ext-rel
tinidazole **(C)**	**Tindamax**	*Tab:* 250*, 500*mg
Aminoglycosides		
amikacin **(C)(G)**	**Amikin**	*Vial:* 500 mg, 1 gm (2 ml)
gentamicin **(C)(G)**	**Garamycin**	*Vial:* 20, 80 mg/2 ml (2 ml)
streptomycin **(D)(G)**	**Streptomycin**	*Amp:* 1 g/2.5 ml <u>or</u> 400 mg/ml (2.5 ml)
Antifungals		
atovaquone **(C)**	**Mepron**	*Susp:* 750 mg/5ml (210 ml)
clotrimazole **(B)(G)**	**Mycelex Troche**	10 mg (70, 40/bottle)
fluconazole **(C)(G)**	**Diflucan**	*Tab:* 50, 100, 150, 200 mg; *Oral susp:* 10, 40 mg/ml (35 ml) (orange)
griseofulvin, microsize **(C)**	**Grifulvin V**	*Tab:* 250, 500 mg; *Oral susp:* 125 mg/5 ml (120 ml) (alcohol 0.02%)
	Gris-PEG	*Tab:* 125, 250 mg

(*continued*)

(*continued*)

Systemic Anti-infectives by Drug Class		
Generic Name	**Brand Name**	**Dose Form/Volume**
itraconazole (C)(G)	**Sporanox**	*Cap:* 100 mg; *Soln:* 10 mg/ml (150 ml); *Pulse Pack*: 100 mg caps (7/pck)
ketoconazole (C)(G)	**Nizoral**	*Tab:* 200 mg
nystatin (C)(G)	**Mycostatin**	*Pastille:* 200,000 units/pastille (30 pastilles/pck); *Oral susp:* 100,000 units/ml (60 ml w. dropper)
terbinafine (B)(G)	**Lamisil**	*Tab:* 250 mg
voriconazole (D)(G)	**Vfend**	*Tab:* 50, 200 mg
Anthelmintics		
albendazole (C)(G)	**Albenza**	*Tab:* 200 mg
ivermectin (C)(G)	**Stromectol**	*Tab:* 3 mg
mebendazole (C)(G)	**Emverm, Vermox**	*Chew tab:* 100 mg
pyrantel pamoate (C)(G)	**Antiminth** **Pin-X**	*Cap:* 180 mg; *Liq:* 50 mg/ml (30 ml); 144 mg/ml (30 ml); *Oral susp:* 50 mg/ml (30 ml) (caramel) (sodium benzoate, tartrazine-free)
thiabendazole (C)(G)	**Mintezol** (currently not available in the United States)	*Chew tab:* 500*mg (orange); *Oral susp:* 500 mg/5 ml (120 ml) (orange)
Antimalarials		
atorvaquone (C)	**Mepron**	*Susp:* 750 mg/5 ml
atovaquone+ proguanil (C)	**Malarone**	*Tab:* atov 250 mg+proq 100 mg
	Malarone Pediatric	*Tab:* atov 62.5 mg+proq 25 mg
chloroquine phosphate (C)(G)	**Aralen**	*Tab:* 500 mg; *Amp:* 50 mg/ml (5 ml)
doxycycline (D)(G)	**Acticlate**	*Tab:* 75, 150**mg
	Adoxa	*Tab:* 50, 75, 100, 150 mg ent-coat
	Doryx	*Cap:* 100 mg; *Tab:* 50, 75, 100, 150, 200 mg
	Doxteric	*Tab:* 50 mg del-rel

(*continued*)

(*continued*)

Systemic Anti-infectives by Drug Class		
Generic Name	**Brand Name**	**Dose Form/Volume**
	Monodox	*Cap*: 50, 75, 100 mg
	Oracea	*Cap*: 40 mg del-rel
	Vibramycin	*Cap*: 50, 100 mg; *Syr*: 50 mg/5 ml (raspberry-apple) (sulfites); *Oral susp*: 25 mg/5 ml (raspberry)
	Vibra-Tab	*Tab*: 100 mg film-coat
hydroxychloroquine **(C)(G)**	**Plaquenil**	*Tab*: 200 mg
mefloquine **(C)**	**Lariam**	*Tab*: 250 mg
minocycline **(D)(G)**	**Dynacin**	*Cap*: 50, 100 mg
	Minocin	*Cap*: 50, 75, 100 mg; *Oral susp*: 50 mg/5 ml (60 ml) (custard) (sulfites, alcohol 5%)
	Minolira	*Tab*: 105, 135 mg ext-rel
	Solodyn	*Tab*: 55, 65, 80, 105, 115 mg ext-rel
Antiprotozoal/Antibacterials		
quinine sulfate **(C)(G)**	**Qualaquin**	*Cap*: 324 mg
metronidazole **(not for use in 1st; B in 2nd, 3rd)(G)**	**Flagyl, Protostat**	*Tab*: 250*, 500*mg
	Flagyl 375	*Cap*: 375 mg
	Flagyl ER	*Tab*: 750 mg ext-rel
nitazoxanide **(C)(G)**	**Alinia**	*Tab*: 500 mg; *Oral susp*: 100 mg/5 ml (60 ml) (strawberry)
tinidazole **(C)**	**Tindamax**	*Tab*: 250*, 500*mg
Antituberculars		
ethambutol (EMB) **(B)(G)**	**Myambutol**	*Tab*: 100, 400*mg
isoniazid (INH) **(C)(G)**	*generic only*	*Tab*: 100, 300*mg; *Syr*: 50 mg/5 ml; *Inj*: 100 mg/ml
pyrazinamide (PZA) **(C)(G)**	*generic only*	*Tab*: 500*mg

(*continued*)

(*continued*)

Systemic Anti-infectives by Drug Class		
Generic Name	**Brand Name**	**Dose Form/Volume**
rifapentine **(C)**	**Priftin**	*Tab:* 150 mg
rifampin **(C)(G)**	**Rifadin**	*Cap:* 150, 300 mg
rifampin+isoniazid **(C)**	**Rifamate**	*Cap:* rif 300 mg+iso 150 mg
rifampin+isoniazid+ pyrazinamide **(C)**	**Rifater**	*Tab:* rif 120 mg+iso 50 mg+pyr 300 mg
Antivirals *(for HIV-specific antiviral drugs see page 562)*		
acyclovir **(C)(G)**	**Zovirax**	*Cap:* 200 mg; *Tab:* 400, 800 mg; *Oral susp:* 200 mg/5 ml (banana)
amantadine **(C)(G)**	**Symmetrel**	*Tab:* 100 mg; *Syr:* 50 mg/5ml (16 oz) (raspberry)
famciclovir **(B)**	**Famvir**	*Tab:* 125, 250, 500 mg
lamivudine **(C)**	**Epivir-HBV**	*Tab:* 100 mg; *Oral soln:* 5 mg/ml (240 ml) (strawberry-banana)
oseltamivir **(C)(G)**	**Tamiflu**	*Cap:* 75 mg
rimantadine **(C)**	**Flumadine**	*Tab:* 100 mg
valacyclovir **(B)**	**Valtrex**	*Tab:* 500 mg; 1 gm
zanamivir	**Relenza**	*Tab:* lami 150+zido 300 mg
Cephalosporins		
1st Generation Cephalosporins		
cefadroxil **(B)**	**Duricef**	*Cap:* 500 mg; *Tab:* 1 gm; *Oral susp:* 250 mg/5 ml (100 ml); 500 mg/5 ml (75, 100 ml) (orange-pineapple)
cefazolin **(B)**	**Ancef, Zolicef**	*Vial:* 500 mg; 1, 10 gm
cephalexin **(B)(G)**	**Keflex**	*Cap:* 250, 333, 500, 750 mg; *Oral susp:*125, 250 mg/5 ml (100, 200 ml)
2nd Generation Cephalosporins		
cefaclor **(B)(G)**	*generic only*	*Tab:* 500 mg; *Cap:* 250, 500 mg; *Susp:* 125 mg/5 ml (75, 150 ml) (strawberry); 187 mg/5 ml (50, 100 ml) (strawberry); 250 mg/5 ml (75, 150 ml) (strawberry); 375 mg/5 ml (50, 100 ml) (strawberry)

(*continued*)

(*continued*)

Systemic Anti-infectives by Drug Class		
Generic Name	**Brand Name**	**Dose Form/Volume**
cefaclor ext-rel **(B)(G)**	**Cefaclor Extended Release**	*Tab:* 375, 500 mg ext-rel
cefamandole **(B)(G)**	**Mandol**	*Vial:* 1, 2 gm
cefotetan **(B)**	**Cefotan**	*Vial:* 1, 2 gm
cefoxitin **(B)**	**Mefoxin**	*Vial:* 1, 2 gm
cefprozil **(B)(G)**	**Cefzil**	*Tab:* 250, 500 mg; *Oral susp:* 125, 250 mg/5 ml (50, 75, 100 ml) (bubble gum) (phenylalanine)
ceftaroline fosamil **(B)**	**Teflaro**	*Vial:* 400, 600 mg
cefuroxime sodium **(B) (G)**	**Zinacef**	*Vial:* 750 mg; 1.5 gm
loracarbef **(B)**	**Lorabid**	*Pulvule:* 200, 400 mg; *Oral susp:* 100 mg/5 ml (50, 100 ml); 200 mg/5 ml (50, 75, 100 ml) (strawberry bubble gum)
3rd Generation Cephalosporins		
cefoperazone **(B)**	**Cefobid**	*Vial:* 1, 2 gm pwdr for reconstitution
cefotaxime **(B)**	**Claforan**	*Vial:* 500 mg; 1, 2 gm pwdr for reconstitution
cefpodoxime proxetil **(B)**	**Vantin**	*Tab:* 100, 200 mg; *Oral susp:* 50, 100 mg/5 ml (50, 75, 100 ml) (lemon creme)
ceftazidime **(B)**	**Ceptaz**	*Vial:* 1, 2 gm pwdr for reconstitution
	Fortaz	*Vial:* 500 mg; 1, 2 gm pwdr for reconstitution
	Tazicef	*Vial:* 1, 2 gm pwdr for reconstitution
	Tazidime	*Vial:* 1, 2 gm pwdr for reconstitution
ceftazidime+ avibactam **(B)**	**Avycaz**	*Vial:* 2.5 gm pwdr for reconstitution
ceftibuten **(B)**	**Cedax**	*Cap:* 400 mg; *Oral susp:* 90 mg/5 ml (30, 60, 90, 120 ml); 180 mg/5 ml (30, 60, 120 ml) (cherry)

(*continued*)

(*continued*)

Systemic Anti-infectives by Drug Class		
Generic Name	**Brand Name**	**Dose Form/Volume**
3rd/4th Generation Cephalosporins		
cefdinir **(B)**	**Omnicef**	*Cap:* 300 mg; *Oral susp:* 125 mg/5 ml (60, 100 ml) (strawberry)
cefditoren pivoxil **(C)**	**Spectracef**	*Tab:* 200 mg
cefepime **(B)**	**Maxipime**	*Vial:* 1 gm pwdr for reconstitution
cefixime **(B)**	**Suprax**	*Tab/Cap:* 400 mg; *Oral Susp:* 100 mg/5 ml (50, 75, 100 ml) (strawberry)
ceftaroline fosamil **(B)**	**Teflaro**	*Vial:* 400, 600 mg
ceftriaxone **(B)(G)**	**Rocephin**	*Vial:* 250, 500 mg; 1, 2 gm
cytolozane+ tazobactam **(B)**	**Zerbaxa**	*Vial:* 1.5 gm pwdr for reconstitution
Penicillins		
amoxicillin **(B)(G)**	**Amoxil**	*Cap:* 250, 500 mg; *Tab:* 500, 875*mg; *Chew tab:* 125, 200, 250, 400 mg (cherry-banana-peppermint) (phenylalanine); *Oral susp:*125, 250 mg/ml (80, 100, 150 ml) (bubble gum); 200, 400 mg/5 ml (50, 75, 100 ml) (bubble gum); *Oral drops:* 50 mg/ml (30 ml) (bubble gum)
	Moxatag	*Tab:* 775 mg ext-rel
	Trimox	*Cap:* 250, 500 mg; *Oral susp:* 125, 250 mg/5ml (80, 100, 150 ml) (raspberry-strawberry)
amoxicillin+ clavulanate **(B)(G)**	**Augmentin**	*Tab:* 250, 500, 875 mg; *Chew tab:* 125, 250 mg (lemon lime); 200, 400 mg (cherry-banana; phenylalanine); *Oral susp:* 125 mg/5 ml (banana), 250 mg/5 ml (orange) (75, 100, 150 ml); 200, 400 mg/5 ml (50, 75, 100 ml) (orange)
	Augmentin ES-600	*Oral susp:* 600 mg/5 ml (50, 75, 100, 125, 150, 200 ml) (strawberry cream) (phenylalanine)
	Augmentin XR	*Tab:* 1000*mg ext-rel

(*continued*)

(*continued*)

Systemic Anti-infectives by Drug Class		
Generic Name	**Brand Name**	**Dose Form/Volume**
ampicillin **(B)(G)**	**Omnipen**	*Cap:* 250, 500 mg; *Oral susp:* 125, 250 mg/ml (100, 150, 200 ml)
	Principen	*Cap:* 250, 500 mg; *Syr:* 125, 250 mg/5 ml
ampicillin+sulbactam **(B)(G)**	**Unasyn**	*Vial:* 1.5, 3 gm
carbenicillin **(B)**	**Geocillin**	*Tab:* 382 mg film-coat
dicloxacillin **(B)(G)**	**Dynapen**	*Cap:* 125, 250, 500 mg; *Oral susp:* 62.5 mg/5 ml (80, 100, 200 ml)
ertapenem **(B)**	**Invanz**	*Vial:* 1 gm pwdr for reconstitution
meropenem **(B)(G)**	**Merrem**	*Vial:* 500 mg; 1 gm pwdr for reconstitution (sodium 3.92 mEq/gm)
penicillin g benzathine **(B)(G)**	**Bicillin LA, Bicillin C-R**	*Cartridge-needle unit:* 600,000 million units (1 ml); 1.2 million units (2 ml); 2.4 million units (4 ml)
	Permapen	*Prefilled syringe:* 1.2 million units
penicillin g potassium **(B)(G)**	*generic only*	***Vial: 5, 20 MU pwdr for reconstitution; Premixed: 1, 2, 3 MU (50 ml)***
penicillin g procaine **(B)(G)**	*generic only*	*Prefilled syringe:* 1.2 million units
penicillin v potassium **(B)(G)**	**Pen-Vee K**	*Tab:* 250, 500 mg; *Oral soln:* 125 mg/5 ml (100, 200 ml); 250 mg/5 ml (100, 150, 200 ml)
piperacillin+ tazobactam **(B)(G)**	**Zosyn**	*Vial:* 2, 3, 4 gm pwdr for reconstitution
Quinolone and Fluoroquinolones		
1st Generation Quinolone		
enoxacin **(C)**	**Penetrex**	*Tab:* 200, 400 mg
1st Generation Fluoroquinolones		
ciprofloxacin **(C)(G)**	**Cipro**	*Tab:* 250, 500, 750 mg; *Oral susp:* 250, 500 mg/5 ml (100 ml) (strawberry); *IV conc:* 10 mg/ml after dilution (20, 40 ml); *IV premixed:* 2 mg/ml (100, 200 ml)

(*continued*)

(*continued*)

Systemic Anti-infectives by Drug Class		
Generic Name	**Brand Name**	**Dose Form/Volume**
	Cipro XR	*Tab:* 500, 1000 mg ext-rel
	ProQuin XR	*Tab:* 500 mg ext-rel
lomefloxacin (C)	**Maxaquin**	*Tab:* 400 mg
norfloxacin (C)(G)	**Noroxin**	*Tab:* 400 mg
ofloxacin (C)(G)	**Floxin**	*Tab:* 200, 300, 400 mg
3rd Generation Fluoroquinolone		
levofloxacin (C)(G)	**Levaquin**	*Tab:* 250, 500, 750 mg
4th Generation Fluoroquinolone		
delafloxacin (C)	**Baxdela**	*Tab:* 400 mg; *Vial:* 300 mg pwdr for reconstitution
gemifloxacin (C)(G)	**Factive**	*Tab:* 320*mg
moxifloxacin (C)(G)	**Avelox**	*Tab:* 400 mg
Ketolide		
telithromycin (C)	**Ketek**	*Tab:* 300, 400 mg
Macrolides		
azithromycin (B)	**Zithromax**	*Tab:* 250, 500, 600 mg; *Granules:* 1 gm/pck for reconstitution (cherry-banana)
	ZithPed Syr	*Oral susp:* 100 mg/5 ml, (15 ml); 200 mg/5 ml (15, 22.5, 30 ml) (cherry)
	Zithromax Tri-Pak	*Tab:* 3 x 500 mg tabs/pck
	Zithromax Z-Pak	*Tab:* 6 x 250 mg tabs/pck
	Zmax	*Granules:* 2 gm/pkt for reconstitution (cherry-banana)
clarithromycin (C)(G)	**Biaxin**	*Tab:* 250, 500 mg; *Oral susp:* 125, 250 mg/5 ml (50, 100 ml) (fruit punch)
	Biaxin XL	*Tab:* 500 mg ext-rel

(*continued*)

(continued)

Systemic Anti-infectives by Drug Class		
Generic Name	**Brand Name**	**Dose Form/Volume**
dirithromycin **(C)(G)**	*generic only*	*Tab:* 250 mg
erythromycin base **(B)(G)**	**Ery-Tab**	*Tab:* 250, 333, 500 mg ent-coat
	PCE	*Tab:* 333, 500 mg
erythromycin estolate **(B)(G)**	**Ilosone**	*Pulvule:* 250 mg; *Tab:* 500 mg; *Liq:* 125, 250 mg/5 ml (100 ml)
erythromycin ethylsuccinate **(B)(G)**	**E.E.S.**	*Tab:* 400 mg; *Oral susp:* 200 mg/5 ml (100, 200 ml) (cherry); 200, 400 mg/5 ml (100 ml) (fruit)
erythromycin ethylsuccinate **(B)(G)**	**EryPed**	*Oral susp:* 200 mg/5 ml (100, 200 ml) (fruit); 400 mg/5 ml (60, 100, 200 ml) (banana); *Oral drops:* 200, 400 mg/5 ml (50 ml) (fruit); *Chew tab:* 200 mg wafer (fruit)
erythromycin stearate **(B)(G)**	**Erythrocin**	*Film tab:* 250, 500 mg
Macrolide+Sulfonamide		
erythromycin ethylsuccinate+ sulfisoxazole **(C)(G)**	**Pediazole**	*Oral susp:* eryth 200 mg+sulf 600 mg per 5 ml (100, 150, 200 ml) (strawberry-banana)
Sulfonamides		
sulfamethoxazole **(B/D)(G)**	**Gantrisin Pediatric**	*Oral susp:* 500 mg/5 ml; *Syr:* 500 mg/5 ml
trimethoprim **(C)(G)**	**Primsol**	*Oral soln:* 50 mg/5 ml (bubble gum) (dye-free, alcohol-free)
	Trimpex	*Tab:* 100 mg
	Proloprim	*Tab:* 100, 200 mg
trimethoprim+ sulfamethoxazole **(D)(G)**	**Bactrim, Septra**	*Tab:* trim 80 mg+sulfa 400 mg*
	Bactrim DS, Septra DS	*Tab:* trim 160 mg+sulfa 800 mg*; *Oral susp:* trim 40 mg+sulfa 200 mg per 5 ml (100 ml) (cherry) (alcohol 0.3%)

(continued)

(*continued*)

Systemic Anti-infectives by Drug Class		
Generic Name	**Brand Name**	**Dose Form/Volume**
Tetracyclines		
demeclocycline **(D)**	**Declomycin**	*Tab:* 300 mg
doxycycline **(D)(G)**	**Adoxa**	*Tab:* 50, 100 mg ent-coat
	Doryx	*Cap:* 100 mg
	Monodox	*Cap:* 50, 100 mg
doxycycline **(D)(G)**	**Vibramycin**	*Cap:* 50, 100 mg; *Syr:* 50 mg/5 ml; (raspberry) (sulfites); *Oral susp:* 25 mg/5 ml (raspberry-apple); *IV conc:* doxy 100 mg+asc acid 480 mg after dilution; doxy 200 mg+asc acid 960 mg after dilution
	Vibra-Tab	*Tab:* 100 mg film-coat
minocycline **(D)(G)**	**Dynacin**	*Cap:* 50, 100 mg
	Minocin	*Cap:* 50, 100 mg; *Oral susp:* 50 mg/5 ml (60 ml) (custard) (sulfites, alcohol 5%); *Vial:* 100 mg soln for inj
	Minolira	*Tab:* 105, 135 mg ext-rel
tetracycline **(D)(G)**	**Achromycin V**	*Cap:* 250, 500 mg
	Sumycin	*Tab:* 250, 500 mg; *Oral susp:* 125 mg/5 ml (fruit) (sulfites)
Unclassified/Miscellaneous		
aztreonam **(B)**	**Cayston**	*Vial:* 75 mg pwdr for reconstitution (preservative-free)
chloramphenicol **(C)(G)**	**Chloromycetin**	*Vial:* 1 gm
clindamycin **(B)(G)**	**Cleocin**	*Cap:* 75 (tartrazine), 150 (tartrazine), 300 mg; *Oral susp*: 75 mg/5 ml (100 ml) (cherry); *Vial:* 150 mg/l (2, 4 ml) (benzyl alcohol)
dalbavancin **(C)**	**Dalvance**	*Vial:* 500 mg pwdr for reconstitution (preservative-free)

(*continued*)

(*continued*)

Systemic Anti-infectives by Drug Class		
Generic Name	**Brand Name**	**Dose Form/Volume**
daptomycin (B)(G)	**Cubicin**	*Vial:* 500 mg pwdr for reconstitution
doripenem (B)	**Doribax**	*Vial:* 500 mg pwdr for reconstitution
fosfomycin tromethamine (B)	**Monurol**	*Sachet:* 3 gm single-dose (mandarin orange) (sucrose)
imipenem+cilastatin (C)(G)	**Primaxin**	*Vial:* imip 500 mg+cila 500 mg; imip 750 mg+cila 750 mg pwdr for reconstitution
lincomycin (B)(G)	**Lincocin**	*Vial:* 300 mg/ml (10 ml)
linezolid (C)(G)	**Zyvox**	*Tab:* 400, 600 mg; *Oral susp:* 100 mg/5 ml (orange) (phenylalanine); *IV:* 2 mg ml (100, 200, 300 ml)
meropenem (B)	**Merrem**	*Vial:* 500 mg; 1 gm (sodium 3.92 mEq/gm)
meropenem+ vaborbactam	**Vabomere**	*Vial:* mero 1 gm+vabor 1 gm pwdr for reconstitution, single dose
nitrofurantoin (B)(G)	**Furadantin**	*Oral susp:* 25 mg/5 ml (60 ml)
	Macrobid	*Cap:* 100 mg
	Macrodantin	*Cap:* 25, 50, 100 mg
quinupristin+ dalfopristin (B)	**Synercid**	*Vial:* quin 150 mg+dalf 350 mg, quin180 mg+dalf 420 mg
tigecycline (D)(G)	**Tygacil**	*Vial:* 50 mg pwdr for reconstitution
rifaximin (C)	**Xifaxan**	*Tab:* 200, 550 mg
telavancin (C)	**Vibativ**	*Vial:* 250, 750 mg pwdr for reconstitution for IV infusion (preservative-free)
vancomycin (C)(G)	**Vancocin**	*Cap:* 125, 250 mg; *Vial:* 500 mg, 1 gm pwdr for reconstitution

APPENDIX P.1. ACYCLOVIR (ZOVIRAX SUSPENSION)

Weight												
Pounds	15	20	25	30	35	40	45	50	55	60	65	70
Kilograms	6.8	9	11.4	13.6	15.9	18.2	20.5	22.7	25	27.3	29.5	31.8
Single Dose (ml)/Frequency/Strength/5-Day Volume (ml)												
20 mg/kg/d ml/dose qid	3.5	4.5	5.5	6.5	8	9	10	11.5	12.5	13.5	14.5	16
mg/5 ml	200	200	200	200	200	200	200	200	200	200	200	200
Volume (ml)	70	90	110	130	160	180	200	230	250	270	290	320

Zovirax Oral Suspension <2 years: not recommended; >2 years, <40 kg: 20 mg/kg dosed qid x 5 days; ≥2 years, >40 kg: 800 mg dosed qid x 5 days; *Oral susp*: 200 mg/5 ml (banana).

APPENDIX P.2. AMANTADINE (SYMMETREL SYRUP)

Weight												
Pounds	15	20	25	30	35	40	45	50	55	60	65	70
Kilograms	6.8	9	11.4	13.6	15.9	18.2	20.5	22.7	25	27.3	29.5	31.8
Single Dose (ml)/Frequency/Strength/10-Day Volume (ml)												
4 mg/kg/d ml/dose bid	3	4	5	6	7	8	9	10	11	12	13	14
mg/5 ml	50	50	50	50	50	50	50	50	50	50	50	50
Volume (ml)	30	40	50	60	70	80	90	100	110	120	130	140
8 mg/lb/d ml/dose bid	6	8	10	12								
mg/5 ml	50	50	50	50								
Volume (ml)	60	80	100	60								

Symmetrel Suspension (C)(G) Symmetrel <1 year: not recommended; 1-8 years: max 150 mg/day; 9-12 years: 2 tsp bid; >12 years: 100 mg bid or 200 mg once daily; *Syr:* 50 mg/5 ml (raspberry).

APPENDIX P.3. AMOXICILLIN (AMOXIL SUSPENSION, TRIMOX SUSPENSION)

Weight												
Pounds	15	20	25	30	35	40	45	50	55	60	65	70
Kilograms	6.8	9	11.4	13.6	15.9	18.2	20.5	22.7	25	27.3	29.5	31.8
Single Dose (ml)/Frequency/Strength/10-Day Volume (ml)												
20 mg/kg/d ml/ dose tid	2	2.5	3	3.5	4	5	5.5	6	7	7.5	8	9
mg/5 ml	125	125	125	125	125	125	125	125	125	125	125	125
Volume (ml)	60	75	90	105	120	150	165	180	210	225	240	270
30 mg/kg/d ml/ dose tid	3	3.5	2.5	3	3	3.5	4	4.5	5	5.5	6	6.5
mg/5 ml	125	125	250	250	250	250	250	250	250	250	250	250
Volume (ml)	90	105	75	90	90	105	120	135	150	165	180	195
40 mg/kg/d ml/ dose bid	5	7	4.5	5	6	7	8	9	10	11	12	13
mg/5 ml	125	125	250	250	250	250	250	250	250	250	250	250
Volume (ml)	100	140	90	100	120	140	160	180	200	220	240	250
45 mg/kg/d ml/ dose bid	4	2.5	3	4	4.5	5	6	6.5	7	7.5	8.5	9

(continued)

APPENDIX P.3. AMOXICILLIN (AMOXIL SUSPENSION, TRIMOX SUSPENSION) (*continued*)

mg/5 ml	200	400	400	400	400	400	400	400	400	400	400	400
Volume (ml)	80	50	60	80	90	100	120	130	140	150	170	180
90 mg/kg/d ml/ dose bid	8	5	6	7	9	10	12	13	14	15	17	18
mg/5 ml	200	400	400	400	400	400	400	400	400	400	400	400
Volume (ml)	160	100	120	140	180	200	240	260	280	300	340	360

<40 kg (88 lb): 20-30 mg/kg/day in 3 divided doses or 40-90 mg/kg/day in 2 divided doses.
Amoxil Suspension (B)(G) 125, 250 mg/5 ml (80, 100, 150 ml) (strawberry); 200, 400 mg/5 ml (50, 75, 100 ml) (bubble gum).
Trimox Suspension (B)(G) 125, 250 mg/5 ml (80, 100, 150 ml) (raspberry-strawberry).

APPENDIX P.4. AMOXICILLIN+CLAVULANATE (AUGMENTIN SUSPENSION)

Weight												
Pounds	15	20	25	30	35	40	45	50	55	60	65	70
Kilograms	6.8	9	11.4	13.6	15.9	18.2	20.5	22.7	25	27.3	29.5	31.8
Single Dose (ml)/Frequency/Strength/10-Day Volume (ml)												
40 mg/kg/d ml/ dose bid	5.5	7	4.5	5.5	6.5	7	8	9	10	11	12	13
mg/5 ml	125	125	250	250	250	250	250	250	250	250	250	250
Volume (ml)	110	140	90	110	130	140	160	180	200	220	240	260
45 mg/kg/d ml/dose bid	3	4	5	6	7	8	9	10	11.5	12.5	13.5	14.5
mg/5 ml	250	250	250	250	250	250	250	250	250	250	250	250
Volume (ml)	60	80	100	120	140	160	180	200	230	250	270	290
45 mg/kg/d ml/dose bid	4	2.5	3	4	4.5	5	6	6.5	7	7.5	8.5	9
mg/5 ml	200	400	400	400	400	400	400	400	400	400	400	400
Volume (ml)	80	50	60	80	90	100	120	130	140	150	170	180
90 mg/kg/d ml/ dose bid	4	5	6.5	8	9	10	11.5	13	14	15.5	16.5	18
mg/5 ml	400	400	400	400	400	400	400	400	400	400	400	400
Volume (ml)	80	100	130	160	180	200	240	260	280	300	340	360

Augmentin Suspension (B)(G) 40-45 mg/kg/day divided tid or 90 mg/kg/day divided bid; 125 mg/5 ml (75, 100, 150 ml) (banana); 250 mg/5 ml (75, 100, 150 ml) (orange); 200, 400 mg/5 ml (50, 75, 100 ml) (orange-raspberry) (phenylalanine).

APPENDIX P.5. AMOXICILLIN+CLAVULANATE (AUGMENTIN ES 600 SUSPENSION)

Weight												
Pounds	15	20	25	30	35	40	45	50	55	60	65	70
Kilograms	6.8	9	11.4	13.6	15.9	18.2	20.5	22.7	25	27.3	29.5	31.8
Single Dose (ml)/Frequency/Strength/10-Day Volume (ml)												
40 mg/kg/d ml/dose bid	1	1.5	2	2	2.5	3	3.5	4	4	4.5	5	5
mg/5 ml	600	600	600	600	600	600	600	600	600	600	600	600
Volume (ml)	30	40	40	40	50	60	70	80	80	90	100	100
45 mg/kg/d ml/dose bid	1.25	1.5	2	2.5	3	3.5	4	4.5	5	5	5.5	6
mg/5 ml	600	600	600	600	600	600	600	600	600	600	600	600
Volume (ml)	25	30	40	50	60	70	80	90	100	100	110	120
90 mg/kg/d ml/dose bid	2.5	3.5	4	5	6	7	8	8.5	9.5	10	11	12
mg/5 ml	600	600	600	600	600	600	600	600	600	600	600	600
Volume (ml)	50	70	80	100	120	140	160	170	190	200	220	240

Augmentin ES 600 Suspension (B) <3 months: not recommended; ≥3 months, <40 kg: 90 mg/kg/day in 2 divided doses; ≥40 kg: not recommended; 600 mg/5 ml (50, 75, 100, 125, 150, 200 ml) (strawberry cream) (phenylalanine).

APPENDIX P.6. AMPICILLIN (OMNIPEN SUSPENSION, PRINCIPEN SUSPENSION)

Weight												
Pounds	15	20	25	30	35	40	45	50	55	60	65	70
Kilograms	6.8	9	11.4	13.6	15.9	18.2	20.5	22.7	25	27.3	29.5	31.8
Single Dose (ml)/Frequency/Strength/10-Day Volume (ml)												
50 mg/kg/d ml/dose q6h	3.5	4.5	3	3.5	4	4.5						
mg/5 ml	125	125	250	250	250	250						
Volume (ml)	140	180	120	140	160	180						
100 mg/kg/d ml/dose q6h	3.5	4.5	6	7	8	9						
mg/5 ml	250	250	250	250	250	250						
Volume (ml)	140	180	240	280	320	360						

Omnipen Suspension, Principen Suspension (B)(G) >20 kg: 250-500 mg q 6 h 125, 250 mg/5 ml (100, 150, 200 ml) (fruit).

APPENDIX P.7. AZITHROMYCIN (ZITHROMAX SUSPENSION, ZMAX SUSPENSION)

Weight								
Pounds	11	22	33	44	55	66	77	88
Kilograms	5	10	15	20	25	30	35	40
Single Dose (ml)/Frequency/Strength/Volume (ml)								
3-Day Regimen								
10 mg/kg qd	2.5	5	7.5	5	6	7.5	9	10
mg/5 ml	100	100	100	200	200	200	200	200
Volume (ml)	7.5	15	22.5	15	18	22.5	27	30
5-Day Regimen								
10 mg/kg qd								
Day 1	2.5	5	7.5	5	6	7.5	7.5	10
Days 2–5	1.25	2.5	4	2.5	3	4	4	5
mg/5 ml	100	100	100	200	200	200	200	200
Volume (ml)	10	15	23.5	15	18	23.5	23.5	30

Zithromax ES 600 Suspension (B)(G) 100 mg/5 ml (15 ml), 200 mg/5 ml (15, 22.5, 30 ml) (cherry-vanilla-banana).

APPENDIX P.8. CEFACLOR (CECLOR SUSPENSION)

Weight												
Pounds	15	20	25	30	35	40	45	50	55	60	65	70
Kilograms	6.8	9	11.4	13.6	15.9	18.2	20.5	22.7	25	27.3	29.5	31.8
Single Dose (ml)/Frequency/Strength/10-Day Volume (ml)												
20 mg/kg/d ml/dose tid	2	2.5	3	3.5	4	5	5.5	6	7	7.5	8	8.5
mg/5 ml	125	125	125	125	125	125	125	125	125	125	125	125
Volume (ml)	60	75	90	105	120	150	165	180	210	225	240	255
20 mg/kg/d ml/dose tid	1.5	1.5	2	2.5	3	3	4	4	4.5	5	5.5	6
mg/5 ml	187	187	187	187	187	187	187	187	187	187	187	187
Volume (ml)	45	45	60	75	90	90	105	120	135	150	165	180
40 mg/kg/d ml/dose tid	2	2.5	3	3.5	4	5	5.5	6	6.5	7	8	8.5
mg/5 ml	250	250	250	250	250	250	250	250	250	250	250	250
Volume (ml)	60	75	90	105	120	150	165	180	195	210	240	255
40 mg/kg/d ml/dose tid	1.5	1.5	2	2.5	3	3	3.5	4	4.5	5	5	5.5
mg/5 ml	375	375	375	375	375	375	375	375	375	375	375	375
Volume (ml)	45	45	60	75	90	90	105	120	135	150	150	165

Ceclor Suspension (B) <6 months: not recommended; 125, 250 mg/5 ml (75, 150 ml) (strawberry); 187, 375 mg/5 ml (50, 100 ml) (strawberry).

APPENDIX P.9. CEFADROXIL (DURICEF SUSPENSION)

Weight												
Pounds	15	20	25	30	35	40	45	50	55	60	65	70
Kilograms	6.8	9	11.4	13.6	15.9	18.2	20.5	22.7	25	27.3	29.5	31.8
Single Dose (ml)/Frequency/Strength/10-Day Volume (ml)												
30 mg/kg/d ml/ dose bid	2	3	3.5	4	5	5.5	6	7	7.5	8	9	9.5
mg/5 ml	250	250	250	250	250	250	250	250	250	250	250	250
Volume (ml)	40	60	75	80	100	110	120	140	150	160	180	190
30 mg/kg/d ml/ dose qd	2	3	3.5	4	5	5.5	6	7	7.5	8	9	9.5
mg/5 ml	500	500	500	500	500	500	500	500	500	500	500	500
Volume (ml)	20	30	35	40	50	55	60	70	75	80	90	95

Duricef Suspension (B) 250 mg/5 ml (100 ml) (orange-pineapple); 500 mg/5 ml (75, 100 ml) (orange-pineapple).

APPENDIX P.10. CEFDINIR (OMNICEF SUSPENSION)

Weight												
Pounds	15	20	25	30	35	40	45	50	55	60	65	70
Kilograms	6.8	9	11.4	13.6	15.9	18.2	20.5	22.7	25	27.3	29.5	31.8
Single Dose (ml)/Frequency/Strength/10-Day Volume (ml)												
7 mg/kg/d ml/dose bid	2	2.5	3	4	4.5	5	6	6.5	7	7.5	8	9
mg/5 ml	125	125	125	125	125	125	125	125	125	125	125	125
Volume (ml)	40	50	60	80	90	100	120	130	140	150	160	180
14 mg/kg ml/dose bid	4	5	6	8	9	10	12	13	14	15	16	18
mg/5 ml	125	125	125	125	125	125	125	125	125	125	125	125
Volume (ml)	40	50	60	80	90	100	120	130	140	150	160	180

Omnicef Suspension (B) <6 months: not recommended; 125 mg/5 ml (60, 100 ml) (strawberry).

APPENDIX P.11. CEFIXIME (SUPRAX ORAL SUSPENSION)

Weight												
Pounds	15	20	25	30	35	40	45	50	55	60	65	70
Kilograms	6.8	9	11.4	13.6	15.9	18.2	20.5	22.7	25	27.3	29.5	31.8
Single Dose (ml)/Frequency/Strength/10-Day Volume (ml)												
8 mg/kg/d ml/ dose bid	1.3	1.8	2.2	2.5	3.1	3.5	4	4.5	5	5.5	6	6.5
mg/5 ml	100	100	100	100	100	100	100	100	100	100	100	100
8 mg/kg/d ml/dose qd	2.7	3.6	4.5	5.5	6.3	7.2	8.2	9	10	11	12	13
mg/5 ml	100	100	100	100	100	100	100	100	100	100	100	100
Volume (ml)	27	36	45	55	65	70	80	90	100	110	120	130

Supra Oral Suspension (B)(G) <6 months: not recommended; 100 mg/5 ml (50, 75, 100 ml) (strawberry).

APPENDIX P.12. CEFPODOXIME PROXETIL

Weight												
Pounds	15	20	25	30	35	40	45	50	55	60	65	70
Kilograms	6.8	9	11.4	13.6	15.9	18.2	20.5	22.7	25	27.3	29.5	31.8
Single Dose (ml)/Frequency/Strength/10-Day Volume (ml)												
5 mg/kg/d ml/dose bid	3.5	4.5	5.5	7	8	9	10	11	12.5	13.5	15	16
mg/5 ml	50	50	50	50	50	50	50	50	50	50	50	50
Volume (ml)	70	90	110	140	160	180	200	220	250	270	300	320
5 mg/kg/d ml/dose bid	2	2	3	3.5	4	4.5	5	5.5	6	7	7.5	8
mg/5 ml	100	100	100	100	100	100	100	100	100	100	100	100
Volume (ml)	40	40	60	70	80	90	100	110	120	140	150	160

Vantin Suspension (B) <2 months: not recommended; 50, 100 mg/5 ml (50, 75, 100 ml) (lemon-crème).

APPENDIX P.13. CEFPROZIL (CEFZIL SUSPENSION)

Weight												
Pounds	15	20	25	30	35	40	45	50	55	60	65	70
Kilograms	6.8	9	11.4	13.6	15.9	18.2	20.5	22.7	25	27.3	29.5	31.8
Single Dose (ml)/Frequency/Strength/10-Day Volume (ml)												
7.5 mg/kg/d ml/dose bid	2	3	3.5	4	5	5.5	6	7	7.5	4	4.5	5
mg/5 ml	125	125	125	125	125	125	125	125	125	250	250	250
Volume (ml)	40	60	70	80	100	110	120	140	150	80	90	100
15 mg/kg/d ml/dose bid	2	3	3.5	4	5	5	6	7	7.5	8	9	9.5
mg/5 ml	250	250	250	250	250	250	250	250	250	250	250	250
Volume (ml)	40	60	70	80	100	100	120	140	150	160	180	190
20 mg/kg/d ml/dose qd	3	3.5	4.5	5.5	6.5	7	8	9	10	11	12	13
mg/5 ml	250	250	250	250	250	250	250	250	250	250	250	250
Volume (ml)	60	70	90	110	130	140	160	180	200	220	240	260

Cefzil Suspension (B) ≤6 months: not recommended; 2-12 years: 7.5-20 mg/kg bid >12 years: 250-500 mg bid or 500 mg once daily; 125, 250 mg/5 ml (50, 75, 100 ml) (bubble gum) (phenylalanine).

APPENDIX P.14. CEFTIBUTEN (CEDAX SUSPENSION)

Weight												
Pounds	15	20	25	30	35	40	45	50	55	60	65	70
Kilograms	6.8	9	11.4	13.6	15.9	18.2	20.5	22.7	25	27.3	29.5	31.8
Single Dose (ml)/Frequency/Strength/10-Day Volume (ml)												
9 mg/kg/d ml/dose qd	3.5	4.5	6	7	8	9	10	11.5	12.5	13.5	15	16
mg/5 ml	90	90	90	90	90	90	90	90	90	90	90	90
Volume (ml)	35	45	60	70	80	90	100	115	125	135	150	160
9 mg/kg/d ml/dose qd	1.75	2.3	3	3.5	4	4.5	5	5.4	6.2	6.6	7.5	8
mg/5 ml	180	180	180	180	180	180	180	180	180	180	180	180
Volume (ml)	20	25	30	35	40	45	50	55	60	65	70	80

Cefzil Suspension (B) 90 mg/5 ml (30, 60, 90, 120 ml) (cherry); 180 mg/5 ml (30, 60, 120 ml) (cherry).

APPENDIX P.15. CEPHALEXIN (KEFLEX SUSPENSION)

Weight												
Pounds	15	20	25	30	35	40	45	50	55	60	65	70
Kilograms	6.8	9	11.4	13.6	15.9	18.2	20.5	22.7	25	27.3	29.5	31.8
Single Dose (ml)/Frequency/Strength/10-Day Volume (ml)												
25 mg/kg/d ml/dose tid	1	1.5	2	2	3	3	3.5	4	4	4.5	5	5
mg/5 ml	125	125	125	125	125	125	125	125	125	125	125	125
Volume (ml)	30	45	60	60	90	90	105	120	120	135	150	150
25 mg/kg/d ml/dose qid	1	1	1.5	2	2	2.5	2.5	3	3	3.5	4	4
mg/5 ml	250	250	250	250	250	250	250	250	250	250	250	250
Volume (ml)	40	40	60	80	80	100	100	120	120	140	160	160
50 mg/kg/d ml/dose tid	2	3	4	4.5	5	6	7	7.5	8	9	10	10.5
mg/5 ml	250	250	250	250	250	250	250	250	250	250	250	250
Volume (ml)	60	90	120	135	150	180	210	225	240	270	300	315
50 mg/kg/d ml/dose qid	2	2	3	3.5	4	4.5	5	6	6	7	7.5	8
mg/5 ml	250	250	250	250	250	250	250	250	250	250	250	250
Volume (ml)	80	80	120	140	160	180	200	240	240	280	300	320

Keflex Suspension (B)(G) <2 months: not recommended; 125, 250 mg/5 ml (100, 200 ml) (strawberry).

APPENDIX P.16. CLARITHROMYCIN (BIAXIN SUSPENSION)

Weight												
Pounds	15	20	25	30	35	40	45	50	55	60	65	70
Kilograms	6.8	9	11.4	13.6	15.9	18.2	20.5	22.7	25	27.3	29.5	31.8
Single Dose (ml)/Frequency/Strength/10-Day Volume (ml)												
7.5 mg/kg/d ml/ dose bid	2	3	3.5	4	5	5.5	6	7	7.5	8	9	10
mg/5 ml	125	125	125	125	125	125	125	125	125	125	125	125
Volume (ml)	40	60	70	80	100	110	120	140	150	160	180	200
7.5 mg/kg/d ml/ dose bid	1	1.5	2	2	2.5	3	3	3.5	4	4	4.5	5
mg/5 ml	250	250	250	250	250	250	250	250	250	250	250	250
Volume (ml)	20	30	40	40	50	60	60	70	80	80	90	100

Biaxin Suspension (B) <6 months: not recommended; 125, 250 mg/5 ml (50, 100 ml) (fruit punch).

APPENDIX P.17. CLINDAMYCIN (CLEOCIN PEDIATRIC GRANULES)

Weight												
Pounds	15	20	25	30	35	40	45	50	55	60	65	70
Kilograms	6.8	9	11.4	13.6	15.9	18.2	20.5	22.7	25	27.3	29.5	31.8
Single Dose (ml)/Frequency/Strength/10-Day Volume (ml)												
8 mg/kg/d ml/dose tid	1	1.5	2	2.5	3	3	3.5	4	4.5	5	5	5.5
mg/5 ml	75	75	75	75	75	75	75	75	75	75	75	75
Volume (ml)	30	45	60	75	90	90	105	120	135	150	150	165
16 mg/kg/d ml/dose tid	2.5	3	4	5	5.5	6.5	7	8	9	9.5	10.5	11
mg/5 ml	75	75	75	75	75	75	75	75	75	75	75	75
Volume (ml)	75	90	120	150	165	105	210	240	270	285	315	330

Cleocin Pediatric Granules (B)(G) 75 mg/5 ml (100 ml) (cherry).

APPENDIX P.18. DICLOXACILLIN (DYNAPEN SUSPENSION)

Weight												
Pounds	15	20	25	30	35	40	45	50	55	60	65	70
Kilograms	6.8	9	11.4	13.6	15.9	18.2	20.5	22.7	25	27.3	29.5	31.8
Single Dose (ml)/Frequency/Strength/10-Day Volume (ml)												
12.5 mg/kg/d ml/dose qid	2	2.5	3	3.5	4	4.5	5	6	6	7	7.5	8
mg/5 ml	62.5	62.5	62.5	62.5	62.5	62.5	62.5	62.5	62.5	62.5	62.5	62.5
Volume (ml)	80	100	120	140	160	180	200	240	240	280	300	320
25 mg/kg/d ml/dose qid	3.5	4.5	6	7	8	9	10	11.5	12.5	13.5	15	16
mg/5 ml	62.5	62.5	62.5	62.5	62.5	62.5	62.5	62.5	62.5	62.5	62.5	62.5
Volume (ml)	140	180	240	280	320	360	400	460	500	540	600	640

Dynapen Suspension (B)(G) 6.25 mg/5 ml (80, 100 ml) (raspberry-strawberry).

APPENDIX P.19. DOXYCYCLINE (VIBRAMYCIN SYRUP/SUSPENSION)

Weight												
Pounds	15	20	25	30	35	40	45	50	55	60	65	70
Kilograms	6.8	9	11.4	13.6	15.9	18.2	20.5	22.7	25	27.3	29.5	31.8
Single Dose (ml)/Frequency/Strength/10-Day Volume (ml)												
1 mg/lb/d ml/dose qd	1.5	2	2.5	3	3.5	4	4.5	5	5.5	6	6.5	7
50 mg/5 ml	50	50	50	50	50	50	50	50	50	50	50	50
Volume (ml)	15	20	25	30	35	40	45	50	55	60	65	70
1 mg/lb/d ml/dose qd	3	4	5	6	7	8	9	10	11	12	13	14
25 mg/5 ml	25	25	25	25	25	25	25	25	25	25	25	25
Volume (ml)	30	40	50	60	70	80	90	100	110	120	130	140

Vibramycin Syrup (B)(G) <8 years: not recommended; double dose first day; 50 mg/5 ml (80, 100, ml) (raspberry-apple) (sulfites).
Vibramycin Suspension (B)(G) <8 years: not recommended; double dose first day; 25 mg/5 ml (80, 100, ml) (raspberry).

APPENDIX P.20. ERYTHROMYCIN ESTOLATE (ILOSONE SUSPENSION)

Weight												
Pounds	15	20	25	30	35	40	45	50	55	60	65	70
Kilograms	6.8	9	11.4	13.6	15.9	18.2	20.5	22.7	25	27.3	29.5	31.8
Dose/Volume (10 days) in ml												
10 mg/kg/d ml/dose bid	3	3.5	4.5	5.5	6	7	8	9	10	5.5	6	6.5
mg/5 ml	125	125	125	125	125	125	125	125	125	250	250	250
Volume (ml)	60	70	90	110	120	140	160	180	200	110	120	130
15 mg/kg/d ml/dose bid	4	5.5	7	8	9.5	5.5	6	7	7.5	8	9	9.5
mg/5 ml	125	125	125	125	125	250	250	250	250	250	250	250
Volume (ml)	80	110	140	160	190	110	120	140	150	160	180	190
20 mg/kg/d ml/dose bid	3	3.5	4.5	5.5	6.5	7	8	9	10	11	12	13
mg/5 ml	250	250	250	250	250	250	250	250	250	250	250	250
Volume (ml)	60	70	90	110	120	140	160	180	200	220	240	260
25 mg/kg/d ml/dose bid	3.5	4.5	5.5	7	8	9	10	11.5	12.5	13.5	15	16
mg/5 ml	250	250	250	250	250	250	250	250	250	250	250	250
Volume (ml)	70	90	110	140	160	180	200	230	250	280	300	320

Ilosone Suspension (B)(G) 125, 250 mg/5 ml (100 ml).

APPENDIX P.21. *ERYTHROMYCIN ETHYLSUCCINATE* (E.E.S. SUSPENSION, ERY-PED DROPS/SUSPENSION)

Weight												
Pounds	15	20	25	30	35	40	45	50	55	60	65	70
Kilograms	6.8	9	11.4	13.6	15.9	18.2	20.5	22.7	25	27.3	29.5	31.8
Single Dose (ml)/Frequency/Strength/10-Day Volume (ml)												
30 mg/kg/d ml/dose qid	1.5	2	2	2.5	3	3.5	4	4	4.5	5	5.5	6
mg/5 ml	200	200	200	200	200	200	200	200	200	200	200	200
Volume (ml)	60	80	80	100	120	140	160	160	180	200	220	240
30 mg/kg/d ml/dose qid			1	1.5	1.5	2	2	2	2.5	2.5	3	3
mg/5 ml			400	400	400	400	400	400	400	400	400	
Volume (ml)			60	60	80	80	80	100	100	120	120	
50 mg/kg/d ml/dose qid	2	3	3.5	4.5	5	5.5	6.5	7	8	8.5	9	10
mg/5 ml	200	200	200	200	200	200	200	200	200	200	200	200
Volume (ml)	80	120	140	180	200	220	260	280	320	340	360	400
50 mg/kg/d ml/dose qid	1	1.5	2	2	2.5	3	3	3.5	4	4.5	4.5	5

(*continued*)

APPENDIX P.21. *ERYTHROMYCIN ETHYLSUCCINATE* (E.E.S. SUSPENSION, ERY-PED DROPS/SUSPENSION) (*continued*)

mg/5 ml	400	400	400	400	400	400	400	400	400	400	400	400
Volume (ml)	40	60	80	80	100	120	140	140	160	180	180	200

Ery-Ped Drops/Suspension (B)(G) 200 mg/5 ml (100, 200 ml) (fruit); 400 mg/5 ml (60, 100, 200 ml) (banana); Oral drops: 200, 400 mg/5 ml (50 ml) (fruit).

E.E.S. Suspension (B)(G) 200 mg/5 ml, 400 mg/5 ml (100 ml) (fruit).
E.E.S. Granules (B)(G) 200 mg/5 ml (100, 200 ml) (cherry).

APPENDIX P.22. ERYTHROMYCIN+SULFISOXAZOLE (ERYZOLE, PEDIAZOLE)

Weight												
Pounds	15	20	25	30	35	40	45	50	55	60	65	70
Kilograms	6.8	9	11.4	13.6	15.9	18.2	20.5	22.7	25	27.3	29.5	31.8
Single Dose (ml)/Frequency/Strength/10-Day Volume (ml)												
10 mg/kg/d ml/dose bid	3	4	5	6	6.5	7.5	8.5	9.5	10	11	12	13.5
mg/5 ml	200	200	200	200	200	200	200	200	200	200	200	200
Volume (ml)	90	120	150	180	200	225	255	285	300	330	360	400

Eryzole (C)(G) <2 months: not recommended; *eryth* 200 mg/*sulf* 600 mg/5 ml (100, 150, 200, 250 ml).
Pediazole (C)(G) <2 months: not recommended; *eryth* 200 mg/*sulf* 600 mg/5 ml (100, 150, 200 ml) (strawberry-banana).

APPENDIX P.23. FLUCONAZOLE (DIFLUCAN SUSPENSION)

Weight												
Pounds	15	20	25	30	35	40	45	50	55	60	65	70
Kilograms	6.8	9	11.4	13.6	15.9	18.2	20.5	22.7	25	27.3	29.5	31.8
Single Dose (ml)/Frequency/Strength/21-Day Volume (ml)												
3 mg/kg/d ml/dose qd	2	3	3.5	4	5	5.5	6	7	7.5	8	9	9.5
mg/ml	10	10	10	10	10	10	10	10	10	10	10	10
Volume (ml)	44	66	77	88	110	121	132	154	165	176	198	209
6 mg/kg/d ml/dose qd	4	5.5	2	2	2.5	3	3	3.5	4	4	4.5	5
mg/ml	10	10	40	40	40	40	40	40	40	40	40	40
Volume (ml)	88	121	44	44	55	66	66	77	88	88	99	110

Diflucan Suspension (B)(G) double dose first day; 10, 40 mg/5 ml (35 ml) (orange).

APPENDIX P.24. FURAZOLIDONE (FUROXONE LIQUID)

Weight												
Pounds	15	20	25	30	35	40	45	50	55	60	65	70
Kilograms	6.8	9	11.4	13.6	15.9	18.2	20.5	22.7	25	27.3	29.5	31.8
Single Dose (ml)/Frequency/Strength/7-Day Volume (ml)												
5 mg/kg/d ml/dose qid	2.5	3.5	4	5	6	7	8	8.5	9.5	10	11	12
mg/15 ml	50	50	50	50	50	50	50	50	50	50	50	50
Vol	100	140	160	200	240	280	320	340	380	400	440	480

Furoxone Liquid (C)(G) double dose first day; 50 mg/15 ml (35 ml).

APPENDIX P.25. GRISEOFULVIN, MICROSIZE (GRIFULVIN V SUSPENSION)

Weight												
Pounds	15	20	25	30	35	40	45	50	55	60	65	70
Kilograms	6.8	9	11.4	13.6	15.9	18.2	20.5	22.7	25	27.3	29.5	31.8
Single Dose (ml)/Frequency/Strength/30-Day Volume (ml)												
5 mg/lb/d ml/dose day	3	4	5	6	7	8	9	10	11	12	13	14
mg/5 ml	125	125	125	125	125	125	125	125	125	125	125	125
Volume (ml)	90	120	150	180	210	240	270	300	330	360	390	420

Grifulvin V Suspension (C)(G) double dose first day; 125 mg/5 ml (120 ml) (orange) (alcohol 0.02%).

APPENDIX P.26. ITRACONAZOLE (SPORANOX SOLUTION)

Weight												
Pounds	15	20	25	30	35	40	45	50	55	60	65	70
Kilograms	6.8	9	11.4	13.6	15.9	18.2	20.5	22.7	25	27.3	29.5	31.8
Single Dose (ml)/Frequency/Strength/7-Day Volume (ml)												
5 mg/kg/d ml/dose qd	3.5	4.5	6	7	8	9	10	11.5	12.5	14	15	16
mg/ml	10	10	10	10	10	10	10	10	10	10	10	10
Volume (ml)	25	32	42	49	56	63	70	71	88	98	105	112

Sporanox V Solution (C)(G) double dose first day; 10 mg/ml (150 ml) (cherry-caramel).

APPENDIX P.27. LORACARBEF (LORABID SUSPENSION)

Weight												
Pounds	15	20	25	30	35	40	45	50	55	60	65	70
Kilograms	6.8	9	11.4	13.6	15.9	18.2	20.5	22.7	25	27.3	29.5	31.8
Single Dose (ml)/Frequency/Strength/10-Day Volume (ml)												
15 mg/kg/d ml/dose bid	2.5	3.5	4	5	3	3.5	4	4	5	5	5.5	6
mg/5 ml	100	100	100	100	200	200	200	200	200	200	200	200
Volume (ml)	50	70	80	100	60	70	80	80	100	100	110	120
30 mg/kg/d ml/dose bid	2.5	3.5	4	5	6	7	8	8.5	9.5	10	11	12
mg/5 ml	200	200	200	200	200	200	200	200	200	200	200	200
Volume (ml)	50	70	80	100	120	140	160	170	190	200	220	240

Lorabid Suspension (B) 100 mg/5 ml (50, 100 ml) (strawberry bubble gum); 200 mg/5 ml (50, 75, 100 ml) (strawberry bubble gum).

APPENDIX P.28. NITROFURANTOIN (FURADANTIN SUSPENSION)

Weight											
Pounds	15	20	25	30	35	40	45	50	55	60	65	70
Kilograms	6.8	9	11.4	13.6	15.9	18.2	20.5	22.7	25	27.3	29.5	31.8
Single Dose (ml)/Frequency/Strength/10-Day Volume (ml)												
5 mg/kg ml/dose qid	1.5	2.5	3	3.5	4	4.5	5	5.5	6	7	7.5	8
mg/5 ml	25	25	25	25	25	25	25	25	25	25	25	25
Volume (ml)	60	100	120	140	160	190	200	220	240	280	300	320

Furadantin Suspension (B)(G) 25 mg/5 ml (60 ml).

APPENDIX P.29. PENICILLIN V POTASSIUM (PEN-VEE K SOLUTION, VEETIDS SOLUTION)

Weight												
Pounds	15	20	25	30	35	40	45	50	55	60	65	70
Kilograms	6.8	9	11.4	13.6	15.9	18.2	20.5	22.7	25	27.3	29.5	31.8
Single Dose (ml)/Frequency/Strength/10-Day Volume (ml)												
25 mg/kg/d ml/dose qid	2	2.5	3	3.5	4	4.5	5	5.5	6	7	7.5	8
mg/5 ml	125	125	125	125	125	125	125	125	125	125	125	125
Volume (ml)	80	90	120	140	160	180	200	220	240	280	300	320
25 mg/kg/d ml/dose qid	1	1	1.5	2	2	2.5	2.5	3	3	3.5	4	4
mg/5 ml	250	250	250	250	250	250	250	250	250	250	250	250
Volume (ml)	40	40	60	80	80	100	100	120	120	140	160	160
50 mg/kg/d ml/dose qid	2	2.5	3	3.5	4	4.5	5	6	6.5	7	7.5	8
mg/5 ml	250	250	250	250	250	250	250	250	250	250	250	250
Volume (ml)	80	100	120	140	160	180	200	240	260	280	300	320

Pen-Vee K Solution (B)(G) 125 mg/5 ml (100, 200 ml); 250 mg/5 ml (100, 150, 200 ml).
Veetids Solution (B)(G) 125, 250 mg/5 ml (100, 200 ml).

APPENDIX P.30. RIMANTADINE (FLUMADINE SYRUP)

Weight												
Pounds	15	20	25	30	35	40	45	50	55	60	65	70
Kilograms	6.8	9	11.4	13.6	15.9	18.2	20.5	22.7	25	27.3	29.5	31.8
Single Dose (ml)/Frequency/Strength/10-Day Volume (ml)												
5 mg/kg/d ml/dose qd	3.5	4.5	6	7	8	9	10	11.5	12.5	13.5	15	16
mg/5 ml	50	50	50	50	50	50	50	50	50	50	50	50
Volume (ml)	35	45	60	70	80	90	100	115	125	135	150	160

Flumadine Syrup (B) 50 mg/5 ml (2, 8, 16 oz) (raspberry).

APPENDIX P.31. TETRACYCLINE (SUMYCIN SUSPENSION)

Weight												
Pounds	15	20	25	30	35	40	45	50	55	60	65	70
Kilograms	6.8	9	11.4	13.6	15.9	18.2	20.5	22.7	25	27.3	29.5	31.8
Single Dose (ml)/Frequency/Strength/10-Day Volume (ml)												
25 mg/kg/d ml/dose qid	1.5	2.5	3	3.5	4	4.5	5	6	6.5	7	7.5	8
mg/5 ml	125	125	125	125	125	125	125	125	125	125	125	125
Volume (ml)	60	100	120	140	160	180	200	240	260	280	300	320
50 mg/kg/d ml/dose qid	3.5	4.5	6	7	8	9	10	11.5	12.5	13.5	15	16
mg/5 ml	125	125	125	125	125	125	125	125	125	125	125	125
Volume (ml)	140	180	240	280	320	360	400	460	500	540	600	640

Sumycin Suspension (D)(G) <8 years: not recommended; 125 mg/5 ml (100, 200 ml) (fruit) (sulfites).

APPENDIX P.32. TRIMETHOPRIM (PRIMSOL SUSPENSION)

Weight												
Pounds	15	20	25	30	35	40	45	50	55	60	65	70
Kilograms	6.8	9	11.4	13.6	15.9	18.2	20.5	22.7	25	27.3	29.5	31.8
Single Dose (ml)/Frequency/Strength/10-Day Volume (ml)												
5 mg/kg/d ml/dose bid	3.5	4.5	6	7	8	9	10	11.5	12.5	13.5	15	16
mg/5 ml	50	50	50	50	50	50	50	50	50	50	50	50
Volume (ml)	70	90	120	140	160	180	200	230	250	270	300	320

Primsol Suspension (C)(G) 50 mg/5 ml (50 mg/5 ml) (bubble gum) (dye-free, alcohol-free).

APPENDIX P.33. TRIMETHOPRIM+SULFAMETHOXAZOLE (BACTRIM SUSPENSION, SEPTRA SUSPENSION)

Weight												
Pounds	15	20	25	30	35	40	45	50	55	60	65	70
Kilograms	6.8	9	11.4	13.6	15.9	18.2	20.5	22.7	25	27.3	29.5	31.8
Single Dose (ml)/Frequency/Strength/10-Day Volume (ml)												
10 mg/kg/d ml/dose bid	2	2	3	3.5	4	4.5	5	5.5	6	7	7.5	8
mg/5 ml	200	200	200	200	200	200	200	200	200	200	200	200
Volume (ml)	40	40	60	70	80	90	100	110	120	140	150	160
20 mg/kg/d ml/dose bid	4	4	6	7	8	9	10	11	12	14	15	16
mg/5 ml	200	200	200	200	200	200	200	200	200	200	200	200
Volume (ml)	80	80	120	140	160	180	200	220	240	280	300	320

Bactrim Pediatric Suspension, Septra Pediatric Suspension (C)(G) *trim* 40 mg/*sulfa* 200 mg/5 ml (100 ml) (cherry) (alcohol 0.3%).

APPENDIX P.34. VANCOMYCIN SOLUTION

Weight												
Pounds	15	20	25	30	35	40	45	50	55	60	65	70
Kilograms	6.8	9	11.4	13.6	15.9	18.2	20.5	22.7	25	27.3	29.5	31.8
Single Dose (ml)/Frequency/Strength/10-Day Volume (ml)												
40 mg/kg/d ml/dose tid	2	2.5	3	3.5	4.5	5	5.5	6	7	7.5	8	8.5
mg/5 ml	250	250	250	250	250	250	250	250	250	250	250	250
Volume (ml)	60	75	90	105	135	150	165	180	210	225	240	255
40 mg/kg/d ml/dose qid	1.5	2	2.5	3	3	3.5	4	4.5	5	5.5	6	6.5
mg/5 ml	250	250	250	250	250	250	250	250	250	250	250	250
Volume (ml)	60	80	100	120	120	140	160	180	200	220	240	260
40 mg/kg/d ml/dose tid	1	1	1.5	2	2	2.5	3	3	3.5	3.5	4	4
mg/5 ml	500	500	500	500	500	500	500	500	500	500	500	500
Volume (ml)	30	30	45	60	60	75	90	90	105	105	120	120

(continued)

APPENDIX P.34. VANCOMYCIN SOLUTION (*continued*)

40 mg/kg/d ml/dose qid	1	1	1.5	1.5	1.5	2	2	2.5	2.5	3	3	3.5
mg/5 ml	500	500	500	500	500	500	500	500	500	500	500	500
Volume (ml)	40	40	60	60	60	80	80	100	100	120	120	140

Vancomycin Suspension (C)(G) Suspension or solution currently not available in the United States.; however, a **Vancomycin** oral solution compounding kit is available and a solution may be prepared by pharmacist on request; <12 years: not established; >12 years: usually 40 mg/kg/day in 3-4 divided doses; max 2 gm/day; ≥40 kg: 500 mg to 2 gm in 3-4 divided doses; max 2 gm/day.

2017 ACC/AHA/AAPA/ABC/ACPM/AGS/APhA/ASH/ASPC/NMA/PCNA Guideline for the Prevention, Detection, Evaluation, and Management of High Blood Pressure in Adults: A report of the American College of Cardiology/ American Heart Association Task Force on Clinical Practice Guidelines
http://hyper.ahajournals.org/content/hypertensionaha/early/2017/11/10/HYP.0000000000000065.full.pdf

ACR Guidelines on Prevention & Treatment of Glucocorticoid-induced Osteoporosis [press release, June 7, 2017]. Atlanta, GA. American College of Rheumatology.
https://www.rheumatology.org/About-Us/Newsroom/Press-Releases/ID/812/ACR-Releases-Guideline-on-Prevention-Treatment-of-Glucocorticoid-Induced-Osteoporosis

Advance for Nurse Practitioners
http://nurse-practitioners.advanceweb.com

Advanced Practice Education Associates
www.apea.com

Ake, JA, Schuetz, A, Pegu, P, *et al.* Safety and immunogenicity of PENNVAX-G DNA prime administered by biojector 2000 or CELLECTRA electroporation device with modified vaccinia Ankara-CMDR boost. *J Infect Dis*. 2017:216(9), 1080–1090. doi:10.1093/infdis/jix456

American Academy of Dermatology
https://www.aad.org/home

American Academy of Pediatrics (AAP)
http://aapexperience.org/

American Association of Nurse Practitioners
www.aanp.org

American College of Cardiology. Then and Now: ATP III vs. IV: Comparison of ATP III and ACC/AHA Guidelines
http://www.acc.org/latest-in-cardiology/articles/2014/07/18/16/03/then-and-now-atp-iii-vs-iv

American Diabetes Association (ADA), Professional Diabetes Resources Online
http://professional.diabetes.org/content/clinical-practice-recommendations/?loc=rp-slabnav

American Diabetes Association. (2018). Children and adolescents: Standards of medical care in diabetes—2018. *Diabetes Care, 41*(Supplement 1), S126–S136. doi:10.2337/dc18-S012

American Diabetes Association. (2018). Management of diabetes in pregnancy: Standards of medical care in diabetes—2018. *Diabetes Care, 41*(Supplement 1), S137–S143. doi:10.2337/dc18-S013

American Diabetes Association. (2018). Microvascular complications and foot care: Standards of medical care in diabetes—2018. *Diabetes Care, 41*(Supplement 1), S105–S118. doi:10.2337/dc18-S010

American Diabetes Association. (2018). Pharmacologic approaches to glycemic treatment: Standards of medical care in diabetes—2018. *Diabetes Care, 41*(Supplement 1), S73–S85. doi:10.2337/dc18-S008

American Diabetes Association. (2018). Summary of revisions: Standards of medical care in diabetes—2018. *Diabetes Care, 41*(Supplement 1), S4–S6. doi:10.2337/dc18-Srev01

American Family Physician
http://www.aafp.org/online/en/home.html

American Headache Society
www.americanheadachesociety.org
American Pain Society
http://americanpainsociety.org/
American Pharmacists Association. (2018). *Pediatric and neonatal dosage handbook: A universal resource for clinicians treating pediatric and neonatal patients* (25th ed.). Hudson, OH: Lexicomp.
American Trypanosomiasis Centers for Disease Control and Prevention. *Parasites—American Trypanosomiasis (also known as Chagas disease). Resources for health professionals.*
Anderson, E, Fantus, RJ, & Haddadin, RI. (2017). Diagnosis and management of herpes zoster ophthalmicus. *Disease-a-Month*, *63*(2), 38–44.
Andorf, S, Purington, N, Block, WM, *et al.* (2018). Anti-IgE treatment with oral immunotherapy in multi-food allergic participants: A double-blind, randomised, controlled trial [published online December 11, 2017]. *The Lancet Gastroenterology & Hepatology*, *3*(2), 85–94. doi:10.1016/S2468-1253(17)30392-8
Aronow, WS. (2017). *Initiation of antihypertensive therapy*. Presented at the American Heart Association (AHA) Scientific Sessions 2017: November 11–15, 2017. Anaheim, CA. http://www.abstractsonline.com/pp8/-!/4412/presentation/55060
ATP III and ACC/AHA guidelines.
http://www.acc.org/latest-in-cardiology/articles/2014/07/18/16/03/then-and-now-atp-iii-vs-iv
Auron, M, & Raissouni, N. (2015). Adrenal insufficiency. *Pediatric Review*, *36*(3), 92–102.
Belknap, R, Holland, D, Feng, PJ, *et al.* (2017). Self-administered versus directly observed once-weekly isoniazid and rifapentine treatment of latent tuberculosis infection: A randomized trial. [Published online ahead of print November 7, 2017]. *Annals of Internal Medicine*, *167*(10), 689–697. doi:10.7326/M17-1150
Bosworth, T. (4/11/17) Testosterone Deficiency Treatment Recommendation
https://www.medpagetoday.com/resource-center/hypogonadism/treatment- recommendations/a/64511
Bradley, JS, & Nelson, JD. *2018 Nelson's pediatric antimicrobial therapy* (24th ed.). American Academy of Pediatrics.
Brody, AA, Gibson, B, & Tresner-Kirsch, D, *et al.* (2016). High prevalence of medication discrepancies between home health referrals and Centers for Medicare and Medicaid Services home health certification and plan of care and their potential to affect safety of vulnerable elderly adults. *Journal of the American Geriatrics Society*, *64*(11), e166–e170.
Brunk, D. Learn 'four Ds' approach to heart failure in diabetes. *Clinician Reviews*. Posted online January 28, 2018 https://www.mdedge.com/clinicalendocrinologynews/article/157198/diabetes/learn-four-ds-approach-heart-failure-diabetes
Canestaro, WJ, Forrester, SH, Raghu, G, *et al.* (2016). Drug treatment of idiopathic pulmonary fibrosis: Systematic review and network meta-analysis. *Chest*, *149*, 756–766.
CDC 2015 Sexually Transmitted Diseases Treatment Guidelines
http://www.cdc.gov/std/tg2015/default.htm
CDC Guidelines for Conception in HIV Positive Women Stress the Use of PrEP in Sexual Partners
https://www.medpagetoday.com/resource-centers/contemporary-hiv-prevention/cdc-guide-lines-conception-hiv-positive-women-stress-use-prep-sexual-partners/775?xid=NL_MPT_MPT_HIV_2017-09-26&eun=g766320d0r

CDC Guideline for Prescribing Opioids for Chronic Pain—United States. (2016).
https://jamanetwork.com/learning/article-quiz/10.1001/jama.2016.1464#qundefined

CDC: Morbidity and Mortality Weekly Report (MMWR)
http://www.cdc.gov/mmwr/mmwr_wk.html

CDC Provider Information Sheet–PrEP during conception, pregnancy, and breast-feeding information for clinicians counseling patients about PrEP use during conception, pregnancy, and breastfeeding.
https://www.cdc.gov/hiv/pdf/prep_gl_clinician_factsheet_pregnancy_english.pdf

CDC Recommended Immunization Schedule for Children and Adolescents Aged 18 Years or Younger, United States 2017
https://www.cdc.gov/vaccines/schedules/downloads/child/0-18yrs-child-combined-schedule.pdf

Centers for Disease Control and Prevention
www.cdc.gov

Centers for Disease Control and Prevention. Diphtheria, tetanus, and pertussis vaccine recommendations. 2016.
http://www.cdc.gov/vaccines/vpd/dtap-tdap-td/hcp/recommendations.htm

Centers for Disease Control and Prevention. (2016). *Facts about ADHD.*
www.cdc.gov/ncbddd/adhd/facts.html

Centers for Disease Control and Prevention. Pneumococcal vaccination: summary of who and when to vaccinate. 2016.
http://www.cdc.gov/vaccines/vpd/pneumo/hcp/who-when-to-vaccinate.html

Chang, AY, Martins, KAO, Encinales, L, *et al.* (2018). Chikungunya arthritis mechanisms in the Americas: A cross-sectional analysis of Chikungunya arthritis patients twenty-two months after infection demonstrating no detectable viral persistence in synovial fluid. *Arthritis & Rheumatology, 70*(4), 585–593. doi:10.1002/art.40383

Chang, AY, Encinales, L, Porras, A, *et al.* (2018). Frequency of chronic joint pain following Chikungunya virus infection. *Arthritis & Rheumatology, 70*(4), 578–584. doi:10.1002/art.40384

Chow, AW, Benninger, MS, & Brook, I, *et al.* (2012). IDSA clinical practice guideline for acute and bacterial rhinosinusitis in children and adults. *Clinical Infectious Diseases, 54*(8), e72–e112.
http://www.clinicianreviews.com/

Clinician Reviews
http://www.clinicianreviews.com/

Cohen, JD, Wang, Y, Thoburn, C, *et al.* (2018). Detection and localization of surgically resectable cancers with a multi-analyte blood test. *Science, 359*(6378), 926–930. doi:10.1126/science.aar3247

Coker, TJ, & Dierfeldt, DM. (2016). Acute bacterial prostatitis: Diagnosis and management. *American Family Physician, 93*(2), 114–120.

Consultant 360
http://www.consultant360.com/home

Daily Med: NIH. US Library of Medicine
https://dailymed.nlm.nih.gov/dailymed/index.cfm

Davis, MC, Miller, BJ, Kalsi, JK, *et al.* (2017). Efficient trial design—FDA approval of valbenazine for tardive dyskinesia. *The New England Journal of Medicine, 376*(26), 2503–2506. doi:10.1056/NEJMp1704898

Dhadwal, G, & Kirchhof, MG. (2017). The risks and benefits of cannabis in the dermatology clinic. [Published online ahead of print October 23, 2017]. *Journal of Cutaneous Medicine and Surgery, 22*(2), 194–199. doi:10.1177/1203475417738971

Dietrich, EA, & Davis, K. (2017). Antibiotics for acute bacterial prostatitis: Which agent, and for how long? *Consultant*, *57*(9), 564–565.

Domino, FJ, Baldor, RA, Golding, J, & Stephens, MB. The 5-minute clinical consult standard *2018 (26th ed.)*. Philadelphia, PA: Wolters Kluwer.

Dowell, D, Haegerich, TM, & Chou, R. (2016). CDC Guidelines for prescribing opioids for chronic pain. *JAMA*, *315*(15), 1624–1645. doi:10.1001/jama.2016.1464

DRUGS.COM
www.drugs.com

DRUGS.COM: Drugs Interaction Checker
https://www.drugs.com/drug_interactions.php

DRUGS at FDA: FDA Approved Drug Products
http://www.accessdata.fda.gov/scripts/cder/drugsatfda/index.cfm

Durkin, MJ, Jafarzadeh, SR, Hsueh, K, *et al.* Outpatient antibiotic prescription trends in the United States: A national cohort study [Published online February 27, 2018]. *Infection Control & Hospital Epidemiology*, *39*(5), 584–589. doi:10.1017/ice.2018.26

Emer, JJ, Bernardo, SG, Kovalerchik, O, & Ahmad, M. (2013). Urticaria multiforme. *The Journal of Clinical and Aesthetic Dermatology*, *6*(31), 34–39.

eMPR. Monthly Prescribing Reference (new FDA approved products, new generics, new drug withdrawals, safety alerts)
http://www.empr.com

Endocrinology on the comprehensive type 2 diabetes management algorithm— 2017 executive summary. *Endocr Pract*. 2017:23(2),207–238. doi:10.4158/ep161682.cs

epocrates
https://online.epocrates.com/drugs

FDA Drug Safety Communication. FDA review finds additional data supports the potential for increased long-term risks with antibiotic clarithromycin (Biaxin) in patients with heart disease. (02/22/18)
https://www.fda.gov/downloads/Drugs/DrugSafety/ucm597723.pdf

FDA News Release: FDA approves drug to treat Duchenne muscular dystrophy. (2017).
https://www.fda.gov/NewsEvents/Newsroom/PressAnnouncements/ucm540945.htm

FDA. PLR Requirements for Prescribing Information.
https://www.fda.gov/Drugs/GuidanceComplianceRegulatoryInformation/LawsActsandRules/ucm084159.htm

FDA. Recalls, Market Withdrawals, and Safety Alerts
http://www.fda.gov/Safety/Recalls/default.htm

Fleming, JE, & Lockwood, S. (2017). Cannabinoid hyperemesis syndrome. *Federal Practitioner*, *34*(10), 33–36.

Flynn, JT, Kaelber, DC, Baker-Smith, CM, *et al.* (2017). Clinical practice guideline for screening and management of high blood pressure in children and adolescents. [Published online ahead of print August 22, 2017]. *Pediatrics*, *140*(3), e20171904.

Freedberg, DE, Kim, LS, & Yang, Y-X. (2017). The risks and benefits of long-term use of proton pump inhibitors: expert review and best practice advice from the American Gastroenterological Association. *Gastroenterology*, *152*(4), 706–715. doi:10.1053/j.gastro.2017.01.031

Garber, AJ, Abrahamson, MJ, Barzilay, JI, *et al.* (2017). Consensus statement by the American Association of Clinical Endocrinologists and American College of Endocrinology on the comprehensive type 2 diabetes management algorithm–2017 executive summary. *Endocrine Practice*, *23*(2), 207–238. doi:10.4158/ep161682.cs

Gilbert, DN, Chambers, HF, Eliopoulos, GM, *et al.* (2018). The Sanford guide to antimicrobial therapy, 2016 (48th ed.). Sperryville, VA: Sanford Guide.

Greenhawt, M, Turner, PJ, & Kelso, JM. (2018). Administration of influenza vaccines to egg allergic recipients: A practice parameter update 2017 [Published online December 19, 2017]. *Annals of Allergy, Asthma & Immunology, 120*(1), 49–52. doi:10.1016/j.anai.2017.10.020.

Groot, N, de Graaff, N, Avcin, T, *et al.* (2017). European evidence-based recommendations for diagnosis and treatment of childhood-onset systemic lupus erythematosus: The SHARE initiative. *Annals of the Rheumatic Diseases, 76*(11), 1788–1796. doi:10.1136/annrheumdis-2016-210960

Groot, N, de Graeff, N, Avcin, T, *et al.* (2017). European evidence-based recommendations for the diagnosis and treatment of childhood-onset lupus nephritis: the SHARE initiative. *Annals of the Rheumatic Diseases, 76*(12), 1965–1973. doi.org/10.1136/annrheumdis-2017-211898

Guidelines updated for thyroid disease in pregnancy and postpartum. *American Journal of Nursing*, April, 2017, 117(4), 16.

Handbook of antimicrobial therapy, 2015 (20th ed.). New Rochelle, NY: The Medical Letter.

Harrison's infectious diseases (3rd ed.). New York, NY: McGraw Hill Education.

Hughes, HK, & Kahl, K. (Eds.). (2018). The Johns Hopkins Hospital: The Harriet Lane handbook for pediatric house officers (21st ed.). Philadelphia, PA: Elsevier.

International Diabetes Federation (IDF) Clinical Practice Guidelines http://www.idf.org/guidelines

Inzucchi, SE, Iliev, H, Pfarr, E, & Zinman, B. (2017) Empagliflozin and assessment of lower-limb amputations in the EMPA-REG OUTCOME Trial [published online November 13, 2017]. *Diabetes Cares, 41*(1), e4–e5. doi.org/10.2337/dc17-1551

Jarrett, JB, & Moss, D. (2017). Oral agent offers relief from generalized hyperhidrosis--An inexpensive and well-tolerated anticholinergic reduces sweating in patients with localized—and generalized—hyperhidrosis [posted online]. *Clinician Reviews, 27*(7), 30–31.
https://www.mdedge.com/sites/default/files/Document/June-2017/CR02707024.PDF

JNC 8 Guideline Summary. *Pharmacist's Letter/Prescriber's Letter* https://www.scribd.com/doc/290772273/JNC-8-guideline-summary

Journal of the American Academy of Nurse Practitioners https://www.aanp.org/publications/jaanp

Journal of the American Medical Association (JAMA) Internal Medicine http://archinte.jamanetwork.com/journal.aspx

Justesen, K, & Prasad, S. (2016). On-demand pill protocol protects against HIV. *Clinician Reviews, 26*(9), 18–19, 22.

Khera, M, Adaikan, G, Buvat, J, *et al.* (2016). Diagnosis and treatment of testosterone deficiency: Recommendations from the Fourth International Consultation for Sexual Medicine (ICSM 2015). *The Journal of Sexual Medicine, 13*, 1787–1804.

Kim, DK, Riley, LE, Harriman, KH, *et al.* (2017). Advisory Committee on Immunization Practices recommended immunization schedule for adults aged 19 years or older—United States, 2017. *MMWR. Morbidity and Mortality Weekly Report, 66*, 136–138. doi:10.15585/mmwr.mm6605e2

Kumar, S, Yegneswaran, B, & Pitchumoni, CS. (2017). Preventing the adverse effects of glucocorticoids: A reminder. *Consultant, 57*(12), 726–728.

Lieberthal, AS, Carroll, AE, Chonmaitree, T, *et al.* (2013). The diagnosis and management of acute otitis media. *Pediatrics, 131*(3), e964–e999.
Lortscher, D, Admani, S, Satur, N, & Eichenfield, LF. (2016). Hormonal contraceptives and acne: a retrospective analysis of 2147 patients. *Journal of Drugs in Dermatology, 15*(6), 670–674. http://jddonline.com/articles/dermatology/S1545961616P0670X
Malesker, MA, Callahan-Lyon, P, Ireland, B, *et al.* (2017). Pharmacological and non-pharmacological treatment for acute cough associated with the common cold. *Chest, 152*(5), 1021–1037. doi:10.1016/j.chest.2017.08.009
Mallick, J, Devi, L, & Malik, PK, *et al.* (2016). Update on normal tension glaucoma. *Journal of Ophthalmic and Vision Research, 11*(2), 204–208. doi:10.4103/2008-322X.183914
Manchikanti, L, Kaye, AM, Knezevic, NN, *et al.* (2017). Responsible, safe, and effective prescription of opioids for chronic non-cancer pain: American Society of Interventional Pain Physicians (ASIPP) guidelines. *Pain Physician, 20*(2S), S3–S92.
McDonald, J, & Mattingly, J. (2016). Chagas disease: Creeping into family practice in the United States. *Clinician Reviews, 26*(11), 38–45.
McMillan, JA, Lee, CKK., Siberry, GK, *et al.* (2013). *The Harriet Lane handbook of pediatric antimicrobial therapy*. Philadelphia, PA: Elsevier Saunders.
McNeill, C, Sisson, W, & Jarrett, A. (2017). Listerosis: A resurfacing menace. The Journal for Nurse Practitioners, 13(10), 647–654.
MDedge: Family Practice News
https://www.mdedge.com/familypracticenews/
MedlinePlus
https://www.nlm.nih.gov/medlineplus/ency/article/000165.htm
MedPage Today
http://www.medpagetoday.com
Medscape
http://www.medscape.com
Medscape: Drug Interaction Checker
http://reference.medscape.com/drug-interactionchecker?src=wnl_druggu-ide_170410_mscpref &uac=123859AY&impID=1324737&faf=1
Molina, JM, Capitant, C, Spire, B, *et al.* (2015). On-demand preexposure prophylaxis in men at high risk for HIV-1 infection. *The New England Journal of Medicine, 373*, 2237–2246.
National Academy of Medicine
http://nam.edu
National Heart, Lung, and Blood Institute (NHLBI)
http://www.nhlbi.nih.gov/
National Institute of Diabetes and Digestive and Kidney Diseases. Adrenal insufficiency and Addison's disease
http://www.nidk.nih.gov/health-infromation/health-topics/endocrine/adren [Accessed May 31, 2016]
New England Journal of Medicine (NEJM) Journal Watch General Medicine
http://www.jwatch.org/general-medicine
Ostergaard, L, Vesikari, T, Absalon, J, *et al.* 2017. A bivalent meningococcal B vaccine in adolescents and young adults [published online December 14, 2017]. *The New England Journal of Medicine, 377*(24), 2349–2362. doi:10.1056/NEJMoa1614474
Paz-Bailey, G, *et al. Zika virus persistence in body fluids, final report in body fluids:mFinal report.* ASTMH 2017. Paper presented at the 66th Annual Meeting of the American Society of Tropical Medicine and Hygiene, November 5-9, Baltimore, MD.

Pharmacist's Letter
www.pharmacistsletter.com
Physicians' Desk Reference (PDR)
http://www.pdr.net/
Pregnancy and Lactation Labeling Final Rule (PLLR)
https://www.drugs.com/pregnancy-categories.html
Prescriber's Letter
http://prescribersletter.therapeuticresearch.com/pl/sample.aspx?cs=&s=PRL&AspxAutoDetectCookieSupport=1
Psychopharmacology. Official Journal of the European Behavioural Pharmacology Society (EBPS)
http://link.springer.com/journal/213
Reference for Interpretation of Hepatitis C Virus (HCV) Test Results
www.cdc.gov/hepatitis
Robinson, CL, Romero, JR, Kempe, A, *et al.* (2017). Advisory Committee on Immunization Practices recommended immunization schedule for children and adolescents aged 18 years or younger—United States, 2017. *MMWR. Morbidity and Mortality Weekly Report*, *66*, 134–135. doi:10.15585/mmwr.mm6605e1
Rosenberg, E, *et al.* (2017, November 5–9). *Prevalence and incidence of Zika virus infection among household contacts of Zika patients, Puerto Rico, 2016-2017.* ASTMH 2017. Paper presented at the 66th Annual Meeting of the American Society of Tropical Medicine and Hygiene, November 5–9, Baltimore, MD.
RxLIST
http://www.rxlist.com/script/main/hp.asp
RxLIST: Drugs A-Z
http://www.rxlist.com/drugs/alpha_a.htm
Saag, MS, Pavia, AT, Chambers, HF, *et al.* (2017). The Sanford guide to antimicrobial therapy (25th ed.). Sperryville, VA: Sanford Guide.
Sáez-Llorens, X, Tricou, V, Yu, D, *et al.* (2018) Immunogenicity and safety of one versus two doses of tetravalent dengue vaccine in healthy children aged 2–17 years in Asia and Latin America: 18-month interim data from a phase 2, randomised, placebo-controlled study. *The Lancet Infectious Diseases*, *18*(2), 162–170. doi:10.1016/S1473-3099 (17)30632-1
Sanford Guide Web Edition
https://webedition.sanfordguide.com
Saunders, KH, Shukla, AP, Igel, LI, *et al.* (2017, September). Obesity: When to con-sider medication. The Journal of Family Practice.
http://www.mdedge.com/sites/default/files/Document/September-2017/JFP06610608.PDF
Schwartz, SR, Magit, AE, Rosenfeld, RM, *et al.* (2017). Clinical practice guideline (update): Earwax (cerumen impaction). *Otolaryngology–Head and Neck Surgery*, *156*(1S), S1–S29. Accessed January 10, 2017.
Solutions for Safer ER/LA Opioid Prescribing in a New Era of Health Care. American Nurses Credentialing Center, Post Graduate Institute of Medicine
www.cmeuniversity.com
Sterling, TR, Villarino, ME, Borisov, AS, *et al.* (2011). Three months of rifapentine and isoniazid for latent tuberculosis infection. *New England Journal of Medicine*, *365*, 2155–2166. doi:10.1056/NEJMoa1104875
Sun, T, Liu, J, & Zhao, DW. (2016). Efficacy of n-acetylcysteine in idiopathic pulmonary fibrosis. *Medicine*, *95*(19), e3629. doi:10.1097/md.0000000000003629

Taipale, H, Mittendorfer-Rutz, E, Alexanderson, K, *et al.* Antipsychotics and mortality in a nationwide cohort of 29,823 patients with schizophrenia [published online December 20, 2017]. *Schizophrenia Research*, doi.org/10.1016/j.schres.2017.12.010

Taketomo, CK, Hodding, JH, & Kraus, DM. (2015). *Pediatric and neonatal dosage handbook: A universal resource for clinicians treating pediatric and neonatal patients* (22nd ed.). Wolters Kluwer.

Tebas, P, Roberts, CC, Muthumani, K, *et al.* (2017). Safety and immunogenicity of an anti-Zika virus DNA vaccine: Preliminary report. *New England Journal of Medicine*. doi:10.1056/NEJMoa1708120

The American Congress of Obstetrics and Gynecology (ACOG)
http://www.acog.org/

The JAMA Network.com
www.jamanetwork.com

The Journal for Nurse Practitioners
www.elsevier.com/locate/tjnp

The Medical Letter on Drugs and Therapeutics
http://secure.medicalletter.org

The Nurse Practitioner Journal
www.tnpj.com

Tomaselli, GF, Mahaffey, KW, Cuker, A, *et al.* (2017). 2017 ACC expert consensus decision pathway on management of bleeding in patients on oral anticoagulants. *Journal of the American College of Cardiology, 70*(24), 3042–3067. doi:10.1016/j.jacc.2017.09.1085

Treatment Guidelines [Annual Volume]: The Medical Letter

Turner, PJ, Southern, J, Andrews, NJ, *et al.* (2015). Influenza vaccine found safe in children with egg allergy. *The Journal of Allergy and Clinical Immunology, 136*(2), 376–381. doi:10.1016/j.jaci.2014.12.1925

Updated CDC guidance: Superbugs threaten hospital patients. *Medscape Education Clinical Briefs* (March 31, 2016).
http://www.medscape.org/viewarticle/859361?nlid=105320_2713&src=wnl_cmemp_160523_mscpedu_nurs&impID=1106718&faf=1

UpToDate.com
http://www.uptodate.com

U.S. Pharmacist Weekly Newsletter
http://www.uspharmacist.com

Vail, B. (2015). Chapter 36: Diabetes mellitus. In J. E. South-Paul, S. E. Matheny, & E. L. Lewis (Eds.), Current diagnosis & treatment: family medicine (4th ed.). New York, NY: McGraw-Hill Education.

Vogt, C. New AHA/ACC guidelines lower high BP threshold. *Consultant360*. November 14, 2017.
https://www.consultant360.com/exclusives/new-ahaacc-guidelines-lower-high-bp-threshold

Wald, ER, Applegate, KE, Bordley, C, *et al.* (2013). Clinical practice guidelines for the diagnosis and management of acute bacterial sinusitis in children 1 to 18 years. *Pediatrics, 132*(1), e262–280. http://www.ncbi.nlm.nih.gov/pubmed/23796742

Wallace, DV, Dykewicz, MS, Oppenheimer, J, *et al.* (2017). Pharmacologic treatment of seasonal allergic rhinitis: Synopsis of guidance from the 2017 Joint Task Force on Practice Parameters. [Published online ahead of print November 28, 2017]. *Annals of Internal Medicine, 167*(12), 876–881. doi:10.7326/M17-2203

Watkins, SL, Glantz, SA, & Chaffee, BW. (2018). Association of noncigarette tobacco product use with future cigarette smoking among youth in the population assessment of tobacco and health (PATH) study, 2013–2015 [Published online January 2, 2018]. *JAMA Pediatrics, 172*(2), 181–187. doi:10.1001/jamapediatrics.2017.4173

Watson, T, Hickok, J, Fraker, S, *et al.* (2017). Evaluating the risk factors for hospital-onset Clostridium difficile infections in a large healthcare system [published online December 20, 2017]. *Clinical Infectious Diseases.* doi.org/10.1093/cid/cix1112

WebMD: Drugs and Medications A to Z. Latest Drug News http://www.webmd.com/drugs

Winkel, P, Hilden, J, Fischer Hansen, J, *et al.* (2015). Clarithromycin for stable coronary heart disease increases all-cause and cardiovascular mortality and cerebrovascular morbidity over 10 years in the CLARICOR randomised, blinded clinical trial. *International Journal of Cardiology, 182*, 459–465.

World Health Organization. (2016, August 30) *Growing antibiotic resistance forces updates to recommended treatments for sexually transmitted infections.*
http://www.who.int/mediacentre/news/releases/2016/antibiotics-sexual-infections/en

World Health Organization. (2016) WHO guidelines for the treatment of *Chlamydia trachomatis.*
http://www.who.int/reproductivehealth/publications/rtis/chlamydia-treatment-guidelines/en/

World Health Organization. (2016). *WHO guidelines for the treatment of* Neisseria gonorrhoeae.
http://www.who.int/reproductivehealth/publications/rtis/gonorrhoea-treatment-guidelines/en/

World Health Organization. (2016). *WHO guidelines for the treatment of* Treponema pallidum *(syphilis).*
http://www.who.int/reproductivehealth/publications/rtis/syphilis-treatment-guidelines/en/

World Health Organization. (2017, March). *WHO model list of essential medicines (20th list).* Geneva, Switzerland: World Health Organization.
http://www.who.int/medicines/publications/essentialmedicines/20th_EML2017.pdf?ua=1

World Health Organization. (2017, March). *WHO model list of essential medicines for Children* (6th list). Geneva, Switzerland: World Health Organization.
http://www.who.int/medicines/publications/essentialmedicines/6th_EMLc2017.pdf?ua=1

World Health Organization. (2017, June 6). *WHO updates essential medicines list with new advice on use of antibiotics, and adds medicines for hepatitis C, HIV, tuberculosis and cancer.* Geneva, Switzerland: World Health Organization.
http://www.who.int/mediacentre/news/releases/2017/essential-medicines-list/en

Xie, Y, Bowe, B, Li, T, *et al.* (2017). Long-term kidney outcomes among users of proton pump inhibitors without intervening acute kidney injury [published online February 22, 2017]. *Kidney International, 91*(6), 1482–1494. doi:10.1016/j.kint.2016.12.021

Yılmaz, D, Heper, Y, & Gözler, L. (2017). Effect of the use of buzzy during phlebotomy on pain and individual satisfaction in blood donors. *Pain Management Nursing, 18*(4), 260–267.

Yoon, I-K, & Thomas, SJ. (2017). Encouraging results but questions remain for dengue vaccine. *The Lancet Infectious Diseases, 18*(2), 125–126. doi:10.1016/S1473-3099(17)30634-5

Zarrabi, H, Khalkhali, M, Hamidi, A, *et al.* (2016). Clinical features, course and treatment of methamphetamine-induced psychosis in psychiatric inpatients. *BMC Psychiatry, 16*, 44. doi:10.1186/s12888-016-0745-5

INDEX

NOTE: Generic names are in italics; FDA pregnancy categories and controlled drug categories appear in parentheses after the entry. * indicates no assigned pregnancy category.